The American Psychiatric Association Publishing

TEXTBOOK OF MOOD DISORDERS

SECOND EDITION

The American Psychiatric Association Publishing

TEXTBOOK OF
MOOD DISORDERS

SECOND EDITION

EDITED BY

Charles B. Nemeroff, M.D., Ph.D.
Natalie Rasgon, M.D., Ph.D.
Alan F. Schatzberg, M.D.
Stephen M. Strakowski, M.D.

AMERICAN
PSYCHIATRIC
ASSOCIATION
PUBLISHING

Note: The authors have worked to ensure that all information in this book is accurate at the time of publication and consistent with general psychiatric and medical standards, and that information concerning drug dosages, schedules, and routes of administration is accurate at the time of publication and consistent with standards set by the U.S. Food and Drug Administration and the general medical community. As medical research and practice continue to advance, however, therapeutic standards may change. Moreover, specific situations may require a specific therapeutic response not included in this book. For these reasons and because human and mechanical errors sometimes occur, we recommend that readers follow the advice of physicians directly involved in their care or the care of a member of their family.

Books published by American Psychiatric Association Publishing represent the findings, conclusions, and views of the individual authors and do not necessarily represent the policies and opinions of American Psychiatric Association Publishing or the American Psychiatric Association.

If you wish to buy 50 or more copies of the same title, please go to www.appi.org/specialdiscounts for more information.

Second Edition

Manufactured in the United States of America on acid-free paper

26 25 24 23 22 5 4 3 2 1

American Psychiatric Association Publishing
800 Maine Avenue SW
Suite 900
Washington, DC 20024-2812
www.appi.org

Library of Congress Cataloging-in-Publication Data
A CIP record is available from the Library of Congress.

British Library Cataloguing in Publication Data
A CIP record is available from the British Library.

To Gayle, Gigi, Ross, Mandy, Michael, Emily, Callie, Rylie, and Finn,
for your support during the long hours, which made this volume possible.

C.B.N

To Alex, for all your love and support.
To the loving memory of my parents.

N.R.

To my wife,
Nancy,
and my daughters,
Melissa Dassori and Lindsey Cedillos.

A.F.S.

To Stacy, Andy, Alexis, Lucas, and Sue,
for all your love and support.

S.M.S.

Contents

PART II
Pathogenesis of Mood Disorders

PART III
Investigating Mood Disorders

PART V
Psychotherapy of Mood Disorders

PART VI
Integrative Management of Mood Disorders

PART VII
Subtypes of Mood Disorders

PART VIII
Additional Perspectives on Mood Disorder

Contributors

Joan Asarnow, Ph.D.
Professor of Psychiatry and Biobehavioral Science, David Geffen School of Medicine, Los Angeles, California

Yuanhan Bai, M.D., M.S.
Attending Physician, Division of Mood Disorders in Shenzhen Kangning Hospital, Shenzhen, Guangdong, China; Research Fellow, Department of Psychiatry, University Hospitals Cleveland Medical Center, Cleveland, Ohio

Wade Berrettini, M.D., Ph.D.
Karl E. Rickels Professor, Department of Psychiatry, Perelman School of Medicine, University of Pennsylvania, Philadelphia, Pennsylvania

Michele A. Bertocci, Ph.D.
Research Assistant Professor of Psychiatry, Department of Psychiatry, University of Pittsburgh, Western Psychiatric Institute and Clinic, Pittsburgh, Pennsylvania

Pierre Blier, M.D., Ph.D.
Professor, Departments of Psychiatry and Cellular and Molecular Medicine, University of Ottawa, Royal Ottawa Institute of Mental Health Research, Ottawa, Ontario, Canada

Martin Brüne, M.D., Ph.D.
Professor of Psychiatry, LWL University Hospital Bochum, Department of Psychiatry, Psychotherapy and Preventive Medicine, Division of Social Neuropsychiatry and Evolutionary Medicine, Ruhr University Bochum, Bochum, Germany

Joseph R. Calabrese, M.D.
Emeritus Professor of Psychiatry, Former Director of Bipolar Disorder Research Center, Case Western Reserve University; Former Director of Mood Disorders Program, Department of Psychiatry, University Hospitals Cleveland Medical Center, Cleveland, Ohio

Kenneth Carpenter, Ph.D.
Associate Professor of Clinical Psychology (in Psychiatry) Department of Psychiatry, Columbia University Irving Medical Center and New York State Psychiatric Institute, New York, New York

Linda L. Carpenter, M.D.
Professor, Department of Psychiatry and Human Behavior, Brown University, Providence, Rhode Island

Frances A. Champagne, Ph.D.
Professor, Department of Psychology, The University of Texas at Austin

Adora Choquette, B.A.
Clinical Psychology doctoral student, Department of Psychology, University of Memphis, Memphis, Tennessee

Teresa Lanza di Scalea, M.D., Ph.D.
Assistant Professor of Psychiatry and Women's Health, Department of Psychiatry, Dell Medical School, The University of Texas at Austin

David A. Lewis, M.D.
Distinguished Professor of Psychiatry and Neuroscience, Thomas Detre Professor of Academic Psychiatry, Translational Neuroscience Program, Department of Psychiatry, University of Pittsburgh, Pittsburgh, Pennsylvania

John T.P. Liggins, M.D., M.S.
Staff Psychiatrist, Palo Verde Behavioral Health, Tucson, Arizona

Elizabeth T.P. Lippard, Ph.D.
Assistant Professor, Department of Psychiatry and Behavioral Sciences, Institute of Early Life Adversity Research, Mulva Clinic for Neuroscience, Dell Medical School; Assistant Professor of Psychiatry, Waggoner Center for Alcohol and Addiction Research, Department of Psychology, University of Texas, Austin, Texas

Matthew Macaluso, D.O., DFAPA
Bee McWane Reid Professor, Department of Psychiatry and Behavioral Neurobiology, and Clinical Director, UAB Depression and Suicide Center, The University of Alabama at Birmingham School of Medicine, Birmingham, Alabama

Dean F. MacKinnon, M.D.
Associate Professor, Department of Psychiatry and Behavioral Sciences, Johns Hopkins University School of Medicine, Baltimore, Maryland

J. John Mann, M.D.
Paul Janssen Professor of Translational Neuroscience in Psychiatry and Radiology, Department of Psychiatry, Columbia University, New York, New York

John C. Markowitz, M.D.
Professor of Clinical Psychiatry, Columbia University; Research Psychiatrist, New York State Psychiatric Institute, New York, New York

William V. McCall, M.D., M.S.
Professor and Case Distinguished University Chair, Department of Psychiatry and Health Behavior, Medical College of Georgia, Augusta University, Augusta, Georgia

William McDonald, M.D.
J.B. Fuqua Chair and Professor of Psychiatry and Behavioral Sciences, Emory University School of Medicine, Atlanta, Georgia

Dora M. Meyer, M.Sc.
Research Scientist, Division of Interventional Biological Psychiatry, Department of Psychiatry and Psychotherapy Medical Center, University of Freiburg Faculty of Medicine, University of Freiburg, Germany

David J. Miklowitz, Ph.D.
Distinguished Professor of Psychiatry and Biobehavioral Sciences, UCLA School of Medicine, Los Angeles, California

Melissa P.H. Miller, M.Sc.
Doctoral Student, Department of Psychology & Interdisciplinary Life Sciences, The University of Texas at Austin

Trevor Mooney, M.D.
Psychiatry Resident, Department of Psychiatry and Health Behavior, Medical College of Georgia, Augusta University, Augusta, Georgia

Christine Yu Moutier, M.D.
Chief Medical Officer, American Foundation for Suicide Prevention, New York, New York

Dominique Musselman, M.D., M.S.C.R.
Associate Professor, Department of Psychiatry and Behavioral Sciences, University of Miami Leonard Miller School of Medicine, Miami, Florida

Alison Myoraku, M.S.
Clinical Research Coordinator Associate, Department of Psychiatry and Behavioral Sciences, Stanford School of Medicine, Stanford, California

Henry A. Nasrallah, M.D.
Professor of Psychiatry, Neurology, and Neuroscience; Vice-Chair for Faculty Development and Mentorship; Director of Neuropsychiatry Program, University of Cincinnati College of Medicine, Cincinnati, Ohio

Charles B. Nemeroff, M.D., Ph.D.
Matthew P. Nemeroff Endowed Chair and Professor, Department of Psychiatry and Behavioral Sciences, Mulva Clinic for the Neurosciences; Director, Institute of Early Life Adversity Research, Dell Medical School, The University of Texas at Austin

Maria Antonietta Nettis, M.D., Ph.D.
Department of Psychological Medicine, Institute of Psychiatry, Psychology and Neuroscience, King's College London; National Institute for Health and Research Biomedical Research Centre at South London and Maudsley NHS Foundation Trust and King's College London, London, United Kingdom

D. Jeffrey Newport, M.D., M.S.
Professor and Associate Chair for Research, Department of Psychiatry, Dell Medical School, The University of Texas at Austin, Texas

Andrew A. Nierenberg, M.D.
Thomas P. Hackett, MD, Endowed Chair in Psychiatry, Department of Psychiatry, Massachusetts General Hospital, Boston, Massachusetts

Edward Nunes, M.D.
Professor of Psychiatry, Department of Psychiatry, Columbia University Irving Medical Center and New York State Psychiatric Institute, New York, New York

Lexi Nutkiewicz, B.A.
Department of Psychiatry and Behavioral Sciences, Stanford School of Medicine, Stanford, California

Lisa A. O'Donnell, Ph.D.
Assistant Professor, Wayne State University, Detroit, Michigan

Dan A. Oren, M.D.
Associate Professor of Psychiatry (Adjunct), Yale University, New Haven, Connecticut

Vanessa Padilla, M.D.
Assistant Professor, Department of Psychiatry and Behavioral Sciences, University of Miami Leonard Miller School of Medicine, Miami, Florida

Carmine Maria Pariante, M.D., Ph.D., FRCPsych
Department of Psychological Medicine, Institute of Psychiatry, Psychology and Neuroscience, King's College London; National Institute for Health and Research Biomedical Research Centre at South London and Maudsley NHS Foundation Trust and King's College London, London, United Kingdom

Brenda W.J.H. Penninx, M.D., Ph.D.
Professor of Psychiatric Epidemiology, Department of Psychiatry, Amsterdam Neuroscience and Amsterdam Public Health Research Institute, Amsterdam UMC, Vrije Universiteit, Amsterdam, The Netherlands

Mary L. Phillips, M.D., M.D. (Cantab)
Pittsburgh Foundation–Emmerling Endowed Chair in Psychotic Disorders and Professor in Psychiatry and Clinical and Translational Science; Director of Center for Translational and Developmental Affective Neuroscience, Collaborative on Mood Disorders Research, and Mood and Brain Laboratory; Department of Psychiatry, University of Pittsburgh School of Medicine, Pittsburgh, Pennsylvania

Grazyna Rajkowska, Ph.D.
Professor, Department of Psychiatry and Human Behavior, University of Mississippi Medical Center, Jackson, Mississippi

Natalie Rasgon, M.D., Ph.D.
Professor, Departments of Psychiatry and Behavioral Sciences and Obstetrics & Gynecology, Stanford University School of Medicine, Stanford, California; Director of the Stanford Center for Neuroscience in Women's Health; Associate Dean of Academic Affairs

Darrel A. Regier, M.D., M.P.H.
Adjunct Professor in Psychiatry, Department of Psychiatry, Uniformed Services University of the Health Sciences, Bethesda, Maryland; and Senior Scientist, Center for the Study of Traumatic Stress, Henry M. Jackson Foundation for the Advancement of Military Medicine, Inc., Bethesda, Maryland

Mina M. Rizk, M.B.B.Ch., M.Sc.
Postgraduate Year 1, Department of Psychiatry, Icahn School of Medicine at Mount Sinai, New York, New York; Postdoctoral Fellow, Research Foundation for Mental Hygiene, New York State Psychiatric Institute, New York, New York

Norman E. Rosenthal, M.D.
Clinical Professor of Psychiatry, Georgetown University Medical School, Washington, DC

Mitchell Rovner, M.D.
Assistant Professor, Department of Psychiatry and Behavioral Sciences, University of Miami Leonard Miller School of Medicine, Miami, Florida

Eric Rubin, M.D., Ph.D.
Associate Clinical Professor of Psychiatry, Columbia University College of Physicians and Surgeons, Harlem Hospital, New York, New York

James K. Rustad, M.D.
Psychiatrist, Department of Mental Health and Behavioral Sciences, White River Junction VA Medical Center, White River Junction, Vermont; Assistant Professor of Psychiatry, Department of Psychiatry, Geisel School of Medicine at Dartmouth, Lebanon, New Hampshire

Gerard Sanacora, M.D., Ph.D.
Professor of Psychiatry, Yale University, New Haven, Connecticut

Alan F. Schatzberg, M.D.
Kenneth T. Norris Jr. Professor, Department of Psychiatry and Behavioral Sciences, Stanford University School of Medicine, Stanford, California; Director, Stanford Mood Disorders Center

Thomas E. Schlaepfer, M.D.
Head, Division of Interventional Biological Psychiatry, Department of Psychiatry and Psychotherapy Medical Center, University of Freiburg Faculty of Medicine, University of Freiburg, Germany; Associate Professor, The Johns Hopkins Hospital, Department of Psychiatry and Behavioral Medicine, Baltimore, Maryland

Marianne Seney, Ph.D.
Assistant Professor, Translational Neuroscience Program, Department of Psychiatry, University of Pittsburgh, Pittsburgh, Pennsylvania

Luca Sforzini, M.D.
Department of Psychological Medicine, Institute of Psychiatry, Psychology and Neuroscience, King's College London, London, United Kingdom

David V. Sheehan, M.D., M.B.A.
Distinguished University Health Professor Emeritus, University of South Florida College of Medicine, Tampa, Florida

Richard C. Shelton, M.D.
Charles Byron Ireland Professor, Department of Psychiatry and Behavioral Neurobiology, School of Medicine, The University of Alabama at Birmingham

Manpreet K. Singh, M.D., M.S.
Associate Professor of Psychiatry and Behavioral Sciences and Director of the Stanford Pediatric Mood Disorders Program and the Pediatric Emotion and Resilience Lab, Stanford University, Stanford, California

David C. Steffens, M.D., M.H.S.
Professor and Chairman, Department of Psychiatry, University of Connecticut School of Medicine, Farmington, Connecticut

Stephen M. Strakowski, M.D.
Vice Dean of Research and Associate Vice President of Regional Mental Health, Dell Medical School, The University of Texas at Austin; Professor of Psychiatry & Behavioral Sciences, Psychology, and Educational Psychology, University of Texas, Austin

Caroline Symcox, B.Sc.
Postbaccalaureate Research Assistant, Department of Psychology, The University of Texas at Austin

Michael E. Thase, M.D.
Professor of Psychiatry, Perelman School of Medicine, University of Pennsylvania, Corporal Michael J. Crescenz Veterans Affairs Medical Center, Philadelphia, Pennsylvania

Martha C. Tompson, Ph.D.
Associate Professor, Department of Psychological and Brain Sciences, Boston University, Boston, Massachusetts

Marisa Toups, M.D.
Assistant Professor of Psychiatry, Dell Medical School, University of Texas at Austin

Philip S. Wang, M.D., Dr.P.H.
Chair and Chief of Psychiatry, Cambridge Health Alliance, and Professor of the Practice of Psychiatry, Harvard Medical School, Cambridge, Massachusetts

Frances Isabella Weston, B.Sc.
Department of Psychological Medicine, Institute of Psychiatry, Psychology and Neuroscience, King's College London, London, United Kingdom

Daniel R. Wilson, M.D., Ph.D.
President Emeritus, Western University of Health Sciences, Pomona, California

Hans-Ulrich Wittchen, Ph.D.
Professor of Clinical Psychology and Psychotherapy, Department of Psychiatry and Psychotherapy, Ludwig-Maximilians-Universität, Munich, Germany

Tyler Wright, M.D., M.P.H.
Chief Resident Physician, University of Southern California, Los Angeles, California

Brian W. Wu, M.D., Ph.D.
Resident Physician, University of Southern California, Los Angeles, California

Zhixing Yao, M.D.
Psychiatry Resident, Department of Psychiatry and Health Behavior, Medical College of Georgia, Augusta University, Augusta, Georgia

Lakshmi N. Yatham, M.B.B.S., FRCPC
Professor and Head, Department of Psychiatry, University of British Columbia, Vancouver, British Columbia, Canada

Shiwen Yuan, M.D.
Clinical Instructor, Department of Psychiatry and Human Behavior, Brown University, Providence, Rhode Island

Kristina F. Zdanys, M.D.
Associate Professor, Department of Psychiatry, University of Connecticut School of Medicine, Farmington, Connecticut

Hannah N. Ziobrowski, Ph.D., M.P.H.
Research Associate, Department of Health Care Policy, Harvard Medical School, Boston, Massachusetts

Disclosure of Interests

The following contributors to this textbook have indicated a financial interest in or other affiliation with a commercial supporter, manufacturer of a commercial product, and/or provider of a commercial service as listed below:

Joan R. Asarnow, Ph.D. Dr. Asarnow has received grant funding and/or other support from the National Institute of Mental Health, the Substance Abuse and Mental Health Services Administration, the American Foundation for Suicide Prevention, the Association for Child and Adolescent Mental Health, the American Psychological Association, and the Society of Clinical Child and Adolescent Psychology. She has also served as a consultant on quality improvement interventions for depression and suicidal/self-harm behavior and on Data Safety and Monitoring and noncommercial Advisory Boards/Expert Panels, as well as on the scientific advisory board for the Klingenstein Third Generation Foundation.

Pierre Blier, M.D., Ph.D. Dr. Blier received honoraria for giving lectures and/or for participating in advisory boards and/or providing expert testimony for Allergan, Bristol Myers Squibb, Janssen, Lundbeck/Otsuka, and Pfizer. He received research grants from the Canadian Institute of Health Research, Canadian Biomarkers for Depression, and Ontario Brain Institute.

Linda L. Carpenter, M.D. *Research Support:* Affect Neuro (formerly Feelmore Labs), Janssen, NeoSync, Neuronetics, and Nexstim; *Consultant:* Janssen, Magstim, and Nexstim.

W. Edward Craighead, Ph.D. Dr. Craighead is a board member of Hugarheill ehf, an Icelandic company dedicated to the prevention of depression; receives book royalties from John Wiley & Sons (Hoboken, NJ, USA); is supported by National Institutes of Health funding, the Mary and John Brock Foundation, and the Fuqua Family Foundations; and is a consultant to the George West Mental Health Foundation, a member of the Scientific Advisory Board (SAB) of the Anxiety and Depression Association of America, and a member of the SAB for AIM for Mental Health Foundation.

Charles DeBattista, M.D. *Grant Support:* Abbott, Biolite, Compass, and Jansen; *Consultant:* Alkermes and Corcept Therapeutics.

Charles F. Gillespie, M.D., Ph.D. *Consultant:* Cohen Veterans Bioscience.

Benjamin Goldstein, M.D., Ph.D. Dr. Goldstein received grant or research support from the Brain and Behavior Research Foundation, Brain Canada, the Canadian Institutes of Health Research, the Heart & Stroke Foundation, the National Institute of Mental Health, the Ontario Ministry of Research & Innovation, and the University of Toronto Department of Psychiatry.

Jennifer L. Hughes, Ph.D., M.P.H. Dr. Hughes receives royalties from Guilford Press for the following book: Kennard BD, Hughes JL, Foxwell AF: *CBT for Depression in Children and Adolescents: A Guide to Relapse Prevention.* New York, Guilford Press, 2016. Research studies that contributed to the development of this treatment (and subsequent book) are presented in Chapter 27 of the Textbook, and this book is cited.

Ronald C. Kessler, Ph.D. In the past 3 years, Dr. Kessler received support for his epidemiological studies from Sanofi Aventis; was a consultant for Johnson & Johnson Wellness and Prevention, Sage Pharmaceuticals, Shire, and Takeda; and served on an advisory board for the Johnson & Johnson Services Inc. Lake Nona Life Project. Dr. Kessler is a co-owner of DataStat Inc., a market research firm that carries out healthcare research.

Brandon M. Kitay, M.D., Ph.D. In the last 12 months, Dr. Kitay has provided consulting services to Janssen Pharmaceuticals and has also received salary support from Janssen Pharmaceuticals and Sage Therapeutics for the conduct of research administered through Yale University and the Yale Depression Research Program. In addition, Dr. Kitay's employer, Yale University, has a financial relationship with Janssen Pharmaceuticals, and may in the future receive financial benefits from this relationship. The University has put multiple measures in place to mitigate this institutional conflict of interest. Questions about the details of these measures should be directed to Yale University's Conflict of Interest office.

Matthew Macaluso, D.O., DFAPA Dr. Macaluso has conducted clinical trials research as principal investigator for the following pharmaceutical companies over the last 12 months: Acadia, Allergan, AssureRx, Eisai, Lundbeck, Janssen, Naurex/Aptinyx, Neurim, and Suven. All clinical trial and study contracts were with and payments made to the Kansas University Medical Center Research Institute, a research institute affiliated with Kansas University School of Medicine–Wichita (KUSM-W).

J. John Mann, M.D. Dr. Mann receives royalties from the Research Foundation for Mental Hygiene for commercial use of the Columbia–Suicide Severity Rating Scale (C-SSRS).

John C. Markowitz, M.D. Dr. Markowitz receives minor royalties for books related to interpersonal psychotherapy from American Psychiatric Association Publishing, Basic Books, and Oxford University Press.

William V. McCall, M.D., M.S. *Research Support:* Merck, MECTA, and Vistagen; *Scientific Advisory Board:* Jazz Pharmaceuticals and Sage Therapeutics; *Royalties:* Wolters Kluwer Publishing; *Speakers Bureau:* CME Outfitters; *Consultant:* Anthem Insurance.

William McDonald, M.D. Dr. McDonald has research contracts from the Stanley Foundation, Soterix, Neuronetics, NeoSync, and Cervel Neurotherapeutics. He is an ad hoc member of several National Institute of Mental Health and National Institute of Neurological Disorders and Stroke study sections. He is a member of the American Psychiatric Association Council on Research and Quality representing Electroconvulsive and Neuromodulation Therapies. Dr. McDonald is compensated as the chair of the Data and Safety Monitoring Board for the National Institute on Aging multicenter study. He receives royalties from Oxford University Press from co-editing a book on the Clinical Guide to Transcranial Magnetic Stimulation in the Treatment of Depression. He is a paid consultant for Signant Health. He holds an endowed chair funded by the JB Fuqua Foundation. He is an employee of Emory University School of Medicine.

David J. Miklowitz, Ph.D. Dr. Miklowitz has received research funding from the National Institute of Mental Health (grants MH093676, MH097007, and MH117200) and from the Deutsch and Kayne Family Foundations, AIM for Mental Health, the Attias Foundation, the Danny Alberts Foundation, and the Max Gray Foundation.

Charles B. Nemeroff, M.D., Ph.D. *Research Grants:* National Institutes of Health (NIH), Stanley Medical Research Institute; *Consultant:* Bracket (Clintara), Fortress Biotech, Gerson Lehrman Group (GLG) Healthcare and Biomedical Council, Janssen Research and Development LLC, Magstim Inc, Prismic Pharmaceuticals, Sumitomo Dainippon Pharma, Sunovion Pharmaceuticals Inc, Taisho Pharmaceutical Inc, Takeda, Total Pain Solutions (TPS), and Xhale; *Stock Holdings:* Abbvie, OPKO Health Inc, Antares, Bracket Intermediate Holding Corp, Celgene, Network Life Sciences Inc, Seattle Genetics, and Xhale; *Scientific Advisory Board:* American Foundation for Suicide Prevention (AFSP), Anxiety Disorders Association of America (ADAA), Bracket (Clintara), Brain and Behavior Research Foundation (BBRF) (formerly named National Alliance for Research on Schizophrenia and Depression [NARSAD]), Laureate Institute for Brain Research Inc, RiverMend Health LLC, Skyland Trail, and Xhale; *Board of Directors:* ADAA, AFSP, and Gratitude America; *Income or Equity ($10,000 or more):* American Psychiatric Publishing, Bracket (Clintara), CME Outfitters, Takeda, and Xhale; *Patents:* U.S. 6,375,990B1 (method and devices for transdermal delivery of lithium) and U.S. 7,148,027B2 (method of assessing antidepressant drug therapy via transport inhibition of monoamine neurotransmitters by ex vivo assay).

D. Jeffrey Newport, M.D., M.S. Dr. Newport has received research support from Eli Lilly, Glaxo Smith Kline (GSK), Janssen, the National Alliance for Research on Schizophrenia and Depression, the National Institutes of Health, Takeda Pharmaceuticals, and Wyeth. He has served on speakers' bureaus and/or received honoraria from AstraZeneca, Eli Lilly, GSK, Pfizer, and Wyeth. He has served on advisory boards for GSK, Janssen, and Sage Therapeutics. He has never served as a consultant to any biomedical or pharmaceutical corporations. Neither he nor his family members have ever held equity positions in biomedical or pharmaceutical corporations.

Andrew A. Nierenberg, M.D. *Consulting:* Acadia Pharm, Eisai, Ginger, Merck, Myriad, and Protogenics; *Scientific Advisory Board:* Alkermes, Jazz Pharma, Neuronetics, Otsuka, and Sage Pharma; *Honoraria:* Sunovion and Neurostar.

Edward Nunes, M.D. Dr. Nunes has received grant funding from the National Institute on Drug Abuse and the National Institute on Alcohol Abuse and Alcoholism.

Carmine Pariante, M.D., Ph.D., FRCPsych Prof. Pariante has received research funding from Johnson & Johnson as part of a program of research on depression and inflammation, and research funding from the Medical Research Council (U.K.) and the Wellcome Trust for research on depression and inflammation as part of two large consortia that also include Johnson & Johnson, Glaxo Smith Kline, and H. Lundbeck.

Gerard Sanacora, M.D., Ph.D. In the last 12 months Dr. Sanacora has provided consulting services to Allergan, Axsome Therapeutics, Biohaven Pharmaceuticals, Boehringer Ingelheim International, Bristol-Myers Squibb, Celexio Biosciences, EMA Wellness, Epiodyne, Intra-Cellular Therapies, Janssen, Lundbeck, Minerva Pharmaceuticals, Navitor Pharmaceuticals, Neurocrine Biosciences, NeuroRx, Noven Pharmaceuticals, Otsuka, Perception Neuroscience, Praxis, Seelos Pharmaceuticals, and Vistagen Therapeutics. He has received funds for contracted research from Janssen Pharmaceuticals, Merck, and Usona Institute. He is holds equity in Biohaven Pharmaceuticals and has received royalties from Yale University paid from patent licenses with Biohaven Pharmaceuticals. In addition, he holds shares in Biohaven Pharmaceuticals Holding Company and is a co-inventor on a patent, "Glutamate agents in the treatment of mental disorders" (Patent number: 8778979), and a U.S. Provisional Patent Application (No. 047162-7177P1 [00754]) filed on August 20, 2018, by Yale University Office of Cooperative Research (OCR 7451 US01). Dr. Sanacora's employer, Yale University, has a financial relationship with Janssen Pharmaceuticals, and may in the future receive financial benefits from this relationship. The University has put multiple measures in place to mitigate this institutional conflict of interest. Questions about the details of these measures should be directed to Yale University's Conflict of Interest office.

Richard C. Shelton, M.D. Dr. Shelton's institution has received grant support from Acadia Pharmaceuticals, Agency for Healthcare Research and Quality, Alkermes, Allergan, Avanir Pharmaceuticals, Cerecor, Genomind, Intracellular Therapies, Janssen Pharmaceutica, Myriad Genetics, National Institute of Mental Health, Navitor Pharmaceuticals, NeuroRx, Novartis, Otsuka Pharmaceuticals, Patient-Centered Outcomes Research Institute, Sage Therapeutics, and Takeda Pharmaceuticals. Dr. Shelton has served as a consultant to Acadia Pharmaceuticals, Allergan, Cerecor, Janssen Pharmaceutica, MSI Methylation Sciences, Naurex, and Takeda Pharmaceuticals.

Manpreet K. Singh, M.D., M.S. Dr. Singh receives research support from Stanford's Maternal Child Health Research Institute and Department of Psychiatry, the National Institute of Mental Health, the National Institute on Aging, Johnson & Johnson, Allergan, PCori, and the Brain and Behavior Foundation. She is on the advisory board for Sunovion and is a consultant for Google X and Limbix.

David C. Steffens, M.D., M.H.S. *Consultant:* Janssen Research and Development.

Michael E. Thase, M.D. Dr. Thase reports the following relationships over the past 3 years: *Advisor/Consultant:* Acadia, Akili, Alkermes, Allergan (Forest, Naurex), Axsome Therapeutics, Boehringer-Ingelheim, Calla, Clexio Biosciences, H. Lundbeck, Jazz Pharmaceuticals, Janssen (Johnson & Johnson), Otsuka, Perception Neuroscience, Sage Therapeutics, Seelos

Pharmaceuticals, and Takeda; *Grant Support:* Acadia, Allergan (Forest, Naurex), Axsome Therapeutics, Intracellular, Janssen Pharmaceutica (Johnson & Johnson), Myriad (Assurex), Otsuka, and Takeda; *Royalties:* American Psychiatric Association Publishing, Guilford Publications, Herald House, and W.W. Norton. *Spouse's Employment:* Peloton Advantage, which does business with a number of pharmaceutical companies. *Disclosure of Intellectual Conflicts of Interest (all prior to 2012):* paid consultant to Depression Guideline Panel, Agency for Health Care Policy and Research; unpaid consultant to Canadian Mood and Anxiety Treatment Guidelines (1st & 2nd Editions) and American Psychiatric Association (DSM-III-R, DSM-IV, and DSM-5); unpaid Work Group member, American Psychiatric Association Practice Guideline for Treatment of Patients With Bipolar Disorder (2nd Edition and, from 2006–2010, work in preparation of 3rd Edition) and American Psychiatric Association Practice Guideline for Treatment of Patients with Major Depressive Disorder (3rd Edition).

Martha C. Tompson, Ph.D. Dr. Tompson received research support from the National Institute of Mental Health, the Patient Centered Outcomes Research Institute, and the Smith Family Foundation; book royalties from Guilford Press and BVT Publishing; and honoraria from the American Psychological Association.

Lakshmi N. Yatham, M.B.B.S., FRCPC Dr. Yatham has received research grants from or has been a consultant or on speaker/advisory boards for Allergan, AstraZeneca, Alkermes, Bristol Myers Squibb, Canadian Institutes of Health Research, Canadian Network for Mood and Anxiety Treatments, Dainippon Sumitomo, Eli Lilly, Forrest, Glaxo Smith Kline, Janssen, Lundbeck, Michael Smith Foundation for Health Research, Novartis, Otsuka, Pfizer, Ranbaxy, Servier, Sunovion, Teva, the Stanley Foundation, and Valeant Pharmaceuticals.

The following contributors stated that they had no competing interests during the year preceding manuscript submission:

Jorge Renner Cardoso de Almeida, M.D., Ph.D.; Yuanhan Bai, M.D., M.S.; Michelle A. Bertocci, Ph.D.; Joseph R. Calabrese, M.D.; Frances A. Champagne, Ph.D.; Adora Choquette, B.A.; Samuel J. Collier, M.D.; William Coryell, M.D.; Adel Farah, M.D., M.Sc.; Andrew A. Fukuda, M.D., Ph.D.; Keming Gao, M.D., Ph.D.; Ana Gomez-Carrillo, M.D.; Ilang M. Guiroy, M.D.; G. Eric Jarvis, M.D., M.Sc.; Brian C. Kavanaugh, Psy.D.; Laurence J. Kirmayer, M.D.; Teresa Lanza di Scalea, M.D., Ph.D.; David A. Lewis, M.D.; Elizabeth T.C. Lippard, Ph.D.; Dean F. MacKinnon, M.D.; Melissa P.H. Miller, M.Sc.; Trevor Mooney, M.D.; Alison Myoraku, M.S.; Maria Antoinetta Nettis, M.D., Ph.D.; Lisa O'Donnell, Ph.D.; Dan A. Oren, M.D.; Vanessa Padilla, M.D.; Brenda W. J. H. Penninx, M.D., Ph.D.; Grazyna Rajkowska, Ph.D.; Mina M. Rizk, M.B.B.Ch., M.Sc.; Mitchell Rovner, M.D.; James K. Rustad, M.D.; Marianne Seney, Ph.D.; Luca Sforzini, M.D.; Marisa Toups, M.D.; Philip S. Wang, M.D., Dr.P.H.; Daniel R. Wilson, M.D., Ph.D.; Hans-Ulrich Wittchen, Ph.D.; Tyler Wright, M.D., M.P.H.; Zhixing Yao, M.D.; Shiwen Yuan, M.D.; Kristina F. Zdanys, M.D.; Hannah N. Ziobrowski, Ph.D., M.P.H.

Acknowledgments

Dr. Nemeroff would like to acknowledge Kelly Puzdrak for getting this volume put together and for everything else as well.

Dr. Rasgon would like to acknowledge Alison Myoraku, M.S., for her contributions.

Dr. Schatzberg would like to acknowledge Adrienne Bronfeld for her contributions.

Dr. Strakowski would like to acknowledge Chiara Onyett and Alison Barajas for their contributions.

PART I

Symptomatology and Epidemiology

CHAPTER 1

Historical Aspects of Mood Disorders

Dean F. MacKinnon, M.D.
J. Raymond DePaulo Jr., M.D.

Depression and mania have been enduring aspects of the human condition, but the idea that they are pathologies of mood is relatively new. Historical/mythological figures in the Bible (Ben-Noun 2004), Homer's writings (Angst and Marneros 2001; Berrios and Schioldann 2019), and other ancient texts are often depicted experiencing what a modern reader might interpret as symptoms of depression and mania, but these narratives describe spiritual agonies and divine afflictions, not medical illness. The history of a diagnostic concept begins with the birth of medicine.

The history of mood disorders illustrates the complex relationship between clinic and theory, because descriptions of manic and depressive symptoms have crossed paths with theories about their nature but have yet to converge on a pathogenic model. In this chapter, we focus on the following: 1) how the phenomena we now associate with mood disorders were described throughout the history of medicine, 2) what physicians have thought were the causes of those disorders, and 3) how therapeutic developments have informed diagnosis and theory. By tracking how we came to our present state of knowledge, we may glimpse its replacement.

Descriptions of Mood Disorders

The first medical descriptions in which we might now recognize mood disorder symptoms emerged in ancient Greek Hippocratic texts and as part of a broader set of problems associated with perturbations of bodily "humors." While "melancholic" described fear and despondency associated with "black bile," it also referred to delusional ideation, insomnia, poor appetite, paralysis, and epilepsy. "Mania" was used to refer to a form of melancholic disease, a strong emotional response, a divine state, or a kind of temperament (Angst and Marneros 2001). In philosophy, meanwhile, the ancient Greek concept of a melancholic temperament denoted not mental illness but a propensity to sad emotions, sometimes linked with creativity (Bos 2009; Pies 2007). These two aspects of melancholy would meld together, much later, to attach the multifaceted disease melancholia more firmly to melancholic emotional disposition.

Physicians in classical Rome also recognized despondency and fear as common symptoms in melancholic patients. Galen wrote of such patients, "They find fault with life and hate people; but not all want to die. For some the fear of death is of principal concern [whereas others] dread death and desire to die at the same time" (quoted in Jackson 1986, p. 42). But the "mania" and "melancholia" of Hippocrates and Galen, and for that matter of Philippe Pinel and Benjamin Rush in the eighteenth and nineteenth centuries, implied not only emotional suffering but also disturbed thought—that is, insanity. Galen mentions melancholic patients "who think to have become a sort of snail so that they must escape everyone in order to avoid having their shell crushed, while others fear that Atlas, who supports the world, may grow weary and vanish" (Telles-Correia and Marques 2015, p. 1). Centuries later, Paul of Aegina similarly described patients who "fancy themselves to be, some, brute animals, and imitate their cries; and others, earthen-vessels, and are frightened lest they be broken.... some believe themselves impelled by higher powers, and foretell what is to come, as if under divine influence; and these are, therefore, properly called demoniacs, or possessed persons" (quoted in Jackson 1986, p. 54).

Somatic symptoms also were often emphasized in Roman depictions of melancholia. Soranus of Ephesus, for example, considered flatulence, coldness in the extremities, diaphoresis, head heaviness, and greenish-black complexion to be signs of melancholia (Jackson 1986). Rufus, a contemporary of Soranus, suggested that the gastrointestinal symptoms defined a "hypochondriacal" form of melancholia localized to the abdomen (*hypo* meaning "below," and *chondria* referring to the diaphragm), whereas the psychological symptoms pointed to melancholic disturbance in the brain. This notion of several different forms of melancholia proved to be a robust idea that could still be found in textbooks nearly two millennia later.

Medieval physicians preserved some ancient elements of melancholic illness for another 1,500 years. In the seventeenth century, in the full bloom of the Renaissance, Felix Platter (sometimes spelled "Plater") in Basel, Switzerland, continued to emphasize abnormal thought over abnormal mood when he described melancholia as "a kind of mental alienation [*mentis alienatio*] in which imagination and judgment are so perverted that without any cause the victims become very sad and fearful" (quoted in Jackson 1986, p. 91). In contrast to Galen's examples concerning snails and Atlas, Platter's examples of false ideation include themes more familiar to modern psychiatrists: patients with melancholia "have felt themselves driven toward blaspheming God and committing many horrible things...out of an involuntary compulsion.... Others... falsely imagine that they are in bad grace with princes and magistrates and that they have done something wrong and are being summoned to punishment" (quoted in Jackson 1986, p. 92).

Themes of guilt were seldom described in ancient texts on melancholia, and their emergence seems to point to an expanding dimension of conscientiousness in the culture. From the earliest Christian era, when Paul differentiated the "godly sorrow" that motivated repentance from "the sorrow of the world" that led one away from salvation (Altschule 1967), introspection to gauge the quality of one's sorrows became a spiritual habit for many, and ultimately, perhaps, the precursor to seeing mood as a phenomenon of clinical significance on its own.

Problems we might now associate with nonpsychotic depression, such as sluggish work and sour attitude, were particularly hard to conceal in a medieval monastery, where such problems called for diagnosis and correction. A fifth-century scholar, John Cassian, attributed these phenomena to the sin of *acedia* (Altschule 1965); a later observer, David of Augsburg, a German mystic and Franciscan friar, noted a spectrum of acedia from vice to mental illness. Whereas acedia could result from mere slothfulness, or from a selective loss of zeal in religious duties, the most severe forms shaded into melancholia: "a certain bitterness of the mind which cannot be pleased by anything cheerful or wholesome. It feeds upon disgust and loathes human intercourse.... It inclines to despair, diffidence, and suspicions, and sometimes drives its victim to suicide when he is oppressed by unreasonable grief. Such sorrow arises sometimes...from the abundance of melancholic humors, in which case it behooves the physician rather than the priest to prescribe a remedy" (quoted in Jackson 1986, p. 72).

Published in England during the Renaissance, Robert Burton's *The Anatomy of Melancholy* invoked the ancient Greek philosophical view of melancholic temperament as a prelude to his exhaustive treatise on melancholic illness. The melancholic temperament, or disposition, is familiar and common, perhaps even normal, until it becomes habitual: "We call him melancholy that is dull, sad, sour, lumpish, ill-disposed, solitary, any way moved, or displeased. And from these melancholy dispositions, no man living is free" (Burton 1652, p. 127). He goes on, "This melancholy of which, we are to treat, is a habit,...a chronic or continuate disease, a settled humour,...not errant, but fixed" (Burton 1652, p. 128).

Turning to the symptoms of melancholic disease, Burton emphasizes delusions, some bizarre, recorded in ancient medical literature: "Some are afraid that heaven will fall on their heads: some they are damned, or shall be.... Fear of devils, death, that they shall be so sick of some such...disease, ready to tremble at every object, they shall die themselves forthwith, or that some of their dear friends or near allies are certainly dead; imminent danger, loss, disgrace, still torment others...that they are all glass, and therefore will suffer no man to come near them: that they are all cork, as light as feathers; others as heavy as lead; some are afraid their heads will fall off their shoulders, that they have frogs in their bellies" (Burton 1652, p. 317).

Only after listing these delusions does Burton turn to descriptions of the mood in melancholic patients: "Sorrow...is an inseparable companion.... [T]he remembrance of some disgrace, loss, injury, abuse, etc. troubles them.... [T]hey are weary of their own lives, and feral thoughts to offer violence to their own persons come into their minds...they are soon tired with all things" (Burton 1652, pp. 319–320).

The traditional emphasis on insanity in descriptions of melancholia did not reflect the experience of physicians in practice, who rarely saw frank insanity but often saw sad patients. Analysis of the copious records kept by one seventeenth-century English physician, Charles Napier, demonstrates his practical linkage of melancholy mood to fear, sadness, troubled mind, and "mopishness" more than to false ideas and sensory disturbances (McDonald 1983).

The interplay of temperament, habit, and insanity in the Renaissance idea of melancholy informed medicine until the nineteenth century. The physician William Cullen, of Edinburgh, Scotland, in his influential medical writings and lectures from the late eighteenth century, describes the melancholic temperament as "slow, disposed to gravity, caution, and timidity, with little sensibility or irritability, but…liable to melancholia, hypochondriasis" (Cullen 1789/1827, vol. I, pp. 217–218). Cullen considered melancholia a "partial insanity" (as opposed to the general insanity of mania) and contrasted it with the health preoccupations in hypochondriasis: "When an anxious fear and despondency arises from a mistaken judgment with respect to other circumstances than those of health…it is what I would strictly name Melancholia" (Cullen 1779/1827, vol. II, p. 533). Cullen also vividly describes mania, again emphasizing the primacy of abnormal thought over abnormal emotion: "What for the most part more especially distinguishes the disease, is a hurry of mind, in pursuing any thing like a train of thought, and in running from one train of thought to another. Maniacal persons are in general very irascible; but what more particularly produces their angry emotions is, that their false judgments lead to some action which is always pushed with impetuosity and violence; when this is interrupted or restrained, they break out into violent anger and furious violence against every person near them, and upon every thing that stands in the way of their impetuous will" (Cullen 1779/1827, vol. II, p. 522).

By the mid-nineteenth century, the idea of melancholia as a disorder primarily of mood, rather than a distressing disorder of ideation and judgment, had begun to take hold among psychiatric thinkers (Kendler 2020). In his textbook, German psychiatrist and neurologist Wilhelm Griesinger lucidly illustrates the change of emphasis. In melancholia, the mental pain precedes both false ideation and altered function: "A state of mental pain becomes always more dominant and persistent, but is increased by every external mental impression. This is the essential mental disorder in melancholia, and, so far as the patient himself is concerned, the mental pain consists in a profound feeling of ill-being, of inability to do anything, of suppression of the physical powers, of depression and sadness, and of total abasement of self-consciousness" (Griesinger 1861, p. 223).

As ideas about the affective nature of melancholia took shape, medicine as a whole was undergoing a radical renovation. One can get a quick sense regarding how thoroughly changed the understanding of medicine was across the nineteenth century simply by contrasting the section headings in one of Cullen's texts (Cullen 1779/1827, vol. II, pp. v–viii) with, say, an early edition of William Osler's *The Principles and Practice of Medicine* (Osler 1896). Cullen had three main sections on diseases: "Pyrexiae," "Nervous Diseases," and "Cachexie." A century later, Osler organized his text into "Specific Infectious Diseases," "Constitutional Diseases," and then a series of sections for pathologies in each organ system (Osler 1896, pp. vii–xvi). In contrast to Cullen's broad categorization of diseases by their major presenting symptom, Osler's reflected the modern idea that diseases arise from organic pathology.

By the end of the nineteenth century, major psychiatric textbooks had largely coalesced around a definition of melancholia as a disorder of depressed mood accompanied by a number of other symptoms, on average about twice as many as would later make up the DSM criteria for a major depressive episode (Kendler 2017). Mania, however, was generally thought of not as an episodic disorder of elevated mood but more as a chronic, variable insanity ultimately leading to intellectual deterioration (Hare 1981).

At about the same time that Osler was linking pathology and nosology, German psychiatrist Emil Kraepelin had begun to take note of patterns in the symptoms and course of illness in the severely ill patients under his care, and to conceive of manic-depressive insanity as an episodic disorder of affect regulation.

In the chapter "Manic-Depressive Insanity" in his seminal general textbook of psychiatry, Kraepelin (1920) posits a predisposition to episodic pathological mood states: "Manic-depressive insanity runs its course in attacks, whose appearance is in general independent of external influences. This fact shows us that the real, the deeper cause of the malady is to be sought in a permanent morbid state which must also continue to exist in the intervals between the attacks" (p. 117). These fundamental "permanent morbid states" consist of depressive, manic, irritable, and cyclothymic temperaments.

For Kraepelin, the depressive temperament, reminiscent of the melancholic disposition of old, "is characterized by a *permanent gloomy emotional stress in all the experiences of life*" (Kraepelin 1920, p. 118, emphasis his). Such patients, from youth onward, are tormented by guilt; are sexually unsatisfied, anxious and avoidant, indecisive, and lacking in self-confidence; are prone to suicidal thoughts and sometimes actions; and tend to have "nervous" or psychosomatic complaints. Manic temperament, in contrast, is one of "constitutional excitement" with a permanently "exalted, careless, confident" mood, a sense of superiority to one's surroundings, and unsteadiness or restlessness in actions, but a lack of perseverance that hinders progress in life. Such patients "live in constant feud. They interfere in everything, overstep their rights, make arrangements which they are not entitled to make" (Kraepelin 1920, p. 128). The irritable temperament is a mixture of the manic and depressive temperaments, whereas the cyclothymic temperament is characterized by frequent flux between the two.

Kraepelin's work suggested that in psychiatry, as in the rest of medicine, classifying diseases by shared clinical features beyond common symptoms could help clinicians to prognosticate, to test therapeutic approaches, and to investigate causes. However, this approach has left open an important question: Who decides where to draw the boundaries, and for what purpose? "The clinician wants classes into which he can put his patient's illness after a reasonably brief period of investigation, and which will assist him to make a prognosis and decide on treatment.... [The researcher] wants his classes, and his words, to have some fixity, so that he can generalize and summarize and communicate his observations: he cannot work in circumstances where the case that he calls an endogenous melancholia another man may call a reactive depression, and a third man call a paranoid schizophrenic" (Lewis 1938).

Government agencies also had use for reliable diagnostic classification of mental impairment. The U.S. Census had counted "idiocy" and "insanity" in households between 1840 and 1880. After that, the Census initiated an enumeration specifically of institutionalized people, and in analyzing these data aimed for a more nuanced typology than "idiocy" and "insanity," arriving at five diagnoses that would be somewhat familiar to modern psychiatry: melancholia, mania, monomania, dementia, and dipsomania, along with two that the modern reader might not consider primarily mental disorders: paresis and epilepsy. A more detailed Census classification scheme to track institutionalized patients emerged in 1918, with input from the psychiatric profession, adding "involutional melancholia" and "manic-depressive psychosis" along with other serious disorders, and was in use into the 1940s (Grob 1991). By the mid-twentieth century, the psychiatric profession had begun to grasp that advancement of the field would entail developing its own, more clinically relevant classification scheme; the American Psychiatric Association (1952) updated the Census nomenclature, and thus developed a system that included not only the diagnoses of institutionalized patients, but also the problems of outpatients, and thus added descriptions of a "psychoneurotic" depressive reaction and a "cyclothymic" personality along with many other non-mood-disorder diagnoses.

In spite of the effort to promote diagnostic reliability, in clinical practice diagnostic inconsistency remained endemic (Spitzer and Fleiss 1974) and strongly influenced by local custom. For example, many patients who would have been diagnosed with an affective psychosis by a British psychiatrist in 1970 would have received a diagnosis of schizophrenia by an American psychiatrist (Kendell et al. 1971). Clinical investigators were thus moved to develop their own sets of operationalized diagnostic criteria. The Feigner criteria (Feighner et al. 1972; Kendler et al. 2010) and the Research Diagnostic Criteria (Spitzer et al. 1978) provided what were essentially early drafts of the criteria for affective disorders that appeared in DSM-III (American Psychiatric Association 1980). Notably, during the process of cleanly delineating affective disorders for DSM-III, the old concept of manic-depressive illness (which sometimes had been applied to patients who had only depressive episodes) evolved into "bipolar" and "unipolar" disorders contingent on the presence of mania or hypomania (Pichot 1995).

Systems such as the Feigner criteria and the Research Diagnostic Criteria, as well as DSM-III, dropped many symptoms that were commonly described but hard to assess reliably, such as depersonalization and vague somatic complaints. While these omissions might have improved diagnostic reliability, they arguably impoverished the clinical concept of what constitutes a mood disorder (Kendler 2016). DSM diagnostic rules for mania and major depressive disorder have remained largely unchanged since 1980, but there have been two notable updates to the larger classification scheme. One update from DSM-III-R to DSM-IV in 1994 was the adoption of criteria for bipolar II disorder (American Psychiatric Association 1987, 1994). The most significant change for the purposes of a textbook on mood disorders was the removal, between DSM-IV and DSM-5 in 2013, of "mood disorders" as a general category of illness in favor of two separate diagnostic classes for depressive disorders and bipolar and related disorders (American Psychiatric Association 2013).

Theories of Mood Disorders

The current concept of "mood disorders," therefore, applies to a subset of the patients with psychosis whom the ancients would have called "melancholic" or "manic"; to a group of anguished patients without psychosis who present with various physical complaints considered as the "hypochondriacal" subtype of melancholia or perhaps as "neurasthenia" by nineteenth-century medicine (Ware and Weiss 1994); and to some sad and unproductive souls who committed the "sin" of acedia, but whom non-theologians might have thought of as expressing the melancholic disposition described by ancient philosophers.

Developments in nosology and in theory have crossed paths at times but have rarely if ever moved along together (Ghaemi and Goodwin 2009). Whereas diagnostic concepts evolved glacially from Hippocrates to Kraepelin, theories to explain mood disorders have advanced in a more discontinuous fashion, starting with the ancient and resilient humoral theory and abruptly changing course in the Renaissance as scientific approaches to knowledge took hold and expanded. We know much more now about the biological correlates of mood disorders, and how to alter their course, but this knowledge has not yet informed stable nosological concepts.

The humoral theory applied ancient concepts of four essential qualities—hot versus cold, wet versus dry—and substances—earth, fire, air, water—to explain abnormal internal bodily processes. Disease was thought to represent a perturbation or imbalance of four bodily fluids, or humors (each with its own qualities)—blood, phlegm, and two different kinds of bile, or "choler": yellow and black (i.e., melancholic). Philosophers also employed this rubric in an early psychology of temperament (Bos 2009). Aside from the view common both to ancient Greeks and modern physicians that medical disorders, including melancholia, are essentially problems in bodily functioning, little of humoralism remains today in medicine.

Nothing much challenged the humoral theory of melancholia until Renaissance physicians began to apply each new scientific theory from chemistry (Paracelsus), anatomy (Andreas Vesalius), and physiology (William Harvey) to understand the nature of melancholic illness, without altering the clinical definition of melancholia. Seventeenth-century English physician Thomas Willis saw the body as composed of a limited number of essential chemicals, including salt, water, earth, sulfur, and spirit. In combination and under various circumstances, the chemicals could mix and ferment, in health giving rise to a "transparent, subtle, and lucid" quality, and in melancholy becoming "obscure, thick, and dark,...as it were in a shadow, or covered with darkness" (both Willis quotes from Jackson 1986, p. 111).

A few generations later, around the turn of the eighteenth century, Dutchman Herman Boerhaave based his theory of melancholia on Harvey's model of circulatory physiology, and saw it as a result of slowing or congestion of blood flow. Albrecht von Haller, in eighteenth-century Switzerland, in his work on the nature and anatomy of nerves, opined that the qualities of sensibility and irritability were essential to understanding diseases such as melancholia and that these qualities arose from variations in the motion of a "nerve fluid" flowing through axons. In contrast, other theorists saw a Newtonian source of melancholia in the (putative) mechanical oscillatory and vibratory motions of the nervous system (Jackson 1986).

The nineteenth-century conceptual metamorphosis from melancholia to mood disorders began, perhaps, with the advent of Romanticism and its regard for feeling over reason, but its widespread incorporation into scientific medicine followed developments in psychological science, such as the counterintuitive idea expounded by the American philosopher William James (and refined by later experiments [Schachter and Singer 1962]) that affect emerges not merely from thoughts but also from actions motivated by provocative circumstances: "Common-sense says, we lose our fortune, are sorry and weep; we meet a bear, are frightened and run; we are insulted by a rival, are angry and strike.... [T]he more rational statement is that we feel sorry because we cry, angry because we strike, afraid because we tremble" (James 1884, p. 190). So if a mood disorder made one sad, angry, or fearful without external cause, this theory implies that in order to make sense of the experience, the mind could invent such a cause—and so a primary emotional disturbance can create false or even delusional ideas.

The emerging science of psychology in the twentieth century offered alternatives to the Kraepelinian assumption that the clinical syndromes of mania and depression arose from a specific disease process in the body. Johns Hopkins psychiatrist Adolf Meyer proposed in his "psychobiological" approach that what others had considered to be discrete disease entities could more dynamically be understood as reaction patterns (Lidz 1966). For example, as cogently summarized by Aubrey Lewis (1934), "depressive states may appear as reactions (protective at any rate in intention, designed to withdraw the individual from an ill-adjusted situation), with concomitant phenomena on various levels—vegetative, kinetic, and topical mental.... There may be sadness, with feelings of difficulty and dearth of ideas and activity, or actual retardation" (p. 33).

Sigmund Freud (1917/1957), in contrasting melancholia with mourning, saw melancholia as complicated by ambivalence, which is either "an element of every love-relation formed by this particular ego, or else it proceeds precisely from those experiences that involved the threat of losing the object" (p. 256). He noted that mania often travels with melancholia when with its resolution "a large expenditure of psychical energy, long maintained or habitually occurring, has at last become unnecessary, so that it is available for numerous applications and possibilities of discharge.... All such situations are characterized by high spirits, by the signs of discharge of joyful emotion and by increased readiness for all kinds of action" (p. 254).

The third wave of modern psychological theories of mood disorder, after Meyerian reactive withdrawal and Freudian ambivalent mourning, came in the behavioral model of "learned helplessness" (Seligman 1972), in which animals subjected to stressful situations entered a depression-like state with symptoms reminiscent of human depression—withdrawal, inertia, diminished appetite, disinterest in mating, and so forth. Although limited as a model of human depression (Henkel et al. 2002), it has proved useful as a means to assess the likely therapeutic efficacy of antidepressant medications (McArthur and Borsini 2006).

DSM-III's unification of mood disorders into a small number of diagnostic categories (albeit with the ability to subtype them) obviated the debate over whether there was a "melancholic" type of illness that arose de novo (or endogenously) from a biological vulnerability, as well as a "reactive" or "neurotic" type of depression that had its basis more in psychological maladjustment to stressful circumstances (Nelson and Charney 1980; Taylor and Fink 2008). The concept had proven intuitively attractive, and gibed with clinical experience: some patients seem clearly to be suffering from adversity, whereas others are ill (and sometimes very severely ill) for no discernible external reason. However, judging whether a patient has sufficient reason to feel depressed introduces a degree of interpretation that weakens diagnostic objectivity: "If the physician can enter into the patient's feelings and understand the illness as the natural outcome of situations in which the patient has been, then he calls it psychogenic or reactive; if he cannot then he calls it autonomous.... No doubt this too is a personally valuable way of reviewing the illness, but it has the disadvantages...[associated with] such subjective judgments" (Lewis 1938, p. 877).

There has remained among many thoughtful psychiatrists the sense that DSM's lumping of all mood disorders into a few symptom-defined categories overlooks something essential about the nature of mental illness (Coryell 2007; Taylor and Fink 2008); however, (for better or worse) this did not lead the developers of DSM-5 to re-establish a melancholic/endogenous versus neurotic/reactive distinction. Temperamental vulnerability, life events, losses, and adjustments to adversity play a limited role in a limited number of DSM-5 diagnoses and none whatsoever in a diagnosis of major depressive or bipolar disorder.

Therapy and Theory

Prior to the modern era, there were essentially three things a physician could do about someone with melancholia: 1) wait and hope for the best; 2) provide commonsense, supportive care in the form of rest, reassurance, and healthy living; or 3) try the sorts of interventions indicated by the prevailing theory, technology, and practice ethos. The latter included purging, trepanning, bloodletting, herbal or nutritional additives, physiological stress (e.g., heat or cold), coitus (or avoidance of coitus, depending on the authority), and so on. The unpleasantness of some of these interventions could help explain why someone suffering with depressive or manic symptoms but still in possession of rational faculties might have chosen not to consult with a physician.

Compounds extracted from nature were the earliest sedatives and stimulants, and also served as tools to alter a patient's mood, if only transiently. These include the medicinal plants belladonna and mandrake, which produce anticholinergic calming effects; the ephedra plant, which yields a prototypical form of our modern amphetamine stimulants; and the more familiar and self-administered intoxicants ethanol, coca, and morphia. Any of these, of course, might worsen melancholia over the long run, but could potentially quell anxiety or arouse action in someone with a not-too-severe case of mania or depression (Shorter 2009).

Treatments demonstrated to alter the course of illness all began with serendipitous observations. Stories behind the discovery of the therapeutic effects on mood disorder of lithium, imipramine, chlorpromazine, iproniazid, and valproic acid share a common theme in that all of the treatments were developed or used for other purposes before their antipsychotic, antidepressant, or antimanic properties were discovered: lithium as a treatment for gout, imipramine as a neuroleptic, chlorpromazine as an antihistamine, iproniazid as an antituberculosis drug, and valproic acid as an antiepileptic (Cade 1949). The dozens of medications currently marketed for mood disorders are essentially extrapolations from these discoveries.

Theories of the pathological basis of mood disorder have sometimes been reverse-engineered to fit the putative mechanism of action of an agent in the treatment of a particular kind of mood disorder. Thus, the discovery that the early antidepressants seemed to work through their influence on monoaminergic receptors led to a resilient hypothesis of affective disorder pathophysiology (Lambert et al. 2000; van Enkhuizen et al. 2015) and even to the leakage into popular culture of people speaking of their depression as being a deficiency of serotonin. Although there is abundant evidence that serotonin perturbations are associated with depression and that altering serotonin activity leads to resolution of the depressive syndrome (in some patients), there are some weak spots in the hypothesis (Baumeister et al. 2003; Hirschfeld 2000). Nevertheless, the monoamine hypothesis has generated a robust research framework (Mulinari 2012) and is thus a model for how therapeutic success can inform the search for an etiology.

Conclusion: Past and Future

We have traced the evolution of diagnostic concepts for a set of medical disorders characterized by anguished mood and several other pervasive symptoms, starting from ancient medical descriptions of melancholia and mania and philosophical models of temperament, the medieval "vice" of spiritual exhaustion, and the psychosomatic notion of a hypochondriacal melancholia and "nervous disorders" presenting in ways that resemble modern depression. We have also observed that developments in the theory of mind, disease, and bodily function have contributed very little to our understanding of these disorders—indeed when explaining them to patients, we still tend to fall back on the vaguely humoral rubric of "chemical imbalance." Through serendipity—and a pharmaceutical industry poised to capitalize on serendipitous findings—we have some empirical validation of the (imperfect and imprecise) diagnostic schema that emerged; however, we still do not have a good working theory of the nature of mood disorders. As Lewis (1938) noted, "No doubt increasing knowledge will bring an improved, eventually even a stable classification based on aetiology, and pointing, it may be hoped, to treatment: Whether it comes by way of genetics, psychology, or somatic pathology, it will be welcome so long as it is useful and valid" (p. 878). The ultimate goal of efforts to identify causes of mood disorders would therefore be to no longer classify mania and depression as mood disorders, but rather as specific deficits in mental functioning that affect individual patients in more complex ways than can be encapsulated by a simple diagnostic label.

References

Altschule MD: Acedia: its evolution from deadly sin to psychiatric syndrome. Br J Psychiatry 111:117–119, 1965 14274176

Altschule MD: The two kinds of depression according to St. Paul. Br J Psychiatry 113(500):779–780, 1967 4860435

American Psychiatric Association: Mental Disorders: Diagnostic and Statistical Manual. Washington, DC, American Psychiatric Association, 1952

American Psychiatric Association: Diagnostic and Statistical Manual of Mental Disorders, 3rd Edition. Washington, DC, American Psychiatric Association, 1980

American Psychiatric Association: Diagnostic and Statistical Manual of Mental Disorders, 3rd Edition Revised. Washington, DC, American Psychiatric Association, 1987

American Psychiatric Association: Diagnostic and Statistical Manual of Mental Disorders, 4th Edition. Washington, DC, American Psychiatric Association, 1994

American Psychiatric Association: Diagnostic and Statistical Manual of Mental Disorders, 5th Edition. Arlington, VA, American Psychiatric Association, 2013

Angst J, Marneros A: Bipolarity from ancient to modern times: conception, birth and rebirth. J Affect Disord 67(1-3):3–19, 2001 11869749

Baumeister AA, Hawkins MF, Uzelac SM: The myth of reserpine-induced depression: role in the historical development of the monoamine hypothesis. J Hist Neurosci 12(2):207–220, 2003 12953623

Ben-Noun L: Mental disorder that afflicted King David the Great. Hist Psychiatry 15(60 Pt 4):467–476, 2004 15628039

Berrios GE, Schioldann J: 'Insanity in Classical Antiquity', by JL Heiberg (1913). Hist Psychiatry 30(4):489–505, 2019 31328570

Bos J: The rise and decline of character: humoral psychology in ancient and early modern medical theory. Hist Human Sci 22(3):29–50, 2009 20213950
Burton R: The Anatomy of Melancholy: What It Is, With All the Kinds, Causes, Symptoms, Prognostics, and Several Cures of It in Three Partitions; With Their Several Sections, Members, and Subsections, Philosophically, Medicinally, Historically Opened and Cut Up (6th Edition, 1652; reprinted by Chatto and Windus, London, 1883). Available at: https://www.exclassics.com/anatomy/anatomy1.pdf. Accessed July 14, 2021.
Cade JFJ: Lithium salts in the treatment of psychotic excitement. Med J Aust 2(10):349–352, 1949 18142718
Coryell W: The facets of melancholia. Acta Psychiatr Scand Suppl 115(433):31–36, 2007 17280568
Cullen W: First lines of the practice of physic (1779), in The Works of William Cullen, M.D., Vol II. Edited by Thomson J. Edinburgh, Scotland, William Blackwood, 1827, pp 467–671
Cullen W: Of temperaments (extracted from the treatise of materia medica [1789]), in The Works of William Cullen, M.D., Vol I. Edited by Thomson J. Edinburgh, Scotland, William Blackwood, 1827, pp 214–224
Feighner JP, Robins E, Guze SB, et al: Diagnostic criteria for use in psychiatric research. Arch Gen Psychiatry 26(1):57–63, 1972 5009428
Freud S: Mourning and melancholia (1917), in The Standard Edition of the Complete Psychological Works of Sigmund Freud, Volume XIV. Translated by Strachey J. London, Hogarth, 1957, pp 243–258
Ghaemi SN, Goodwin FK: Diagnostic classifications of mood disorders: historical context and implications for neurobiology, in Neurobiology of Mental Illness, 3rd Edition. Edited by Charney DS, Nestler EJ. New York, Oxford University Press, 2009, pp 351–359
Griesinger W: Mental Pathology and Therapeutics, 2nd Edition. Translated by Robertson CL, Rutherford J. London, The New Sydenham Society, 1861
Grob GN: Origins of DSM-I: a study in appearance and reality. Am J Psychiatry 148(4):421–431, 1991 2006685
Hare E: The two manias: a study of the evolution of the modern concept of mania. Br J Psychiatry 138(2):89–99, 1981 7020819
Henkel V, Bussfeld P, Möller H-J, Hegerl U: Cognitive-behavioural theories of helplessness/hopelessness: valid models of depression? Eur Arch Psychiatry Clin Neurosci 252(5):240–249, 2002 12451467
Hirschfeld RM: History and evolution of the monoamine hypothesis of depression. J Clin Psychiatry 61 (suppl 6):4–6, 2000 10775017
Jackson SW: Melancholia and Depression: From Hippocratic Times to Modern Times. New Haven, CT, Yale University Press, 1986
James W: What is an emotion? Mind 9(34).188–205, 1884. Available at: https://academic.oup.com/mind/article-abstract/os-IX/34/188/2870785. Accessed July 14, 2021.
Kendell RE, Cooper JE, Gourlay AJ, et al: Diagnostic criteria of American and British psychiatrists. Arch Gen Psychiatry 25(2):123–130, 1971 5569450
Kendler KS: The phenomenology of major depression and the representativeness and nature of DSM criteria. Am J Psychiatry 173(8):771–780, 2016 27138588
Kendler KS: The genealogy of major depression: symptoms and signs of melancholia from 1880 to 1900. Mol Psychiatry 22(11):1539–1553, 2017 28785109
Kendler KS: The origin of our modern concept of depression: the history of melancholia from 1780–1880. A review. JAMA Psychiatry 77(8):863–868, 2020 31995137
Kendler KS, Muñoz RA, Murphy G: The development of the Feighner criteria: a historical perspective. Am J Psychiatry 167(2):134–142, 2010 20008944
Kraepelin E: Manic Depressive Insanity and Paranoia. Translated by Barclay RM. Edited by Robertson GM. Chicago, IL, Chicago Medical Book, 1920
Lambert G, Johansson M, Agren H, Friberg P: Reduced brain norepinephrine and dopamine release in treatment-refractory depressive illness: evidence in support of the catecholamine hypothesis of mood disorders. Arch Gen Psychiatry 57(8):787–793, 2000 10920468

Lewis AJ: Melancholia: a historical review. Journal of Mental Science 80(328):1–42, 1934
Lewis A: States of depression. BMJ 2(4060):875–878, 1938 20781840
Lidz T: Adolf Meyer and the development of American psychiatry. Am J Psychiatry 123(3):320–332, 1966 5331215
McArthur R, Borsini F: Animal models of depression in drug discovery: a historical perspective. Pharmacol Biochem Behav 84(3):436–452, 2006 16844210
McDonald M: Mystical Bedlam. Cambridge, UK, Cambridge University Press, 1983
Mulinari S: Monoamine theories of depression: historical impact on biomedical research. J Hist Neurosci 21(4):366–392, 2012 22947380
Nelson JC, Charney DS: Primary affective disorder criteria and the endogenous-reactive distinction. Arch Gen Psychiatry 37(7):787–793, 1980 7396656
Osler W: The Principles and Practice of Medicine, 2nd Edition. New York, D. Appleton & Company, 1896
Pichot P: The birth of the bipolar disorder. Eur Psychiatry 10(1):1–10, 1995 19698309
Pies R: The historical roots of the "bipolar spectrum": did Aristotle anticipate Kraepelin's broad concept of manic-depression? J Affect Disord 100(1–3):7–11, 2007 17224187
Schachter S, Singer JE: Cognitive, social, and physiological determinants of emotional state. Psychol Rev 69:379–399, 1962 14497895
Seligman ME: Learned helplessness. Annu Rev Med 23:407–412, 1972 4566487
Shorter E: Before Prozac: The Troubled History of Mood Disorders in Psychiatry. New York, Oxford University Press, 2009
Spitzer RL, Fleiss JL: A re-analysis of the reliability of psychiatric diagnosis. Br J Psychiatry 125(578):341–347, 1974 4425771
Spitzer RL, Endicott J, Robins E: Research diagnostic criteria: rationale and reliability. Arch Gen Psychiatry 35(6):773–782, 1978 655775
Taylor MA, Fink M: Restoring melancholia in the classification of mood disorders. J Affect Disord 105(1–3):1–14, 2008 17659352
Telles-Correia D, Marques JG: Melancholia before the twentieth century: fear and sorrow or partial insanity? Front Psychol 6:81, 2015 25691879
van Enkhuizen J, Janowsky DS, Olivier B, et al: The catecholaminergic-cholinergic balance hypothesis of bipolar disorder revisited. Eur J Pharmacol 753:114–126, 2015 25107282
Ware NC, Weiss MG: Neurasthenia and the social construction of psychiatric knowledge. Transcultural Psychiatric Research Review 31(2):101–124, 1994

CHAPTER 2

Classifications of Mood Disorders

Darrel A. Regier, M.D., M.P.H.

Developmental History of Mood Disorder Classification

The focus in this chapter is on classifications of mood disorders by the World Health Organization (WHO) and the American Psychiatric Association (APA). The discussion will cover a period of approximately 70 years, from 1948 to 2020. During this time period, there was a gradual evolution of etiological concepts about mental disorders that affected the organizational structure of mood disorders within the overall classification of mental disorders.

In the sixth edition of the *International Classification of Diseases* (ICD-6) (World Health Organization 1948) and in DSM-I (American Psychiatric Association 1952), both published in the post–World War II era, mental disorders were most prominently considered to be "reactions" either to internal psychodynamic conflicts or to external exposures to environmental stresses, such as combat, interpersonal conflict,

Disclaimers:
The opinions and assertions expressed herein are those of the author and do not reflect the official policy or position of the Uniformed Services University of the Health Sciences or the Department of Defense.

The contents of this publication are the sole responsibility of the author and do not necessarily reflect the views, opinions, or policies of The Henry M. Jackson Foundation for the Advancement of Military Medicine, Inc. Mention of trade names, commercial products, or organizations does not imply endorsement by the U.S. Government.

or the breakdown of social supports. The mood disorder diagnoses in DSM-I included manic-depressive reactions, cyclothymic personality (in the personality disorder section), involutional psychotic reaction, psychotic depressive reaction, and depressive reaction.

As more biologically focused psychopharmacological treatments emerged in the late 1950s and early 1960s, a shift to a more biopsychosocial understanding of mental disorder etiology began (Engel 1980). By the time of DSM-II in 1968, the term *reaction* was dropped from almost all of these disorders and more elaborative descriptions were added, including manic-depressive illness, circular type; manic-depressive illness, depressed type; other major affective illness; involutional melancholia; psychosis with childbirth; psychotic depressive reaction; and depressive neurosis (American Psychiatric Association 1968). In this DSM edition, however, the conceptual approach to psychoses and neuroses remained essentially the same. Also in DSM-II, cyclothymic personality remained in the personality disorder section with an added parenthetical descriptor (affective personality). The psychoses were split between organic brain syndromes and "functional psychoses." The former included disorders in which clear etiological factors, such as Alzheimer's disease, strokes, infections, nutritional deficiencies, or substance exposure, were involved. The functional psychoses—those not attributed to physical conditions—included manic-depressive illness (manic, depressed, and circular types) and involutional melancholia (affective psychosis). Anxiety was considered to be the chief characteristic of all of the neuroses that could be expressed directly, or controlled unconsciously and automatically (by psychological defense mechanisms). In the case of depressive neurosis, there was no gross distortion or falsification of external reality (e.g., delusions or hallucinations); this diagnosis was considered to be "an excessive reaction of depression due to an internal conflict or to an identifiable event such as the loss of a love object or cherished possession" (American Psychiatric Association 1968, p. 40).

Although DSM-I and DSM-II were developed jointly by APA and WHO's Division of Mental Health, there was a clear break in that collaboration with DSM-III (American Psychiatric Association 1980). The psychoanalytic (psychodynamic) and the social psychiatry (stress exposure) mental disorder etiological theories had lost some of their valence in both U.S. and European psychiatry. WHO had commissioned an international review of the "Classification of Mental Disorders" by Erwin Stengel. This included a review of the existing ICD and the American DSM, as well as Canadian, French, German, Dutch, Danish, Soviet, Japanese, Spanish, and Norwegian classifications. In addition, there were classifications named after the U.S. War Department and leading psychiatrists, including Klaus Conrad, Erik Essen-Möller, Carl Gustav Jung, Juan José López Ibor, Gabriel Langfeldt, Henrik Sjögren, Henricus Cornelius Rümke, Adolf Meyer, and Kurt Schneider. In fact, it appeared that every major department or "school" of psychiatry needed to have its own classification and followers. To bypass theoretical debates about the variations in mental disorder etiological concepts represented in these various classification schemes, Stengel (1959) recommended that "many of the difficulties created by lack of knowledge regarding pathology and etiology may be overcome by the use of 'operational definitions'" (p. 601), and then outlined the basic principles on which a generally acceptable international classification might be constructed. He noted that "this approach should lead to a greater measure of agreement regarding the value of specific treatments for mental disorders and greatly facilitate a broad epidemiological approach to psychiatric research" (Stengel 1959, p. 601).

As a result of the international collaboration of the U.S. National Institute of Mental Health (NIMH), APA, and WHO on DSM and ICD revisions from 1948 to 1968, there was also a focus on the statistical application of classifications to mental hospital admission diagnostic prevalence rates. Two U.S. mental health statisticians, Morton Kramer at NIMH and Joseph Zubin at Columbia University in New York, noted that there were marked differences in the reported admission rates of individuals with schizophrenia versus manic-depressive illness in London and New York City, with higher rates of schizophrenia diagnoses in New York and higher rates of manic-depressive disorder in London. To test whether there were true differences in risk factors for these disorders or simply differences in diagnostic criteria, the U.S./U.K. study of mental disorders was initiated with NIMH support (Cooper et al. 1972). By using a common glossary of diagnostic criteria incorporated into a structured diagnostic interview, the researchers demonstrated that the true prevalence rates were almost identical. Their findings led to adoption of a glossary of diagnostic terms that was added to DSM-II, ICD-8, and ICD-9 (American Psychiatric Association 1968; World Health Organization 1968, 1977).

In the United States, a more fundamental change was taking place in the late 1960s and early 1970s at Washington University in St. Louis, Missouri, where Eli Robins and Samuel Guze were leading a more biologically focused department of psychiatry that did not agree with either the psychodynamic or the social psychiatry theories about the etiology of mental disorders. With the assistance of one of their chief residents, John Feighner, they systematically studied the symptom profiles of patients admitted to their inpatient units and established diagnostic criteria for 16 different disorders (Feighner et al. 1972). Because this descriptive approach and underlying theory of a biological etiology was similar to that of Emil Kraepelin's classification approach in the late nineteenth and early twentieth centuries, it was referred to as a neo-Kraepelinian classification. Robins and Guze also recommended a series of criteria-validating steps, which included the development of laboratory studies to follow the natural clinical course of the illness, examine family genetic aggregation and risks, and assess whether there would be strict boundaries that would separate these disorders (Robins and Guze 1970). In contrast, the predominant psychodynamic formulation was that all "functional disorders" were on a continuum, and all were caused by different levels of psychodynamic conflicts (Menninger et al. 1963).

At NIMH in the early 1970s, there was also a growing emphasis on psychopharmacology. NIMH staff had to deal with conflicts between the psychoanalysts, who thought that these medications were interfering with their treatments, and the more biologically oriented psychiatrists, who viewed medications—such as the neuroleptic thorazine, mood stabilizer lithium, antidepressant imipramine, and anxiolytic benzodiazepine—as treating different specific illnesses. NIMH decided to conduct a collaborative depression study to test the "validity" of specific mood disorders that would include a biological laboratory study component and a longitudinal clinical course component, as recommended by Robins and Guze (1970). To devise a common diagnostic approach for the multiple sites used in this collaborative study, NIMH asked Robert Spitzer, who had trained under Joseph Zubin at Columbia University and then developed his own structured psychiatric interview (Spitzer et al. 1970), to work with Robins to incorporate the Feighner criteria into his interview for the NIMH study. The resultant Research Diagnostic Criteria (RDC) (Spitzer et al. 1978) and the Schedule for Affective Disorders and Schizophrenia (SADS) (Endicott and Spitzer 1987) were developed and used for this study, which was conceptualized as the longitudinal "Framingham Study" of these mental disorders. To separate the mood disorders from all other mental disorders, the SADS interview covered the full range of mental disorders, and also included a lifetime version (SADS-L) that was used in a Yale epidemiological study (Weissman and Myers 1978) and an early primary mental health care study of the NIMH primary care research program (Regier et al. 1985).

When WHO was ready to develop ICD-9, with a publication date of 1977, the APA also planned to issue the third edition of DSM (American Psychiatric Association 1980). Robert Spitzer applied to be the chair of the APA task force that would develop DSM-III, with the clear intent of using his experience with the RDC as a prototype for the entire mental disorder classification (Decker 2013). The intent was to use explicit descriptive diagnostic criteria for all disorders, with an announcement that the classification would be agnostic about any psychodynamic, social psychiatry, or biological etiology. By closely following the guidance that had been given to WHO by Stengel in 1960, Spitzer did indeed make the diagnostic criteria amenable to a new generation of epidemiological studies initiated by the NIMH Epidemiologic Catchment Area (ECA) project—using the Diagnostic Interview Schedule (DIS) that incorporated the DSM-III criteria (Regier et al. 1993; Robins and Regier 1991; Robins et al. 1981). This approach also made it possible to describe diagnostic groups for clinical treatment studies, including psychopharmacological and psychotherapy clinical trials. In the United States, clinical trials started to be conducted using the RDC-based SADS interview, which was then modified after publication of DSM-III by Robert Spitzer to become the Structured Clinical Interview for DSM (SCID) (Kay et al. 1991).

The DSM-III classification introduced bipolar disorder as a replacement term for manic-depressive illness and included circular, manic, mixed, and depressed subtypes. Of particular importance was the introduction of explicit criteria (A–E), with a required duration of at least 1 week (or hospitalization) during which at least three of seven symptomatic B criteria needed to be present, or four of seven if the mood was only irritable. DSM-III also introduced the concept of a hypomanic episode that was similar to but not as severe as a full manic episode. In addition to providing explicit criteria for a manic episode, similar A–E criteria were specified for a major depressive episode. The B criteria included a duration of at least 2 weeks and at least four of eight symptomatic criteria. There was also a specifier "with melancholia" that required at least three of six symptoms relating to diurnal sleep and depressed mood cycles, as well as significant anorexia, excessive guilt, and a qualitatively different type of depressed mood that is distinct from a grief reaction. As a precursor of a bipolar II diagnosis, there was an "atypical bipolar disorder" residual category that included features of a past major depressive episode with a current hypomanic episode that did not reach manic episode criteria.

Very significantly, cyclothymic disorder, requiring at least a 2-year duration of numerous periods of depression and hypomania, was moved from personality disorders into mood disorders; the hypomanic and depressive periods could not be of sufficient severity and duration to meet the criteria for a manic episode or a major depressive episode. The hypomanic periods needed to include at least 3 of 12 symptoms, and the depressive periods also required 3 of 12 different symptoms, with an absence of psychotic features of delusions, hallucinations, incoherence, or loosening of associations. Also with a 2-year duration criterion, dysthymic disorder (replacing depressive neurosis) was introduced, requiring at least 3 of 13 symptoms and an absence of psychotic features. With regard to the relationship of these disorders to the 1977 ICD-9 statistical coding conventions, both bipolar disorder and major depressive disorder were classified in the ICD-9 psychotic disorders section (296 [affective psychoses]), whereas dysthymic disorder (300.4 [neurotic depression]) and cyclothymic disorder (301.13 [affective personality disorder]) were classified in the neurotic disorders section of ICD-9.

The APA was encouraged to evaluate and update DSM-III just a few years after the 1980 publication, and changes to the mood disorders classification appeared in DSM-III-R (American Psychiatric Association 1987; Tischler 1987). The major depressive episode was modified to require five of nine symptoms, the melancholic subtype required five of nine slightly different symptoms, and a seasonal pattern subtype was introduced in which either manic or depressive symptoms regularly appeared in a particular 60-day period of the year.

Following publication of DSM-III in 1980, the "operational criteria" approach embodied in this edition rapidly became adopted for research purposes on an international level (Spitzer et al. 1983). This was facilitated by support for WHO from the U.S Alcohol, Drug Abuse, and Mental Health Administration (ADAMHA), which included NIMH, the National Institute on Alcohol Abuse and Alcoholism (NIAAA), and the National Institute on Drug Abuse (NIDA). The administrator of ADAMHA, Gerald Klerman, initiated a contract with the WHO Division of Mental Health (under Norman Sartorius) to review international classifications of mental disorders, which led to a 1982 Copenhagen conference where these reviews were reported (Sartorius 1983–2001)—with the result that there was broad international agreement to use DSM-III as the model for the tenth revision of ICD, set for 1992 (Jablensky et al. 1983). A cooperative agreement established between the ADAMHA institutes and WHO supported the development of three standardized interviews of mental disorders as a means of obtaining international agreement on the diagnostic criteria that would be incorporated into ICD-10. These interviews included the Composite International Diagnostic Interview (CIDI) (Robins et al. 1988), an epidemiological interview developed as an international version of the DIS used in the ECA project; the Schedules for Clinical Assessment in Neuropsychiatry (SCAN) (Wing et al. 1990), based on the Present State Examination (PSE; Wing et al. 1967) used in the U.S./U.K. project (Cooper et al. 1972); and the International Personality Disorders Examination (IPDE) (Loranger et al. 1991), based on the U.S. Personality Disorder Examination of Loranger (1988). Once all ICD-10 disorders were required to have explicit criteria that could be measured using these instruments, it was possible to obtain international agreement on criteria for this 1992 ICD edition that closely matched DSM-IV, which was published in 1994 (American Psychiatric Association 1994). A legal agreement between the APA and WHO permitted this close approximation without violation of the APA copyright on DSM-III, DSM-III-R, and DSM-IV.

The 1994 DSM-IV section on mood disorders reflected the changes in criteria recommended in the 1987 DSM-III-R, which included these disorders: major depressive disorder, dysthymic disorder, depressive disorder not otherwise specified (NOS), bi-

substituted for the current categorical approach to diagnosis, 5) increasing compatibility between DSM-5 and ICD-11, 6) assessing the applicability of criteria across different cultures, and 7) facilitating the diagnostic process in nonpsychiatric primary care settings. Discussions about these issues guided much of the DSM-5 developmental process and the coordination with the ICD-11 development until publication of DSM-5 in 2013. The major harmonization effort between the two classifications occurred in the overall reorganization of the entire mental health classification to reflect a more developmentally grounded and disorder spectrum–based organizational structure (Andrews et al. 2009). There was also the introduction of more dimensional measures in DSM-5, particularly in the sections on the following: neurodevelopmental disorders, schizophrenia spectrum and other psychotic disorders, bipolar and related disorders, depressive disorders, substance-related and addictive disorders, somatic symptom and related disorders, and personality disorders.

With regard to the mood disorders in DSM-5, the placement of bipolar disorder in a separate chapter from the depressive disorders constituted a significant structural change. The rationale for this move entailed a careful evaluation of 11 different validation criteria for the classification of schizophrenia, schizoaffective illness, bipolar disorder, major depressive disorder, and anxiety disorders. Relevant literature reviews for each of these disorder groups were performed to assess the following validating correlates: genetics, familiality, early environment, neural substrate, biomarkers, temperament, cognitive and emotional processing, symptomatology, comorbidity, course of illness, and treatment response (Goldberg et al. 2009a). Based on these correlates, it appeared that bipolar disorder was more closely related to schizophrenia than to unipolar major depressive disorder—with the latter more closely related to the anxiety disorder spectrum. All of the mental disorders consisting of states with increased levels of anxiety, depression, fear, and somatic symptoms were conceptualized as emotional or internalizing disorders (Goldberg et al. 2009b). As a result of the remaining clinical and validating distinctions between these conditions, the DSM-5 committee decided to maintain separate categories for bipolar disorder, depressive disorders, and anxiety disorders (Goldberg et al. 2010). However, the ICD-11 committee continued to group bipolar disorder with the mood disorders (Reed et al. 2019).

The bipolar and related disorders chapter of DSM-5 includes bipolar I disorder, bipolar II disorder, cyclothymic disorder, substance/medication-induced bipolar and related disorder, bipolar and related disorder due to another medical condition, other specified bipolar and related disorder, and unspecified bipolar and related disorder. In DSM-5, the definition of a component manic episode has been changed from DSM-IV Criterion A to read (additions underlined): "A distinct period of abnormally and persistently elevated, expansive, or irritable mood <u>and abnormally and persistently increased goal-directed activity or energy</u>, lasting at least 1 week, <u>and present most of the day, nearly every day</u> (or any duration if hospitalization is necessary)" (American Psychiatric Association 2013, p. 124). Criterion B of the manic episode criteria is largely unchanged from DSM-IV and requires three or more of seven symptoms or four of seven if the mood is only irritable. DSM-IV Criterion C, which excluded a mixed episode, was dropped in DSM-5 in favor of including a mixed features specifier among 10 specifiers for the bipolar and depressive disorder conditions. Criterion D in DSM-IV and Criterion C in DSM-5 require that the mood disturbance is sufficiently severe to cause marked impairment in social or occupational functioning or to necessitate hospitalization to prevent harm to self or others, or that psychotic features are present.

The definition of a major depressive episode in the DSM-5 bipolar and depressive disorder chapters is very similar to that in DSM-IV and requires five of nine symptoms occurring over the same 2-week period. DSM-IV symptom A1 has been changed to read (DSM-5 addition underlined) "depressed mood most of the day, nearly every day, as indicated by either subjective report (e.g., feels sad, empty, or hopeless) or observation made by others (e.g., appears tearful)." It is interesting to note that the "hopeless" symptom was previously included only in the dysthymia criteria of DSM-IV but had been included in the Patient Health Questionnaire–9 screening interview for major depressive disorder that was developed by Robert Spitzer; this 27-point instrument is recommended as a severity measure in DSM-5 (Spitzer et al. 1994). Criterion E, known as the bereavement exclusion in DSM-IV, was replaced in DSM-5 with a note requiring clinical judgment to distinguish major depressive disorder from a normal grief response to a significant loss. In addition, DSM-5 includes an extensive footnote describing the difference between a major depressive episode and a normal grief response. This modification in the criteria for a major depressive episode received a great deal of attention and attracted controversy during the development of DSM-5, and is dealt with somewhat differently in ICD-11 (Zachar et al. 2017). In ICD-11, the diagnosis of major depressive disorder is not excluded in a person who is bereaved, but it requires a longer duration (i.e., at least 1 month) and the presence of symptoms unlikely to be associated with a normal grief response, such as low self-worth, guilt not related to the lost loved one, psychotic symptoms, suicidal ideation, or psychomotor retardation (Stein et al. 2020). These additional requirements in ICD-11 for the diagnosis in bereaved persons are similar to but less complete than the description differentiating normal grief from a major depressive episode in the DSM-5 criteria note and footnote.

Bipolar I disorder in DSM-5 requires the presence of a manic episode that may have been preceded by and may be followed by a hypomanic episode or a major depressive episode. *Bipolar II disorder* requires a current or past hypomanic episode and a current or past major depressive episode. *Cyclothymic disorder* criteria are much more long term and require at least 2 years (1 year in children and adolescents) of numerous periods with hypomanic symptoms that never meet criteria for a hypomanic episode and numerous periods with depressive symptoms that fail to meet criteria for a major depressive episode. The hypomanic or depressive symptoms must cause clinically significant distress or impairment; they must be present for at least half of the 2- or 1-year time frame and must never be absent for more than 2 months at a time. *Substance/medication-induced bipolar and related disorder* requires prior exposure to a substance or medication capable of producing bipolar symptoms; ICD-10-CM coding instructions are provided for the various types of precipitating substances or medications (Centers for Medicare & Medicaid Services 2021). Likewise, *bipolar and related disorder due to another medical condition* requires that the syndrome be the direct pathophysiological consequence of another medical condition. Following ICD-10 conventions, there are also *other specified bipolar and related disorders*, with examples of subthreshold combinations of symptoms, and *unspecified bipolar and related disorders*, for use in cases where the clinician opts not to specify the reasons why criteria are not met for specific bipolar and related disorders.

DSM-5 includes 10 similar specifiers that—with the exception noted below—can be applied to either bipolar or depressive disorders:

1. With anxious distress
2. With mixed features
3. With rapid cycling (**Note:** applicable only to bipolar disorders)
4. With melancholic features
5. With atypical features
6. With mood-congruent psychotic features
7. With mood-incongruent psychotic features
8. With catatonia
9. With peripartum onset
10. With seasonal pattern

The added symptom profiles provided by the specifiers are intended to allow a more dimensional description of the bipolar and depressive disorders without producing the expanded number of separate categorical disorders that would otherwise result from multiplying the number of specifiers by the number of separately identified disorders. ICD-11 uses the term *qualifiers* instead of *specifiers* to include refined (more dimensional) descriptions of current mood episodes, including prominent anxiety, melancholy, current perinatal episode, seasonal patterns, and rapid cycling. Although ICD-11 does not include a mixed features qualifier for either bipolar or depressive disorders, it has retained the DSM-IV and ICD-10 "mixed-episode" category for bipolar I disorder—most recent episode mixed, which was eliminated in DSM-5 (Stein et al. 2020).

The DSM-5 section on depressive disorders includes, for the first time, *disruptive mood dysregulation disorder*, a condition that should not be diagnosed before age 6 or after age 18 years. It requires severe recurrent temper outbursts and either verbal or physical rage episodes (which can include physical aggression) that are out of proportion in intensity or duration to the situation or provocation. These outbursts occur three or more times per week, and irritable or angry mood persists between outbursts for most of the day, nearly every day, for 12 or more months. The major debate in developing criteria for this disorder was that it was not considered to be bipolar disorder, conduct disorder, or intermittent explosive disorder, although it shares multiple symptoms with each of these conditions. Disruptive mood dysregulation disorder was not included in ICD-11, which considered it to be more similar to conduct disorder. Following publication of DSM-5, the borderline personality disorder advocacy community expressed concern that this symptom profile may reflect a childhood onset of borderline personality disorder.

Major depressive disorder is largely unchanged from DSM-IV, with the exception of the addition in DSM-5 of hopelessness as an example of depressed mood and the elimination of the bereavement criteria for depressive episode. The addition of the specifier "with anxious distress" requires at least two of five symptoms that include feeling keyed up or tense, feeling unusually restless, difficulty concentrating because of worry, fear that something awful may happen, and feeling that the individual might lose control of himself or herself. Severity is rated according to number of symptoms as mild (2/5), moderate (3/5), moderate-severe (4–5/5), or severe (4–5/5 with motor agitation) (American Psychiatric Association 2013, p. 184). This severity specifier was added when it was found in the DSM-5 field trials that a separate diagnosis of anxious depression was not reliably diagnosed, even though a majority of people with major depressive disorder are found to have significant anxiety (Regier et al. 2013).

Persistent depressive disorder (dysthymia) was introduced into DSM-5 to combine DSM-IV dysthymia that required a 2-year duration and DSM-IV chronic major depressive episode that also required a 2-year duration. Several key studies had been unable to find any difference in correlates or outcomes for these two conditions.

Premenstrual dysphoric disorder, which was included in the DSM-IV appendix "Conditions for Further Study," was studied extensively between 1994 and 2012 and shown to have the requisite syndrome pattern and clinical distress and disability to be recognized as a disorder, as well as a good response to recognized treatments. The treatment responses were sufficient to receive an FDA indication for antidepressant medications—a rare accomplishment for a mental disorder not recognized in DSM-IV.

Substance/medication-induced depressive disorder, depressive disorder due to another medical condition, other specified depressive disorder, and *unspecified depressive disorder* have a structure and rationale similar to the bipolar disorders with identical modifiers discussed above.

Future of Mood Disorder Classification

Although the current DSM and ICD classifications of mood disorder have largely retained specific categorical diagnoses with explicit diagnostic criteria, the many overlaps in criteria produce very porous boundaries across spectra of disorders in the depressive and bipolar disorder groups. The requirement for clinically significant distress or impairment for almost all other DSM and ICD disorders means that some combination of depressive and anxiety symptoms is inevitably present in most mental disorders. The research screening instrument that is most frequently used in epidemiological and many clinical studies to detect the clinical significance criteria is the Kessler Psychological Distress Scale (either the 6-item [K6] or the 10-item [K10] version), which covers a broad range of depressive and anxiety symptoms (Andrews and Slade 2001). The presence of depressive and anxiety symptoms in virtually all clinically significant mental disorders is widely understood to result in high levels of comorbidity between specific mental and addictive disorders. This finding also results in spectra disorders, with porous instead of the strict boundaries between categorical disorders envisioned by the Robins and Guze (1970) validation criteria.

As genetic research has advanced with genome-wide association studies (GWASs) of specific mental disorders, there have been increasing requirements for linking the large number of genetic variants with component traits and symptom profiles of thousands of people diagnosed with these disorders (Lee et al. 2013). The very heterogeneous nature of specific mental disorders has led NIMH to establish the Research Domain Criteria (RDoC), a research program that supports a dimensional characterization of research subjects (Insel et al. 2010). The cross-diagnostic symptom domains of interest include negative valence systems, positive valence systems, cognitive systems, systems for social processes, and arousal/modulatory systems. Both animal and human subjects may be assessed in these domains using progressively more complex units of analysis, including genetic, molecular, cellular, neurocircuitry, physiological, and behavioral studies. Ideally, results from such studies should be linked to the clinical patient profiles that are routinely assessed for the thousands of patients in genetic studies with DSM and ICD diagnostic criteria (Cuthbert 2014; Regier 2015; Vaidyanathan et al. 2015). Unfortunately, such linkages are not routinely leaping the bench-to-bedside implementation hurdles. By taking a more clinically informed empirical approach to dimensional diagnoses of mental disorders, the Hierarchical Typology of Psychopathology (HiTOP) has initiated a much more detailed description of traits, symptoms, and syndromes that has a better chance of linking to GWAS and RDoC correlates than the current heterogeneous DSM and ICD disorder groups (Kotov et al. 2017). Nonetheless, application of dimensional trait and symptom profiles to patients is difficult in routine clinical settings, and further automation of such assessments will be needed before DSM and ICD diagnostic practices are replaced in such settings (Ruggero et al. 2019).

In the immediate future, DSM-5 is the standard classification system for clinical diagnosis of mental disorders in the United States, with diagnostic codes drawn from ICD-10-CM for all medical records. DSM-5 is also the standard classification system for clinical trials research in the United States and much of the international scientific community.

ICD-11 was approved by the World Health Assembly in May 2019 (World Health Organization 2019) but will not be available for official adoption in any WHO member country until 2022. Each member state of the United Nations and WHO must decide when it will transition from ICD-10 to the new ICD-11 classification and coding system. For the United States, this transition will require the federal government to discontinue use of the ICD-10-CM alphanumeric coding system (A00.00–Z99.99) and adopt the ICD-11 numeric-alpha-numeric system (01A00.00–99Z99.99). Considering that it took 23 years of negotiations from the WHO release of ICD-10 in 1992 to the U.S. adoption of ICD-10-CM in 2015, it is unclear how long it will take to negotiate resistance from electronic health record and health insurance companies to reprogram their coding systems and adopt ICD-11.

Nevertheless, DSM-5 is largely similar to ICD-11 in organization and content (Regier et al. 2020). Because DSM-5 maintains this compatibility with the ICD-10-CM codes, one can expect that the annual ICD-10-CM coding updates will gradually adopt many of the ICD-11 substantive revisions over the next decade. This is similar to how ICD-9-CM, issued in 1979 with numeric codes (000.00–999.99), gradually changed to adopt the DSM-III disorders in 1980 and the DSM-IV disorders in 1994. By 2015, when the United States discontinued ICD-9-CM and adopted ICD-10-CM, all of the DSM-IV diagnoses had been incorporated into ICD-10, and some of the DSM-5 disorder changes were ready for incorporation into the first annual revisions of ICD-10-CM. Because each ICD edition coding change substantially increased the number of coding options, the major problem with adopting new, more complex substantive diagnoses while continuing to use older ICD codes is that there are insufficient coding options to fully capture the new disorders. The same will be true until ICD-11 and its associated codes become the international standard for clinical mental disorder diagnoses.

To develop phenotypic diagnoses for research that can be linked more closely with genotype-validating criteria, there will still need to be a paradigm shift in clinical descriptions of large patient populations. This shift will inevitably require a greater degree of dimensional assessments to match the dimensional complexity of genetic risk profiles (e.g., Manhattan plots). A step in this direction was provided by the DSM-5 Alternative Model for Personality Disorders (in DSM-5 Section III, "Emerging Measures and Models"), which enabled a more dimensional assessment of component traits and impairments of personality disorders that could be matched with genetic traits.

It remains to be seen whether the RDoC approach to classifying biological traits or the HiTOP approach of classifying phenotypic traits and symptoms will ultimately lead to an international research standard (Krueger and Bezdjian 2009). How future DSM and ICD revisions adapt to such paradigm changes will depend on the explanatory power that these approaches bring to the development of new treatments for mood and all other mental disorders.

References

American Psychiatric Association: Diagnostic and Statistical Manual: Mental Disorders. Washington, DC, American Psychiatric Association, 1952

American Psychiatric Association: Diagnostic and Statistical Manual of Mental Disorders, 2nd Edition. Washington, DC, American Psychiatric Association, 1968

American Psychiatric Association: Diagnostic and Statistical Manual of Mental Disorders, 3rd Edition. Washington, DC, American Psychiatric Association, 1980

American Psychiatric Association: Diagnostic and Statistical Manual of Mental Disorders, 3rd Edition, Revised. Washington, DC, American Psychiatric Association, 1987

American Psychiatric Association: Diagnostic and Statistical Manual of Mental Disorders, 4th Edition. Washington, DC, American Psychiatric Association, 1994

American Psychiatric Association: Diagnostic and Statistical Manual of Mental Disorders, 5th Edition. Arlington, VA, American Psychiatric Association, 2013

Andrews G, Slade T: Interpreting scores on the Kessler Psychological Distress Scale (K10). Aust N Z J Public Health 25(6):494–497, 2001 11824981

Andrews G, Henderson S, Hall W: Prevalence, comorbidity, disability and service utilisation. Overview of the Australian National Mental Health Survey. Br J Psychiatry 178:145–153, 2001 11157427

Andrews G, Goldberg DP, Krueger RF, et al: Exploring the feasibility of a meta-structure for DSM-V and ICD-11: could it improve utility and validity? Psychol Med 39(12):1993–2000, 2009 19796425

Centers for Medicare & Medicaid Services: The International Classification of Diseases, 10th Revision, Clinical Modification (ICD-10-CM): The Complete Official Codebook. January 2021 Integrated Outpatient Code Editor (I/OCE) Specifications, Version 22.0. Available at: https://www.cms.gov/Medicare/Coding/OutpatientCodeEdit/OCEQtrReleaseSpecs. Accessed September 27, 2021.

Cooper JE, Kendell RE, Gurland BJ, et al: Psychiatric Diagnosis in New York and London: A Comparative Study of Mental Hospital Admissions. London, Oxford University Press, 1972

Cuthbert BN: The RDoC framework: facilitating transition from ICD/DSM to dimensional approaches that integrate neuroscience and psychopathology. World Psychiatry 13(1):28–35, 2014 24497240

Decker H: The Making of DSM-III: A Diagnostic Manual's Conquest of American Psychiatry. New York, Oxford University Press, 2013

Endicott J, Spitzer RL: [Schedule for Affective Disorders and Schizophrenia (SADS) [in French]]. Acta Psychiatr Belg 87(4):361–516, 1987 3434318

Engel GL: The clinical application of the biopsychosocial model. Am J Psychiatry 137(5):535–544, 1980 7369396

Feighner JP, Robins E, Guze SB, et al: Diagnostic criteria for use in psychiatric research. Arch Gen Psychiatry 26(1):57–63, 1972 5009428

Goldberg DP, Andrews G, Hobbs MJ: Where should bipolar disorder appear in the meta-structure? Psychol Med 39(12):2071–2081, 2009a 19796430

Goldberg DP, Krueger RF, Andrews G, Hobbs MJ: Emotional disorders: cluster 4 of the proposed meta-structure for DSM-V and ICD-11. Psychol Med 39(12):2043–2059, 2009b 19796429

Goldberg D, Kendler KS, Sirovatka PJ, Regier DA (eds): Diagnostic Issues in Depression and Generalized Anxiety Disorder. Refining the Research Agenda for DSM-V. Washington, DC, American Psychiatric Publishing, 2010

Insel T, Cuthbert B, Garvey M, et al: Research Domain Criteria (RDoC): developing a valid diagnostic framework for research on mental disorders. Am J Psychiatry 167:748–751, 2010 20595427

Jablensky A, Sartorius N, Hirschfeld R, et al: Diagnosis and classification of mental disorders and alcohol- and drug-related problems: a research agenda for the 1980s. Psychol Med 13(4):907–921, 1983 6665106

Kay SR, Opler LA, Spitzer RL, et al: SCID-PANSS: two-tier diagnostic system for psychotic disorders. Compr Psychiatry 32(4):355–361, 1991 1935026

Kotov R, Krueger RF, Watson D, et al: The Hierarchical Taxonomy of Psychopathology (HiTOP): a dimensional alternative to traditional nosologies. J Abnorm Psychol 126(4):454–477, 2017 28333488

Krueger RF, Bezdjian S: Enhancing research and treatment of mental disorders with dimensional concepts: toward DSM-V and ICD-11. World Psychiatry 8(1):3–6, 2009 19293948

Kupfer DJ, First MB, Regier DA: Introduction, in A Research Agenda for DSM-V. Edited by Kupfer DJ, First MB, Regier DA. Arlington, VA, American Psychiatric Association, 2002, pp xv–xxiii

Lee SH, Ripke S, Neale BM, et al; Cross-Disorder Group of the Psychiatric Genomics Consortium; International Inflammatory Bowel Disease Genetics Consortium (IIBDGC): Genetic relationship between five psychiatric disorders estimated from genome-wide SNPs. Nat Genet 45(9):984–994, 2013 23933821

Loranger AW: Personality Disorder Examination (PDE) Manual. Yonkers, NY, DV Communications, 1988

Loranger AW, Hirschfeld RMA, Sartorius N, Regier DA: The WHO/ADAMHA International Pilot Study of Personality Disorders: background and purpose. Journal of Personality Disorders 5(3):296–306, 1991. Available at: https://guilfordjournals.com/doi/10.1521/pedi.1991.5.3.296. Accessed September 27, 2021.

Menninger K, Mayman M, Pruyser P: The Vital Balance: The Life Process in Mental Health and Illness. New York, Viking Press, 1963

Reed GM, First MB, Kogan CS, et al: Innovations and changes in the ICD-11 classification of mental, behavioural and neurodevelopmental disorders. World Psychiatry 18(1):3–19, 2019 30600616

Regier DA: Potential DSM-5 and RDoC synergy for mental health research, treatment, and health policy advances. Psychol Inq 26:268–271, 2015

Regier DA, Burke JD Jr, Manderscheid RW, Burns BJ: The chronically mentally ill in primary care. Psychol Med 15(2):265–273, 1985 4023131

Regier DA, Narrow WE, Rae DS, et al: The de facto U.S. mental and addictive disorders service system. Epidemiologic Catchment Area prospective 1-year prevalence rates of disorders and services. Arch Gen Psychiatry 50(2):85–94, 1993 8427558

Regier DA, Narrow WE, Clarke DE, et al: DSM-5 field trials in the United States and Canada, II: test-retest reliability of selected categorical diagnoses. Am J Psychiatry 170(1):59–70, 2013 23111466

Regier DA, Goldberg DP, Reed GM, Ustün T: DSM-5 and ICD-11 classifications, in New Oxford Textbook of Psychiatry. London, Oxford University Press, 2020, pp 51–61

Robins E, Guze SB: Establishment of diagnostic validity in psychiatric illness: its application to schizophrenia. Am J Psychiatry 126(7):983–987, 1970 5409569

Robins E, Regier DA: Psychiatric Disorders in America: The Epidemiologic Catchment Area Study. New York, Free Press, 1991

Robins LN, Helzer JE, Croughan J, Ratcliff KS: National Institute of Mental Health Diagnostic Interview Schedule. Its history, characteristics, and validity. Arch Gen Psychiatry 38(4):381–389, 1981 6260053

Robins LN, Wing J, Wittchen HU, et al: The Composite International Diagnostic Interview. An epidemiologic instrument suitable for use in conjunction with different diagnostic systems and in different cultures. Arch Gen Psychiatry 45(12):1069–1077, 1988 2848472

Rounsaville BJ, Alarcon RD, Andrews G, et al: Basic nomenclature issues for DSM-V, in A Research Agenda for DSM-V. Edited by Kupfer DJ, First MB, Regier DA. Arlington, VA, American Psychiatric Association, 2002, pp 1–29

Ruggero CJ, Kotov R, Hopwood CJ, et al: Integrating the Hierarchical Taxonomy of Psychopathology (HiTOP) into clinical practice. J Consult Clin Psychol 87(12):1069–1084, 2019 31724426

Sartorius N (principal investigator): The WHO/Alcohol, Drug Abuse, and Mental Health Administration Joint Project on Diagnosis and Classification. Cooperative agreement U01MH035883, from the National Institute of Mental Health to the World Health Organization, 1983–2001

Slade T, Andrews G: DSM-IV and ICD-10 generalized anxiety disorder: discrepant diagnoses and associated disability. Soc Psychiatry Psychiatr Epidemiol 36(1):45–51, 2001 11320807

Spitzer RL, Endicott J, Fleiss JL, Cohen J: The Psychiatric Status Schedule. A technique for evaluating psychopathology and impairment in role functioning. Arch Gen Psychiatry 23(1):41–55, 1970 4911363

Spitzer RL, Endicott J, Robins E: Research Diagnostic Criteria: rationale and reliability. Arch Gen Psychiatry 35(6):773–782, 1978 655775

Spitzer RL, Williams JBW, Skodol AE: International Perspectives on DSM-III. Washington, DC, American Psychiatric Press, 1983

Spitzer RL, Williams JB, Kroenke K, et al: Utility of a new procedure for diagnosing mental disorders in primary care. The PRIME-MD 1000 study. JAMA 272(22):1749–1756, 1994 7966923

Stein DJ, Szatmari P, Gaebel W, et al: Mental, behavioral and neurodevelopmental disorders in the ICD-11: an international perspective on key changes and controversies. BMC Med 18(1):21, 2020 31983345

Stengel E: Classification of mental disorders. Bull World Health Organ 21(4–5):601–663, 1959 13834299

Tischler GL (ed): Diagnosis and Classification in Psychiatry: A Critical Appraisal of DSM-III. New York, Cambridge University Press, 1987

Ustün TB, Goldberg D, Cooper J, et al: New classification for mental disorders with management guidelines for use in primary care: ICD-10 PHC chapter five. Br J Gen Pract 45(393):211–215, 1995 7612324

Vaidyanathan U, Vrieze SI, Iacono WG: The art of smart science: weaving theory and risky study design into psychopathology research and RDoC. Psychol Inq 26(3):286–292, 2015 27019570

Weissman MM, Myers JK: Affective disorders in a U.S. urban community: the use of Research Diagnostic Criteria in an epidemiological survey. Arch Gen Psychiatry 35(11):1304–1311, 1978 708194

Wing JK, Birley JL, Cooper JE: Reliability of a procedure for measuring and classifying "present psychiatric state." Br J Psychiatry 113(498):499–515, 1967 6033492

Wing JK, Babor T, Brugha T, et al; SCAN: Schedules for Clinical Assessment in Neuropsychiatry. Arch Gen Psychiatry 47(6):589–593, 1990 2190539

World Health Organization: International Classification of Diseases, 6th Revision. Geneva, World Health Organization, 1948

World Health Organization: International Classification of Diseases, 8th Revision. Geneva, World Health Organization, 1968
World Health Organization: International Classification of Diseases, 9th Revision. Geneva, World Health Organization, 1977
World Health Organization: International Classification of Diseases, 9th Revision, Clinical Modification. Ann Arbor, MI, Commission on Professional and Hospital Activities, 1978
World Health Organization: ICD-10 Classification of Mental and Behavioural Disorders: Clinical Descriptions and Diagnostic Guidelines. Geneva, World Health Organization, 1992a
World Health Organization: Manual of the International Statistical Classification of Diseases, Injuries, and Causes of Death. Geneva, World Health Organization, 1992b
World Health Organization: The ICD-10 Classification of Mental and Behavioral Disorders: Diagnostic Criteria for Research. Geneva, World Health Organization, 1993
World Health Organization: Diagnostic and Management Guidelines for Mental Disorders in Primary Care: ICD-10 Chapter V Primary Care Version. Göttingen, Germany, Hogrefe and Huber, 1996
World Health Organization: International Classification of Diseases, 11th Revision. Geneva, World Health Organization, 2019
Zachar P, First MB, Kendler KS: The bereavement exclusion debate in the DSM-5: a history. Clinical Psychological Science 5(5):890–906, 2017. Available at: https://journals.sagepub.com/doi/abs/10.1177/2167702617711284. Accessed September 27, 2021.

CHAPTER 3

Epidemiology and Burden of Mood Disorders

Ronald C. Kessler, Ph.D.
Andrew A. Nierenberg, M.D.
Brenda W.J.H. Penninx, M.D., Ph.D.
Philip S. Wang, M.D., Dr.P.H.
Hans-Ulrich Wittchen, Ph.D.
Hannah N. Ziobrowski, Ph.D., M.P.H.

In this chapter, we review the literature on the descriptive epidemiology and burden of mood disorders worldwide. Data on these topics have increased substantially over the past two decades as governments have implemented epidemiological surveys to provide guidance for mental health policy planning (Kawakami et al. 2020; Stagnaro et al. 2018), meta-analyses have been conducted using these epidemiological surveys (Charlson et al. 2016; Whiteford et al. 2016), and policy proposals have been developed based on the results of these meta-analyses (Patel et al. 2016; Vigo et al. 2016). The realizations that mood disorders are highly prevalent and that they have substantial costs to the individuals experiencing them, as well as to their families and society emerged for the first time among health policy analysts as a result of the World Health Organization's (WHO's) 1996 Global Burden of Disease (GBD) Study (Murray and Lopez 1996). In that study, researchers attempted to quantify the relative importance of diverse illnesses with a metric other than mortality by taking into consideration the comparative effects of different illnesses on impaired role functioning. After considering the data in this way, the GBD researchers concluded that mental and substance use disorders, which do not figure prominently as causes of mortality, are the most burdensome class of disorders in the world, accounting for nearly one-fourth of all years lived with disability (Alonso et al. 2013; James et al. 2018). Mood disorders are the most important mental or substance use disorders in this respect, as they account for more than 40% of all years lived with disability due to these disorders (Whiteford et al. 2013). Other epidemiological studies have found that mood disorders contribute to an even greater burden than the role-related burdens examined in the GBD studies (Alonso et al. 2013). But why are mood disorders so burdensome from a societal perspective? We review the major factors contributing to an answer in this chapter.

We will not review the epidemiological data on mood disorders among children or among the elderly in this chapter, because significant methodological and conceptual problems exist in estimating the prevalence and burden of mood disorders in both of these populations. These issues are discussed elsewhere (Arean et al. 2017; Powell et al. 2017; Richards and Bearden 2017; see also Chapter 37, "Pediatric Mood Disorders," and Chapter 38, "Geriatric Mood Disorders," in this volume). We also will not discuss epidemiological risk factors for mood disorders, which are reviewed elsewhere (Johnson et al. 2017; Monroe and Cummins 2017).

Epidemiology of Mood Disorders

Prevalence

The many forms of mood disorders are typically divided into two groups: 1) unipolar depressive disorders, which include various forms of major depressive disorder and dysthymia (the latter term is used in DSM-IV and DSM-IV-TR [American Psychiatric Association 1994, 2000], whereas persistent depressive disorder is the term used in DSM-5 [American Psychiatric Association 2013]), and 2) bipolar and related disorders, including bipolar I and bipolar II disorders as well as cyclothymia. The epidemiological evidence presented in this chapter is almost exclusively based on DSM-IV criteria due to the lack of available epidemiological data on DSM-5 disorders.

Depressive disorders of various degrees of severity are by far the most frequent mood disorders. An estimated 4.4%–5.0% of the world's population experience an episode of major depressive disorder (MDD) in any given 12-month period (Ferrari et al. 2013; World Health Organization 2018), although there is substantial variation by country and region. Perhaps the most accurate 12-month MDD prevalence estimate for adults in the United States before the increase caused by the coronavirus disease 2019 (COVID-19) pandemic was 7.7% (Kessler et al. 2012b). Similar estimates have been reported in European Union countries (Wittchen et al. 2011). Much less information exists on lifetime MDD prevalence, with the most comprehensive data coming from the WHO's World Mental Health (WMH) Survey Initiative (Bromet et al. 2018), which conducted coordinated adult community epidemiological surveys in 28 countries. In those surveys, retrospectively reported lifetime MDD prevalence rates averaged 10.6% across countries, with an interquartile range (IQR) of 6%–14%. It is likely that these retrospective self-reports underestimate true lifetime MDD prevalence (Moffitt et al. 2010).

Bipolar I disorder (which requires the occurrence of a full manic episode) and bipolar II disorder (which requires the occurrence of a hypomanic episode or a major depressive episode [MDE] in a person with a lifetime history of the other type of episode) are less prevalent than MDD. For example, the WMH surveys estimated that the 12-month prevalence of broad bipolar spectrum disorders was 1.2%, with estimates for bipolar I disorder, bipolar II disorder, and subthreshold bipolar disorder (i.e., either a hypomanic episode by a person with no lifetime history of MDE or a subthreshold hypomanic episode by a person with a lifetime history of MDE) of 0.4%, 0.3%, and 0.8%, respectively (Merikangas et al. 2011). Across countries, retrospectively reported lifetime broad bipolar spectrum disorder prevalence was 1.9% in the WMH surveys, although this estimate varied widely across surveys (IQRs of 0.6–2.5; Kessler et al. 2018). Aggregate lifetime prevalence estimates were 0.6% for bipolar I disorder, 0.4% for bipolar II disorder, and 1.4% for subthreshold bipolar disorder (Merikangas et al. 2011). As with MDD, these retrospective lifetime prevalence estimates likely underestimate true lifetime prevalence (Moffitt et al. 2010).

Point prevalence estimates of dysthymia (i.e., chronic minor depression with a duration of more than 2 years that has never met diagnostic criteria for MDD) average about 1.5% in the epidemiological studies in which such estimates have been assessed (Charlson et al. 2013). Reliable estimates for cyclothymic disorder—as part of the bipolar spectrum—are not available.

Available nationally representative data from adults in the United States suggest that about 30% of MDD cases in the population at a point in time are severe, 50% moderate, and 20% mild using conventional clinical severity thresholds (Kessler et al. 2005). The great majority of bipolar disorder cases at a point in time, in comparison, are estimated to be serious (82%) and the remainder moderate. Among adolescents, nationally representative U.S. data suggest that about one-third of mood disorder cases are severe and the remainder are moderate or mild (Kessler et al. 2012a).

In addition to the prevalence of mood disorders, another useful metric for describing the magnitude of the burden of mood disorders is the *lifetime morbid risk*. The latter is an estimate of the proportion of individuals in the population who will ever experience a mood disorder in their lifetime. This estimate is considerably higher than the proportion of the population that has ever experienced a mood disorder to date because of the relatively high proportion of all mood disorders, especially MDD, with first onsets in middle or old age (Kessler et al. 2012b).

Beyond the established DSM diagnoses, there is also substantial interest in clinically significant *mood syndromes* that do not meet established diagnostic criteria (Angst and Merikangas 1997; Ayuso-Mateos et al. 2010). Although no broad agreement exists on the best way to define these syndromes, prevalence estimates of "minor depression" (i.e., when individuals experience fewer symptoms or a shorter duration of symptoms, typically less than 2 weeks) and of "recurrent brief depression" (i.e., when individuals experience depressive episodes that last only a few days at a time but recur on a periodic basis over 1 or more years) have been as high as 17% (Rodríguez et al. 2012; Vandeleur et al. 2017). Epidemiological studies of these syndromes have only assessed current prevalence, and therefore no research is available on their lifetime prevalence. However, we know from available research that the prevalence of minor depression, unlike MDD, is high among children (Wesselhoeft et al. 2013) and adolescents (Carrellas et al. 2017). We also know that minor depressive syndromes can be associated with substantial distress and impairment, indicating that they are clinically significant (Ayuso-Mateos et al. 2010; Merikangas et al. 1994). Furthermore, individuals with subthreshold depressive syndromes have an elevated risk for subsequently developing MDD (Angst and Merikangas 1997; Forsell 2007) and bipolar disorder, which suggests that people with subthreshold depressive disorders might particularly benefit from early intervention (Angst and Merikangas 1997; Judd et al. 2002).

A syndrome referred to as mixed anxiety-depression disorder (MADD) has also been studied as a cross-sectional diagnosis of clinical interest. ICD-10 defined MADD as the co-occurrence of subsyndromal depression with subsyndromal anxiety disorder (World Health Organization 1992). Prevalence estimates for MADD, which require that the person never meet full criteria for either MDD or an anxiety disorder, are highly variable due to different definitions and study designs (Batelaan et al. 2012). A key question, however, is whether it is important to distinguish between MADD and minor depression. The small amount of research that has investigated this issue suggests that this distinction is not important, because the persistence-progression and severity are comparable in the two syndromes (Spijker et al. 2010). This is a different matter from the new ICD-11 category of threshold anxious depression (which requires full criteria for MDD and a reduced duration requirement for anxiety symptoms from the several months required for a diagnosis of generalized anxiety disorder to the same 2 weeks as MDD), as the evidence is clear that this subtype of MDD is much more impairing than non-anxious MDD (Ziebold et al. 2019).

Course

Prospective evidence from both clinical and community epidemiological studies shows that MDD tends to be an intermittent recurrent disorder over the life course (Coryell et al. 2009; Klein et al. 2008; Ten Have et al. 2019), with a variable number, type, and duration of episodes. However, there is great heterogeneity in the natural course of MDD. Persistence and length of episodes are lower in the general population than among individuals who seek treatment, with the latter often exhibiting only partial remission between episodes (Coryell et al. 2009; Klein et al. 2008; Ten Have et al. 2019). Most depressive episodes remit within 1 year. However, a large minority of individuals in community samples (Eaton et al. 2008; Hardeveld et al. 2013; Mattisson et al. 2007; Ten Have et al. 2018) and a majority in clinical samples (Conradi et al. 2017; Gopinath et al. 2007; Hardeveld et al. 2013; Holma et al. 2008; Mueller et al. 1999; Paterniti et al. 2017; Ramana et al. 1995; Riihimäki et al. 2014) experience a recurrence of MDD after an initial remission of symptoms. Moreover, chronic episodes, characterized by symptoms persisting for at least 2 consecutive years, are relatively common (Comijs et al. 2015; Judd et al. 1998; Penninx et al. 2013; Rhebergen et al. 2010; Ten Have et al. 2018; Verduijn et al. 2017). Especially if individuals with MDD are followed up over longer periods of time, recurrent and chronic episodes are more often the rule than the exception (Verduijn et al. 2017).

The course of bipolar disorder is also very heterogeneous but is typically characterized by distinct periods of mania, hypomania, depression, and mixed mood episodes of variable duration and severity interspersed with periods of euthymia (i.e., a relatively stable mood state) (Alvarez Ariza et al. 2009; Judd et al. 2008; Miller et al. 2004; Paykel et al. 2006). Manic/hypomanic, depressive, and mixed periods can switch rapidly from one pole to the other (i.e., have great polarity) or can be separated by periods of subsyndromal symptoms rather than euthymia. The polarity, frequency, duration, and intensity of manic and depressive periods (which may include episodes of psychosis) are highly variable, both within and between individuals (Alvarez Ariza et al. 2009; Judd et al. 2008; Miller et al. 2004; Paykel et al. 2006).

Clinical studies in people with bipolar disorder show that depressive episodes typically have first onsets earlier than manic or hypomanic episodes; that these depressive episodes are typically more frequent than mania/hypomania or mixed episodes; that mixed episodes typically have the longest durations, followed by depressive episodes; and that depressive and mixed episodes are associated with more impairment than manic/hypomanic episodes (Saunders and Goodwin 2010). In addition, rapid cycling between manic and depressive periods in clinical samples has been associated with earlier age at onset and greater disease burden (Bauer et al. 1994). Individuals with rapid cycling are likely to experience greater distress and disturbance in everyday functioning (Bauer et al. 1994; Coryell et al. 2003) and therefore may be more likely to seek treatment than individuals without rapid cycling (Demyttenaere et al. 2004). Estimates of the relative prevalence and correlates of rapid cycling in clinical samples (Oepen et al. 2004) thus may provide a biased portrait of patterns in the population.

True prevalence and correlates of rapid cycling are unknown in the general population because it is difficult to date the onset and offset of manic and depressive episodes or to delineate clear periods of partial or full remission in community samples. However, some relevant information has been reported on frequent mood episodes, defined as self-reports of four or more separate major depressive episodes or mania/hypomania episodes within a year, as a proxy measure for rapid cycling, in the WMH surveys (Lee et al. 2010; Nierenberg et al. 2010). About 40% of WMH survey respondents with 12-month bipolar disorder and close to one-third of those with lifetime bipolar disorder reported a history of frequent mood episodes. These respondents reported an earlier age at onset, higher persistence, more severe depressive symptoms, greater impairment associated with depressive symptoms, more days out-of-role associated with mania/hypomania, more anxiety disorders, and an increased likelihood of using health services in comparison with respondents without frequent mood episodes.

Age at Onset

Recently, the literature on age at onset of MDD (Yalin and Young 2019) and of bipolar disorder (Dagani et al. 2019) was reviewed comprehensively. Age at onset is an important but often neglected aspect of the epidemiology of mood disorders. Early age at onset is associated with delays in initial help-seeking and increased disorder persistence and severity (de Girolamo et al. 2019). For MDD, the median age at onset was found to be in the mid-20s. This is later than the median age at onset for several other psychiatric disorders that are highly comorbid with MDD (Kessler et al. 2007b, 2011), which means that MDD is typically the (temporally) secondary disorder in commonly occurring multivariate disorder profiles. This relatively late age at onset also means that when comparing estimates of lifetime disorder burden, adjustments must be made for between-disorder differences in future onsets, because relative estimated lifetime prevalence (i.e., the proportion of the population who have experienced the disorder to date) will be lower than relative estimated lifetime morbid risk (i.e., the projected proportion of the population who will experience the disorder at some time in their life, as estimated using actuarial methods with life tables [Kessler et al. 2007c,

2012b]) for disorders with later-age-at-onset distributions. The situation is similar for bipolar disorder, in which the median age at onset—that is, in the mid-20s—was estimated to be similar to that of MDD.

Comorbidities With Other Mental Disorders and the Higher-Order Structure of Comorbidity

The majority of people with a history of a mood disorder also meet lifetime criteria for at least one other mental disorder (Kessler and Ustün 2008; Merikangas et al. 2011). This comorbidity—confirmed by prospective and retrospective longitudinal data (Beesdo et al. 2010; Beesdo-Baum et al. 2015)—is particularly strong for MDD with anxiety and substance use disorders, as observed in both community-based epidemiological studies (Hasin et al. 2018; Wanders et al. 2016) and clinical studies with patients from both primary care (Aillon et al. 2014; Kotiaho et al. 2019) and specialty care settings (Lamers et al. 2011). Community-based epidemiological studies have similarly observed that bipolar disorder is highly comorbid with anxiety disorders (particularly panic attacks) as well as with behavior and substance use disorders (Johnson et al. 2000; Lewinsohn et al. 1995; Merikangas et al. 2011).

There has been some controversy over how best to approach the complexity of comorbid disorders among patients and community cases. In time-pressured clinical settings, assigning a broad principal diagnosis rather than multiple single diagnoses may be most clinically useful, but doing so neglects the fact that information about comorbidity is often of prognostic value. Although a number of clinical and methodological concerns have been expressed (Wittchen et al. 2009), numerous studies have suggested that latent predispositions to two broad classes of internalizing and externalizing disorders account for most of the bivariate associations between hierarchy-free pairs of mood, anxiety, behavior, and substance use disorders (de Jonge et al. 2018; Eaton et al. 2012; Krueger and Markon 2006; Lahey et al. 2008). The internalizing disorders have been further divided into fear disorders (e.g., panic, phobia) and distress disorders (e.g., major depressive episodes, generalized anxiety disorder, posttraumatic stress disorder). A stable structure of this sort has been documented cross-nationally (de Jonge et al. 2018). Researchers have also investigated clustering of symptoms in ways that define syndromes that are more consistent with the actual structure of psychopathology than those in the existing DSM and ICD classifications, although this work is still preliminary (Kotov et al. 2018; Krueger et al. 2018).

An important line of investigation involving the evolving structure of comorbidity has examined the temporal progression across lifetime comorbid mental disorders and considered whether risk factors for individual disorders are more accurately conceptualized as risk factors for the latent dimensions underlying these disorders. Kramer et al. (2008), in an early study of this sort, found that significant gender differences in MDD became statistically insignificant when latent internalizing and externalizing dimensions were controlled for statistically (Kramer et al. 2008). A broader analysis of a similar sort, based on cross-national self-reported data using retrospective age-at-onset reports in cross-sectional community epidemiological surveys to mimic temporal progression, found that essentially all temporally primary lifetime mood, anxiety, behavior, and substance use disorders were significantly associated with subsequent secondary mental disorders (Kessler et al. 2011). Within-domain (i.e., internalizing or externalizing) associations were for the most part stronger than between-domain associations. Also, virtually all time-lagged associations between pairs of disorders were explained by a model that assumed the existence of mediating latent internalizing and externalizing variables. Importantly, MDD and bipolar disorder were not found in this analysis to be more important than other internalizing disorders in defining these latent variables. In line with these studies, Wittchen et al. (2014) proposed "symptom progression models" for diagnosing and treating mental disorders, similar to approaches used in somatic medicine for hypertension, cardiovascular disease, and diabetes.

Applying the same basic logic as in the comorbidity study by Kessler et al. (2011), a more recent cohort study, using information about age at first treatment of common mental disorders from health registries for the entire population of Denmark, found that all temporally primary mental disorders were associated with elevated risk of subsequent onset of all temporally secondary mental disorders (Plana-Ripoll et al. 2019). Decays in these associations were found as a function of number of years since onset of the primary disorders. Early-onset (i.e., diagnosis before age 20 years) mood disorders were associated with an especially high absolute risk of subsequent neurotic disorders (ICD-10 codes F40–F48 [Neurotic, stress-related, and somatoform disorders; includes phobic, anxiety, obsessive-compulsive, and dissociative disorders]) over the next 5 years among both men (30.6%) and women (38.4%). Another noteworthy result was that the time-lagged associations of temporally primary mood disorders with subsequent secondary other mental disorders were consistently higher than the time-lagged associations of the other mental disorders with subsequent onset of temporally secondary mood disorders.

Disease Burden of Mood Disorders

Evidence has accumulated that mood disorders, including MDD (Broadhead et al. 1990; Coryell et al. 1993; Greenberg et al. 2015; Kessler et al. 2006a, 2007a; Rohde et al. 1990; Tweed 1993; Wells et al. 1989; Zeiss and Lewinsohn 1988), bipolar disorder (Calabrese et al. 2003; Coryell et al. 1993; Dion et al. 1988; Kessler et al. 2006b; Lish et al. 1994; MacQueen et al. 2001), and dysthymia (Cassano et al. 1990; Ferrari et al. 2016; Hays et al. 1995; Hellerstein et al. 2010; Klein et al. 1988, 2008), impose substantial societal burdens. The 2017 GBD Study estimated, for example, that MDD was the third leading cause of years lived with disability (YLD) among women and the fifth leading cause of YLD among men out of 354 types of disease and injury considered (James et al. 2018). Although bipolar disorder is relatively rare, the early onset, severity, and chronicity of bipolar disorder in comparison with most serious chronic physical disorders make it a substantially debilitating illness (Ferrari et al. 2016). The 2013 GBD Study estimated that bipolar disorder explained 1.3% of the total YLD, ranking it the sixteenth leading cause of YLD (Ferrari et al. 2016). Although not examined in the GBD Study, even highly prevalent subsyndromal levels of affective symptomatology have been found in other studies to be associated with significant reductions in role functioning (Backenstrass et al. 2006; da Silva Lima and de Almeida Fleck 2007; Judd et al. 1994, 1996, 2012; Rapaport and Judd 1998). Mood disorders may impair several aspects of life, including educational attainment, marriage, parental functioning, working ability, and physical health, as discussed below, all of which may contribute to the high burden and economic costs associated with mood disorders (Alonso et al. 2013).

Education

Numerous studies have demonstrated that early-onset mental disorders are associated with the premature termination of education (Breslau et al. 2008, 2011b, 2013; Kessler et al. 1995; Lee et al. 2009; McLeod and Kaiser 2004; Porche et al. 2011; Vaughn et al. 2011). The WMH surveys found that in comparison with peers without mood disorders, individuals with childhood-onset mood disorders in high-income countries had twice the odds of not completing primary school and 1.5 times the odds of not completing secondary education (Breslau et al. 2013). Other community-based epidemiological surveys have also found that early-onset mood disorders were associated with lower odds of graduating from high school (Breslau et al. 2008, 2011b; Lee et al. 2009; Porche et al. 2011) and higher odds of being disengaged while in school (Vaughn et al. 2011).

Marital Timing, Stability, and Quality

Associations between pre-existing mental disorders and subsequent marriage have been examined in a number of studies (Breslau et al. 2011a; Forthofer et al. 1996; Whisman et al. 2007). These studies consistently show that early-onset mental disorders confer a lower probability of ever marrying (Breslau et al. 2011a; Forthofer et al. 1996), with these associations largely the same for men and women and across countries. Mood disorders are among the most important pre-existing mental disorders in these respects. Premarital history of mental disorders also predicts divorce (Butterworth and Rodgers 2008; Kessler et al. 1998), with MDD and bipolar disorder among the most important mental disorders in this regard (Breslau et al. 2011a). Again, associations are quite similar for men and women across countries.

MDD and bipolar disorder are also related to marital dissatisfaction (Whisman 1999) and distress (Whisman 2007). Using nationally representative data from a U.S. epidemiological survey, one study found that bipolar disorder was the strongest predictor of marital distress out of 11 mental disorders considered (Whisman 2007). Longitudinal studies show that the association of depressive symptoms with marital quality is bidirectional (Mamun et al. 2009; Whisman and Uebelacker 2009), but with a stronger time-lagged association of marital discord predicting depressive symptoms than vice versa (Proulx et al. 2007). The relatively fewer studies that considered the effects of clinical depression or bipolar disorder on marital functioning consistently documented significant negative associations (Coyne et al. 2002; Grover et al. 2017; Kronmüller et al. 2011; Pearson et al. 2010).

Although many studies have examined the presumed mental health consequences of relationship violence (Afifi et al. 2009; Kim et al. 2008; Renner 2009), some research suggests that marital violence is partly a consequence of preexisting mental disorders (Kessler et al. 2001; Lorber and O'Leary 2004; O'Leary et al. 2008; Riggs et al. 2000). A WMH survey found that whereas bipolar disorder and depression were not individually associated with marital violence, premarital externalizing disorders (i.e., disruptive behaviour disorders [ADHD, oppositional defiant disorder, conduct disorder], intermittent explosive disorder, and substance use disorders) among men were significantly associated with marital violence perpetration (Miller et al. 2011). This study also found that premarital internalizing disorders (i.e., mood disorders, anxiety disorders, and PTSD) among women were significantly associated with being in a violent relationship. The causal mechanisms involved are unclear but warrant further investigation.

Parental Functioning and Offspring Health

It is well established that depression runs in families (Lieb et al. 2002) and that parental depression is associated with negative outcomes for offspring during infancy, prepubescence, adolescence, and adulthood (Gelaye and Koenen 2018; Goodman et al. 2011; Tronick and Reck 2009; Weissman et al. 2016). Findings include associations of parental depression with low offspring birth weight, poor school performance, physical health problems, depression, anxiety, substance abuse, and suicidal behavior. These associations are stronger when parents experience persistent depression, live in poverty, or both (Netsi et al. 2018; Santavirta et al. 2018; Stein et al. 2014; Weissman 2018). Research suggests that, like MDD, parental bipolar disorder is associated with worse psychosocial functioning in children (Bella et al. 2011; Henin et al. 2005; Hirshfeld-Becker et al. 2006; Maciejewski et al. 2018). Children with parents with bipolar disorder have been found to have cognitive deficits (de la Serna et al. 2016; Diwadkar et al. 2011; Klimes-Dougan et al. 2006), difficult temperaments (Bruder-Costello et al. 2007; Duffy et al. 2007; Sanches et al. 2014), worse coping skills (Jones et al. 2006; Nijjar et al. 2014; Silk et al. 2006), and an elevated risk of developing mental disorders (Birmaher et al. 2009; DelBello and Geller 2001; Henin et al. 2005; Lapalme et al. 1997), including mood, anxiety, and behavior disorders.

Both observational studies (Garber et al. 2011; Pilowsky et al. 2008; Weissman et al. 2006) and randomized trials (Swartz et al. 2016; Weissman et al. 2015) have found that children's psychosocial functioning may improve when their mother's depressive symptoms remit and maternal depression is treated. In one 12-week randomized clinical trial (Weissman et al. 2015), mothers with depression were randomly assigned to receive treatment with either escitalopram (a selective serotonin reuptake inhibitor), bupropion (a norepinephrine and dopamine reuptake inhibitor), or the combination of the two medications. This study found that depressive symptoms improved over the 12 weeks across all treatment groups. However, a reduction in depressive symptoms in mothers was significantly associated with improvement in their child's depressive symptoms only among the escitalopram monotherapy group. The authors hypothesized that this association may have been due in part to the fact that mothers in the escitalopram monotherapy group showed improvements in self-reported parental functioning, whereas mothers in the other treatment groups did not. A number of studies have documented significant associations of both maternal (Lovejoy et al. 2000) and paternal (Wilson and Durbin 2010) depression with negative parenting behaviors. In another study that randomly assigned mothers with depression to nine sessions of either brief interpersonal psychotherapy for mothers or brief supportive psychotherapy, an improvement in the mothers' depressive symptoms was associated with improved psychosocial functioning in their children (Swartz et al. 2016). This effect was not different between treatment groups. However, other clinical trials that included younger children have not observed an association between an improvement in maternal depressive symptoms and child psychosocial outcomes (Coiro et al. 2012; Verduyn et al. 2003).

Physical Morbidity

Mood disorders are associated with myriad chronic physical disorders, including arthritis, asthma, cancer, cardiovascular disease, diabetes, hypertension, cognitive impairment, and a variety of chronic pain conditions (Buist-Bouwman et al. 2005; Derogatis et al. 1983; Ferro 2016; Forty et al. 2014; McWilliams et al. 2003; Ortega et al. 2006; Scott et al. 2007; Smith et al. 2013). These associations may be due to causal effects of mental disorders on physical health, causal effects of physical disorders on mental disorders, or shared antecedents. Spurious associations between mental and physical disorders may also occur when the same set of symptoms is counted twice to arrive at both psychiatric and physical diagnoses (Dowrick et al. 2005). This sort of confounding, however, would not likely explain time-lagged associations (Penninx et al. 2013) that are also observed.

In a study using WMH survey data from 10 countries, Scott et al. (2011) examined time-lagged associations of early-onset (before age 21 years) mental disorders (including MDD, but not bipolar disorder) with the subsequent onset of a range of adult-onset chronic physical health conditions. Early-onset MDD was associated with heart disease, asthma, osteoarthritis, chronic spinal pain, and frequent or severe headaches, but not with diabetes mellitus. Associations of early-onset mental disorders with these conditions remained statistically significant, although the magnitudes of association were slightly attenuated, after further adjusting for childhood adversities, a potentially strong confounding variable in these associations. A recent nationwide study from Denmark also observed an increased risk for onset of a range of somatic disorders among persons with mood disorders (Momen et al. 2020). The association between the presence of a mental disorder and an increased risk of subsequent medical conditions was present for all mental disorders examined, however, suggesting that the association was not specific to mood disorders.

Several plausible mechanisms have been proposed to explain time-lagged associations of mood disorders with subsequent physical conditions. One possible pathway is through poor health behaviors. Individuals with mood disorders are more likely to smoke, be sedentary, drink heavily, use drugs, and be less adherent to medication or treatment regimens, all of which may contribute to the development of physical conditions across the life course (Davidson et al. 2001; Scott et al. 2006). Another possible pathway is through dysregulation of endocrinological, immune, or stress response systems, which are associated with both mental disorders and chronic disease development (Gibney and Drexhage 2013; Goodyer 2007; Juster et al. 2010; Pawelec et al. 2014; Watson and Mackin 2006). In line with these mechanisms, MDD has been linked to an accelerated cellular biological aging process (Han et al. 2018; Verhoeven et al. 2014).

Comparative Impairments

The comparative associations of diverse diseases with various aspects of role functioning have been examined in community surveys. Results typically show that musculoskeletal disorders and mood disorders are associated with the highest levels of disability at the individual level among all commonly occurring disorders. For example, a study of 15 national surveys in the WMH Survey Initiative compared disorder-specific self-reported role impairment scores among people who experienced each of 10 chronic physical disorders and 10 mental disorders in the year before being interviewed (Ormel et al. 2008). MDD and bipolar disorder were the mental disorders most often rated "severely impairing." Even when including such severe conditions as cancer, diabetes, and heart disease, none of the physical disorders considered had impairment levels as high as those associated with MDD or bipolar disorder. Comparable results were observed when analyses were limited to subsamples of cases in treatment and when comparisons were restricted to respondents who had both disorders in a pair (e.g., respondents who had both a mood disorder and cancer or both a mood disorder and heart disease).

Individuals with mood disorders also report experiencing a high number of days out of role. For example, in the WMH surveys, 62,971 respondents across 24 countries reported on a wide range of common physical and mental disorders as well as days out of role, defined as being totally unable to work or carry out normal activities because of problems with physical health, mental health, or use of alcohol or drugs, in the 30 days before the interview (Alonso et al. 2011). Individuals with MDD and bipolar disorder experienced, on average, 34.4 and 41.2 days out of role per year, respectively. In comparison, the average number of days out of role for physical disorders was 24.5 days per year. MDD was associated with 5.1% of all days out of role, which was the fourth-highest population attributable risk proportion of all the disorders considered (exceeded only by headache/migraine, other chronic pain conditions, and cardiovascular disorders) and by far the largest among the mental disorders. This large population attributable risk proportion is due to the comparatively high prevalence and strong individual-level effect of MDD on days out of role (Collins et al. 2005; Munce et al. 2007; Wang et al. 2003). The population attributable risk proportion for bipolar disorder, in comparison, was 1.4%.

Economic Costs

Estimates of the economic burden attributable to mood disorders are staggering. For example, Greenberg et al. (2015) estimated that the annual cost of adults in the United States with MDD was $210.5 billion in 2010. Approximately 47% of this cost was attributable to direct treatment costs, 5% to suicide-related costs, and the remaining 48% to workplace costs. Of the total costs, only 38% were due to MDD itself, as opposed to comorbid conditions. This analysis also found that every dollar spent on MDD direct costs (including both medical and pharmaceutical services directly related to MDD treatment) was associated with an additional $1.90 in MDD-related indirect costs (e.g., suicide-related, workplace) and another $4.70 in direct and workplace comorbidity costs. In a parallel study on the costs of bipolar I disorder in the United States, Cloutier et al. (2018) estimated a total annual cost of $81,559 per individual with bipolar I disorder. They estimated that the excess cost, defined as the difference between costs incurred by individuals with bipolar I disorder and individuals in the general population, was $48,333 per individual with bipolar I disorder. The largest contributors to bipolar I disorder costs were caregiving costs, direct health care costs, and unemployment costs. Another study estimated that in 2010 in Europe, 33 million individuals suffered from mood disorders, costing €113 billion in *purchasing power parity*—a measure designed to allow for price comparisons across countries (Gustavsson et al. 2011). In this study, mood disorders were estimated to be the costliest of brain disorders, due mainly to indirect costs from individuals being unable to work.

The true economic costs of mood disorders to society are almost certainly larger than those suggested in the paragraph above, because these estimates do not capture the potentially devastating long-term consequences of mood disorders on educational and occupational attainments (Breslau et al. 2013; Kessler et al. 1995). Current cost-of-illness studies are also predicated on assigning a value to life that is limited to the person's productive contribution to society (i.e., a human capital model). In addition to not accounting for non-monetary costs, such as pain, suffering, and decrements in quality of life, such models place no value on the contributions of individuals not employed in the labor market, such as children, those engaged primarily in non-wage household work, and elderly retirees.

Taken together, these results point to three broad factors accounting for the high estimated costs of mood disorders from a societal perspective. The first is that mood disorders are among the most commonly occurring chronic diseases in the population, with a much earlier age at onset than the chronic physical disorders that have relatively comparable prevalence and individual-level effects (Kessler et al. 2007c).

The second set of factors accounting for the high estimated costs of mood disorders from a societal perspective is that these disorders have powerful negative impacts on work performance (Alonso et al. 2011; Kessler et al. 2006a, 2006b). As mentioned in the preceding section on comparative impairments, both MDD and bipolar disorder are associated with substantial numbers of days out of role each year (Alonso et al. 2011). MDD in particular was associated in the WMH surveys with by far the highest population attributable risk proportion of days out of role among all mental and substance use disorders (Kessler et al. 2006a). In addition, MDD and bipolar disorder were associated in these surveys, as well as in other studies, with the highest numbers of days across conditions in which the respondent was at work but performing poorly (Stewart et al. 2003). Other research additionally has shown that unemployment and disability are predicted by prior mood disorders (Birnbaum et al. 2010).

The third set of factors accounting for the high estimated costs of mood disorders from a societal perspective is related to the fact that few people with mood disorders receive adequate treatment despite the availability of effective treatments that could otherwise lead to improved clinical and work outcomes. A WMH survey with more than 50,000 participants across 21 countries found that only a minority of individuals with MDD receive adequate treatment (Thornicroft et al. 2017). The majority (71%) of individuals who reported that they felt they needed treatment made at least one visit to some type of service provider. However, only 41% of these individuals received treatment consistent with established treatment guidelines. The reasons that such a large proportion of individuals with mental disorders receive inadequate care may be related to high dropout from mental health care treatment (Fernández et al. 2020).

There is also evidence that bipolar disorder is often unrecognized and inadequately treated (Keck et al. 2008). Individuals with bipolar disorder are more likely to present to treatment for depressive symptoms than for mania/hypomania, and therefore they are often inaccurately diagnosed with and treated for unipolar depression (Keck et al. 2008). The WMH surveys found that a substantial proportion of people with bipolar spectrum disorders do not receive treatment for these disorders (Merikangas et al. 2011). The proportion of respondents who reported treatment was higher in high-income countries (50% for lifetime and 28% for 12-month prevalence) than in middle-income countries (33% for lifetime and 15% for 12-month prevalence) and low-income countries (25% for lifetime and 13% for 12-month prevalence). Most individuals who received treatment used mental health specialty sectors. Individuals with bipolar I disorder and bipolar II disorder had greater odds of reporting treatment compared with individuals with subthreshold bipolar disorders.

Addressing the Burdens

Preventive interventions and best-practice treatments could reduce the burdens of mood disorders. Prevention is an underdeveloped area that requires improved methods of early detection and interventions (Malhi et al. 2018). Increased use of best-practice treatments, in comparison, is possible but would require new investments and, to be cost-effective, changes in the organization of treatment to implement an evidence-based stepped-care approach (Murray 2019; Parikh 2014; van Straten et al. 2015). The decision to implement such an approach will require an increased understanding of the costs to society as well as to institutional payers (most notably, employers) of untreated and undertreated mood disorders (Chisholm et al. 2016), an understanding that will be necessary to motivate payers to carry out rigorous large-scale demonstration projects that evaluate the return on investment of best-practice treatment systems (Levin and Chisholm 2016). Initial efforts along these lines are promising (Clark 2018) but require expansion and refinement.

References

Afifi TO, MacMillan H, Cox BJ, et al: Mental health correlates of intimate partner violence in marital relationships in a nationally representative sample of males and females. J Interpers Violence 24(8):1398–1417, 2009 18718882

Aillon JL, Ndetei DM, Khasakhala L, et al: Prevalence, types and comorbidity of mental disorders in a Kenyan primary health centre. Soc Psychiatry Psychiatr Epidemiol 49(8):1257–1268, 2014 23959589

Alonso J, Petukhova M, Vilagut G, et al: Days out of role due to common physical and mental conditions: results from the WHO World Mental Health Surveys. Mol Psychiatry 16(12):1234–1246, 2011 20938433

Alonso J, Chatterji S, He Y (eds): The Burdens of Mental Disorders: Global Perspectives From the WHO World Mental Health Surveys. New York, Cambridge University Press, 2013

Alvarez Ariza M, Mateos Alvarez R, Berrios GE: A review of the natural course of bipolar disorders (manic-depressive psychosis) in the pre-drug era: review of studies prior to 1950. J Affect Disord 115(3):293–301, 2009 19041142

American Psychiatric Association: Diagnostic and Statistical Manual of Mental Disorders, 4th Edition. Washington, DC, American Psychiatric Association, 1994

American Psychiatric Association: Diagnostic and Statistical Manual of Mental Disorders, 4th Edition, Text Revision. Washington, DC, American Psychiatric Association, 2000

American Psychiatric Association: Diagnostic and Statistical Manual of Mental Disorders, 5th Edition. Arlington, VA, American Psychiatric Association, 2013

Angst J, Merikangas K: The depressive spectrum: diagnostic classification and course. J Affect Disord 45(1–2):31–39, discussion 39–40, 1997 9268773

Arean P, Lenze E, Anguera J: Mood disorders in late life, in The Oxford Handbook of Mood Disorders. Edited by DeRubeis R, Strunk D. New York, Oxford University Press, 2017, pp 299–309

Ayuso-Mateos JL, Nuevo R, Verdes E, et al: From depressive symptoms to depressive disorders: the relevance of thresholds. Br J Psychiatry 196(5):365–371, 2010 20435961

Backenstrass M, Frank A, Joest K, et al: A comparative study of nonspecific depressive symptoms and minor depression regarding functional impairment and associated characteristics in primary care. Compr Psychiatry 47(1):35–41, 2006 16324900

Batelaan NM, Spijker J, de Graaf R, Cuijpers P: Mixed anxiety depression should not be included in DSM-5. J Nerv Ment Dis 200(6):495–498, 2012 22652614

Bauer MS, Calabrese J, Dunner DL, et al: Multisite data reanalysis of the validity of rapid cycling as a course modifier for bipolar disorder in DSM-IV. Am J Psychiatry 151(4):506–515, 1994 8147448

Beesdo K, Pine DS, Lieb R, Wittchen HU: Incidence and risk patterns of anxiety and depressive disorders and categorization of generalized anxiety disorder. Arch Gen Psychiatry 67(1):47–57, 2010 20048222

Beesdo-Baum K, Knappe S, Asselmann E, et al: The "Early Developmental Stages of Psychopathology (EDSP) study": a 20-year review of methods and findings. Soc Psychiatry Psychiatr Epidemiol 50(6):851–866, 2015 25982479

Bella T, Goldstein T, Axelson D, et al: Psychosocial functioning in offspring of parents with bipolar disorder. J Affect Disord 133(1–2):204–211, 2011 21463899

Birmaher B, Axelson D, Monk K, et al: Lifetime psychiatric disorders in school-aged offspring of parents with bipolar disorder: the Pittsburgh Bipolar Offspring study. Arch Gen Psychiatry 66(3):287–296, 2009 19255378

Birnbaum HG, Kessler RC, Kelley D, et al: Employer burden of mild, moderate, and severe major depressive disorder: mental health services utilization and costs, and work performance. Depress Anxiety 27(1):78–89, 2010 19569060

Breslau J, Lane M, Sampson N, Kessler RC: Mental disorders and subsequent educational attainment in a U.S. national sample. J Psychiatr Res 42(9):708–716, 2008 18331741

Breslau J, Miller E, Jin R, et al: A multinational study of mental disorders, marriage, and divorce. Acta Psychiatr Scand 124(6):474–486, 2011a 21534936

Breslau J, Miller E, Joanie Chung WJ, Schweitzer JB: Childhood and adolescent onset psychiatric disorders, substance use, and failure to graduate high school on time. J Psychiatr Res 45(3):295–301, 2011b 20638079

Breslau J, Lee S, Tsang A, et al: Associations between mental disorders and early termination of education, in The Burdens of Mental Disorders: Global Perspectives From the WHO World Mental Health Surveys. Edited by Alonso J, Chatterji S, He Y. New York, Cambridge University Press, 2013, pp 56–65

Broadhead WE, Blazer DG, George LK, Tse CK: Depression, disability days, and days lost from work in a prospective epidemiologic survey. JAMA 264(19):2524–2528, 1990 2146410

Bromet E, Andrade L, Bruffaerts R, Williams DR: Major depressive disorder, in Mental Disorders Around the World: Facts and Figures From the WHO World Mental Health Surveys. Edited by Scott KM, de Jonge P, Stein DJ, Kessler RC. New York, Cambridge University Press, 2018, pp 41–56

Bruder-Costello B, Warner V, Talati A, et al: Temperament among offspring at high and low risk for depression. Psychiatry Res 153(2):145–151, 2007 17651814

Buist-Bouwman MA, de Graaf R, Vollebergh WA, Ormel J: Comorbidity of physical and mental disorders and the effect on work-loss days. Acta Psychiatr Scand 111(6):436–443, 2005 15877710

Butterworth P, Rodgers B: Mental health problems and marital disruption: is it the combination of husbands and wives' mental health problems that predicts later divorce? Soc Psychiatry Psychiatr Epidemiol 43(9):758–763, 2008 18478168

Calabrese JR, Hirschfeld RM, Reed M, et al: Impact of bipolar disorder on a U.S. community sample. J Clin Psychiatry 64(4):425–432, 2003 12716245

Carrellas NW, Biederman J, Uchida M: How prevalent and morbid are subthreshold manifestations of major depression in adolescents? A literature review. J Affect Disord 210:166–173, 2017 28049101

Cassano GB, Perugi G, Maremmani I, Akiskal HS: Social adjustment in dysthymia, in Dysthymic Disorder. Edited by Burton SW, Akiskal HS. London, Gaskell/ Royal College of Psychiatrists, 1990, pp 78–85

Charlson FJ, Ferrari AJ, Flaxman AD, Whiteford HA: The epidemiological modelling of dysthymia: application for the Global Burden of Disease Study 2010. J Affect Disord 151(1):111–120, 2013 23806588

Charlson FJ, Baxter AJ, Dua T, et al: Excess mortality from mental, neurological, and substance use disorders in the Global Burden of Disease Study 2010, in Mental, Neurological, and Substance Use Disorders (Disease Control Priorities, 3rd Edition, Vol 4). Edited by Patel V, Chisholm D, Dua T, et al. Washington, DC, The International Bank for Reconstruction and Development/The World Bank, 2016, pp 41–66

Chisholm D, Johansson KA, Raykar N, et al: Universal health coverage for mental, neurological, and substance use disorders: an extended cost-effectiveness analysis, in Mental, Neurological, and Substance Use Disorders (Disease Control Priorities, 3rd Edition, Vol 4). Edited by Patel V, Chisholm D, Dua T, et al. Washington, DC, The International Bank for Reconstruction and Development/The World Bank, 2016, pp 237–252

Clark DM: Realizing the mass public benefit of evidence-based psychological therapies: the IAPT program. Annu Rev Clin Psychol 14:159–183, 2018 29350997

Cloutier M, Greene M, Guerin A, et al: The economic burden of bipolar I disorder in the United States in 2015. J Affect Disord 226:45–51, 2018 28961441

Coiro MJ, Riley A, Broitman M, Miranda J: Effects on children of treating their mothers' depression: results of a 12-month follow-up. Psychiatr Serv 63(4):357–363, 2012 22388476

Collins JJ, Baase CM, Sharda CE, et al: The assessment of chronic health conditions on work performance, absence, and total economic impact for employers. J Occup Environ Med 47(6):547–557, 2005 15951714

Comijs HC, Nieuwesteeg J, Kok R, et al: The two-year course of late-life depression; results from the Netherlands study of depression in older persons. BMC Psychiatry 15:20, 2015 25775143

Conradi HJ, Bos EH, Kamphuis JH, de Jonge P: The ten-year course of depression in primary care and long-term effects of psychoeducation, psychiatric consultation and cognitive behavioral therapy. J Affect Disord 217:174–182, 2017 28411506

Coryell W, Scheftner W, Keller M, et al: The enduring psychosocial consequences of mania and depression. Am J Psychiatry 150(5):720–727, 1993 8480816

Coryell W, Solomon D, Turvey C, et al: The long-term course of rapid-cycling bipolar disorder. Arch Gen Psychiatry 60(9):914–920, 2003 12963673

Coryell W, Solomon D, Leon A, et al: Does major depressive disorder change with age? Psychol Med 39(10):1689–1695, 2009 19296865

Coyne JC, Thompson R, Palmer SC: Marital quality, coping with conflict, marital complaints, and affection in couples with a depressed wife. J Fam Psychol 16(1):26–37, 2002 11915407

Dagani J, Baldessarini RJ, Signorini G, et al: The age of onset of bipolar disorders, in Age of Onset of Mental Disorders. Edited by de Girolamo G, McGorry P, Sartorius N. New York, Springer, 2019, pp 75–110

da Silva Lima AF, de Almeida Fleck MP: Subsyndromal depression: an impact on quality of life? J Affect Disord 100(1–3):163–169, 2007 17126913

Davidson S, Judd F, Jolley D, et al: Cardiovascular risk factors for people with mental illness. Aust N Z J Psychiatry 35(2):196–202, 2001 11284901

de Girolamo G, McGorry P, Sartorius N: Introduction: Relevance of the age of onset of mental disorders to research in psychiatry and to the organization of services for people with mental illness, in Age of Onset of Mental Disorders. Edited by de Girolamo G, McGorry P, Sartorius N. New York, Springer, 2019, pp 1–14

de Jonge P, Wardenaar KJ, Lim CCW, et al: The cross-national structure of mental disorders: results from the World Mental Health Surveys. Psychol Med 48(12):2073–2084, 2018 29254513

de la Serna E, Vila M, Sanchez-Gistau V, et al: Neuropsychological characteristics of child and adolescent offspring of patients with bipolar disorder. Prog Neuropsychopharmacol Biol Psychiatry 65:54–59, 2016 26343306
DelBello MP, Geller B: Review of studies of child and adolescent offspring of bipolar parents. Bipolar Disord 3(6):325–334, 2001 11843782
Demyttenaere K, Bruffaerts R, Posada-Villa J, et al; WHO World Mental Health Survey Consortium: Prevalence, severity, and unmet need for treatment of mental disorders in the World Health Organization World Mental Health Surveys. JAMA 291(21):2581–2590, 2004 15173149
Derogatis LR, Morrow GR, Fetting J, et al: The prevalence of psychiatric disorders among cancer patients. JAMA 249(6):751–757, 1983 6823028
Dion GL, Tohen M, Anthony WA, Waternaux CS: Symptoms and functioning of patients with bipolar disorder six months after hospitalization. Hosp Community Psychiatry 39(6):652–657, 1988 3402925
Diwadkar VA, Goradia D, Hosanagar A, et al: Working memory and attention deficits in adolescent offspring of schizophrenia or bipolar patients: comparing vulnerability markers. Prog Neuropsychopharmacol Biol Psychiatry 35(5):1349–1354, 2011 21549798
Dowrick C, Katona C, Peveler R, Lloyd H: Somatic symptoms and depression: diagnostic confusion and clinical neglect. Br J Gen Pract 55(520):829–830, 2005 16281997
Duffy A, Alda M, Trinneer A, et al: Temperament, life events, and psychopathology among the offspring of bipolar parents. Eur Child Adolesc Psychiatry 16(4):222–228, 2007 17136299
Eaton NR, Keyes KM, Krueger RF, et al: An invariant dimensional liability model of gender differences in mental disorder prevalence: evidence from a national sample. J Abnorm Psychol 121(1):282–288, 2012 21842958
Eaton WW, Shao H, Nestadt G, et al: Population-based study of first onset and chronicity in major depressive disorder. Arch Gen Psychiatry 65(5):513–520, 2008 18458203
Fernández D, Vigo D, Sampson NA, et al: Patterns of care and dropout rates from outpatient mental healthcare in low-, middle- and high-income countries from the World Health Organization's World Mental Health Survey Initiative. Psychol Med 51(12):2104–2116, 2020 32343221
Ferrari AJ, Somerville AJ, Baxter AJ, et al: Global variation in the prevalence and incidence of major depressive disorder: a systematic review of the epidemiological literature. Psychol Med 43(3):471–481, 2013 22831756
Ferrari AJ, Stockings E, Khoo JP, et al: The prevalence and burden of bipolar disorder: findings from the Global Burden of Disease Study 2013. Bipolar Disord 18(5):440–450, 2016 27566286
Ferro MA: Major depressive disorder, suicidal behaviour, bipolar disorder, and generalised anxiety disorder among emerging adults with and without chronic health conditions. Epidemiol Psychiatr Sci 25(5):462–474, 2016 26347304
Forsell Y: A three-year follow-up of major depression, dysthymia, minor depression and subsyndromal depression: results from a population-based study. Depress Anxiety 24(1):62–65, 2007 16947910
Forthofer MS, Kessler RC, Story AL, Gotlib IH: The effects of psychiatric disorders on the probability and timing of first marriage. J Health Soc Behav 37(2):121–132, 1996 8690874
Forty L, Ulanova A, Jones L, et al: Comorbid medical illness in bipolar disorder. Br J Psychiatry 205(6):465–472, 2014 25359927
Garber J, Ciesla JA, McCauley E, et al: Remission of depression in parents: links to healthy functioning in their children. Child Dev 82(1):226–243, 2011 21291439
Gelaye B, Koenen KC: The intergenerational impact of prenatal stress: time to focus on prevention? Biol Psychiatry 83(2):92–93, 2018 29223219
Gibney SM, Drexhage HA: Evidence for a dysregulated immune system in the etiology of psychiatric disorders. J Neuroimmune Pharmacol 8(4):900–920, 2013 23645137
Goodman A, Joyce R, Smith JP: The long shadow cast by childhood physical and mental problems on adult life. Proc Natl Acad Sci USA 108(15):6032–6037, 2011 21444801
Goodyer IM: The hypothalamic-pituitary-adrenal axis: cortisol, DHEA and mental and behavioral function, in Depression and Physical Illness. Edited by Steptoe A. London, Cambridge University Press, 2007, pp 280–298

Gopinath S, Katon WJ, Russo JE, Ludman EJ: Clinical factors associated with relapse in primary care patients with chronic or recurrent depression. J Affect Disord 101(1–3):57–63, 2007 17156852

Greenberg PE, Fournier AA, Sisitsky T, et al: The economic burden of adults with major depressive disorder in the United States (2005 and 2010). J Clin Psychiatry 76(2):155–162, 2015 25742202

Grover S, Nehra R, Thakur A: Bipolar affective disorder and its impact on various aspects of marital relationship. Ind Psychiatry J 26(2):114–120, 2017 30089956

Gustavsson A, Svensson M, Jacobi F, et al; CDBE2010Study Group: Cost of disorders of the brain in Europe 2010. Eur Neuropsychopharmacol 21(10):718–779, 2011 21924589

Han LKM, Aghajani M, Clark SL, et al: Epigenetic aging in major depressive disorder. Am J Psychiatry 175(8):774–782, 2018 29656664

Hardeveld F, Spijker J, De Graaf R, et al: Recurrence of major depressive disorder and its predictors in the general population: results from the Netherlands Mental Health Survey and Incidence Study (NEMESIS). Psychol Med 43(1):39–48, 2013 23111147

Hasin DS, Sarvet AL, Meyers JL, et al: Epidemiology of adult DSM-5 major depressive disorder and its specifiers in the United States. JAMA Psychiatry 75(4):336–346, 2018 29450462

Hays RD, Wells KB, Sherbourne CD, et al: Functioning and well-being outcomes of patients with depression compared with chronic general medical illnesses. Arch Gen Psychiatry 52(1):11–19, 1995 7811158

Hellerstein DJ, Agosti V, Bosi M, Black SR: Impairment in psychosocial functioning associated with dysthymic disorder in the NESARC study. J Affect Disord 127(1–3):84–88, 2010 20471093

Henin A, Biederman J, Mick E, et al: Psychopathology in the offspring of parents with bipolar disorder: a controlled study. Biol Psychiatry 58(7):554–561, 2005 16112654

Hirshfeld-Becker DR, Biederman J, Henin A, et al: Laboratory-observed behavioral disinhibition in the young offspring of parents with bipolar disorder: a high-risk pilot study. Am J Psychiatry 163(2):265–271, 2006 16449480

Holma KM, Holma IA, Melartin TK, et al: Long-term outcome of major depressive disorder in psychiatric patients is variable. J Clin Psychiatry 69(2):196–205, 2008 18251627

James SL, Abate D, Abate KH, et al; GBD 2017 Disease and Injury Incidence and Prevalence Collaborators: Global, regional, and national incidence, prevalence, and years lived with disability for 354 diseases and injuries for 195 countries and territories, 1990–2017: a systematic analysis for the Global Burden of Disease Study 2017. Lancet 392(10159):1789–1858, 2018 30496104

Johnson JG, Cohen P, Brook JS: Associations between bipolar disorder and other psychiatric disorders during adolescence and early adulthood: a community-based longitudinal investigation. Am J Psychiatry 157(10):1679–1681, 2000 11007724

Johnson SL, Gershon A, McMaster KJ: Environmental risk and protective factors in bipolar disorder, in The Oxford Handbook of Mood Disorders. Edited by DeRubeis R, Strunk D. New York, Oxford University Press, 2017, pp 132–141

Jones SH, Tai S, Evershed K, et al: Early detection of bipolar disorder: a pilot familial high-risk study of parents with bipolar disorder and their adolescent children. Bipolar Disord 8(4):362–372, 2006 16879137

Judd LL, Rapaport MH, Paulus MP, Brown JL: Subsyndromal symptomatic depression: a new mood disorder? J Clin Psychiatry 55 (suppl):18–28, 1994 8077164

Judd LL, Paulus MP, Wells KB, Rapaport MH: Socioeconomic burden of subsyndromal depressive symptoms and major depression in a sample of the general population. Am J Psychiatry 153(11):1411–1417, 1996 8890673

Judd LL, Akiskal HS, Maser JD, et al: A prospective 12-year study of subsyndromal and syndromal depressive symptoms in unipolar major depressive disorders. Arch Gen Psychiatry 55(8):694–700, 1998 9707379

Judd LL, Schettler PJ, Akiskal HS: The prevalence, clinical relevance, and public health significance of subthreshold depressions. Psychiatr Clin North Am 25(4):685–698, 2002 12462855

Judd LL, Schettler PJ, Akiskal HS, et al: Residual symptom recovery from major affective episodes in bipolar disorders and rapid episode relapse/recurrence. Arch Gen Psychiatry 65(4):386–394, 2008 18391127

Judd LL, Schettler PJ, Akiskal H, et al: Prevalence and clinical significance of subsyndromal manic symptoms, including irritability and psychomotor agitation, during bipolar major depressive episodes. J Affect Disord 138(3):440–448, 2012 22314261

Juster RP, McEwen BS, Lupien SJ: Allostatic load biomarkers of chronic stress and impact on health and cognition. Neurosci Biobehav Rev 35(1):2–16, 2010 19822172

Kawakami N, Yasuma N, Watanabe K, et al: Association of response rate and prevalence estimates of common mental disorders across 129 areas in a nationally representative survey of adults in Japan. Soc Psychiatry Psychiatr Epidemiol 55(10):1373–1382, 2020 32047970

Keck PE Jr, Kessler RC, Ross R: Clinical and economic effects of unrecognized or inadequately treated bipolar disorder. J Psychiatr Pract 14 (suppl 2):31–38, 2008 18677197

Kessler RC, Ustün TB (eds): The WHO World Mental Health Surveys: Global Perspectives on the Epidemiology of Mental Disorders. New York, Cambridge University Press, 2008

Kessler RC, Foster CL, Saunders WB, Stang PE: Social consequences of psychiatric disorders, I: educational attainment. Am J Psychiatry 152(7):1026–1032, 1995 7793438

Kessler RC, Walters EE, Forthofer MS: The social consequences of psychiatric disorders, III: probability of marital stability. Am J Psychiatry 155(8):1092–1096, 1998 9699699

Kessler RC, Molnar BE, Feurer ID, Appelbaum M: Patterns and mental health predictors of domestic violence in the United States: results from the National Comorbidity Survey. Int J Law Psychiatry 24(4–5):487–508, 2001 11521422

Kessler RC, Chiu WT, Demler O, et al: Prevalence, severity, and comorbidity of 12-month DSM-IV disorders in the National Comorbidity Survey Replication. Arch Gen Psychiatry 62(6):617–627, 2005 15939839

Kessler RC, Akiskal HS, Ames M, et al: Prevalence and effects of mood disorders on work performance in a nationally representative sample of U.S. workers. Am J Psychiatry 163(9):1561–1568, 2006a 16946181

Kessler RC, Akiskal H, Angst J, et al: The workplace costs of mood disorders: bringing bipolar spectrum disorder into the equation. Journal of Health and Productivity 1:3–8, 2006b

Kessler RC, Akiskal HS, Ames M, et al: Considering the costs of bipolar depression. Behav Healthc 27(1):45–47, 2007a 17310917

Kessler RC, Amminger GP, Aguilar-Gaxiola S, et al: Age of onset of mental disorders: a review of recent literature. Curr Opin Psychiatry 20(4):359–364, 2007b 17551351

Kessler RC, Angermeyer M, Anthony JC, et al: Lifetime prevalence and age-of-onset distributions of mental disorders in the World Health Organization's World Mental Health Survey Initiative. World Psychiatry 6(3):168–176, 2007c 18188442

Kessler RC, Ormel J, Petukhova M, et al: Development of lifetime comorbidity in the World Health Organization World Mental Health Surveys. Arch Gen Psychiatry 68(1):90–100, 2011 21199968

Kessler RC, Avenevoli S, Costello J, et al: Severity of 12-month DSM-IV disorders in the National Comorbidity Survey Replication Adolescent Supplement. Arch Gen Psychiatry 69(4):381–389, 2012a 22474106

Kessler RC, Petukhova M, Sampson NA, et al: Twelve-month and lifetime prevalence and lifetime morbid risk of anxiety and mood disorders in the United States. Int J Methods Psychiatr Res 21(3):169–184, 2012b 22865617

Kessler RC, Karam EG, Lee S, et al: Bipolar spectrum disorder, in Mental Disorders Around the World: Facts and Figures From the WHO World Mental Health Surveys. Edited by Scott KM, de Jonge P, Stein DL, Kessler RC. New York, Cambridge University Press, 2018, pp 57–58

Kim HK, Laurent HK, Capaldi DM, Feingold A: Men's aggression toward women: a 10-year panel study. J Marriage Fam 70(5):1169–1187, 2008 19122790

Klein DN, Taylor EB, Dickstein S, Harding K: Primary early-onset dysthymia: comparison with primary nonbipolar nonchronic major depression on demographic, clinical, familial, personality, and socioenvironmental characteristics and short-term outcome. J Abnorm Psychol 97(4):387–398, 1988 3204224

Klein DN, Shankman SA, Rose S: Dysthymic disorder and double depression: prediction of 10-year course trajectories and outcomes. J Psychiatr Res 42(5):408–415, 2008 17466334

Klimes-Dougan B, Ronsaville D, Wiggs EA, Martinez PE: Neuropsychological functioning in adolescent children of mothers with a history of bipolar or major depressive disorders. Biol Psychiatry 60(9):957–965, 2006 16934765

Kotiaho S, Korniloff K, Vanhala M, et al: Psychiatric diagnosis in primary care patients with increased depressive symptoms. Nord J Psychiatry 73(3):195–199, 2019 30929594

Kotov R, Krueger RF, Watson D: A paradigm shift in psychiatric classification: the Hierarchical Taxonomy of Psychopathology (HiTOP). World Psychiatry 17(1):24–25, 2018 29352543

Kramer MD, Krueger RF, Hicks BM: The role of internalizing and externalizing liability factors in accounting for gender differences in the prevalence of common psychopathological syndromes. Psychol Med 38(1):51–61, 2008 17892625

Kronmüller KT, Backenstrass M, Victor D, et al: Quality of marital relationship and depression: results of a 10-year prospective follow-up study. J Affect Disord 128(1–2):64–71, 2011 20674034

Krueger RF, Markon KE: Reinterpreting comorbidity: a model-based approach to understanding and classifying psychopathology. Annu Rev Clin Psychol 2:111–133, 2006 17716066

Krueger RF, Kotov R, Watson D, et al: Progress in achieving quantitative classification of psychopathology. World Psychiatry 17(3):282–293, 2018 30229571

Lahey BB, Rathouz PJ, Van Hulle C, et al: Testing structural models of DSM-IV symptoms of common forms of child and adolescent psychopathology. J Abnorm Child Psychol 36(2):187–206, 2008 17912624

Lamers F, van Oppen P, Comijs HC, et al: Comorbidity patterns of anxiety and depressive disorders in a large cohort study: the Netherlands Study of Depression and Anxiety (NESDA). J Clin Psychiatry 72(3):341–348, 2011 21294994

Lapalme M, Hodgins S, LaRoche C: Children of parents with bipolar disorder: a meta-analysis of risk for mental disorders. Can J Psychiatry 42(6):623–631, 1997 9288425

Lee S, Tsang A, Breslau J, et al: Mental disorders and termination of education in high-income and low- and middle-income countries: epidemiological study. Br J Psychiatry 194(5):411–417, 2009 19407270

Lee S, Tsang A, Kessler RC, et al: Rapid-cycling bipolar disorder: cross-national community study. Br J Psychiatry 196(3):217–225, 2010 20194545

Levin C, Chisholm D: Cost-effectiveness and affordability of interventions, policies, and platforms for the prevention and treatment of mental, neurological, and substance use disorders, in Mental, Neurological, and Substance Use Disorders (Disease Control Priorities, 3rd Edition, Vol 4). Edited by Patel V, Chisholm D, Dua T, et al. Washington, DC, The International Bank for Reconstruction and Development/The World Bank, 2016, pp 219–236

Lewinsohn PM, Klein DN, Seeley JR: Bipolar disorders in a community sample of older adolescents: prevalence, phenomenology, comorbidity, and course. J Am Acad Child Adolesc Psychiatry 34(4):454–463, 1995 7751259

Lieb R, Isensee B, Höfler M, et al: Parental major depression and the risk of depression and other mental disorders in offspring: a prospective-longitudinal community study. Arch Gen Psychiatry 59(4):365–374, 2002 11926937

Lish JD, Dime-Meenan S, Whybrow PC, et al: The National Depressive and Manic-Depressive Association (DMDA) survey of bipolar members. J Affect Disord 31(4):281–294, 1994 7989643

Lorber MF, O'Leary KD: Predictors of the persistence of male aggression in early marriage. Journal of Family Violence 19(6):329–338, 2004. Available at: https://link.springer.com/article/10.1007/s10896-004-0678-5. Accessed October 26, 2021.

Lovejoy MC, Graczyk PA, O'Hare E, Neuman G: Maternal depression and parenting behavior: a meta-analytic review. Clin Psychol Rev 20(5):561–592, 2000 10860167

Maciejewski D, Hillegers M, Penninx B: Offspring of parents with mood disorders: time for more transgenerational research, screening and preventive intervention for this high-risk population. Curr Opin Psychiatry 31(4):349–357, 2018 29708895

MacQueen GM, Young LT, Joffe RT: A review of psychosocial outcome in patients with bipolar disorder. Acta Psychiatr Scand 103(3):163–170, 2001 11240572

Malhi GS, Outhred T, Morris G, et al: Primary prevention of mood disorders: a primary concern that requires urgent action. J Am Acad Child Adolesc Psychiatry 57(9):629–631, 2018 30196864

Mamun AA, Clavarino AM, Najman JM, et al: Maternal depression and the quality of marital relationship: a 14-year prospective study. J Womens Health (Larchmt) 18(12):2023–2031, 2009 20044866

Mattisson C, Bogren M, Horstmann V, et al: The long-term course of depressive disorders in the Lundby Study. Psychol Med 37(6):883–891, 2007 17306047

McLeod JD, Kaiser K: Childhood emotional and behavioral problems and educational attainment. American Sociological Review 69(5):636–658, 2004. Available at: https://journals.sagepub.com/doi/10.1177/000312240406900502. Accessed October 26, 2021.

McWilliams LA, Cox BJ, Enns MW: Mood and anxiety disorders associated with chronic pain: an examination in a nationally representative sample. Pain 106(1–2):127–133, 2003 14581119

Merikangas KR, Wicki W, Angst J: Heterogeneity of depression. Classification of depressive subtypes by longitudinal course. Br J Psychiatry 164(3):342–348, 1994 8199787

Merikangas KR, Jin R, He JP, et al: Prevalence and correlates of bipolar spectrum disorder in the World Mental Health Survey Initiative. Arch Gen Psychiatry 68(3):241–251, 2011 21383262

Miller E, Breslau J, Petukhova M, et al: Premarital mental disorders and physical violence in marriage: cross-national study of married couples. Br J Psychiatry 199(4):330–337, 2011 21778172

Miller IW, Uebelacker LA, Keitner GI, et al: Longitudinal course of bipolar I disorder. Compr Psychiatry 45(6):431–440, 2004 15526253

Moffitt TE, Caspi A, Taylor A, et al: How common are common mental disorders? Evidence that lifetime prevalence rates are doubled by prospective versus retrospective ascertainment. Psychol Med 40(6):899–909, 2010 19719899

Momen NC, Plana-Ripoll O, Agerbo E, et al: Association between mental disorders and subsequent medical conditions. N Engl J Med 382(18):1721–1731, 2020 32348643

Monroe SM, Cummins LF: Environmental risk and protection in unipolar depression, in The Oxford Handbook of Mood Disorders. Edited by DeRubeis R, Strunk D. New York, Oxford University Press, 2017, pp 120–131

Mueller TI, Leon AC, Keller MB, et al: Recurrence after recovery from major depressive disorder during 15 years of observational follow-up. Am J Psychiatry 156(7):1000–1006, 1999 10401442

Munce SE, Stansfeld SA, Blackmore ER, Stewart DE: The role of depression and chronic pain conditions in absenteeism: results from a national epidemiologic survey. J Occup Environ Med 49(11):1206–1211, 2007 17993924

Murray CJ, Lopez AD (eds): The Global Burden of Disease: A Comprehensive Assessment of Mortality and Disability From Diseases, Injuries, and Risk Factors in 1990 and Projected to 2020: Summary. Geneva, Switzerland, World Health Organization, 1996

Murray G: What would digital early intervention for bipolar disorder look like? Theoretical and translational considerations for future therapies. Front Psychiatry 10:599, 2019 31507467

Netsi E, Pearson RM, Murray L, et al: Association of persistent and severe postnatal depression with child outcomes. JAMA Psychiatry 75(3):247–253, 2018 29387878

Nierenberg AA, Akiskal HS, Angst J, et al: Bipolar disorder with frequent mood episodes in the National Comorbidity Survey Replication (NCS-R). Mol Psychiatry 15(11):1075–1087, 2010 19564874

Nijjar R, Ellenbogen MA, Hodgins S: Personality, coping, risky behavior, and mental disorders in the offspring of parents with bipolar disorder: a comprehensive psychosocial assessment. J Affect Disord 166:315–323, 2014 25012447

Oepen G, Baldessarini RJ, Salvatore P, Slater E: On the periodicity of manic-depressive insanity, by Eliot Slater (1938): translated excerpts and commentary. J Affect Disord 78(1):1–9, 2004 14672791

O'Leary KD, Tintle N, Bromet EJ, Gluzman SF: Descriptive epidemiology of intimate partner aggression in Ukraine. Soc Psychiatry Psychiatr Epidemiol 43(8):619–626, 2008 18360731

Ormel J, Petukhova M, Chatterji S, et al: Disability and treatment of specific mental and physical disorders across the world. Br J Psychiatry 192(5):368–375, 2008 18450663

Ortega AN, Feldman JM, Canino G, et al: Co-occurrence of mental and physical illness in U.S. Latinos. Soc Psychiatry Psychiatr Epidemiol 41(12):927–934, 2006 17013767

Parikh SV: Brief versus intensive psychosocial treatments for bipolar disorder: time for stepped care? Am J Psychiatry 171(12):1335, 2014 25756769

Patel V, Chisholm D, Parikh R, et al: Global priorities for addressing the burden of mental, neurological, and substance use disorders, in Mental, Neurological, and Substance Use Disorders (Disease Control Priorities, 3rd Edition, Vol 4). Edited by Patel V, Chisholm D, Dua T, et al. Washington, DC, The International Bank for Reconstruction and Development/The World Bank, 2016, pp 1–28

Paterniti S, Sterner I, Caldwell C, Bisserbe JC: Childhood neglect predicts the course of major depression in a tertiary care sample: a follow-up study. BMC Psychiatry 17(1):113, 2017 28351403

Pawelec G, Goldeck D, Derhovanessian E: Inflammation, ageing and chronic disease. Curr Opin Immunol 29:23–28, 2014 24762450

Paykel ES, Abbott R, Morriss R, et al: Sub-syndromal and syndromal symptoms in the longitudinal course of bipolar disorder. Br J Psychiatry 189:118–123, 2006 16880480

Pearson KA, Watkins ER, Kuyken W, Mullan EG: The psychosocial context of depressive rumination: ruminative brooding predicts diminished relationship satisfaction in individuals with a history of past major depression. Br J Clin Psychol 49(Pt 2):275–280, 2010 20109277

Penninx BW, Milaneschi Y, Lamers F, Vogelzangs N: Understanding the somatic consequences of depression: biological mechanisms and the role of depression symptom profile. BMC Med 11:129, 2013 23672628

Pilowsky DJ, Wickramaratne P, Talati A, et al: Children of depressed mothers 1 year after the initiation of maternal treatment: findings from the STAR*D-Child Study. Am J Psychiatry 165(9):1136–1147, 2008 18558646

Plana-Ripoll O, Pedersen CB, Holtz Y, et al: Exploring comorbidity within mental disorders among a Danish national population. JAMA Psychiatry 76(3):259–270, 2019 30649197

Porche MV, Fortuna LR, Lin J, Alegria M: Childhood trauma and psychiatric disorders as correlates of school dropout in a national sample of young adults. Child Dev 82(3):982–998, 2011 21410919

Powell A, Ocean S, Stanick C: Depressive disorders, in Handbook of DSM-5 Disorders in Children and Adolescents. Edited by Goldstein S, DeVries M. New York, Springer, 2017, pp 151–172

Proulx CM, Helms HM, Buehler C: Marital quality and personal well-being: a meta-analysis. Journal of Marriage and Family 69(3):576–593, 2007. Available at: https://onlinelibrary.wiley.com/doi/10.1111/j.1741-3737.2007.00393.x. Accessed October 26, 2021.

Ramana R, Paykel ES, Cooper Z, et al: Remission and relapse in major depression: a two-year prospective follow-up study. Psychol Med 25(6):1161–1170, 1995 8637946

Rapaport MH, Judd LL: Minor depressive disorder and subsyndromal depressive symptoms: functional impairment and response to treatment. J Affect Disord 48(2–3):227–232, 1998 9543213

Renner LM: Intimate partner violence victimization and parenting stress: assessing the mediating role of depressive symptoms. Violence Against Women 15(11):1380–1401, 2009 19809099

Rhebergen D, Beekman AT, de Graaf R, et al: Trajectories of recovery of social and physical functioning in major depression, dysthymic disorder and double depression: a 3-year follow-up. J Affect Disord 124(1–2):148–156, 2010 19945171

Richards M, Bearden C: Bipolar disorder in children, in Handbook of DSM-5 Disorders in Children and Adolescents. Edited by Goldstein S, DeVries M. New York, Springer, 2017, pp 125–150

Riggs DS, Caulfield MB, Street AE: Ris2k for domestic violence: factors associated with perpetration and victimization. J Clin Psychol 56(10):1289–1316, 2000 11051060

Riihimäki KA, Vuorilehto MS, Melartin TK, Isometsä ET: Five-year outcome of major depressive disorder in primary health care. Psychol Med 44(7):1369–1379, 2014 22085687

Rodríguez MR, Nuevo R, Chatterji S, Ayuso-Mateos JL: Definitions and factors associated with subthreshold depressive conditions: a systematic review. BMC Psychiatry 12:181, 2012 23110575

Rohde P, Lewinsohn PM, Seeley JR: Are people changed by the experience of having an episode of depression? A further test of the scar hypothesis. J Abnorm Psychol 99(3):264–271, 1990 2212276

Sanches M, Scott-Gurnell K, Patel A, et al: Impulsivity in children and adolescents with mood disorders and unaffected offspring of bipolar parents. Compr Psychiatry 55(6):1337–1341, 2014 24889339

Santavirta T, Santavirta N, Gilman SE: Association of the World War II Finnish evacuation of children with psychiatric hospitalization in the next generation. JAMA Psychiatry 75(1):21–27, 2018 29188292

Saunders KE, Goodwin GM: The course of bipolar disorder. Advances in Psychiatric Treatment 16(5):318–328, 2010. Available at: https://www.cambridge.org/core/journals/advances-in-psychiatric-treatment/article/course-of-bipolar-disorder/58EDBBA7422C12C4D4FB5230646E971. Accessed October 26, 2021.

Scott KM, Oakley Browne MA, McGee MA, Wells JE; New Zealand Mental Health Survey Research Team: Mental-physical comorbidity in Te Rau Hinengaro: the New Zealand Mental Health Survey. Aust N Z J Psychiatry 40(10):882–888, 2006 16959014

Scott KM, Bruffaerts R, Tsang A, et al: Depression-anxiety relationships with chronic physical conditions: results from the World Mental Health Surveys. J Affect Disord 103(1–3):113–120, 2007 17292480

Scott KM, Von Korff M, Angermeyer MC, et al: Association of childhood adversities and early-onset mental disorders with adult-onset chronic physical conditions. Arch Gen Psychiatry 68(8):838–844, 2011 21810647

Silk JS, Shaw DS, Skuban EM, et al: Emotion regulation strategies in offspring of childhood-onset depressed mothers. J Child Psychol Psychiatry 47(1):69–78, 2006 16405643

Smith DJ, Martin D, McLean G, et al: Multimorbidity in bipolar disorder and undertreatment of cardiovascular disease: a cross sectional study. BMC Med 11:263, 2013 24359325

Spijker J, Batelaan N, de Graaf R, Cuijpers P: Who is MADD? Mixed anxiety depressive disorder in the general population. J Affect Disord 121(1–2):180–183, 2010 19577307

Stagnaro JC, Cía AH, Aguilar Gaxiola S, et al: Twelve-month prevalence rates of mental disorders and service use in the Argentinean Study of Mental Health Epidemiology. Soc Psychiatry Psychiatr Epidemiol 53(2):121–129, 2018 29302708

Stein A, Pearson RM, Goodman SH, et al: Effects of perinatal mental disorders on the fetus and child. Lancet 384(9956):1800–1819, 2014 25455250

Stewart WF, Ricci JA, Chee E, et al: Cost of lost productive work time among U.S. workers with depression. JAMA 289(23):3135–3144, 2003 12813119

Swartz HA, Cyranowski JM, Cheng Y, et al: Brief psychotherapy for maternal depression: impact on mothers and children. J Am Acad Child Adolesc Psychiatry 55(6):495–503.e2, 2016 27238068

Ten Have M, de Graaf R, van Dorsselaer S, et al: Recurrence and chronicity of major depressive disorder and their risk indicators in a population cohort. Acta Psychiatr Scand 137(6):503–515, 2018 29577236

Ten Have M, de Graaf R, van Dorsselaer S, et al: Recurrence and chronicity of major depressive disorder in the general population: results from the Netherlands Mental Health Survey and Incidence Study-2 [in Dutch]. Tijdschr Psychiatr 61(1):22–31, 2019 30640403

Thornicroft G, Chatterji S, Evans-Lacko S, et al: Undertreatment of people with major depressive disorder in 21 countries. Br J Psychiatry 210(2):119–124, 2017 27908899

Tronick E, Reck C: Infants of depressed mothers. Harv Rev Psychiatry 17(2):147–156, 2009 19373622

Tweed DL: Depression-related impairment: estimating concurrent and lingering effects. Psychol Med 23(2):373–386, 1993 8332654

Vandeleur CL, Fassassi S, Castelao E, et al: Prevalence and correlates of DSM-5 major depressive and related disorders in the community. Psychiatry Res 250:50–58, 2017 28142066 van Straten A, Hill J, Richards DA, Cuijpers P: Stepped care treatment delivery for depression: a systematic review and meta-analysis. Psychol Med 45(2):231–246, 2015 25065653

Vaughn MG, Wexler J, Beaver KM, et al: Psychiatric correlates of behavioral indicators of school disengagement in the United States. Psychiatr Q 82(3):191–206, 2011 20957435

Verduijn J, Verhoeven JE, Milaneschi Y, et al: Reconsidering the prognosis of major depressive disorder across diagnostic boundaries: full recovery is the exception rather than the rule. BMC Med 15(1):215, 2017 29228943

Verduyn C, Barrowclough C, Roberts J, et al: Maternal depression and child behaviour problems. Randomised placebo-controlled trial of a cognitive-behavioural group intervention. Br J Psychiatry 183:342–348, 2003 14519613

Verhoeven JE, Révész D, Epel ES, et al: Major depressive disorder and accelerated cellular aging: results from a large psychiatric cohort study. Mol Psychiatry 19(8):895–901, 2014 24217256

Vigo D, Thornicroft G, Atun R: Estimating the true global burden of mental illness. Lancet Psychiatry 3(2):171–178, 2016 26851330

Wanders RB, van Loo HM, Vermunt JK, et al: Casting wider nets for anxiety and depression: disability-driven cross-diagnostic subtypes in a large cohort. Psychol Med 46(16):3371–3382, 2016 27624913

Wang PS, Beck A, Berglund P, et al: Chronic medical conditions and work performance in the Health and Work Performance Questionnaire calibration surveys. J Occup Environ Med 45(12):1303–1311, 2003 14665817

Watson S, Mackin P: HPA axis function in mood disorders. Psychiatry 5(5):166–170, 2006. Available at: https://www.sciencedirect.com/science/article/abs/pii/S1476179306700374?via%3Dihub. Accessed October 26, 2021.

Weissman MM: Postpartum depression and its long-term impact on children: many new questions. JAMA Psychiatry 75(3):227–228, 2018 29387871

Weissman MM, Pilowsky DJ, Wickramaratne PJ, et al; STAR*D-Child Team: Remissions in maternal depression and child psychopathology: a STAR*D–Child report. JAMA 295(12):1389–1398, 2006 16551710

Weissman MM, Wickramaratne P, Pilowsky DJ, et al: Treatment of maternal depression in a medication clinical trial and its effect on children. Am J Psychiatry 172(5):450–459, 2015 25615566

Weissman MM, Berry OO, Warner V, et al: A 30-year study of 3 generations at high risk and low risk for depression. JAMA Psychiatry 73(9):970–977, 2016 27532344

Wells KB, Stewart A, Hays RD, et al: The functioning and well-being of depressed patients. Results from the Medical Outcomes Study. JAMA 262(7):914–919, 1989 2754791

Wesselhoeft R, Sørensen MJ, Heiervang ER, Bilenberg N: Subthreshold depression in children and adolescents—a systematic review. J Affect Disord 151(1):7–22, 2013 23856281

Whisman MA: Marital dissatisfaction and psychiatric disorders: results from the National Comorbidity Survey. J Abnorm Psychol 108(4):701–706, 1999 10609435

Whisman MA: Marital distress and DSM-IV psychiatric disorders in a population-based national survey. J Abnorm Psychol 116(3):638–643, 2007 17696721

Whisman MA, Uebelacker LA: Prospective associations between marital discord and depressive symptoms in middle-aged and older adults. Psychol Aging 24(1):184–189, 2009 19290750

Whisman MA, Tolejko N, Chatav Y: Social consequences of personality disorders: probability and timing of marriage and probability of marital disruption. J Pers Disord 21(6):690–695, 2007 18072869

Whiteford HA, Degenhardt L, Rehm J, et al: Global burden of disease attributable to mental and substance use disorders: findings from the Global Burden of Disease Study 2010. Lancet 382(9904):1575–1586, 2013 23993280

Whiteford HA, Ferrari AJ, Degenhardt L, et al: Global burden of mental, neurological, and substance use disorders: an analysis from the Global Burden of Disease Study 2010, in Mental, Neurological, and Substance Use Disorders (Disease Control Priorities, 3rd Edition, Vol 4). Edited by Patel V, Chisholm D, Dua T, et al. Washington, DC, The International Bank for Reconstruction and Development/The World Bank, 2016, pp 29–40

Wilson S, Durbin CE: Effects of paternal depression on fathers' parenting behaviors: a meta-analytic review. Clin Psychol Rev 30(2):167–180, 2010 19926376

Wittchen HU, Beesdo K, Gloster AT: A new meta-structure of mental disorders: a helpful step into the future or a harmful step back to the past? Psychol Med 39(12):2083–2089, 2009 19796434

Wittchen HU, Jacobi F, Rehm J, et al: The size and burden of mental disorders and other disorders of the brain in Europe 2010. Eur Neuropsychopharmacol 21(9):655–679, 2011 21896369

Wittchen HU, Knappe S, Andersson G, et al: The need for a behavioural science focus in research on mental health and mental disorders. Int J Methods Psychiatr Res 23 (suppl 1):28–40, 2014 24375534

World Health Organization: International Statistical Classification of Diseases and Related Health Problems, 10th Revision. Geneva, Switzerland, World Health Organization, 1992

World Health Organization: WHO Global Health Observatory Data Repository, 2018. Available at: https://apps.who.int/gho/data/node.main. Accessed July 21, 2021.

Yalin N, Young AH: The age of onset of unipolar depression, in Age of Onset of Mental Disorders. Edited by de Girolamo G, McGorry P, Sartorius N. New York, Springer, 2019, pp 111–124

Zeiss AM, Lewinsohn PM: Enduring deficits after remissions of depression: a test of the scar hypothesis. Behav Res Ther 26(2):151–158, 1988 3365205

Ziebold C, Mari JJ, Goldberg DP, et al: Diagnostic consequences of a new category of anxious depression and a reduced duration requirement for anxiety symptoms in the ICD-11 PHC. J Affect Disord 245:120–125, 2019 30368071

CHAPTER 4

Rating Scales and Structured Diagnostic Interviews for Mood Disorders

David V. Sheehan, M.D., M.B.A.

"If something exists, it can be measured," according to Edward L. Thorndike. If something cannot be measured, it is very difficult to study.

If you want to use rating scales and related assessment instruments, you should first be clear on your goals. The most common goals are these:

1. You are following someone else's ("just do it") directive.
2. You have a genuine interest in integrating more targeted and precise measurement into your clinical practice for assessment and follow-up monitoring.
3. You need to choose rating scales to address specific questions in your planned research studies.

The solutions to these goals are different.

The author thanks Janet Williams and Mark Zimmerman for contributions to the descriptions of their scales in the manuscript.

- **Solution to Goal 1:** Someone in your management thinks there is value in measurement-based care. They should be commended. Some managers are genuinely interested in improving the quality of care in their systems. They may even intend to do so in the best way possible. They may hire expert consultants to advise in these choices. For this group there is hope.

  Others may have more mercenary reasons; for example, they have been told by a payor that they will not be reimbursed unless they assess treatment outcomes. Alternately, they may need to justify why they should be the prime beneficiary in a competitive bid for services. Unless the evaluators of such a process are sophisticated, this leads to a scramble to meet this need in the cheapest, easiest way possible, without serious regard for quality. They delegate responsibility for the selection of outcome measures to juniors in their systems "to make it happen." This in turn leads to the uninitiated frantically trolling search engines in a quest for quick, cheap, easy solutions. I confess to little sympathy with this latter group. If following another's directive is your only goal, you can skip the rest of this chapter and instead use Google or Bing or social media. Good luck.
- **Solution to Goal 2:** If you have this goal, I can give you some useful guidance. You should choose assessment instruments that are simple, brief, easy to use, and well tried, and that meet your own specific goals for assessment. In general, instruments that are self-rated are better choices. In fact, several scales designed as clinician-rated scales can often be self-rated by patients in a clinic. These include the Montgomery-Åsberg Depression Rating Scale (MADRS) (Montgomery and Åsberg 1979) and the Hamilton Depression Rating Scale (HAM-D) (Hamilton 1960, 1967). Clinicians rarely spend time completing these rating scales at the first visit and then at each follow-up visit in the clinic; the best initial intentions will soon fall apart under visit time pressure.

  Have the patient input this information in the waiting room or on a digital platform just before the visit. Front office staff need to be trained to routinely provide these scales to patients on arrival. Clinicians should explain the need and value of such scales and train patients to use them properly. The scales are completed before the face-to-face clinician-patient visit begins. This practice helps eliminate the often-heard clinician complaint "I don't have enough time to implement assessment tools," and provides the clinician with much fresh, precise information at the start of each visit. The clinician can then check the data for accuracy and focus on already reported information. In addition to saving time, this procedure also provides some medicolegal protection because the clinician has a record of patient-provided information at each visit, in addition to the clinician's progress notes, which could be deemed as either misleading or self-serving.

  Some patients who fear that a human rater is judging them are often more honest with a self-report form on paper or a digital platform. The paper or digital platform is judgment neutral, particularly for assessments of suicidality and substance use.
- **Solution to Goal 3:** Design your research studies to answer your research question(s) in a clear, precise, and very focused manner. All too often researchers try to address too many unresolved questions in one study. Accordingly, they adopt the "let's throw the kitchen sink" clutter of scales into the study, in the hope that "something will stick." The added clutter, however, distracts from the main focus.

> It is always better to spend more time at each research visit on the measure that addresses the primary question. Purge the clutter that detracts from the time available to properly address the central question. The more research experience that you accumulate, the more you grasp the importance of this.
>
> Too little time and attention are given to selecting the scale that could most accurately address the research question. Priority is often given to choosing an older scale on which there are many "validation" studies or publications, when a newer revised and improved version of the same scale or another scale with fewer associated publications would be a better choice. This lack of attention and lack of thoughtful selection is not restricted to those who design such research studies or to those who make these choices for clinical settings. Often the choice is driven by pushback from study sponsors or clinicians, who have their own biases, or from those who adjudicate the merits of such research protocols or clinical choices, who are so focused on "validation" that they miss the forest for the trees. More on this later in the section on validation.

I have seen many examples of sponsors choosing wrong versions of scales they found on the internet (or at any rate not the proper version approved by the scale author). Then the administration of the scale is not properly implemented, leading to failures in studies that would have otherwise succeeded. This is a particular problem with the accurate digital implementation of scales and the failure to follow author guidance.

A Simple Model for Measurement-Based Care Assessments

The following is a simple formula to apply in selecting assessment instruments in clinical and research settings for any psychiatric disorder. It has emerged from decades of experience in designing clinical research studies.

1. Confirm and document the diagnosis using a structured diagnostic interview.
2. Measure and track severity using dimensional rating scales.
3. Use one or more dimensional symptom scales to measure the severity of the central cluster(s) of the primary disorder's symptoms of interest. This may be the cluster of depressive symptoms in major depressive disorder (MDD) or the mania symptoms in bipolar disorder, or both.
4. Use a dimensional scale to measure the level of functional impairment associated with the disorder.
5. Use a dimensional scale to measure the seriousness of suicidality associated with the disorder.
6. Use a dimensional scale to measure the global improvement in the disorder over time in response to treatment.

In addition, you can choose whatever you need or deem necessary. However, these additional scales are usually not central, unless they are included to very specifically measure a target not otherwise captured.

Role of Structured Diagnostic Interviews

As a first step, you need to confirm your diagnosis accurately. This cannot be done using a rating scale. No, you did not misread the last sentence. Let me repeat it, because there is so much misunderstanding around this point. You CANNOT confirm a psychiatric diagnosis using a rating scale.

Attempting to make a diagnosis using a rating scale that assesses the symptoms of one syndrome, without gathering similar information on other potential psychiatric diagnoses, is a mistake and potentially dangerous. This practice is regrettably rampant and has even been recommended by some august bodies. The 9-item Patient Health Questionnaire (PHQ-9) (Spitzer et al. 1999), for example, cannot and should not be used to confirm a diagnosis of MDD. It should only be used as a first-step screening instrument. Using it for confirmation of a diagnosis would be like using a mammogram to confirm a diagnosis of breast cancer and then proceeding directly to doing a mastectomy. However, all too often primary care physicians who find an elevated PHQ-9 score after a brief discussion with the patient immediately start an antidepressant. Some of these patients have bipolar disorder; they often fail to improve from any of a series of antidepressants, have rapid cycling induction, and become more suicidal. PHQ-9 scores can be elevated in patients with various psychiatric and medical conditions. To confirm and accurately document the diagnosis, you need to do a structured (or, more accurately, semistructured) diagnostic interview that maps directly to diagnostic criteria from DSM-5 (American Psychiatric Association 2013) or ICD-11 (World Health Organization 2019).

The Difference Between Structured and Semistructured Diagnostic Interviews

In a semistructured diagnostic interview, the interviewer begins by following the scripted wording in the questions provided, but then is allowed to ask follow-up questions. In addition, the interviewer makes the final call on how to most accurately code (score) the response, based on clinical judgment, experience, and training. Because the semistructured diagnostic interview gives the interviewer more latitude, it is more suitable for clinically experienced and trained interviewers. In contrast, strictly structured diagnostic interviews give the interviewer no latitude and must be strictly adhered to. Fully structured diagnostic interviews are used only in rare situations, such as in epidemiology studies when only lay interviewers with limited training are available. For the great majority of situations in health care settings, the semistructured interview is the preferred choice.

The Difference Between a Structured Diagnostic Interview and a Rating Scale

A structured diagnostic interview uses very carefully worded questions that map closely to the DSM or ICD diagnostic criteria being probed. The response options are binary (yes/no). The algorithms that navigate through criteria rules are usually integrated into the sequence of questions. A patient's symptoms may meet criteria for one or more diagnostic categories (in which case these separate disorders are considered comorbid diagnoses). Each structured interview handles the navigation and the algorithms in a different and more or less efficient way. Some structured diagnostic interviews are shorter to implement than others. Each covers a different number of diagnoses from DSM-IV (American Psychiatric Association 1994), DSM-5, or ICD-10 (World Health Organization 1992). Some have several different versions (for different sets of disorders) to accommodate different clinical settings and different research populations. For this purpose, some make customized variants available to accommodate different needs in the most time-efficient manner for each setting and study. For example, the standard (time-efficient) Mini International Neuropsychiatric Interview (MINI) (Lecrubier et al. 1997; Sheehan 2020; Sheehan et al. 1997, 1998) has an abbreviated psychotic disorders module to rule out all psychotic disorders of all kinds from most outpatient studies. However, for schizophrenia studies when it is necessary to identify and precisely differentiate all of the psychotic disorders from each other, the shorter psychotic disorders module of the MINI should be swapped out for a more expanded psychotic disorders module. This latter version is called the MINI for Psychotic Disorders (Amorim et al. 1998).

Examples of Semistructured Diagnostic Interviews

The principal semistructured diagnostic interviews used for adults are the MINI, the Structured Clinical Interview for DSM-5 (SCID-5) (First 2015), and the Composite International Diagnostic Interview (CIDI) for ICD-10 (World Health Organization 1990) or CIDI 3.0 for DSM-IV (Haro et al. 2006). There is also a SCID-5-PD for the evaluation of personality disorders (First et al. 2016). The principal semistructured diagnostic interviews for children and adolescents are the Mini International Neuropsychiatric Interview for Children and Adolescents (MINI-KID) (Sheehan et al. 2010) and the Kiddie Schedule for Affective Disorders and Schizophrenia (Kiddie SADS, K-SADS-PL-DSM-5) (Kaufman et al. 2016).

Both the MINI and the SCID (and their several variants) are organized into separate disorder- or episode-specific modules. Both cover the most common disorders seen in clinical and research settings. The CIDI does not map exactly to DSM-5.

Variants of the SCID include the Clinician Version (SCID-CV) (First et al. 2015b) and the Clinical Trials version (SCID-CT) (First et al. 2015a).

Variants of the MINI include the MINI for Psychotic Disorders (Amorim et al. 1998), which has an enhanced psychotic disorders module to disaggregate all the psychotic disorder subtypes from each other; the MINI KID (Sheehan et al. 2010); the MINI KID for Psychotic Disorders Studies (Sheehan 2016a); the MINI Screen (Sheehan 2016b), which has all the screening questions on one page (two sides) for use in primary care settings; and the MINI Tracking (Sheehan 2016c), which provides dimensional (0–4 Likert scale) response options for all the key symptoms of each disorder in the MINI and can be used as a collection of symptom severity outcome measures.

Earlier versions of the MINI, the SCID, and the CIDI have been validated against each other (Lecrubier et al. 1997; Sheehan et al. 1997, 1998). Additionally, an earlier version of the MINI KID was validated against an earlier version of the K-SADS (Sheehan et al. 2010). Typically, the decision to choose one or another of these interviews is driven by practical matters such as brevity, simplicity of use, and ease of navigation through the questions. Some take several hours to administer correctly, whereas others can be done in 15–20 minutes on average, and the final information yield may not be substantially different. Your best option is to get evaluation copies of each, test them out on real patients, and make a selection based on the needs of your setting.

Depression Rating Scales

Adult Depression Rating Scales

Hamilton Depression Rating Scale

The HAM-D (Hamilton 1960, 1967) is a 17-item clinician-administered questionnaire designed to assess the severity of depression in research and clinical practice. Over the last 50 years, many variants have evolved, including versions with 6, 21, 24, 27, and 31 items—the HAM-D6, HAM-D21, HAM-D24, HAM-D27, and HAM-D31 (Williams 2001).

The HAM-D6, pioneered by Per Bech and his team, was found to capture the items most sensitive in assessing the severity of depression (Bech et al. 1975, 1981, 2009). Maier and Philipp (1985) reported similar results, using a six-item version that has five items in common with the version proposed by Bech and colleagues. Maier and Philipp reported that their 6-item HAM-D was as sensitive as the 17-, 21-, and 24-item versions. One study found that the 6-, 17-, 21-, and 24-item versions correlated strongly with each other at baseline and at study endpoint (O'Sullivan et al. 1997). Other authors reported that the shorter version of the scale assesses depression severity with comparable sensitivity to the longer versions (Williams 2001).

In a systematic review of the clinimetric properties of the HAM-D6 in comparison to the HAM-D17 and the MADRS, Timmerby et al. (2017) identified 51 articles that met their inclusion criteria from a universe of 681 unique search records on the HAM-D6 in the PubMed, PsycInfo, and EMBASE databases. The review followed the Preferred Reporting Items for Systematic Reviews and Meta-Analyses guidelines (Moher et al. 2009). The authors concluded that the HAM-D6 was "superior to both HAM-D17 and MADRS in terms of scalability (each item contains unique information regarding syndrome severity), transferability (scalability is constant over time and irrespective of sex, age, and depressive subtypes), and responsiveness (sensitivity to change in severity during treatment)" (Timmerby et al. 2017, p. 141).

The longer 24-item version assesses helplessness, hopelessness, pessimism, and worthlessness (Williams 1988). The 27- and 31-item versions accommodate what are referred to as symptoms of "atypical depression" (Williams 1988). These include items such as increased appetite, hypersomnia, feelings of heaviness in the arms and legs, and sensitivity to rejection or criticism. It is not unusual for authors to fail to identify which "version" of the HAM-D they used in a study.

Hamilton's original 17-item scale yields a maximum total score of 52; nine of the items are scored 0–4, and eight items are scored 0–2. Hamilton did not assign these different dimensional ratings based on differential weighting. He thought that the eight items were more difficult to anchor dimensionally and elected to use fewer response options for these items. The result is that the nine items contribute more to the total score than the other eight (Hamilton 1967). In addition, there are three insomnia items, two anxiety items, and two somatic items. The result is that these seven items contribute disproportionately to the total score. These considerations and others have led some reviewers to conclude that the instrument is psychometrically and conceptually flawed (Bagby et al. 2004).

There was a significant period of time during which it was reported that benzodiazepines, notably alprazolam, had "significant antidepressant effects" (Warner et al. 1988), although they most definitely do not. These reports were based on misinterpretation of the HAM-D total score. Benzodiazepines do impact the insomnia, anxiety, and somatic items of the HAM-D (and therefore the total score), but they have little or no concurrent effect on the depressed mood or suicide items. To assert that they have antidepressant effects based on the total is a mistake (Sheehan et al. 1980).

Some HAM-D items lack interval constancy between response options. For example, sexual symptoms can be rated as absent, mild, and severe, but not moderate. There is a similar lack of interval constancy across the suicide response options. The suicide item lacks sensitivity in detecting treatment effects.

Zimmerman et al. (2013b) provided an empirical basis for a severity of depression classification using the 17-item HAM-D. In a study of 627 outpatients, the authors recommended the following score ranges for each of the major severity categories: no depression (0–7); mild depression (8–16); moderate depression (17–23); and severe depression (≥24).

Reynolds and Kobak (1995) developed a self-report version of the HAM-D called the Hamilton Depression Inventory (HDI). This measure consists of a 23-item full form, a 17-item form, and a 9-item short form. The 17-item HDI corresponds in content to the HAM-D17. Substantial psychometric data support its value and use in outpatients.

Despite its wide use, the HAM-D is not optimally designed to be easily learned or reliably administered. Indeed, clinicians often develop their own idiosyncratic interpretations of items. As a result, reliability is compromised. Williams's (1988) Structured Interview Guide for the Hamilton Depression Rating Scale (SIGH-D) was developed to improve item reliability and facilitate rater training so that inexperienced clinicians are not left to devise their own questions to assess each item. The SIGH-D provides the rater with helpful parenthetical qualifications and semistructured follow-up questions for individual items. This guide encourages more standard administration and has been shown to result in improved levels of interrater agreement for most of the HAM-D17 items (Williams 1988).

Given the growing frequency of scale administration by telephone, video, and virtual conferencing, several studies have examined the accuracy of clinical assessments obtained from face-to-face, in-person administration compared with telephone and video administration, yielding results that favor the continued use of remote administration in training and research (Amarendran et al. 2011; Hubley et al. 2016; Kobak et al. 2008a; Shore et al. 2007). The COVID-19 pandemic has increased the need to improve the consistency, accuracy, and comparability of scale administration between face-to-face and remote video and virtual conferencing. This goal can be accomplished provided that the necessary accommodations are made in planning and implementing the virtual administration.

Montgomery-Åsberg Depression Rating Scale

The MADRS is a 10-item clinician-administered questionnaire designed to assess the severity of depression (Montgomery and Åsberg 1979). Each of the 10 items has seven possible response option scores (0–6), with four descriptive anchors for item scores of 0, 2, 4, and 6. Interim anchor points (1, 3, 5) may be used but are not specifically defined. Some believe the extended scale points facilitate the use of the scale, as compared with the more restricted range for each item in the HAM-D (Hamilton 1967). The scores on each MADRS item are added to yield a single total score; the maximum total score possible is 60. Individual total scores are often used as a cutoff for admission to a clinical trial. The scale was developed by selecting most of the items that were found to be sensitive to change in an antidepressant trial from a larger rating scale and symptoms that were not associated with side effects of antidepressants. This approach provides a more empirical foundation than many contemporary rating scales. Correlation with the 17-item HAM-D tends to be high (Hamilton 1967).

Questions have been raised about some of the MADRS item scale points. Item 10 for suicidal thoughts, for example, has been identified as not being reflective of contemporary evaluations of suicidal thoughts or intent. In addition, the verbal descriptive anchor for a score of 0 ("Enjoys life or takes it as it comes") on the suicide item is problematic. One consequence of this unfortunate wording is that most patients in most studies do not match this descriptive anchor and therefore strictly cannot get a score of 0 on this item even if they have no suicidality. The verbal anchor for a score of 0 on this item should instead read "No suicidality at all" or "No suicidal thoughts, suicidal plan, suicidal intent, suicidal impulses, or suicidal behaviors at all." Consequently, most patients in a research study will score in the range of 1–3 or maybe 1–4, which substantially reduces the sensitivity to change of this item in any research study and narrows the drug versus placebo differences on this item and, by extension, on the total score.

The MADRS is one of the two most widely used depression rating scales (the other being the HAM-D). Its use has become more frequent in the past two decades, and it is now used often to measure the depressive symptoms in patients with bipolar depression, treatment-resistant depression, and schizoaffective disorder.

The MADRS was designed to be easily learned and administered. However, clinicians often develop their own, frequently idiosyncratic, interpretations of many of the items, and interrater reliability can be compromised. Some of the language may be unfamiliar to U.S. mental health professionals. For example, the word "lassitude" is rarely used in the United States. Likewise, it is more common to refer to "anhedonia" than "inability to feel." For these reasons, the Structured Interview Guide for the MADRS (SIGMA) (Williams and Kobak 2008) was developed to guide the clinical inquiry by providing a group of semistructured questions that should be used for each of the 10 MADRS items. The improved standardization increases interrater reliability of the MADRS and can facilitate video or telephone administration. The SIGMA facilitates training on the scale because inexperienced clinicians are not left to devise their own questions to assess each item. Because of the growing frequency of scale administration by telephone and video, a study was conducted to compare face-to-face versus remote administration of the SIGMA using videoconference and telephone, yielding results that favored the continued use of remote administration in training and research (Kobak et al. 2008b).

Although the MADRS is a clinician-rated scale, for the most part it lends itself well to use as a patient-rated scale, with minimal patient training. I am surprised that the scale is not more frequently used in this way.

Quick Inventory of Depressive Symptomatology

The Quick Inventory of Depressive Symptomatology (QIDS) (Rush et al. 2003) is a 16-item rating scale for depression. It is available in clinician (QIDS-C) and self-rated formats (QIDS-SR). Both formats map to the nine core depressive symptoms of a major depressive episode in DSM-5. The QIDS measures severity of depressive symptoms on a four-point (0–3) severity scale. It is a shortened version of the 30-item Inventory of Depressive Symptomatology (IDS). A score of 5 or less is declared a "remission," whereas a score of 21 or higher suggests a very severe depressive episode. One QIDS study in adolescents recommended that a total score of 5 or less be considered as "no depression," 6–10 as mild depression, 11–15 as moderate, 16–20 as severe, and 21 or higher as very severe (Bernstein et al. 2010). The maximum total score is 27. A score of 5 on the QIDS corresponds to a total score of 7 on the HAM-D17. A QIDS-SR score multiplied by 1.3 is a close predictor of the concurrent HAM-D17 score. Unlike the HAM-D17, the QIDS-SR and the QIDS-C restrict themselves to more pure depressive symptoms and avoid contamination with other symptom clusters such as anxiety. They can usually be completed in about 5 minutes. The QIDS has much to recommend it for use in both clinical and research settings and is used with increasing frequency. It is successful in detecting efficacy signals in clinical trials. The 16-item QIDS-SR is as sensitive to symptom change as the 30-item QIDS-SR and the HAM-D17. It has acceptable psychometric properties (Bernstein et al. 2010; Rush et al. 2003; Trivedi et al. 2004). In my opinion, it is a better choice than the PHQ-9. The QIDS has been translated into many languages; translated versions are available from Mapi Research Trust in Lyon, France.

Patient Health Questionnaire–9

The PHQ-9 is a nine-item self-report inventory of depressive symptoms used for screening (Kroenke et al. 2001). The nine items map to the nine key symptoms associated with a major depressive episode in DSM-IV and DSM-5. Patients who endorse at least five of the nine symptoms at a frequency level of "more than half the days" should then be evaluated in more depth for a mood or other disorder using a structured diagnostic interview. Treatment "response" is said to be a score of 10 or less and a 50% or greater reduction of the baseline score. The PHQ-9 has some value in tracking the treatment response for the core depressive symptoms of an independently confirmed major depressive disorder; however, it is not as sensitive to change or efficacy signal detection as the MADRS, HAM-D, IDS, or QIDS. The suicide item is not an adequate screening question for suicidality and could place a clinician in medicolegal jeopardy for having relied on it if an adverse outcome occurs. Some health care groups have recommended that their providers use a "PHQ-8" (the PHQ-9 minus the suicide question) in a "don't ask, don't tell" strategy. Participating in such a charade is irresponsible of a mental health care provider and potentially harmful.

(0=not at all true/0 days; 1=rarely true/1–2 days; 2=sometimes true/3–4 days; 3=usually true/5–6 days; 4=almost always true/every day). Zimmerman et al. (2008a) chose an ordinal rating of the symptom statements to keep the CUDOS brief. In contrast, scales such as the BDI and IDS, described above, assess symptoms with groups of four or five statements and are thus composed of 80 or more statements. These scales take respondents 10–15 minutes to complete, and Zimmerman and colleagues considered this time to be too long for regular use in clinical practice, in which the scale would be routinely administered at every follow-up appointment.

One study found that in comparison with the BDI, the CUDOS took less time to complete (<2 minutes on average, and >95% of patients were able to complete it in <3 minutes), the CUDOS was less of a burden to complete, and the patients preferred to complete the CUDOS at every visit in order to monitor the outcome of treatment (Zimmerman and McGlinchey 2008). Patients did not find scale completion burdensome and were willing to complete the CUDOS on a regular basis.

Later versions of CUDOS include brief subscales assessing the DSM-5 anxious distress and mixed features subtypes of MDD (Zimmerman et al. 2014a, 2014b) and modifications to enable the scale to be administered to assess depressive symptoms across other time frames, including daily and shorter time frames, so that it can be used to evaluate the efficacy of rapidly effective treatments for depression (Zimmerman et al. 2018). One such version lends itself well to use in ecological momentary assessment (Zimmerman et al. (2018). The CUDOS and its modifications have undergone the usual psychometric analyses and have been found to be reliable and valid instruments.

Remission From Depression Questionnaire

Experts agree that remission is the desired outcome when treating depression (American Psychiatric Association 2000b; Anderson et al. 2000; Stahl 1999; Thase 1999). In most studies, *remission* is defined as a score below a cutoff value on a symptom severity scale. Determination of treatment efficacy focuses on *symptom* improvement; however, depressed patients consider several factors in addition to symptom resolution as critically important in determining whether a depressive episode is in remission (Zimmerman et al. 2006). These factors, which include a return to premorbid functioning, having positive mental health, and good quality of life, were more frequently rated as very important in determining remission from depression than was symptom resolution (Zimmerman et al. 2008b).

Zimmerman and colleagues (2013a) designed a new outcome measure to assess the domains that depressed patients considered important in evaluating treatment outcome. In contrast to most measures of depression that assess only symptom presence during the past 1 or 2 weeks, the Remission from Depression Questionnaire (RDQ) assesses multiple factors (Zimmerman et al. 2013a). The domains covered on the RDQ were based on a literature review, a study of depressed patients' ratings of the relative importance of 16 factors in determining remission from depression, and meetings with two focus groups of depressed patients. During the focus group meetings, a list of items was generated and reviewed by patients as to the items' understandability, redundancy, and relevance in determining whether treatment for depression was addressing important treatment targets. An initial pool of 77 items that were generated was reduced to 41 items after pilot testing. The domains assessed are symptoms of depression, other symptoms that are often present in depressed patients such as anxiety and irritability, features of positive mental health, coping ability, functioning, life satisfaction, and a general sense of well-being. The items are rated based on the prior week using a three-point rating scale (not at all or rarely true; sometimes true; often or almost always true). The items are scored 0, 1, and 2, with higher item values reflecting greater pathology. Thus, for symptom items (e.g., "I felt sad or depressed"), a rating of often or almost always true was scored as 2, whereas for the positive mental health items (e.g., "When I woke up I looked forward to the day"), a rating of not at all or rarely true was scored as 2.

In a study of 102 depressed outpatients in ongoing treatment, the patients completed the RDQ and QIDS-SR and a nine-item measure of patient preference (Zimmerman et al. 2011). The patients indicated that the RDQ was a better indicator of their overall state and their goals in treatment. The patients also judged the RDQ to be a more accurate and preferred measure to determine the outcome of treatment, and a more accurate indicator of remission.

In a second study, including nearly 300 depressed outpatients, both the RDQ and QIDS were significantly associated with patients' self-reported remission status (Zimmerman et al. 2013a). However, the RDQ remained significantly associated with remission status after controlling for QIDS scores (r=–0.32, P<0.001), whereas the QIDS was not associated with remission status after controlling for RDQ scores (r=–0.06). This finding supported the hypothesis that the RDQ measures constructs other than depressive symptoms that patients consider important in determining remission. A third study replicated the finding that the RDQ was significantly associated with patient self-reported remission status after controlling for QIDS scores, whereas the QIDS was not associated with remission status after controlling for RDQ scores (Zimmerman et al. 2014c).

The RDQ is a reliable and valid measure that assesses the multiple domains that depressed patients consider important in evaluating treatment efficacy and particularly remission. The findings of the studies of the RDQ are consistent with prior research suggesting that depressed patients' perspectives of treatment efficacy and remission go beyond symptom improvement and resolution.

Rapid-Acting Antidepressant Scales

Although no scales have been specifically developed to measure rapid action of antidepressants, researchers are using one or a few items (e.g., depressed mood, anhedonia, concentration problems) from the MDD scales to conduct repeated assessments (e.g., every few minutes, hourly, or daily) over short periods of time to detect the onset of the antidepressant effect. There is still no consensus about how best to measure this effect, but many alternative approaches are currently under study, which vary depending on the specific research question or treatment target. The optimal solution will differ by target. For example, the best way to measure an antidepressant's effect on suicidality will be different from the best way to measure its effect on depression.

Pediatric Depression Rating Scales

The Children's Depression Rating Scale—Revised (CDRS-R) (Poznanski and Mokros 1996) is the most widely used depression scale for children ages 6–12 years. It is a clinician-rated scale, based on a semistructured interview taking about 10–15 minutes.

The original CDRS (Poznanski et al. 1984) had 15 items, with a total score of up to 61 points. The CDRS-R has 17 items, with a total score of up to 113 points. The response options range from 1 to 5 in the CDRS (normal, doubtful, mild, moderate, severe) and from 1 to 7 in the CDRS-R; the CDRS-R has additional response options between mild and moderate and between moderate and severe. In a study of depressed children, the CDRS-R was found to show greater effect size for differentiating drug and placebo than the MADRS (Jain et al. 2007).

The majority of depression scales for children are self-rated. These self-rated children's depression scales include the Birleson Depression Self-Rating Scale for Children (DSRS-C) (Birleson 1981), the Children's Depression Inventory (CDI) (Kovacs 1981, 1983; Saylor et al. 1984; Zalsman et al. 2005), and the Children's Affective Rating Scale (CARS) (McKnew et al. 1979). The DSRS-C has 18 items rated on a 3-point scale for severity. The CDI has 27 items rated on a 3-point scale for severity. The CARS is a 27-symptom checklist rated on a 10-point scale for severity without subcategory definitions.

Personal Favorites Among the Many Depression Scales

My favorites among the depression scales are the MADRS and the 16-item QIDS-SR. The DID also shows great promise, and its development has been very sophisticated.

Mania Rating Scales

The Young Mania Rating Scale

The 11-item clinician-rated Young Mania Rating Scale (YMRS) (Young et al. 1978) is the most widely used scale to assess manic/hypomanic symptoms in clinical trials for bipolar disorder. This scale has been extensively studied psychometrically and is available in many translations. It is sensitive in detecting the efficacy signal of antimanic medications and remains the first choice for this purpose in the United States and the United Kingdom. It lends itself well to use in clinical settings as well as research because of its brevity.

Bipolar Inventory of Symptoms Scale

The Bipolar Inventory of Symptoms Scale (BISS) is a 44-item scale that was designed to assess the comprehensive domains and wide spectrum of symptoms in bipolar disorders (Bowden et al. 2007). It discriminates well between depressed, manic/hypomanic, and mixed episodes and remission status specifiers for bipolar disorders. It has acceptable psychometric properties. It compares very favorably with the combination of the MADRS and the YMRS (Bowden et al. 2007; Gonzalez et al. 2008).

I have long thought that "bipolar disorder" was a *quadri*polar disorder rather than a *bi*polar disorder, with mania, depression, anxiety, and irritability as the four domains. These domains do not track each other synchronously in their progression over time or in their response to the same treatments. One of the most common clinical presentations in outpatients with bipolar disorder (particularly in episodes with mixed features) is anxiety, which prompted us to conduct several double-blind studies on "bipolar anxiety." We found that the anxiety domain responded differently to treatment than would have been predicted from the expected responses to the other domains (Sheehan et al. 2013). Consistent with this line of thinking, Thompson et al. (2010), in an exploratory factor analytic study of the BISS that used the maximum likelihood factor extraction method, followed by oblique rotation of the extracted factor loadings, found five factors: mania, depression, irritability, anxiety, and psychosis. Using the Pearson correlation coefficient to determine the strength of the relationship, the authors found that the mania factor score correlated only weakly with the other four factors. This makes very good clinical sense and challenges the clinician to monitor the response to treatment in all five of these domains. That the BISS can identify each of these domains makes this scale unique and deserving of much more widespread use. Its development was very thoughtful, and I highly recommend it.

Singh et al. (2013) found that a small subset of symptoms captured in the BISS, several of which are absent in the DSM-IV-TR (American Psychiatric Association 2000a) and DSM-5 criteria and traditional rating scales for bipolar disorder studies, help in distinguishing mixed episodes from depressive or manic/hypomanic episodes.

Bech-Rafaelsen Mania and Melancholia Scales

The Bech-Rafaelsen Mania Scale (BRMaS) (Bech 2002a; Bech et al. 1978) is an 11-item clinician-rated scale. Items are rated from 0 to 4; the sum is used to assess the severity of manic symptoms. A score of less than 15 suggests hypomania, scores around 20 suggest moderate mania, and scores around 28 suggest severe mania. This scale has been found to be superior to the Clinical Global Impression—Severity scale (Guy 1976) (see later section "Global Severity and Improvement Scales") in detecting responsiveness to treatment and has been very sensitive in detecting placebo-drug differences in a wide range of studies of antimania treatments. The items on the companion six-item clinician-rated Bech-Rafaelsen Melancholia Scale (BRMeS) (Bech 2002b) are a subset of items from the BDI. The BRMeS is very sensitive in detecting efficacy signals of antidepressants in the depressive melancholic cluster of symptoms. Both Bech-Rafaelsen scales have been widely used and studied, especially in Europe (Bech 1981, 2002a, 2002b; Bech et al. 1978).

Mood Disorder Questionnaire

The Mood Disorder Questionnaire (MDQ) (Hirschfeld et al. 2000) is a 13-item self-rated questionnaire with binary (yes/no) response options. It maps well to DSM-IV and DSM-5 symptom criteria for a manic/hypomanic episode. A score of 7 or higher has good sensitivity (0.73) and specificity (0.9) as a quick one-page pencil-and-paper test in screening for bipolar I disorder, bipolar II disorder, and bipolar disorder not otherwise specified. The MDQ is useful in clinical practice settings but is not designed for use in efficacy signal detection as a treatment outcome measure. Because bipolar disorders are so frequently missed in clinical practice, the MDQ should be used more frequently, especially when any depression scale is used in mental health screening.

There are several good reviews of mood scales in bipolar disorders (Berk et al. 2007; Miller et al. 2009; Sajatovic et al. 2015; Vieta 2011). They are all worth reading.

Irritability and Anhedonia Scales

Irritability Scales

Irritability is a troublesome symptom that is often comorbid with mood disorders, especially bipolar disorders. It can continue to cause impairment as a residual symptom following treatment. For some families and in work and social settings, it can cause substantial disruption. In some cases, irritability is the most disruptive symptom to other people. Effective monitoring and treatment of the irritability are often critical in restoring family social and workplace harmony. Validated scales that specifically assess the severity of irritability include the Concise Associated Symptom Tracking (CAST) scale (Jha et al. 2018, 2019) and the Sheehan Irritability Scale (SIS) (Khan et al. 2016; Mannix et al. 2016).

Anhedonia Scales

Measuring anhedonia and apathy is of principal interest in schizophrenia. More recently, anhedonia is being studied as a treatment target in mood disorders. Some medications may have more ability than others to improve apathy and anhedonia. For example, monoamine oxidase inhibitors (MAOIs) have long been believed to be more effective than tricyclic antidepressants or selective serotonin reuptake inhibitors or serotonin-norepinephrine reuptake inhibitors in improving anhedonia and apathy. This effect is believed to be due to the dopamine uptake–inhibiting effects of MAOIs. Triple reuptake inhibitors—which inhibit the uptake of norepinephrine and serotonin in addition to the uptake of dopamine—are being studied for the treatment of anhedonia, because the additional dopaminergic effect is hypothesized to play a central role in improving anhedonia (Sharma et al. 2015). Although there are several candidate anhedonia scales, it is not yet clear which scale is the most sensitive in discriminating between drug and placebo on the anhedonia domain in mood disorders (Chapman et al. 1976; Leventhal et al. 2006; Nakonezny et al. 2010).

Functional Impairment Scales

Including functional impairment in the assessment of mood disorder symptoms is important for two reasons. First, improvement in functional impairment does not align exactly at any one point in time or in its progression over time with symptom improvement. In fact, it is often *desynchronous* with symptom improvement. One patient may have severe symptoms but function fairly well. The next patient may have mild symptoms, but function poorly. Patients can have impairment of functioning even when they have no symptoms and can have symptoms even when they have no impairment (Samara et al. 2014).

Second, although employers and governments may or may not care about suffering related to mental illness, they do care about days lost from work, days underproductive at work, and impairment in social life, leisure activities, and family life/home responsibilities. After all, these have direct economic and financial impacts. Improvement in functional impairment is also high on patients' lists of important factors in recovery and remission. Table 4–1 lists the most commonly used functional impairment scales in order of their length.

The Global Assessment of Functioning (GAF) scale (American Psychiatric Association 1994) is well known because it was used as Axis V of DSM-IV-TR. Consisting of only one item, it is scored from 0 to 100, with high scores indicating good functioning and low scores reflecting poor functioning. The GAF has the advantage of simplicity. The instrument, however, has well-documented issues. A modification of the Global Assessment Scale (GAS) (Endicott et al. 1976), a measure of overall severity of psychiatric disturbance, the GAF does not specifically assess *functioning*. Rather, it assesses a concurrent mixture of several domains that include symptoms, signs, behaviors, suicidality, and functioning as well as psychotic symptoms and signs. In my opinion, it would have been better named the Global Psychological Symptoms Scale. Other drawbacks are psychometric problems related to its reliability as well as its concurrent and predictive validity (Aas 2011). The lack of interval constancy across the scale's spectrum of response options created problems for clinicians trying to score it in everyday clinical practice. In spite of many attempts to remedy these issues, the GAF was never able to circumvent its innate drawbacks and was abandoned in DSM-5. It makes no sense to use the GAF or to resuscitate it in its DSM-IV form.

In contrast, the one-item Social and Occupational Functioning Assessment Scale (SOFAS) in DSM-IV has much to recommend it as a single-score, single-domain global measure of social and occupational functioning. Like the GAF, it is scored from 0 to 100, but unlike the GAF, SOFAS focuses exclusively on an individual's social and occupational functioning (American Psychiatric Association 1994; Goldman et al. 1992; Samara et al. 2014). The Personal and Social Performance (PSP) scale (Morosini et al. 2000) attempts to improve on the SOFAS, using a similar 100-point, single-item scale that is subdivided into 10 equal intervals. The PSP scale is said to have better face validity and psychometric properties than the SOFAS and is therefore a good choice for a quick and valid measure of personal and social functioning.

The GAF was replaced in DSM-5 by the World Health Organization Disability Assessment Schedule (WHODAS 2.0) (Üstün et al. 2010), a scale that more closely measures functioning. However, with 36 items, the WHODAS 2.0 is too lengthy and unwieldy for routine clinical use and is now rarely used in clinical settings in the way that the GAF was. The WHODAS 2.0 violates the brevity and simplicity rule. It covers seven domains of functioning: understanding and communicating, getting around, self-care, getting along with people, life activities—household, life activities—school/work, and participation in society. The standard WHODAS 2.0 has 36 items, although there is a 12-item version of the instrument. Both versions of the WHODAS 2.0 are designed not just for mental health settings but also for use across all diseases. They are linked to the International Classification of Functioning, Disability and Health (World Health Organization 2001). The WHODAS 2.0 is well thought out, is well designed, is useful for epidemiology studies, and has much to recommend it in cross-sectional research studies. Its value and utility as a sensitive change measure or research efficacy signal detector is less clear at this time (Üstün et al. 2010).

The three-item Sheehan Disability Scale (SDS) (Sheehan and Sheehan 2008; Sheehan et al. 1996) is now the most widely used measure of functional impairment in

TABLE 4–1. Validated functional impairment scales

Validated scales	No. of items	Domains
Social and Occupational Functioning Assessment Scale (SOFAS) and the related Personal and Social Performance (PSP) scale	1	Social, occupational
Global Assessment of Functioning (GAF) scale	1	Severity of symptoms and functional alteration
Sheehan Disability Scale (SDS)	3	Work/school, social life and leisure activities, family life/home responsibilities
Work and Social Adjustment Scale (WSAS)	5	Work, home management, social and personal leisure activities, relationships
Longitudinal Interval Follow-Up Evaluation Range of Impaired Functioning Tool (LIFE-RIFT)	9	Work, interpersonal relations, general satisfaction with functioning, recreation
Assessment of Impairment of Functioning/Disability from the Mini International Neuropsychiatric Interview for DSM-5	12	Work, social life, leisure activities, family life/home responsibilities, relationships, getting along with others, ability to communicate, self-care ability, interpersonal aggression/disruption, financial impairment, physical impairment, spiritual/religious impairment, impairment of family by symptoms
Life Functioning Questionnaire (LFQ)	14	Tasks at work/school, tasks in the home, leisure time with family and friends
Endicott Work Productivity Scale (EWPS)	25	Work efficiency and productivity
World Health Organization Disability Assessment Schedule (WHODAS 2.0)	36	Cognition, mobility, self-care, interpersonal actions, activities, participation in society
Social Adjustment Scale (SAS)	48	Work, leisure and social activities, marital role, parent role, family role

international clinical trials. The SDS is very sensitive to change effects and is very sensitive as an efficacy signal detector, often detecting such signals when the other outcome measures fail. It has been used as the key measure for regulatory agency approvals for improving functional impairment with several medications for mood disorders. The SDS, which has been translated into more than 80 languages/language variants, assesses the three most important domains of functioning: work and school, social life/leisure activities, and family life/home responsibilities. It captures days lost and days underproductive at work. It accommodates 13 different time frames. It is very short, simple, and clear, appearing on one page. The SDS can be rated by patient or clinician, although it is much more frequently used as a patient-rated scale. It uses a unique discretized-analog (Discan) metric that was specifically designed to be sensitive in detecting efficacy signals in treatment studies. The Discan metric is anchored numerically (0–10), verbally-descriptively, and visually-spatially to enhance sensitivity across a population of subjects. Several variants of the scale with additional domains, including a child and adolescent version, are available for specific settings and needs (Sheehan and Sheehan 2008; Sheehan et al. 1996). The SDS has been expanded to cover 12 domains in an add-on module to the MINI 7.0.2 for DSM-5 (Sheehan 2020).

The five-item Work and Social Adjustment Scale (WSAS) (Mundt et al. 2002) is very similar to the SDS, and its design was largely based on an earlier SDS. It assesses five domains and uses a 0–8 scale of response options. It has acceptable internal consistency, test-retest reliability, and sensitivity to change.

The nine-item Longitudinal Interval Follow-up Evaluation Range of Impaired Functioning Tool (LIFE-RIFT; P. Fisher, A.C. Leon, and M.E. Coles, unpublished manuscript, New York, New York State Psychiatric Institute, 2002) assesses functioning in the domains of work, interpersonal relations, life satisfaction, and recreation. This scale has been found to have good reliability and validity (Leon et al. 1999). It has been used in a longitudinal study of bipolar I disorder with good results (Leon et al. 2000) and has been adapted for children and adolescents (P. Fisher, A.C. Leon, and M.E. Coles, "The Longitudinal Interval Follow-up Evaluation Range of Impaired Functioning Tool (LIFE-RIFT) Adapted for Children and Adolescents," unpublished manuscript, New York, New York State Psychiatric Institute, 2002).

The 14-item Life Functioning Questionnaire (LFQ) (Altshuler et al. 2002) was designed to assess functioning in four domains: workplace, duties at home, leisure time with family, and leisure time with friends. It was found to be a reliable, consistent, and valid assessment of function at work and home in a study of patients with a mood disorder.

The 25-item Endicott Work Productivity Scale (EWPS) (Endicott and Nee 1997) focuses on work productivity and efficiency.

The 48-item self-rated Social Adjustment Scale (SAS) (Weissman and Bothwell 1976) is the oldest and most detailed of the functioning scales. It was used in many epidemiology studies and found to be very informative across a wide range of domains. However, because of its length, it is less suitable for routine clinical use or as an outcome measure in treatment studies. However, it remains the mother of most functional impairment scales.

Assessment Instruments for Suicidal Ideation and Behavior

More attention has been paid to the development of assessment instruments for suicidal ideation and behavior in the past decade than to scale development in any other area of mood disorders. Meyer et al. (2010) reviewed the status of the 29 most important assessment scales following a large international consensus conference on suicidality and suicide risk in 2009. Nine of the 29 scales were considered to have achieved a higher level of development than the others. Several of the more important scales in that review have undergone significant updates and revisions since then. The standards against which they were judged were the categories in the 2010 Draft Guidance of the U.S. Food and Drug Administration (2010). This guidance underwent significant revisions in 2012 (U.S. Food and Drug Administration, Center for Drug Evaluation and Research 2012) and is undergoing further revision at the time of this writing in 2021.

Some of these scales were developed for adults, others for adolescents, and still others for children. Some are self-report measures, others are clinician administered, and some accommodate both routes of administration. Some focus on the assessment of suicidal ideation, others evaluate suicidal behaviors or self-injury, and others assess a wider range of suicidality phenomena across the spectrum of suicidality.

To be acceptable for use in a clinical trial or as an outcome measure of safety or efficacy, a suicidality assessment scale must map closely or precisely to the categories outlined in the 2012 FDA draft guidance document (U.S. Food and Drug Administration, Center for Drug Evaluation and Research 2012). In 2021, the following five scales were deemed to meet this standard: the Columbia–Suicide Severity Rating Scale (C-SSRS) (Posner et al. 2011), the Suicide Ideation and Behavior Assessment Tool (SIBAT) (Alphs et al. 2017), the Sheehan–Suicidality Tracking Scale (S-STS) (Sheehan et al. 2014b), the Sheehan–Suicidality Tracking Scale Clinically Meaningful Change Measure (S-STS CMCM) version (Sheehan et al. 2014a), and the InterSePT Scale for Suicidal Thinking (ISST Plus) (Lindenmayer et al. 2003). All five scales can be clinician rated. The S-STS and the S-STS CMCM can also be patient rated. The SIBAT has some patient-rated components. The S-STS is the only suicidality assessment scale that has been linguistically validated for children and adolescents (Amado et al. 2014). It is available in three versions for three different age groups.

The C-SSRS was originally developed as a safety assessment questionnaire with binary (yes/no) response options. It is therefore a questionnaire rather than a dimensional rating scale and consequently does not lend itself to use as a sensitive treatment outcome measure capable of detecting an efficacy signal. Although it was a welcome improvement at the time over preexisting suicidality assessment methods in assessing treatment-emergent suicidality in clinical trials, it has many well-documented limitations (Giddens and Sheehan 2014b; Giddens et al. 2014).

The Beck Scale for Suicidal Ideation (BSI) (Beck et al. 1979) has also been used as an efficacy outcome measure. The BSI assesses a narrower range of the spectrum of suicidality than many of the other suicidality scales. One result is that it does not detect some important treatment-emergent suicidality phenomena. Overall, the BSI has been the least sensitive assessment in detecting treatment effects and in discriminating between active treatment and placebo for suicidality. Both item 10 on the MADRS and the S-STS have been more sensitive in detecting these efficacy signals in double-blind, placebo-controlled trials (Canuso et al. 2018; Khan et al. 2011). Suicidality assessment measures continue to evolve rapidly (Chappell et al. 2014).

There is much more to suicidality than suicidal ideation and behavior. Suicidality also includes suicidal impulses, suicidal hallucinations, delusional suicidality, and suicidal dreams. A good suicidality assessment scale should ask about the full range of suicidality phenomena. It should be sensitive in simultaneously detecting treatment efficacy and treatment-emergent safety effects (e.g., increased suicidality) and in detecting differences between drug and placebo. Such sensitivity is ethically necessary to identify efficacy and safety signals in as small a sample size as possible, while exposing the fewest possible number of patients to risk in clinical trials.

Using one or two suicidality items from a depression scale (e.g., item 3 of the HAM-D, item 10 of the MADRS, or item 9 on the PHQ-9) to screen for suicidality is a mistake. If you want to screen for suicidality, screen for suicidality directly rather than screening for one of its proxies, and assess the full range of suicidality phenomena in the process (Preti et al. 2013). This matters because the progression of any one suicidality phenomenon over time is not related to any other in a precise linear fashion (Sheehan and Giddens 2015). Their relationship to each other is almost always polynomial to the fourth order or higher. You cannot accurately predict the presence or magnitude of one by the presence or absence of another (Sheehan and Giddens 2015). As a result, you cannot rely on any one phenomenon to tell you whether any other suicidality phenomenon is present or absent or to what extent within a time frame. Time spent per day in suicidal ideation/behavior and the total S-STS score may be more accurate and sensitive measures of global suicidality than a global severity of suicidality measure, especially at the more serious end of the spectrum (Giddens and Sheehan 2014a, 2014c).

When using a suicidality assessment scale, you should adopt the mindset that you are assessing the presence or absence of suicidal phenomena within a recent *past* time frame while at the same time avoiding the temptation to make predictions about *future* suicidality. You cannot accurately predict suicidality at the individual level within a narrow time frame. The reason is that the progression of suicidality over time within a single individual is nonlinear when mathematically modeled (Sheehan and Giddens 2015). You do not use a schizophrenia scale to predict if and when someone is going to get a future hallucination or delusion, and you do not use a panic disorder scale to predict if or when someone is going to have another panic attack. Instead, you measure what has already occurred and you make your management decisions accordingly. Assessment of suicidality calls for the same approach as assessment of other areas of mental health. My recommendation is that you get copies of the various scales, try them out with patients, get patient feedback on them, and see whether they meet your needs and address your clinical and research questions.

Global Severity and Improvement Scales

The Clinical Global Impression—Severity (CGI-S) and Clinical Global Impression—Improvement (CGI-I) scales have been widely used to assess illness severity and global improvement or change. Both are seven-point scales. The CGI-S rates severity from 1 (normal) through 7 (among the most severely ill patients) (Guy 1976). On the CGI-I, there are three points of deterioration and three points of improvement, with a point denoting no change in between (Guy 1976). The CGI-I met the needs for an improvement scale when it was first developed and used. However, with increasing numbers of treatments and an increasing need to detect smaller differences in efficacy between multiple treatments in the same study, it became necessary to develop more sensitive global improvement scales. To meet this need, the Sheehan Clinical Global Improvement (S-CGI) scale and the Sheehan Patient Global Improvement (S-PGI) scale were developed. These measures of improvement are 21-point scales using a Discan metric for the response options. There are 10 points of improvement (1–10) and 10 points of deterioration (–1 to –10), with a zero (0) point in the middle, reflecting the baseline starting point score in the study or no change at any visit (Sheehan et al. 1988).

Comparison of Patient-Rated and Clinician-Rated Scales of Mood Disorders

Self-rated scales take less clinician time, but are they comparable to clinician-rated scales? Early comparisons in the adult depression scale literature (Carroll et al. 1973; Prusoff et al. 1972) found only moderate correlation between self-rated scales and clinician-rated scales (r=0.11–0.63 and r=0.42, respectively); this may be because different scales were used in the comparisons. The Carroll (Depression) Rating Scale (CRS) is a scale specifically designed to correspond with the 17-item Hamilton Depression Rating Scale (HAM-D). Even though they are very closely related instruments, a comparison between the two yielded a correlation that was still far from ideal, although it was higher (r=0.67) than that usually found between self-rated and clinician-rated scales. The conclusion was that self-rated depression scales are less reliable than clinician-rated depression scales (Carroll et al. 1981). That conclusion is open to debate. Biases (sometimes self-serving) are inherent in clinician-rated scales. Clinicians using a clinician scale sometimes have their own rating prejudices and preconceived ideas that are at variance with other raters. Similarly, patients using a patient-rated scale may not be able to accurately rate the severity of their symptoms in relation to how other patients rate the same symptoms. In the absence of information about how other people experience depression, one patient may overvalue or underestimate the severity of one or another symptom in the depressive cluster, compared with another patient's ratings. However, both clinician and patient perspectives have merits and limitations.

Experience has taught me that as patients became more familiar over time with completing these scales and reviewing and discussing them with their clinicians, their scores grow closer to the clinicians' ratings. I have more confidence in patient ratings than many other clinicians do. Clinicians should use them more frequently and should spend more time up front training patients in the proper and accurate completion of rating scales.

Interpretation of Scale Scores

Use and Misuse of Factor Scores

Factor scores have been extracted from existing scales based on factor analytic studies. For example, somatic anxiety/somatization, psychic anxiety, pure depression, and anorexia factors have been identified for the HAM-D. However, these factors are not stable across different samples in different settings. Identifying items belonging to these named factors and then studying the effect of treatments on them in subsequent studies is a misleading process. For example, in a very large dataset used to investigate anxiety in clinical trials with depressed patients, we (Goldberger et al. 2011) found that the "use of Cleary and Guy's anxiety/somatisation factor from the HAMD_{17} is unstable across studies and is not an appropriate routine measure of anxiety in depressed patients" (p. 48). We suggested that "in clinical trials, other scales specifically designed and validated for anxiety assessment should be used. An alternative strategy is to assess the factorial structure of the $HAMD_{17}$ scale for each studied sample and use for outcome assessment the factors identified by this analysis [within each study sample]. Such 'tailored' factor analysis would retrospectively allow the identification of the set of items appropriate for each specific study sample" (p. 48).

Response and Remission Cutoffs

Response for each individual on any scale is usually defined as a 50% or greater reduction from the baseline score. *Remission* for each individual on any scale is usually defined as a 70% or greater reduction from the baseline score. Remission is typically anchored to a reduction of 2 standard deviations from the baseline mean. Patients are said to be in remission when their scores reflect their own expectations of a good outcome, even if the score is less than perfect. Remission is also said to reflect an experienced clinician's expectations of a good treatment result, even if the outcome is not yet perfect. In mood disorders there is remarkable confluence and consistency across all four of these anchors of remission. These four anchors of remission line up with remission scores of 7 or lower on the HAM-D17 and 10 or lower on the MADRS.

In recent years, some pharmaceutical companies and researchers have used a score of 12 or lower on the MADRS as a remission cutoff score. Clinicians should beware of cutoffs like this. Such reports can be self-serving, instigated without justification by marketing divisions so that a larger percentage of patients can be declared in remission in the interest of making an investigational product appear more effective than it really is. Instead, such reports have the opposite effect by diminishing the companies' image in the eyes of the reader. Inflating results in this way has negative consequences. These include reducing interest in investing in new treatments by suggesting 1) that existing treatments are better than they are, 2) that we do not have unmet treatment needs, and 3) that we do not have a long way to go in improving the efficacy of current treatments. No clinicians should participate in these charades.

Challenges in Developing Scales

Based on my experience in developing several scales, at least $2 million is spent per scale before it is widely adopted, translated into many languages, and used and accepted internationally. If a scale is good, it takes about 7 years of work before it gains traction in the field and 15 years before its use grows exponentially. The hurdles involve psychometric testing, validation and reliability studies, extensive patient and expert opinion input, cognitive debriefing, overcoming hurdles and expectations of regulatory agencies, and linguistic validation and cognitive debriefing for all translations into other languages. That is why there are so few very good and widely used scales across the entire field of mental health. Many developers give up long before they reach the goal, because they get discouraged at the time and/or expense involved. Scale development requires a thick skin and endless persistence. The results are rewarding, however. What is important is to get started and to stick with it. The biggest progress is made in the first 2–3 years, if the scale developer stays focused on designing a scale that is "fit for purpose."

Advice on Use of Scales in Clinical Practice

You as a clinician may hope to administer scales and structured diagnostic interviews during clinic visits, but you will not have enough time. If you expect success, then have the patient complete a self-report scale before the start of the visit. Schedule patients early so they have time to complete the battery of scales before they see you. Arrange for front office staff to hand these scales to patients on a clipboard to complete in the waiting room before their appointments. Alternatively, email the patients the battery of scales individualized for them to complete on the day before their appointments. Ask patients to bring their completed scales to the visit. Let them know they *must* complete the scales before seeing the clinician. This practice will significantly improve the success and adherence rate. At the start of the visit, quickly review the completed scales, thank patients for completing them, and tell them how helpful this information is to you in your decision making. Use the scale responses as a basis for more in-depth probing or follow-up questions.

Ecological Momentary Assessment

Ecological momentary assessment (EMA) involves repeated sampling of an individual's symptoms, behaviors, functioning, and cognitions in real time. This can be done using mobile devices or microprocessors to sample subjects in their real-world and natural environment for a few moments during their day, often using random timing. It minimizes recall bias and maximizes ecological validity—that is in the individuals' ability to relate to themselves, to other people, and to their environment.

EMA most frequently utilizes mobile phones or wearable devices like heart monitors, electronic wrist bands, or rings with built-in technology. The information is often linked to a mobile phone app, which in turn synchronizes data to remote sites, where the data are gathered across large study samples. The use of EMA is rising rapidly.

Advice on Use of Scales in Research Settings

Number of Scales

A common problem in a research study is using too many scales. As you do more research across time, you will learn to minimize the number of scales you will use. In your early-career studies, try to resist participating in "fishing expedition studies" with a wide range of scales. Stay focused on addressing your narrow research questions.

Statistical Analysis

When you plan a study involving rating scales and structured diagnostic interviews, you need to clearly state your plans for how to collect and analyze your scale data. Your study design and analysis should be precisely aligned to address your research question. Your hypotheses should be clearly and explicitly stated a priori. If you have several hypotheses, they should be prioritized. All this is best done in consultation with an experienced statistician. Presenting your dataset for the first time to statisticians after the study is completed and then expecting them to find something of interest by fishing around in your dataset elicits sighs of despair and is an all-too-frequent occurrence. You cannot rescue by analysis what you have already damaged in your research design. There are many fine books on this topic. My favorite is Krathwohl's superb classic on preparing a research proposal (Krathwohl and Smith 2005).

Reporting Results

It is important for clinical researchers to follow the Consolidated Standards of Reporting Trials (CONSORT) statement proposed by the *Journal of the American Medical Association* when reporting results of studies that use rating scales as endpoints (American Educational Research Association 2014). The figures and tables in a research report should clearly identify the specific statistical test and the dataset—whether it is a completer analysis, an observed case, a last observation carried forward, or a modeled dataset (as in MMRM [Mallinckrodt et al. 2001] or ET Rank analysis [Entsuah 1996]). There are different levels of scientific confidence associated with each (Begg et al. 1996). In addition to the sources cited above, readers seeking further guidance on these different datasets are referred to Elobeid et al. (2009).

Validation

Validation is a fundamental and necessary step in scale development. It refers to the evidence in support of the interpretation of the scale scores for the proposed use and the extent to which it is "fit for purpose." However, there can be an overemphasis on validating any new scale against some existing "gold standard" scale. The problem is that there may not be gold in any so-called gold standard scale. When two scales are compared or "validated against" each other in this manner, it is like studying the correlation or agreement between two clouds floating across the sky. Neither cloud is anchored to anything on the ground. If the so-called gold standard is itself flawed, then showing a high agreement or correlation with it is not necessarily a positive attribute. When I am contacted about one of my scales or structured interviews and the first question is "Has your scale been validated?" I know I am dealing with someone who is not sophisticated in scale selection or evaluation. Many scales in mental health are flawed in one way or another and need to be improved. In the validation testing of a new scale, being able to demonstrate discrepancies or nonagreement with a preexisting standard may be a positive attribute rather than a negative one. Indeed, it may indicate that the new scale has improved on an older reference scale in an area of known weakness in the earlier scale. When there is no standard scale in a new area of investigation, it is difficult to validate a new scale in this way. *Standards for Educational and Psychological Testing* (American Educational Research Association 2014) is mandatory reading for everyone involved in scale development and evaluation.

Reliability

In contrast to the tendency to overemphasize validation in scale development, there is an underemphasis, in my opinion, on the importance of reliability testing. Interrater, intrarater, and test-retest reliability are all critically important properties in the use of scales in mental health research. Good reliability lends confidence to administering a scale in a large multisite study involving many raters over time. For a detailed discussion of reliability, readers are referred to the *Standards for Educational and Psychological Testing* (American Educational Research Association 2014).

Linguistic Validation

Linguistic validation is also too often neglected, misunderstood, and undervalued. It needs to be much more highly valued and much more frequently included in the planning of scale development and international study planning. Linguistic validation is very expensive and time consuming, but it is a necessary step to ensure good interrater reliability across collaborating study sites and international investigators. This process is well delineated in publications by the International Society for Pharmacoeconomics and Outcomes Research (ISPOR) Task Force for Translation and Cultural Adaptation (Wild et al. 2005, 2009). The process involves a forward translation of the source scale by one research team. A second team, blind to the original language's source scale, then back-translates the forward translation into the original source language. The back-translation is then compared with the original source language scale by a third team, which includes expert bilingual consultants who have expertise in the mental health specialties in collaboration with input and consultation from a consultant at a translation and linguistic validation service, such as Mapi Research Trust in Lyon, France. Final reconciliation between all involved, including the scale author or developer, completes the process. Every step by all involved in every stage of the process is documented in a spreadsheet. For example, a typical spreadsheet for the translation and linguistic validation of the MINI into one language is six columns wide and 10,000–15,000 rows deep. When the process is complete, the linguistic validation service provides certification of the process. This documentation is then available for audit and review by regulatory agencies, research organizations, and sponsors with oversight responsibilities for the study.

Importance of Sensitivity in Detecting Change Over Time and in Identifying Differences Between Effective Medications and Placebo

Efficacy signal detection, or the ability to detect a statistically significant difference between an active medication and placebo in a clinical trial, is a highly valued and essential property of any scale used in monitoring treatment outcomes. Scales that are consistently successful in this regard are more widely used, are more highly regarded, and survive longer than scales that do not have this property. When scales are found to lack this property, their use thereafter goes into decline.

Virtual Administration of Scales and Structured Diagnostic Interviews During Pandemics Such as COVID-19

During the COVID-19 pandemic, I regularly encountered problems while consulting on the use of scales and structured interviews during virtual administration. These issues merit further attention, investigation, and study to restore confidence in the integrity of the process. The following are some concerns regarding and recommendations for improving the issues that became apparent in virtual administration of scales and structured interviews:

1. The strengths, weaknesses, limitations, sensitivity, and specificity of administration of scales and structured interviews conducted during virtual administration versus live face-to-face interviews need to be carefully studied. Researchers need to investigate telephone interviewing; virtual interviewing on Zoom, Doximity, Skype, and WhatsApp; and the different technologies on which apps are used, such as mobile devices (phones) or desktops, laptops, or tablet computers. The use of the various platforms may result in alterations in sensitivity, specificity, and efficacy and safety signal detection. Screen sharing on several of these platforms may come very close to in-person interviews in sensitivity and specificity. There may even be some advantages in signal detection during virtual administration. However, there may be a loss of sensitivity and efficacy and safety signal detection while using information technology (IT) versions or during virtual administration of rating scales.
2. Because these virtual modes of administration are likely to become more common in the future, we need more data to justify the pooling of data captured in these diverse ways across sites and over time in a single study in order to have confidence in the integrity of the process.
3. During the pandemic, restrictions on security concerns in the collection of health care information were relaxed in the interest of safety and to ensure proper social distancing. Policies to ensure proper compliance with the Health Insurance Portability and Accountability Act of 1996 (HIPAA) and the General Data Protection Regulation (GDPR) (Politou et al. 2018; see also Pew Research Center 2014) need to be reviewed and revised for future research studies.
4. The IT version of a scale or interview on a software platform may not be exactly the same as a paper or PDF version. The layout of a scale on a page can affect both response and error rates.
5. In reviewing software implementations of scales and structured interviews, I regularly encountered software coding errors by IT developers and have learned that the scale authors are frequently not involved or consulted in the certification of the IT versions. Closer collaboration is necessary.
6. The use of scales and structured interviews in data entry/capture software has too frequently fallen short of ideal implementation. IT developers and their sponsors have frequently refused to update or to correct updated versions of the scales and structured interviews and have failed to update these to the correct and current linguistically validated translations. This is a particular problem in ensuring consistency with updates to DSM.
7. Training of raters in the use of remote data entry software is incomplete when versions of scales suitable for virtual administration are used. During a pandemic, it is not possible to have safe in-person investigator meetings to ensure good reliability and consistent implementation across sites.
8. Missing data, double entries, and input errors can be avoided by careful software design on the platform used for data capture and entry. Many data capture software programs are not designed to minimize these problems.

Intellectual Property Issues and Violations

Concern about intellectual property violations in the use of scales and structured diagnostic interviews is growing. The extent of this problem is massive. Many software companies have profited by using the intellectual property of scale developers without permission and enriched themselves at the owners' expense and without their knowledge. Several universities, health care organizations, and government agencies have also used and posted on their websites the intellectual property of scale developers without permission. Some of these violations are due to lack of training or awareness, some are due to sloppiness or not having policies and procedures in place to reduce the likelihood of these transgressions, and some are due to outright mischief on the part of the perpetrators. My own experience is that most of the perpetrators are not in foreign countries, as is popularly believed, but are within the United States. Pharmaceutical companies, in my experience, are by far the most adherent to correct procedure in this arena. Increasingly, pharmaceutical companies, clinical research organizations, and university institutional review boards (IRBs) are putting policies, procedures, and checks in place to reduce the chance of such transgressions occurring. Federal and state funding agencies, the National Institutes of Health, universities, clinical research organizations, pharmaceutical companies, and IRBs are also now frequently checking their clinical and research audits and monitoring procedures to ensure that intellectual property licenses are current and consistent with usage. If your institution does not have such procedures in place, I recommend that you make an effort to correct this to preclude the institution's wandering inadvertently into this dangerous minefield. The easiest way to do this is to anchor these checks to routine IRB renewals and research committee reviews in research settings and to annual reviews in clinical settings.

Summary

Select the scales to use by matching your choice precisely to your needs. In the arena of scale development, brevity, simplicity, clarity, and sensitivity in efficacy signal detection always win.

References

Aas IH: Guidelines for rating Global Assessment of Functioning (GAF). Ann Gen Psychiatry 10:2, 2011 21251305

Alphs L, Fu DJ, Canuso C: Patient and clinician acceptance of the Suicide Ideation and Behavior Assessment Tool (SIBAT). Biol Psychiatry 81 (10 suppl):s210–s211, 2017

Altshuler L, Mintz J, Leight K: The Life Functioning Questionnaire (LFQ): a brief, gender-neutral scale assessing functional outcome. Psychiatry Res 112(2:161–182, 2002

Amado DM, Beamon DA, Sheehan DV: The linguistic validation of the pediatric versions of the Sheehan-Suicidality Tracking Scale (S-STS). Innov Clin Neurosci 11(9-10):141–163, 2014 25520893

Amarendran V, George A, Gersappe V, et al: The reliability of telepsychiatry for a neuropsychiatric assessment. Telemed J E Health 17(3):223–225, 2011 21443440
American Educational Research Association (American Psychological Association, National Council on Measurement in Education, Joint Committee on Standards for Educational, and Psychological Testing): Standards for Educational and Psychological Testing. Washington, DC, American Educational Research Association, 2014
American Psychiatric Association: Diagnostic and Statistical Manual of Mental Disorders, 4th Edition. Washington, DC, American Psychiatric Association, 1994
American Psychiatric Association: Diagnostic and Statistical Manual of Mental Disorders, 4th Edition, Text Revision. Washington, DC, American Psychiatric Association, 2000a
American Psychiatric Association: Practice Guideline for the Treatment of Patients with Major Depressive Disorder (Revision). Washington, DC, American Psychiatric Association, 2000b
American Psychiatric Association: Diagnostic and Statistical Manual of Mental Disorders, 5th Edition. Arlington, VA, American Psychiatric Association, 2013
Amorim P, Lecrubier Y, Weiller E, et al: DSM-III-R psychotic disorders: procedural validity of the Mini International Neuropsychiatric Interview (MINI). Concordance and causes for discordance with the CIDI. Eur Psychiatry 13(1):26–34, 1998 19698595
Anderson IM, Nutt DJ, Deakin JF; British Association for Psychopharmacology: Evidence-based guidelines for treating depressive disorders with antidepressants: a revision of the 1993 British Association for Psychopharmacology guidelines. J Psychopharmacol 14(1):3–20, 2000 10757248
Bagby RM, Ryder AG, Schuller DR, Marshall MB: The Hamilton Depression Rating Scale: has the gold standard become a lead weight? Am J Psychiatry 161(12):2163–2177, 2004 15569884
Bech P: Rating scales for affective disorders: their validity and consistency. Acta Psychiatr Scand 64 (suppl 295):11–101, 1981 7044046
Bech P: The Bech-Rafaelsen Mania Scale in clinical trials of therapies for bipolar disorder: a 20-year review of its use as an outcome measure. CNS Drugs 16(1):47–63, 2002a 11772118
Bech P: The Bech-Rafaelsen Melancholia Scale (MES) in clinical trials of therapies in depressive disorders: a 20-year review of its use as outcome measure. Acta Psychiatr Scand 106(4):252–264, 2002b 12225492
Bech P, Gram LF, Dein E, et al: Quantitative rating of depressive states. Acta Psychiatr Scand 51(3):161–170, 1975 1136841
Bech P, Rafaelsen OJ, Kramp P, Bolwig TG: The Mania Rating Scale: scale construction and inter-observer agreement. Neuropharmacology 17(6):430–431, 1978 673161
Bech P, Allerup P, Gram LF, et al: The Hamilton Depression Scale. Evaluation of objectivity using logistic models. Acta Psychiatr Scand 63(3):290–299, 1981 7015793
Bech P, Wilson P, Wessel T, et al: A validation analysis of two self-reported HAM-D6 versions. Acta Psychiatr Scand 119(4):298–303, 2009 19032701
Beck AT, Beck RW: Screening depressed patients in family practice. A rapid technic. Postgrad Med 52(6):81–85, 1972 4635613
Beck AT, Ward CH, Mendelson M, et al: An inventory for measuring depression. Arch Gen Psychiatry 4:561–571, 1961 13688369
Beck AT, Kovacs M, Weissman A: Assessment of suicidal intention: the Scale for Suicide Ideation. J Consult Clin Psychol 47(2):343–352, 1979 469082
Beck AT, Steer RA, Carbin MG: Psychometric properties of the Beck Depression Inventory: twenty-five years of evaluation. Clin Psychol Rev 8(1):77–100, 1988
Beck AT, Steer RA, Brown GK: Beck Depression Inventory-II (BDI-II). London, Pearson, 1996
Begg C, Cho M, Eastwood S, et al: Improving the quality of reporting of randomized controlled trials. The CONSORT statement. JAMA 276(8):637–639, 1996 8773637
Berk M, Malhi GS, Cahill C, et al: The Bipolar Depression Rating Scale (BDRS): its development, validation and utility. Bipolar Disord 9(6):571–579, 2007 17845271
Bernstein IH, Rush AJ, Trivedi MH, et al: Psychometric properties of the Quick Inventory of Depressive Symptomatology in adolescents. Int J Methods Psychiatr Res 19(4):185–194, 2010 20683845

Sheehan DV, Lecrubier Y, Sheehan KH, et al: The Mini-International Neuropsychiatric Interview (M.I.N.I.): the development and validation of a structured diagnostic psychiatric interview for DSM-IV and ICD-10. J Clin Psychiatry 59 (suppl 20):22–33, quiz 34–57, 1998 9881538

Sheehan DV, Sheehan KH, Shytle RD, et al: Reliability and validity of the Mini International Neuropsychiatric Interview for Children and Adolescents (MINI-KID). J Clin Psychiatry 71(3):313–326, 2010 20331933

Sheehan DV, Harnett-Sheehan K, Hidalgo RB, et al: Randomized, placebo-controlled trial of quetiapine XR and divalproex ER monotherapies in the treatment of the anxious bipolar patient. J Affect Disord 145(1):83–94, 2013 22920718

Sheehan DV, Alphs LD, Mao L, et al: Comparative validation of the S-STS, the ISST-Plus, and the C-SSRS for assessing the suicidal thinking and behavior FDA 2012 suicidality categories. Innov Clin Neurosci 11(9–10):32–46, 2014a 25520887

Sheehan DV, Giddens JM, Sheehan IS: Status update on the Sheehan-Suicidality Tracking Scale (S-STS) 2014. Innov Clin Neurosci 11(9–10):93–140, 2014b 25520892

Sheehan KH, Sheehan DV: Assessing treatment effects in clinical trials with the Discan metric of the Sheehan Disability Scale. Int Clin Psychopharmacol 23(2):70–83, 2008 18301121

Shore JH, Savin D, Orton H, et al: Diagnostic reliability of telepsychiatry in American Indian veterans. Am J Psychiatry 164(1):115–118, 2007 17202552

Singh V, Bowden CL, Gonzalez JM, et al: Discriminating primary clinical states in bipolar disorder with a comprehensive symptom scale. Acta Psychiatr Scand 127(2):145–152, 2013 22774941

Spitzer RL, Kroenke K, Williams JB; Patient Health Questionnaire Primary Care Study Group: Validation and utility of a self-report version of PRIME-MD: the PHQ primary care study. JAMA 282(18):1737–1744, 1999 10568646

Stahl SM: Why settle for silver, when you can go for gold? Response vs. recovery as the goal of antidepressant therapy. J Clin Psychiatry 60(4):213–214, 1999 10221279

Thase ME: Summary: defining remission in patients treated with antidepressants. J Clin Psychiatry 60 (3–6 suppl 22):35–36, 1999 10634354

Thompson PM, Gonzalez JM, Singh V, et al: Principal domains of behavioral psychopathology identified by the Bipolar Inventory of Signs and Symptoms Scale (BISS). Psychiatry Res 175(3):221–226, 2010 20022384

Timmerby N, Andersen JH, Søndergaard S, et al: A systematic review of the clinimetric properties of the 6-item version of the Hamilton Depression Rating Scale (HAM-D6). Psychother Psychosom 86(3):141–149, 2017 28490031

Trivedi MH, Rush AJ, Ibrahim HM, et al: The Inventory of Depressive Symptomatology, Clinician Rating (IDS-C) and Self-Report (IDS-SR), and the Quick Inventory of Depressive Symptomatology, Clinician Rating (QIDS-C) and Self-Report (QIDS-SR) in public sector patients with mood disorders: a psychometric evaluation: psychometrics of the QIDS in public sector patients. Psychol Med 34(1):73–82, 2004 14971628

U.S. Food and Drug Administration: Guidance for Industry: Suicidality: Prospective Assessment of Occurrence in Clinical Trials, Draft Guidance. September 9, 2010. Available at: https://www.federalregister.gov/documents/2010/09/09/2010-22404/draft-guidance-for-industry-on-suicidality-prospective-assessment-of-occurrence-in-clinical-trials. Accessed October 26, 2021.

U.S. Food and Drug Administration, Center for Drug Evaluation and Research: Guidance for Industry: Suicidality: Prospective Assessment of Occurrence in Clinical Trials, Draft Guidance. August 2012. Revision 1. Available at: https://www.fda.gov/regulatory-information/search-fda-guidance-documents/guidance-industry-suicidal-ideation-and-behavior-prospective-assessment-occurrence-clinical-trials. Accessed October 26, 2021.

Üstün TB, Kostanjsek N, Chatterji S, Rehm J (eds): Measuring Health and Disability: Manual for WHO Disability Assessment Schedule (WHODAS 2.0). Geneva, World Health Organization, 2010

Vaccarino AL, Evans KR, Kalali AH, et al: The Depression Inventory Development Workgroup: a collaborative, empirically driven initiative to develop a new assessment tool for major depressive disorder. Innov Clin Neurosci 13(9–10):20–31, 2016 27974997

Vaccarino AL, Kalali AH, Blier P, et al: The Depression Inventory Development Scale: assessment of psychometric properties using classical and modern measurement theory in a CAN-BIND trial. Innov Clin Neurosci 17(7–9):30–40, 2020 33520402
Vieta E: Guide to Assessment Scales in Bipolar Disorder. New York, Springer Science and Business Media, 2011
Warner MD, Peabody CA, Whiteford HA, Hollister LE: Alprazolam as an antidepressant. J Clin Psychiatry 49(4):148–150, 1988 3281931
Weissman MM, Bothwell S: Assessment of social adjustment by patient self-report. Arch Gen Psychiatry 33(9):1111–1115, 1976 962494
Wild D, Grove A, Martin M, et al; ISPOR Task Force for Translation and Cultural Adaptation: Principles of good practice for the translation and cultural adaptation process for patient-reported outcomes (PRO) measures: report of the ISPOR task force for translation and cultural adaptation. Value Health 8(2):94–104, 2005 15804318
Wild D, Eremenco S, Mear I, et al: Multinational trials—recommendations on the translations required, approaches to using the same language in different countries, and the approaches to support pooling the data: the ISPOR Patient-Reported Outcomes Translation and Linguistic Validation Good Research Practices Task Force report. Value Health 12(4):430–440, 2009 19138309
Williams JB: A structured interview guide for the Hamilton Depression Rating Scale. Arch Gen Psychiatry 45(8):742–747, 1988 3395203
Williams JB: Standardizing the Hamilton Depression Rating Scale: past, present, and future. Eur Arch Psychiatry Clin Neurosci 251 (2 suppl 2):II6–II12, 2001 11824839
Williams JB, Kobak KA: Development and reliability of a structured interview guide for the Montgomery-Asberg Depression Rating Scale (SIGMA). Br J Psychiatry 192(1):52–58, 2008 18174510
World Health Organization: Composite International Diagnostic Interview (WHO WMH-CIDI). Geneva, World Health Organization, 1990
World Health Organization: International Statistical Classification of Diseases and Related Health Problems, 10th Edition. Geneva, World Health Organization, 1992
World Health Organization: International Classification of Functioning, Disability and Health. Geneva, World Health Organization, 2001
World Health Organization: International Statistical Classification of Diseases and Related Health Problems, 11th Edition. Geneva, World Health Organization, 2019
Young RC, Biggs JT, Ziegler VE, Meyer DA: A rating scale for mania: reliability, validity and sensitivity. Br J Psychiatry 133(5):429–435, 1978 728692
Zalsman G, Misgav S, Sommerfeld E, et al: Children's Depression Inventory (CDI) and the Children's Depression Rating Scale-Revised (CDRS-R): reliability of the Hebrew version. Int J Adolesc Med Health 17(3):255–257, 2005 16231477
Zickar MJ, Broadfoot AA: The partial revival of a dead horse? Comparing classical test theory and item response theory, in Statistical and Methodological Myths and Urban Legends: Doctrine, Verity and Fable in Organizational and Social Sciences. Edited by Lance CE, Vandenberg RJ. New York, Routledge/Taylor & Francis Group, 2009, pp 37–59
Zimmerman M, McGlinchey JB: Depressed patients' acceptability of the use of self-administered scales to measure outcome in clinical practice. Ann Clin Psychiatry 20(3):125–129, 2008 18633738
Zimmerman M, McGlinchey JB, Posternak MA, et al: How should remission from depression be defined? The depressed patient's perspective. Am J Psychiatry 163(1):148–150, 2006 16390903
Zimmerman M, Chelminski I, McGlinchey JB, Posternak MA: A clinically useful depression outcome scale. Compr Psychiatry 49(2):131–140, 2008a 18243884
Zimmerman M, McGlinchey JB, Posternak MA, et al: Remission in depressed outpatients: more than just symptom resolution? J Psychiatr Res 42(10):797–801, 2008b 17986389
Zimmerman M, Galione JN, Attiullah N, et al: Depressed patients' perspectives of two measures of outcome: the Quick Inventory of Depressive Symptomatology (QIDS) and the Remission from Depression Questionnaire (RDQ). Ann Clin Psychiatry 23(3):208–212, 2011 21808753

Zimmerman M, Martinez JH, Attiullah N, et al: A new type of scale for determining remission from depression: the Remission from Depression Questionnaire. J Psychiatr Res 47(1):78–82, 2013a 23102820
Zimmerman M, Martinez JH, Young D, et al: Severity classification on the Hamilton Depression Rating Scale. J Affect Disord 150(2):384–388, 2013b 23759278
Zimmerman M, Chelminski I, Young D, et al: A clinically useful self-report measure of the DSM-5 anxious distress specifier for major depressive disorder. J Clin Psychiatry 75(6):601–607, 2014a 24813209
Zimmerman M, Chelminski I, Young D, et al: A clinically useful self-report measure of the DSM-5 mixed features specifier of major depressive disorder. J Affect Disord 168:357–362, 2014b 25103631
Zimmerman M, Martinez JH, Attiullah N, et al: The Remission from Depression Questionnaire as an outcome measure in the treatment of depression. Depress Anxiety 31(6):533–538, 2014c 24115164
Zimmerman M, Harris L, Martin J, McGonigal P: Reliability and validity of a self-report scale for daily assessments of the severity of depressive symptoms. Psychiatry Res 270:581–586, 2018 30368164

PART II

Pathogenesis of Mood Disorders

CHAPTER 5

Neurochemistry of Mood Disorders

Charles F. Gillespie, M.D., Ph.D.

Depression and mania are ancient diseases. Contemporary descriptions of the clinical phenomenology of depression and mania resonate with the antiquarian writings of the Greek physician Hippocrates (ca. 460–377 B.C.), the Roman physician Galen (ca. 129–199 A.D.), the Turkish physician Aretaeus of Cappadocia (fl. ca. 150 A.D.), and the Arabic physician Ishaq Ibn Imran (ca. 848–906 A.D.). Independent of culture, the central features of depression, or rather depressive disorders, include profound feelings of despondency paired with a loss of will and of the capacity to experience pleasure. By contrast, mania is characterized by feelings of elation or irritability, accompanied by elevated energy and drive coupled with a radically enhanced sense of personal agency.

Historical conceptualizations of the biology of depression, then called *melancholia*, and states of mania were rooted in the humoral theory of disease and emphasized imbalances of the four humors, such as an excess of black bile leading to melancholia, the historical description of a present-day subtype of severe depression. Modern-era theories, beginning in the 1950s, of the neurochemical pathophysiology of mood disorders have been structured predominantly around a core of monoamine neurotransmitters: norepinephrine and dopamine, which are catecholamines, and serotonin, which is an indoleamine. In more recent decades, clinical investigation has extended to the role of a neuropeptide, corticotropin-releasing hormone, and two amino acid neurotransmitters, GABA and glutamate, in the pathophysiology of mood disorders. Comprehensive and critical treatment of this topic, which spans nearly seven decades of clinical studies of patients with unipolar depression and bipolar disorders, is impossible in the space available. Therefore, emphasis in this chapter is placed on coverage of replicated findings and outcomes assessed by meta-analyses.

tory of depression responsive to serotonergic or noradrenergic antidepressants (reviewed in Delgado 2004). Considered as a whole, these investigations produced mixed results. A meta-analysis of 45 acute tryptophan depletion and 8 acute phenylalanine/tyrosine depletion studies (Ruhé et al. 2007) found no support for an effect of 5-HT or NE/DA depletion on mood in healthy controls. Conversely, depletion of 5-HT or NE/DA acutely reduced mood by a small but significant degree in healthy controls with a family history of depression. In drug-free patients with remitted depression, depletion of 5-HT resulted in a moderate decrease in mood, but no effect on mood was observed following NE/DA depletion. Finally, depletion of 5-HT was found to result in relapse of depressed mood only in patients with remitted depression who previously responded to serotonergic antidepressants.

Corticotropin-Releasing Hormone

In addition to its role in regulation of the hypothalamic-pituitary-adrenal axis, corticotropin-releasing hormone (CRH) also acts as a neurotransmitter coordinating the behavioral, autonomic, endocrine, and immune responses to stress and has a central role in the pathogenesis of major depressive disorder (reviewed in Waters et al. 2015). Elevated CSF concentrations of CRH have been reported in patients with depression (Nemeroff et al. 1984) and reviewed in Hartline et al. (1996). Postmortem findings from individuals who died by suicide include increased transcription (Raadsheer et al. 1995) and expression (Raadsheer et al. 1994) of CRH, elevated concentrations of CSF CRH (Arató et al. 1989), decreased expression of CRH_1 receptor mRNA within the frontal cortex (Merali et al. 2004), and increased CRH concentrations and decreased density of CRH receptors within the frontal cortex (Merali et al. 2006; Nemeroff et al. 1988b). Successful treatment of depression using either electroconvulsive therapy (Nemeroff et al. 1991) or antidepressants (De Bellis et al. 1993; Veith et al. 1993) reduces the high pretreatment concentrations of CSF CRH. Conversely, persistently elevated CSF CRH in depressed patients with symptomatic improvement is associated with early relapse of depression (Banki et al. 1992).

Gamma-Aminobutyric Acid

GABA is an amino acid derivative of glutamate and is the primary inhibitory neurotransmitter within the brain. Several lines of imaging, physiological, and postmortem data are consistent with a pivotal role for altered GABAergic neurotransmission in the pathophysiology of mood disorders (reviewed in Duman et al. 2019; Prévot and Sibille 2021). Reduced levels of GABA were first observed in the CSF of patients with unipolar depression 40 years ago (Gold et al. 1980). This finding was subsequently replicated (Gerner and Hare 1981; Gerner et al. 1984; Kasa et al. 1982) and extended to medication-free, euthymic patients with bipolar disorder (Berrettini et al. 1983). More recently, data from two meta-analyses (Godfrey et al. 2018; Schür et al. 2016) of in vivo magnetic resonance spectroscopy (MRS) studies indicate that levels of GABA are reduced in the cortex of patients with depression. In addition, functional studies of GABAergic neurotransmission using transcranial magnetic stimulation (TMS) in patients with depression have demonstrated impairment of GABAergic neurotransmission using analysis of short- and long-interval cortical inhibition and the cortical silent period (Bajbouj et al. 2006; Levinson et al. 2010), implicating both ionotropic ($GABA_A$) and metabotropic ($GABA_B$) receptors in this process (Fee et al. 2017; Radhu et al. 2013). Furthermore, reduced levels of the GABA synthetic enzyme glutamic acid decarboxylase 67 (GAD67) have been reported in the prefrontal cortex of individuals with major depressive disorder (Karolewicz et al. 2010). Finally, data from large gene expression studies of individuals who died by suicide have demonstrated changes in the expression of GABA and glutamate receptors associated with depression (Choudary et al. 2005; Klempan et al. 2009: Sequeira et al. 2007, 2009).

Glutamate

Glutamate is the principal excitatory neurotransmitter in the brain. A growing body of evidence suggests that disruption in glutamatergic neurotransmission plays a central role in the pathophysiology of depression (reviewed in Duman et al. 2019; Lener et al. 2017; Sanacora et al. 2012). Stress reactivity may be one pathway through which this occurs. Exposure to acute stress results in increased levels of extracellular glutamate within the prefrontal cortex and hippocampus, and it has been hypothesized that this in turn leads to excitotoxicity driven by glutamatergic activation of extrasynaptic *N*-methyl-D-aspartate (NMDA) receptors, resulting in atrophy of the prefrontal cortex and hippocampus (reviewed in Popoli et al. 2011).

Data from a systematic review and meta-analysis of in vivo proton MRS studies indicate that glutamate and related metabolites are reduced within the frontal cortex of individuals with major depressive disorder (Moriguchi et al. 2019). Reduction in the level of cortical glutamate may be related to the loss of glial cells, which play a key role in the reuptake and recycling of glutamate (Hamidi et al. 2004; Ongür et al. 1998; Rajkowska and Miguel-Hidalgo 2007). Imaging studies combining MRS and functional MRI have demonstrated that glutamate levels in the medial prefrontal cortex are associated with the extent of connectivity to subcortical regions (Duncan et al. 2013) and that reduced glutamate levels in the subgenual anterior cingulate cortex are associated with reduced connectivity in the insula (Horn et al. 2010) and reduced responses to emotionally salient stimuli in depressed patients with predominant anhedonia (Walter et al. 2009). Data from postmortem studies have demonstrated reduced levels of the NR2A and NR2B subunits of the NMDA receptor (Feyissa et al. 2009) and reductions in synaptic markers and increased loss of synapses (Kang et al. 2012) within the dorsolateral prefrontal cortex of patients with unipolar depression.

Conclusion

In this brief chapter, I have provided an overview of clinical and experimental research findings related to the neurochemical pathophysiology of unipolar and bipolar mood disorders. Despite the enormous volume of translational and clinical research on the biological basis of mood disorders, the fundamental causes of these disorders remain unclear. Philosophically, there has been a shift from reductionist, single-neurotransmitter models of mood disorder pathophysiology to complex and hierarchical models of pathophysiology emphasizing the impact of genetics, developmental and adult exposure to environmental stress, sex differences, role of neuroplasticity and neurotrophic processes, and contributions from the immune and endocrine systems (reviewed in Duman et al. 2019; Miller et al. 2017). Broadly speaking, challenges to progress have included the variety of mood states (and their putative subtypes) to study—that is, euthymic (unipolar vs. bipolar), depressed (unipolar vs. bipolar), manic, and mixed—along with a reliance, driven by practical considerations, on cross-sectional instead of longitudinal studies. Future research in the form of interdisciplinary "team science," involving the recruitment of large samples, use of consistent case definitions, and use of longitudinal methods, may have a transformative impact on the understanding of mood disorders.

References

Anisman H, Du L, Palkovits M, et al: Serotonin receptor subtype and p11 mRNA expression in stress-relevant brain regions of suicide and control subjects. J Psychiatry Neurosci 33(2):131–141, 2008 18330459

Arango V, Ernsberger P, Marzuk PM, et al: Autoradiographic demonstration of increased serotonin 5-HT2 and beta-adrenergic receptor binding sites in the brain of suicide victims. Arch Gen Psychiatry 47(11):1038–1047, 1990 2173513

Arató M, Bánki CM, Bissette G, Nemeroff CB: Elevated CSF CRF in suicide victims. Biol Psychiatry 25(3):355–359, 1989 2536563

Asberg M: Neurotransmitters and suicidal behavior. The evidence from cerebrospinal fluid studies. Ann NY Acad Sci 836:158–181, 1997 9616798

Asberg M, Träskman L, Thorén P: 5-HIAA in the cerebrospinal fluid. A biochemical suicide predictor? Arch Gen Psychiatry 33(10):1193–1197, 1976 971028

Ashok AH, Marques TR, Jauhar S, et al: The dopamine hypothesis of bipolar affective disorder: the state of the art and implications for treatment. Mol Psychiatry 22(5):666–679, 2017 28289283

Bajbouj M, Lisanby SH, Lang UE, et al: Evidence for impaired cortical inhibition in patients with unipolar major depression. Biol Psychiatry 59(5):395–400, 2006 16197927

Banki CM, Karmacsi L, Bissette G, Nemeroff CB: CSF corticotropin-releasing hormone and somatostatin in major depression: response to antidepressant treatment and relapse. Eur Neuropsychopharmacol 2(2):107–113, 1992 1352999

Berrettini WH, Nurnberger JI Jr, Hare TA, et al: Reduced plasma and CSF gamma-aminobutyric acid in affective illness: effect of lithium carbonate. Biol Psychiatry 18(2):185–194, 1983 6403063

Briley MS, Langer SZ, Raisman R, et al: Tritiated imipramine binding sites are decreased in platelets of untreated depressed patients. Science 209(4453):303–305, 1980 7384806

Bunney WE Jr, Davis JM: Norepinephrine in depressive reactions. A review. Arch Gen Psychiatry 13(6):483–494, 1965 5320621

Camardese G, Di Giuda D, Di Nicola M, et al: Imaging studies on dopamine transporter and depression: a review of literature and suggestions for future research. J Psychiatr Res 51:7–18, 2014 24433847

Choudary PV, Molnar M, Evans SJ, et al: Altered cortical glutamatergic and GABAergic signal transmission with glial involvement in depression. Proc Natl Acad Sci USA 102(43):15653–15658, 2005 16230605

Coppen AJ: Depressed states and indolealkylamines. Adv Pharmacol 6(Pt B):283–291, 1968 5301640

Cottingham C, Wang Q: α2 adrenergic receptor dysregulation in depressive disorders: implications for the neurobiology of depression and antidepressant therapy. Neurosci Biobehav Rev 36(10):2214–2225, 2012 22910678
Crane GE: The psychiatric side-effects of iproniazid. Am J Psychiatry 112(7):494–501, 1956 13283130
De Bellis MD, Gold PW, Geracioti TD Jr, et al: Association of fluoxetine treatment with reductions in CSF concentrations of corticotropin-releasing hormone and arginine vasopressin in patients with major depression. Am J Psychiatry 150(4):656–657, 1993 8465888
Delgado PL: How antidepressants help depression: mechanisms of action and clinical response. J Clin Psychiatry 65 (suppl 4):25–30, 2004 15046538
De Paermentier F, Cheetham SC, Crompton MR, et al: Brain beta-adrenoceptor binding sites in depressed suicide victims: effects of antidepressant treatment. Psychopharmacology (Berl) 105(2):283–288, 1991 1686657
Duman RS, Sanacora G, Krystal JH: Altered connectivity in depression: GABA and glutamate neurotransmitter deficits and reversal by novel treatments. Neuron 102(1):75–90, 2019 30946828
Duncan NW, Wiebking C, Tiret B, et al: Glutamate concentration in the medial prefrontal cortex predicts resting-state cortical-subcortical functional connectivity in humans. PLoS One 8(4):e60312, 2013 23573246
Dunlop BW, Nemeroff CB: The role of dopamine in the pathophysiology of depression. Arch Gen Psychiatry 64(3):327–337, 2007 17339521
Ellis PM, Salmond C: Is platelet imipramine binding reduced in depression? A meta-analysis. Biol Psychiatry 36(5):292–299, 1994 7993955
Fee C, Banasr M, Sibille E: Somatostatin-positive gamma-aminobutyric acid interneuron deficits in depression: cortical microcircuit and therapeutic perspectives. Biol Psychiatry 82(8):549–559, 2017 28697889
Feyissa AM, Chandran A, Stockmeier CA, Karolewicz B: Reduced levels of NR2A and NR2B subunits of NMDA receptor and PSD-95 in the prefrontal cortex in major depression. Prog Neuropsychopharmacol Biol Psychiatry 33(1):70–75, 2009 18992785
Freis ED: Mental depression in hypertensive patients treated for long periods with large doses of reserpine. N Engl J Med 251(25):1006–1008, 1954 13214379
Gerner RH, Hare TA: CSF GABA in normal subjects and patients with depression, schizophrenia, mania, and anorexia nervosa. Am J Psychiatry 138(8):1098–1101, 1981 7258390
Gerner RH, Fairbanks L, Anderson GM, et al: CSF neurochemistry in depressed, manic, and schizophrenic patients compared with that of normal controls. Am J Psychiatry 141(12):1533–1540, 1984 6209989
Godfrey KEM, Gardner AC, Kwon S, et al: Differences in excitatory and inhibitory neurotransmitter levels between depressed patients and healthy controls: a systematic review and meta-analysis. J Psychiatr Res 105:33–44, 2018 30144668
Gold BI, Bowers MB Jr, Roth RH, Sweeney DW: GABA levels in CSF of patients with psychiatric disorders. Am J Psychiatry 137(3):362–364, 1980 7356067
Hamidi M, Drevets WC, Price JL: Glial reduction in amygdala in major depressive disorder is due to oligodendrocytes. Biol Psychiatry 55(6):563–569, 2004 15013824
Hartline KM, Owens MJ, Nemeroff CB: Postmortem and cerebrospinal fluid studies of corticotropin-releasing factor in humans. Ann NY Acad Sci 780:96–105, 1996 8602742
Horn DI, Yu C, Steiner J, et al: Glutamatergic and resting-state functional connectivity correlates of severity in major depression—the role of pregenual anterior cingulate cortex and anterior insula. Front Syst Neurosci 4:33, 2010 20700385
Kambeitz JP, Howes OD: The serotonin transporter in depression: meta-analysis of in vivo and post mortem findings and implications for understanding and treating depression. J Affect Disord 186:358–366, 2015 26281039
Kang HJ, Voleti B, Hajszan T, et al: Decreased expression of synapse-related genes and loss of synapses in major depressive disorder. Nat Med 18(9):1413–1417, 2012 22885997
Kaplan RD, Mann JJ: Altered platelet serotonin uptake kinetics in schizophrenia and depression. Life Sci 31(6):583–588, 1982 7132568

Karolewicz B, Maciag D, O'Dwyer G, et al: Reduced level of glutamic acid decarboxylase-67 kDa in the prefrontal cortex in major depression. Int J Neuropsychopharmacol 13(4):411–420, 2010 20236554

Kasa K, Otsuki S, Yamamoto M, et al: Cerebrospinal fluid gamma-aminobutyric acid and homovanillic acid in depressive disorders. Biol Psychiatry 17(8):877–883, 1982 7115838

Kaufman J, DeLorenzo C, Choudhury S, Parsey RV: The 5-HT1A receptor in major depressive disorder. Eur Neuropsychopharmacol 26(3):397–410, 2016 26851834

Klempan TA, Sequeira A, Canetti L, et al: Altered expression of genes involved in ATP biosynthesis and GABAergic neurotransmission in the ventral prefrontal cortex of suicides with and without major depression. Mol Psychiatry 14(2):175–189, 2009 17938633

Knorr U, Simonsen AH, Zetterberg H, et al: Biomarkers in cerebrospinal fluid of patients with bipolar disorder versus healthy individuals: a systematic review. Eur Neuropsychopharmacol 28(7):783–794, 2018 29802040

Kuhn R: [Treatment of depressive states with an iminodibenzyl derivative (G 22355)]. Schweiz Med Wochenschr 87(35–36):1135–1140, 1957 13467194

Lapin IP, Oxenkrug GF: Intensification of the central serotoninergic processes as a possible determinant of the thymoleptic effect. Lancet 1(7586):132–136, 1969 4178247

Lemieux G, Davignon A, Genest J: Depressive states during Rauwolfia therapy for arterial hypertension; a report of 30 cases. Can Med Assoc J 74(7):522–526, 1956 13304797

Lener MS, Niciu MJ, Ballard ED, et al: Glutamate and gamma-aminobutyric acid systems in the pathophysiology of major depression and antidepressant response to ketamine. Biol Psychiatry 81(10):886–897, 2017 27449797

Lesch KP, Wolozin BL, Murphy DL, Reiderer P: Primary structure of the human platelet serotonin uptake site: identity with the brain serotonin transporter. J Neurochem 60(6):2319–2322, 1993 7684072

Lester D: The concentration of neurotransmitter metabolites in the cerebrospinal fluid of suicidal individuals: a meta-analysis. Pharmacopsychiatry 28(2):45–50, 1995 7542785

Levinson AJ, Fitzgerald PB, Favalli G, et al: Evidence of cortical inhibitory deficits in major depressive disorder. Biol Psychiatry 67(5):458–464, 2010 19922906

Li Z, He Y, Tang J, et al: Molecular imaging of striatal dopamine transporters in major depression—a meta-analysis. J Affect Disord 174:137–143, 2015 25497470

Lin Z, Madras BK: Human genetics and pharmacology of neurotransmitter transporters. Handb Exp Pharmacol (175):327–371, 2006 16722243

Mann JJ, Stanley M, McBride PA, McEwen BS: Increased serotonin2 and beta-adrenergic receptor binding in the frontal cortices of suicide victims. Arch Gen Psychiatry 43(10):954–959, 1986 3019268

Merali Z, Du L, Hrdina P, et al: Dysregulation in the suicide brain: mRNA expression of corticotropin-releasing hormone receptors and GABA(A) receptor subunits in frontal cortical brain region. J Neurosci 24(6):1478–1485, 2004 14960621

Merali Z, Kent P, Du L, et al: Corticotropin-releasing hormone, arginine vasopressin, gastrin-releasing peptide, and neuromedin B alterations in stress-relevant brain regions of suicides and control subjects. Biol Psychiatry 59(7):594–602, 2006 16197926

Meyerson LR, Wennogle LP, Abel MS, et al: Human brain receptor alterations in suicide victims. Pharmacol Biochem Behav 17(1):159–163, 1982 6289359

Miller AH, Haroon E, Felger JC: Therapeutic implications of brain-immune interactions: treatment in translation. Neuropsychopharmacology 42(1):334–359, 2017 27555382

Moriguchi S, Yamada M, Takano H, et al: Norepinephrine transporter in major depressive disorder: a PET study. Am J Psychiatry 174(1):36–41, 2017 27631962

Moriguchi S, Takamiya A, Noda Y, et al: Glutamatergic neurometabolite levels in major depressive disorder: a systematic review and meta-analysis of proton magnetic resonance spectroscopy studies. Mol Psychiatry 24(7):952–964, 2019 30315224

Müller-Oerlinghausen B, Roggenbach J, Franke L: Serotonergic platelet markers of suicidal behavior—do they really exist? J Affect Disord 79(1–3):13–24, 2004 15023476

Mulvihill KG: Presynaptic regulation of dopamine release: role of the DAT and VMAT2 transporters. Neurochem Int 122:94–105, 2019 30465801

Murrough JW, Henry S, Hu J, et al: Reduced ventral striatal/ventral pallidal serotonin1B receptor binding potential in major depressive disorder. Psychopharmacology (Berl) 213(2–3):547–553, 2011 20480149
Nemeroff CB, Widerlöv E, Bissette G, et al: Elevated concentrations of CSF corticotropin-releasing factor-like immunoreactivity in depressed patients. Science 226(4680):1342–1344, 1984 6334362
Nemeroff CB, Knight DL, Krishnan RR, et al: Marked reduction in the number of platelet-tritiated imipramine binding sites in geriatric depression. Arch Gen Psychiatry 45(10):919–923, 1988a 2844132
Nemeroff CB, Owens MJ, Bissette G, et al: Reduced corticotropin releasing factor binding sites in the frontal cortex of suicide victims. Arch Gen Psychiatry 45(6):577–579, 1988b 2837159
Nemeroff CB, Bissette G, Akil H, Fink M: Neuropeptide concentrations in the cerebrospinal fluid of depressed patients treated with electroconvulsive therapy. Corticotrophin-releasing factor, beta-endorphin and somatostatin. Br J Psychiatry 158:59–63, 1991 1673078
Ongür D, Drevets WC, Price JL: Glial reduction in the subgenual prefrontal cortex in mood disorders. Proc Natl Acad Sci USA 95(22):13290–13295, 1998 9789081
Pacholczyk T, Blakely RD, Amara SG: Expression cloning of a cocaine- and antidepressant-sensitive human noradrenaline transporter. Nature 350(6316):350–354, 1991 2008212
Pandey GN: Biological basis of suicide and suicidal behavior. Bipolar Disord 15(5):524–541, 2013 23773657
Pech J, Forman J, Kessing LV, Knorr U: Poor evidence for putative abnormalities in cerebrospinal fluid neurotransmitters in patients with depression versus healthy non-psychiatric individuals: a systematic review and meta-analyses of 23 studies. J Affect Disord 240:6–16, 2018 30041075
Popoli M, Yan Z, McEwen BS, Sanacora G: The stressed synapse: the impact of stress and glucocorticoids on glutamate transmission. Nat Rev Neurosci 13(1):22–37, 2011 22127301
Prévot T, Sibille E: Altered GABA-mediated information processing and cognitive dysfunctions in depression and other brain disorders. Mol Psychiatry 26(1):151–167, 2021 32346158
Raadsheer FC, Hoogendijk WJ, Stam FC, et al: Increased numbers of corticotropin-releasing hormone expressing neurons in the hypothalamic paraventricular nucleus of depressed patients. Neuroendocrinology 60(4):436–444, 1994 7824085
Raadsheer FC, van Heerikhuize JJ, Lucassen PJ, et al: Corticotropin-releasing hormone mRNA levels in the paraventricular nucleus of patients with Alzheimer's disease and depression. Am J Psychiatry 152(9):1372–1376, 1995 7653697
Racagni G, Popoli M: Cellular and molecular mechanisms in the long-term action of antidepressants. Dialogues Clin Neurosci 10(4):385–400, 2008 19170396
Radhu N, de Jesus DR, Ravindran LN, et al: A meta-analysis of cortical inhibition and excitability using transcranial magnetic stimulation in psychiatric disorders. Clin Neurophysiol 124(7):1309–1320, 2013 23485366
Rajkowska G, Miguel-Hidalgo JJ: Gliogenesis and glial pathology in depression. CNS Neurol Disord Drug Targets 6(3):219–233, 2007 17511618
Ressler KJ, Nemeroff CB: Role of norepinephrine in the pathophysiology and treatment of mood disorders. Biol Psychiatry 46(9):1219–1233, 1999 10560027
Ressler KJ, Nemeroff CB: Role of serotonergic and noradrenergic systems in the pathophysiology of depression and anxiety disorders. Depress Anxiety 12 (suppl 1):2–19, 2000 11098410
Rivero G, Gabilondo AM, García-Sevilla JA, et al: Increased α2- and β1-adrenoceptor densities in postmortem brain of subjects with depression: differential effect of antidepressant treatment. J Affect Disord 167:343–350, 2014 25020269
Ruhé HG, Mason NS, Schene AH: Mood is indirectly related to serotonin, norepinephrine and dopamine levels in humans: a meta-analysis of monoamine depletion studies. Mol Psychiatry 12(4):331–359, 2007 17389902
Sanacora G, Treccani G, Popoli M: Towards a glutamate hypothesis of depression: an emerging frontier of neuropsychopharmacology for mood disorders. Neuropharmacology 62(1):63–77, 2012 21827775

Savitz JB, Drevets WC: Neuroreceptor imaging in depression. Neurobiol Dis 52:49–65, 2013 22691454

Schildkraut JJ: The catecholamine hypothesis of affective disorders: a review of supporting evidence. Am J Psychiatry 122(5):509–522, 1965 5319766

Schür RR, Draisma LW, Wijnen JP, et al: Brain GABA levels across psychiatric disorders: a systematic literature review and meta-analysis of (1) H-MRS studies. Hum Brain Mapp 37(9):3337–3352, 2016 27145016

Sequeira A, Klempan T, Canetti L, et al: Patterns of gene expression in the limbic system of suicides with and without major depression. Mol Psychiatry 12(7):640–655, 2007 17353912

Sequeira A, Mamdani F, Ernst C, et al: Global brain gene expression analysis links glutamatergic and GABAergic alterations to suicide and major depression. PLoS One 4(8):e6585, 2009 19668376

Stockmeier CA: Involvement of serotonin in depression: evidence from postmortem and imaging studies of serotonin receptors and the serotonin transporter. J Psychiatr Res 37(5):357–373, 2003 12849929

Svenningsson P, Chergui K, Rachleff I, et al: Alterations in 5-HT1B receptor function by p11 in depression-like states. Science 311(5757):77–80, 2006 16400147

Svenningsson P, Kim Y, Warner-Schmidt J, et al: p11 and its role in depression and therapeutic responses to antidepressants. Nat Rev Neurosci 14(10):673–680, 2013 24002251

Tiger M, Farde L, Rück C, et al: Low serotonin1B receptor binding potential in the anterior cingulate cortex in drug-free patients with recurrent major depressive disorder. Psychiatry Res Neuroimaging 253:36–42, 2016 27269199

Tiger M, Varnäs K, Okubo Y, Lundberg J: The 5-HT1B receptor—a potential target for antidepressant treatment. Psychopharmacology (Berl) 235(5):1317–1334, 2018 29546551

Veith RC, Lewis N, Langohr JI, et al: Effect of desipramine on cerebrospinal fluid concentrations of corticotropin-releasing factor in human subjects. Psychiatry Res 46(1):1–8, 1993 8464952

Walter M, Henning A, Grimm S, et al: The relationship between aberrant neuronal activation in the pregenual anterior cingulate, altered glutamatergic metabolism, and anhedonia in major depression. Arch Gen Psychiatry 66(5):478–486, 2009 19414707

Wang L, Zhou C, Zhu D, et al: Serotonin-1A receptor alterations in depression: a meta-analysis of molecular imaging studies. BMC Psychiatry 16(1):319, 2016 27623971

Waters RP, Rivalan M, Bangasser DA, et al: Evidence for the role of corticotropin-releasing factor in major depressive disorder. Neurosci Biobehav Rev 58:63–78, 2015 26271720

Yatham LN, Sossi V, Ding YS, et al: A positron emission tomography study of norepinephrine transporter occupancy and its correlation with symptom response in depressed patients treated with quetiapine XR. Int J Neuropsychopharmacol 21(2):108–113, 2018 29016993

CHAPTER 6

Psychoneuroendocrinology of Mood Disorders

Luca Sforzini, M.D.
Maria Antonietta Nettis, M.D., Ph.D.
Frances Isabella Weston, B.Sc.
Carmine Maria Pariante, M.D., Ph.D., FRCPsych

The body and mind are profoundly linked. Underpinning this link is the neuroendocrine system, which is the major route of communication between body and mind and results from the interaction between the endocrine system and the nervous system (Toni 2004). The endocrine system comprises several glands throughout the body; these glands release hormones, which in turn can affect many physiological processes. The interaction between the endocrine and nervous systems helps to maintain homeostasis—that is, the equilibrium among all organs and systems in the body. It is therefore conceivable that everything that affects the mind could also affect the body, and vice versa. In fact, each time homeostasis deviates from its optimal functioning, an imbalance is caused, which could result in several pathological signs and symptoms.

Psychoneuroendocrinology is the study of the relationship between the neuroendocrine system and psychiatric symptoms. Compelling evidence indicates that endocrine dysregulations are frequently associated in a bidirectional link with psychiatric conditions, including mood disorders. In particular, neuroendocrine alterations are

This research was funded by the National Institute for Health Research (NIHR) Maudsley Biomedical Research Centre (BRC), London, United Kingdom. This work was also supported by the Wellcome Trust strategic award (104025) to the Neuroimmunology of Mood Disorders and Alzheimer's Disease (NIMA) Consortium, which is also funded by Janssen, GlaxoSmithKline, Lundbeck, and Pfizer. Dr. Sforzini and Prof. Pariante report grant funding from the European Commission (IMI2 853966).

among the biological alterations most consistently reported in both major depressive disorder (MDD) and bipolar disorder (Belvederi Murri et al. 2014; Daban et al. 2005; Delvecchio et al. 2017). In this chapter, we discuss in detail the psychoneuroendocrinology of mood disorders by describing different neuroendocrine systems, their interactions, and their clinical relevance to the development of psychiatric symptoms.

Physiology of the Neuroendocrine System

Our review focuses on four major components of the neuroendocrine system: the hypothalamic-pituitary-adrenal (HPA), the hypothalamic-pituitary-thyroid (HPT), and the hypothalamic-pituitary-gonadal (HPG) axes, and the hypothalamic-neurohypophysial system (HNS). The HPA, HPT, and HPG axes show similar functioning. The coordinating center is the hypothalamus, which receives numerous cortical and peripheral inputs and communicates directly with the pituitary gland. In particular, the hypothalamus produces neurohormones—also called *releasing hormones* because of their ability to regulate the secretion of hormones from the pituitary gland (also called the *hypophysis*). The pituitary gland stimulates production of hormones in peripheral glands. Notably, within each axis, there is a negative feedback system that self-regulates hormonal production: peripheral hormones act upstream in each axis, inhibiting the release of the respective hypothalamic and pituitary hormones. In contrast, the HNS involves hypothalamic neurons and their axonal projection to the posterior pituitary (or *neurohypophysis*), where hormones are then released into the bloodstream. The physiology of the neuroendocrine system is graphically summarized in Figure 6–1.

Hypothalamic-Pituitary-Adrenal Axis

The HPA axis is pivotal in modulating immune responses and, together with the autonomic system, it is also the main center involved in stress response (Ulrich-Lai and Herman 2009). Following stressful stimuli, the autonomic sympathetic system represents the most rapid response, whereas the HPA axis is responsible for more complex and both acute and longer-term biological modifications, modulating homeostasis in the whole body, including the brain. These biological effects aim to promote the fight-or-flight response—that is, the physiological changes that occur in the body in response to stressful and potentially harmful stimuli.

The final products of the HPA axis are glucocorticoid (GC) hormones, mainly cortisol in humans. The paraventricular nucleus of the hypothalamus produces corticotropin-releasing hormone (CRH), leading to the release of adrenocorticotropic hormone (ACTH) in the pituitary gland. This stimulates the cortical region of the adrenal glands, which are two endocrine glands located on top of the kidneys. Finally, the adrenal cortex stimulation induces the discharge of GC hormones.

GC hormones are a class of steroid hormones synthesized from cholesterol and then capable of passing through lipid membranes and acting on nuclear receptors. GC hormones act on two different types of receptors: the GC receptor (GR), encoded by the NR3C1 (nuclear receptor subfamily 3, group C, member 1) gene, and the mineralocorticoid receptor (MR). Cortisol binds with low affinity to GRs and with high affinity to MRs. This is consistent with the hypothesis that MR binding is mainly in-

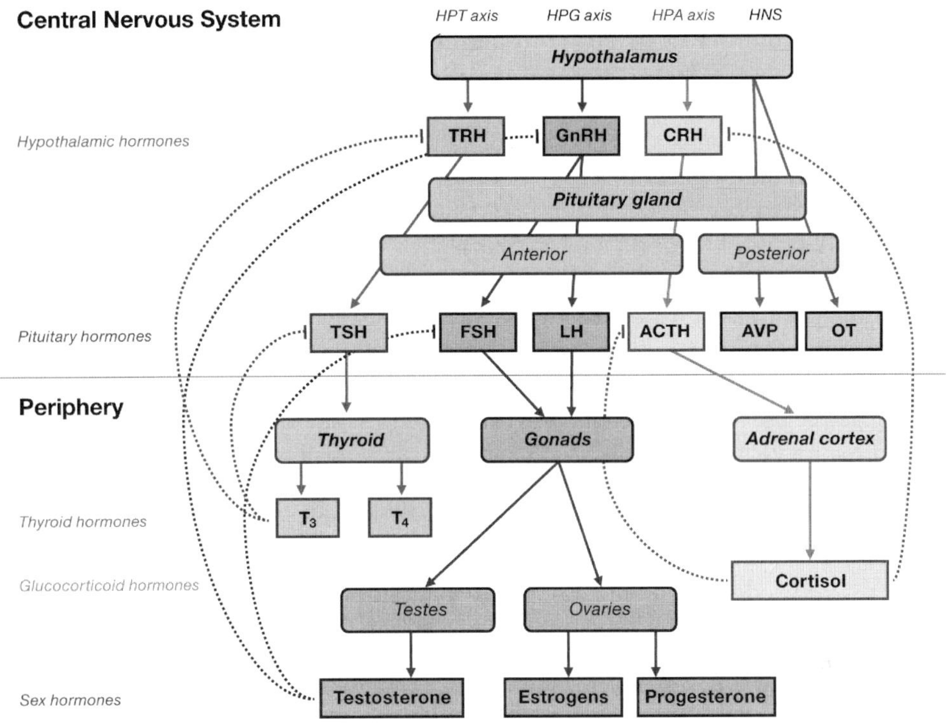

FIGURE 6–1. Physiology of the neuroendocrine system.

To view this figure in color, see Plate 1 in Color Gallery in middle of book.

Schematic representation of the four major components of the neuroendocrine system: the HPA, HPT, and HPG axes and the HNS. Hypothalamic neurons produce releasing hormones and HNS hormones. Releasing hormones act on the anterior pituitary gland, causing the release of stimulating hormones. HNS hormones are released from hypothalamic axons in the posterior pituitary, also called the neurohypophysis. The stimulating hormones produced in the pituitary gland then stimulate peripheral organs (thyroid, gonads, and adrenal cortex) to produce specific hormones, which in turn exert several biological functions (T_3, T_4; testosterone, progesterone, estrogens; and cortisol, respectively). These peripheral hormones also act backward within each axis, self-controlling their production via a negative feedback. The hypothalamic-pituitary-thyroid (HPT) axis is represented in *red*, the hypothalamic-pituitary-gonadal (HPG) axis in *blue*, the hypothalamic-pituitary-adrenal (HPA) axis in *yellow*, the hypothalamus and the hypothalamic-neurohypophysial system (HNS) in *black*, and the pituitary gland in *green*. *Arrows* indicate a stimulation, and *dotted lines* an inhibition. Hormone-producing organs are shown in *rounded boxes*, and hormonal products in *rectangles*.

ACTH=adrenocorticotropic hormone; AVP=arginine vasopressin; CRH=corticotropin-releasing hormone; FSH=follicle-stimulating hormone; GnRH=gonadotropin-releasing hormone; LH=luteinizing hormone; OT=oxytocin; T_3=triiodothyronine; T_4=thyroxine; TRH=thyrotropin-releasing hormone; TSH=thyroid-stimulating hormone.

volved in the homeostatic basal function, whereas cortisol-GR binding is more clearly related to stress response, when cortisol levels are raised (Pariante 2004).

GRs are the main modulators of HPA axis activity; they are necessary for life after birth and are expressed in nearly every cell of the body. Following GC binding, through different isoforms and diverse signaling cascades, GRs regulate the transcription of target genes and mediate composite biological actions (Oakley and Cidlowski 2013). Central in GR functioning and sensitivity is the *FKBP5* gene, encoding FK506-binding protein 51 or FKBP51, a co-chaperone protein (Alhajji and Nemeroff

2015) that physiologically binds to the GR complex, reducing the receptor affinity for GC. The increased transcription and translation of *FKBP5* following the activation of GRs by GC hormones further reduce the GR sensitivity in an overall ultrashort negative feedback loop (Binder 2009; Menke 2019).

Cortisol production is a highly controlled process, optimized to maintain GC hormone levels in the perfect range. As for other neuroendocrine systems, in normal individuals, cortisol regulates the synthesis of CRH by exerting negative feedback that controls its own production (Zunszain et al. 2013). Interestingly, this negative feedback is mediated by GR and thus is impaired when GR is disrupted, such as in chronic GC stimulation. This phenomenon, called GC resistance, in turn leads to HPA axis hyperactivity (Pariante and Lightman 2008; Pariante and Miller 2001). The most diffused clinical tests for assessing HPA axis function, namely suppression tests, assess the efficacy of the negative feedback mechanism. In the dexamethasone suppression test, cortisol levels are measured after the injection of the exogenous steroid dexamethasone, which binds to GR. The prednisolone suppression test has the advantage of probing both GR and MR (Juruena et al. 2009). Cortisol levels show a marked circadian rhythm; they peak in the morning shortly after a person wakes (around 8 A.M.), in what is defined as the cortisol awakening response (Elder et al. 2014), and then progressively decline during the day, reaching the nadir in the middle of the night, about 3–5 hours after a person falls asleep (roughly from midnight to 4 A.M.).

Hypothalamic-Pituitary-Thyroid Axis

The HPT axis is pivotal in the regulation of metabolism. Thyroid hormones affect basal metabolic rate, energy balance, protein synthesis, and cell growth. The hypothalamus produces thyrotropin-releasing hormone (TRH), thus stimulating the anterior pituitary to release thyroid-stimulating hormone (TSH). TSH acts on the thyroid, an endocrine gland located in the anterior part of the neck, to produce the thyroid hormones, namely triiodothyronine (T_3) and thyroxine (T_4), together with the peptide hormone calcitonin. The thyroid mainly releases T_4 into the bloodstream, where it is then enzymatically converted to T_3, which has a much higher affinity for the thyroid hormone receptor, a nuclear receptor (Baek et al. 2014). When the HPT axis is balanced, a person has a condition of euthyroidism. The HPT axis can be disrupted in two main directions, resulting in increased or reduced thyroid functioning, referred to as hyperthyroidism or hypothyroidism, respectively. Moreover, TSH levels may be altered in the presence of normal thyroid hormones levels, resulting in what is called subclinical hypo- or hyperthyroidism. T_3 and T_4 inhibit TRH and TSH secretion via a negative feedback similar to the one described in the HPA axis.

Hypothalamic-Pituitary-Gonadal Axis

The HPG axis is the main regulator of reproductive functions. The hormones estrogen, progesterone, and testosterone are secreted from gonads, and are differently represented according to sex. The hypothalamus secretes gonadotropin-releasing hormone (GnRH), which stimulates the anterior pituitary to produce luteinizing hormone (LH) and follicle-stimulating hormone (FSH). These two hormones, each with precise and different roles, exert their action on the gonads. In females, they act together on the ovaries to produce estrogen and progesterone, thus regulating menstrual and ovarian cycles. In males, they act chiefly on testes to induce the production of testosterone and regulate spermatogenesis. Sex hormones could inhibit their own production, acting on the hypothalamus or hypophysis via a negative feedback. Circulating sex hormones are largely bound to carrier proteins, mainly albumin and sex hormone–binding globulin; thus, only very small percentages of estrogens and testosterone (approximately 1%–2%) are unbound (i.e., free) and bioactive.

Sex hormones exert their function by acting on specific nuclear receptors. There are two main types of estrogen receptors, alpha (ER-α) and beta (ER-β). Androgens act primarily on the androgen receptor. Estrogen levels change widely in relation to life stages and menstrual and ovarian cycles. Testosterone levels can also vary according to an individual's age, even if in a less dramatic way. Interestingly, however, androgen levels also may vary within the same day, similar to cortisol, with significant diurnal variations (Long et al. 2015). In addition to its obvious function of regulating the life cycle and reproduction, the HPG axis affects several other biological functions, including the activity of the immune system, which in turn affects brain development, structure, and functioning.

Hypothalamic-Neurohypophysial System

In addition to the three main axes discussed above, a fourth part of the neuroendocrine system that is important for mood disorders is the HNS, which includes projections of hypothalamic neurons to the posterior pituitary, or neurohypophysis. These neurons produce two structurally related neurohypophysial hormones, oxytocin (OT) and arginine vasopressin (AVP), which are then released into the bloodstream. OT facilitates lactation and parturition by acting on mammalian glands and uterus smooth muscles. It also plays an important and widespread role in social functioning (Jones et al. 2017). Interestingly, OT promotes affiliation and both mother-child and pair bonding and modulates fear and anxiety behavior (Zik and Roberts 2015). AVP, also called antidiuretic hormone (ADH), regulates body water balance and fluid homeostasis by regulating blood pressure, osmotic balance, and kidney function. The release of AVP can be pathologically increased, as observed in the syndrome of inappropriate ADH secretion (SIADH), or decreased, causing diabetes insipidus, with inability to concentrate urine (Verbalis 2014). AVP acts on three different receptors (V1a, V1b [also known as V3], and V2), whereas OT has a unique receptor (Surget and Belzung 2008). Of note, there is cross-reactivity in the binding of AVP and OT with their respective receptors, with a higher bonding affinity observed for OT (Kimura et al. 1994; Lach et al. 2018; Surget and Belzung 2008).

Cross Talk Between Endocrine and Immune Systems

In the wide-ranging and multifaceted field of psychoneuroendocrinology, the immune system also plays a central role. Indeed, the neuroendocrine system is firmly connected to the immune system in a complex neuroimmune-endocrine interaction (Ashley and Demas 2017), which influences both hormonal functioning and the immune response in order to maintain homeostasis. Immune system cells can produce low levels of different hormones, and neuroendocrine system cells can release cytokines (Verburg-van Kemenade et al. 2017). Remarkably, alterations of the immune system have been widely linked to several psychiatric diseases, including mood disorders (Pariante 2017; Stetler and Miller 2011). The immune system and its response, inflammation, are therefore important factors in the relationship between the neuroendocrine system and mood disorders.

Particularly important in the endocrine-immune cross talk is the HPA axis, which directly controls the immune system, and vice versa. Indeed, immune cells express both GRs and adrenergic receptors (Ménard et al. 2017). In addition, a number of proinflammatory cytokines, such as interleukin-1, interleukin-6, and tumor necrosis factor alpha, can activate the HPA axis. On the other hand, cortisol has an extremely powerful anti-inflammatory effect. Therefore, the HPA axis acts as a modulator of the inflammatory responses that occur throughout the whole body, including the CNS (Otmishi et al. 2008). The hyperactivation of the HPA axis, which is typical under chronic conditions, can induce persistent GC resistance. The lack of GR-mediated negative feedback leads to HPA axis hyperactivity, and at the same time the lack of GR-mediated restraint of inflammation leads to increased inflammation (Pariante 2014). Finally, an excess of cortisol may activate the kynurenine pathway (Menke 2019). This catabolic pathway for tryptophan is enhanced both in inflammation and depression; therefore, it has been proposed as a potential biological shared mechanism for depression comorbid with immune-related diseases (Sforzini et al. 2019).

The HPT axis also is linked to the immune system (Masek et al. 2003). In fact, thyroid function is fundamental for the normal development of the thymus, which is a specialized organ of the immune system in which hematopoietic precursors from the bone marrow, called thymocytes, mature into the immune cells, called T-lymphocytes. Again, this relationship is bidirectional; activated immune cells are able to synthesize and secrete small quantities of TRH (Masek et al. 2003). Furthermore, the thyroid is the organ that is most commonly affected by autoimmune diseases (McLeod and Cooper 2012). Autoimmunity is a fascinating concept: it is the process involving the activation of the immune system against the individual's own healthy cells. Three different thyroid proteins can be targeted by specific autoantibodies: thyroid peroxidase antibody (TPOAb), thyroglobulin antibody (TGAb), and TSH receptor antibody (TRAb).

The same bidirectional link with the immune system characterizes both the HPG axis and the HNS. This is demonstrated by the expression of both estrogen receptors (ER-α and ER-β) and androgen receptors (Taub 2008) in the immune cells and by the ability of inflammatory cytokines such as interleukin-1 to stimulate the release of both AVP and OT (Landgraf et al. 1995). Because this chapter focuses specifically on psychoneuroendocrinology, we will not explore the function of immune processes further, and we will mention them only when directly related to the neuroendocrine system.

Role of Neuroendocrine and Immune Systems in Mood Disorders

Just as a disruption at any level within the neuroendocrine and immune systems could result in severe consequences for a person's health, including mental health, a person's neuroendocrine and immune systems may be altered by different psychiatric diseases. Disruptions in homeostatic balance could follow both external and internal stressors, or basically everything that causes stress to an organism. An appropriate response to stress involves both the immune and the neuroendocrine systems (McEwen et al. 2015; Ulrich-Lai and Herman 2009). Under physiological conditions, body and mind are able to face even massive perturbations. Yet, at times, homeostasis is disrupted.

Most research available on mood disorders focuses on unipolar depression. Characteristics intrinsic to bipolar disorder complicate the recognition of specific etiopathogenetic mechanisms. Indeed, the clinical picture, with depressive and manic or hypomanic episodes, is often unstable, and the clinical presentation could be extremely wide ranging. Misdiagnosis of patients with bipolar disorder is unfortunately a frequent event (Angst et al. 2003), due to potential overlap with depressive disorders, as well as with psychotic disorders. Moreover, even in patients diagnosed with bipolar disorder, most data are collected in depressive episodes, and less evidence is available on manic, hypomanic, and mixed episodes. Bearing in mind these challenges, we discuss the available evidence on the relationship between each of the four components of the neuroendocrine system and depression and bipolar disorder, respectively.

Hypothalamic-Pituitary-Adrenal Axis

Depression

The HPA axis has been demonstrated to be crucial in the pathophysiology of depressive disorders. This is not surprising, given the role of this axis in mediating between stress responses and brain functioning (Pariante and Lightman 2008). Hyperactivity of the HPA axis is probably the most prominent and consistent neuroendocrine abnormality found in depression (Min et al. 2012; Pariante and Lightman 2008). Patients with depression typically exhibit higher baseline cortisol levels, altered responses to the dexamethasone suppression test, and reduced GR mRNA expression (Palazidou 2012). HPA axis hyperactivity has also been proposed as a biological mechanism explaining the high prevalence of comorbid medical illnesses during depression (Stetler and Miller 2011). In a large meta-analysis, Stetler and Miller (2011) confirmed this evidence of HPA axis hyperactivity in depressed individuals. Specifically, they found increased levels of cortisol and ACTH, but no difference in CRH, in patients with depression compared with healthy control subjects. They found that the degree of HPA axis hyperactivity was variable across groups of patients with depression, being the most marked in older hospitalized individuals and in patients with depression with melancholic or psychotic features. Therefore, interestingly, HPA biological correlates of depression may be different based on clinical features, such as depression subtype or age.

Consistently, increased cortisol levels have been found in patients who have depression with psychotic features compared with healthy subjects and with patients with nonpsychotic depression (Cherian et al. 2019). Moreover, Lamers et al. (2013) found that the HPA axis was hyperactive in patients with depression with melancholic features; they also observed a lower diurnal slope in patients with depression with atypical features compared with subjects without atypical depression. In a recent systematic review exploring the evidence to date on the HPA axis in depression with seasonal pattern, Agustini et al. (2019) found some evidence of an attenuated cortisol awakening response in these patients during winter, but not in summer, compared with healthy control subjects, even though the evidence on this specific subtype of depression is still insufficient. Focusing on age, in a meta-analysis on elderly patients (older than 60 years), Belvederi Murri et al. (2014) found significantly higher cortisol levels in patients with depression compared with healthy control subjects, and this effect was even higher when analyzing cortisol levels after patients took dexamethasone. As the authors suggest, this effect could be due to a number of different mechanisms related to aging and may be only collaterally linked to depression. In addition to patients' depression subtype and age, their sex may partly mediate neuroendocrine dysfunctions, even though results are sometimes conflicting. Sanches et al. (2013) found significantly higher cortisol levels in depressed males, but not females, compared with healthy control subjects. This finding further confirms the complexity of the relationship between the HPA axis and depression, which may involve other neuroendocrine mechanisms, including the HPG axis.

It is widely recognized that women in the perinatal period, including both pregnancy and postpartum, have a higher risk of developing depression (Sawyer et al. 2019). This could be due to the massive HPA axis alterations that are typical in this period. During a normal pregnancy, the HPA axis is hyperactive, mainly due to placental production of CRH, with reduced GR function and GC resistance (Glynn et al. 2013). Notably, these alterations are more marked when depressive symptoms occur during pregnancy (Katz et al. 2012; Pariante 2014). In the postpartum period, there is a drop in CRH levels, leading to low levels of ACTH. This HPA "refractory period" may represent a risk factor for the development of depression, and may persist for weeks, months, or even years (Dickens and Pawluski 2018; Glynn et al. 2013). This lingering refractory period could be due to the HPA axis modifications during pregnancy, and especially to the fall in cortisol and CRH levels in the postpartum period. Furthermore, depression during pregnancy is associated with increased cortisol response to stress in the offspring at 1 year of age (Osborne et al. 2018).

Another intriguing topic is the predictive value of HPA axis alterations in mediating the development of depression. Pariante and Lightman (2008) proposed that HPA axis alterations are not simply a consequence or epiphenomenon of depression, but also a risk factor predisposing to it. In an interesting 10-year study of patients hospitalized for MDD, Tsuru et al. (2013) found no correlation between baseline measures of HPA axis activity (combined dexamethasone and CRH [DEX/CRH] levels) and the future recurrence of depressive symptoms (within 10 years). However, an increased cortisol awakening response has been associated with the recurrence of MDD, suggesting an increased vulnerability to depression (Hardeveld et al. 2014). Dysfunctions in the HPA axis also could predict nonresponse to treatment. Juruena et al. (2009), in addition to confirming higher cortisol levels in patients with depression compared with control subjects, found higher cortisol levels after a prednisolone suppression test and a lower percentage of suppression in patients with depression who did not respond to subsequent treatment compared with responders.

Finally, early life stress, including childhood maltreatment, can chronically activate the HPA axis (Cousins and Goodyer 2015). This sustained hyperactivation, with increased CRH and impaired GR-mediated negative feedback, may be an independent predisposing factor in the development of depression during adolescence and adulthood (Cousins and Goodyer 2015; Pariante and Lightman 2008; van Bodegom et al. 2017). In this context, *NR3C1* has been found to be susceptible to epigenetic modification, specifically DNA methylation (Smart et al. 2015). Early life adversities could also influence cortisol regulation during pregnancy, with a larger cortisol awakening response, and also moderate the effect of depressive symptoms on diurnal slope (Epstein et al. 2020).

Bipolar Disorder

Growing evidence also suggests a hyperactive HPA axis in patients with bipolar disorder (Daban et al. 2005). In a study using the combined DEX/CRH suppression test, Schmider et al. (1995) found a significantly increased ACTH response in patients with bipolar disorder in both manic and depressive phases compared with control subjects. A significantly increased cortisol response to the DEX/CRH test was reported even in remitted patients with bipolar disorder (Watson et al. 2004). A more recent comprehensive meta-analysis (Belvederi Murri et al. 2016) supported these findings, confirming significantly higher basal cortisol—at awakening, and similarly when measured over 12 or 24 hours—and higher ACTH levels in patients with bipolar disorder compared with control subjects. Although the majority of evidence points toward an increased cortisol response in patients with bipolar disorder, opposite results have been reported as well. For example, Yatham (1996) found no difference in cortisol response to fenfluramine (a serotonin-releasing agent formerly used as an appetite suppressor) in a comparison of patients with bipolar disorder and healthy control subjects.

Importantly, HPA axis activity has been shown to change in accordance with the different phases of bipolar disorder, which could account for the inconsistencies in research findings on these patients. In a fascinating study, Feng et al. (2019) compared measures of neuroendocrine function between untreated first-episode patients with MDD and those with bipolar disorder. The authors found significantly higher cortisol and ACTH levels in patients with MDD than in patients with bipolar disorder. Even if patients with MDD were consistently more numerous than patients with bipolar disorder, and patients with bipolar disorder were mostly in depressive episodes, these findings confirm a difference in neuroendocrine functioning between unipolar and bipolar depression. A possible explanation for these findings is that either melancholic or atypical symptoms are common in bipolar depression (Belvederi Murri et al. 2016). As we discussed in the previous subsection on depression, melancholic and atypical depression present with opposing biological correlates and HPA axis activity (Lamers et al. 2013). Therefore, when evaluating the role of the endocrine system, one needs to consider that changes will differ during mania, depression and its subtypes, and mixed episodes.

As also seen in patients with depression, the changes in HPA axis activity in patients with bipolar disorder is due to decreased GR function, seen through decreased levels of GR protein (Bei et al. 2009) or GR-α mRNA (Matsubara et al. 2006). Decreased GR-α mRNA was also identified in healthy first-degree relatives of patients with bipolar disorder, and it has been linked to irregular GR splicing and transcriptional activity (Bei et al. 2009; Watanuki et al. 2008), altered heat shock proteins (Bei et al. 2013), and epigenetic modulation of the *FKBP5* gene (Fries et al. 2014).

Longitudinal studies further support these findings, suggesting that HPA axis abnormalities might also influence and predict the development of bipolar disorder, and vice versa. Previously high mean daytime cortisol levels significantly predicted the development of depression and bipolar disorder in a 3-year follow-up study of young adults (Ellenbogen et al. 2011). This relationship could be bidirectional; in fact, another study showed that patients with bipolar disorder who had more previous manic or depressive episodes had higher mean cortisol levels and a blunted response and flatter diurnal slopes compared with those with fewer previous episodes (Havermans et al. 2011).

Finally, salivary cortisol levels were found to be higher in offspring of parents with bipolar disorder compared with offspring of parents with no mental health disorder (Ellenbogen et al. 2004, 2010). The findings were not influenced by confounders such as medication or differences in affective diagnosis, but sex was not accounted for. However, findings have not been consistent within research, and there is also evidence of no significant difference in cortisol levels between the offspring of patients with bipolar disorder and offspring of healthy control subjects (Deshauer et al. 2006).

Hypothalamic-Pituitary-Thyroid Axis

Depression

Another well-established neuroendocrine alteration in patients with depression involves abnormalities in the HPT axis (Nemeroff and Evans 1989). Even if no conclusive data support an overt thyroid dysfunction in depression, it is clear that thyroid abnormalities are often present in patients with depression (Fountoulakis et al. 2006). Thyroid function generally appears to be hypoactive in depression (Swaab et al. 2005). Literature data show patients with depression may have a disruption of the HPT axis at different levels. Central alterations—hypothalamic and pituitary—have been reported, mainly with reduced TSH secretion and increased TRH activity, and therefore an abnormal TSH response to TRH (Hage and Azar 2012). Alterations in thyroid functioning also may occur at the peripheral level, with elevated T_4 levels, low T_3, and positive antithyroid antibodies (Hage and Azar 2012). Moreover, serotonin (5-hydroxytryptamine [5-HT]) plays an important role in HPT axis regulation, mainly inhibiting TRH secretion. Accordingly, the 5-HT depletion typical of depression could lead to increased secretion of TRH and blunted TSH response (Duval et al. 2002), confirming the extensive interconnections between neuroendocrine systems and mood disorders. However, the majority of patients with depression have no overt abnormalities in thyroid function, even though they probably have a greater prevalence of subclinical hypothyroidism compared with the general population (Bauer et al. 2008). Brouwer et al. (2005) reported higher TSH levels in depressed outpatients compared with matched control subjects, suggesting a dysregulation of TSH levels rather than a clear decrease or increase. Interestingly, Tsuru et al. (2013) found significantly higher TSH responses to TRH in patients whose clinical depression later recurred within 10 years after remission.

The relationship between depression and thyroid illness is bidirectional, as we can observe by also analyzing the high prevalence rates of depression in thyroid illnesses. Classically, hypothyroidism has been associated with an increased risk of depression. However, there is also evidence showing an increased risk of depression in patients with hyperthyroidism (Bauer et al. 2008). Results are more controversial regarding subclinical hypothyroidism. In their meta-analysis, Zhao et al. (2018) showed an association between subclinical hypothyroidism and depression only in younger patients. On the other hand, low TSH levels that are still within the normal range have been linked to future development of depression in elderly patients (Medici et al. 2014). In addition, in a recent cross-sectional study in patients with MDD, Shen et al. (2019) found higher serum levels of TSH, TGAb, and TPOAb in suicide attempters compared with non–suicide attempters.

Autoimmunity may also be involved in HPT axis disruption in depression. TPOAbs have been extensively associated with a higher prevalence of depression. These findings were also confirmed by analyzing specific clinical subgroups, such as those with postnatal depression (Wesseloo et al. 2018) and subclinical hypothyroidism (Jucevičiūtė et al. 2019). However, there are discrepancies; some studies did not find any association between TPOAbs and depression, but also higher concentration of TRAbs have been reported in patients with depression compared with control subjects (Fam et al. 2015).

Lastly, it has been proposed that thyroid dysfunction in depression may result from an impairment of the thyroid hormone receptor. A preclinical study found that mice with receptor-mediated hypothyroidism—caused by an unliganded thyroid hormone receptor alpha 1—presented a depressive phenotype that was responsive to continuous T_3 substitution (Pilhatsch et al. 2010).

Bipolar Disorder

Despite the absence of clear evidence for a direct causal relationship, patients with bipolar disorder may have an increased risk of thyroid abnormalities compared with healthy individuals, and thyroid alterations have been reported in patients with bipolar disorder (Barbuti et al. 2017). Patients with bipolar disorder have been reported to be particularly sensitive to variations in thyroid function within the normal range, and lower thyroid function may predict slower response to treatment for bipolar depression (Cole et al. 2002). Hypothyroidism is a frequent finding in patients with bipolar disorder, and it has been associated with more severe clinical presentations, such as rapid cycling (Bauer et al. 1990). Patients with bipolar disorder had higher mean thyroid volumes and TSH levels in comparison with healthy control subjects (Ezzaher et al. 2011; Ozsoy et al. 2010), as well as higher TSH levels compared with patients with unipolar depression and schizophrenia (Wysokiński and Kloszewska 2014). Moreover, increased TSH is associated with increased risk of manic relapse (Amann et al. 2017), and low T_4 is associated with mood instability (more mood episodes, both manic and depressive) and severity of mania (Frye et al. 1999). In addition, an association between bipolar disorder and increased T_3 has been found (Krishna et al. 2013). These findings suggest that an imbalance in thyroid function may be related to all phases of bipolar disorder.

As we discuss later (see "Clinical Implications"), lithium treatment is well known to cause a significant disruption in thyroid functionality and thyroid volume, causing hypothyroidism. However, HPT changes were also demonstrated in lithium-naïve patients with bipolar disorder. Compared with healthy control subjects, lithium-free patients with bipolar disorder had significantly higher mean thyroid volumes and lower T_4 levels (Ozsoy et al. 2010). Kraszewska et al. (2019) showed that the rates of hypothyroidism in lithium-treated and untreated patients were similar, suggesting that changes within the HPT axis may have other causes, and possibly are directly related to bipolar disorder itself.

Increased circulating thyroid autoantibodies are frequently seen in patients with bipolar disorder. As in studies of patients with unipolar depression, TPOAbs are the most consistently studied in patients with bipolar disorder (Bocchetta et al. 2016); however, there is an evident increase in both TGAbs and TPOAbs in patients with bipolar disorder compared with healthy control subjects (Barbuti et al. 2017). The majority of these increases were seen in specific subtypes of patients with bipolar disorder—that is, in those with rapid cycling, mixed features, or bipolar depression. Prevalence of TPOAbs has also been compared in twin studies, which further suggest an inherited risk of bipolar disorder and thyroid autoimmunity. In one such study (Vonk et al. 2007), patients with bipolar disorder had significantly higher levels of TPOAbs compared with their co-twins without bipolar disorder. This suggests that thyroid immunity may act as an endophenotype for bipolar disorder. However, results are contradictory, as other studies did not find the same results (Cobo et al. 2015). Children of parents with bipolar disorder have been shown to be more susceptible to thyroid autoimmunity. According to a study from Hillegers et al. (2007), a larger percentage of offspring of parents with bipolar disorder were positive for TPOAbs compared with healthy control subjects, and the majority of these TPOAbs-positive offspring also had raised TSH. The susceptibility to thyroid autoimmunity appeared to be independent from the child's risk of developing a psychiatric disorder, but further research is needed. In addition, there was increased statistical significance when comparing female offspring with control subjects, suggesting that females are at higher risk than males for developing thyroid autoimmunity. However, conflicting evidence exists on the role of sex in the incidence of thyroid autoimmunity in patients with bipolar disorder. For example, Cobo et al. (2015) found that TSH and T_4 levels were not affected by sex; however, women had a higher presence of TGAb and TPOAb positivization. Other authors have not found a significant relationship between sex and the presence of thyroid autoantibodies (Kupka et al. 2002).

In summary, HPT axis abnormalities are quite common among patients with bipolar disorder. However, the biological mechanisms behind this evidence are still unclear, and the role of lithium in inducing HPT axis dysfunction is an important confounder.

Hypothalamic-Pituitary-Gonadal Axis

Depression

A correct balance in the levels of sex hormones appears to be crucial in mental health. Estrogens are directly and indirectly implicated in the neurobiology of depression. Estrogens regulate the synthesis, metabolism, receptor concentration, and trafficking of neurotransmitters that are implicated in depression, including 5-HT, dopamine, and norepinephrine. Moreover, estrogens regulate the neuroplasticity acting on the levels of brain-derived neurotrophic factor (BDNF) (Schiller et al. 2016). Testosterone also has been widely linked to depression. Overall, an imbalance in testosterone levels has been associated with an increased risk for depression, in both men and women (Rohr 2002). In male patients with depression, lower levels of testosterone, mainly free testosterone, have been reported (Almeida et al. 2008). Even though results are sometimes conflicting, a recent meta-analysis confirmed significantly lower testosterone levels in men with depression compared with healthy control subjects (Fischer et al. 2019a).

One hypothesis on how sex hormones could affect mood involves the interaction between the HPG and the HPA axes. There is a reciprocal relationship between these two axes, as each one plays a role in the regulation and functioning of the other. Increased GC levels suppress the release of GnRH and synthesis of gonadotropins, while estrogen and testosterone regulate levels of cortisol (Toufexis et al. 2014). For example, a common symptom of Cushing's syndrome is amenorrhea (Zada et al. 2015); moreover, HPA axis hypoactivity may lead to chronic high testosterone levels (Ludwig et al. 2019).

Women are more likely than men to develop depression, and this sex difference is more evident during the reproductive years, peaking in adolescence and then declining and remaining stable in adulthood (Salk et al. 2017). These findings suggest a potential role of sex hormones in the pathogenesis of depression, even if a clear relation-ship has not yet been established (Brummelte and Galea 2016; Hammarström et al. 2009). Perinatal depression clearly occurs together with great changes in levels of sex hormones. During pregnancy and postpartum, estrogen and progesterone levels dramatically fluctuate from high to hypogonadal status after parturition. Earlier in this chapter, we discussed the relevance of HPA axis alterations in perinatal depression. Additionally, Pařízek et al. (2014) found that levels of both estrogens and androgens during pregnancy were involved in the development of mental changes in the postpartum period. The onset of depression-like behaviors in postpartum rats may be partly attenuated by a complex estrogen-mediated mechanism, mainly ER-α (Furuta et al. 2013). Using combined mouse and human data, Guintivano et al. (2014) identified epigenetic alterations in estradiol-mediated signaling genes that are implicated in postpartum depression. These results confirm once again the firm connection between the HPA and HPG axes and suggest that sex hormones may be of etiological importance in perinatal depression. Another well-known clinical condition that could affect women of reproductive age is premenstrual dysphoric disorder. In this disorder women experience affective symptoms specifically during the luteal phase of the menstrual cycle (with complete remission before and after it). The most supported etiopathological theory suggests that women with premenstrual dysphoric disorder have higher sensitivity to hormonal changes, particularly the fall in progesterone levels. In support of this hypothesis, selective serotonin reuptake inhibitors (SSRIs) are rapidly effective in this disorder; even if the exact mechanism is not completely clear, this effectiveness is probably due to the action of SSRIs on sex hormones, neuromodulating estrogen or progesterone levels (Lanza di Scalea and Pearlstein 2017; Yonkers and Simoni 2018).

Bipolar Disorder

High rates of reproductive disorders have been reported in women with bipolar disorder. Early-onset menstrual cycle dysfunction is significantly more likely to occur in patients with bipolar disorder compared with patients with unipolar depression and healthy control subjects, and this dysfunction occurs more commonly before the onset of bipolar disorder (Joffe et al. 2016). In their pilot study, Rasgon et al. (2000) suggested that menstrual dysfunction preceded the diagnosis and treatment of bipolar disorder, thus implying a role for HPG axis dysfunction in bipolar disorder. In a larger study from the same group, the authors confirmed this hypothesis in 50% of these women (Rasgon et al. 2005). Additionally, the study found that preexisting menstrual abnormalities were associated with increases in 17-α-hydroxyprogesterone, LH/FSH ratio, and free testosterone, which suggest HPG axis dysfunction in these patients. However, most of these studies have reported small sample and effect sizes, limiting the translational impact of these data in a clinical setting. Menstrual cycle dysfunction in patients with bipolar disorder has also been associated with changes in testosterone levels (O'Donovan et al. 2002; Rasgon et al. 2005). Interestingly, testosterone levels were found to be positively correlated with the number of manic episodes and the number of suicide attempts, in both males and females (Sher et al. 2012). This latter finding was further confirmed in a longitudinal study of the same group. In female patients with bipolar disorder, higher baseline testosterone levels predicted suicide attempts in a 2.5-year follow-up period (Sher et al. 2014). However, results are conflicting. Indeed, in the study by Feng et al. (2019) discussed earlier in the subsection on the role of the HPA axis in mood disorders, the authors found that untreated first-episode patients with bipolar disorder had reduced testosterone secretion.

Obviously, there is a substantial difference between male and female hormonal physiologies. Wooderson et al. (2015) reported that women with bipolar disorder had significantly higher testosterone levels compared with female control subjects, whereas men with bipolar disorder had lower testosterone levels compared with male control subjects. Thus, sex differences need to be considered for further research.

Hypothalamic-Neurohypophysial System

HNS hormones also are important in mood disorders. Arginine vasopressin (AVP) has been demonstrated to influence several CNS-related functions, including cognitive and behavioral ones (Surget and Belzung 2008). It has also been hypothesized to have a depressogenic effect. In fact, higher AVP plasma levels (van Londen et al. 1998) and increased AVP mRNA expression (Meynen et al. 2006) have been reported in patients with depression compared with control subjects. Interestingly, a major single-nucleotide polymorphism (SNP) haplotype of the AVP receptor has been found to be protective against recurrent MDD (van West et al. 2004). Very few studies have analyzed AVP in patients with bipolar disorder, and no significant results have been reported (Rutigliano et al. 2016).

Oxytocin (T) may be involved in the development or maintenance of depression (McQuaid et al 2014). Decreased OT levels have been associated with depression (Lach et al. 2018). Ozsoy et al. (2009) found significantly lower OT levels in patients with depression (unipolar and bipolar) compared with healthy control subjects, but only in females. Also, perinatal depression and OT levels have been found to have a reciprocal link: low OT levels during pregnancy are associated with risk of postnatal depression, and antenatal depression is associated with low OT levels after birth (Sawyer et al. 2019). Epigenetic studies showed that DNA methylation in the OT receptor gene was associated with postpartum depression (Kimmel et al. 2016), and specifically with persistent symptoms (King et al. 2017). Also, studies in patients with bipolar disorder reported heightened OT levels (Lien et al. 2017; Turan et al. 2013). In a postmortem study of patients with a major psychiatric disorder, the authors found that diagnoses of MDD or bipolar disorder were associated with significantly increased OT receptor mRNA levels in the dorsolateral prefrontal cortex (Lee et al.

2018). Notably, in subjects with either MDD or bipolar disorder, a specific SNP of the OT receptor gene was associated with suicide attempt history (Parris et al. 2018).

Interestingly, both neurohypophysial hormones can affect HPA axis activity (Engelmann et al. 2004) and consequently act on mood. AVP stimulates ACTH production synergistically with CRH, thus activating the HPA axis (Salata et al. 1988). This has been proposed as a main depressogenic mechanism (Neumann and Landgraf 2012). OT may differently regulate HPA axis activity, by inhibiting basal HPA axis activity and potentiating it under conditions of stress (Neumann et al. 2000).

Clinical Implications

Overall, neuroendocrine functioning is crucial in mood disorders and has therefore been studied for its clinical implications. The recognition of specific neuroendocrine alterations in mood disorders may offer new possibilities for diagnosis, treatment, and prevention of both depression and bipolar disorder. Several therapies currently available for mood disorders act to varying extents on neuroendocrine systems, several treatments specifically targeting neuroendocrine systems at different levels are currently being investigated for mood disorders, and new treatments may be developed in the upcoming years. Even if this is a promising field, we still do not have conclusive results, and further research is needed.

Hypothalamic-Pituitary-Adrenal Axis

Several studies have been focused on the HPA axis as a potential target for treatment of mood disorders. Different anti-GC compounds have been studied as antidepressants, although findings are not univocal and systematic research is still limited. In their review, Holsboer and Ising (2008) reported the results of clinical studies on two CRH type 1 receptor antagonists, NBI-30775/R121919 and NBI-34041. Results were encouraging: the first compound demonstrated a clinical profile comparable to that of the antidepressant paroxetine, whereas the second one reduced the stress-elicited secretion of cortisol. In contrast, Ferrier et al. (2015) reported negative findings in their clinical trial of metyrapone augmentation in patients with treatment-refractory depression. They found that this compound—a competitive inhibitor of 11β-hydroxylase (with resulting inhibition of cortisol)—was ineffective in the treatment of depression. Mifepristone, a potent competitive GR antagonist, has been evaluated both as augmentation and as monotherapy in the treatment of MDD (Maric and Adzic 2013). Interestingly, this compound has demonstrated effectiveness in reducing psychotic symptoms in depression with psychotic features (Block et al. 2018). Treatment with the mifepristone has been investigated in bipolar depression as well, as an adjuvant to current treatment (with mood stabilizers, antidepressants, and antipsychotics) (Young et al. 2004). A significant improvement in depression rating scores was seen in patients taking mifepristone compared to placebo. Furthermore, significant improvements in neurocognitive functioning were observed. A recent meta-analysis by our research group (Lombardo et al. 2019) involving both patients with depression and patients with bipolar disorder highlighted that among those treated with cortisol synthesis inhibitors, responders had significantly higher peripheral baseline cortisol levels compared with nonresponders, supporting a potential role for cortisol as a predictive biomarker for treatment with cortisol synthesis inhibitors in patients with mood disorders.

The firm connection between the HPA axis and mood disorders is further supported by the fact that almost every psychotropic drug has an effect on the HPA axis, as confirmed by a recent review (Subramaniam et al. 2019). Antidepressants are mainly, but not always, associated with a reduction in both basal and post-DEX/CRH cortisol levels, whereas psychostimulant medications are more frequently associated with an increase (or no change) in basal cortisol levels (Subramaniam et al. 2019). It is particularly important to highlight that antidepressants require the GR to exert their action (Anacker et al. 2011). Whereas antidepressants activate the GR in order to increase neurogenesis, cortisol exerts the opposite effect (Pariante 2017). GR function is therefore crucial to achieving an effective antidepressant response. In fact, Binder et al. (2004) found *FKBP5* SNPs to be associated with treatment response in patients with depression. Ising et al. (2019) confirmed these findings, demonstrating increased expression levels of the *FKBP5* gene, and specifically its product FKBP51, to be associated with nonresponse to antidepressant treatment in patients with depression. Another recent systematic review (Fischer et al. 2019b) found that specific SNPs and haplotypes in genes related to CRH (*CRHBP, CRHR1*) and melanocortins (*POMC*) were predictive of nonresponse to antidepressants. However, the authors reported equivocal findings on GR- and MR-related genes. Moreover, both antidepressants and the HPA axis act on 5-HT receptors. Therefore, long-term treatment with antidepressants could modulate serotonergic transmission and lead to activation of the HPA axis, which in turn unfavorably affects 5-HT receptor functioning. This mechanism could cause, at least partly, sensitization and/or tolerance to treatment (Fornaro et al. 2019).

Finally, we have to mention the gut microbiota, which are profoundly linked to the HPA axis and have an important clinical value. The gut microbiota, which include all the indigenous microorganisms that live in the human gut, have an important role in mediating the response to stress (Farzi et al. 2018; Sudo 2014). Hence, probiotics are now emerging as a new potential adjunctive treatment for depression, also acting through modulation of the HPA axis (Butler et al. 2019; Vlainić et al. 2016).

Hypothalamic-Pituitary-Thyroid Axis

Every clinician should be aware of the importance of evaluating thyroid function when assessing a patient with mood disorder. Thyroid hormone supplementation is beneficial in improving depressive symptoms in patients with hypothyroidism and may also benefit patients with normal thyroid function. Augmentation of conventional treatments for depression with T_3 has been proven to be effective in treatment-resistant depression (Carvalho et al. 2009). Very few studies have examined the use of T_3 in bipolar depression, but results are promising (Parmentier and Sienaert 2018). Evidence suggests that T_4 also may act as a neuroprotective agent in the CNS by acting on BDNF, similarly to antidepressants (Hung et al. 2013). In this regard, Baek et al. (2014) found higher TSH levels to be associated with lower baseline, as well as a reduced increase in, BDNF levels during antidepressant treatment, thus suggesting that the HPT axis is crucial in mediating the antidepressant response. In clinical trials in patients with bipolar disorder, treatment of rapid cycling with levothyroxine (L-T_4) has resulted in significantly less time in a depressed or mixed state, and greater time euthymic, compared with placebo (Walshaw et al. 2018). In addition, subclinical hypothyroidism—and also higher TSH levels within the normal range (>2.5 μIU/mL)—has been associated with poorer antidepressant response in both unipolar and bipolar depression (Cohen et al. 2018). Thus, optimizing TSH levels with thyroid hormone supplementation may be an effective treatment strategy in depressed patients with high-normal TSH levels and poor antidepressant response (Cohen et al. 2018).

One of the most common side effects of long-term use of lithium—probably still the most effective treatment for bipolar disorder—is hypothyroidism. Because lithium treatment has been seen to affect the level of thyroid hormones, it could also be suggested that lithium plays a role in increasing thyroid autoantibodies in patients with bipolar disorder. However, some studies (Barbuti et al. 2017; Kupka et al. 2002) reported that the increased presence of TPOAbs in patients with bipolar disorder compared with control subjects was not associated with lithium exposure. Also, other psychotropic medications have been demonstrated to affect thyroid function. In a recent study in patients with bipolar disorder, Li et al. (2019) found no differences in thyroid profiles among patients with different types of mood episodes, but they found quetiapine treatment to affect thyroid function, significantly reducing levels of thyroid hormones.

Hypothalamic-Pituitary-Gonadal Axis

Obviously, sex differences are crucial when analyzing the role of sex hormones in mood disorders. However, there is some evidence regarding the effects of both testosterone and estrogens on mood, independent of a person's sex. In their review, McHenry et al. (2014) reported that testosterone has antidepressant effects in women, men, and animals. The hippocampal mitogen-activated protein kinase pathway may be the mediator of such protective effects. Supplementation with testosterone—administered in an intramuscular, transdermal, or oral formulation—has been proposed as an adjunctive treatment for depressed men, especially for partial responders with low or borderline testosterone levels (Kanayama et al. 2007). Pope et al. (2003) reported that a testosterone transdermal gel was effective in reducing depressive symptoms in male patients with refractory depression and low or borderline testosterone levels. In a subsequent larger study by the same group (Pope et al. 2010), however, testosterone supplementation failed to achieve a significant reduction in depressive symptoms compared with placebo. Despite conflicting findings, a recent meta-analysis including 27 randomized placebo-controlled clinical trials confirmed the efficacy and effectiveness of testosterone in reducing depressive symptoms in men, particularly in higher-dosage regimens (Walther et al. 2019). Interestingly, low-dose transdermal testosterone was found to improve depressive symptoms in women with treatment-resistant depression (Miller et al. 2009). These findings suggest that women may be more sensitive to androgens compared with men. Huang et al. (2008) reported that menopausal status and ovarian steroid levels, but not age, were the main determinants of the antidepressant efficacy of repetitive transcranial magnetic stimulation in women with treatment-resistant depression, both in MDD and in bipolar disorder. Interestingly, depression occurring in perimenopausal women may be directly related to the decline in ovarian estrogen production (estradiol withdrawal), and hormone replacement therapy with estradiol may therefore be protective against the development of depression in susceptible patients (Schmidt and Rubinow 2009; Schmidt et al. 2015).

Several psychotropic medications commonly prescribed for mood disorders, chiefly antipsychotics and antidepressants, but also mood stabilizers, may affect the HPG axis (Drobnis and Nangia 2017). Both first- and second-generation antipsychotics can indeed block the dopamine receptors (mainly D_2) and increase the levels of prolactin, decreasing gonadotropin release. This effect is less frequent with the use of some second-generation compounds, such as aripiprazole and cariprazine, which have a partial agonist effect on dopamine receptors. Prolactin levels also may be increased by several antidepressants, again through their effect on dopamine (inhibition of the reuptake). Additionally, lithium has been shown to increase prolactin and LH levels and decrease sex hormones. Anticonvulsants generally decrease free or bioavailable testosterone and have variable effects on the other reproductive hormones (Drobnis and Nangia 2017). Valproate has been clearly linked with high rates of menstrual abnormalities, hyperandrogenism, and polycystic ovary syndrome in patients with bipolar disorder (O'Donovan et al. 2002).

As discussed, the clinical relevance of the HPG axis in mood disorders may lie in its overlap with the HPA axis. Interestingly, the ginsenoside Rg1—one of the active compounds of the plant genus *Panax* (ginseng)—has several biological functions, including sex hormone–like activities and GR modulation. Mou et al. (2017) reported that Rg1 had antidepressant effects in mice, by modulating both the HPA and HPG axes; specifically, mice treated with Rg1 presented significantly lessened depressive-like symptoms, together with reduced GC levels and increased testosterone levels.

Hypothalamic-Neurohypophysial System

Due to the role of the neurohypophysial system in depression and its intricate connections with other neuroendocrine and immune pathways, it is not surprising that AVP and OT have been studied for their therapeutic potential. Antagonists of the AVP receptor V1b have been demonstrated to have antidepressant effects (Neumann and Landgraf 2012). However, Griebel et al. (2012) reported results from three randomized, double-blind, placebo-controlled studies of patients with depression who were taking SSR149415—an AVP V1b receptor antagonist—for 8 weeks, with no univocal results. Of note, SIADH could be caused by several drugs commonly prescribed for mood disorders, such as many antidepressants (mainly SSRIs, but also tricyclics, monoamine oxidase inhibitors, and venlafaxine) and anticonvulsants (e.g., valproic acid, carbamazepine, oxcarbazepine) (Liamis et al. 2008; Spasovski et al. 2014). Even if the precise mechanisms have not been completely clarified, SIADH could be due to an increase in ADH secretion caused by 5-HT and norepinephrine (De Picker et al. 2014) or to a direct effect on renal sensitivity to ADH (Sachdeo et al. 2002).

Preclinical and clinical evidence indicate that OT, administered either peripherally or centrally, may counteract depression (Matsuzaki et al. 2012; Neumann and Landgraf 2012). These antidepressant effects are not blocked by the administration of an OT receptor antagonist (Acevedo-Rodriguez et al. 2015), suggesting that they are differently mediated, probably through the AVP receptors (Manning et al. 2012). Interestingly, OT could exert an antidepressant effect by increasing dopaminergic transmission, via D_1 receptor activation, in the medial prefrontal cortex (Li et al. 2020). The administration of OT to prevent postpartum depression is still under debate. Some studies found that OT may negatively impact maternal mood (Kroll-Desrosiers et al. 2017; Mah 2016), although other evidence suggests a protective role for future development of postpartum depression, even without immediate effects on maternal mood (Takács et al. 2019).

Conclusion

Mood disorders are profoundly linked to biological alterations in the body. We should therefore think of mental health as a part of the whole individual's well-being. The human organism is a complex orchestra in which all the instruments play together in order to maintain homeostasis; an imbalance within one system could cause the disruption of others. Through the investigation of the interface between body and mind, psychoneuroendocrinology provides a broader perspective for approaching mental health. Even though current findings are not definitive and some critical issues remain, research in this field may shed light on the biological mechanisms underpinning mood disorders, identify new paths for diagnosis and treatment, and ultimately lead to delivery of better patient care.

References

Acevedo-Rodriguez A, Mani SK, Handa RJ: Oxytocin and estrogen receptor beta in the brain: an overview. Front Endocrinol (Lausanne) 6:160, 2015 26528239

Agustini B, Bocharova M, Walker AJ, et al: Has the sun set for seasonal affective disorder and HPA axis studies? A systematic review and future prospects. J Affect Disord 256:584–593, 2019 31299439

Alhajji L, Nemeroff CB: Personalized medicine and mood disorders. Psychiatr Clin North Am 38(3):395–403, 2015 26300030

Almeida OP, Yeap BB, Hankey GJ, et al: Low free testosterone concentration as a potentially treatable cause of depressive symptoms in older men. Arch Gen Psychiatry 65(3):283–289, 2008 18316674

Amann BL, Radua J, Wunsch C, et al: Psychiatric and physical comorbidities and their impact on the course of bipolar disorder: a prospective, naturalistic 4-year follow-up study. Bipolar Disord 19(3):225–234, 2017 28544558

Anacker C, Zunszain PA, Cattaneo A, et al: Antidepressants increase human hippocampal neurogenesis by activating the glucocorticoid receptor. Mol Psychiatry 16(7):738–750, 2011 21483429

Angst J, Gamma A, Benazzi F, et al: Diagnostic issues in bipolar disorder. Eur Neuropsychopharmacol 13 (suppl 2):S43–S50, 2003 12957719

Ashley NT, Demas GE: Neuroendocrine-immune circuits, phenotypes, and interactions. Horm Behav 87:25–34, 2017 27765499

Baek JH, Kang ES, Fava M, et al: Thyroid stimulating hormone and serum, plasma, and platelet brain-derived neurotrophic factor during a 3-month follow-up in patients with major depressive disorder. J Affect Disord 169:112–117, 2014 25189990

Barbuti M, Carvalho AF, Köhler CA, et al: Thyroid autoimmunity in bipolar disorder: a systematic review. J Affect Disord 221:97–106, 2017 28641149

Bauer MS, Whybrow PC, Winokur A: Rapid cycling bipolar affective disorder, I: association with grade I hypothyroidism. Arch Gen Psychiatry 47(5):427–432, 1990 2109970

Bauer M, Goetz T, Glenn T, Whybrow PC: The thyroid-brain interaction in thyroid disorders and mood disorders. J Neuroendocrinol 20(10):1101–1114, 2008 18673409
Bei E, Salpeas V, Pappa D, et al: Phosphorylation status of glucocorticoid receptor, heat shock protein 70, cytochrome c and Bax in lymphocytes of euthymic, depressed and manic bipolar patients. Psychoneuroendocrinology 34(8):1162–1175, 2009 19359101
Bei ES, Salpeas V, Alevizos B, et al: Pattern of heat shock factor and heat shock protein expression in lymphocytes of bipolar patients: increased HSP70-glucocorticoid receptor heterocomplex. J Psychiatr Res 47(11):1725–1736, 2013 23938235
Belvederi Murri M, Pariante C, Mondelli V, et al: HPA axis and aging in depression: systematic review and meta-analysis. Psychoneuroendocrinology 41:46–62, 2014 24495607
Belvederi Murri M, Prestia D, Mondelli V, et al: The HPA axis in bipolar disorder: systematic review and meta-analysis. Psychoneuroendocrinology 63:327–342, 2016 26547798
Binder EB: The role of FKBP5, a co-chaperone of the glucocorticoid receptor in the pathogenesis and therapy of affective and anxiety disorders. Psychoneuroendocrinology 34 (suppl 1):S186–S195, 2009 19560279
Binder EB, Salyakina D, Lichtner P, et al: Polymorphisms in FKBP5 are associated with increased recurrence of depressive episodes and rapid response to antidepressant treatment. Nat Genet 36(12):1319–1325, 2004 15565110
Block TS, Kushner H, Kalin N, et al: Combined analysis of mifepristone for psychotic depression: plasma levels associated with clinical response. Biol Psychiatry 84(1):46–54, 2018 29523415
Bocchetta A, Traccis F, Mosca E, et al: Bipolar disorder and antithyroid antibodies: review and case series. Int J Bipolar Disord 4(1):5, 2016 26869176
Brouwer JP, Appelhof BC, Hoogendijk WJ, et al: Thyroid and adrenal axis in major depression: a controlled study in outpatients. Eur J Endocrinol 152(2):185–191, 2005 15745924
Brummelte S, Galea LAM: Postpartum depression: etiology, treatment and consequences for maternal care. Horm Behav 77:153–166, 2016 26319224
Butler MI, Sandhu K, Cryan JF, Dinan TG: From isoniazid to psychobiotics: the gut microbiome as a new antidepressant target. Br J Hosp Med (Lond) 80(3):139–145, 2019 30860919
Carvalho AF, Machado JR, Cavalcante JL: Augmentation strategies for treatment-resistant depression. Curr Opin Psychiatry 22(1):7–12, 2009 19122528
Cherian K, Schatzberg AF, Keller J: HPA axis in psychotic major depression and schizophrenia spectrum disorders: cortisol, clinical symptomatology, and cognition. Schizophr Res 213:72–79, 2019 31307859
Cobo J, Giménez-Palop O, Patró E, et al: Lack of confirmation of thyroid endophenotype in bipolar disorder type I and their first-degree relatives. Psychoneuroendocrinology 51:351–364, 2015 25462907
Cohen BM, Sommer BR, Vuckovic A: Antidepressant-resistant depression in patients with comorbid subclinical hypothyroidism or high-normal TSH levels. Am J Psychiatry 175(7):598–604, 2018 29961367
Cole DP, Thase ME, Mallinger AG, et al: Slower treatment response in bipolar depression predicted by lower pretreatment thyroid function. Am J Psychiatry 159(1):116–121, 2002 11772699
Cousins L, Goodyer IM: Antidepressants and the adolescent brain. J Psychopharmacol 29(5):545–555, 2015 25744620
Daban C, Vieta E, Mackin P, Young AH: Hypothalamic-pituitary-adrenal axis and bipolar disorder. Psychiatr Clin North Am 28(2):469–480, 2005 15826743
Delvecchio G, Altamura AC, Soares JC, Brambilla P: Pituitary gland in bipolar disorder and major depression: evidence from structural MRI studies. J Affect Disord 218:446–450, 2017 28412090
De Picker L, Van Den Eede F, Dumont G, et al: Antidepressants and the risk of hyponatremia: a class-by-class review of literature. Psychosomatics 55(6):536–547, 2014 25262043
Deshauer D, Duffy A, Meaney M, et al: Salivary cortisol secretion in remitted bipolar patients and offspring of bipolar parents. Bipolar Disord 8(4):345–349, 2006 16879135

Dickens MJ, Pawluski JL: The HPA axis during the perinatal period: implications for perinatal depression. Endocrinology 159(11):3737–3746, 2018 30256957

Drobnis EZ, Nangia AK: Psychotropics and male reproduction. Adv Exp Med Biol 1034:63–101, 2017 29256128

Duval F, Mokrani MC, Monreal J, et al: Interaction between the serotonergic system and HPA and HPT axes in patients with major depression: implications for pathogenesis of suicidal behavior. Dialogues Clin Neurosci 4(4):417, 2002 22033833

Elder GJ, Wetherell MA, Barclay NL, Ellis JG: The cortisol awakening response—applications and implications for sleep medicine. Sleep Med Rev 18(3):215–224, 2014 23835138

Ellenbogen MA, Hodgins S, Walker CD: High levels of cortisol among adolescent offspring of parents with bipolar disorder: a pilot study. Psychoneuroendocrinology 29(1):99–106, 2004 14575732

Ellenbogen MA, Santo JB, Linnen AM, et al: High cortisol levels in the offspring of parents with bipolar disorder during two weeks of daily sampling. Bipolar Disord 12(1):77–86, 2010 20148869

Ellenbogen MA, Hodgins S, Linnen AM, Ostiguy CS: Elevated daytime cortisol levels: a biomarker of subsequent major affective disorder? J Affect Disord 132(1–2):265–269, 2011 21329985

Engelmann M, Landgraf R, Wotjak CT: The hypothalamic-neurohypophysial system regulates the hypothalamic-pituitary-adrenal axis under stress: an old concept revisited. Front Neuroendocrinol 25(3-4):132–149, 2004 15589266

Epstein CM, Houfek JF, Rice MJ, et al: Early life adversity and depressive symptoms predict cortisol in pregnancy. Arch Women Ment Health 23(3):379–389, 2020 31289940

Ezzaher A, Haj Mouhamed D, Mechri A, et al: Thyroid function and lipid profile in bipolar I patients. Asian J Psychiatr 4(2):139–143, 2011 23051081

Fam J, Rush AJ, Burt T, et al: Thyroid autoimmune antibodies and major depressive disorder in women. Ann Acad Med Singapore 44(8):284–289, 2015 26477960

Farzi A, Fröhlich EE, Holzer P: Gut microbiota and the neuroendocrine system. Neurotherapeutics 15(1):5–22, 2018 29380303

Feng G, Kang C, Yuan J, et al: Neuroendocrine abnormalities associated with untreated first episode patients with major depressive disorder and bipolar disorder. Psychoneuroendocrinology 107:119–123, 2019 31125758

Ferrier IN, Anderson IM, Barnes J, et al; ADD Study Team: Randomised controlled trial of Antiglucocorticoid augmentation (metyrapone) of antiDepressants in Depression (ADD Study). Efficacy and Mechanism Evaluation (Southampton [UK]: NIHR Journals Library) 2(4), 2015 26086063

Fischer S, Ehlert U, Amiel Castro R: Hormones of the hypothalamic-pituitary-gonadal (HPG) axis in male depressive disorders—a systematic review and meta-analysis. Front Neuroendocrinol 55:100792, 2019a 31557486

Fischer S, Gardini ES, Haas F, Cleare AJ: Polymorphisms in genes related to the hypothalamic-pituitary-adrenal axis and antidepressant response—systematic review. Neurosci Biobehav Rev 96:182–196, 2019b 30465786

Fornaro M, Anastasia A, Novello S, et al: The emergence of loss of efficacy during antidepressant drug treatment for major depressive disorder: an integrative review of evidence, mechanisms, and clinical implications. Pharmacol Res 139:494–502, 2019 30385364

Fountoulakis KN, Kantartzis S, Siamouli M, et al: Peripheral thyroid dysfunction in depression. World J Biol Psychiatry 7(3):131–137, 2006 16861138

Fries GR, Vasconcelos-Moreno MP, Gubert C, et al: Hypothalamic-pituitary-adrenal axis dysfunction and illness progression in bipolar disorder. Int J Neuropsychopharmacol 18(1):pyu043, 2014 25522387

Frye MA, Denicoff KD, Bryan AL, et al: Association between lower serum free T4 and greater mood instability and depression in lithium-maintained bipolar patients. Am J Psychiatry 156(12):1909–1914, 1999 10588404

Furuta M, Numakawa T, Chiba S, et al: Estrogen, predominantly via estrogen receptor alpha, attenuates postpartum-induced anxiety- and depression-like behaviors in female rats. Endocrinology 154(10):3807–3816, 2013 23913447

Glynn LM, Davis EP, Sandman CA: New insights into the role of perinatal HPA-axis dysregulation in postpartum depression. Neuropeptides 47(6):363–370, 2013 24210135

Griebel G, Beeské S, Stahl SM: The vasopressin V(1b) receptor antagonist SSR149415 in the treatment of major depressive and generalized anxiety disorders: results from 4 randomized, double-blind, placebo-controlled studies. J Clin Psychiatry 73(11):1403–1411, 2012 23146246

Guintivano J, Arad M, Gould TD, et al: Antenatal prediction of postpartum depression with blood DNA methylation biomarkers. Mol Psychiatry 19(5):560–567, 2014 23689534

Hage MP, Azar ST: The link between thyroid function and depression. J Thyroid Res 2012:590648, 2012 22220285

Hammarström A, Lehti A, Danielsson U, et al: Gender-related explanatory models of depression: a critical evaluation of medical articles. Public Health 123(10):689–693, 2009 19853877

Hardeveld F, Spijker J, Vreeburg SA, et al: Increased cortisol awakening response was associated with time to recurrence of major depressive disorder. Psychoneuroendocrinology 50:62–71, 2014 25179322

Havermans R, Nicolson NA, Berkhof J, deVries MW: Patterns of salivary cortisol secretion and responses to daily events in patients with remitted bipolar disorder. Psychoneuroendocrinology 36(2):258–265, 2011 20732746

Hillegers MHJ, Reichart CG, Wals M, et al: Signs of a higher prevalence of autoimmune thyroiditis in female offspring of bipolar parents. Eur Neuropsychopharmacol 17(6–7):394–399, 2007 17140771

Holsboer F, Ising M: Central CRH system in depression and anxiety—evidence from clinical studies with CRH1 receptor antagonists. Eur J Pharmacol 583(2–3):350–357, 2008 18272149

Huang CC, Wei IH, Chou YH, Su TP: Effect of age, gender, menopausal status, and ovarian hormonal level on rTMS in treatment-resistant depression. Psychoneuroendocrinology 33(6):821–831, 2008 18468810

Hung PL, Huang CC, Huang HM, et al: Thyroxin treatment protects against white matter injury in the immature brain via brain-derived neurotrophic factor. Stroke 44(8):2275–2283, 2013 23715956

Ising M, Maccarrone G, Brückl T, et al: FKBP5 gene expression predicts antidepressant treatment outcome in depression. Int J Mol Sci 20(3):485, 2019 30678080

Joffe H, Kim DR, Foris JM, et al: Menstrual dysfunction prior to onset of psychiatric illness is reported more commonly by women with bipolar disorder than by women with unipolar depression and healthy controls. J Clin Psychiatry 67(2):297–304, 2006 16566627

Jones C, Barrera I, Brothers S, et al: Oxytocin and social functioning. Dialogues Clin Neurosci 19(2):193–201, 2017 28867943

Jucevičiūtė N, Žilaitienė B, Aniulienė R, Vanagienė V: The link between thyroid autoimmunity, depression and bipolar disorder. Open Med (Wars) 14:52–58, 2019 30775452

Juruena MF, Pariante CM, Papadopoulos AS, et al: Prednisolone suppression test in depression: prospective study of the role of HPA axis dysfunction in treatment resistance. Br J Psychiatry 194(4):342–349, 2009 19336786

Kanayama G, Amiaz R, Seidman S, Pope HG Jr: Testosterone supplementation for depressed men: current research and suggested treatment guidelines. Exp Clin Psychopharmacol 15(6):529–538, 2007 18179305

Katz ER, Stowe ZN, Newport DJ, et al: Regulation of mRNA expression encoding chaperone and co-chaperone proteins of the glucocorticoid receptor in peripheral blood: association with depressive symptoms during pregnancy. Psychol Med 42(5):943–956, 2012 21995950

Kimmel M, Clive M, Gispen F, et al: Oxytocin receptor DNA methylation in postpartum depression. Psychoneuroendocrinology 69:150–160, 2016 27108164

Kimura T, Makino Y, Saji F, et al: Molecular characterization of a cloned human oxytocin receptor. Eur J Endocrinol 131(4):385–390, 1994 7921228

King L, Robins S, Chen G, et al: Perinatal depression and DNA methylation of oxytocin-related genes: a study of mothers and their children. Horm Behav 96:84–94, 2017 28918249
Kraszewska A, Ziemnicka K, Sowiński J, et al: No connection between long-term lithium treatment and antithyroid antibodies. Pharmacopsychiatry 52(5):232–236, 2019 30731477
Krishna VN, Thunga R, Unnikrishnan B, et al: Association between bipolar affective disorder and thyroid dysfunction. Asian J Psychiatr 6(1):42–45, 2013 23380316
Kroll-Desrosiers AR, Nephew BC, Babb JA, et al: Association of peripartum synthetic oxytocin administration and depressive and anxiety disorders within the first postpartum year. Depress Anxiety 34(2):137–146, 2017 28133901
Kupka RW, Nolen WA, Post RM, et al: High rate of autoimmune thyroiditis in bipolar disorder: lack of association with lithium exposure. Biol Psychiatry 51(4):305–311, 2002 11958781
Lach G, Schellekens H, Dinan TG, Cryan JF: Anxiety, depression, and the microbiome: a role for gut peptides. Neurotherapeutics 15(1):36–59, 2018 29134359
Lamers F, Vogelzangs N, Merikangas KR, et al: Evidence for a differential role of HPA axis function, inflammation and metabolic syndrome in melancholic versus atypical depression. Mol Psychiatry 18(6):692–699, 2013 23089630
Landgraf R, Neumann I, Holsboer F, Pittman QJ: Interleukin-1beta stimulates both central and peripheral release of vasopressin and oxytocin in the rat. Eur J Neurosci 7(4):592–598, 1995 7620610
Lanza di Scalea T, Pearlstein T: Premenstrual dysphoric disorder. Psychiatr Clin North Am 40(2):201–216, 2017 28477648
Lee MR, Sheskier MB, Farokhnia M, et al: Oxytocin receptor mRNA expression in dorsolateral prefrontal cortex in major psychiatric disorders: a human post-mortem study. Psychoneuroendocrinology 96:143–147, 2018 29940428
Li C, Lai J, Huang T, et al: Thyroid functions in patients with bipolar disorder and the impact of quetiapine monotherapy: a retrospective, naturalistic study. Neuropsychiatr Dis Treat 15:2285–2290, 2019 31496710
Li Q, Zhang B, Cao H, et al: Oxytocin exerts antidepressant-like effect by potentiating dopaminergic synaptic transmission in the mPFC. Neuropharmacology 162:107836, 2020 31682854
Liamis G, Milionis H, Elisaf M: A review of drug-induced hyponatremia. Am J Kidney Dis 52(1):144–153, 2008 18468754
Lien YJ, Chang HH, Tsai HC, et al: Plasma oxytocin levels in major depressive and bipolar II disorders. Psychiatry Res 258:402–406, 2017 28865715
Lombardo G, Enache D, Gianotti L, et al: Baseline cortisol and the efficacy of antiglucocorticoid treatment in mood disorders: a meta-analysis. Psychoneuroendocrinology 110:104420, 2019 31499391
Long N, Nguyen L, Stevermer J: Priority Updates from the Research Literature (PURLs): it's time to reconsider early-morning testosterone tests. J Fam Pract 64(7):418–419, 2015 26324959
Ludwig B, Roy B, Dwivedi Y: Role of HPA and the HPG axis interaction in testosterone-mediated learned helpless behavior. Mol Neurobiol 56(1):394–405, 2019 29704202
Mah BL: Oxytocin, postnatal depression, and parenting: a systematic review. Harv Rev Psychiatry 24(1):1–13, 2016 26735320
Manning M, Misicka A, Olma A, et al: Oxytocin and vasopressin agonists and antagonists as research tools and potential therapeutics. J Neuroendocrinol 24(4):609–628, 2012 22375852
Maric NP, Adzic M: Pharmacological modulation of HPA axis in depression—new avenues for potential therapeutic benefits. Psychiatr Danub 25(3):299–305, 2013 24048401
Masek K, Slánský J, Petrovický P, Hadden JW: Neuroendocrine immune interactions in health and disease. Int Immunopharmacol 3(8):1235–1246, 2003 12860179
Matsubara T, Funato H, Kobayashi A, et al: Reduced glucocorticoid receptor alpha expression in mood disorder patients and first-degree relatives. Biol Psychiatry 59(8):689–695, 2006 16458268
Matsuzaki M, Matsushita H, Tomizawa K, Matsui H: Oxytocin: a therapeutic target for mental disorders. J Physiol Sci 62(6):441–444, 2012 23007624

McEwen BS, Gray JD, Nasca C: 60 years of neuroendocrinology: redefining neuroendocrinology: stress, sex and cognitive and emotional regulation. J Endocrinol 226(2):T67–T83, 2015 25934706
McHenry J, Carrier N, Hull E, Kabbaj M: Sex differences in anxiety and depression: role of testosterone. Front Neuroendocrinol 35(1):42–57, 2014 24076484
McLeod DS, Cooper DS: The incidence and prevalence of thyroid autoimmunity. Endocrine 42(2):252–265, 2012 22644837
McQuaid RJ, McInnis OA, Abizaid A, Anisman H: Making room for oxytocin in understanding depression. Neurosci Biobehav Rev 45:305–322, 2014 25025656
Medici M, Direk N, Visser WE, et al: Thyroid function within the normal range and the risk of depression: a population-based cohort study. J Clin Endocrinol Metab 99(4):1213–1219, 2014 24564323
Ménard C, Pfau ML, Hodes GE, Russo SJ: Immune and neuroendocrine mechanisms of stress vulnerability and resilience. Neuropsychopharmacology 42(1):62–80, 2017 27291462
Menke A: Is the HPA axis as target for depression outdated, or is there a new hope? Front Psychiatry 10:101, 2019 30890970
Meynen G, Unmehopa UA, van Heerikhuize JJ, et al: Increased arginine vasopressin mRNA expression in the human hypothalamus in depression: a preliminary report. Biol Psychiatry 60(8):892–895, 2006 16499879
Miller KK, Perlis RH, Papakostas GI, et al: Low-dose transdermal testosterone augmentation therapy improves depression severity in women. CNS Spectr 14(12):688–694, 2009 20394176
Min W, Liu C, Yang Y, et al: Alterations in hypothalamic-pituitary-adrenal/thyroid (HPA/HPT) axes correlated with the clinical manifestations of depression. Prog Neuropsychopharmacol Biol Psychiatry 39(1):206–211, 2012 22750689
Mou Z, Huang Q, Chu SF, et al: Antidepressive effects of ginsenoside Rg1 via regulation of HPA and HPG axis. Biomed Pharmacother 92:962–971, 2017 28618657
Nemeroff CB, Evans DL: Thyrotropin-releasing hormone (TRH), the thyroid axis, and affective disorder. Ann NY Acad Sci 553:304–310, 1989 2497676
Neumann ID, Landgraf R: Balance of brain oxytocin and vasopressin: implications for anxiety, depression, and social behaviors. Trends Neurosci 35(11):649–659, 2012 22974560
Neumann ID, Krömer SA, Toschi N, Ebner K: Brain oxytocin inhibits the (re)activity of the hypothalamo-pituitary-adrenal axis in male rats: involvement of hypothalamic and limbic brain regions. Regul Pept 96(1–2):31–38, 2000 11102649
Oakley RH, Cidlowski JA: The biology of the glucocorticoid receptor: new signaling mechanisms in health and disease. J Allergy Clin Immunol 132(5):1033–1044, 2013 24084075
O'Donovan C, Kusumakar V, Graves GR, Bird DC: Menstrual abnormalities and polycystic ovary syndrome in women taking valproate for bipolar mood disorder. J Clin Psychiatry 63(4):322–330, 2002 12000206
Osborne S, Biaggi A, Chua TE, et al: Antenatal depression programs cortisol stress reactivity in offspring through increased maternal inflammation and cortisol in pregnancy: the Psychiatry Research and Motherhood—Depression (PRAM-D) Study. Psychoneuroendocrinology 98:211–221, 2018 30033161
Otmishi P, Gordon J, El-Oshar S, et al: Neuroimmune interaction in inflammatory diseases. Clin Med Circ Respirat Pulm Med 2:35–44, 2008 21157520
Ozsoy S, Esel E, Kula M: Serum oxytocin levels in patients with depression and the effects of gender and antidepressant treatment. Psychiatry Res 169(3):249–252, 2009 19732960
Ozsoy S, Mavili E, Aydin M, et al: Ultrasonically determined thyroid volume and thyroid functions in lithium-naïve and lithium-treated patients with bipolar disorder: a cross-sectional and longitudinal study. Hum Psychopharmacol 25(2):174–178, 2010 20196184
Palazidou E: The neurobiology of depression. Br Med Bull 101:127–145, 2012 22334281
Pariante CM: Glucocorticoid receptor function in vitro in patients with major depression. Stress 7(4):209–219, 2004 16019586
Pariante CM: Depression during pregnancy: molecular regulations of mothers' and children's behaviour. Biochem Soc Trans 42(2):582–586, 2014 24646281

Pariante CM: Why are depressed patients inflamed? A reflection on 20 years of research on depression, glucocorticoid resistance and inflammation. Eur Neuropsychopharmacol 27(6):554–559, 2017 28479211

Pariante CM, Lightman SL: The HPA axis in major depression: classical theories and new developments. Trends Neurosci 31(9):464–468, 2008 18675469

Pariante CM, Miller AH: Glucocorticoid receptors in major depression: relevance to pathophysiology and treatment. Biol Psychiatry 49(5):391–404, 2001 11274650

Pařízek A, Mikešová M, Jirák R, et al: Steroid hormones in the development of postpartum depression. Physiol Res 63 (suppl 2):S277–S282, 2014 24908233

Parmentier T, Sienaert P: The use of triiodothyronine (T3) in the treatment of bipolar depression: a review of the literature. J Affect Disord 229:410–414, 2018 29331701

Parris MS, Grunebaum MF, Galfalvy HC, et al: Attempted suicide and oxytocin-related gene polymorphisms. J Affect Disord 238:62–68, 2018 29860184

Pilhatsch M, Winter C, Nordström K, et al: Increased depressive behaviour in mice harboring the mutant thyroid hormone receptor alpha 1. Behav Brain Res 214(2):187–192, 2010 20580649

Pope HG Jr, Cohane GH, Kanayama G, et al: Testosterone gel supplementation for men with refractory depression: a randomized, placebo-controlled trial. Am J Psychiatry 160(1):105–111, 2003 12505808

Pope HG Jr, Amiaz R, Brennan BP, et al: Parallel-group placebo-controlled trial of testosterone gel in men with major depressive disorder displaying an incomplete response to standard antidepressant treatment. J Clin Psychopharmacol 30(2):126–134, 2010 20520285

Rasgon NL, Altshuler LL, Gudeman D, et al: Medication status and polycystic ovary syndrome in women with bipolar disorder: a preliminary report. J Clin Psychiatry 61(3):173–178, 2000 10817101

Rasgon NL, Altshuler LL, Fairbanks L, et al: Reproductive function and risk for PCOS in women treated for bipolar disorder. Bipolar Disord 7(3):246–259, 2005 15898962

Rohr UD: The impact of testosterone imbalance on depression and women's health. Maturitas 41 (suppl 1):S25–S46, 2002 11955793

Rutigliano G, Rocchetti M, Paloyelis Y, et al: Peripheral oxytocin and vasopressin: biomarkers of psychiatric disorders? A comprehensive systematic review and preliminary meta-analysis. Psychiatry Res 241:207–220, 2016 27183106

Sachdeo RC, Wasserstein A, Mesenbrink PJ, D'Souza J: Effects of oxcarbazepine on sodium concentration and water handling. Ann Neurol 51(5):613–620, 2002 12112108

Salata RA, Jarrett DB, Verbalis JG, Robinson AG: Vasopressin stimulation of adrenocorticotropin hormone (ACTH) in humans. In vivo bioassay of corticotropin-releasing factor (CRF) which provides evidence for CRF mediation of the diurnal rhythm of ACTH. J Clin Invest 81(3):766–774, 1988 2830315

Salk RH, Hyde JS, Abramson LY: Gender differences in depression in representative national samples: meta-analyses of diagnoses and symptoms. Psychol Bull 143(8):783–822, 2017 28447828

Sanches M, Zunta-Soares GB, Hatch JP, et al: Gender differences in serum cortisol levels among patients with major depressive disorder. Neuropsychiatria Neuropsychologia 8:89–93, 2013

Sawyer KM, Zunszain PA, Dazzan P, Pariante CM: Intergenerational transmission of depression: clinical observations and molecular mechanisms. Mol Psychiatry 24(8):1157–1177, 2019 30283036

Schiller CE, Johnson SL, Abate AC, et al: Reproductive steroid regulation of mood and behavior. Compr Physiol 6(3):1135–1160, 2016 27347888

Schmider J, Lammers CH, Gotthardt U, et al: Combined dexamethasone/corticotropin-releasing hormone test in acute and remitted manic patients, in acute depression, and in normal controls: I. Biol Psychiatry 38(12):797–802, 1995 8750037

Schmidt PJ, Rubinow DR: Sex hormones and mood in the perimenopause. Ann NY Acad Sci 1179:70–85, 2009 19906233

Schmidt PJ, Ben Dor R, Martinez PE, et al: Effects of estradiol withdrawal on mood in women with past perimenopausal depression: a randomized clinical trial. JAMA Psychiatry 72(7):714–726, 2015 26018333

Sforzini L, Nettis MA, Mondelli V, Pariante CM: Inflammation in cancer and depression: a starring role for the kynurenine pathway. Psychopharmacology (Berl) 236(10):2997–3011, 2019 30806743

Shen Y, Wu F, Zhou Y, et al: Association of thyroid dysfunction with suicide attempts in first-episode and drug naïve patients with major depressive disorder. J Affect Disord 259:180–185, 2019 31446378

Sher L, Grunebaum MF, Sullivan GM, et al: Testosterone levels in suicide attempters with bipolar disorder. J Psychiatr Res 46(10):1267–1271, 2012 22858352

Sher L, Grunebaum MF, Sullivan GM, et al: Association of testosterone levels and future suicide attempts in females with bipolar disorder. J Affect Disord 166:98–102, 2014 25012416

Smart C, Strathdee G, Watson S, et al: Early life trauma, depression and the glucocorticoid receptor gene—an epigenetic perspective. Psychol Med 45(16):3393–3410, 2015 26387521

Spasovski G, Vanholder R, Allolio B, et al; Hyponatraemia Guideline Development Group: Clinical practice guideline on diagnosis and treatment of hyponatraemia. Eur J Endocrinol 170(3):G1–G47, 2014 24569125

Stetler C, Miller GE: Depression and hypothalamic-pituitary-adrenal activation: a quantitative summary of four decades of research. Psychosom Med 73(2):114–126, 2011 21257974

Subramaniam A, LoPilato A, Walker EF: Psychotropic medication effects on cortisol: implications for research and mechanisms of drug action. Schizophr Res 213:6–14, 2019 31307858

Sudo N: Microbiome, HPA axis and production of endocrine hormones in the gut. Adv Exp Med Biol 817:177–194, 2014 24997034

Surget A, Belzung C: Involvement of vasopressin in affective disorders. Eur J Pharmacol 583(2–3):340–349, 2008 18255056

Swaab DF, Bao AM, Lucassen PJ: The stress system in the human brain in depression and neurodegeneration. Ageing Res Rev 4(2):141–194, 2005 15996533

Takács L, Seidlerová JM, Štěrbová Z, et al: The effects of intrapartum synthetic oxytocin on maternal postpartum mood: findings from a prospective observational study. Arch Women Ment Health 22(4):485–491, 2019 30306269

Taub DD: Neuroendocrine interactions in the immune system. Cell Immunol 252(1–2):1–6, 2008 18619587

Toni R: The neuroendocrine system: organization and homeostatic role. J Endocrinol Invest 27(6 suppl):35–47, 2004 15481802

Toufexis D, Rivarola MA, Lara H, Viau V: Stress and the reproductive axis. J Neuroendocrinol 26(9):573–586, 2014 25040027

Tsuru J, Ishitobi Y, Ninomiya T, et al: The thyrotropin-releasing hormone test may predict recurrence of clinical depression within ten years after discharge. Neuroendocrinol Lett 34(5):409–417, 2013 23922049

Turan T, Uysal C, Asdemir A, Kılıç E: May oxytocin be a trait marker for bipolar disorder? Psychoneuroendocrinology 38(12):2890–2896, 2013 24080188

Ulrich-Lai YM, Herman JP: Neural regulation of endocrine and autonomic stress responses. Nat Rev Neurosci 10(6):397–409, 2009 19469025

van Bodegom M, Homberg JR, Henckens MJAG: Modulation of the hypothalamic-pituitary-adrenal axis by early life stress exposure. Front Cell Neurosci 11:87, 2017 28469557

van Londen L, Kerkhof GA, van den Berg F, et al: Plasma arginine vasopressin and motor activity in major depression. Biol Psychiatry 43(3):196–204, 1998 9494701

van West D, Del-Favero J, Aulchenko Y, et al: A major SNP haplotype of the arginine vasopressin 1B receptor protects against recurrent major depression. Mol Psychiatry 9(3):287–292, 2004 15094789

Verbalis JG: Disorders of water metabolism: diabetes insipidus and the syndrome of inappropriate antidiuretic hormone secretion. Handb Clin Neurol 124:37–52, 2014 25248578

Verburg-van Kemenade BML, Cohen N, Chadzinska M: Neuroendocrine-immune interaction: evolutionarily conserved mechanisms that maintain allostasis in an ever-changing environment. Dev Comp Immunol 66:2–23, 2017 27296493
Vlainić JV, Šuran J, Vlainić T, Vukorep AL: Probiotics as an adjuvant therapy in major depressive disorder. Curr Neuropharmacol 14(8):952–958, 2016 27226112
Vonk R, van der Schot AC, Kahn RS, et al: Is autoimmune thyroiditis part of the genetic vulnerability (or an endophenotype) for bipolar disorder? Biol Psychiatry 62(2):135–140, 2007 17141745
Walshaw PD, Gyulai L, Bauer M, et al: Adjunctive thyroid hormone treatment in rapid cycling bipolar disorder: a double-blind placebo-controlled trial of levothyroxine (L-T4) and triiodothyronine (T3). Bipolar Disord 20(7):594–603, 2018 29869405
Walther A, Breidenstein J, Miller R: Association of testosterone treatment with alleviation of depressive symptoms in men: a systematic review and meta-analysis. JAMA Psychiatry 76(1):31–40, 2019 30427999
Watanuki T, Funato H, Uchida S, et al: Increased expression of splicing factor SRp20 mRNA in bipolar disorder patients. J Affect Disord 110(1–2):62–69, 2008 18281098
Watson S, Gallagher P, Ritchie JC, et al: Hypothalamic-pituitary-adrenal axis function in patients with bipolar disorder. Br J Psychiatry 184:496–502, 2004 15172943
Wesseloo R, Kamperman AM, Bergink V, Pop VJM: Thyroid peroxidase antibodies during early gestation and the subsequent risk of first-onset postpartum depression: a prospective cohort study. J Affect Disord 225:399–403, 2018 28850854
Wooderson SC, Gallagher P, Watson S, Young AH: An exploration of testosterone levels in patients with bipolar disorder. BJPsych Open 1(2):136–138, 2015 27703738
Wysokiński A, Kłoszewska I: Level of thyroid-stimulating hormone (TSH) in patients with acute schizophrenia, unipolar depression or bipolar disorder. Neurochem Res 39(7):1245–1253, 2014 24723220
Yatham LN: Prolactin and cortisol responses to fenfluramine challenge in mania. Biol Psychiatry 39(4):285–288, 1996 8645775
Yonkers KA, Simoni MK: Premenstrual disorders. Am J Obstet Gynecol 218(1):68–74, 2018 28571724
Young AH, Gallagher P, Watson S, et al: Improvements in neurocognitive function and mood following adjunctive treatment with mifepristone (RU-486) in bipolar disorder. Neuropsychopharmacology 29(8):1538–1545, 2004 15127079
Zada G, Carmichael JD, Selman WR: Introduction: Cushing's disease: a century of evolving diagnostics and therapeutics for an often elusive entity. Neurosurg Focus 38(2):E1, 2015 25639311
Zhao T, Chen BM, Zhao XM, Shan ZY: Subclinical hypothyroidism and depression: a meta-analysis. Transl Psychiatry 8(1):239, 2018 30375372
Zik JB, Roberts DL: The many faces of oxytocin: implications for psychiatry. Psychiatry Res 226(1):31–37, 2015 25619431
Zunszain PA, Hepgul N, Pariante CM: Inflammation and depression. Curr Top Behav Neurosci 14:135–151, 2013 22553073

CHAPTER 7

Role of the Immune System in Mood Disorders

Marisa Toups, M.D.
Charles B. Nemeroff, M.D., Ph.D.

Although significant advances in treating mood disorders have been made using drugs and other therapies that target the brain, significant progress remains to be made in developing personalized treatments. Increasing understanding of the complexity of mental disorders has expanded the view of them as diseases of "neurotransmitters" to diseases of brain circuits and to, in some cases, diseases that involve the entire living system (Akil et al. 2018). Psychoneuroimmunology is a growing field that takes a systems approach to understanding behavior after modulating the function of the immune system and, therefore, its interconnection with the nervous system (Ader et al. 1995). Over the last few decades, our understanding of the role of immune function in mood disorders has grown, and psychoneuroimmunology is likely to make major contributions to clinical practice in the next few decades. In this chapter, we outline the essentials of immune function, describe the current evidence supporting a role for immune function dysregulation in mood disorders, and explore emerging evidence that interventions that impact the immune system may be useful in treatment.

Thanks to Alyssa Marron for assistance with the figure and to Margaret Balfour for editorial input.

The Immune System

The immune system recognizes and protects self-cells while eliminating invading pathogens, infected cells, or cancerous cells (Nathan 2002). This is achieved via four main functions that occur as part of an immune response to infection or injury: 1) recognition, 2) response, 3) resolution, and 4) memory. The immune system is divided into innate and adaptive arms, which work together in all four functions. The cells of the innate immune system, which include macrophages, dendritic cells, and natural killer cells, among others, monitor the blood and tissue and respond to any insults through production of cytokines or presentation of antigens to the adaptive immune system (Akira et al. 2006). Cells of the adaptive immune system, B lymphocytes and T lymphocytes, primarily reside in lymph nodes and related tissue, although some also circulate in the blood. The adaptive response temporally lags behind the innate, especially for new infections, and also activates various strategies to eliminate the insults. In addition, it is responsible for the memory function of the immune system and thus is critical for maintaining lifelong immunity to infections (Iwasaki and Medzhitov 2015). Figure 7–1 shows the major classes of immune cells and their roles in responding to infection.

A major component of the immune response is the generation of cytokines and chemokines, which attract immune cells to infected or damaged tissue, activate other immune cells, amplifying the response to the insult, direct the development of immune cells, activate the differentiation of T and B cells, participate in the immune memory formation, and promote the clearance of the insult. Several of these cytokines, particularly those driving the immediate short-term response to infection, appear to be dysregulated in depression. These include interleukin-6 (IL-6), IL-1β, and tumor necrosis factor-α (TNF-α), as well as the anti-inflammatory cytokine IL-10. Table 7–1 summarizes the most studied cytokines, their main functions, and associations with depression and bipolar disorder.

Immune Responses Inside the Central Nervous System

The CNS has specialized immune cells (Norris and Kipnis 2019). Because the blood-brain barrier (BBB) restricts the infiltration of peripheral immune cells, the brain possesses microglia—specialized macrophage-like cells that perform innate immune functions and account for up to 10% of brain cells (Kim and de Vellis 2005). Microglial ancestor cells enter the brain during embryonic development and sustain their population throughout life. In health, they perform "housekeeping," such as assisting with synaptic plasticity by eliminating synapses. However, they can be activated into distinct states, such as promoting inflammation or enhancing tissue repair, which may be associated with neurodegenerative and neuropsychiatric disease (Yirmiya 2000). Under pathological circumstances—CNS infection, severe systemic infection (e.g., sepsis), or profound stress—when the BBB is compromised, circulating cells from the periphery enter the brain parenchyma, damaging the brain (Varatharaj and Galea 2017). Whether this process is a significant contributor to mental disorders is an active area of study.

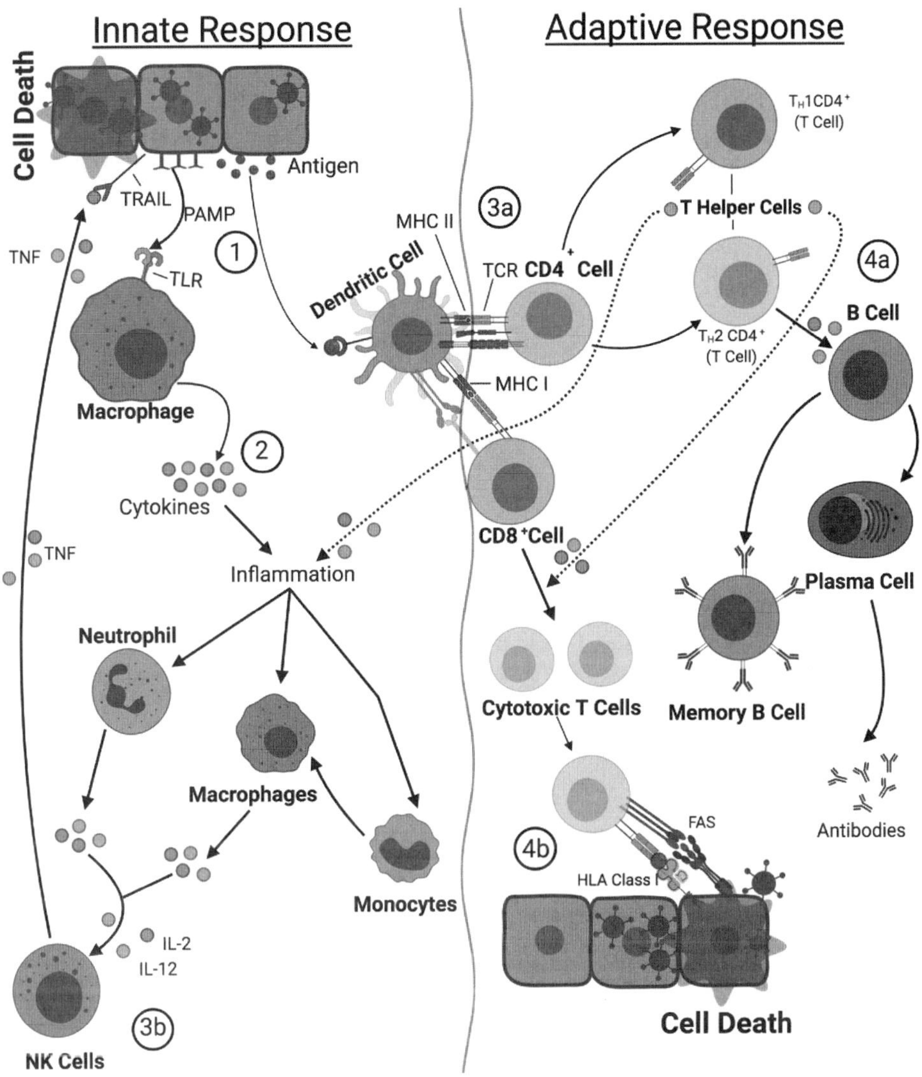

Figure 7–1. Immune cells and their roles in the immune response.
To view this figure in color, see Plate 2 in Color Gallery in middle of book.

(1) *Immune recognition:* A monocyte recognizes pathogen-associated molecular patterns (PAMPs) on an infected cell using a toll-like receptor (TLR). **(2)** *Activation:* Inflammatory cytokines are produced by cells at the site of infection, and this draws other innate immune cells. **(3a)** *Antigen presentation:* A dendritic cell presents fragments of pathogen to T cells, looking for a match. **(3b)** Meanwhile, innate immune cells such as natural killer (NK) cells and neutrophils directly and indirectly attack the infected cells, inducing apoptosis or cell death. **(4a)** B cells that can make antibodies effective against the pathogen mature into plasma cells for immediate production and memory cells to facilitate response if the same pathogen is encountered again. Mature lymphocytes will direct resolution of the response as it completes. **(4b)** Matching T cells mature into helper T cells and cytotoxic T cells that integrate the immune response and directly attack infected cells, respectively.

$CD8^+$ cell=a critical subpopulation of MHC class I restricted T cells; FAS=a type II membrane protein within the tumor necrosis family; HLA=human leukocyte antigen; IL=interleukin; MHC=major histocompatibility complex; TCR=T cell receptor; T_H1 $CD4^+$=a type of lymphocyte that helps coordinate the immune response by stimulating other immune cells; T_H2 $CD4^+$=a type of lymphocyte that helps coordinate the immune response by stimulating other immune cells; TNF=tumor necrosis factor; TRAIL=TNF-related apoptosis-inducing ligand.

TABLE 7–1. Commonly studied cytokines in mental health and their main functions, as well as mood-related findings

Cytokine	Type	Main function	Clinical findings
IL-1β	Inflammatory	Coordinates/activates inflammatory cascade	Activated in MDD
IL-2	Differentiator	Promotes T cell survival	Increased in MDD
IL-4	Differentiator	Promotes Th2-associated allergic responses	Decreased in MDD
IL-6	Inflammatory	Activates the acute phase response	Increased in MDD; increased in mania
IL-10	Anti-inflammatory	Inhibits the production of proinflammatory cytokines	Increased in MDD
IFN-γ	Inflammatory	Responds to infection, especially viral	Decreased in MDD
TNF-α	Inflammatory	Plays a critical role in multiple cellular functions: survival, proliferation, differentiation, and death	Increased in MDD; increased in mania
Other			
C-reactive protein[a]	Acute phase reactant	Participates in the complement pathway activation or promotes phagocytosis pathogens by macrophages	Increased in MDD

IFN=interferon, IL=interleukin; MDD=major depressive disorder; Th2=T helper type 2 cells; TNF=tumor necrosis factor.
[a]C-reactive protein is an acute-phase reactant, not a cytokine.

Communication Between the Brain and the Immune System

The brain receives signals from the immune system in several ways. As mentioned above, when the immune cells enter the CNS, they also produce cytokines, which can be detected in the cerebrospinal fluid (Banks and Erickson 2010) and enhance damage. Peripherally produced and circulating cytokines may enter the CNS through openings of the BBB, such as the circumventricular organs (Quan and Banks 2007). Cytokine signals are also received via direct detection by nerves, particularly those of the autonomic nervous system (Dantzer et al. 2000). The existence of a lymphatic system within the meninges of the brain has been validated and represents another potential route by which cells and circulating cytokines may reach the CNS (Sandrone et al. 2019).

Reciprocally, the brain communicates with and modulates the immune system (Qiu et al. 1996). Both the hypothalamic-pituitary-adrenal (HPA) axis and the autonomic nervous system contribute to control of immune cells (Sternberg 2006), and both are involved in suppressing cytokine production as well as in resolving the immune response (Rosas-Ballina and Tracey 2009). The peripheral anti-inflammatory effects of cortisol, which is a major component of the stress response, include inhibition of the infiltration of the immune cells around the body as well as the release of cytokines (Dhabhar 2009; Silverman and Sternberg 2012). The catecholamines norepinephrine and epinephrine also modulate the activity of the immune system, in particular by directly impacting immune cells.

Evidence of Immune Dysfunction in Mood Disorders

Although it appears that a range of psychiatric illnesses may involve immune dysfunction, the most promising potential for future treatment applications exists for mood disorders, particularly major depressive disorder (MDD). Overall, the existing literature supports an immune dysregulation in MDD with the following characteristics: 1) mild but chronic elevations of proinflammatory cytokines, 2) chronic elevations in some anti-inflammatory cytokines, and 3) suppressed immune cell response. Similar patterns of dysregulation of the immune system have been found in other diseases (e.g., diabetes, cardiovascular disease, obesity), underlying some of the potential mechanisms mediating the high rates of comorbidity between these diseases and depression.

There are several important clinical contributors to immune dysregulation in depressed patients, including stress, particularly early in life. Additionally, at least in some cases, a primary immune cause, such as a drug therapy or an autoimmune disease, may be associated with depression development. Few data exist on the immune response in patients with bipolar disorder. Although mania is considered to be associated with increased inflammation, there is less evidence linking bipolar depression with immune dysfunction (Goldsmith et al. 2016).

The finding that clinically depressed subjects exhibit elevated markers of inflammation when compared with healthy subjects has been extensively replicated (Haapakoski et al. 2015). C-reactive protein (CRP) is one of the most studied inflammatory markers in MDD because, empirically, CRP has been used as a marker of cardiovascular disease risk and can be obtained from most clinical labs, making it ideal for clinicians. CRP in healthy adults is less than 1–3 mg/L. Levels greater than 3 mg/L indicate chronic inflammation, and levels greater than 100 mg/L are associated with active severe bacterial infection (D'Agostino et al. 2008). In samples of patients with MDD, the mean CRP value is elevated compared with that of healthy subjects, and depressed patients are more likely to have levels greater than 3 mg/L. Some severely depressed patients may have CRP levels elevated into the range associated with chronic inflammation (Raison et al. 2013).

In addition to laboratory findings, there is substantial epidemiological evidence linking depression and immune dysfunction. Epidemiologists have noted the high rate of medical comorbidity in depressed patients for decades, and chronic disorders such as metabolic syndrome and cardiovascular disease carry up to a doubled risk of depression (Anderson et al. 2001; Evans et al. 2005; Heiskanen et al. 2006). Similarly, autoimmune disorders and severe infections increase future risk of depression by about 50% (Benros et al. 2013). Interestingly, depression increases the longitudinal risk of developing many of these same medical disorders, as well as cancer, over time (Currier and Nemeroff 2014; Goldbacher et al. 2009), suggesting bidirectionality of underlying mechanisms. One might guess that the association of depression with increased inflammation would protect patients with MDD from infection, but paradoxically they are at greater risk of minor infections (Cohen 1995) and may not respond successfully to vaccines (Irwin et al. 2011). Depression is also associated with a significant increase in longitudinal risk for serious infection (Andersson et al. 2016) and with increased infection-related mortality (Davydow et al. 2016).

Clinical Contributors to Immune Dysfunction in Depression

To realize the goal of advancing mood disorder treatment, we as researchers and clinicians need to understand the etiology of the co-occurring immune dysfunction and identify patients for whom psychoneuroimmunology-based therapies might be beneficial. For example, it is not yet clear whether immune dysfunction is universal or impacts only a subset of patients (Glassman and Miller 2007). We also lack a clear understanding of the "which came first?" directionality of these associations; although data support the conclusion that the depressed population has signs of immune dysregulation, many of these patients may have preexisting factors that contribute to their mood disorder.

Diet

In a study by Lucas et al. (2014), diet that was associated with elevated inflammatory markers was also associated with depression symptoms, with a relative risk of approximately 1.3 for the highest inflammatory quintile. Although this study was limited by the inclusion of only female subjects, these results suggest that diet increases depression risk primarily through chronic inflammation, and that the high prevalence of poor-quality diet and associated obesity among psychiatric patients is a likely contributor to depression-associated inflammation.

Psychological Stress

The relationship between stress and immune response is dependent on the nature of the stressor and the population under study (Segerstrom and Miller 2004). Occupational or interpersonal stress may be associated with an increase in inflammatory cytokines (Maes et al. 1998). A greater inflammatory stress response is observed in individuals with higher chronic or baseline stress, and this effect may be most pronounced in those with depression or anxiety. This increase in inflammatory markers may explain the increased vulnerability to infection (Cohen 1995), because psychosocial stress has been associated with a decrease in the gene expression associated with antiviral immunity (Miller et al. 2008).

Early-life stress or trauma may be the major contributor to inflammation in mood disorders. Early-life adversity—a well-known risk factor for adult psychopathology—also substantially increases risk of metabolic and inflammatory illness in adulthood (Ehlert 2013; Su et al. 2015), including obesity and elevated CRP (Baumeister et al. 2016; Coelho et al. 2014). Survivors of childhood trauma have epigenetic changes in genes regulating HPA axis function (Danese et al. 2011; Nemeroff 2016) and also exhibit behavior changes impairing cortisol sensitivity, such as insomnia (Miller et al. 2011). There is at least some evidence that the effects of childhood and later-life trauma on inflammation are additive (Hostinar et al. 2015; Lin et al. 2016).

Iatrogenic Inflammation

Mood episodes induced by medications impacting immune responses have been in the scope of psychiatric practice for many years. Corticosteroids and related immunosuppressants cause mania in susceptible individuals upon acute administration, and depression after prolonged exposure (Warrington and Bostwick 2006). Perhaps the best evidence relates to interferon-α (IFN-α) therapy for hepatitis C virus infection, melanoma, or other illness; IFN-α induces depressive symptoms in approximately 45% of the patients receiving this treatment. Exogenous immune stimulation is sufficient to induce sickness behavior. Amazingly, close to half may go on to develop a full major depressive episode, including symptoms such as worthlessness and suicidal ideation (Capuron and Miller 2004). Having a history of depression is a risk factor for interferon-induced depression (Schlaak et al. 2012). The depressive effects of interferon therapy provided some of the first evidence that altering the immune system is capable of causing depression.

Autoimmune and Other Illnesses

Given the overlap between medical illnesses and mood disorders, the population of patients with an obviously immune diathesis to their disorder is important to consider. In particular, individuals with autoimmune disorders have extremely high rates of comorbid MDD, reportedly as high as 40% (Benros et al. 2013). This overlap might be attributed to the direct impact of immune activity in the brain (e.g., cytokines or immune cell infiltration [Pryce and Fontana 2017]). Patients with cancer also often experience increased inflammation from the cancer as well as tissue-destructive therapies (Mantovani et al. 2008) and have high rates of comorbid depression that is associated with poor outcomes (Bortolato et al. 2017), suggesting that inflammation is the common theme associated with the development of depression. Thus, consideration of the particular vulnerability of these patients may warrant measures to screen for and treat mood symptoms in these patients.

Interventions for Inflammatory Depression

In this section, we discuss three interesting questions related to treatment of mood disorders and immune responses. First, is there an association between antidepressant treatment and normalization of immune system function? Next, does restoring immune function result in a therapeutic mood effect? And finally, can immune markers be used to select patients for specific antidepressant treatments, regardless of whether those treatments are immune related?

Data on whether antidepressant treatment improves immune dysfunction, as assessed via meta-analysis (Köhler et al. 2018), are mixed. Part of this heterogeneity is likely attributable to treatment with different modalities and drugs; however, more work needs to be done to examine this question. The latest analysis specifically failed to find a connection between the observed decreases in IL-6, the cytokine most consistently elevated in MDD, and improvement in symptoms with treatment (Köhler et al. 2018). Other therapies, such as exercise, mindfulness, and even psychotherapies such as cognitive-behavioral therapy, have also been associated with reductions in inflammatory markers, and thereby provide broader support for a nonspecific effect based more on ameliorating the disease state than on mechanism of treatment (Eyre et al. 2013; Lopresti 2017; Morgan et al. 2014).

Two major sets of data examine treating the immune dysfunction in depression directly with cytokine-inhibiting drugs or nonsteroidal anti-inflammatory drugs (NSAIDs). Anticytokine therapy is typically in the form of manufactured monoclonal antibodies that target cytokines or related molecules. Most of the relevant trials include subjects treated for an autoimmune disease with comorbid depression and show consistently positive results (Kappelmann 2018). One study in a sample of patients with severe unipolar depression without medical comorbidity had negative results overall, but found that the subjects with the highest levels of inflammation, as assessed with CRP level, appeared to benefit from treatment with the TNF-α antagonist infliximab (Raison et al. 2013). A similar trial enrolling subjects with bipolar depression showed no effect, perhaps because bipolar depression is less related to immune dysfunction than is unipolar depression (McIntyre et al. 2019). It remains to be seen, given the risks associated with these drugs and the mixed results, whether cytokine inhibitors will find use outside of the niche of patients with comorbid inflammatory illnesses. NSAIDs have also been studied as primary or augmentation treatments, with mostly positive findings (O. Köhler et al. 2014). In particular, selective cyclooxygenase-2 (COX-2) inhibitor drugs have been found to be effective treatments for MDD. Unfortunately, other studies have found no effect, and chronic NSAID use is not without risks (Eyre et al. 2015).

Finally, we consider whether there is any recommendation for matching currently accepted therapies with patients with the goal of improving the remission rate by identifying patients who may benefit from targeted therapy (e.g., patients with medical comorbidity or patients with a history of childhood trauma). A few secondary analyses of large studies found evidence that inflammation, as assessed with CRP level, is associated with a poorer response to treatment with selective serotonin reuptake inhibitors (Hedayati et al. 2017; O'Brien et al. 2007) compared with dopamine reuptake inhibitors (Jha et al. 2017; Uher et al. 2014). However, more research on the topic is needed. Some trials also suggest that exercise may be especially beneficial for depressed patients with elevated cytokines (Greer and Trivedi 2009; Rethorst et al. 2013), although researchers do not yet understand which types of exercise are most effective in reducing inflammation, and therefore depression symptoms (Eyre and Baune 2014).

Conclusion

As of this writing, we can conclude that mood disorders involve abnormal immune responses. Major depressive disorder shows substantial associations with poorer outcomes when combined with medical illness involving inflammation. Nevertheless, work remains to better understand how the multiple clinical phases of bipolar disorders relate to immune and medical outcomes. Given the rapid increase in the understanding of immune responses and technological advances allowing the development of new assays and treatments, it is likely that psychiatrists will soon see major new therapies applying the knowledge base of psychoneuroimmunology to treatment of mood disorders in the clinic.

References

Ader R, Cohen N, Felten D: Psychoneuroimmunology: interactions between the nervous system and the immune system. Lancet 345(8942):99–103, 1995 7815892

Akil H, Gordon J, Hen R, et al: Treatment resistant depression: a multi-scale, systems biology approach. Neurosci Biobehav Rev 84:272–288, 2018 28859997

Akira S, Uematsu S, Takeuchi O: Pathogen recognition and innate immunity. Cell 124(4):783–801, 2006 16497588

Anderson RJ, Freedland KE, Clouse RE, Lustman PJ: The prevalence of comorbid depression in adults with diabetes: a meta-analysis. Diabetes Care 24(6):1069–1078, 2001 11375373

Andersson NW, Goodwin RD, Okkels N, et al: Depression and the risk of severe infections: prospective analyses on a nationwide representative sample. Int J Epidemiol 45(1):131–139, 2016 26708840

Banks WA, Erickson MA: The blood-brain barrier and immune function and dysfunction. Neurobiol Dis 37(1):26–32, 2010 19664708

Baumeister D, Akhtar R, Ciufolini S, et al: Childhood trauma and adulthood inflammation: a meta-analysis of peripheral C-reactive protein, interleukin-6 and tumour necrosis factor-alpha. Mol Psychiatry 21(5):642–649, 2016 26033244

Benros ME, Waltoft BL, Nordentoft M, et al: Autoimmune diseases and severe infections as risk factors for mood disorders: a nationwide study. JAMA Psychiatry 70(8):812–820, 2013 23760347

Bortolato B, Hyphantis TN, Valpione S, et al: Depression in cancer: the many biobehavioral pathways driving tumor progression. Cancer Treat Rev 52:58–70, 2017 27894012

Capuron L, Miller AH: Cytokines and psychopathology: lessons from interferon-alpha. Biol Psychiatry 56(11):819–824, 2004 15576057

Coelho R, Viola TW, Walss-Bass C, et al: Childhood maltreatment and inflammatory markers: a systematic review. Acta Psychiatr Scand 129(3):180–192, 2014 24205846

Cohen S: Psychological stress and susceptibility to upper respiratory infections. Am J Respir Crit Care Med 152(4 Pt 2):S53–S58, 1995 7551414

Currier MB, Nemeroff CB: Depression as a risk factor for cancer: from pathophysiological advances to treatment implications. Annu Rev Med 65:203–221, 2014 24215332

D'Agostino RB Sr, Vasan RS, Pencina MJ, et al: General cardiovascular risk profile for use in primary care: the Framingham Heart Study. Circulation 117(6):743–753, 2008 18212285

Danese A, Caspi A, Williams B, et al: Biological embedding of stress through inflammation processes in childhood. Mol Psychiatry 16(3):244–246, 2011 20157309

Dantzer R, Konsman JP, Bluthé RM, Kelley KW: Neural and humoral pathways of communication from the immune system to the brain: parallel or convergent? Auton Neurosci 85(1–3):60–65, 2000 11189027

Davydow DS, Ribe AR, Pedersen HS, et al: The association of unipolar depression with thirty-day mortality after hospitalization for infection: a population-based cohort study in Denmark. J Psychosom Res 89:32–38, 2016 27663108

Dhabhar FS: A hassle a day may keep the pathogens away: the fight-or-flight stress response and the augmentation of immune function. Integr Comp Biol 49(3):215–236, 2009 21665815

Ehlert U: Enduring psychobiological effects of childhood adversity. Psychoneuroendocrinology 38(9):1850–1857, 2013 23850228

Evans DL, Charney DS, Lewis L, et al: Mood disorders in the medically ill: scientific review and recommendations. Biol Psychiatry 58(3):175–189, 2005 16084838

Eyre HA, Baune BT: Assessing for unique immunomodulatory and neuroplastic profiles of physical activity subtypes: a focus on psychiatric disorders. Brain Behav Immun 39:42–55, 2014 24269526

Eyre HA, Papps E, Baune BT: Treating depression and depression-like behavior with physical activity: an immune perspective. Front Psychiatry 4:3, 2013 23382717

Eyre HA, Air T, Proctor S, et al: A critical review of the efficacy of non-steroidal anti-inflammatory drugs in depression. Prog Neuropsychopharmacol Biol Psychiatry 57:11–16, 2015 25455584

Glassman AH, Miller GE: Where there is depression, there is inflammation…sometimes! Biol Psychiatry 62(4):280–281, 2007 17678943

Goldbacher EM, Bromberger J, Matthews KA: Lifetime history of major depression predicts the development of the metabolic syndrome in middle-aged women. Psychosom Med 71(3):266–272, 2009 19188528

Goldsmith DR, Rapaport MH, Miller BJ: A meta-analysis of blood cytokine network alterations in psychiatric patients: comparisons between schizophrenia, bipolar disorder and depression. Mol Psychiatry 21(12):1696–1709, 2016 26903267

Greer TL, Trivedi MH: Exercise in the treatment of depression. Curr Psychiatry Rep 11(6):466–472, 2009 19909669

Haapakoski R, Mathieu J, Ebmeier KP, et al: Cumulative meta-analysis of interleukins 6 and 1beta, tumour necrosis factor alpha and C-reactive protein in patients with major depressive disorder. Brain Behav Immun 49:206–215, 2015 26065825

Hedayati SS, Gregg LP, Carmody T, et al: Effect of sertraline on depressive symptoms in patients with chronic kidney disease without dialysis dependence: the CAST randomized clinical trial. JAMA 318(19):1876–1890, 2017 29101402

Heiskanen TH, Niskanen LK, Hintikka JJ, et al: Metabolic syndrome and depression: a cross-sectional analysis. J Clin Psychiatry 67(9):1422–1427, 2006 17017829

Hostinar CE, Lachman ME, Mroczek DK, et al: Additive contributions of childhood adversity and recent stressors to inflammation at midlife: findings from the MIDUS study. Dev Psychol 51(11):1630–1644, 2015 26389605

Irwin MR, Levin MJ, Carrillo C, et al: Major depressive disorder and immunity to varicella-zoster virus in the elderly. Brain Behav Immun 25(4):759–766, 2011 21329753

Iwasaki A, Medzhitov R: Control of adaptive immunity by the innate immune system. Nat Immunol 16(4):343–353, 2015 25789684

Jha MK, Minhajuddin A, Gadad BS, et al: Can C-reactive protein inform antidepressant medication selection in depressed outpatients? Findings from the CO-MED trial. Psychoneuroendocrinology 78:105–113, 2017 28187400

Kappelmann N, Lewis G, Dantzer R, et al: Antidepressant activity of anti-cytokine treatment: a systematic review and meta-analysis of clinical trials of chronic inflammatory conditions. Mol Psychiatry 23(2):335–343, 2018 27752078

Kim SU, de Vellis J: Microglia in health and disease. J Neurosci Res 81(3):302–313, 2005 15954124

Köhler CA, Freitas TH, Stubbs B, et al: Peripheral alterations in cytokine and chemokine levels after antidepressant drug treatment for major depressive disorder: systematic review and meta-analysis. Mol Neurobiol 55(5):4195–4206, 2018 28612257

Köhler O, Benros ME, Nordentoft M, et al: Effect of anti-inflammatory treatment on depression, depressive symptoms, and adverse effects: a systematic review and meta-analysis of randomized clinical trials. JAMA Psychiatry 71(12):1381–1391, 2014 25322082

Lin JE, Neylan TC, Epel E, O'Donovan A: Associations of childhood adversity and adulthood trauma with C-reactive protein: a cross-sectional population-based study. Brain Behav Immun 53:105–112, 2016 26616398

Lopresti AL: Cognitive behaviour therapy and inflammation: a systematic review of its relationship and the potential implications for the treatment of depression. Aust N Z J Psychiatry 51(6):565–582, 2017 28382827

Lucas M, Chocano-Bedoya P, Schulze MB, et al: Inflammatory dietary pattern and risk of depression among women. Brain Behav Immun 36:46–53, 2014 24095894
Maes M, Song C, Lin A, et al: The effects of psychological stress on humans: increased production of pro-inflammatory cytokines and a Th1-like response in stress-induced anxiety. Cytokine 10(4):313–318, 1998 9617578
Mantovani A, Allavena P, Sica A, Balkwill F: Cancer-related inflammation. Nature 454(7203):436–444, 2008 18650914
McIntyre RS, Subramaniapillai M, Lee Y, et al: Efficacy of adjunctive infliximab vs placebo in the treatment of adults with bipolar I/II depression: a randomized clinical trial. JAMA Psychiatry 76(8):783–790, 2019 31066887
Miller GE, Chen E, Sze J, et al: A functional genomic fingerprint of chronic stress in humans: blunted glucocorticoid and increased NF-kappaB signaling. Biol Psychiatry 64(4):266–272, 2008 18440494
Miller GE, Chen E, Parker KJ: Psychological stress in childhood and susceptibility to the chronic diseases of aging: moving toward a model of behavioral and biological mechanisms. Psychol Bull 137(6):959–997, 2011 21787044
Morgan N, Irwin MR, Chung M, Wang C: The effects of mind-body therapies on the immune system: meta-analysis. PLoS One 9(7):e100903, 2014 24988414
Nathan C: Points of control in inflammation. Nature 420(6917):846–852, 2002 12490957
Nemeroff CB: Paradise lost: the neurobiological and clinical consequences of child abuse and neglect. Neuron 89(5):892–909, 2016 26938439
Norris GT, Kipnis J: Immune cells and CNS physiology: microglia and beyond. J Exp Med 216(1):60–70, 2019 30504438
O'Brien SM, Scully P, Fitzgerald P, et al: Plasma cytokine profiles in depressed patients who fail to respond to selective serotonin reuptake inhibitor therapy. J Psychiatr Res 41(3–4):326–331, 2007 16870211
Pryce CR, Fontana A: Depression in autoimmune diseases. Curr Top Behav Neurosci 31:139–154, 2017 27221625
Qiu Y, Peng Y, Wang J: Immunoregulatory role of neurotransmitters. Adv Neuroimmunol 6(3):223–231, 1996 8968422
Quan N, Banks WA: Brain-immune communication pathways. Brain Behav Immun 21(6):727–735, 2007 17604598
Raison CL, Rutherford RE, Woolwine BJ, et al: A randomized controlled trial of the tumor necrosis factor antagonist infliximab for treatment-resistant depression: the role of baseline inflammatory biomarkers. JAMA Psychiatry 70(1):31–41, 2013 22945416
Rethorst CD, Toups MS, Greer TL, et al: Pro-inflammatory cytokines as predictors of antidepressant effects of exercise in major depressive disorder. Mol Psychiatry 18(10):1119–1124, 2013 22925832
Rosas-Ballina M, Tracey KJ: The neurology of the immune system: neural reflexes regulate immunity. Neuron 64(1):28–32, 2009 19840545
Sandrone S, Moreno-Zambrano D, Kipnis J, van Gijn J: A (delayed) history of the brain lymphatic system. Nat Med 25(4):538–540, 2019 30948855
Schlaak JF, Trippler M, Hoyo-Becerra C, et al: Selective hyper-responsiveness of the interferon system in major depressive disorders and depression induced by interferon therapy. PLoS One 7(6):e38668, 2012 22701688
Segerstrom SC, Miller GE: Psychological stress and the human immune system: a meta-analytic study of 30 years of inquiry. Psychol Bull 130(4):601–630, 2004 15250815
Silverman MN, Sternberg EM: Glucocorticoid regulation of inflammation and its functional correlates: from HPA axis to glucocorticoid receptor dysfunction. Ann NY Acad Sci 1261:55–63, 2012 22823394
Sternberg EM: Neural regulation of innate immunity: a coordinated nonspecific host response to pathogens. Nat Rev Immunol 6(4):318–328, 2006 16557263
Su S, Jimenez MP, Roberts CT, Loucks EB: The role of adverse childhood experiences in cardiovascular disease risk: a review with emphasis on plausible mechanisms. Curr Cardiol Rep 17(10):88, 2015 26289252

Uher R, Tansey KE, Dew T, et al: An inflammatory biomarker as a differential predictor of outcome of depression treatment with escitalopram and nortriptyline. Am J Psychiatry 171(12):1278–1286, 2014 25017001

Varatharaj A, Galea I: The blood-brain barrier in systemic inflammation. Brain Behav Immun 60:1–12, 2017 26995317

Warrington TP, Bostwick JM: Psychiatric adverse effects of corticosteroids. Mayo Clin Proc 81(10):1361–1367, 2006 17036562

Yirmiya R: Depression in medical illness: the role of the immune system. West J Med 173(5):333–336, 2000 11069873

CHAPTER 8

Evolutionary Contributions to the Understanding of Mood and Mood Disorders

Martin Brüne, M.D., Ph.D.
Daniel R. Wilson, M.D., Ph.D.

After the mind has suffered from an acute paroxysm of grief, and the cause still continues, we fall into a state of low spirits; or we may be utterly cast down and dejected. Prolonged bodily pain, if not amounting to an agony, generally leads to the same state of mind. If we expect to suffer, we are anxious; if we have no hope of relief, we despair.

Charles Darwin (1872)

Mood manages much of mammalian motivation. This is especially so in the eusocial domain that operates above more ancient reptilian modes of agonic competition. Behavior of primates, particularly humans, is guided by brain systems that evolved over millions of years. Yet mood disorders, notably depression, are among the most common noncommunicable medical problems worldwide. How can this reality be reconciled with the view that the human body and mind were shaped by natural selection over eons of adaptation? Our answer is that neither the brain nor behavior was "designed" so much as accrued as a collection of all and sundry evolutionary adaptations to address diverse selective pressures. Thus, it is not surprising that regulation of mood is far from perfect. (We are unable to recap millions of years of evolutionary sculpting of mood and its disorders in a short chapter, so we posit some basic concepts. For more information, readers may consult other references, both supportive [as cited herein] and critical of our viewpoint [e.g., Confer et al. 2010; Plotkin 2004]).

In 2006 the World Health Organization predicted that by 2030, depression will constitute the second most burdensome disease (as measured in "years lived with disability"), surpassed only by HIV/AIDS but ranking before cardiovascular disease (Mathers and Loncar 2006; see also Chapter 3, "Epidemiology and Burden of Mood Disorders," in this text). Notably, however, in contrast to cardiovascular disease, mood disorders usually affect people in the prime of life. What is low mood good for? Why is depression so widespread that in high-income countries, about one in four adults at some point will suffer a depressive episode? Why does depression commonly occur at an age at which the influence of selection is greatest—that is, near the peak of reproductive potential—unlike most other noncommunicable diseases, which increase with advanced age? Why is depression so readily elicited by the experience of adverse life events? Is there an intrinsic connection between rising incidence rates of depression worldwide and the decline of communicable (i.e., infectious) diseases, and if so, how can we make sense of it?

These are not the questions usually asked by clinicians or neuroscientists. Instead, low mood, or "spirit" as Darwin called it, is conventionally considered a psychologically painful condition that needs to be prevented because it is unpleasant and harmful. Accordingly, when studying more extreme forms of low mood, clinically labeled "depression," neuroscientists seek to identify mechanisms that cause dysregulation of neurotransmission (e.g., low serotonin turnover in relation to genetic variation) and to determine functional and structural abnormalities in the brain (see Chapter 5, "Neurochemistry of Mood Disorders"; Chapter 9, "Anatomical Pathology"; and Chapter 11, "Brain Imaging"). Similarly, when neuroscientists ask why many psychiatric disorders emerge during adolescence and early adulthood, they typically attribute such risk to reorganization of the brain and/or hormonal changes, rather than considering the broader ramifications of what makes adolescence and young adulthood so special (Paus et al. 2008). Third, losses of important relationships and declines in social status are well known to precipitate depression, which, according to the conventional diathesis-stress model (Monroe and Simons 1991), unfolds pathogenic potential via genetic vulnerability. But an important question is why these genes are so prevalent in the human gene pool. Finally, although the association of low mood and mood disorders with immunological activity has been well known for some time (Rook and Lowry 2009), inflammatory responses in depression are usually not considered in relation to epidemiological issues pertaining to infectious diseases. In sum, while clinical neuroscience explores important questions about the mechanistic causation of low mood and depression, it has paid insufficient attention to the evolved nature of the human mind.

This discrepancy in inquiry between neuroscience and evolutionary biology was long ago pointed out in a now famous article by Nobel Laureate Nicolaas Tinbergen (1963). Tinbergen made the distinction between "proximate" causation (mechanism and ontogeny) and "ultimate" or evolutionary causation (phylogeny and adaptive value), each of which needs to be studied to fully understand any anatomical, physiological, or behavioral trait. Originally conceptualized to analyze animal anatomy and behavior, Tinbergen's framework has been adopted to account for physical and psychological traits, including traits that at first sight appear dysfunctional (Brüne 2014). Thus, contrary to the view that an evolutionary approach to mood and mood disorders is reductionistic, such an approach is actually in full accord with a biopsychosocial model of health and disease (Engel 1977). Therefore, to give "ultimate" or evolutionary questions full credit, we emphasize in this chapter adaptationist perspectives on excessively low and high mood (Nesse 2009; Wilson 2001). Specifically, we aim to review the most widely discussed evolutionary theories of mood and mood disorders, particularly the ones involving attachment and social competition; we further explore the association of low mood with inflammation, discuss common genetic risk factors from an evolutionary vantage point, and present special aspects of mood disorders, including bereavement and suicidal behavior.

Evolutionary Principles for Understanding Mood and Mood Disorders

Ancestral Conditions and "Goals" of Evolution

To appreciate what evolutionary biology can contribute to the understanding of mood and mood disorders—particularly the lingering question of why nature has left us vulnerable to depression, mania, and other psychiatric disorders—one needs to consider several issues. First, considering an evolutionary time frame is of particular importance. The human mind is endowed with cognitive, emotional, and behavioral capacities that emerged by natural and sexual selection at a time when our forebears lived as hunter-gatherers in close-knit communities, commonly referred to as an "environment of evolutionary adaptedness" (Bowlby 1969; Tooby and Cosmides 1990). This does not contradict recent evidence for ongoing selection in *Homo sapiens* (Stearns et al. 2010), but our emotional life has probably changed very little since the Stone Age (Panksepp 2006). Ancestral environments were fraught with dangers, against which humans (and indeed our primate and mammalian ancestors) developed a broad array of defense mechanisms. These dangers ranged from microbial pathogens (even though—counterintuitively at first sight—the diversity of pathogens was probably smaller than after domestication of animals) (Barnes 2005) to social threats, including competition for status and mates, as well as intertribal conflict (Gilbert et al. 2004). Therefore, evolved defenses include ones to fight infectious diseases, such as cough, fever, and inflammatory responses, as well as ones to minimize damage from social threats, including withdrawal, appeasement, and submission—or, conversely, to defend by way of social dominance. Whatever ancestral environments were specifically like, however, they were in many respects fundamentally different from contemporary conditions, and therefore our species experiences a range of phenotypic reactivity (Wilson 1998).

Second, although natural and sexual selection operate on the phenotype of any given trait, there is no "goal" in evolution apart from an anagenic tendency (an evolutionary trend from simpler to more complex forms) (Mayr 2001). Organisms do maximize replication of genes, whereby the concept of kin selection refers to the replication of an individual's genes shared with relatives of varying degree (Hamilton 1964). These technical statements have at least two important implications for the present chapter: 1) evolution does not specifically favor well-being or health, and 2) evolved traits are not optimal by design but rather are compromises of sometimes opposing selection pressures. Accordingly, low mood can be regarded as a defense against real or perceived environmental threats (i.e., a rescue strategy to preserve one's reproductive potential), whereas high mood can be viewed as an effort to attain reproductive success via higher social rank. In the next section, we illustrate this principle of "design compromise" by describing the compromise with the furthest-reaching consequences for human mental life.

Life History Patterns and Human Attachment as a Design Compromise

Life history theory makes the point that organisms can invest in either somatic growth or reproduction, but not both simultaneously (Stearns 1992). Accordingly, there are two fundamentally different reproductive "strategies" (which here does not imply conscious choice): K-selected and r-selected strategies. Humans are among K-selected life forms, which grow larger-bodied, are slow to develop, reproduce repetitively, have few offspring per litter, care intensely for their young over long periods of time (which includes a long gestation period), and have relatively low death rates in infancy and childhood. The onset of reproductive activity is delayed, and K-selected species usually enjoy long lives. Typically, social competition among adults is high, because—due to prolonged lifespans—success in intrasexual competition determines survival and reproductive success. K-selected species also usually live in conditions with little random environmental variation. A K-selected pattern is characteristic for primates, as well as for whales and elephants. In contrast, an r-selected strategy, which has characteristics that are opposite those described above, is the reproductive strategy for most insect and fish species, as well as (among mammals) small rodents (Stearns 1992).

In humans, the typical primate pattern is extended in all stages of development from infancy to adolescence and adulthood (Bogin 1999). It is important to note, however, that there is also within-species variation in life history strategies, commonly referred to as the "pace of life." In other words, some human life histories appear to be slightly more pushed to an r-selected-like pattern ("fast" life history), whereas others have a more extreme K-selected pattern ("slow" life history). Indeed, humans differ with regard to timing of biological maturation, age at onset of sexual activity and reproduction, mating, number of offspring, and care provided for offspring (Ellis et al. 2011). These differences in "pace of life" critically depend on the nature of attachment patterns that develop during infancy and early childhood, whereby the special quality of dyadic and triadic bonds between infant, mother, and father in terms of intensity and duration can be regarded as a design compromise *par excellence*.

Indeed, some 2.5 million years ago, environmental changes in East Africa were the starting point for a new way of locomotion in a clade of primates: bipedalism. Although the selection pressures that caused upright walking are still debated (Preuschoft 2004), as selection favored the evolution of larger brains in bipedal hominins, probably due to the demands of increasingly complex social structures (Dunbar and Shultz 2007), giving birth to immature offspring emerged as a design compromise to accommodate a narrow pelvis, a situation termed the "obstetric dilemma" (Wells et al. 2012). However, not only brain size (and hence head circumference) mattered, but also the nutritional demands of a large brain that could not be supplied by the maternal placenta for longer than 9 months (Campbell 2010). These circumstances, in turn, created new selective pressures on parenting and mating. If humans were born as maturely as our closest extant relatives, the great apes, pregnancy would last 22 months. Human immaturity at birth necessitated particular adaptations in mother-infant bonding; because mothers were less capable of foraging when caring for immature babies, there was a need for increasing paternal and close kin investment, allowing "cooperative breeding" (Hrdy 2000).

The mechanism through which dyadic and triadic relationships between infant, mother, and father develop is known as "attachment." Bowlby (1969) discovered that human newborns, like other primates and perhaps all mammals, are "preprogrammed" to seek proximity to caregivers as a way to secure their own survival. Evolutionarily speaking, it is in the genetic interest of mothers and fathers to be highly responsive to their babies' needs (Hamilton 1964). However, attachment is not only about food and security. Rather, it is also about the caregiver's emotional availability, which is decisive for the development of a child's "internal working model" about the world. A child who can rely on trustworthy and responsive care is more likely to perceive the world as a safe place. Conversely, if caregivers are less willing or able to emotionally respond to infants' needs, insecure attachment may cause infants to perceive the world as dangerous (Bowlby 1969). Impending abandonment is a life-threatening condition in the environment of evolutionary adaptedness, in which young infants typically display separation distress and anxiety. If separation continues, infants go through phases of protest, despair, and detachment, typically associated with low mood. Prolonged separation, such as for hospitalized infants, may cause "anaclitic" depression (Spitz 1945).

Although Bowlby (1969) believed that only secure attachment could be adaptive, more recent work suggests that fluctuations in ancestral environmental conditions in terms of resource availability have selected for a set of flexible adaptive behavioral responses to accomplish important biosocial goals (Simpson 1999). For example, when confronting harsh environmental conditions, which may include food scarcity or lack of emotional availability of caregivers, an individual is more likely to develop an internal working model that the world is unsafe and future resources are uncertain, so that immediate resource extraction might be the best strategy. Such strategies may include exploitation of others with an opportunistic interpersonal style, more risk-prone behaviors, early mating efforts with limited investment in offspring, and even the acceleration of biological maturation, thus driving the "pace of life" slightly into a "faster" direction (Belsky 1999). Insecure attachment therefore reflects, to some extent, a proximate adaptive strategy evolved to ensure survival and to maximize reproductive success under unpredictable environmental conditions. However, as the likelihood of not reaching significant goals also increases, it is plausible to assume that a "faster" pace of life is associated with an increased risk for psychopathology, including depression and mania (Brüne 2016a; Del Giudice 2014; Hurst and Kavanagh 2017). Such individual differences are observable to the present day, in that poverty and social inequality leave their marks on individual pace of life (Hochberg and Belsky 2013).

Biosocial Goals

In addition to care-eliciting and caregiving (the major concerns of attachment and bonding), humans pursue other biosocial goals that, from an evolutionary point of view, are critical for the sake of survival and reproductive success (Gilbert and Allan 1998). These goals embrace mate selection and mating, formation of alliances, and rank in the social hierarchy. This formulation is so general that it applies to virtually all social species; however, the increasing complexity of human sociality has brought about a sophisticated set of emotions and cognitive abilities that evolved to maintain cooperation and reciprocal relationships in tribal societies (Trivers 1971). In fact, mutual dependence (including food sharing), caring for sick or otherwise incapacitated individuals, sharing of knowledge, and other forms of altruistic behaviors were so imperative in ancestral societies that tendencies of "free riding" or cheating had to be controlled. Such a scenario has most likely contributed to the evolution of rewarding emotions such as friendship, sympathy, trust, and gratitude; in addition, negative emotions, including shame and guilt, emerged in response to the need for reconciliation when cooperation was violated (Trivers 1971). Given the complexity of human social life, it is almost inconceivable that biosocial goals and rules of cooperation and reciprocity are never thwarted or violated. Instead, the experience of social goals obstructed by one's own or others' failure is so common that low mood is an inevitable part of human nature. Moreover, as evolutionary analysis of low mood and mood disorders suggests, guilt and shame are intricately linked with phenotypic expressions of depression (Panksepp 2006).

In summary, there are several evolutionary explanations as to why the human mind is left vulnerable to developing low mood and mood disorders (Gilbert and Allan 1998; Wilson 1998): 1) environmental mismatch and phenotypic plasticity (i.e., ancestral environments, including the pathogenic landscape, are different from contemporary ones); 2) selection favors reproductive success but not well-being; 3) psychological features, like anatomical traits, are design compromises; 4) moods (including some extreme variants) are defense mechanisms and thus part of human nature; and 5) the thwarting of biosocial goals is inevitable. All of this leads to the question of what low and high mood could be good for.

Evolutionary Theories of Mood and Mood Disorders

The concept of "mood" is intricately linked to the concepts of "emotions" and "feelings," and the terms are often used interchangeably. However, the difference between the concepts of "mood" and "emotions" is more akin to that between "climate" and "weather." That is, in contrast to acute emotions, mood is a more pervasive state, partly detached from immediate environmental stimuli (Nettle and Bateson 2012). As mood emerges from recurrent experiences of emotional responses to specific triggers associated with reward or punishment, it can adjust the threshold for detection of future incentives or threats. Possessing a "mood system" is thus adaptive, because it can direct attention and vigilance toward the approach of rewarding events or avoidance of punishing events. The absence of reward, for example, causes low (or depressed) mood and raises the threshold for reward-seeking behavior, whereas repeated punishment (or continuous exposure to danger) initiates avoidance behavior through anxious mood states (Nettle and Bateson 2012), and avidity for reward can drive hypomania and mania (Wilson 1998). Emotions are commonly elicited by exteroceptive input (i.e., vision, audition, odor, taste, or tactile sensation) that can elicit feelings—that is, the subjective experiences accompanying emotional states. Conversely, some feelings (e.g., hunger and thirst) need not necessarily be caused by emotions (Damasio and Carvalho 2013).

Mood is a phylogenetically old adaptation that helps guide organismic behavior based on the estimated likelihood that a particular situation will recur. More specifically, low mood can be regarded as an evolved defense mechanism that protects the organism against ongoing exposure to fitness-reducing environmental contingencies. Although low mood is subjectively unpleasant and undesirable, it is an important signal to the organism to pause, save energy, and reevaluate the situation in order to recuperate homeostasis. On the other end of the scale, high mood can propel organisms toward resources and social rank.

Excessive low mood is commonly associated with a diagnosis of clinical depression, and excessive high mood with mania. The excess can pertain to the intensity, duration, or both. Evolutionary perspectives on mood disorders would argue that there is no clear boundary between "normal" mood and pathological extremes (Brüne 2016b; Nettle and Bateson 2012). However, even though it is disputed by some evolutionary scientists, our standpoint is that at least severe states of clinical depression and mania are maladaptive in the Darwinian sense. Moreover, these likely are more common in the modern ontogenic environment than they were in the environment of evolutionary adaptedness. The analogy to cough and fever may illustrate this stance: these defenses against attacks of pathogenic agents are clearly adaptive if they help expel or kill viruses or microbes. Excessive cough or septic fever, however, can cause severe damage or even death. Likewise, (severe) depression or mania is detrimental to biological fitness and may cause significant disability (Wilson 1998). Given the vast number of life events that can cause mood variation, depression, or mania, we look at specific evolutionary explanations for mood and mood disorders.

Attachment Theory Perspective

Darwin's statement heading this chapter alluded to a common cause of depression, namely the loss of an important relationship. Darwin's deep insights foreshadowed the typical stages of low mood following separation from an attachment figure (Bowlby 1969). In fact, young mammals, when abandoned, are exposed to several risks, such as predation, starvation, or perishing from cold. Accordingly, a first response to abandonment is protest, by which the young signal distress to reinforce reunion with the attachment figure. This response is typically associated with communicative signals of low mood—vocally by crying, and facially by the expression of anger. In addition, locomotor activity in search of the attachment figure can occur. Prolonged protesting, however, is perilous itself, because it may attract predators or lead to exhaustion. Therefore, after some time, protest ceases, giving way to a phase of despair. Despair is adaptive in situations in which rapid reunion is precluded. The young thus stops signaling. Instead, it immobilizes, turns mute, and changes facial expression to sadness/despair (for an overview, see Gilbert 2006). Darwin already noted "the oblique drawing up of the eyebrows, the puckering of their inner ends, and the formation of rectangular furrows on the middle of the forehead" as a species-typical expression of this kind of low mood (Darwin 1872, p. 192).

Clinicians will immediately notice the similarities of the behavioral correlates of protest and despair to signs and symptoms of agitated (protest) and retarded (despair) depression, respectively. In that attachment styles are "transposed" over the lifespan to important relationships other than the primary caregiver (Bowlby 1969), separation or loss can trigger low mood and depressive responses by activating evolutionarily and developmentally "primitive" mechanisms that originally evolved as coping strategies for impending or real abandonment. Depression in response to social losses is more likely to occur in individuals who as children were exposed to neglectful or inconsistent parenting and hence developed insecure attachment. Arguably, attachment insecurity results in individuals having greater difficulties in eliciting social support, while their mistrustful inner working models promote the subjective experience of social isolation and emotional distance from others (Gilbert 2006), potentially creating a vicious circle from which there is no escape without therapeutic support. This interpretation is compatible with ethological work showing that poor maternal care predicts an unfavorable subsequent course of depression (Geerts et al. 2009). Bereavement is another typical response associated with low mood in reaction to the loss of an important attachment figure; it is not to be pathologized and mistaken for depression (Nesse 2005). Aside from attachment issues, however, mood extremes of depression or mania can emerge from other potential social hazards, such as ones relating to social hierarchy.

Social Competition

Interpersonal tension is another common source of low mood and depression, whereas ingratiation and dominance are drivers of high mood and mania. In social animals, conflict can arise over any one of the above-described biosocial goals. Indeed, disputes over access to mates, social status, and reciprocal relationships occur in every primate society, including human social groups (de Waal 1989). Succinctly put, competition for mates, resources, and status is so inevitably linked to human social life that everybody is exposed to it at some point (Wilson 1998). Accordingly, there are several evolutionary theories about the role of social competition in relation to excessive mood states (Price et al. 1994). These theories differ in nuances—that is, whether the focus is on the chosen strategy to negotiate social hierarchy (escalating vs. deescalating social conflict) (Gardner 1982), the role of defeat (Price 1967), or involuntary subordination in relation to social rank (Gilbert 1992), which includes the expression of arrested anger (Gilbert et al. 2004), entrapment in situations where submission is ineffective (Gilbert 1992; Price and Wilson 2011), or the reduction of social risk (Allen and Badcock 2003), including the functional role of ruminative thinking (Watson and Andrews 2002). For its part, mania can be seen as an unconstrained acquisitive drive (Wilson 1998).

In a now-classic contribution, Price (1967) was the first to highlight similarities in behavior between nonhuman primates negotiating social rank and the signs and symptoms of human depression. He argued that dominant individuals display aggression overtly or more subtly to subordinates in response to challenges to, or to simply maintain, their social rank. Submissive behavior and defeat, in contrast, are typical behavioral responses by the subordinate to deescalate social conflict (i.e., signal appeasement) (Price et al. 2007). Changes in rank usually cause elation when climbing up the social ladder, or depression when slipping (Sloman et al. 2011). The former is an equivalent to (hypo)mania, which can also include challenging behavior (Sloman et al. 2011). The latter is protective because it prevents subordinates from fighting back (although irritable mood may be redirected against "inferior" subjects) (Price 1967). In human depression, as Price and colleagues subsequently argued, not only do individuals signal social defeat by withdrawing from the social arena, but they also actively deescalate conflict through manifest submission, such as hunched body posture, gaze aversion, and avoidance of movements that could be interpreted as competitive (reviewed in Hagen 2011). In addition, loss of appetite and libido indicate abstention from competition for resources or mates. Internal signals or subjective appraisals of defeat comprise feelings of inferiority, shame or guilt, loss of self-esteem, self-criticism, and powerlessness, altogether contributing to low mood (Carvalho et al. 2013; Gilbert 2006). This is entirely consistent with ethological work on nonverbal behavior showing that depressed individuals avoid eye-to-eye contact, manifest reduced facial expressivity and speech production, and frequently make use of species-specific child behaviors (traditionally labeled "regression"), thus reducing the risk of being attacked (Geerts and Brüne 2009). Conversely, mania is associated with the activation of evolutionarily ancient systems involved in the regulation of arousal and ambition (Wilson 1998).

In an extension to the social rank theory of depression, Gilbert et al. (2002) have pointed out that in situations in which signaling defeat is ineffective, social support is lacking, or control over social resources is poor, feelings of entrapment and arrested anger may occur, and are associated with persistent high arousal. In such circumstances, feelings of inferiority necessitate holding upward aggression against dominant individuals in check (Carvalho et al. 2013). Behaviorally, conflicting motivation involving fight-or-flight responses is expressed through so-called displacement activities, such as self-grooming, locomotor activity, or "nervousness," any of which may present in what is clinically called "agitated depression" (Troisi 2002). As Gilbert and Allan (1998) have noted, subjective feelings of entrapment can be amplified by internal processes such as intrusive thoughts and ruminations. For example, continuous rumination about one's inferiority may enhance perceptions that there is no escape from the situation, which may ultimately lead to suicidal ideation or actions. In contrast, Andrews and Thomson (2009) ascribe to rumination associated with low mood a functional role, which helps direct one's attention away from distracting and unattainable goals and reallocate energy to solving problems entailed in the precipitation of the current situation (Durisko et al. 2015).

The social competition hypothesis is in full accord with the broader concept of low mood and depression as a risk-averse strategy for coping with social threat (Allen and Badcock 2003). This version of the same theme emphasizes that whereas people with a functional social network can engage in some risk-taking activities, individuals with less supportive social relationships are reluctant to take social risks. Thus, this view emphasizes the role of social adversity in depression, implying that subjects who are risk averse are also more vigilant toward social threats and avoidance of their own failure.

In essence, the multiple versions of the social competition hypothesis are by no means mutually exclusive. Moreover, the attachment perspective and the social competition approach converge on findings that the association between insecure attachment and depression is mediated by one's perceived social rank, which is not the case for individuals with secure attachment patterns, even though the picture is less clear for people with bipolar disorder (Gilbert et al. 2007). On the other hand, Keller and Nesse (2005) noted some interesting differences in symptomatology between depressed subjects who experienced loss and depressed subjects who failed to achieve important biosocial goals. Indeed, the former more often display crying and sadness (akin to Bowlby's [1969] protest-despair stages following loss or abandonment), whereas the latter more frequently experience subjective feelings of pessimism and fatigue. Low mood in response to social losses or thwarted biosocial goals can serve as an honest signal to elicit help from one's social environment, but also can express a (nonconscious) dishonest strategy of extracting "unearned" resources from others, especially when disguised as "learned helplessness" (Watson and Andrews 2002). This interpretation is consistent with ethological research analyzing nonverbal behavior of depressed patients and their interlocutors during clinical interviews, in which high levels of nonverbal support-seeking on the part of the depressed patient and high levels of received nonverbal support from the interviewer were found to be associated with an unfavorable prognosis. Indeed, Segrin (2000) found that even mild symptoms of depression can induce rejection responses in other people, particularly if the depressive symptomatology persists over extended periods of time. Thus, ethological perspectives on depression suggest that depression can also be the consequence of malfunctioning interpersonal processes, rather than a strategy to ameliorate interpersonal social stress (Geerts and Brüne 2009). It is something of a paradox that members of an altruistic and empathic species like ours sometimes reject those who need help.

Sickness Behavior, the Immune System, and Depression

Natural selection has endowed all living creatures with defense mechanisms against pathogenic agents. Higher vertebrates possess an innate and adaptive immune system that activates when the body is attacked by viruses, bacteria, fungi, or prions. Proinflammatory states are associated with a behavioral response, known as "sickness behavior." Sickness behavior is characterized by lethargy, fatigue, loss of appetite, psychomotor retardation, and social withdrawal. This evolutionarily conserved defense reaction to infection is adaptive, because it helps the organism recuperate by saving energy and by reducing the risk of being attacked in times of enhanced vulnerability (Eisenberger et al. 2017; Raison and Miller 2017). In fact, in gregarious species, sick individuals not only are at risk of predation but also are susceptible to decline in social rank, and to suffering a reduction in reproductive success, as their sexual attractiveness decreases (Schaller 2011). Thus, sickness behavior is also associated with heightened vigilance toward social threats (Eisenberger et al. 2017). In addition, kin selection theory (Hamilton 1964) suggests that social withdrawal may reduce the risk of infection for genetically related individuals, even though the costly side of social avoidance may be the loss of provisionary care (Schaller 2011). Interestingly, animals, including humans, are well able to recognize even subtle signs of sickness in others, which activates an immune response in the observer, and often fosters rejection and avoidance of the sick individual (Schaller 2011). In humans, however, sickness behavior is usually associated with approaching close others and avoiding contact with strangers (Eisenberger et al. 2017).

Because sickness behavior is associated with low mood and anhedonia, depression can be seen as an evolved state of "pathogen defense readiness" (Raison and Miller 2017). Aside from the behavioral similarities between sickness behavior and depression, abundant evidence from immunological research supports the idea that depression can be associated with a proinflammatory state (Dantzer and Kelley 2007; see also Chapter 7, "Role of the Immune System in Mood Disorders," in this text). In addition, precipitating conditions of low mood and depression, including parental separation, loss, childhood trauma, intense social competition, loneliness, or social disconnectedness, are accompanied by increased immune activation. In other words, evolved environmental contingencies identified as potentially dangerous for survival and reproduction—for example, loss of important attachment figures or thwarted biosocial goals—cause the organism to take preparatory action by activating the immune system. Notably, in terms of causality, proinflammatory states, such as ones induced by the experimental application of lipopolysaccharide, a bacterial agent that triggers an inflammatory response, induce not only low mood and anhedonia but also feelings of social disconnectedness, loneliness, and desire for closeness to familiar others, as well as greater vigilance toward social threat (Eisenberger et al. 2017).

Together, the evidence strongly suggests that evolution by natural selection has produced powerful mechanisms that protect organisms against a broad variety of threats, including infectious and social ones. Immunological response patterns seem to be designed in ways that bodies do not discriminate between different causes of threats, but instead uniformly react with proinflammatory states. With regard to depression, it has been debated as to whether the increase in prevalence, particularly in urban areas of developed countries, could be related to alterations of the immune system caused by a diminished exposure to pathogens early in life. According to the "old friends" hypothesis, exposure to some pathogenic agents early in life is necessary for normal development of immunoregulation. In the absence of the acquisition of normal immunocompetence, a person's risk for chronic proinflammatory states increases, as well as risk for autoimmune disease. Due to space limitations, this perspective on epidemiological aspects of depression cannot be dealt with in greater detail here (for further discussion, see Rook and Lowry 2009, as well as Chapter 7 in this text). It is noteworthy, however, that recent research indicates that the picture is even more complex, with both elevated pro- and anti-inflammatory markers in treatment-naïve patients with major depressive disorder (Syed et al. 2018). Interestingly, lack of response to treatment was associated with a pervasive upregulation of proinflammatory cytokines, suggesting that a downregulation of defense mechanisms at both somatic and psychological levels is vital for the improvement of depressed mood states.

Evolutionary Genetics, Depression, and Mania

Excessive mood states of depression and mania are so common across the globe that it is implausible to assume that genes associated with the condition are wholly disadvantageous in terms of survival and reproduction, or even selectively neutral. The crucial question is why genes conferring risk for depression and mania have been preserved in the human gene pool (Wilson 1998). A meta-analysis in about 250,000 individuals with depression and 560,000 control subjects revealed 102 independently segregating genes and another 269 genes associated with depression (Howard et al. 2019); however, even though the analysis indicated some interesting inverse correlations of depression with age of menarche and menopause, it failed to examine potential evolutionary implications of these findings. As with many other genetic studies, the basic misconception is that genes associated with disorder are maladaptive (Wilson 1998). The prevailing view on gene-environment interaction concerning psychopathological conditions (also known as the "diathesis-stress model," per Monroe and Simons 1991) suggests that individuals carrying certain genetic variants who are exposed to negative life events are vulnerable to developing clinically relevant signs and symptoms. In contrast, individuals not possessing the "risk allele" are genetically protected or resilient (Feder et al. 2009). For example, the short (S) allele of the serotonin transporter gene predisposes to depression if accompanied by stressful life events (Caspi et al. 2003); however, variation at the corticotropin-releasing hormone receptor may prevent depression even in the presence of childhood maltreatment (Polanczyk et al. 2009).

A pervasive theoretical problem associated with the diathesis-stress model concerns the observation that many of the supposed "vulnerability genes" have undergone positive selection in human evolution. It is simply implausible to assume that natural selection has favored the preservation of alleles in the human gene pool that increase vulnerability to adversity, particularly when considering that the environment of evolutionary adaptedness was probably fraught with negative life events occurring throughout the entire life span. Instead, positive selection of such alleles strongly suggests that these genes exert hitherto undetected or overlooked beneficial effects on reproductive fitness (which is not the same as being "good for health") (Ellis et al. 2011). For example, the S allele of the serotonin transporter gene predisposes to depression if associated with adverse life events, but it is also linked to cognitive performance and social conformity, which may compensate for its disadvantageous effect on mood in a "balanced polymorphism" fashion (Homberg and Lesch 2011). Along similar lines, there is evidence to suggest that genes predisposing to depression and mania may play an important role in immune function, potentially being involved in the defense against pathogens that were more prevalent in our evolutionary past (Raison and Miller 2017). Such a proposition would be compatible with seasonal peaks of depression during winter and spring, when exposure to pathogens is high (Anders et al. 2013).

In addition, a given genetic variation that predisposes to psychopathology if associated with adverse life events can have beneficial effects when environmental contingencies are developmentally more supportive; this variability is known as "differential susceptibility" or "phenotypic plasticity." Put another way, the idea that genes confer responsivity to both positive and negative conditions can explain why they persist in human gene pools (Boyce and Ellis 2005). Consistent with this conceptualization, the S allele of the serotonin transporter gene confers a *lower* risk for depression in individuals who grow up in favorable early environments (Taylor et al. 2006).

In any event, because the search for so-called risk alleles for psychopathological conditions has been criticized for methodological reasons, and especially because the role of the serotonin transporter gene in depression has come under attack, with meta-analyses both in favor of and against its involvement (e.g., Clarke et al. 2010; Culverhouse et al. 2018), we need to emphasize that the heritability of mood disorders is polygenic, with individual candidate genes contributing only small effects to the phenotypic expression (Howard et al. 2019). It may nevertheless be fruitful to reframe research into the relevance of gene-environment interaction for mood disorders in a broader Darwinian perspective.

Conclusion

In this chapter, we set out to explore the evolutionary or "ultimate" dimensions of mood and mood disorders, while leaving aside the "proximate" factors, including the neurophysiological and endocrinological foundations of mood disorders, which are discussed in other chapters of this text (see Chapter 5, "Neurochemistry of Mood Disorders"; and Chapter 6, "Psychoneuroendocrinology of Mood Disorders"). We also skipped the increasing evidence for a role of epigenetic changes in mood disorders (see Chapter 13, "Epigenetics of Mood Disorders") and shed only a sketchy light on immunological and genetic aspects of mood disorders (see Chapter 7, "Role of the Immune System in Mood Disorders"; and Chapter 12, "Genetics of Mood Disorders"), as well as the impact of coevolutionary processes of the human microbiota on brain function (Cryan and Dinan 2012). Instead, we have focused on the role of low mood as a defense mechanism against abandonment and social threats, and on its protective role for organisms in times of increased vulnerability, in contrast to high mood, which is a mechanism for resource and/or social attainment.

At a general level, symptoms associated with clinical depression such as avolition and anergia can be understood as imbalances between active and passive responses to threat (LeDoux and Daw 2018). However, it is a common misconception to believe that positive mood states are superior to low mood states simply because the latter are associated with potentially disadvantageous situations and subjectively bad feelings. Even suicidal behavior may be interpreted, under specific circumstances, as biologically advantageous (in the evolutionary sense). For example, "perceived burdensomeness" toward kin may undermine self-preservation motives, such that sacrificing one's own life may eventually foster survival of one's genes (Joiner et al. 2002). From an evolutionary point of view, killing oneself is, however, such a tremendously costly behavior (aside from being a personal tragedy, of course) that eusocial motives or entrapment can certainly not fully account for such a multifaceted phenomenon that is putatively human specific (even though self-sacrificial behavior is widespread in eusocial animals) (Chiurliza et al. 2018). Although an evolutionary analysis of suicidality is beyond the scope of this chapter, we assert that severe clinical depression does not serve adaptive purposes. However, the boundaries between adaptive low or high mood and maladaptive depression or mania may wax and wane with individual ecological contingencies and have likely become more prominent as the modern environment differs from the environment of evolutionary adaptedness, and hence are difficult to determine (Wilson 1998). Recent calculations suggest that the global prevalence of unipolar depression is about 8 times that of bipolar disorder, 14 times that of schizophrenia, and 34 times that of autism spectrum disorder, and therefore is too frequent to conclude that it is always associated with biological malfunction. Moreover, mood disorders may be the only major psychiatric condition to be associated with increased biological fitness (i.e., fecundity), especially in women (Durisko et al. 2015). This idea is consistent with evolutionary explanations for sex differences in prevalence of depression as well as hypersexuality in mania. Women are twice as vulnerable to developing depression as men, which could relate to the biological fact that they invest much more in offspring and thus are more dependent on support from their mates and close kin (Troisi 2001). Therefore, the risk of losing important social connections when engaging in conflict-escalating strategies may be more relevant for women than men, even though this is not reflected in differences in the prevalence of bipolar disorder. In contrast, the preservation of genes predisposing to (hypo)mania may, in part, relate to the enhanced creativity, charisma, and leadership found in first-degree relatives of patients with bipolar disorder, all of which likely serve as proxies for reproductive success (Wilson 1998).

Understanding mood and mood disorders in an evolutionary perspective can also be informative with regard to therapy. One conclusion could be that it might not always be useful to suppress low mood, just as it is not always helpful to block cough, fever, or pain. Instead, it might be more appropriate to analyze individual needs in terms of mood regulation systems, including motivation, affiliation, and safeness, as conceptualized in compassion-focused therapy (Gilbert 2014).

Evolutionary accounts of psychopathology, including this abbreviated consideration of mood and mood disorders, have limitations and certainly many critics. Nevertheless, because nothing in biology really makes sense except from an evolutionary perspective, additional research on the evolved bases of mood and its disorders will surely make further and significant contributions (Dobzhansky 1973).

References

Allen NB, Badcock PB: The social risk hypothesis of depressed mood: evolutionary, psychosocial, and neurobiological perspectives. Psychol Bull 129(6):887–913, 2003 14599287

Anders S, Tanaka M, Kinney DK: Depression as an evolutionary strategy for defense against infection. Brain Behav Immun 31:9–22, 2013 23261774

Andrews PW, Thomson JA Jr: The bright side of being blue: depression as an adaptation for analyzing complex problems. Psychol Rev 116(3):620–654, 2009 19618990

Barnes E: Diseases and Human Evolution. Albuquerque, University of New Mexico Press, 2005

Belsky J: Modern evolutionary theory and patterns of attachment, in Handbook of Attachment: Theory, Research, and Clinical Applications. Edited by Cassidy J, Shaver PR. New York, Guilford, 1999, pp 141–180

Bogin B: Evolutionary perspective on human growth. Annu Rev Anthropol 28:109–153, 1999 12295621

Bowlby J: Attachment and Loss, Vol. 1: Attachment. London: Hogarth Press/Institute of Psycho-Analysis, 1969

Boyce WT, Ellis BJ: Biological sensitivity to context, I: an evolutionary-developmental theory of the origins and functions of stress reactivity. Dev Psychopathol 17(2):271–301, 2005 16761546

Brüne M: On aims and methods of psychiatry—a reminiscence of 50 years of Tinbergen's famous questions about the biology of behavior. BMC Psychiatry 14(1):1695, 2014 25528560

Brüne M: Borderline personality disorder: why "fast and furious"? Evol Med Public Health 2016(1):52–66, 2016a 26929090

Brüne M: Textbook of Evolutionary Psychiatry and Psychosomatic Medicine: The Origins of Psychopathology, 2nd Edition. Oxford, UK, Oxford University Press, 2016b
Campbell BC: Human biology, energetics, and the human brain, in Human Evolutionary Biology. Edited by Muehlenbein MP. Cambridge, UK, Cambridge University Press, 2010, pp 425–438
Carvalho S, Pinto-Gouveia J, Pimentel P, et al: Entrapment and defeat perceptions in depressive symptomatology: through an evolutionary approach. Psychiatry 76(1):53–67, 2013 23458115
Caspi A, Sugden K, Moffitt TE, et al: Influence of life stress on depression: moderation by a polymorphism in the 5-HTT gene. Science 301(5631):386–389, 2003 12869766
Chiurliza B, Rogers ML, Schneider ME, et al: Evolutionary processes in suicide. Curr Opin Psychol 22:84–88, 2018 28961457
Clarke H, Flint J, Attwood AS, Munafò MR: Association of the 5-HTTLPR genotype and unipolar depression: a meta-analysis. Psychol Med 40(11):1767–1778, 2010 20380781
Confer JC, Easton JA, Fleischman DS, et al: Evolutionary psychology: controversies, questions, prospects, and limitations. Am Psychol 65(2):110–126, 2010 20141266
Cryan JF, Dinan TG: Mind-altering microorganisms: the impact of the gut microbiota on brain and behaviour. Nat Rev Neurosci 13(10):701–712, 2012 22968153
Culverhouse RC, Saccone NL, Horton AC, et al: Collaborative meta-analysis finds no evidence of a strong interaction between stress and 5-HTTLPR genotype contributing to the development of depression. Mol Psychiatry 23(1):133–142, 2018 28373689
Damasio A, Carvalho GB: The nature of feelings: evolutionary and neurobiological origins. Nat Rev Neurosci 14(2):143–152, 2013 23329161
Dantzer R, Kelley KW: Twenty years of research on cytokine-induced sickness behavior. Brain Behav Immun 21(2):153–160, 2007 17088043
Darwin C: The Expression of the Emotions in Man and Animals. London, John Murray, 1872, p 178
Del Giudice M: An evolutionary life history framework for psychopathology. Psychological Inquiry 25:261–300, 2014
de Waal FBM: Chimpanzee Politics: Power and Sex Among Apes. Baltimore, MD, Johns Hopkins University Press, 1989
Dobzhansky T: Nothing in biology makes sense except in the light of evolution. American Biology Teacher 35(3):125–129, 1973
Dunbar RI, Shultz S: Understanding primate brain evolution. Philos Trans R Soc Lond B Biol Sci 362(1480):649–658, 2007 17301028
Durisko Z, Mulsant BH, Andrews PW: An adaptationist perspective on the etiology of depression. J Affect Disord 172:315–323, 2015 25451432
Eisenberger NI, Moieni M, Inagaki TK, et al: In sickness and in health: the co-regulation of inflammation and social behavior. Neuropsychopharmacology 42(1):242–253, 2017 27480575
Ellis BJ, Shirtcliff EA, Boyce WT, et al: Quality of early family relationships and the timing and tempo of puberty: effects depend on biological sensitivity to context. Dev Psychopathol 23(1):85–99, 2011 21262041
Engel GL: The need for a new medical model: a challenge for biomedicine. Science 196(4286):129–136, 1977 847460
Feder A, Nestler EJ, Charney DS: Psychobiology and molecular genetics of resilience. Nat Rev Neurosci 10(6):446–457, 2009 19455174
Gardner R Jr: Mechanisms in manic-depressive disorder: an evolutionary model. Arch Gen Psychiatry 39(12):1436–1441, 1982 7149905
Geerts E, Brüne M: Ethological approaches to psychiatric disorders: focus on depression and schizophrenia. Aust N Z J Psychiatry 43(11):1007–1015, 2009 20001396
Geerts E, van Os T, Gerlsma C: Nonverbal communication sets the conditions for the relationship between parental bonding and the short-term treatment response in depression. Psychiatry Res 165(1–2):120–127, 2009 19042029
Gilbert P: Depression: The Evolution of Powerlessness. London, Routledge & Kegan Paul, 1992

Gilbert P: Evolution and depression: issues and implications. Psychol Med 36(3):287–297, 2006 16236231
Gilbert P: The origins and nature of compassion focused therapy. Br J Clin Psychol 53(1):6–41, 2014 24588760
Gilbert P, Allan S: The role of defeat and entrapment (arrested flight) in depression: an exploration of an evolutionary view. Psychol Med 28(3):585–598, 1998 9626715
Gilbert P, Allan S, Brough S, et al: Relationship of anhedonia and anxiety to social rank, defeat and entrapment. J Affect Disord 71(1–3):141–151, 2002 12167510
Gilbert P, Gilbert J, Irons C: Life events, entrapments and arrested anger in depression. J Affect Disord 79(1–3):149–160, 2004 15023489
Gilbert P, McEwan K, Irons JHC, Cheung M: Social rank and attachment in people with a bipolar disorder. Clinical Psychology and Psychotherapy 14:48–53, 2007
Hagen EH: Evolutionary theories of depression: a critical review. Can J Psychiatry 56(12):716–726, 2011 22152640
Hamilton WD: The genetical evolution of social behaviour, I. J Theor Biol 7(1):1–16, 1964 5875341
Hochberg Z, Belsky J: Evo-devo of human adolescence: beyond disease models of early puberty. BMC Med 11:113, 2013 23627891
Homberg JR, Lesch KP: Looking on the bright side of serotonin transporter gene variation. Biol Psychiatry 69(6):513–519, 2011 21047622
Howard DM, Adams MJ, Clarke TK, et al; 23andMe Research Team; Major Depressive Disorder Working Group of the Psychiatric Genomics Consortium: Genome-wide meta-analysis of depression identifies 102 independent variants and highlights the importance of the prefrontal brain regions. Nat Neurosci 22(3):343–352, 2019 30718901
Hrdy SB: Mother Nature: Maternal Instincts and How They Shape the Human Species. London, Vintage, 2000
Hurst JE, Kavanagh PS: Life history strategies and psychopathology: the faster the life strategies, the more symptoms of psychopathology. Evolution and Human Behavior 38(1):1–8, 2017
Joiner TE, Pettit JW, Walker RL, et al: Perceived burdensomeness and suicidality: two studies on the suicide notes of those attempting and those completing suicide. Journal of Social and Clinical Psychology 21(5):531–545, 2002
Keller MC, Nesse RM: Is low mood an adaptation? Evidence for subtypes with symptoms that match precipitants. J Affect Disord 86(1):27–35, 2005 15820268
LeDoux J, Daw ND: Surviving threats: neural circuit and computational implications of a new taxonomy of defensive behaviour. Nat Rev Neurosci 19(5):269–282, 2018 29593300
Mathers CD, Loncar D: Projections of global mortality and burden of disease from 2002 to 2030. PLoS Med 3(11):e442, 2006 17132052
Mayr E: What Evolution Is. New York, Basic Books, 2001
Monroe SM, Simons AD: Diathesis-stress theories in the context of life stress research: implications for the depressive disorders. Psychol Bull 110(3):406–425, 1991 1758917
Nesse RM: An Evolutionary Framework for the Understanding of Grief. New York, Springer, 2005
Nesse RM: Explaining depression: neuroscience is not enough, evolution is essential, in Understanding Depression: A Translational Approach. Edited by Pariente CM, Nesse RM, Nutt DJ, Wolpert L. Oxford, UK, Oxford University Press, 2009, pp 17–36
Nettle D, Bateson M: The evolutionary origins of mood and its disorders. Curr Biol 22(17):R712–R721, 2012 22975002
Panksepp J: Emotional endophenotypes in evolutionary psychiatry. Prog Neuropsychopharmacol Biol Psychiatry 30(5):774–784, 2006 16554114
Paus T, Keshavan M, Giedd JN: Why do many psychiatric disorders emerge during adolescence? Nat Rev Neurosci 9(12):947–957, 2008 19002191
Plotkin H: Evolutionary Thought in Psychology: A Brief History. London, Blackwell, 2004
Polanczyk G, Caspi A, Williams B, et al: Protective effect of CRHR1 gene variants on the development of adult depression following childhood maltreatment: replication and extension. Arch Gen Psychiatry 66(9):978–985, 2009 19736354
Preuschoft H: Mechanisms for the acquisition of habitual bipedality: are there biomechanical reasons for the acquisition of upright bipedal posture? J Anat 204(5):363–384, 2004 15198701

Price J: The dominance hierarchy and the evolution of mental illness. The Lancet 290(7509):243–246, 1967
Price JS, Wilson DR: Male Philopatry, Female Entrapment, and Sex Difference in the Incidence of Depressive Illness. Athens, GA, University of Athens Press, 2011, pp 36–41
Price J, Sloman L, Gardner R Jr, et al: The social competition hypothesis of depression. Br J Psychiatry 164(3):309–315, 1994 8199784
Price JS, Gardner RJ, Wilson DR, et al: Territory, rank and mental health: the history of an idea. Evolutionary Psychology 5(3):531–554, 2007
Raison CL, Miller AH: Pathogen-host defense in the evolution of depression: insights into epidemiology, genetics, bioregional differences and female preponderance. Neuropsychopharmacology 42(1):5–27, 2017 27629366
Rook GAW, Lowry CA: The hygiene hypothesis and affective and anxiety disorders, in The Hygiene Hypothesis and Darwinian Medicine. Edited by Rook GAW. Birkhäuser Verlag, Basel, Switzerland, 2009, pp 189–220
Schaller M: The behavioural immune system and the psychology of human sociality. Philos Trans R Soc Lond B Biol Sci 366(1583):3418–3426, 2011 22042918
Segrin C: Social skills deficits associated with depression. Clin Psychol Rev 20(3):379–403, 2000 10779900
Simpson JA: Attachment theory in modern evolutionary perspectives, in Handbook of Attachment: Theory, Research, and Clinical Applications. Edited by Cassidy J, Shaver PR. New York, Guilford, 1999, pp 115–140
Sloman L, Gardner R, Price J: Biology of family systems and mood disorders. Fam Process 28(4):387–398, 1989 2599065
Sloman L, Sturman ED, Price JS: Winning and losing: an evolutionary approach to mood disorders and their therapy. Can J Psychiatry 56(6):324–332, 2011 21756446
Spitz RA: Hospitalism: an inquiry into the genesis of psychiatric conditions in early childhood, in The Psychoanalytic Study of the Child, Vol 1. Edited by Eissler R. New York, International Universities Press, 1945, pp 53–74
Stearns SC: The Evolution of Life Histories. Oxford, UK, Oxford University Press, 1992
Stearns SC, Byars SG, Govindaraju DR, Ewbank D: Measuring selection in contemporary human populations. Nat Rev Genet 11(9):611–622, 2010 20680024
Syed SA, Beurel E, Loewenstein DA, et al: Defective inflammatory pathways in never-treated depressed patients are associated with poor treatment response. Neuron 99(5):914–924.e3, 2018 30146307
Taylor SE, Way BM, Welch WT, et al: Early family environment, current adversity, the serotonin transporter promoter polymorphism, and depressive symptomatology. Biol Psychiatry 60(7):671–676, 2006 16934775
Tinbergen N: On aims and methods of ethology. Zeitschrift für Tierpsychologie 20(4):410–433, 1963
Tooby J, Cosmides L: The past explains the present: emotional adaptations and the structure of ancestral environments. Ethology and Sociobiology 11(4–5):375–424, 1990
Trivers RL: Evolution of reciprocal altruism. The Quarterly Review of Biology 46(1):35–57, 1971
Troisi A: Gender differences in vulnerability to social stress: a Darwinian perspective. Physiol Behav 73(3):443–449, 2001 11438373
Troisi A: Displacement activities as a behavioral measure of stress in nonhuman primates and human subjects. Stress 5(1):47–54, 2002 12171766
Watson PJ, Andrews PW: Toward a revised evolutionary adaptationist analysis of depression: the social navigation hypothesis. J Affect Disord 72(1):1–14, 2002 12204312
Wells JC, DeSilva JM, Stock JT: The obstetric dilemma: an ancient game of Russian roulette, or a variable dilemma sensitive to ecology? Am J Phys Anthropol 149 (suppl 55):40–71, 2012 23138755
Wilson DR: Evolutionary epidemiology and manic depression. Br J Med Psychol 71(Pt 4):375–395, 1998 9875952
Wilson DR: Depression is an adaptation. Arch Gen Psychiatry 58(11):1086–1087, author reply 1085–1086, 2001 11695962

PART III

Investigating Mood Disorders

CHAPTER 9

Anatomical Pathology

Grazyna Rajkowska, Ph.D.

In people with mood disorders such as major depressive disorder (MDD) and bipolar disorder, brain imaging studies show reductions in volume, blood flow, and metabolism and altered connectivity in frontolimbic brain regions (see Chapter 11, "Brain Imaging," in this text). Changes in the number and density of neurons and glial cells in people with mood disorders represent a potential cellular and molecular basis for the aberrant in vivo morphology and functions of the frontolimbic brain regions.

Glial Pathology

Prominent decreases in the number and density of glial cells have been the most consistent cellular abnormality identified in mood disorders. As discussed in this section, early studies reported postmortem pathology of a nonspecific Nissl-stained population of glial cells in MDD and bipolar disorder, and subsequent studies using immunohistochemistry found morphometric alterations in specific types of glial cells such as astrocytes, oligodendrocytes, and microglia.

General Population of Glial Cells

Decreases in the number and density of a general or nonspecific population of Nissl-stained glial cells were reported by independent laboratories in frontolimbic brain regions in MDD and bipolar disorder. A significant decrease in the number of glial cells was found in the subgenual anterior cingulate cortex in a small subgroup of subjects with either familial MDD or familial bipolar disorder, in comparison with controls (Ongür et al. 1998). Cell number in this study was estimated across all six cortical layers, with no information on laminar specificity of glial loss. In finer detail, reductions in glial cell density were observed in layer VI of the supragenual anterior cingulate cortex (Cotter et al. 2001), in layers III and V of the dorsolateral prefrontal cortex (Cotter et al. 2002b; Rajkowska et al. 1999, 2001), and in layers III–VI of the caudal orbitofrontal cortex (Rajkowska et al. 1999) in subjects with mood disorders. Another study found decreases in glial cell density in layers II–VI of the anterior cingulate cortex (Gittins and Harrison 2011). However, glial cell pathology in mood disorders is not noted throughout the cerebral cortex. Ongür et al. (1998) found no changes in the number of glial cells in the sensorimotor cortex in either MDD or bipolar disorder, whereas other researchers reported no changes in glial density in the supragenual part of the anterior cingulate cortex or the entorhinal cortex in bipolar disorder or MDD, or in the rostral orbitofrontal cortex in MDD (Bowley et al. 2002; Chana et al. 2003; Rajkowska et al. 1999).

Glial pathology in mood disorders has also been studied in subcortical structures. Two studies found a significant decrease in glial cell density in the amygdala in subjects with MDD and unmedicated subjects with bipolar disorder (Bowley et al. 2002; Hamidi et al. 2004). However, other studies of the amygdala found no changes in the total number or density of glial cells in subjects with MDD or bipolar disorder (Bezchlibnyk et al. 2007; Rubinow et al. 2016). Likewise, in the hippocampus there was no significant difference between MDD and control subjects in total number or density of glial cells (Cobb et al. 2013).

Astrocytes

Astrocytes are the most numerous and versatile type of glial cells in the CNS. They are crucial to the neuronal microenvironment because of their role in regulating glucose metabolism, glutamate uptake, synaptic development and maturation, and the blood-brain barrier. Astrocytes have been suggested to be major contributors to general pathology of glial cells in mood disorders, as observed in postmortem studies (Rajkowska and Stockmeier 2013).

Decreases in astrocyte cell density and disruption in the cells' integrity have been reported in frontolimbic brain regions in MDD or bipolar disorder. Immunohistochemical examination of astrocytes using an antibody to glial fibrillary acidic protein (GFAP) in the gray matter of the dorsolateral prefrontal cortex revealed significant decreases in the density of astrocytes in a subgroup of younger patients (ages 30–45 years) with MDD as compared with younger control subjects and older patients (ages 46–86 years) with MDD (Miguel-Hidalgo et al. 2000). GFAP is a marker of astrocytes and an indicator of their integrity. Subsequently, GFAP levels were reduced in the same cortical region in these younger subjects with MDD as compared to age-matched control subjects, and GFAP levels were positively correlated with both age at onset of depression and age at time of death (Si et al. 2004). Together, these studies suggest that astrocyte pathology is characteristic of early-onset depression. Another study noted that later-onset depression features neuronal pathology (Rajkowska et al. 2005).

In addition to studies that examined astrocytes in cortical gray matter, other studies reported alterations in astrocyte pathology in frontal white matter in mood disorders. Reduced GFAP, detected autoradiographically, was observed in the white matter of the anterior cingulate cortex in a cohort including subjects with mood disorder (MDD or bipolar disorder) (Gittins and Harrison 2011). Enlarged cell bodies of white matter astrocytes were detected in the anterior cingulate cortex in depressed subjects who died by suicide (Torres-Platas et al. 2011). In another study, in the white matter of orbitofrontal cortex, no changes in the size of astrocyte cell bodies were noted; however, the density of GFAP-positive astrocytes and area fraction was decreased in MDD (Rajkowska et al. 2018). Decreased area fraction, but not density of GFAP immunostaining, was reported in the white matter adjacent to the dorsolateral prefrontal cortex in subjects with bipolar disorder (Hercher et al. 2014). Astrocyte pathology in cortical white matter may affect the changes in axon integrity that have been seen in neuroimaging studies in mood disorders, and thereby interfere with signal conduction.

Subcortical structures also exhibit astrocyte pathology. A decrease in the density of astrocytes positive for S100 calcium-binding protein B (S100B), a marker that is abundant in astrocytes, was identified in the hippocampus in subjects with MDD or bipolar disorder (Gos et al. 2013). The density of astrocytes labeled with GFAP, a marker of astrocyte integrity, was decreased in the hippocampus in MDD (Müller et al. 2001), but this decrease was only in MDD in the absence of an antidepressant drug (Cobb et al. 2016). This latter observation is supported by the study of an animal model of depression, suggesting that antidepressants can prevent an astrocyte deficit in the hippocampus in MDD (Czéh and Nagy 2018). The density of GFAP-positive astrocytes was also decreased in the amygdala in MDD but not in bipolar disorder (Altshuler et al. 2010). In addition, reduced GFAP expression was observed in the locus coeruleus (Chandley et al. 2013) and in the cerebellum (Fatemi et al. 2004) in MDD. Finally, the expression of GFAP mRNA and protein was decreased in the thalamus and caudate nucleus of depressed subjects who died by suicide, indicating dysfunction in astrocytes and their genes in these brain structures (Torres-Platas et al. 2016).

Furthermore, pathology in astrocytes in MDD is evident in studies on astrocytic endfeet, astrocytic gap junction channels, and astrocytic glutamate transporters. Each of these measures provides an assessment of the quantity and health of astrocytes. The coverage of blood vessels by astrocytic endfeet expressing aquaporin-4 was reduced in the orbitofrontal cortex in MDD, suggesting impaired blood flow and glucose uptake by astrocytes (Rajkowska et al. 2013). Decreased density and size of gap junctions and levels of connexin 43, the main protein subunit of astrocyte gap junctions, were detected in the orbitofrontal cortex in MDD (Miguel-Hidalgo et al. 2014). Furthermore, there was a downregulation of connexin 43 and connexin 30 mRNA in several brain regions of depressed subjects who died by suicide (Nagy et al. 2017); downregulation of these mRNAs suggests that decreases in astrocyte connexins are related to a decrease in the gene expression of these connexins. Changes in connexins in MDD likely alter the diffusion of ions and small molecules between astrocytes via gap junctions and may alter neurotransmission. Other proteins expressed by astrocytes, such as glutamate transporters and glutamine synthetase, were also decreased in the prefrontal cortex in MDD (Choudary et al. 2005; Miguel-Hidalgo et al. 2010), supporting the hypothesis of glutamatergic dysfunction in depression noted in clinical studies and animal models (Arnone et al. 2015).

Astrocyte dysfunction was reported in a molecular study investigating genome-wide differential methylation associated with depression and suicide (Nagy et al. 2015). Significant differences in the methylation patterns specific to astrocytic dysfunction were observed in the dorsolateral prefrontal cortex in subjects with MDD who died by suicide. Thus, astrocyte dysfunction in depression could involve epigenetic factors, such as DNA methylation, that modulate gene expression.

Oligodendrocytes

Oligodendrocytes support and insulate axons by creating the myelin sheath. Consequently, oligodendrocyte pathology can cause abnormal development, demyelination, or reduction of myelinated axons, which can alter neuronal circuitry in mood disorders. The involvement of oligodendrocytes in glial pathology is suggested in MDD and bipolar disorder.

Reductions in the level of myelin basic protein, a marker for mature oligodendrocytes, were found in the anterior frontal cortex of depressed subjects who died by suicide (Honer et al. 1999). In other studies, ultrastructural changes in oligodendrocytes suggestive of apoptosis and necrosis were observed in the anterior frontal cortex in bipolar disorder (Uranova et al. 2001), and there were significant decreases in the cell density of Nissl-stained oligodendrocytes in layer VI of the dorsolateral prefrontal cortex in MDD and bipolar disorder (Uranova et al. 2004). In addition, there was a prominent reduction in the number of perineuronal oligodendrocytes in layer III in the dorsolateral prefrontal cortex in MDD and bipolar disorder (Vostrikov et al. 2007). Reduced density of oligodendrocytes was also found in the anterior frontal cortex in MDD (Hayashi et al. 2011).

Oligodendrocyte morphometry in frontal white matter has also been examined in mood disorders. Increased density of Nissl-stained oligodendrocytes was reported in the white matter of the dorsolateral prefrontal cortex in bipolar disorder (Hercher et al. 2014). Reductions in soma size of CNPase-positive oligodendrocytes, but not cell density, were observed in the white matter underlying the ventral prefrontal cortex in MDD (Rajkowska et al. 2015). Finally, greater thickness of myelinated fibers was detected in the genu of the corpus callosum in MDD (Williams et al. 2015).

Oligodendrocyte pathology was also reported in subcortical structures in mood disorders. In a study in the amygdala, in which oligodendrocytes were identified solely by morphometry in Nissl-stained sections, the density of oligodendrocytes was decreased in subjects with MDD and in unmedicated subjects with bipolar disorder (Bowley et al. 2002). In bipolar disorder, the density of oligodendrocytes immunostained with S100B, a marker of oligodendrocyte integrity, was decreased in the hippocampus (Gos et al. 2013).

Molecular pathology of oligodendrocytes has been reported in mood disorders. The expression of key oligodendrocyte-specific and myelin-associated genes is decreased in the dorsolateral prefrontal cortex in bipolar disorder (Tkachev et al. 2003) and in the temporal cortex in MDD (Aston et al. 2005). Another study found increased or decreased expression of similar genes (per Aston et al.) in the white matter of the ventral prefrontal cortex in MDD (Rajkowska et al. 2015). Cellular and molecular pathology of oligodendrocytes may underlie the altered frontolimbic connectivity seen with diffusion tensor imaging in MDD and bipolar disorder (reviewed in Czéh and Nagy 2018).

Microglia

Microglia, the third type of glial cells, are the primary immune cells of the CNS and are functionally similar to peripheral macrophages. Microglia act as the major inflammatory cell type in the brain, so abnormalities in microglia support the hypothesis that neuroinflammation contributes to the pathophysiology of depression (Mechawar and Savitz 2016; Rosenblat et al. 2014; Yirmiya et al. 2015). For example, activated microglia are reported in the hippocampus, anterior cingulate cortex, prefrontal cortex, and thalamus of the postmortem brains of depressed subjects and depressed subjects who died by suicide (Bayer et al. 1999; Steiner et al. 2008; Torres-Platas et al. 2014). A recent review of postmortem studies notes changes in microglial neuroinflammatory markers in the frontal cortex, dorsal raphe, and hippocampus in bipolar disorder (Giridharan et al. 2020). Altered neuroinflammatory gene expression has been detected in the prefrontal cortex and hippocampus in MDD (Mahajan et al. 2018; Shelton et al. 2011). Moreover, there is increased density of the translocator protein, a marker of activated microglia and neuroinflammation, in the prefrontal cortex, anterior cingulate cortex, hippocampus, and insula during major depressive episodes (Setiawan et al. 2015). Another in vivo study provides evidence for focal neuroinflammation in the hippocampus but not prefrontal cortex in bipolar disorder (Haarman et al. 2014).

Neuronal Pathology

Neuronal pathology in mood disorders is less obvious than glial pathology because the former is found in fewer brain regions than glial pathology (Bowley et al. 2002; Cotter et al. 2001, 2002b; Ongür et al. 1998). Moreover, if changes in neuronal density and/or size are detected, these changes are smaller in magnitude than those in glial cells. Neuronal pathology is not evident when the general population of Nissl-stained neurons is analyzed (Cotter et al. 2002b; Ongür et al. 1998; Rajkowska et al. 1999, 2001). Significant reductions are found in both MDD and bipolar disorder only when neurons are analyzed in individual cortical layers or in size-dependent or immunohistochemistry-dependent separate subtypes.

Cerebral Cortex

In postmortem studies of mood disorders, reductions in neuronal density and soma size have been found in association cortices but not in the primary sensory cortical regions. The density of large neurons was decreased in layers II–VI of the dorsolateral prefrontal and orbitofrontal cortices in MDD (Rajkowska et al. 1999). In addition, in MDD, smaller sizes of neuronal cell bodies were reported in certain layers in these same brain regions plus the anterior cingulate cortex (Cotter et al. 2001, 2002b; Rajkowska et al. 1999). Decreases in laminar neuronal density were also detected in the dorsolateral prefrontal and anterior cingulate cortices in bipolar disorder (Benes et al. 2001; Bouras et al. 2001; Cotter et al. 2002a; Rajkowska et al. 2001). Moreover, reduced density of layer II nonpyramidal (presumably GABAergic) neurons and of layer III and V pyramidal (presumably glutamatergic) neurons was observed in the same brain regions in bipolar disorder (Benes et al. 2001; Rajkowska et al. 2001). Pathology of layer II GABAergic neurons in bipolar disorder was confirmed by a study using an antibody to calbindin (Cotter et al. 2002a). Calbindin-positive neurons are a subset of GABA neurons. A decrease in calbindin-positive neuron density was also found in the dorsolateral prefrontal and occipital cortices in MDD (Maciag et al. 2010; Rajkowska et al. 2007). A reduction in GABA cell density coincides with clinical evidence of decreased levels of cortical GABA in MDD (Hasler et al. 2007; Sanacora et al. 2000).

Glutamatergic, in addition to GABAergic, neuron pathology has been detected in mood disorders. The density of pyramidal neurons was decreased in cortical layers III, V, and VI of the orbitofrontal cortex and in deep sublayer Vb of the anterior cingulate cortex in mood disorders (Gittins and Harrison 2011; Rajkowska et al. 2005). There may be a deficit in glutamatergic neurotransmission in mood disorders, as pyramidal neurons of layers III, V, and VI use glutamate as a neurotransmitter. The role of the glutamatergic system in the pathophysiology and treatment of mood disorders is further supported by postmortem, clinical, and preclinical studies (e.g., Deschwanden et al. 2011; Duman et al. 2019; Feyissa et al. 2009; Kadriu et al. 2019; Kugaya and Sanacora 2005). Interestingly, the drug ketamine, an antagonist at glutamatergic *N*-methyl-D-aspartate receptors, produces a rapid antidepressant effect in people with treatment-resistant MDD (Kadriu et al. 2019).

Pathology of cortical neurons in mood disorders coincides with a substantial reduction in the number of synapses. The density of dendritic spine synapses was nearly halved in the dorsolateral prefrontal cortex in MDD, as determined by electron microscopy (Kang et al. 2012). In both PET and functional MRI (fMRI) studies, both synaptic density and functional connectivity were decreased in the dorsolateral prefrontal and anterior cingulate cortices in MDD (Holmes et al. 2019). Rodent models of depression and stress have been used to examine synaptic structure and function, because there is evidence of neuronal atrophy, reduced synaptic density, and cell loss (reviewed in Duman and Aghajanian 2012).

Hippocampus

Morphometric studies have examined the hippocampal formation in mood disorders. In a detailed stereological estimation of the total number of neurons in all hippocampal substructures, there were no significant changes in MDD (Cobb et al. 2013). However, an increase in the density of pyramidal neurons with a longer duration of depression may explain the reduction in hippocampal volume in imaging studies of MDD (Sheline et al. 1996). In a study of bipolar disorder, there was a decrease in the density and size of nonpyramidal neurons in a hippocampal subregion (Benes et al. 1998).

Subcortical Structures

Morphometric studies in the hypothalamus, amygdala, and brain stem nuclei in mood disorders reveal mixed and inconsistent findings—namely increases, decreases, or no change in the cell number or density. For example, the numbers of specific populations of immunoreactive neurons in the hypothalamus were increased in mood disorders (Purba et al. 1996; Raadsheer et al. 1994; Swaab et al. 1993), consistent with activation of the hypothalamic-pituitary-adrenal (HPA) axis in some individuals with depression (Holsboer et al. 1992). The number and density of serotonin-immunoreactive neurons were increased in the dorsal raphe of depressed subjects who died by suicide compared with controls (Underwood et al. 1999). There was no difference in the number of noradrenergic neurons in the locus coeruleus between MDD patients and control subjects; however, there was a reduction in the level of noradrenergic transporters on these neurons in subjects with MDD, suggesting a compensatory downregulation of this transporter in response to an insufficient availability of norepinephrine at the synapse (Klimek et al. 1997). Finally, there were no changes in neuronal density or number of neurons in the amygdala in MDD or bipolar disorder (Bowley et al. 2002; Rubinow et al. 2016).

Attempts to Reverse Cell Pathology With Antidepressants and Mood Stabilizers

It remains to be determined whether cellular changes found in mood disorders represent the cause or the consequence of the disease, or are a response to medication (or some combination of all of these mechanisms). Because studies of postmortem tissue are cross-sectional rather than longitudinal, identifying a temporal sequence of cell pathology remains elusive. However, there is strong evidence from an animal model of stress showing that loss of glial cells in the prefrontal cortex induces depression-like behaviors (Banasr and Duman 2008). Interestingly, unpredictable stress-induced glial loss can be reversed by riluzole, a glutamate-modulating drug (Banasr et al. 2010). Earlier stress-related models of depression revealed that loss of glial cells and diminished neurogenesis in the hippocampus and medial prefrontal cortex were reversed by treatment with the antidepressant fluoxetine (Czéh and Nagy 2018; Malberg and Duman 2003). Moreover, it was reported that antidepressant therapies act directly on astrocytes, modifying their function and morphology (Czéh and Nagy 2018; Zhao et al. 2018). In addition to antidepressant drug treatment, electroconvulsive therapy stimulates the proliferation of hippocampal progenitor cells (Madsen et al. 2000; Scott et al. 2000). The mood stabilizer lithium can also increase hippocampal neurogenesis in mice (Chen et al. 2000) and the number of mature neurons and glial cells in the hippocampus (Rajkowska et al. 2016). Hippocampal neurogenesis also occurs in the hippocampus of nonhuman primates and humans and is affected by stress and possibly depression in humans. In monkeys, stress-induced depression-like behavior and reduced hippocampal neurogenesis are prevented by treatment with fluoxetine (Perera et al. 2011). In MDD, cellular changes in the hippocampus suggest less neurogenesis (Boldrini et al. 2019). Subjects with MDD receiving antidepressant drugs that are selective serotonin reuptake inhibitors had more neural progenitor cells in the hippocampus than untreated MDD subjects and control subjects (Boldrini et al. 2012). Thus, at least some of the glial and neuronal cell loss or atrophy observed in mood disorders may be prevented or reversed by antidepressant or mood-stabilizing treatments.

Conclusion: Functional Consequences of Cell Pathology in Mood Disorders

Alterations in the cell number, density, and size of specific populations of brain cells, as well as their molecular pathology, may account for the brain dysfunction observed in MDD and bipolar disorder. For example, deficits in astrocytes may account for the glutamatergic system dysfunction observed in imaging and postmortem studies in MDD. Pathology of oligodendrocytes and myelin-related genes may underlie the disturbed connectivity of frontolimbic brain regions reported using diffusion tensor imaging in MDD and bipolar disorder. Neuroimaging studies implicate microglial alterations related to neuroimmune dysfunction in mood disorders. Pathology of glutamate and GABA neurons in postmortem tissues supports neuroimaging reports of glutamate and GABA changes in mood disorders. Increased numbers of hypothalamic neurons support the evidence for activation of the HPA axis in some depressed individuals.

Postmortem cell pathology in mood disorders suggests changes in cell plasticity and function rather than cell loss. These observations could be relevant to hypothesized stress-induced changes in gene expression related to signal transduction pathways and cell survival (neurotrophic/neuroprotective) factors. If cell loss has occurred in the brain in mood disorders, it can be hypothesized that the loss of neurons would be paralleled by an increase in astrocytes as evidenced in neurodegenerative disorders. Instead, in depression there are decreases in neuronal cell density, and not necessarily neuron loss, which are accompanied by decreases in glial cell density. Glial pathology appears to be more prominent than neuronal alterations in MDD. In addition, glial pathology is preferentially observed in younger versus older subjects with MDD. Lastly, removal of glia but not neurons is sufficient to induce depression-like behavior in animal models of depression. Therefore, we suggest that the cell pathology in depression begins with glia, and specifically astrocytes. With duration and progression of depression, insufficient glial support for neuronal functions may eventually lead to neuronal pathology (Rajkowska and Miguel-Hidalgo 2007).

References

Altshuler LL, Abulseoud OA, Foland-Ross L, et al: Amygdala astrocyte reduction in subjects with major depressive disorder but not bipolar disorder. Bipolar Disord 12(5):541–549, 2010 20712756

Arnone D, Mumuni AN, Jauhar S, et al: Indirect evidence of selective glial involvement in glutamate-based mechanisms of mood regulation in depression: meta-analysis of absolute prefrontal neuro-metabolic concentrations. Eur Neuropsychopharmacol 25(8):1109–1117, 2015 26028038

Aston C, Jiang L, Sokolov BP: Transcriptional profiling reveals evidence for signaling and oligodendroglial abnormalities in the temporal cortex from patients with major depressive disorder. Mol Psychiatry 10(3):309–322, 2005 15303102

Banasr M, Duman RS: Glial loss in the prefrontal cortex is sufficient to induce depressive-like behaviors. Biol Psychiatry 64(10):863–870, 2008 18639237

Banasr M, Chowdhury GM, Terwilliger R, et al: Glial pathology in an animal model of depression: reversal of stress-induced cellular, metabolic and behavioral deficits by the glutamate-modulating drug riluzole. Mol Psychiatry 15(5):501–511, 2010 18825147

Bayer TA, Buslei R, Havas L, et al: Evidence for activation of microglia in patients with psychiatric illnesses. Neurosci Lett 271(2):126–128, 1999 10477118

Benes FM, Kwok EW, Vincent SL, et al: A reduction of nonpyramidal cells in sector CA2 of schizophrenics and manic depressives. Biol Psychiatry 44(2):88–97, 1998 9646890

Benes FM, Vincent SL, Todtenkopf M: The density of pyramidal and nonpyramidal neurons in anterior cingulate cortex of schizophrenic and bipolar subjects. Biol Psychiatry 50(6):395–406, 2001 11566156

Bezchlibnyk YB, Sun X, Wang JF, et al: Neuron somal size is decreased in the lateral amygdalar nucleus of subjects with bipolar disorder. J Psychiatry Neurosci 32(3):203–210, 2007 17476367

Boldrini M, Hen R, Underwood MD, et al: Hippocampal angiogenesis and progenitor cell proliferation are increased with antidepressant use in major depression. Biol Psychiatry 72(7):562–571, 2012 22652019
Boldrini M, Galfalvy H, Dwork AJ, et al: Resilience is associated with larger dentate gyrus, while suicide decedents with major depressive disorder have fewer granule neurons. Biol Psychiatry 85(10):850–862, 2019 30819514
Bouras C, Kövari E, Hof PR, et al: Anterior cingulate cortex pathology in schizophrenia and bipolar disorder. Acta Neuropathol 102(4):373–379, 2001 11603813
Bowley MP, Drevets WC, Ongür D, et al: Low glial numbers in the amygdala in major depressive disorder. Biol Psychiatry 52(5):404–412, 2002 12242056
Chana G, Landau S, Beasley C, et al: Two-dimensional assessment of cytoarchitecture in the anterior cingulate cortex in major depressive disorder, bipolar disorder, and schizophrenia: evidence for decreased neuronal somal size and increased neuronal density. Biol Psychiatry 53(12):1086–1098, 2003 12814860
Chandley MJ, Szebeni K, Szebeni A, et al: Gene expression deficits in pontine locus coeruleus astrocytes in men with major depressive disorder. J Psychiatry Neurosci 38(4):276–284, 2013 23415275
Chen G, Rajkowska G, Du F, et al: Enhancement of hippocampal neurogenesis by lithium. J Neurochem 75(4):1729–1734, 2000 10987856
Choudary PV, Molnar M, Evans SJ, et al: Altered cortical glutamatergic and GABAergic signal transmission with glial involvement in depression. Proc Natl Acad Sci USA 102(43):15653–15658, 2005 16230605
Cobb JA, Simpson J, Mahajan GJ, et al: Hippocampal volume and total cell numbers in major depressive disorder. J Psychiatr Res 47(3):299–306, 2013 23201228
Cobb JA, O'Neill K, Milner J, et al: Density of GFAP-immunoreactive astrocytes is decreased in left hippocampi in major depressive disorder. Neuroscience 316:209–220, 2016 26742791
Cotter D, Mackay D, Landau S, et al: Reduced glial cell density and neuronal size in the anterior cingulate cortex in major depressive disorder. Arch Gen Psychiatry 58(6):545–553, 2001 11386983
Cotter D, Landau S, Beasley C, et al: The density and spatial distribution of GABAergic neurons, labelled using calcium binding proteins, in the anterior cingulate cortex in major depressive disorder, bipolar disorder, and schizophrenia. Biol Psychiatry 51(5):377–386, 2002a 11904132
Cotter D, Mackay D, Chana G, et al: Reduced neuronal size and glial cell density in area 9 of the dorsolateral prefrontal cortex in subjects with major depressive disorder. Cereb Cortex 12(4):386–394, 2002b 11884354
Czéh B, Nagy SA: Clinical findings documenting cellular and molecular abnormalities of glia in depressive disorders. Front Mol Neurosci 11:56, 2018 29535607
Deschwanden A, Karolewicz B, Feyissa AM, et al: Reduced metabotropic glutamate receptor 5 density in major depression determined by [(11)C]ABP688 PET and postmortem study. Am J Psychiatry 168(7):727–734, 2011 21498461
Duman RS, Aghajanian GK: Synaptic dysfunction in depression: potential therapeutic targets. Science 338(6103):68–72, 2012 23042884
Duman RS, Sanacora G, Krystal JH: Altered connectivity in depression: GABA and glutamate neurotransmitter deficits and reversal by novel treatments. Neuron 102(1):75–90, 2019 30946828
Fatemi SH, Laurence JA, Araghi-Niknam M, et al: Glial fibrillary acidic protein is reduced in cerebellum of subjects with major depression, but not schizophrenia. Schizophr Res 69(2–3):317–323, 2004 15469203
Feyissa AM, Chandran A, Stockmeier CA, et al: Reduced levels of NR2A and NR2B subunits of NMDA receptor and PSD-95 in the prefrontal cortex in major depression. Prog Neuropsychopharmacol Biol Psychiatry 33(1):70–75, 2009 18992785
Giridharan VV, Sayana P, Pinjari OF, et al: Postmortem evidence of brain inflammatory markers in bipolar disorder: a systematic review. Mol Psychiatry 25(1):94–113, 2020 31249382

Gittins RA, Harrison PJ: A morphometric study of glia and neurons in the anterior cingulate cortex in mood disorder. J Affect Disord 133(1–2):328–332, 2011 21497910

Gos T, Schroeter ML, Lessel W, et al: S100B-immunopositive astrocytes and oligodendrocytes in the hippocampus are differentially afflicted in unipolar and bipolar depression: a postmortem study. J Psychiatr Res 47(11):1694–1699, 2013 23896207

Haarman BC, Riemersma-Van der Lek RF, de Groot JC, et al: Neuroinflammation in bipolar disorder—a [(11)C]-(R)-PK11195 positron emission tomography study. Brain Behav Immun 40:219–225, 2014 24703991

Hamidi M, Drevets WC, Price JL: Glial reduction in amygdala in major depressive disorder is due to oligodendrocytes. Biol Psychiatry 55(6):563–569, 2004 15013824

Hasler G, van der Veen JW, Tumonis T, et al: Reduced prefrontal glutamate/glutamine and gamma-aminobutyric acid levels in major depression determined using proton magnetic resonance spectroscopy. Arch Gen Psychiatry 64(2):193–200, 2007 17283286

Hayashi Y, Nihonmatsu-Kikuchi N, Yu X, et al: A novel, rapid, quantitative cell-counting method reveals oligodendroglial reduction in the frontopolar cortex in major depressive disorder. Mol Psychiatry 16(12):1155–1158, 2011 21747396

Hercher C, Chopra V, Beasley CL: Evidence for morphological alterations in prefrontal white matter glia in schizophrenia and bipolar disorder. J Psychiatry Neurosci 39(6):376–385, 2014 24936776

Holmes SE, Scheinost D, Finnema SJ, et al: Lower synaptic density is associated with depression severity and network alterations. Nat Commun 10(1):1529, 2019 30948709

Holsboer F, Spengler D, Heuser I: The role of corticotropin-releasing hormone in the pathogenesis of Cushing's disease, anorexia nervosa, alcoholism, affective disorders and dementia. Prog Brain Res 93:385–417, 1992 1336204

Honer WG, Falkai P, Chen C, et al: Synaptic and plasticity-associated proteins in anterior frontal cortex in severe mental illness. Neuroscience 91(4):1247–1255, 1999 10391432

Kadriu B, Musazzi L, Henter ID, et al: Glutamatergic neurotransmission: pathway to developing novel rapid-acting antidepressant treatments. Int J Neuropsychopharmacol 22(2):119–135, 2019 30445512

Kang HJ, Voleti B, Hajszan T, et al: Decreased expression of synapse-related genes and loss of synapses in major depressive disorder. Nat Med 18(9):1413–1417, 2012 22885997

Klimek V, Stockmeier C, Overholser J, et al: Reduced levels of norepinephrine transporters in the locus coeruleus in major depression. J Neurosci 17(21):8451–8458, 1997 9334417

Kugaya A, Sanacora G: Beyond monoamines: glutamatergic function in mood disorders. CNS Spectr 10(10):808–819, 2005 16400244

Maciag D, Hughes J, O'Dwyer G, et al: Reduced density of calbindin immunoreactive GABAergic neurons in the occipital cortex in major depression: relevance to neuroimaging studies. Biol Psychiatry 67(5):465–470, 2010 20004363

Madsen TM, Treschow A, Bengzon J, et al: Increased neurogenesis in a model of electroconvulsive therapy. Biol Psychiatry 47(12):1043–1049, 2000 10862803

Mahajan GJ, Vallender EJ, Garrett MR, et al: Altered neuro-inflammatory gene expression in hippocampus in major depressive disorder. Prog Neuropsychopharmacol Biol Psychiatry 82:177–186, 2018 29175309

Malberg JE, Duman RS: Cell proliferation in adult hippocampus is decreased by inescapable stress: reversal by fluoxetine treatment. Neuropsychopharmacology 28(9):1562–1571, 2003 12838272

Mechawar N, Savitz J: Neuropathology of mood disorders: do we see the stigmata of inflammation? Transl Psychiatry 6(11):e946, 2016 27824355

Miguel-Hidalgo JJ, Baucom C, Dilley G, et al: Glial fibrillary acidic protein immunoreactivity in the prefrontal cortex distinguishes younger from older adults in major depressive disorder. Biol Psychiatry 48(8):861–873, 2000 11063981

Miguel-Hidalgo JJ, Waltzer R, Whittom AA, et al: Glial and glutamatergic markers in depression, alcoholism, and their comorbidity. J Affect Disord 127(1–3):230–240, 2010 20580095

Miguel-Hidalgo JJ, Wilson BA, Hussain S, et al: Reduced connexin 43 immunolabeling in the orbitofrontal cortex in alcohol dependence and depression. J Psychiatr Res 55:101–109, 2014 24774648

Müller MB, Lucassen PJ, Yassouridis A, et al: Neither major depression nor glucocorticoid treatment affects the cellular integrity of the human hippocampus. Eur J Neurosci 14(10):1603–1612, 2001 11860455

Nagy C, Suderman M, Yang J, et al: Astrocytic abnormalities and global DNA methylation patterns in depression and suicide. Mol Psychiatry 20(3):320–328, 2015 24662927

Nagy C, Torres-Platas SG, Mechawar N, et al: Repression of astrocytic connexins in cortical and subcortical brain regions and prefrontal enrichment of H3K9me3 in depression and suicide. Int J Neuropsychopharmacol 20(1):50–57, 2017 27516431

Ongür D, Drevets WC, Price JL: Glial reduction in the subgenual prefrontal cortex in mood disorders. Proc Natl Acad Sci USA 95(22):13290–13295, 1998 9789081

Perera TD, Dwork AJ, Keegan KA, et al: Necessity of hippocampal neurogenesis for the therapeutic action of antidepressants in adult nonhuman primates. PLoS One 6(4):e17600, 2011 21525974

Purba JS, Hoogendijk WJ, Hofman MA, et al: Increased number of vasopressin- and oxytocin-expressing neurons in the paraventricular nucleus of the hypothalamus in depression. Arch Gen Psychiatry 53(2):137–143, 1996 8629889

Raadsheer FC, Hoogendijk WJ, Stam FC, et al: Increased numbers of corticotropin-releasing hormone expressing neurons in the hypothalamic paraventricular nucleus of depressed patients. Neuroendocrinology 60(4):436–444, 1994 7824085

Rajkowska G, Miguel-Hidalgo JJ: Gliogenesis and glial pathology in depression. CNS Neurol Disord Drug Targets 6(3):219–233, 2007 17511618

Rajkowska G, Stockmeier CA: Astrocyte pathology in major depressive disorder: insights from human postmortem brain tissue. Curr Drug Targets 14(11):1225–1236, 2013 23469922

Rajkowska G, Miguel-Hidalgo JJ, Wei J, et al: Morphometric evidence for neuronal and glial prefrontal cell pathology in major depression. Biol Psychiatry 45(9):1085–1098, 1999 10331101

Rajkowska G, Halaris A, Selemon LD: Reductions in neuronal and glial density characterize the dorsolateral prefrontal cortex in bipolar disorder. Biol Psychiatry 49(9):741–752, 2001 11331082

Rajkowska G, Miguel-Hidalgo JJ, Dubey P, et al: Prominent reduction in pyramidal neurons density in the orbitofrontal cortex of elderly depressed patients. Biol Psychiatry 58(4):297–306, 2005 15953590

Rajkowska G, O'Dwyer G, Teleki Z, et al: GABAergic neurons immunoreactive for calcium binding proteins are reduced in the prefrontal cortex in major depression. Neuropsychopharmacology 32(2):471–482, 2007 17063153

Rajkowska G, Hughes J, Stockmeier CA, et al: Coverage of blood vessels by astrocytic endfeet is reduced in major depressive disorder. Biol Psychiatry 73(7):613–621, 2013 23146357

Rajkowska G, Mahajan G, Maciag D, et al: Oligodendrocyte morphometry and expression of myelin-related mRNA in ventral prefrontal white matter in major depressive disorder. J Psychiatr Res 65:53–62, 2015 25930075

Rajkowska G, Clarke G, Mahajan G, et al: Differential effect of lithium on cell number in the hippocampus and prefrontal cortex in adult mice: a stereological study. Bipolar Disord 18(1):41–51, 2016 26842627

Rajkowska G, Legutko B, Moulana M, et al: Astrocyte pathology in the ventral prefrontal white matter in depression. J Psychiatr Res 102:150–158, 2018 29660602

Rosenblat JD, Cha DS, Mansur RB, McIntyre RS: Inflamed moods: a review of the interactions between inflammation and mood disorders. Prog Neuropsychopharmacol Biol Psychiatry 53:23–34, 2014 24468642

Rubinow MJ, Mahajan G, May W, et al: Basolateral amygdala volume and cell numbers in major depressive disorder: a postmortem stereological study. Brain Struct Funct 221(1):171–184, 2016 25287512

Sanacora G, Mason GF, Krystal JH: Impairment of GABAergic transmission in depression: new insights from neuroimaging studies. Crit Rev Neurobiol 14(1):23–45, 2000 11253954
Scott BW, Wojtowicz JM, Burnham WM: Neurogenesis in the dentate gyrus of the rat following electroconvulsive shock seizures. Exp Neurol 165(2):231–236, 2000 10993683
Setiawan E, Wilson AA, Mizrahi R, et al: Role of translocator protein density, a marker of neuroinflammation, in the brain during major depressive episodes. JAMA Psychiatry 72(3):268–275, 2015 25629589
Sheline YI, Wang PW, Gado MH, et al: Hippocampal atrophy in recurrent major depression. Proc Natl Acad Sci USA 93(9):3908–3913, 1996 8632988
Shelton RC, Claiborne J, Sidoryk-Wegrzynowicz M, et al: Altered expression of genes involved in inflammation and apoptosis in frontal cortex in major depression. Mol Psychiatry 16(7):751–762, 2011 20479761
Si X, Miguel-Hidalgo JJ, O'Dwyer G, et al: Age-dependent reductions in the level of glial fibrillary acidic protein in the prefrontal cortex in major depression. Neuropsychopharmacology 29(11):2088–2096, 2004 15238995
Steiner J, Bielau H, Brisch R, et al: Immunological aspects in the neurobiology of suicide: elevated microglial density in schizophrenia and depression is associated with suicide. J Psychiatr Res 42(2):151–157, 2008 17174336
Swaab DF, Hofman MA, Lucassen PJ, et al: Functional neuroanatomy and neuropathology of the human hypothalamus. Anat Embryol (Berl) 187(4):317–330, 1993 8512084
Tkachev D, Mimmack ML, Ryan MM, et al: Oligodendrocyte dysfunction in schizophrenia and bipolar disorder. Lancet 362(9386):798–805, 2003 13678875
Torres-Platas SG, Hercher C, Davoli MA, et al: Astrocytic hypertrophy in anterior cingulate white matter of depressed suicides. Neuropsychopharmacology 36(13):2650–2658, 2011 21814185
Torres-Platas SG, Cruceanu C, Chen GG, et al: Evidence for increased microglial priming and macrophage recruitment in the dorsal anterior cingulate white matter of depressed suicides. Brain Behav Immun 42:50–59, 2014 24858659
Torres-Platas SG, Nagy C, Wakid M, et al: Glial fibrillary acidic protein is differentially expressed across cortical and subcortical regions in healthy brains and downregulated in the thalamus and caudate nucleus of depressed suicides. Mol Psychiatry 21(4):509–515, 2016 26033239
Underwood MD, Khaibulina AA, Ellis SP, et al: Morphometry of the dorsal raphe nucleus serotonergic neurons in suicide victims. Biol Psychiatry 46(4):473–483, 1999 10459396
Uranova N, Orlovskaya D, Vikhreva O, et al: Electron microscopy of oligodendroglia in severe mental illness. Brain Res Bull 55(5):597–610, 2001 11576756
Uranova NA, Vostrikov VM, Orlovskaya DD, et al: Oligodendroglial density in the prefrontal cortex in schizophrenia and mood disorders: a study from the Stanley Neuropathology Consortium. Schizophr Res 67(2–3):269–275, 2004 14984887
Vostrikov VM, Uranova NA, Orlovskaya DD: Deficit of perineuronal oligodendrocytes in the prefrontal cortex in schizophrenia and mood disorders. Schizophr Res 94(1–3):273–280, 2007 17566708
Williams MR, Sharma P, Fung KL, et al: Axonal myelin increase in the callosal genu in depression but not schizophrenia. Psychol Med 45(10):2145–2155, 2015 25712170
Yirmiya R, Rimmerman N, Reshef R: Depression as a microglial disease. Trends Neurosci 38(10):637–658, 2015 26442697
Zhao Y, Lin Z, Chen L, et al: Hippocampal astrocyte atrophy in a mouse depression model induced by corticosterone is reversed by fluoxetine instead of benzodiazepine diazepam. Prog Neuropsychopharmacol Biol Psychiatry 83:99–109, 2018 29369777

CHAPTER 10

Molecular and Cellular Neurobiology

Marianne Seney, Ph.D.
David A. Lewis, M.D.

In this chapter, we focus on studies performed in the human postmortem brain intended to characterize cellular and molecular alterations present in subjects with mood disorders. Although this review cannot be exhaustive of all reported findings, we focus on four overarching themes that have been repeatedly probed: alterations in numbers and morphology of brain cells, imbalances in glutamate and GABA neurotransmission, monoaminergic dysfunction, and disturbances in neurotrophin signaling.

Alterations in Cell Number and Morphology in Mood Disorders

Neurons

In the dorsolateral prefrontal cortex (DLPFC), neuronal density and size in both the supra- and infragranular layers have been reported to be lower in subjects with major depressive disorder (MDD) than in unaffected comparison subjects (Rajkowska et al. 1999). Ongür et al. (1998) reported that in Brodmann area 24 (BA24; also known as subgenual anterior cingulate cortex), overall neuronal number or size was found not to differ between unaffected comparison subjects, subjects with MDD, and subjects with bipolar disorder. Cotter et al. (2001), however, reported smaller neuronal size, specifically in layer VI, in MDD but not in bipolar disorder. Neuronal deficits have also been reported in the orbitofrontal cortex (OFC); these deficits appear to differ by subregion. In the rostral OFC, smaller size and lower density of neurons were found in cortical layers II–IV, whereas in the caudal OFC, smaller neuronal size, without a difference in density, was present in cortical layers V and VI (Rajkowska et al. 1999). In the hippocampus, smaller pyramidal neuron soma size was found in all subfields in subjects with MDD (Stockmeier et al. 2004), and lower numbers of neural progenitor cells and granule neurons in the anterior dentate gyrus were reported for subjects with MDD who died from suicide (Boldrini et al. 2013, 2019). However, in the basolateral amygdala, neuron number, neuron density, or both were reported to be unchanged in MDD (Bowley et al. 2002; Rubinow et al. 2016). Thus, deficits in neuronal number or density and size appear to be present in the brains of subjects with mood disorders, with evidence suggesting that these alterations are specific to certain brain regions. These brain region–specific alterations might be tied to the function of each region, with downstream effects on symptom presentation.

Glia

In the DLPFC, glial density and size were reported to be lower in subjects with MDD (Rajkowska et al. 1999). Numbers of glia in BA24 of subjects with MDD or bipolar disorder were also lower, accompanied by lower glial density in layer VI in subjects with MDD but not in subjects with bipolar disorder (Cotter et al. 2001). Alterations in glia were found in the OFC, with lower densities in upper cortical layers (II–IV) in the rostral OFC and in lower cortical layers (V and VI) in the caudal OFC (Rajkowska et al. 1999); lower glial fibrillary acidic protein (GFAP) expression in the rostral OFC suggests that astrocyte deficits at least partially underlie these glial reductions in the OFC in subjects with MDD (Miguel-Hidalgo et al. 2010). In the hippocampus, although no alterations were found in total glial cell numbers in the dentate gyrus (Boldrini et al. 2019), the total area of GFAP immunoreactivity (a marker of astrocytes) was lower in the dentate gyrus and *Cornu Ammonis* subfields 2/3 (CA2/3) in female but not in male subjects with MDD (Cobb et al. 2016). Additionally, astrocyte density was reported to be lower in the dentate gyrus hilus of unmedicated subjects with MDD (Cobb et al. 2016). Interestingly, although no neuronal alterations were found in the basolateral amygdala (Bowley et al. 2002; Rubinow et al. 2016), glial density was reported to be lower in subjects with MDD (Bowley et al. 2002). Results from a follow-up study by the same research group suggested that the lower total glia density might be due to lower oligodendrocyte density in subjects with MDD (but not bipolar disorder), with no differences in astrocyte or microglia density (Hamidi et al. 2004). When all results are considered, a single pattern of glial-related differences in mood disorders is not present across the brain. Rather, alterations appear to affect specific glial subtypes, often with brain region specificity.

Dendritic Spines

Dendritic spines, small morphological protrusions on pyramidal neuron dendrites, are the primary locations of excitatory synaptic inputs to these neurons (DeFelipe and Fariñas 1992). Given their importance for neuronal signaling, information coding, and memory storage, dendritic spines have been investigated in the context of mood disorders. In the DLPFC, numbers of spine synapses (as measured by electron microscopy) in layers II and III and dendritic processes (as measured by microtubule-associated protein 2 immunoreactivity) in layers III–V were reported to be lower in subjects with MDD (Kang et al. 2012). Two additional studies used Golgi staining to examine dendritic spines and length in DLPFC, both with a focus on basilar dendrites. One of these studies reported no differences in spine density in superficial or deep layer III but shorter dendritic length in deep layer III of 15 psychiatric patients, 12 of whom had MDD or bipolar disorder (Glantz and Lewis 2000). The other study reported lower spine density and shorter dendritic length in deep layer III of subjects with bipolar disorder compared with unaffected comparison subjects (Konopaske et al. 2014). In BA24, subjects with MDD who died from suicide exhibited no differences in length, branching, or spine density for basilar dendritic arbors of layer VI pyramidal neurons compared with unaffected comparison subjects; however, Hercher et al. (2010) reported that subjects with MDD exhibited fewer dendritic branches. In the hippocampus, negative associations were reported between anxiety or depressive symptoms and microtubule-associated protein 2–immunolabeled dendrites as well as synaptopodin-immunolabeled dendritic spines (Soetanto et al. 2010). Together, the available evidence suggests that subjects with mood disorders have lower levels of dendritic spines and/or dendritic complexity. However, possibly due to the technological challenges of examining dendritic spines in the human postmortem brain, only a few brain regions have been examined.

Evidence for Altered Neocortical Glutamate and GABA in Mood Disorders

In humans, 80% of neocortical neurons are excitatory and form 85% of synapses, whereas 20% of neocortical neurons are inhibitory and form 15% of synapses (Douglas and Martin 2007). Excitatory neurons use glutamate as the main excitatory neurotransmitter, sending excitatory signals within and across brain regions (Orrego and Villanueva 1993). Activity of these excitatory neurons is modulated by inhibitory interneurons that use GABA as their main neurotransmitter (DeFelipe et al. 2013; Fino et al. 2013). Postmortem studies of subjects with MDD or bipolar disorder found higher glutamate levels in the frontal cortex, suggesting that excitatory glutamatergic function is elevated in this brain region in both disorders (Hashimoto et al. 2007; Lan et al. 2009). In the OFC of subjects with MDD, lower levels of excitatory amino acid transporters 1 and 2, which are expressed in astrocytes and are responsible for recycling synaptic glutamate, were reported; lower expression of these transporters is consistent with higher levels of glutamate in subjects with MDD (Miguel-Hidalgo et al. 2010). Altered expressions of glutamate receptor genes and of genes related to glutamate recycling were reported in several cortical brain regions and in the amygdala of subjects with MDD who died from suicide (Sequeira et al. 2009), suggesting glutamatergic dysfunction in mood disorders. Evidence also suggests that some of these changes in glutamate-related genes might be sex specific in the DLPFC, with higher expression in females, but not in males, with MDD (Gray et al. 2015).

Several studies have also reported inhibitory GABA-related alterations in mood disorders. Subjects with MDD exhibited lower GABA concentrations in postmortem cortical brain tissue, suggesting that inhibitory GABAergic function is lower in the cortex of subjects with MDD (Honig et al. 1988). In line with findings of lower GABA

cortical microcircuits drives symptom expression in affected individuals. Depending on the brain region affected, shifts in excitation/inhibition balance due to glutamate and GABA deficits might drive particular mood-related symptoms controlled by each brain region.

Evidence for Altered Monoaminergic Function in Mood Disorders

Because many of the drugs used to treat mood-related symptoms modulate monoaminergic function, much research has focused on whether the serotonergic, noradrenergic, and dopaminergic systems are altered in the brains of subjects with mood disorders. We review some of these studies here.

Serotonergic System

Evidence suggests lower levels of serotonin (5-hydroxytryptamine [5-HT]) and 5-hydroxyindoleacetic acid (5-HIAA), a major metabolite of 5-HT, in the brain stem but not in the frontal cortex of subjects who died from suicide (Mann et al. 1989). However, because measuring 5-HT in the postmortem brain is challenging due to cellular and chemical degradation, most of what is known about serotonergic dysfunction in the postmortem brain in mood disorders is based on investigation of 5-HT receptor binding and expression (reviewed in Stockmeier 2003 and summarized here). Evidence suggests higher levels of agonist binding to the postsynaptic 5-HT type 1A (5-HT_{1A}) receptor in the ventrolateral prefrontal cortex (PFC), but no consistent changes elsewhere in the PFC or hippocampus, in individuals who died from suicide. Depending on the methodology used, evidence exists for both higher and lower levels of binding to 5-HT_{1A} autoreceptors in the midbrain dorsal raphe nucleus in depressed individuals who died from suicide; 5-HT_{1A} autoreceptors act to inhibit further release of 5-HT. For the postsynaptic 5-HT_{2A} receptor, higher levels of agonist binding in the dorsal PFC and hippocampus were reported for subjects with MDD as well as for subjects who died from suicide, with no changes in other regions of the PFC. For the 5-HT transporter, evidence in subjects who died from suicide, had MDD, or both suggests lower levels or no differences in binding in cerebral cortex. Studies also suggest no differences in 5-HT transporter binding in the midbrain dorsal raphe nucleus, pontine dorsal raphe, medial raphe, or locus coeruleus. Taken together, consistent results suggest higher binding to the 5-HT_{1A} receptor in the ventrolateral PFC and to the 5-HT_{2A} receptor in the dorsal PFC in subjects who died from suicide. Because the ventrolateral and dorsal PFC are both involved in cognition, alterations in serotonergic processes in subjects who died from suicide might suggest dysfunctional cognitive processes.

Noradrenergic System

Most noradrenergic neurons originate in the locus coeruleus and project throughout the brain. In subjects who died from suicide, had MDD, or both, levels of norepinephrine (also known as noradrenaline) were not found to differ across several brain regions, including the brain stem, hypothalamus, frontal cortex, amygdala, and striatum

(Beskow et al. 1976; Moses and Robins 1975; Pare et al. 1969; Riederer et al. 1980; but see Arango et al. 1993). However, lower levels of the norepinephrine metabolite methoxy-4-hydroxyphenylgycol were reported for some brain regions in subjects with MDD (Riederer et al. 1980). Related to norepinephrine synthesis, higher levels of tyrosine hydroxylase, the rate-limiting enzyme in catecholamine synthesis, were reported in the locus coeruleus of subjects with MDD (Zhu et al. 1999). Levels of the norepinephrine transporter, which removes norepinephrine from the synapse, are lower in the locus coeruleus in subjects with MDD (Klimek et al. 1997). Adrenergic receptor subtypes have differing effects, with α_1- and β-adrenoreceptors tending to have a stimulatory effect on cell signaling and α_2-adrenoreceptors tending to inhibit signaling. Several studies have examined receptor binding in the brains of subjects with mood disorders (reviewed in Cottingham and Wang 2012 and summarized with additional citations here). Higher levels of α_1-adrenoreceptor binding were seen in the frontal cortex in subjects who died from suicide, although no such differences were seen across multiple brain regions in antidepressant-treated subjects who died from suicide or in the PFC of subjects with MDD (Ferrier et al. 1986).

Findings regarding binding and expression of the α_2-adrenoreceptor and β-adrenoreceptors have also been mixed. Some studies reported higher levels of α_2-adrenoreceptor in frontal cortex and hippocampus in subjects who died from suicide, had MDD, or both (Rivero et al. 2014); some studies reported no difference (Ferrier et al. 1986); and one study reported lower levels (Gross-Isseroff et al. 2000). Results for α_2-adrenoreceptor binding in the locus coeruleus appear more consistent, with higher binding levels both in subjects who died from suicide and in subjects with MDD. For the β-adrenoreceptors, higher binding levels were reported for β_1-adrenoreceptors in the PFC of antidepressant-free subjects with MDD (Rivero et al. 2014), although no changes in β_1- or β_2-adrenoreceptors were reported in the hippocampus in subjects with MDD. Thus, with respect to adrenergic receptor subtype binding, results vary by receptor subtype and brain region, with inconsistent findings across studies. Some of these discrepancies may be due to methodology or to subject groups examined (e.g., subjects who died from suicide, subjects with MDD who died from suicide, subjects taking or not taking antidepressants). Moving forward, for greater insight into whether noradrenergic neurotransmission is altered in patients with mood disorders, future postmortem studies should carefully consider cohort design to disentangle effects driven by disease, suicide, and/or psychiatric medications.

Dopaminergic System

Amotivation and anhedonia are frequent symptoms of mood disorders. Given that these are regulated in part by dopamine-related circuits, it is not surprising that researchers have asked whether dopaminergic systems are altered in the brains of subjects with mood disorders. Most dopamine-producing neurons are found in brain stem nuclei, with projections throughout the brain. We summarize findings reviewed in Dunlop and Nemeroff (2007) and include additional reports. Although evidence suggests that dopamine levels are unaltered across multiple brain regions, including the brain stem, hypothalamus, and striatum, levels of dopamine metabolites do appear to be altered. For instance, lower levels of the dopamine metabolite dihydroxyphenylacetic acid were found in the striatum of antidepressant-free subjects with MDD who died from suicide, and higher levels of the dopamine metabolite homovanillic acid were found in the frontal cortex of subjects who died from suicide. Lower levels of tyrosine hydroxylase, the rate-limiting enzyme in catecholamine synthesis, were reported in the striatum of subjects with MDD who died from suicide (Pizzagalli et al. 2019). For the dopamine transporter, which is responsible for removing dopamine from the synapse, lower levels were found in the striatum (Pizzagalli et al. 2019), and lower levels of binding were reported for the central and basal nuclei of the amygdala of subjects with MDD (Klimek et al. 2002). At the dopamine receptor level, no changes in binding to the dopamine type 1 (D_1) receptor (which increases cell signaling) or type 2 (D_2) receptor (which decreases cell signaling) were found in the striatum of antidepressant-free subjects with MDD who died from suicide or in the dorsal striatum of subjects who died from suicide (Fitzgerald et al. 2017). Interestingly, however, although levels of D_1 and D_2 receptor binding are positively correlated in the dorsal striatum in unaffected comparison subjects, these binding levels are not correlated in subjects who died from suicide, suggesting dysregulation of these receptors (Fitzgerald et al. 2017). In the amygdala, higher levels of D_2/D_3 receptor binding were found in the central, basal, and lateral nuclei (Klimek et al. 2002) and higher expression of the dopamine receptor 4 gene *DRD4* was reported for the basal nucleus in subjects with MDD (Xiang et al. 2008) (like D_2 receptors, D_3 and D_4 receptors inhibit cell signaling).

Although D_1 and D_2 binding levels did not differ in the frontal cortex in subjects with mood disorders, investigation of splice variants provides another potential avenue for altered dopamine neurotransmission in these disorders. Splice variants are alternative forms of mRNA produced by the same gene; splice variants can produce different proteins with different functions, even though they are coded for by the same gene. Subjects with affective disorders exhibit lower expression levels of the dopamine receptor 2 gene *DRD2* short variant (thought to act as a presynaptic autoreceptor) and higher expression of the *DRD2* long variant (thought to mediate postsynaptic actions), as well as higher levels of *DRD1* in the DLPFC (Kaalund et al. 2014); these results suggest that altered splicing may play a role in the pathophysiology of affective disorders. Together, most of the evidence for dopaminergic dysfunction in the brains of subjects with mood disorders comes from measuring dopamine synthesis, metabolism, and transport, with less consistent findings for dopamine receptors. The findings suggest that dopaminergic activity is diminished in subjects with mood disorders, and that this deficit occurs through alterations in a variety of receptor variants as well as alterations in neurotransmitter release. Since dopamine is linked to motivation, concentration, and ability to experience pleasure, alterations in dopaminergic activity might underlie deficits in these functions in individuals with mood disorders.

Evidence for Altered Brain-Derived Neurotrophic Factor Function in Mood Disorders

Brain-derived neurotrophic factor (BDNF) is a neurotrophin that regulates neuron survival, plasticity, and synaptic function (Barde 1989; Korte et al. 1995; Linnarsson et al. 1997; Liu et al. 2004; Ma et al. 1998; Patterson et al. 1996). Given the importance of

BDNF to these basic brain functions, it is not surprising that BDNF dysfunction has been linked to psychiatric disorders. Indeed, researchers have found evidence of low levels of BDNF protein in the hippocampus (Banerjee et al. 2013; Dwivedi et al. 2003; Karege et al. 2005) and the PFC (Dwivedi et al. 2003; Karege et al. 2005) of subjects who died from suicide, and in the basolateral amygdala of female subjects with MDD (Guilloux et al. 2012). Similarly, pro-BDNF is lower in the right hippocampus (Dunham et al. 2009) and BDNF is lower in the anterior cingulate in subjects with MDD (Youssef et al. 2018). Gene expression analyses are consistent with protein-level deficits associated with mood disorders. For instance, evidence indicates lower levels of BDNF signaling in the anterior cingulate and entorhinal cortex in subjects with MDD (Thompson Ray et al. 2011; Tripp et al. 2012) and in the basolateral amygdala of female subjects with MDD (Guilloux et al. 2012). Thus, multiple lines of evidence suggest that BDNF signaling is lower in the brains of subjects with mood disorders. Low levels of neurotrophic support might underlie the reduced cell numbers reported in subjects with mood disorders (see section "Alterations in Cell Number and Morphology in Mood Disorders" earlier in this chapter). Because so many factors (e.g., genetics, age, sex, stress) influence BDNF, a number of different pathological pathways might lead to diminished BDNF signaling and subsequent mood-related deficits. Understanding how BDNF interacts with these factors might provide insight into why particular individuals are more susceptible to developing mood disorders.

Conclusion

In summary, human postmortem brain studies suggest that subjects with mood disorders exhibit many differences compared to unaffected comparison subjects. Although this chapter does not discuss all differences found in the postmortem brains of subjects with mood disorders, we have summarized findings from four general themes. In terms of number and morphology of brain cells, subjects with mood disorders appear to have alterations in neurons, glia, dendritic spines, and dendritic complexity; many of these findings are brain region specific. Subjects with mood disorders also exhibit alterations related to glutamate and GABA, potentially with increased glutamate signaling and decreased GABA signaling. Evidence also suggests monoaminergic signaling dysfunction in the postmortem brains of subjects with mood disorders. Finally, BDNF signaling appears to be lower in subjects with mood disorders.

These alterations might define different subtypes of mood disorder subjects (i.e., dysfunction in only one theme might be present in a particular mood disorder subtype). For instance, subjects who died from suicide might represent a subtype exhibiting distinct human postmortem brain pathology. However, a substantial proportion of subjects who die from suicide also have a mood disorder, presenting a challenge to disentangling the two. Studies that include subjects who died from suicide without a mood disorder may provide important insight into suicide-specific brain alterations. Indeed, evidence suggests that this may be the case, at least in terms of lower brain stem levels of 5-HT or 5-HIAA in subjects who died from suicide, independent of psychiatric diagnosis (Mann et al. 1989). Additionally, some postmortem brain differences seem to distinguish MDD and bipolar disorder. For instance, subjects with MDD, but not those with bipolar disorder, appear to exhibit smaller neuronal size in layer VI of the subgenual anterior cingulate (Cotter et al. 2001) and lower oligodendrocyte density in the basolateral amygdala (Hamidi et al. 2004). Also, subjects with bipolar disorder seem to have lower DLPFC levels of both somatostatin and parvalbumin mRNA, whereas subjects with MDD have a lower level of somatostatin mRNA, but not of parvalbumin mRNA, in this cortical region (Sibille et al. 2009); these differences might represent disease specificity in GABA-related alterations.

Another possibility to consider is that psychiatric medications may impact dependent measures investigated in the human postmortem brain. Although it is challenging to tease apart psychiatric medication effects, given that most subjects with mood disorders included in postmortem brain studies were taking at least one of these medications at the time of death, some studies have examined antidepressant-free subjects and still found differences from unaffected comparison subjects. For instance, lower striatal levels of dihydroxyphenylacetic acid were reported in antidepressant-free subjects with MDD who died from suicide, and higher PFC binding levels were reported for β_1-adrenoreceptors in antidepressant-free subjects with MDD (Rivero et al. 2014).

Although we have considered each of the four themes separately, it is likely that these alterations co-occur and interact in the brains of subjects with mood disorders. At this time, it is not possible to conclude whether these alterations co-occur, because most previous studies investigated measures relevant to only one theme. If alterations related to these four themes do co-occur in the brains of subjects with mood disorders, it is possible that one "upstream" factor (e.g., stress exposure, with potential interaction with genetic susceptibility) drives brain alterations related to all described themes. Indeed, evidence from rodent studies suggests that this may be the case, at least with respect to stress exposure. For instance, chronic stress leads to structural changes in brain cells, glutamate- and GABA-related alterations, monoaminergic dysfunction, and lower brain BDNF levels (reviewed in Belleau et al. 2019; Nowacka and Obuchowicz 2013). Researchers have yet to determine whether chronic stress, either during early life or in adulthood, might interact with genes, resulting in the postmortem brain pathology fitting all described themes.

In general, future postmortem studies should carefully consider cohort design, with adequate statistical power, as a strategy for disentangling the effects of disease, suicide, and/or psychiatric medications on brain alterations in mood disorders. Future studies might also examine multiple dependent measures (e.g., systems affected by stress exposures) that cross-cut these general themes.

References

Arango V, Ernsberger P, Sved AF, et al: Quantitative autoradiography of alpha 1- and alpha 2-adrenergic receptors in the cerebral cortex of controls and suicide victims. Brain Res 630(1–2):271–282, 1993 8118693

Banerjee R, Ghosh AK, Ghosh B, et al: Decreased mRNA and protein expression of BDNF, NGF, and their receptors in the hippocampus from suicide: an analysis in human postmortem brain. Clin Med Insights Pathol 6:1–11, 2013 24031163

Barde YA: Trophic factors and neuronal survival. Neuron 2(6):1525–1534, 1989 2697237

Belleau EL, Treadway MT, Pizzagalli DA: The impact of stress and major depressive disorder on hippocampal and medial prefrontal cortex morphology. Biol Psychiatry 85(6):443–453, 2019 30470559

Beskow J, Gottfries CG, Roos BE, et al: Determination of monoamine and monoamine metabolites in the human brain: post mortem studies in a group of suicides and in a control group. Acta Psychiatr Scand 53(1):7–20, 1976 1251756

Boldrini M, Santiago AN, Hen R, et al: Hippocampal granule neuron number and dentate gyrus volume in antidepressant-treated and untreated major depression. Neuropsychopharmacology 38(6):1068–1077, 2013 23303074

Boldrini M, Galfalvy H, Dwork AJ, et al: Resilience is associated with larger dentate gyrus, while suicide decedents with major depressive disorder have fewer granule neurons. Biol Psychiatry 85(10):850–862, 2019 30819514

Bowley MP, Drevets WC, Ongür D, et al: Low glial numbers in the amygdala in major depressive disorder. Biol Psychiatry 52(5):404–412, 2002 12242056

Cobb JA, O'Neill K, Milner J, et al: Density of GFAP-immunoreactive astrocytes is decreased in left hippocampi in major depressive disorder. Neuroscience 316:209–220, 2016 26742791

Cotter D, Mackay D, Landau S, et al: Reduced glial cell density and neuronal size in the anterior cingulate cortex in major depressive disorder. Arch Gen Psychiatry 58(6):545–553, 2001 11386983

Cottingham C, Wang Q: Alpha2 adrenergic receptor dysregulation in depressive disorders: implications for the neurobiology of depression and antidepressant therapy. Neurosci Biobehav Rev 36(10):2214–2225, 2012 22910678

DeFelipe J, Fariñas I: The pyramidal neuron of the cerebral cortex: morphological and chemical characteristics of the synaptic inputs. Prog Neurobiol 39(6):563–607, 1992 1410442

DeFelipe J, López-Cruz PL, Benavides-Piccione R, et al: New insights into the classification and nomenclature of cortical GABAergic interneurons. Nat Rev Neurosci 14(3):202–216, 2013 23385869

Douglas RJ, Martin KA: Mapping the matrix: the ways of neocortex. Neuron 56(2):226–238, 2007 17964242

Douillard-Guilloux G, Lewis D, Seney ML, et al: Decrease in somatostatin-positive cell density in the amygdala of females with major depression. Depress Anxiety 34(1):68–78, 2017 27557481

Dunham JS, Deakin JF, Miyajima F, et al: Expression of hippocampal brain-derived neurotrophic factor and its receptors in Stanley consortium brains. J Psychiatr Res 43(14):1175–1184, 2009 19376528

Dunlop BW, Nemeroff CB: The role of dopamine in the pathophysiology of depression. Arch Gen Psychiatry 64(3):327–337, 2007 17339521

Dwivedi Y, Rizavi HS, Conley RR, et al: Altered gene expression of brain-derived neurotrophic factor and receptor tyrosine kinase B in postmortem brain of suicide subjects. Arch Gen Psychiatry 60(8):804–815, 2003 12912764

Ferrier IN, McKeith IG, Cross AJ, et al: Postmortem neurochemical studies in depression. Ann NY Acad Sci 487:128–142, 1986 2436529

Fino E, Packer AM, Yuste R: The logic of inhibitory connectivity in the neocortex. Neuroscientist 19(3):228–237, 2013 22922685

Fitzgerald ML, Kassir SA, Underwood MD, et al: Dysregulation of striatal dopamine receptor binding in suicide. Neuropsychopharmacology 42(4):974–982, 2017 27402414

Glantz LA, Lewis DA: Decreased dendritic spine density on prefrontal cortical pyramidal neurons in schizophrenia. Arch Gen Psychiatry 57(1):65–73, 2000 10632234

Gray AL, Hyde TM, Deep-Soboslay A, et al: Sex differences in glutamate receptor gene expression in major depression and suicide. Mol Psychiatry 20(9):1057–1068, 2015 26169973

Gross-Isseroff R, Weizman A, Fieldust SJ, et al: Unaltered alpha(2)-noradrenergic/imidazoline receptors in suicide victims: a postmortem brain autoradiographic analysis. Eur Neuropsychopharmacol 10(4):265–271, 2000 10871708

Guilloux JP, Douillard-Guilloux G, Kota R, et al: Molecular evidence for BDNF- and GABA-related dysfunctions in the amygdala of female subjects with major depression. Mol Psychiatry 17(11):1130–1142, 2012 21912391
Hamidi M, Drevets WC, Price JL: Glial reduction in amygdala in major depressive disorder is due to oligodendrocytes. Biol Psychiatry 55(6):563–569, 2004 15013824
Hashimoto K, Sawa A, Iyo M: Increased levels of glutamate in brains from patients with mood disorders. Biol Psychiatry 62(11):1310–1316, 2007 17574216
Hercher C, Canetti L, Turecki G, et al: Anterior cingulate pyramidal neurons display altered dendritic branching in depressed suicides. J Psychiatr Res 44(5):286–293, 2010 19765721
Honig A, Bartlett JR, Bouras N, et al: Amino acid levels in depression: a preliminary investigation. J Psychiatr Res 22(3):159–164, 1988 3225786
Kaalund SS, Newburn EN, Ye T, et al: Contrasting changes in DRD1 and DRD2 splice variant expression in schizophrenia and affective disorders, and associations with SNPs in postmortem brain. Mol Psychiatry 19(12):1258–1266, 2014 24322206
Kang HJ, Voleti B, Hajszan T, et al: Decreased expression of synapse-related genes and loss of synapses in major depressive disorder. Nat Med 18(9):1413–1417, 2012 22885997
Karege F, Vaudan G, Schwald M, et al: Neurotrophin levels in postmortem brains of suicide victims and the effects of antemortem diagnosis and psychotropic drugs. Brain Res Mol Brain Res 136(1–2):29–37, 2005 15893584
Karolewicz B, Maciag D, O'Dwyer G, et al: Reduced level of glutamic acid decarboxylase-67 kDa in the prefrontal cortex in major depression. Int J Neuropsychopharmacol 13(4):411–420, 2010 20236554
Klempan TA, Sequeira A, Canetti L, et al: Altered expression of genes involved in ATP biosynthesis and GABAergic neurotransmission in the ventral prefrontal cortex of suicides with and without major depression. Mol Psychiatry 14(2):175–189, 2009 17938633
Klimek V, Stockmeier C, Overholser J, et al: Reduced levels of norepinephrine transporters in the locus coeruleus in major depression. J Neurosci 17(21):8451–8458, 1997 9334417
Klimek V, Schenck JE, Han H, et al: Dopaminergic abnormalities in amygdaloid nuclei in major depression: a postmortem study. Biol Psychiatry 52(7):740–748, 2002 12372665
Konopaske GT, Lange N, Coyle JT, et al: Prefrontal cortical dendritic spine pathology in schizophrenia and bipolar disorder. JAMA Psychiatry 71(12):1323–1331, 2014 25271938
Korte M, Carroll P, Wolf E, et al: Hippocampal long-term potentiation is impaired in mice lacking brain-derived neurotrophic factor. Proc Natl Acad Sci USA 92(19):8856–8860, 1995 7568031
Lan MJ, McLoughlin GA, Griffin JL, et al: Metabonomic analysis identifies molecular changes associated with the pathophysiology and drug treatment of bipolar disorder. Mol Psychiatry 14(3):269–279, 2009 18256615
Linnarsson S, Björklund A, Ernfors P: Learning deficit in BDNF mutant mice. Eur J Neurosci 9(12):2581–2587, 1997 9517463
Liu IY, Lyons WE, Mamounas LA, et al: Brain-derived neurotrophic factor plays a critical role in contextual fear conditioning. J Neurosci 24(36):7958–7963, 2004 15356210
Ma YT, Hsieh T, Forbes ME, et al: BDNF injected into the superior colliculus reduces developmental retinal ganglion cell death. J Neurosci 18(6):2097–2107, 1998 9482796
Maciag D, Hughes J, O'Dwyer G, et al: Reduced density of calbindin immunoreactive GABAergic neurons in the occipital cortex in major depression: relevance to neuroimaging studies. Biol Psychiatry 67(5):465–470, 2010 20004363
Mann JJ, Arango V, Marzuk PM, et al: Evidence for the 5-HT hypothesis of suicide. A review of post-mortem studies. Br J Psychiatry 155 (suppl 8):7–14, 1989 2692642
Miguel-Hidalgo JJ, Waltzer R, Whittom AA, et al: Glial and glutamatergic markers in depression, alcoholism, and their comorbidity. J Affect Disord 127(1–3):230–240, 2010 20580095
Moses SG, Robins E: Regional distribution of norepinephrine and dopamine in brains of depressive suicides and alcoholic suicides. Psychopharmacol Commun 1(3):327–337, 1975 1224002

Nowacka M, Obuchowicz E: BDNF and VEGF in the pathogenesis of stress-induced affective diseases: an insight from experimental studies. Pharmacol Rep 65(3):535–546, 2013 23950576

Ongür D, Drevets WC, Price JL: Glial reduction in the subgenual prefrontal cortex in mood disorders. Proc Natl Acad Sci USA 95(22):13290–13295, 1998 9789081

Orrego F, Villanueva S: The chemical nature of the main central excitatory transmitter: a critical appraisal based upon release studies and synaptic vesicle localization. Neuroscience 56(3):539–555, 1993 7902967

Packer AM, McConnell DJ, Fino E, et al: Axo-dendritic overlap and laminar projection can explain interneuron connectivity to pyramidal cells. Cereb Cortex 23(12):2790–2802, 2013 22941716

Pare CM, Yeung DP, Price K, et al: 5-Hydroxytryptamine, noradrenaline, and dopamine in brainstem, hypothalamus, and caudate nucleus of controls and of patients committing suicide by coal-gas poisoning. Lancet 2(7612):133–135, 1969 4183246

Patterson SL, Abel T, Deuel TA, et al: Recombinant BDNF rescues deficits in basal synaptic transmission and hippocampal LTP in BDNF knockout mice. Neuron 16(6):1137–1145, 1996 8663990

Pizzagalli DA, Berretta S, Wooten D, et al: Assessment of striatal dopamine transporter binding in individuals with major depressive disorder: in vivo positron emission tomography and postmortem evidence. JAMA Psychiatry 76(8):854–861, 2019 31042280

Rajkowska G, Miguel-Hidalgo JJ, Wei J, et al: Morphometric evidence for neuronal and glial prefrontal cell pathology in major depression. Biol Psychiatry 45(9):1085–1098, 1999 10331101

Rajkowska G, O'Dwyer G, Teleki Z, et al: GABAergic neurons immunoreactive for calcium binding proteins are reduced in the prefrontal cortex in major depression. Neuropsychopharmacology 32(2):471–482, 2007 17063153

Riederer P, Birkmayer W, Seemann D, et al: 4-Hydroxy-3-methoxyphenylglycol as an index of brain noradrenaline turnover in endogenous depression. Acta Psychiatr Scand Suppl 280:251–257, 1980 6996431

Rivero G, Gabilondo AM, García-Sevilla JA, et al: Increased alpha2- and beta1-adrenoceptor densities in postmortem brain of subjects with depression: differential effect of antidepressant treatment. J Affect Disord 167:343–350, 2014 25020269

Rubinow MJ, Mahajan G, May W, et al: Basolateral amygdala volume and cell numbers in major depressive disorder: a postmortem stereological study. Brain Struct Funct 221(1):171–184, 2016 25287512

Seney ML, Tripp A, McCune S, et al: Laminar and cellular analyses of reduced somatostatin gene expression in the subgenual anterior cingulate cortex in major depression. Neurobiol Dis 73:213–219, 2015 25315685

Sequeira A, Klempan T, Canetti L, et al: Patterns of gene expression in the limbic system of suicides with and without major depression. Mol Psychiatry 12(7):640–655, 2007 17353912

Sequeira A, Mamdani F, Ernst C, et al: Global brain gene expression analysis links glutamatergic and GABAergic alterations to suicide and major depression. PLoS One 4(8):e6585, 2009 19668376

Sibille E, Wang Y, Joeyen-Waldorf J, et al: A molecular signature of depression in the amygdala. Am J Psychiatry 166(9):1011–1024, 2009 19605536

Soetanto A, Wilson RS, Talbot K, et al: Association of anxiety and depression with microtubule-associated protein 2- and synaptopodin-immunolabeled dendrite and spine densities in hippocampal CA3 of older humans. Arch Gen Psychiatry 67(5):448–457, 2010 20439826

Stockmeier CA: Involvement of serotonin in depression: evidence from postmortem and imaging studies of serotonin receptors and the serotonin transporter. J Psychiatr Res 37(5):357–373, 2003 12849929

Stockmeier CA, Mahajan GJ, Konick LC, et al: Cellular changes in the postmortem hippocampus in major depression. Biol Psychiatry 56(9):640–650, 2004 15522247

Thompson Ray M, Weickert CS, Wyatt E, et al: Decreased BDNF, trkB-TK+ and GAD67 mRNA expression in the hippocampus of individuals with schizophrenia and mood disorders. J Psychiatry Neurosci 36(3):195–203, 2011 21223646

Tripp A, Oh H, Guilloux JP, et al: Brain-derived neurotrophic factor signaling and subgenual anterior cingulate cortex dysfunction in major depressive disorder. Am J Psychiatry 169(11):1194–1202, 2012 23128924

Wamsley B, Fishell G: Genetic and activity-dependent mechanisms underlying interneuron diversity. Nat Rev Neurosci 18(5):299–309, 2017 28381833

Xiang L, Szebeni K, Szebeni A, et al: Dopamine receptor gene expression in human amygdaloid nuclei: elevated D4 receptor mRNA in major depression. Brain Res 1207:214–224, 2008 18371940

Youssef MM, Underwood MD, Huang YY, et al: Association of BDNF Val66Met polymorphism and brain BDNF levels with major depression and suicide. Int J Neuropsychopharmacol 21(6):528–538, 2018 29432620

Zhu MY, Klimek V, Dilley GE, et al: Elevated levels of tyrosine hydroxylase in the locus coeruleus in major depression. Biol Psychiatry 46(9):1275–1286, 1999 10560033

CHAPTER 11

Brain Imaging

Michele A. Bertocci, Ph.D.
Jorge Renner Cardoso de Almeida, M.D., Ph.D.
Stephen M. Strakowski, M.D.
Mary L. Phillips, M.D., M.D. (Cantab)

Mood (affective) disorders are among the leading causes of disability worldwide. Surveys suggest that depression is the leading cause of disability in high-income countries. Up to 30% of people with mood disorders suffer from chronic, often lifelong illness. Mood disorders include episodes of depressed mood (depression) and elevated mood (mania), both separately and in combination, and are believed to arise from dysregulation in neural network structure and function that can be measured in vivo using brain imaging techniques. These techniques include magnetic resonance imaging (MRI), positron emission tomography (PET), single-photon emission computed tomography (SPECT), computed axial tomography (CT), optical imaging, cranial ultrasound, and magnetoencephalography (MEG), through which measures of structure, function, energy metabolism, and neurotransmitter concentrations can be acquired. In this chapter, we focus on neural abnormalities measured with MRI, PET, and SPECT, because these techniques have the most robust datasets at this time.

To start, we provide a brief review of how these techniques image the brain. MRI takes advantage of the magnetism of atoms—usually hydrogen (a single proton)—in water, tissue, myelin, and other molecules to measure structure, function, and concentrations of neurochemicals. MRI can differentiate gray and white matter and cerebrospinal fluid in the brain, allowing measurement of neural structures that may be important in mood disorder pathology. Gray matter consists mostly of neuronal cell bodies and can be measured by volume and thickness. White matter consists mostly of myelinated axons; measurements of white matter generally reflect the movement of water along the axon and include volume, length, radial diffusivity, longitudinal diffusivity, and fractional anisotropy, as well as newer measures using spectral diffusion. Using the same magnetic characteristic of hydrogen atoms, MRI can be used to acquire proxy measures of neural activity using two approaches, blood oxygen level–

dependent (BOLD) measures and oxygen perfusion using arterial spin labeling (ASL). BOLD imaging essentially measures the amount of oxygenated hemoglobin in the brain as a positive signal; the level of oxygenation increases in regions of activation because the brain is designed to oversupply blood to brain areas that are in use. ASL works by using magnetic pulses to "label" a volume of blood that can then be followed as it travels through the brain. MRI can also measure neurotransmitters and energy sources that allow the brain to function using magnetic resonance spectroscopy (MRS). MRS capitalizes on the magnetic differences of neurochemicals to assess their concentrations. PET and SPECT can be used to measure blood flow, neurotransmitter concentrations, and glucose metabolism by measuring the effects of radioactive metabolites (radiotracers) injected into the bloodstream, although these approaches are less commonly used since MRI technology has rapidly advanced. However, PET and SPECT use labeled isotopes to study specific brain activities (e.g., the number of dopamine receptors or the metabolism of glucose) that cannot yet be studied with MRI. Detailed descriptions of these techniques exceed the scope of this chapter; interested readers are referred to the reviews of Gonul et al. (2009) and Videbech (2000).

These neuroimaging modalities have been used to identify biological markers of mood disorders that may be used for early identification and diagnosis and to develop more effective treatments. At present, however, no neuroimaging techniques have a direct clinical application in the care of people with mood disorders.

In the sections that follow, we introduce the neural networks that are believed to underlie key clinical features of mood disorders—the emotion processing and regulation, reward processing, and resting state networks (Figure 11–1)—and discuss abnormal activity and abnormal functional connectivity within these networks. Most of the findings presented are from research utilizing functional MRI (fMRI), given that these studies dominate the current literature. We then address gray and white matter structural abnormalities associated with mood disorders. Findings from studies using PET and MRS that examined regional neurotransmitter concentration and neuroreceptor density are discussed in relation to larger-scale neural network models of mood disorders. Together, these results contribute to emerging functional neuroanatomical models of mood disorders that may eventually increase diagnostic precision, identify markers of risk for future mood disorders, and lay the foundation for personalized treatments.

Abnormal Activity and Functional Connectivity in Neural Networks Underlying Clinical Features of Mood Disorders

Emotion Processing and Regulation Neurocircuitry

Emotion processing and regulation arise from ventral prefrontal-striatal-thalamic networks and their interactions with the amygdala and other brain regions. More specifically, emotion processing involves a network that includes the ventrolateral and ventromedial, dorsal, and medial prefrontal cortices; anterior cingulate cortex; amygdala; and hippocampus (see Figure 11–1A). Studies of people with major depressive

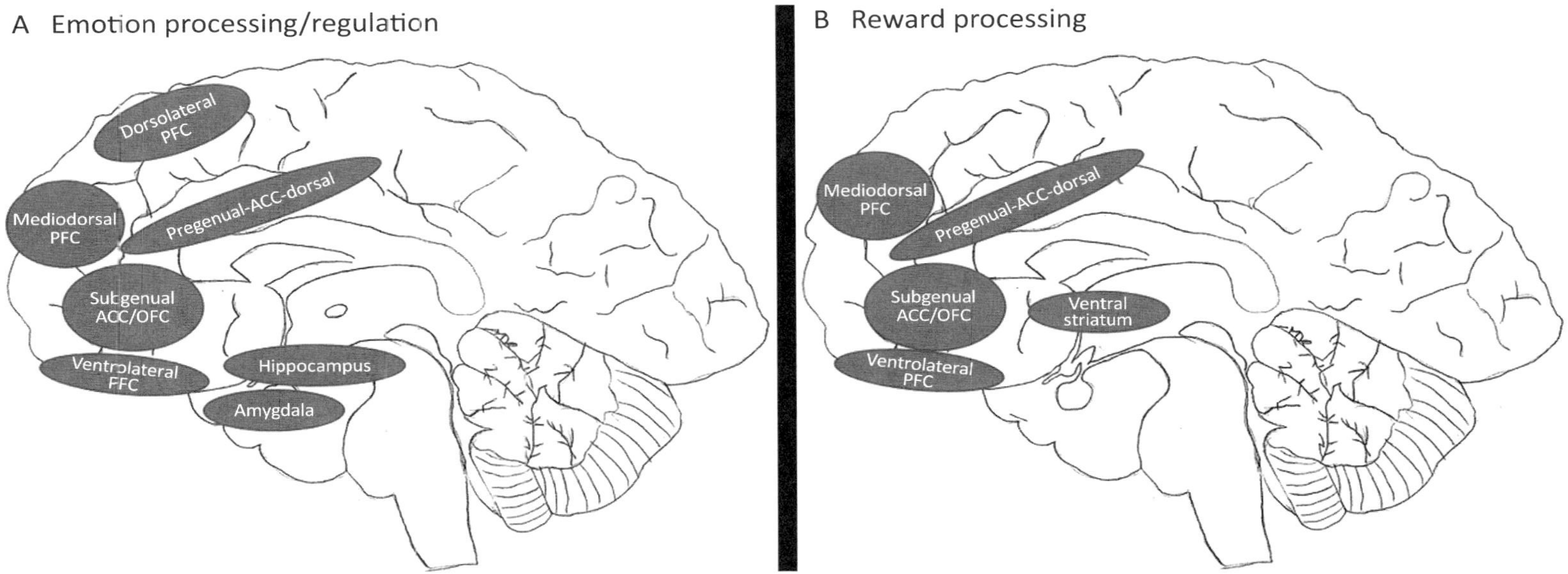

FIGURE 11–1. Key nodes in emotion processing and regulation and in reward processing neural circuitries in healthy individuals.
(A) Key nodes in emotion processing and emotion regulation neural circuitries in healthy individuals. **(B)** Key nodes in reward processing neural circuitry in healthy individuals. ACC=anterior cingulate cortex; OFC=orbitofrontal cortex; PFC=prefrontal cortex.

disorder typically find abnormally reduced activity in these networks during exposure to positive emotional stimuli, and increased activation during exposure to negative emotional stimuli. Specifically, findings include abnormally decreased activity in the lateral, orbital, and medial portions of the prefrontal cortex and elevated activity in the amygdala in depressed individuals during exposure to negative emotional stimuli (Groenewold et al. 2013; Rive et al. 2013). In contrast, activity during exposure to positive emotional stimuli is less predictable (Groenewold et al. 2013; Rive et al. 2013). Overrecruitment of the anterior cingulate cortex in response to both positive and negative emotional stimuli suggests that depressed individuals have difficulty recruiting prefrontal cortical regions to regulate the overactive limbic regions, particularly during exposure to negative emotional stimuli. Functional connectivity studies, which describe patterns of coactivation between two or more neural regions, also support this deficit in amygdala-prefrontal functional connectivity in response to negative emotional stimuli in depressed individuals relative to healthy individuals (Anand et al. 2005).

In individuals with bipolar disorder, this emotion processing neurocircuitry shows heightened emotional salience even during exposure to *nonemotional* content. More specifically, individuals with bipolar disorder show abnormally decreased ventrolateral prefrontal cortical activity during tasks involving emotion processing and emotion regulation, and response inhibition (Chen et al. 2011). These studies report abnormally decreased inferior frontal cortical activity, especially in the ventrolateral prefrontal cortex, and abnormally decreased ventrolateral prefrontal cortex–amygdala functional connectivity during different positive and negative emotion processing and emotion regulation tasks in adults with bipolar disorder across different mood states (Strakowski et al. 2011).

Furthermore, individuals with bipolar disorder also show abnormally increased activity in the amygdala, ventral striatum, and medial prefrontal cortex and decreased functional connectivity between the amygdala and prefrontal cortex, during exposure to positive emotional stimuli (Phillips and Swartz 2014). Here, the studies in bipolar disorder show abnormally increased amygdala and medial prefrontal cortex activity (Almeida et al. 2009; Chen et al. 2011) and abnormally decreased positive bilateral orbitofrontal cortex–amygdala effective connectivity in response to positive emotional stimuli, especially happy faces (Almeida et al. 2009), suggesting a dysregulated emotional network response to these stimuli. These findings may reflect an underlying attentional bias to positive emotional stimuli in bipolar disorder, predisposing to or associated with risk for mania. However, others found that the prefrontal-amygdala-striatal circuit distinguished depressed from manic mood states during processing of negatively valenced information (Grotegerd et al. 2014; Man et al. 2019). In summary, in both (unipolar) major depressive disorder and bipolar disorder, dysregulation of emotion processing and emotion regulation networks has been consistently demonstrated through a variety of neuroimaging approaches and tasks.

Reward Processing Neurocircuitry

Reward-related neurocircuitry is centered on medial and lateral prefrontal cortical modulation of the ventral striatum (Figure 11–1B), primarily through dopaminergic systems. Reward processes are related to mood state, so it is not surprising that there is overlap in the neural networks involved in reward and emotion processing. Reward processing includes periods of motivation, anticipation, and satiety. Consumption of rewards induces feelings of pleasure, leading to reinforcement of reward cues and behaviors (Schultz 2006). Reward-seeking and learning tend to decrease during depressive episodes and are heightened during manic periods. Neuroimaging studies assess the neurocircuitry of reward using a variety of paradigms, including monetary, social, and appetitive rewards. These human studies (Beckmann et al. 2009; Kumar et al. 2008; Ongür and Price 2000) have confirmed the presence of a reward network previously identified in animal studies (Haber 2016), consisting of the ventral striatum with connections to the ventral tegmental area and the ventral pallidum, which then connect (through the thalamus and anterior cingulate) to the orbitofrontal cortex. In animal studies, reward processing tends to localize within the striatum to the nucleus accumbens; however, in humans, this nucleus is less well delineated, so activation occurs at the ventral striatal–putamen junction. This activation is blunted or unsustained in depressed individuals (Zhang et al. 2013), and cortical regions that regulate the ventral striatum, such as the anterior cingulate and middle frontal cortex, show abnormal activation in response to rewarding stimuli and reward anticipation (Zhang et al. 2013). Studies in bipolar disorder have reported abnormally increased left ventrolateral prefrontal cortex and ventral striatal activity during reward anticipation in adults with bipolar disorder in different mood states (Bermpohl et al. 2010; Nusslock et al. 2012; Phillips and Swartz 2014). However, others found no differences in activity in the ventral striatum in response to reward receipt versus omission in manic adults with bipolar disorder (Abler et al. 2008). Collectively, data suggest that depression and mania may be associated with dysfunction of these neural networks that manage rewards and reward learning, but further study is required.

Resting State Neurocircuitry

Studies of resting state functional connectivity examine measures of context-independent neural circuits and may represent fundamental abnormalities in the functional neuroanatomy of mood disorders. Measuring resting state functional connectivity is based on the discovery that low-frequency (<~0.1 Hz) BOLD fluctuations in functionally related gray matter regions show strong temporal correlations at rest (i.e., they vary together over time). Resting state studies are useful in clinical populations because of the ease of image acquisition; however, this technique is vulnerable to individual variations in behavior, arousal, and head motion in the scanner.

Studies during rest have identified distributed regions—including the default mode, salience, attentional, and emotion regulation networks—that are abnormally activated during rest in participants with MDD (Kaiser et al. 2015). The *default mode network*, which comprises coactivation among the hippocampus, medial prefrontal cortex, posterior cingulate cortex, and temporal cortex (Drevets et al. 2008), is normatively activated during rest. The *salience network* consists of coactivation between the anterior cingulate cortex and frontoinsular regions (Chiong et al. 2013). The *attentional network* consists of dorsal and ventral networks that work in concert to orient attention and consists of visual areas, inferior frontal cortex, and parietal and temporal cortices (Vossel et al. 2014). The *emotion regulation network* includes regulatory regions of the anterior cingulate cortex and the lateral and medial prefrontal cortex and subcortical regions of the amygdala, insula, and caudate (Etkin et al. 2015). Findings suggest that interference of other networks during rest may be related to mood disorder pathology. Specifically, in individuals with MDD during rest, abnormally low connectivity within the attentional and emotion regulation networks (Kaiser et al. 2015) and abnormally high connectivity within the default mode and salience networks (Kaiser et al. 2015; Sundermann et al. 2014) have been shown, and these abnormalities may become more pronounced with repeated depressive episodes (Meng et al. 2014).

In individuals with bipolar disorder, Brady et al. (2017) found two patterns of altered functional connectivity that differentiated mood states in bipolar disorder as well as distinguishing bipolar euthymia from a healthy population: 1) dorsal attentional network—the bipolar euthymia group demonstrated hypoconnectivity and the mania group demonstrated hyperconnectivity relative to a healthy control population; 2) default mode network—the bipolar euthymic state demonstrated hypoconnectivity, while bipolar mania demonstrated connectivity comparable to that of a healthy population between the dorsal frontal nodes and the rest of the network. Moreover, Martino et al. (2020) found increased functional connectivity between the sensorimotor network and the thalamus during bipolar mania that was absent during bipolar depression. In summary, mood disorders may be associated with a specific functional neuroanatomic architecture, although the details of this architecture are still incompletely defined.

Abnormal Cerebral Blood Flow

Cerebral blood flow during emotion processing, reward processing, and rest shows hypoperfusion in bipolar participants during both depressed and manic mood episodes (Toma et al. 2018). Both bipolar and unipolar depressed participants showed hypoactive cerebral blood flow during rest, especially in regions involved in emotion processing and cognitive control, such as the anterior cingulate, frontoparietal, and striatal regions (Toma et al. 2018; Vasic et al. 2015).

Neural Structural Abnormalities

Abnormal Gray Matter Structure

In the brain, gray matter measurements are thought to reflect the density of dendrites, short-range axons, and glial cell bodies (Zatorre et al. 2012). Individuals with mood disorders, relative to healthy subjects, showed decreased gray matter in cortical (anterior cingulate cortex and across the prefrontal cortex) and subcortical regions (caudate, putamen, hippocampus, and insula), especially after recurrent affective episodes (Arnone et al. 2012; Bore et al. 2012; Phillips and Swartz 2014). In bipolar disorder, gray matter volume may also be used as a proxy measure of neurotrophic exposure to lithium medication, because several studies and a meta-analysis suggest that individuals with bipolar disorder who are being treated with lithium have a greater global and regional (e.g., anterior cingulate gyrus) gray matter volume than individuals with bipolar disorder who are lithium-free (Sun et al. 2018), although not all investigators have replicated these findings (see, e.g., Eker et al. 2014). These findings provide evidence of structural abnormalities that parallel the functional abnormalities associated with emotion processing, emotion regulation, and reward processing neurocircuitries in mood disorders.

Abnormal White Matter Structure Measured With Diffusion Imaging

Diffusion imaging allows measurement of the architecture of the white matter fiber tracts by approximating the movement of water along the axon. Greater *longitudinal diffusivity* reflects high cohesion along the length of the axis, perhaps reflecting greater myelination and higher tract organization. By contrast, greater *radial diffusivity* reflects greater movement of water molecules perpendicular to the tract length and suggests a less linear structure and may reflect damaged axonal membranes and/or myelin sheaths. Fractional anisotropy is the ratio of longitudinal diffusivity to radial diffusivity, with high fractional anisotropy characterizing densely packed collinear white matter fibers, along with few noncollinear fibers.

Key white matter tracts that connect the prefrontal cortical and subcortical regions involved in emotion regulation and reward processing neural circuits include the superior longitudinal fasciculus, uncinate fasciculus, corpus callosum, and cingulum (Versace et al. 2014). Meta-analyses of studies in depressed patients have shown reductions in fractional anisotropy in the corpus callosum extending to the body of the corpus callosum and the left anterior limb of the internal capsule (Chen et al. 2016; Jiang et al. 2017). Moreover, decreased uncinate fasciculus fractional anisotropy is consistently found in adults with depression (Bracht et al. 2015). Findings of abnormal fractional anisotropy in the medial forebrain bundle and cingulum bundle have also been shown and may be associated with severity of depressive symptoms (Bracht et al. 2015). Abnormally reduced fractional anisotropy in tracts such as the uncinate fasciculus, which connects the prefrontal cortical and subcortical regions, may underlie some of the functional abnormalities in emotion regulation and reward processing observed in depressed individuals. In bipolar disorder, several meta-analyses of white matter volumes converged to identify reductions in the posterior corpus callosum (Arnone et al. 2008; Ganzola and Duchesne 2017; Kempton et al. 2008; Pezzoli et al. 2018), and in one study, reduced volumes extended to the adjacent posterior cingulate cortex (Pezzoli et al. 2018). The observed white matter decrease seems to be a trait marker of disease, because it is not typically correlated with other clinical variables. The white matter region lies adjacent to the posterior cingulate cortex, which is a core region of the default mode network (Greicius et al. 2003). Finally, increased white matter hyperintensities continue to be the most replicated finding in bipolar disorder. However, this finding lacks specificity, given that it is also seen in other psychiatric disorders, including major depressive disorder, as well as in normal aging and in other medical illnesses that impact the brain.

Magnetic Resonance Spectroscopy Studies of Neurotransmitters Implicated in Mood Disorders

Noninvasive detection of metabolites, such as choline, *N*-acetylaspartate, and lactate, can be measured using MRS. Utilizing the chemically specific radiofrequency signals within metabolites and varying the magnetic fields, MRS can estimate neurotransmitter concentrations in neural regions of interest. We describe here two neurotransmitters implicated in mood disorders because of their roles in inhibition and excitation: GABA and glutamate.

GABA is the principal mediator of inhibition in the CNS. GABA concentration deficits have been demonstrated in depressed individuals in occipital, medial prefrontal, and anterior cingulate cortices. These deficits appeared to resolve with remission from depression but to remain low in individuals with recurrent or treatment-resistant depression (Schür et al. 2016). GABA concentrations were also negatively associated with anhedonia severity (Gabbay et al. 2012). These findings suggest that high concentrations of GABA in the cortex are needed to successfully regulate negative symptoms of anhedonia.

Glutamate may also have a relationship with mood disorders. It is the principal excitatory neurotransmitter in the CNS. In depressed individuals, glutamate concentrations have been reported to be increased in the occipital cortex and decreased across the prefrontal cortex and anterior cingulate cortex (Lener et al. 2017). Changes in glutamate levels after treatment for depression were not consistently associated with symptom improvement (Lener et al. 2017). Additional research is needed to understand the relationship between glutamate concentrations in the cortex and depression.

Individuals with bipolar I disorder who were being treated with long-term pharmacotherapy showed increased glutamate and reduced *N*-acetylaspartate concentrations, which, combined, suggested neuronal metabolic dysfunction (Bustillo et al. 2019). Moreover, glutamate and *N*-acetylaspartate concentrations were also relatively lower in the anterior cingulate cortex of bipolar individuals who had experienced multiple episodes compared with those who were experiencing their first episode (Borgelt et al. 2019).

Newer Areas of Neuroimaging Research in Mood Disorders

Neuroimaging studies have focused on specific subgroups of individuals with mood disorders. This research includes studies comparing individuals with major depressive disorder and individuals with bipolar depression, as well as studies of specific mood states, neural correlates, and predictors of treatment response in individuals with mood disorders, risk for the development of mood disorders, and pediatric-onset mood disorders. Although an in-depth discussion is beyond the scope of this chapter, briefly, this research supports findings from studies of adults with mood disorders and suggests that emotion processing and reward processing neurocircuitries are abnormal in mood disorder pathology. It also identifies other neural regions, such as the insula and precuneus, that may be implicated in mood disorders. However, use of these findings as biomarkers of disease is not yet feasible. Machine learning is a promising approach for identifying individual subject–level patterns of neurocircuitry abnormalities in mood disorders. These approaches can identify individuals with mood disorders with 70%–80% accuracy. Improvements in the use of machine learning technologies in conjunction with neuroimaging measures have the potential to improve the diagnosis of psychopathology as well as identification of optimal treatment choices.

Familial Risk and Resilience

Risk for mood disorder development can be elevated by genetic risk (i.e., having a parent or sibling with a mood disorder) or symptomatic risk (i.e., having subthreshold symptoms or a clinically related disorder such as an anxiety disorder). Patients and high-risk relatives showed similar abnormalities in neural activation and functional connectivity during emotional tasks; however, resilient relatives had larger cerebral volumes, enhanced prefrontal connectivity during tasks, and heightened functional coactivation of the default mode network during rest (Frangou 2019). Unaffected relatives also showed a constellation of differences, including greater gray matter volumes in the frontal, prefrontal, and temporal regions and hyperactivation in the amygdala, frontal cortex, and striatum (Cattarinussi et al. 2019), suggesting neural compensation in these individuals. In addition, higher anterior cingulate activity and greater functional connectivity with the amygdala has been highlighted as a potential marker of genetic risk for bipolar disorder (Acuff et al. 2018).

Pediatric Mood Disorders

The emergence of mood disorders during childhood or adolescence often portends more severe symptoms and increased risk of suicide in comparison with mood disorder emergence in adulthood. Neural networks that are implicated in emotion and reward processing are also important in pediatric depression. In depressed youth, patterns of increased activity in the ventrolateral and dorsolateral prefrontal cortex and anterior cingulate cortex have been shown (Miller et al. 2015). In youth with bipolar disorder, abnormal patterns of increased amygdala activity, decreased ventrolateral prefrontal cortical activity, and decreased prefrontal cortical–amygdala functional connectivity during emotion processing were reported (Frank et al. 2015). Corroborating the activity and functional connectivity findings, decreased cortical and subcortical gray and white matter measures have also been observed in youth with pediatric-onset bipolar disorder (Acuff et al. 2019).

Summary

Neuroimaging studies of mood disorders have identified specific patterns of neural network dysfunction and related structural abnormalities. Neural network abnormalities include dysfunction in bilateral prefrontal cortical (especially ventrolateral prefrontal cortex and orbitofrontal cortex)–hippocampal–amygdala emotion processing and emotion regulation networks along with hyperactivity in predominantly left-sided ventrostriatal-ventrolateral prefrontal cortex reward processing neurocircuitry. Additionally, parallel abnormalities in resting-state functional connectivity and gray and white matter structure in these networks have been shown. Bioenergetic abnormalities that may be related to mitochondrial dysfunction, abnormal neuronal glial interactions, and abnormal glucose metabolism in some of the same regions showing gray matter loss have been reported. The combination of these functional and structural abnormalities may underlie the behavioral abnormalities associated with mood disorders, such as emotional lability, emotional dysregulation, and reward processing dysregulation.

Future Directions in Neuroimaging Research in Mood Disorders

Neuroimaging techniques are helping us better understand the neurocircuitry of mood disorders and are making significant contributions to our understanding of mood disorder pathophysiology (Gotlib and Hamilton 2008; Zhang et al. 2016). Many consistencies across neuroimaging studies and methods are reported, although inconsistencies are also seen. Inconsistencies may be the result of imaging parameters or analytic differences but may also represent important differences in subcategories of mood disorders related to symptom dimensions and symptom development. Some approaches to improving current methods include the following:

1. Using dimensional symptomatic approaches to examine pathological behaviors that cut across conventionally defined diagnostic categories of mood disorders
2. Incorporating longitudinal designs to identify developmental trajectories of abnormal neurocircuitry associated with symptoms and with risk
3. Merging multimodal neuroimaging techniques and other biological system–level approaches to examine the impact of genetic variation and molecular-level processes on neurocircuitry development
4. Implementing pattern recognition techniques in combination with neuroimaging methodologies to identify individual-level neurocircuitry markers that not only help classify individuals into present diagnostic groups but also help predict individual-level clinical course

Collectively, these approaches will enhance our understanding of the complex neuropathophysiological processes underlying abnormal behaviors associated with mood disorders, and they may ultimately provide individual-level biological markers that have clinical utility for diagnosis and future illness prediction, and for guiding personalized treatment choices.

References

Abler B, Greenhouse I, Ongur D, et al: Abnormal reward system activation in mania. Neuropsychopharmacology 33(9):2217–2227, 2008 17987058

Acuff HE, Versace A, Bertocci MA, et al: Association of neuroimaging measures of emotion processing and regulation neural circuitries with symptoms of bipolar disorder in offspring at risk for bipolar disorder. JAMA Psychiatry 75(12):1241–1251, 2018 30193355

Acuff HE, Versace A, Bertocci MA, et al: White matter—emotion processing activity relationships in youth offspring of bipolar parents. J Affect Disord 243:153–164, 2019 30243195

Almeida JR, Versace A, Mechelli A, et al: Abnormal amygdala-prefrontal effective connectivity to happy faces differentiates bipolar from major depression. Biol Psychiatry 66(5):451–459, 2009 19450794

Anand A, Li Y, Wang Y, et al: Activity and connectivity of brain mood regulating circuit in depression: a functional magnetic resonance study. Biol Psychiatry 57(10):1079–1088, 2005 15866546

Arnone D, McIntosh AM, Chandra P, et al: Meta-analysis of magnetic resonance imaging studies of the corpus callosum in bipolar disorder. Acta Psychiatr Scand 118(5):357–362, 2008 18644004

Arnone D, McIntosh AM, Ebmeier KP, et al: Magnetic resonance imaging studies in unipolar depression: systematic review and meta-regression analyses. Eur Neuropsychopharmacol 22(1):1–16, 2012 21723712

Beckmann M, Johansen-Berg H, Rushworth MF: Connectivity-based parcellation of human cingulate cortex and its relation to functional specialization. J Neurosci 29(4):1175–1190, 2009 19176826

Bermpohl F, Kahnt T, Dalanay U, et al: Altered representation of expected value in the orbitofrontal cortex in mania. Hum Brain Mapp 31(7):958–969, 2010 19950195

Bora E, Fornito A, Pantelis C, Yücel M: Gray matter abnormalities in major depressive disorder: a meta-analysis of voxel based morphometry studies. J Affect Disord 138(1–2):9–18, 2012 21511342

Borgelt L, Strakowski SM, DelBello MP, et al: Neurophysiological effects of multiple mood episodes in bipolar disorder. Bipolar Disord 21(6):503–513, 2019 31025452

Bracht T, Linden D, Keedwell P: A review of white matter microstructure alterations of pathways of the reward circuit in depression. J Affect Disord 187:45–53, 2015 26318270

Brady RO Jr, Tandon N, Masters GA, et al: Differential brain network activity across mood states in bipolar disorder. J Affect Disord 207:367–376, 2017 27744225

Bustillo JR, Jones T, Qualls C, et al: Proton magnetic resonance spectroscopic imaging of gray and white matter in bipolar-I and schizophrenia. J Affect Disord 246:745–753, 2019 30623820

Cattarinussi G, Di Giorgio A, Wolf RC, et al: Neural signatures of the risk for bipolar disorder: a meta-analysis of structural and functional neuroimaging studies. Bipolar Disord 21(3):215–227, 2019 30444299

Chen C-H, Suckling J, Lennox BR, et al: A quantitative meta-analysis of fMRI studies in bipolar disorder. Bipolar Disord 13(1):1–15, 2011 21320248

Chen G, Hu X, Li L, et al: Disorganization of white matter architecture in major depressive disorder: a meta-analysis of diffusion tensor imaging with tract-based spatial statistics. Sci Rep 6:21825, 2016 26906716

Chiong W, Wilson SM, D'Esposito M, et al: The salience network causally influences default mode network activity during moral reasoning. Brain 136(Pt 6):1929–1941, 2013 23576128

Drevets WC, Price JL, Furey ML: Brain structural and functional abnormalities in mood disorders: implications for neurocircuitry models of depression. Brain Struct Funct 213(1–2):93–118, 2008 18704495

Eker C, Simsek F, Yılmazer EE, et al: Brain regions associated with risk and resistance for bipolar I disorder: a voxel-based MRI study of patients with bipolar disorder and their healthy siblings. Bipolar Disord 16(3):249–261, 2014 24589068

Etkin A, Büchel C, Gross JJ: The neural bases of emotion regulation. Nat Rev Neurosci 16(11):693–700, 2015 26481098

Frangou S: Neuroimaging markers of risk, disease expression, and resilience to bipolar disorder. Curr Psychiatry Rep 21(7):52, 2019 31161278

Frank E, Nimgaonkar VL, Phillips ML, et al: All the world's a (clinical) stage: rethinking bipolar disorder from a longitudinal perspective. Mol Psychiatry 20(1):23–31, 2015 25048003

Gabbay V, Mao X, Klein RG, et al: Anterior cingulate cortex γ-aminobutyric acid in depressed adolescents: relationship to anhedonia. Arch Gen Psychiatry 69(2):139–149, 2012 21969419

Ganzola R, Duchesne S: Voxel-based morphometry meta-analysis of gray and white matter finds significant areas of differences in bipolar patients from healthy controls. Bipolar Disord 19(2):74–83, 2017 28444949

Gonul AS, Coburn K, Kula M: Cerebral blood flow, metabolic, receptor, and transporter changes in bipolar disorder: the role of PET and SPECT studies. Int Rev Psychiatry 21(4):323–335, 2009 20374147

Gotlib IH, Hamilton JP: Neuroimaging and depression: current status and unresolved issues. Curr Dir Psychol Sci 17(2):159–163, 2008

Greicius MD, Krasnow B, Reiss AL, et al: Functional connectivity in the resting brain: a network analysis of the default mode hypothesis. Proc Natl Acad Sci USA 100(1):253–258, 2003 12506194

Groenewold NA, Opmeer EM, de Jonge P, et al: Emotional valence modulates brain functional abnormalities in depression: evidence from a meta-analysis of fMRI studies. Neurosci Biobehav Rev 37(2):152–163, 2013 23206667

Grotegerd D, Stuhrmann A, Kugel H, et al: Amygdala excitability to subliminally presented emotional faces distinguishes unipolar and bipolar depression: an fMRI and pattern classification study. Hum Brain Mapp 35(7):2995–3007, 2014 24038516

Haber SN: Corticostriatal circuitry. Dialogues Clin Neurosci 18(1):7–21, 2016 27069376

Jiang J, Zhao Y-J, Hu X-Y, et al: Microstructural brain abnormalities in medication-free patients with major depressive disorder: a systematic review and meta-analysis of diffusion tensor imaging. J Psychiatry Neurosci 42(3):150–163, 2017 27780031

Kaiser RH, Andrews-Hanna JR, Wager TD, et al: Large-scale network dysfunction in major depressive disorder: a meta-analysis of resting-state functional connectivity. JAMA Psychiatry 72(6):603–611, 2015 25785575

Kempton MJ, Geddes JR, Ettinger U, et al: Meta-analysis, database, and meta-regression of 98 structural imaging studies in bipolar disorder. Arch Gen Psychiatry 65(9):1017–1032, 2008 18762588

Kumar P, Waiter G, Ahearn T, et al: Abnormal temporal difference reward-learning signals in major depression. Brain 131(Pt 8):2084–2093, 2008 18579575

Lener MS, Niciu MJ, Ballard ED, et al: Glutamate and gamma-aminobutyric acid systems in the pathophysiology of major depression and antidepressant response to ketamine. Biological Psychiatry 81(10):886–897, 2017 27449797

Man V, Gruber J, Glahn DC, et al: Altered amygdala circuits underlying valence processing among manic and depressed phases in bipolar adults. J Affect Disord 245:394–402, 2019 30423467

Martino M, Magioncalda P, Conio B, et al: Abnormal functional relationship of sensorimotor network with neurotransmitter-related nuclei via subcortical-cortical loops in manic and depressive phases of bipolar disorder. Schizophr Bull 46(1):163–174, 2020 31150559

Meng C, Brandl F, Tahmasian M, et al: Aberrant topology of striatum's connectivity is associated with the number of episodes in depression. Brain 137(Pt 2):598–609, 2014 24163276

Miller CH, Hamilton JP, Sacchet MD, Gotlib IH: Meta-analysis of functional neuroimaging of major depressive disorder in youth. JAMA Psychiatry 72(10):1045–1053, 2015 26332700
Nusslock R, Almeida JR, Forbes EE, et al: Waiting to win: elevated striatal and orbitofrontal cortical activity during reward anticipation in euthymic bipolar disorder adults. Bipolar Disord 14(3):249–260, 2012 22548898
Ongür D, Price JL: The organization of networks within the orbital and medial prefrontal cortex of rats, monkeys and humans. Cereb Cortex 10(3):206–219, 2000 10731217
Pezzoli S, Emsell L, Yip SW, et al: Meta-analysis of regional white matter volume in bipolar disorder with replication in an independent sample using coordinates, T-maps, and individual MRI data. Neurosci Biobehav Rev 84:162–170, 2018 29162519
Phillips ML, Swartz HA: A critical appraisal of neuroimaging studies of bipolar disorder: toward a new conceptualization of underlying neural circuitry and a road map for future research. Am J Psychiatry 171(8):829–843, 2014 24626773
Rive MM, van Rooijen G, Veltman DJ, et al: Neural correlates of dysfunctional emotion regulation in major depressive disorder. A systematic review of neuroimaging studies. Neurosci Biobehav Rev 37(10 Pt 2):2529–2553, 2013 23928089
Schultz W: Behavioral theories and the neurophysiology of reward. Annu Rev Psychol 57:87–115, 2006 16318590
Schür RR, Draisma LW, Wijnen JP, et al: Brain GABA levels across psychiatric disorders: a systematic literature review and meta-analysis of 1H-MRS studies. Hum Brain Mapp 37(9):3337–3352, 2016 27145016
Strakowski SM, Eliassen JC, Lamy M, et al: Functional magnetic resonance imaging brain activation in bipolar mania: evidence for disruption of the ventrolateral prefrontal-amygdala emotional pathway. Biol Psychiatry 69(4):381–388, 2011 21051038
Sun YR, Herrmann N, Scott CJM, et al: Global grey matter volume in adult bipolar patients with and without lithium treatment: a meta-analysis. J Affect Disord 225:599–606, 2018 28886501
Sundermann B, Olde Lütke Beverborg M, Pfleiderer B: Toward literature-based feature selection for diagnostic classification: a meta-analysis of resting-state fMRI in depression. Front Hum Neurosci 8:692, 2014 25309382
Toma S, MacIntosh BJ, Swardfager W, et al: Cerebral blood flow in bipolar disorder: a systematic review. J Affect Disord 241:505–513, 2018 30149339
Vasic N, Wolf ND, Grön G, et al: Baseline brain perfusion and brain structure in patients with major depression: a multimodal magnetic resonance imaging study. J Psychiatry Neurosci 40(6):412–421, 2015 26125119
Versace A, Andreazza AC, Young LT, et al: Elevated serum measures of lipid peroxidation and abnormal prefrontal white matter in euthymic bipolar adults: toward peripheral biomarkers of bipolar disorder. Mol Psychiatry 19(2):200–208, 2014 23358158
Videbech P: PET measurements of brain glucose metabolism and blood flow in major depressive disorder: a critical review. Acta Psychiatr Scand 101(1):11–20, 2000 10674946
Vossel S, Geng JJ, Fink GR: Dorsal and ventral attention systems: distinct neural circuits but collaborative roles. Neuroscientist 20(2):150–159, 2014 23835449
Zatorre RJ, Fields RD, Johansen-Berg H: Plasticity in gray and white: neuroimaging changes in brain structure during learning. Nat Neurosci 15(4):528–536, 2012 22426254
Zhang K, Zhu Y, Zhu Y, et al: Molecular, functional, and structural imaging of major depressive disorder. Neurosci Bull 32(3):273–285, 2016 27142698
Zhang W-N, Chang S-H, Guo L-Y, et al: The neural correlates of reward-related processing in major depressive disorder: a meta-analysis of functional magnetic resonance imaging studies. J Affect Disord 151(2):531–539, 2013 23856280

CHAPTER 12

Genetics of Mood Disorders

Wade Berrettini, M.D., Ph.D.

In this chapter I summarize some recent advances in genetics of bipolar disorder and recurrent unipolar disorder (RUP). Emphasis is placed on genome-wide association study (GWAS) reports that use a bipolar disorder or RUP diagnosis as the phenotype; these diagnoses may be from a direct semistructured interview, review of medical records, or simple self-report (e.g., an answer to the question "Have you ever been depressed?"). Copy number variants (CNVs) influencing risk for mood disorders are also summarized. This chapter also stresses shared genetic liability across nosological categories. Although future pharmacogenetic studies of bipolar disorder and RUP will identify alleles that predict a good therapeutic response to specific pharmacotherapies, this review does not cover pharmacogenetics of mood disorders. Because independent confirmation has been uncommon for candidate gene association studies not based on previous genome-wide significant data, reviews of such reports have been omitted; reviews of linkage reports have also been omitted. Finally, this chapter does not include a review of epigenetic studies of mood disorders.

General Comments on Genome-Wide Association Studies

GWAS research has been reported since approximately 2005, made possible through technological advances allowing determination of genotypes for common single-nucleotide polymorphisms (SNPs), the great majority of which have two alleles, differing by a single base pair. The less common allele for these biallelic SNPs in a specified population will have an allele frequency of less than 50%. There are several million common SNPs (minor allele frequency >1%) across the human genome, or one common SNP for every 500 or so base pairs of DNA. Modern GWAS technology involves determining genotypes very inexpensively by direct genotyping at approximately 1 million common SNPs for all participants, typically more than 10,000 individuals. Furthermore, alleles for other common (not genotyped) SNPs adjacent to the directly genotyped SNPs can be inferred through a process of imputation (Das et al. 2018), which uses DNA sequence data for large numbers of people to infer the missing alleles.

GWAS research involves testing the statistical significance of allele frequency differences between case subjects and control subjects at these millions of common SNPs. Because there is a multiple hypothesis testing problem, a statistical adjustment must be used for testing each SNP for a case-control difference in allele frequency. A value of $P \approx 5 \times 10^{-8}$ is the equivalent of $P = 0.05$ for a GWAS experiment on a single phenotype. The stringent statistical correction for multiple testing no doubt masks true signals from alleles that confer only very modest risk of disease, although in theory this limitation could be overcome by ever-larger sample sizes. GWAS results for psychiatric disorders have not uncovered single *common* alleles that convey risk greater than an odds ratio (OR) of 1.3. The absolute value of the odds ratio is a measure of the magnitude of risk conveyed by the relevant allele. The sample size required to achieve adequate power for the modest expected effect sizes (OR $\leq$1.3), given the correction for a genome-wide search, is approximately 10,000 case subjects and 10,000 control subjects.

Heritability (h^2) may be defined as that fraction of total risk attributable to inherited factors. For bipolar disorder, h^2 has been estimated recently from a large Swedish sibling study as approximately 55% (Pettersson et al. 2019). For RUP, h^2 has been estimated from this sibling study as ~30% (Pettersson et al. 2019). These sibling estimates agree well with data from twin studies (Polderman et al. 2015). GWAS reports on bipolar disorder and RUP estimate that SNP h^2 (h^2 explained by all common SNPs in a GWAS) explains approximately 20%–35% of total h^2 for these mood disorders (Lee et al. 2013; Pettersson et al. 2019) (Table 12–1).

If common SNPs explain approximately 20%–35% of total h^2 for bipolar disorder and RUP, then what factors might account for the missing h^2 (Manolio et al. 2009)? The remaining h^2 is probably explained by rare variants of large effect and epistasis (the multiplicative risk-increasing effect due to interaction among two or more risk alleles).

Bipolar Disorder Genome-Wide Association Studies

A recent sibling bipolar disorder h^2 estimate of approximately 50% from several million Swedish siblings (Pettersson et al. 2019) agrees well with data from twin studies (Polderman et al. 2015). These and several previous h^2 estimates indicate that environmental and stochastic influences play substantial roles in risk for bipolar disorder. The initial bipolar disorder GWAS reports were seriously underpowered, in retrospect, to detect alleles of small effect, conveying odds ratios of less than 1.3. Baum et al. (2008), Sklar et al. (2008), and the Wellcome Trust Case Control Consortium (2007) each consisted of fewer than 2,000 case subjects. It is noteworthy that the strongest association signals (e.g., the "top 10") in each of these three studies were not confirmed

TABLE 12–1. Heritability (h^2) and single-nucleotide polymorphism (SNP) heritability

Disorder	h^2	SNP h^2
Bipolar disorder	55%	20%
Recurrent unipolar disorder	30%	10%

Source. Data from Pettersson et al. 2019.

in either of the other two, suggesting that the individual sample sizes lacked sufficient power to detect small effects.

This sample size limitation was partially addressed by a collaborative effort including 4,387 case subjects and 6,209 control subjects, which were analyzed jointly using the SNP genotypes from several bipolar disorder GWAS reports (Ferreira et al. 2008). The strongest statistical signal was in the ankyrin 3 (*ANK3*) gene on chromosome 10q21, with single SNP and haplotype (rs4582919—rs10994357—rs7910492, risk haplotype CCT) analyses yielding a *P* of approximately 10^{-9}. This statistical level indicates genome-wide significance. The 10q21 *ANK3* location coincides with a previous report of bipolar disorder genetic susceptibility occurring at this location on chromosome 10 (Segurado et al. 2003). A meta-analysis (Psychiatric GWAS Consortium Bipolar Disorder Working Group 2011) of bipolar disorder GWAS data revealed evidence for risk alleles in *ANK3, CACNA1c, SYNE1,* and *ODZ4*. Confirmation of these alleles in additional samples has been published (e.g., Green et al. 2013).

Stahl et al. (2019) and Mullins et al. (2021) reported on substantial numbers of bipolar disorder case subjects and control subjects of European ancestry (Figure 12–1). With 64 loci of genome-wide significance, the findings of Mullins et al. (2021) provided a wealth of statistically sound data. The loci included ion channels and neurotransmitter transporters (*CACNA1C, GRIN2A, SCN2A, SLC4A1*), as well as synaptic proteins (*RIMS1, ANK3*). In keeping with findings for other psychiatric disorders, the odds ratios were less than 1.2 for each common allele, consistent with hundreds of bipolar disorder risk alleles.

Shared Genetic Susceptibility of Bipolar Disorder With Other Psychiatric Disorders

Twin and family studies indicate that bipolar disorder and RUP share genetic susceptibility alleles (e.g., Gershon et al. 1982; Weissman et al. 1984). Family studies also indicate shared susceptibility for bipolar disorder and schizophrenia (Lichtenstein et al. 2009), as well as shared susceptibility for RUP and schizophrenia (Kendler and Gardner 1997; Lichtenstein et al. 2009). Because all common risk-increasing alleles for psychiatric disorders have small effect sizes (OR $\leq$1.3), very large sample sizes must be ascertained and studied to detect them at genome-wide levels of significance (5×10^{-8}). Thus, there are large numbers of putative risk alleles with odds ratios between 1.01 and 1.05 that remain undetected. One method of assembling such common alleles of small effect in a single statistic is termed a *polygenic risk score* (PRS).

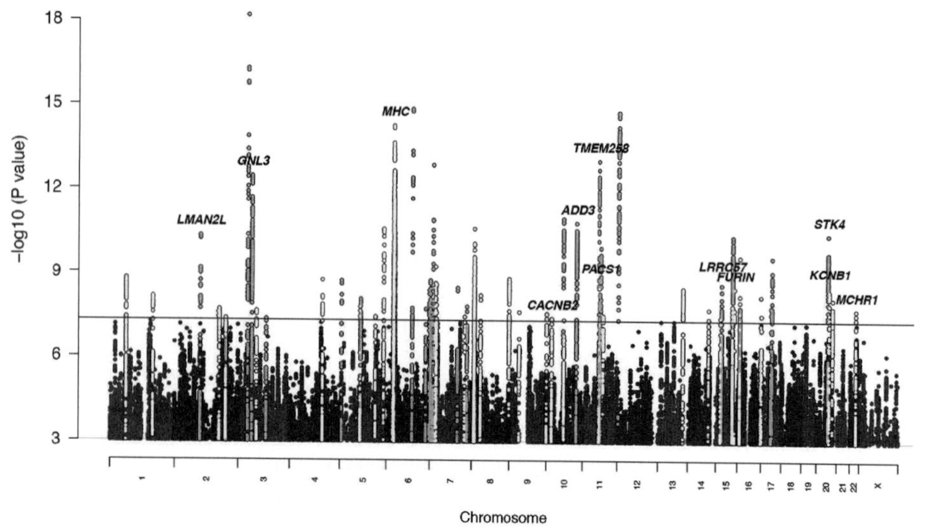

FIGURE 12–1. **Bipolar disorder genome-wide association study (GWAS) meta-analysis reveals many risk loci.**

To view this figure in color, see Plate 4 in Color Gallery in middle of book.

Manhattan plot for the primary GWAS meta-analysis of 41,917 bipolar disorder case subjects and 371,549 control subjects (Mullins et al. 2021). GWAS $-\log_{10}(P)$ values are plotted for all single-nucleotide polymorphisms (SNPs) across chromosomes 1–22. The *red line* shows the genome-wide significance threshold ($P<5\times10^{-8}$). SNPs in genome-wide significant loci are colored *green* for loci previously associated with bipolar disorder and *yellow* for novel associations from this study.

Source. Reprinted from Figure 1 in Mullins N, Forstner AJ, O'Connell KS, et al.: "Genome-Wide Association Study of More Than 40,000 Bipolar Disorder Cases Provides New Insights Into the Underlying Biology." *Nature Genetics* 53(6):817–829, 2021. PMCID: PMC8192451.

A PRS is constructed in the following manner. All alleles with nominal statistical significance in a case-control GWAS (e.g., with a cutoff $P<0.01$) are assembled and weighted by their individual odds ratios into a single PRS, simply a large number of putative risk alleles. In practice, investigators often use P values at five or more levels (e.g., $P<0.1$, 0.05, 0.01, 0.001, and 0.0001), and the number of alleles can vary between ~100,000 at $P<0.1$ and ~1,000 at $P<0.0001$. Most of these alleles are false positives, but some unknown fraction are true positives.

The validity of the PRS can be established by comparing the degree of overlap (percentage of all alleles shared) among genotyped individuals with the disorder (who were not part of the original studies defining the PRS) with that of GWAS-genotyped persons without the disorder. For example, a PRS for bipolar disorder should show a higher degree of overlap than would be expected randomly when studying a PRS derived from individuals with bipolar disorder or RUP. Conversely, there should be only randomly expected overlap (approximately 5%) when a bipolar disorder PRS is compared with a PRS derived from inflammatory bowel disease or some other unrelated illness.

Using a PRS for RUP and schizophrenia, Stahl et al. (2019) and Mullins et al. (2021) confirmed earlier reports (Athanasiu et al. 2010; Lee et al. 2013; Schizophrenia Psychiatric Genome-Wide Association Study Consortium 2011) of substantial overlap in risk alleles among persons carrying a diagnosis of schizophrenia, bipolar disorder, or RUP (Table 12–2). These findings are consistent with the family study reports noted

TABLE 12–2. Genetic correlations (r_g) among schizophrenia, recurrent unipolar disorder, and bipolar disorder

Disorders	r_g
Schizophrenia–bipolar disorder	0.70
Schizophrenia–recurrent unipolar disorder	0.35
Bipolar disorder–recurrent unipolar disorder	0.34

Source. Data from Stahl et al. 2019.

earlier. Given the evidence for overlap in genetic susceptibility for bipolar disorder, RUP, and schizophrenia, bivariate analyses of GWAS reports were hypothesized to reveal novel loci for the shared risk alleles. This indeed was the case, as reported by Amare et al. (2020), confirming the hypothesis that these three nosological categories share a fraction of risk alleles.

The genetic origins of cognitive impairment in schizophrenia remain undefined. To study this issue, Smeland et al. (2019) conducted conditional genetic analyses of assembled GWAS data for general intelligence (*n*=~270,000), schizophrenia (*n*=~82,000), and bipolar disorder (*n*=~52,000). They identified 75 distinct genomic loci associated with both schizophrenia and intelligence and 12 loci associated with both bipolar disorder and intelligence. Of these 87 loci, 20 were novel for schizophrenia and 4 were novel for bipolar disorder. The great majority of the 75 alleles associated with both schizophrenia and intelligence conveyed risk for cognitive impairment. In contrast, 9 of the 12 alleles associated with both bipolar disorder and intelligence were associated with improved cognition. These data suggest that cognitive impairment in schizophrenia is due at least in part to the cognitive effects of some schizophrenia risk alleles.

Conclusions Regarding Bipolar Disorder

The bipolar disorders are a substantially heritable group of disorders, as indicated by results from GWAS reports that confirm the h^2 indicated by family and twin studies (Pettersson et al. 2019; Polderman et al. 2015). There is a distinct absence of common alleles conveying even moderate risk for bipolar disorder, because nearly all have odds ratios of less than 1.2, consistent with a polygenic inheritance, in which hundreds of common alleles increase risk for bipolar disorder. These susceptibility alleles conveying modest amounts of risk require tens of thousands of case subjects and control subjects to achieve adequate power to detect them. In this scenario, it is difficult to imagine that widespread genetic testing for bipolar disorder in symptomatic individuals will become common and useful in establishing diagnosis or predicting course of illness or response to medications. Whole-genome sequencing is not likely to improve on these results for common alleles but may identify rare alleles.

A substantial challenge exists in translating the genetic data into novel treatments for bipolar disorder. Even in Mendelian (single-gene) diseases, this has proved very difficult. For success in this area, it may be necessary to define subgroups of bipolar disorder that have specific environmental contributions, such as *in utero* viral infections or early childhood adversity.

Genome-Wide Association Studies of Recurrent Unipolar Disorder

The h^2 of RUP has been estimated by twin, sibling, and family studies across the past 75 years, with a recent sibling h^2 estimate of approximately 35% from several million Swedish sibling pairs (Pettersson et al. 2019), an estimate that agrees well with twin studies (Polderman et al. 2015). RUP SNP h^2 is ~10%, or one-third of RUP h^2 (Pettersson et al. 2019). These and several previous estimates indicate that environmental and stochastic factors play substantial roles in RUP risk.

Several small RUP GWAS reports were the first to be published, including Muglia et al. (2010), Shyn et al. (2011), Sullivan et al. (2009), and Wray et al. (2012). There were no genome-wide significant results, even in the largest study, which included 2,431 case subjects and 3,673 screened control subjects (Wray et al. 2012). In a study of 5,303 Han Chinese women with RUP and 5,337 screened control subjects, using whole-genome sequencing, two genome-wide significant associations were identified, and were subsequently replicated in an independent Han Chinese sample (CONVERGE Consortium 2015). The two loci contributing to risk for RUP were located on chromosome 10: one near the *SIRT1* gene ($P=2.53\times10^{-10}$) and the other in an intron of the *LHPP* gene ($P=6.45\times10^{-12}$).

A self-reported diagnosis of depression as the phenotype was used in a large RUP GWAS that reported 15 associated loci ($N=459{,}481$; 121,380 case subjects and 338,101 control subjects) from patrons of a commercial genetics company (Hyde et al. 2016). A United Kingdom Biobank GWAS identified 17 variants associated across three definitions of RUP (maximum $N=322{,}580$; 113,769 case subjects and 208,811 control subjects). These three RUP phenotypes included a "broad" definition (RUP based on self-reported help-seeking for problems with nerves, anxiety, tension, or depression), a probable RUP phenotype (based on self-reported depressive symptoms with associated impairment), and definite RUP (defined by hospital records) (Howard et al. 2018a). A meta-analysis of 35 cohorts (130,664 RUP case subjects and 330,470 control subjects) reported 44 genome-wide significant loci, using several RUP phenotypes (Wray et al. 2018).

Howard et al. (2019) reported the largest RUP GWAS meta-analysis to date: 807,553 individuals (246,363 case subjects and 561,190 control subjects) from the three largest GWAS reports of RUP. They described 102 independent variants, 269 genes, and 15 gene sets associated with depression, including genes and gene pathways involving synaptic structure and neurotransmission. In an independent replication sample of 1,306,354 individuals (414,055 case subjects and 892,299 control subjects), 87 of the 102 associated variants were significant after multiple testing correction (Figure 12–2). An enrichment analysis provided specific evidence of the importance of prefrontal brain regions (Howard et al. 2018b).

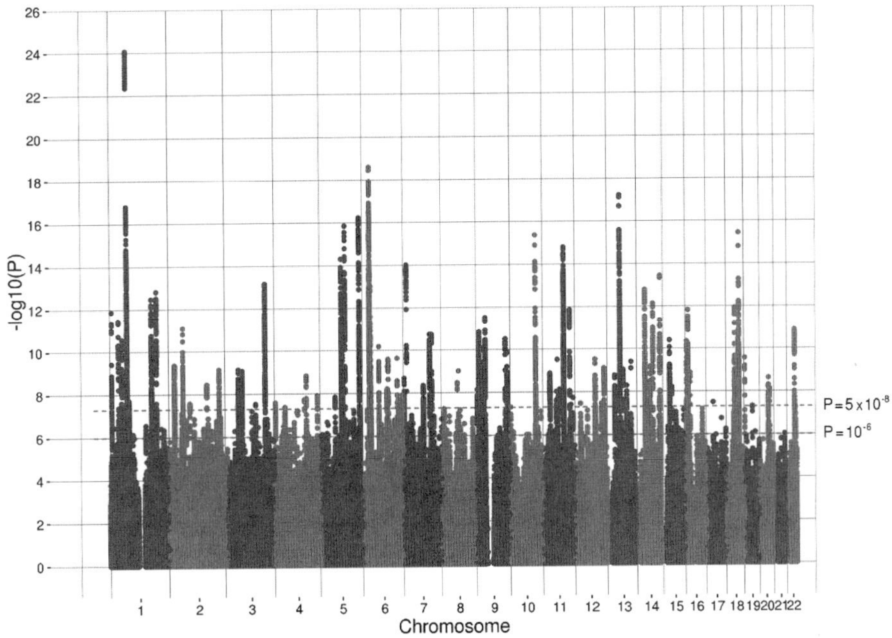

FIGURE 12–2. Manhattan plot of 87 loci for major depressive disorder in a genome-wide association study (GWAS) meta-analysis.

To view this figure in color, see Plate 5 in Color Gallery in middle of book.

Manhattan plot of the observed $-\log_{10} P$ values of each variant for an association with depression in the meta-analysis (see text description). Variants are positioned according to the Genome Reference Consortium Human Build 37 (GRCh37) assembly.

Source. Reprinted from Figure 1 in Howard DM, Adams MJ, Clarke TK, et al.: "Genome-Wide Meta-Analysis of Depression Identifies 102 Independent Variants and Highlights the Importance of the Prefrontal Brain Regions." *Nature Neuroscience* 22(3):343–352, 2019. PMCID: PMC6522363.

Copy Number Variants in Recurrent Unipolar Disorder and Bipolar Disorder

CNVs are often defined as deletions, duplications, or insertions larger than 1,000 base pairs. They may be inherited or arise de novo in the germ cell, in the zygote, or relatively early in neuronal development. In the latter case, the CNV may be somatic and not represented in the germline. Early studies of CNVs were focused on relatively large deletions, insertions, and duplications involving more than 100,000 DNA base pairs. This was partially due to the detection limit in first-generation "tiling arrays" and the relative paucity of genotyped SNPs (~100,000) in these early studies, because the ability to call relatively smaller CNVs with high accuracy was limited. Genome-wide CNV reports have revealed that rare (frequencies <1%) inherited or de novo large CNVs occur in people with idiopathic developmental delay/intellectual disability, autism spectrum disorder, and schizophrenia at a twofold higher rate than in control subjects (Cooper et al. 2011; Sebat et al. 2007). These CNVs have large effect sizes, with odds ratios ranging from 2 to 50. A more recent, larger study of 20,000 schizophrenia case subjects and 20,000 control subjects (Marshall et al. 2017) revealed genome-wide significance for eight CNVs that were overrepresented among the case subjects, including 1q21.1, 2p16.3 (*NRXN1*), 3q29, 7q11.2, 15q13.3, distal 16p11.2, proximal 16p11.2, and 22q11.2. A global enrichment analysis yielded an odds ratio of 1.11 ($P=5.7\times10^{-15}$), providing high-quality evidence that rare CNVs contribute to schizophrenia risk.

In a study of de novo CNVs in a cohort of 788 parent-child trios ($n=185$ for subjects with bipolar disorder, $n=177$ for schizophrenia, and $n=488$ for control subjects), Malhotra et al. (2011) reported that frequencies of de novo CNVs were significantly higher in subjects with bipolar disorder compared with control subjects (OR 4.8; $P=0.009$). De novo CNVs were more common among subjects with bipolar disorder with an age at onset younger than 18 (OR 6.3 [1.7–22.6]; $P=0.006$). Malhotra and colleagues also noted a significant enrichment of de novo CNVs in subjects with schizophrenia (OR 5.0; $P=0.007$).

In contrast to Malhotra et al. (2011), Grozeva et al. (2010) reported no evidence for an increased large CNV burden among 1,697 subjects with bipolar disorder and 2,806 nonpsychiatric control subjects, all of United Kingdom or European ancestry. Green et al. (2016), in a study of large (>100,000 base pairs) CNVs in 2,600 patients with bipolar disorder, reported that three such CNVs (duplications at 1q21.1, deletions at 3q29, and duplications at 16p11.2) previously associated with schizophrenia (Sebat et al. 2007) were also associated with bipolar disorder. However, only the statistical significance of the duplications at 16p11.2 survived correction for a genome-wide search for CNVs.

In a study of short (<100 base pairs) and long (>100 base pairs) CNVs across four cohorts of patients with RUP, Zhang et al. (2019) reported an excess of short CNVs but no excess of long CNVs. Short deletions were also modestly enriched for high-confidence "enhancer regions." Because enhancer regions are thought to bind transcription factors (which regulate mRNA production), such results suggest abnormalities of gene regulation rather than changes in amino acid sequences of proteins. CNVs in these enhancer genomic regions may cause abnormal amounts of mRNA (either increased or decreased), thereby elevating risk for RUP. Charney et al. (2019) noted that CNVs were increased among individuals with a schizoaffective disorder diagnosis, but not among those with a bipolar disorder diagnosis. Depending on the inclusion criteria for CNV studies of bipolar disorder, this diagnostic gray area may help resolve some contradictory studies. Kendall et al. (2019) conducted a large study of CNVs in approximately 466,000 individuals from the UK Biobank. Those with CNVs had a modestly increased risk (odds ratio of 1.34) of a depression diagnosis, using three different definitions, including a diagnosis given by a physician. This small risk increase may indicate that studies of fewer patients may not have had sufficient power.

It is evident that CNVs, documented as more frequent in schizophrenia, autism spectrum disorder, and developmental disabilities, are marginally, if at all, increased in bipolar disorder (Charney et al. 2019) and RUP. Large-scale studies of smaller CNVs in these disorders are expected as whole-genome sequencing is completed in more case subjects. The roles of these shorter CNVs in risk for bipolar disorder and RUP remain to be fully established.

Conclusions Regarding Recurrent Unipolar Disorder

It is clear that RUP risk is polygenic, with hundreds of common alleles contributing to overall risk. The total h^2 of RUP is approximately 35%, and the SNP h^2 is approximately 30% of total h^2. Thus, SNP data explain approximately 10% of the total risk for RUP. In this scenario, given the heterogeneity of an RUP diagnosis, it is unlikely that a PRS for RUP will be clinically useful in confirmation of diagnosis or prediction of course of illness or response to a distinct class of antidepressants.

Genetic Counseling

Families frequently seek advice regarding genetic risk for mood disorders, and heritability is sufficiently substantial that most persons with bipolar disorder or RUP have affected first- or second-degree relatives. Couples from families that have been severely affected may have concerns about reproduction and may request counseling regarding the risks to their children. Although important advances have been made through GWASs and sequencing, DNA data (including PRSs) are not currently used to predict risk, but these may be employed in the future. Most current mood disorder DNA data are derived from common SNPs, which capture only 20%–30% of the total h^2 (Lee et al. 2013) and only 5%–25% of the total phenotypic variance for mood disorders. At present, there is no indication for genetic testing of people at risk for bipolar disorder by virtue of an affected first-degree relative or other positive family history. No diagnostic or therapeutic advantage can be gained by applying a bipolar disorder PRS to a person suspected of or confirmed as having bipolar disorder. Such a PRS does not identify optimal pharmacotherapy or predict course of illness for an affected individual.

Family studies of mood disorders (e.g., Gershon et al. 1982; Weissman et al. 1984) form the basis for estimates of family risk, and several tables of risks have been published. It is important to take a careful family history, because the risks from studies must be interpreted in light of the specific family being counseled. It is strongly recommended that medical records of affected family members be reviewed whenever possible. Family lore and medical record evidence may not coincide. A high familial load suggests a greater risk, as does bilinear transmission (both prospective parents have a personal or family history of bipolar disorder and RUP).

When counseling family members who request risk assessment, emphasize both the recurrent course and the treatable nature of the mood disorder. Individual family members may interpret the available evidence quite differently due, in part, to personal experience, and the psychiatrist's sensitivity to this issue is an essential aspect of genetic counseling for psychiatric disorders. Another key aspect of genetic counseling for psychiatric disorders should include education about the signs and symptoms, as well as recommendations for consultation should such signs and symptoms appear. Providing website URLs for organizations that promote evidence-based evaluation and treatment information (e.g., the International Bipolar Foundation, Depression and Bipolar Support Alliance, Brain and Behavior Research Foundation, National Alliance for the Mentally Ill) is strongly recommended. This is particularly important in this era of widely available misinformation.

Conclusion

Family, twin, and adoption studies of bipolar disorder and RUP consistently indicate that both disorders have substantial heritable components of risk, with bipolar disorder having a higher h^2 (~50%) than RUP (~30%). Dozens of alleles have been implicated by several independent groups in the GWAS reports on bipolar disorder. A picture of bipolar disorder emerges as a polygenic disorder with hundreds of risk-increasing alleles, a substantial fraction of which may be shared by other psychiatric disorders, including schizophrenia and RUP. The genetic architecture of RUP is similar, with hundreds of risk-increasing alleles and a greater contribution (compared with that of bipolar disorder) from environmental factors. Lower h^2 in RUP may also predict greater difficulty in detecting common risk alleles of small effect.

The most recent GWAS reports provide a wealth of data on more than 100 genes containing risk alleles for bipolar disorder and RUP. However, this knowledge does not permit rapid translation to improved diagnosis and treatment. Current state-of-the-art genetic counseling should rely on estimates of common family history configurations (e.g., one or two affected parents), because no current evidence indicates that adding DNA estimates of risk (e.g., through a PRS) produces more predictive data.

References

Amare AT, Vaez A, Hsu YH, et al: Bivariate genome-wide association analyses of the broad depression phenotype combined with major depressive disorder, bipolar disorder or schizophrenia reveal eight novel genetic loci for depression. Mol Psychiatry 25(7):1420–1429, 2020 30626913

Athanasiu L, Mattingsdal M, Kähler AK, et al: Gene variants associated with schizophrenia in a Norwegian genome-wide study are replicated in a large European cohort. J Psychiatr Res 44(12):748–753, 2010 20185149

Baum AE, Akula N, Cabanero M, et al: A genome-wide association study implicates diacylglycerol kinase eta (DGKH) and several other genes in the etiology of bipolar disorder. Mol Psychiatry 13(2):197–207, 2008 17486107

Charney AW, Stahl EA, Green EK, et al: Contribution of rare copy number variants to bipolar disorder risk is limited to schizoaffective cases. Biol Psychiatry 86(2):110–119, 2019 30686506

CONVERGE Consortium: Sparse whole-genome sequencing identifies two loci for major depressive disorder. Nature 523(7562):588–591, 2015 26176920

Cooper GM, Coe BP, Girirajan S, et al: A copy number variation morbidity map of developmental delay. Nat Genet 43(9):838–846, 2011 21841781

Das S, Abecasis GR, Browning BL: Genotype imputation from large reference panels. Annu Rev Genomics Hum Genet 19:73–96, 2018 29799802

Ferreira MA, O'Donovan MC, Meng YA, et al: Collaborative genome-wide association analysis supports a role for ANK3 and CACNA1C in bipolar disorder. Nat Genet 40(9):1056–1058, 2008 18711365

Gershon ES, Hamovit J, Guroff JJ, et al: A family study of schizoaffective, bipolar I, bipolar II, unipolar, and normal control probands. Arch Gen Psychiatry 39(10):1157–1167, 1982 7125846

Green EK, Hamshere M, Forty L, et al: Replication of bipolar disorder susceptibility alleles and identification of two novel genome-wide significant associations in a new bipolar disorder case-control sample. Mol Psychiatry 18(12):1302–1307, 2013 23070075

Green EK, Rees E, Walters JT, et al: Copy number variation in bipolar disorder. Mol Psychiatry 21(1):89–93, 2016 25560756

Grozeva D, Kirov G, Ivanov D, et al: Rare copy number variants: a point of rarity in genetic risk for bipolar disorder and schizophrenia. Arch Gen Psychiatry 67(4):318–327, 2010 20368508

Howard DM, Adams MJ, Shirali M, et al: Genome-wide association study of depression phenotypes in UK Biobank identifies variants in excitatory synaptic pathways. Nat Commun 9(1):1470–1474, 2018a 29662059

Howard DM, Adams MJ, Shirali M, et al: Addendum: Genome-wide association study of depression phenotypes in UK Biobank identifies variants in excitatory synaptic pathways. Nat Commun 9(1):3578, 2018b 30166530

Howard DM, Adams MJ, Clarke TK, et al: Genome-wide meta-analysis of depression identifies 102 independent variants and highlights the importance of the prefrontal brain regions. Nat Neurosci 22(3):343–352, 2019 30718901

Hyde CL, Nagle MW, Tian C, et al: Identification of 15 genetic loci associated with risk of major depression in individuals of European descent. Nat Genet 48(9):1031–1036, 2016 27479909

Kendall KM, Rees E, Bracher-Smith M, et al: Association of rare copy number variants with risk of depression. JAMA Psychiatry 76(8):818–825, 2019 30994872

Kendler KS, Gardner CO: The risk for psychiatric disorders in relatives of schizophrenic and control probands: a comparison of three independent studies. Psychol Med 27(2):411–419, 1997 9089833

Lee SH, Ripke S, Neale BM, et al: Genetic relationship between five psychiatric disorders estimated from genome-wide SNPs. Nat Genet 45(9):984–994, 2013 23933821

Lichtenstein P, Yip BH, Björk C, et al: Common genetic determinants of schizophrenia and bipolar disorder in Swedish families: a population-based study. Lancet 373(9659):234–239, 2009 19150704

Malhotra D, McCarthy S, Michaelson JJ, et al: High frequencies of de novo CNVs in bipolar disorder and schizophrenia. Neuron 72(6):951–963, 2011 22196331

Manolio TA, Collins FS, Cox NJ, et al: Finding the missing heritability of complex diseases. Nature 461(7265):747–753, 2009 19812666

Marshall CR, Howrigan DP, Merico D, et al: Contribution of copy number variants to schizophrenia from a genome-wide study of 41,321 subjects. Nat Genet 49(1):27–35, 2017 27869829

Muglia P, Tozzi F, Galwey NW, et al: Genome-wide association study of recurrent major depressive disorder in two European case-control cohorts. Mol Psychiatry 15(6):589–601, 2010 19107115

Mullins N, Forstner AJ, O'Connell KS, et al: Genome-wide association study of more than 40,000 bipolar disorder cases provides new insights into the underlying biology. Nat Genet 53(6):817–829, 2021 34002096

Pettersson E, Lichtenstein P, Larsson H, et al: Genetic influences on eight psychiatric disorders based on family data of 4 408 646 full and half-siblings, and genetic data of 333 748 cases and controls. Psychol Med 49(7):1166–1173, 2019 30221610

Polderman TJC, Benyamin B, de Leeuw CA, et al: Meta-analysis of the heritability of human traits based on fifty years of twin studies. Nat Genet 47(7):702–709, 2015 25985137

Psychiatric GWAS Consortium Bipolar Disorder Working Group: Large-scale genome-wide association analysis of bipolar disorder identifies a new susceptibility locus near ODZ4. Nat Genet 43(10):977–983, 2011 21926972

Schizophrenia Psychiatric Genome-Wide Association Study Consortium: Genome-wide association study identifies five new schizophrenia loci. Nat Genet 43(10):969–976, 2011 21926974

Sebat J, Lakshmi B, Malhotra D, et al: Strong association of de novo copy number mutations with autism. Science 316(5823):445–449, 2007 17363630

Segurado R, Detera-Wadleigh SD, Levinson DF, et al: Genome scan meta-analysis of schizophrenia and bipolar disorder, part III: bipolar disorder. Am J Hum Genet 73(1):49–62, 2003 12802785

Shyn SI, Shi J, Kraft JB, et al: Novel loci for major depression identified by genome-wide association study of Sequenced Treatment Alternatives to Relieve Depression and meta-analysis of three studies. Mol Psychiatry 16(2):202–215, 2011 20038947

Sklar P, Smoller JW, Fan J, et al: Whole-genome association study of bipolar disorder. Mol Psychiatry 13(6):558–569, 2008 18317468

Smeland OB, Bahrami S, Frei O, et al: Genome-wide analysis reveals extensive genetic overlap between schizophrenia, bipolar disorder, and intelligence. Mol Psychiatry 25(4):844–853, 2020 30610197

Stahl EA, Breen G, Forstner AJ, et al: Genome-wide association study identifies 30 loci associated with bipolar disorder. Nat Genet 51(5):793–803, 2019 31043756

Sullivan PF, de Geus EJ, Willemsen G, et al: Genome-wide association for major depressive disorder: a possible role for the presynaptic protein piccolo. Mol Psychiatry 14(4):359–375, 2009 19065144

Weissman MM, Gershon ES, Kidd KK, et al: Psychiatric disorders in the relatives of probands with affective disorders. The Yale University–National Institute of Mental Health Collaborative Study. Arch Gen Psychiatry 41(1):13–21, 1984 6691780

Wellcome Trust Case Control Consortium: Genome wide association study of 14,000 cases of seven common diseases and 3,000 shared controls. Nature 447:661–678, 2007

Wray NR, Pergadia ML, Blackwood DH, et al: Genome-wide association study of major depressive disorder: new results, meta-analysis, and lessons learned. Mol Psychiatry 17(1):36–48, 2012 21042317

Wray NR, Ripke S, Mattheisen M, et al; Major Depressive Disorder Working Group of the Psychiatric Genomics Consortium: Genome-wide association analyses identify 44 risk variants and refine the genetic architecture of major depression. Nat Genet 50(5):668–681, 2018 29700475

Zhang X, Abdellaoui A, Rucker J, et al: Genome-wide burden of rare short deletions is enriched in major depressive disorder in four cohorts. Biol Psychiatry 85(12):1065–1073, 2019 31003785

CHAPTER 13

Epigenetics of Mood Disorders

Melissa P.H. Miller, M.Sc.
Caroline Symcox, B.Sc.
Frances A. Champagne, Ph.D.

Advances in molecular biology have generated novel perspectives within the study of mood disorders, with particular relevance to understanding the mechanisms that contribute to altered neurobiological structure and function. Epigenetic mechanisms have been increasingly explored, broadly within the context of health and development and more specifically as a molecular interface between the environmental factors that confer physical and psychiatric disease risk and the neural and behavioral outcomes associated with disease. In the case of mood disorders, epigenetic variation in the form of DNA methylation, posttranslational histone modifications, and expression of noncoding RNAs is being increasingly explored in humans and builds on an expansive foundation of studies in animal models that illustrate the role of epigenetics in depressive-like behavior (Peña and Nestler 2018), the epigenetic effects of pharmacological agents used in the treatment of mood disorders (Vialou et al. 2013), and the impact of stress and early life adversity on epigenetic variation in the brain (Alyamani and Murgatroyd 2018).

In this chapter, we describe the current state of knowledge on the role of epigenetics in mood disorders, focusing on research in humans that indicates epigenetic variation in the brain and in peripheral tissues associated with depression and bipolar disorder; epigenetic effects of pharmacological treatments used in depression and bipolar disorder; and the role of stress- and trauma-induced epigenetic variation in predicting the emergence of mood disorders.

Peripheral and Brain Epigenetic Markers of Depression

The regulation of gene expression is a dynamic process involving a broad range of factors that interact with DNA to either increase or decrease transcription (Cheung et al. 2000; Feng and Fan 2009; Meller et al. 2015). Characterization of variation in DNA methylation, posttranslational histone modifications, and noncoding RNAs has illustrated the role of these epigenetic mechanisms in gene regulation and also implicates these mechanisms as either etiologically relevant or as biomarkers for mood disorders. Within this growing literature, variation in DNA methylation within candidate genes or across the genome is most prevalent, primarily due to the stability of DNA methylation and the reliability of methods of assessing differential DNA methylation in the human genome. This literature includes epigenetic analyses of peripheral tissues, such as blood, buccal cells, and saliva, and analyses of postmortem brain tissue.

Given the role of epigenetic mechanisms in shaping the differentiation of cell types, interpretation of the "meaning" of epigenetic variation within peripheral tissues is challenging. Peripheral epigenetic variation associated with mood disorders may be a useful biomarker, but it is unclear whether these epigenetic biomarkers would also be evident in the brain or relevant in the altered brain function associated with mood-related outcomes. Analysis of epigenetic variation in the human brain is limited to postmortem brain tissue of individuals with a history of mood disorder. Although this epigenetic variation could be implied to be etiologically relevant, the confounding effects of treatment, emotional and behavioral phenotypes, and a broad range of limitations associated with molecular analyses in postmortem tissue (Ferrer et al. 2008) need to be carefully considered. Despite these caveats, the analysis of epigenetic variation in the periphery and brain, particularly when coupled with genetic and environment data, has the potential to identify novel pathways and treatment approaches in mood disorders.

Peripheral DNA Methylation Biomarkers of Depression

In addition to a growing literature on genome-wide analyses of DNA methylation in human tissues in cohorts of patients versus control subjects, much of the established work is focused on candidate genes selected based on their role in stress responsivity (e.g., *NR3C1*), neural plasticity (e.g., brain-derived neurotrophic factor [*BDNF*]), or neurotransmitter pathways implicated in depression (e.g., *SLC6A4*). The *NR3C1* gene, which encodes for the glucocorticoid receptor, is implicated in stress reactivity through the role of hippocampal glucocorticoid receptor expression in negative feedback within the hypothalamic-pituitary-adrenal axis (Sapolsky et al. 1985). In a longitudinal study, increased DNA methylation within the *NR3C1* gene in DNA extracted from blood samples was associated with current and follow-up depression as assessed by the Geriatric Mental State Schedule (Kang et al. 2018). Differential DNA methylation of *NR3C1* has also been observed in younger patient populations. In blood samples from patients with major depressive disorder (MDD) and healthy control subjects, DNA methylation of *NR3C1* was significantly positively associated with hippocampal volume within the MDD group, as assessed by MRI (Na et al. 2014).

This type of analysis provides useful insight into the potential relationship between epigenetic biomarkers observed in the periphery and brain structures implicated in the pathology of depression.

Genes involved in neuroplasticity, such as *BDNF*, are also implicated in depression, and analyses of DNA extracted from saliva indicate that decreased *BDNF* DNA methylation is associated with higher depression scores in adults (Song et al. 2014). However, in geriatric populations, an association has been found between increased *BDNF* DNA methylation in promoters I and IV and depression at baseline, as well as chronic late-life depression (Januar et al. 2015). Similar to *NR3C1*, peripheral DNA methylation of *BDNF* is associated with reduced cortical thickness among patients with MDD (Na et al. 2016), indicating the predictive utility of this biomarker in psychiatric phenotypes.

Analysis of DNA methylation in blood within a large cohort of elderly adults (N=1,863) indicated that increased DNA methylation of the angiotensin-converting enzyme (*ACE*) gene, which is a regulator of the stress response via vascular function (Tikellis and Thomas 2012), was inversely correlated with cortisol levels (Lam et al. 2018). Although *ACE* DNA methylation did not significantly correlate with depression in this sample, the relationship between *ACE* DNA methylation was moderated by genetic polymorphisms in *ACE*. These findings highlight the importance of incorporating both genetic and epigenetic analyses in the study of depression and complement a growing literature on gene-by-environment interactions in predicting altered epigenetic states (Liu et al. 2008).

Twin studies offer a methodologically more rigorous approach for incorporating analyses of genetics and shared environment in the relationship between DNA methylation and mood. In a study of 84 monozygotic twin pairs, DNA methylation within the serotonin transporter gene (*SLC6A4*), which is implicated in depression risk, was associated with scores on the Beck Depression Inventory–II using a matched twin-pair analysis and adjusting for lifestyle variables (Zhao et al. 2013).

Genome-wide analyses of DNA methylation in blood samples using the Infinium® HumanMethylation450 BeadChip (Illumina 450K) array indicate differential DNA methylation between World Trade Center first responders with a current diagnosis of MDD and those without a current or past MDD diagnosis (Kuan et al. 2017). However, even with a sample size of 473 participants, these effects did not survive false discovery rate correction. A similar lack of differential DNA methylation between MDD and healthy control subjects has been observed in monozygotic twin studies (examining concordant and discordant twin pairs), although increased *variability* in blood DNA methylation is observed in subjects with MDD (Byrne et al. 2013), a finding that was replicated in an additional cohort of monozygotic twin pairs (Córdova-Palomera et al. 2015).

A critical variable that may contribute to the reduced capacity to detect epigenetic effects in genome-wide analyses is medication status. Profiling of DNA methylation in the blood leukocytes of medication-free patients with MDD and healthy controls revealed that patients with MDD have significantly reduced DNA methylation within 363 cytosines and that patients and control subjects can be distinguished based on these epigenetic markers (Numata et al. 2015). In a community sample of 100 adults, analyses of DNA methylation using the HumanMethylation17 BeadChip array indicated increased and decreased DNA methylation at genomic loci associated with a lifetime history of depression (Uddin et al. 2011). A meta-analysis of epigenome-wide association studies (EWAS) likewise indicated an association between DNA methylation at several genomic loci and the severity of depressive symptomatology (Story Jovanova et al. 2018).

Genome-wide DNA methylation analysis can also be used to assess biological aging, by comparing accelerated "epigenetic age" relative to chronological age based on the DNA methylation status of approximately 300 genes (Horvath 2013). Epigenetic age acceleration is associated with exposure to stress (Wolf et al. 2018) and with mortality rates (even when controlling for chronological age) (Fransquet et al. 2019). Analyses of DNA from blood samples of patients with depression compared with healthy control subjects indicate significant epigenetic age acceleration in depressed patients, with increasing symptom severity associated with increased epigenetic age acceleration (Han et al. 2018). This effect was also replicated in postmortem brain tissue samples of patients with depression and healthy control subjects, confirming the lack of tissue specificity for this particular epigenetic measure (Han et al. 2018; Horvath 2013). Importantly, epigenetic age acceleration can be altered through intervention (Brody et al. 2016) and lifestyle factors (Quach et al. 2017), which may be a promising supplement to pharmacological treatments of depression.

DNA Methylation Variation in the Brain in Depression

In some cases, MDD-associated epigenetic variations in the periphery overlap with those in the brain (Oh et al. 2015). In a comparison of patients with MDD and healthy control subjects, differential DNA methylation within the prefrontal cortex was found to overlap with loci found to be differentially methylated in the blood (Aberg et al. 2020). The differential methylation of genes implicated in depression is more evident with increasing age (McKinney et al. 2019), possibly indicating disruption to molecular processes that control gene regulation.

An important consideration in these postmortem brain studies is the overlap between MDD and suicidality. Suicidal behavior may be associated with a unique epigenomic profile within the brain in comparison with healthy control subjects and patients with MDD without suicidal behavior. Research designs that can disentangle the MDD-specific DNA methylation profiles will be critical to generating fine-tuned hypotheses about the epigenetics of depression.

Histones and Noncoding RNA in Depression

Posttranslational histone modifications are a dynamic mechanism of gene regulation and are themselves regulated by enzymatic processes that add and remove chemical tags to histone proteins. A comparison of blood samples from subjects with MDD and healthy control subjects indicates increased expression of histone deacetylase (HDAC), an enzyme that removes the acetyl group from histone proteins during a depressive state but not during remission (Hobara et al. 2010), in the blood of patients with MDD. Similarly, differential HDAC expression in patients with MDD is normalized following 8 weeks of treatment with paroxetine (Iga et al. 2007). Within the brain, histone acetylation of histone 3 (H3) at lysine 14 (H3K14ac) within the nucleus accumbens is increased in patients with MDD compared with healthy control subjects (Covington et al. 2009). Histone trimethylation within the synapsin I (*SYN1*) gene (which is involved in neurotransmitter release and synaptic plasticity) is increased in the prefrontal cortex of patients with MDD (Cruceanu et al. 2013).

Noncoding RNAs regulate transcription and translation through direct interactions with DNA, RNA, and proteins (Sato et al. 2011). Within the epigenetics literature, microRNAs (miRNAs) have emerged as critical regulators of gene function during development and in response to stress and other environmental exposures (Allen and Dwivedi 2020; Lema and Cunningham 2010). Compared with healthy control subjects, patients with depression have elevated levels of serum miR-132 and miR-182 (Li et al. 2013). These miRNAs may play a significant role in regulating *BDNF* RNA and protein levels, with implications for neuroplasticity. Although other miRNAs have been explored as peripheral biomarkers of depression, inconsistencies among studies limit the generalizability of their findings (Yuan et al. 2018). Within the prefrontal cortex, expression of miR-1202 is decreased in patients with MDD compared with healthy control subjects (Lopez et al. 2014). Within human cell lines, miR-1202 expression was found to increase following a 2-week treatment with citalopram or imipramine (Lopez et al. 2014). These findings suggest that increased understanding of the role of miRNAs in depression can potentially identify novel therapeutic targets.

Brain and Peripheral Epigenetic Markers of Bipolar Disorder

Similar to the work on depression, epigenetic analyses have been increasingly incorporated into the study of bipolar disorder, with the focus on both candidate gene and whole-genome characterization of the epigenome in both the periphery and postmortem brain tissue. A critical question is whether a unique epigenomic signature is associated with different clinical diagnoses within the mood disorders. Although robust clinical epigenetic markers have yet to emerge, the potential of this approach remains and will benefit from prospective study designs and analyses that determine the relationship between specific epigenetic markers and symptom profiles.

Peripheral DNA Methylation Biomarkers in Bipolar Disorder

Within peripheral blood DNA samples of patients with bipolar disorder compared with healthy control subjects, DNA methylation within the long interspersed nuclear element-1 (*LINE-1*), a transposable element within the human genome, is significantly decreased (Li et al. 2018). DNA methylation within *LINE-1* has been demonstrated to be highly correlated with genome-wide DNA methylation levels. Consistent with these *LINE-1* findings, global DNA hypomethylation has been observed in blood samples of patients with bipolar disorder compared with healthy control subjects (Murata et al. 2020). Analyses of DNA methylation levels in genes that have significant overlap between bipolar disorder and schizophrenia (based on genome-wide association studies) indicate that although some overlap in DNA methylation between these disorders occurs (e.g., hypomethylation of *FAM63B*), unique DNA methylation patterns differentiate these candidate genes (e.g., hypermethylation of

TBC1D22A in bipolar disorder; hypomethylation of *TBC1D22A* in schizophrenia) (Sugawara et al. 2018).

Twin studies of bipolar disorder provide additional insights into the epigenetic profiles of mood disorders. Among 11 pairs of monozygotic twins discordant for bipolar disorder, differential DNA methylation was found within blood samples in the gene encoding *ST6GALNAC1*, which was hypomethylated in the affected twin compared with the unaffected sibling (Dempster et al. 2011). Similar to the findings regarding *TBC1D22A*, the *ZNF659* gene (which encodes *ZNF385D*) was found to be hypomethylated in the twin pairs with bipolar disorder but hypermethylated in twin pairs with schizophrenia. Differential methylation of the peptidylprolyl isomerase E-like (*PPIEL*) pseudogene in lymphoblastoid cells has also been observed in bipolar disorder–discordant twin-pair analyses (Kuratomi et al. 2008). Follow-up analyses have indicated decreased DNA methylation of *PPIEL* in patients with bipolar II disorder compared with healthy control subjects and patients with bipolar I disorder, indicating a potential relationship between DNA methylation and specific symptom profiles.

Hypermethylation of the *SLC6A4* gene has been observed in lymphoblastoid cells of patients with bipolar disorder in a twin-pair and a case-control analysis (Sugawara et al. 2011). This effect has also been observed in the postmortem frontal cortex of patients with bipolar disorder. Interestingly, the impact of *SLC6A4* DNA methylation on the expression of the serotonin transporter depends on the *SLC6A4* genotype (Sugawara et al. 2011), illustrating the interdependency of genetic and epigenetic factors.

DNA Methylation in the Brain in Bipolar Disorder

Within the prefrontal cortex, patients with bipolar disorder have been found to have decreased DNA methylation of *KCNQ3* (which encodes for a voltage-gated potassium channel) in comparison with matched control subjects (Kaminsky et al. 2015). Differential DNA methylation of the serotonin receptor type 2 (*HTR2A*) gene between patients with bipolar disorder and healthy control subjects has been observed in the frontal cortex. This epigenetic profile in bipolar disorder is significantly impacted by medication history, with valproate use associated with hypomethylation (Abdolmaleky et al. 2011). Hypomethylation of the membrane-bound catechol-*O*-methyltransferase (*MB-COMT*) gene has been observed in the frontal cortex of patients with bipolar disorder compared with healthy control subjects (Abdolmaleky et al. 2006), and the DNA methylation status of both *MB-COMT* and *HTR2A* is also observed in saliva samples of patients with bipolar disorder (Ghadirivasfi et al. 2011; Nohesara et al. 2011).

Similar to MDD, the *BDNF* gene exhibits differential DNA methylation in patients with bipolar disorder, with increased DNA methylation of the *BDNF* promoter in the frontal cortex in a sample of patients compared with matched control subjects (Rao et al. 2012). Within blood samples, this association between bipolar disorder and *BDNF* hypermethylation has been replicated; however, the differential DNA methylation and expression of *BDNF* were restricted to patients with bipolar II disorder (D'Addario et al. 2012).

Bipolar disorder is associated with indices of premature aging, including decreased cognitive functioning, increased cardiovascular risk, and decreased gray matter volume (Fries et al. 2020b). Analyses of hippocampal tissue from postmortem brains of patients with bipolar disorder and matched nonpsychiatric control subjects indicated epigenetic age acceleration in the patients based on genome-wide DNA methylation levels (Fries et al. 2020a). However, this effect was observed only in the hippocampus of older patients and was not observed in the cerebellum (Fries et al. 2017), although some evidence suggests that the cerebellum is generally slower to age compared with other brain regions (Horvath et al. 2015).

Histones and Noncoding RNA in Bipolar Disorder

The expression of *HDAC4* mRNA is increased during depressive states in patients with bipolar disorder compared with control subjects, whereas the expression of *HDAC6* and *HDAC8* is decreased during both depression and remission (Hobara et al. 2010). In genome-wide association analyses aimed at identifying common pathways across MDD, bipolar disorder, and schizophrenia, genes involved in histone methylation emerge as a convergent gene cluster in these forms of psychiatric illness. Within the frontal cortex of postmortem bipolar disorder brain samples, increased global histone (H3) acetylation and phosphorylation are observed (Fries et al. 2020b). A broad characterization of miRNA expression in the prefrontal cortex indicates that approximately 19% of the variance in expression can be accounted for by a diagnosis of bipolar disorder and its associated decreased expression of miRNAs (Moreau et al. 2011). The association between bipolar disorder and altered histone and miRNA profiles likely has broad implications for gene expression and may also provide insights into treatment response.

Epigenetic Effects of Treatment of Mood Disorders

A consistent theme within the literature on epigenetic variation in mood disorders is the utility of using epigenetic profiles to predict treatment responsiveness and the epigenetic effects of pharmacological treatments with proven antidepressant or mood stabilizing effectiveness. This theme is particularly relevant to compounds such as valproate and sodium butyrate, which are used extensively in preclinical studies to modify histone acetylation and DNA methylation, with consequences for gene expression and behavior (Nicolini and Fahnestock 2018; Schroeder et al. 2007).

In addition to the previously noted effects of paroxetine, citalopram, and imipramine on histones (Iga et al. 2007) and miRNAs (Lopez et al. 2014), differential DNA methylation may be a significant predictor of treatment response. Comparison of antidepressant responders and nonresponders indicates that DNA methylation within *BDNF* is associated with treatment response, such that nonresponders have significantly lower *BDNF* DNA methylation in blood samples (Tadić et al. 2014). Pharmacological treatments for patients with bipolar disorder, including quetiapine and valproate, can induce genome wide changes in DNA methylation (Houtepen et al. 2016). Analyses of DNA methylation in blood samples from patients with bipolar disorder after at least 1 month of treatment using the Illumina 450K array indicate altered DNA methylation levels (compared with baseline) when controlling for immune cell type composition of the blood sample.

Among patients with bipolar disorder, compared with control subjects, global DNA methylation levels in leukocytes were decreased in patients treated with lithium monotherapy, whereas hypermethylation was observed in patients treated with a lithium combination therapy (lithium+valproate) (Backlund et al. 2015). mRNA levels of the prodynorphin (*PDYN*) gene were significantly downregulated, and the *PDYN* promoter was hypermethylated; this effect on *PDYN* DNA methylation was not observed if the patients were being treated with lithium, which is associated with decreased DNA methylation at the *PDYN* promoter (D'Addario et al. 2018). Effects of BPD treatments have also been observed on measures of histone acetylation (Sharma et al. 2006) and miRNA expression (Lim et al. 2016), confirming the broad epigenetic effects of pharmacotherapies that ameliorate bipolar disorder symptoms.

Epigenetic Effects of Stress and Trauma

Early life adversity and later life trauma and stress are established predictors of psychiatric illness. These exposures also induce robust epigenetic changes in both the periphery and the brain that may account for some of the observed epigenetic differences between patients with MDD, patients with bipolar disorder, and healthy control subjects. For example, in blood samples from monozygotic twin pairs, differential DNA methylation of *BDNF* and *NR3C1* was found to account for approximately 20% of the relationship between childhood trauma and depressive symptoms in adulthood (Peng et al. 2018). Elevated DNA methylation within *NR3C1* is also observed in the hippocampus among individuals with a history of childhood maltreatment (McGowan et al. 2009). Adult trauma is also associated with altered DNA methylation in the periphery, and these epigenetic changes, combined with a history of childhood adversity, can predict posttraumatic stress symptomatology (Boks et al. 2016).

Interactions between genetic polymorphisms within MDD and bipolar disorder candidate genes and childhood adversity or adult trauma are also observed in analyses of the epigenome. Comparison of individuals with a diagnosis of MDD with healthy control subjects indicates that among patients with MDD who have the high-risk allele of the glucocorticoid receptor regulator FK506 binding protein 5 (*FKBP5*) gene, childhood adversity predicts lower levels of DNA methylation within *FKBP5* in white blood cells (Tozzi et al. 2018). Moreover, among participants with MDD and control subjects, reduced *FKBP5* DNA methylation levels were associated with reduced gray matter in the inferior frontal orbital gyrus, suggesting a link between peripheral *FKBP5* DNA methylation and neurodevelopmental processes.

Analyses of polymorphisms within *SLC6A4* have indicated that, compared with individuals who have the LL alleles, individuals with the S-allele show increased global DNA methylation associated with early life stress, chronic stress, and recent depressive symptoms (Duman and Canli 2015). Among individuals with the L-allele of the monoamine oxidase A (*MAOA*) gene, history of childhood adversity is a significant risk factor for depression, and decreased DNA methylation within *MAOA* in saliva samples is associated with MDD (Melas et al. 2013). Although disentangling the epigenetic effects of childhood adversity from those associated with MDD or bipolar disorder symptoms, lifestyle, and medication history is challenging, this growing body of literature provides a more integrative viewpoint on risk and resilience for psychiatric disorders.

Conclusion

Epigenetic mechanisms play a fundamental role in basic biological processes that has broad implications for health and development. In the case of mood disorders such as MDD and bipolar disorder, epigenetic processes may be a contributor to disrupted neurodevelopmental trajectories in response to childhood adversity, a significant predictor of treatment response, a mechanism of treatment effects, and a molecular link between mental health and physical health and longevity. With increasing tools to profile the human epigenome, our understanding of the role of epigenetics in mood disorders is poised to expand. Future work in this area should consider study designs that are genetically informed, account for exposures from the physical and psychosocial environment that can impact the epigenome, and provide a detailed analysis of patient medication history.

References

Abdolmaleky HM, Cheng K-H, Faraone SV, et al: Hypomethylation of MB-COMT promoter is a major risk factor for schizophrenia and bipolar disorder. Hum Mol Genet 15(21):3132–3145, 2006 16984965

Abdolmaleky HM, Yaqubi S, Papageorgis P, et al: Epigenetic dysregulation of HTR2A in the brain of patients with schizophrenia and bipolar disorder. Schizophr Res 129(2-3):183–190, 2011 21550210

Aberg KA, Dean B, Shabalin AA, et al: Methylome-wide association findings for major depressive disorder overlap in blood and brain and replicate in independent brain samples. Mol Psychiatry 25(6):1344–1354, 2020 30242228

Allen L, Dwivedi Y: MicroRNA mediators of early life stress vulnerability to depression and suicidal behavior. Mol Psychiatry 25(2):308–320, 2020 31740756

Alyamani RAS, Murgatroyd C: Epigenetic programming by early life stress, in Epigenetics and Psychiatric Disease (Progress in Molecular Biology and Translational Science, Vol 157). Edited by Grayson DR. Cambridge, MA, Academic Press, 2018, pp 133–150

Backlund L, Wei YB, Martinsson L, et al: Mood stabilizers and the influence on global leukocyte DNA methylation in bipolar disorder. Mol Neuropsychiatry 1(2):76–81, 2015 27602359

Boks MP, Rutten BPF, Geuze E, et al: SKA2 methylation is involved in cortisol stress reactivity and predicts the development of posttraumatic stress disorder (PTSD) after military deployment. Neuropsychopharmacology 41(5):1350–1356, 2016 26361058

Brody GH, Yu T, Chen E, et al: Family-centered prevention ameliorates the longitudinal association between risky family processes and epigenetic aging. J Child Psychol Psychiatry 57(5):566–574, 2016 26680699

Byrne EM, Carrillo-Roa T, Henders AK, et al: Monozygotic twins affected with major depressive disorder have greater variance in methylation than their unaffected co-twin. Transl Psychiatry 3:e269, 2013 23756378

Cheung P, Allis CD, Sassone-Corsi P: Signaling to chromatin through histone modifications. Cell 103(2):263–271, 2000 11057899

Córdova-Palomera A, Fatjó-Vilas M, Gastó C, et al: Genome-wide methylation study on depression: differential methylation and variable methylation in monozygotic twins. Transl Psychiatry 5:e557, 2015 25918994

Covington HE 3rd, Maze I, LaPlant QC, et al: Antidepressant actions of histone deacetylase inhibitors. J Neurosci 29(37):11451–11460, 2009 19759294

Cruceanu C, Alda M, Nagy C, et al: H3K4 tri-methylation in synapsin genes leads to different expression patterns in bipolar disorder and major depression. Int J Neuropsychopharmacol 16(2):289–299, 2013 22571925

D'Addario C, Dell'Osso B, Palazzo MC, et al: Selective DNA methylation of BDNF promoter in bipolar disorder: differences among patients with BDI and BDII. Neuropsychopharmacology 37(7):1647–1655, 2012 22353757

D'Addario C, Palazzo MC, Benatti B, et al: Regulation of gene transcription in bipolar disorders: role of DNA methylation in the relationship between prodynorphin and brain derived neurotrophic factor. Prog Neuropsychopharmacol Biol Psychiatry 82:314–321, 2018 28830794

Dempster EL, Pidsley R, Schalkwyk LC, et al: Disease-associated epigenetic changes in monozygotic twins discordant for schizophrenia and bipolar disorder. Hum Mol Genet 20(24):4786–4796, 2011 21908516

Duman EA, Canli T: Influence of life stress, 5-HTTLPR genotype, and SLC6A4 methylation on gene expression and stress response in healthy Caucasian males. Biol Mood Anxiety Disord 5(1):2, 2015 25995833

Feng J, Fan G: The role of DNA methylation in the central nervous system and neuropsychiatric disorders. Int Rev Neurobiol 89:67–84, 2009 19900616

Ferrer I, Martinez A, Boluda S, et al: Brain banks: benefits, limitations and cautions concerning the use of post-mortem brain tissue for molecular studies. Cell Tissue Bank 9(3):181–194, 2008 18543077

Fransquet PD, Wrigglesworth J, Woods RL, et al: The epigenetic clock as a predictor of disease and mortality risk: a systematic review and meta-analysis. Clin Epigenetics 11(1):62, 2019 30975202

Fries GR, Bauer IE, Scaini G, et al: Accelerated epigenetic aging and mitochondrial DNA copy number in bipolar disorder. Transl Psychiatry 7(12):1283, 2017 29225347

Fries GR, Bauer IE, Scaini G, et al: Accelerated hippocampal biological aging in bipolar disorder. Bipolar Disord 22(5):498–507, 2020a 31746071

Fries GR, Zamzow MJ, Andrews T, et al: Accelerated aging in bipolar disorder: a comprehensive review of molecular findings and their clinical implications. Neurosci Biobehav Rev 112:107–116, 2020b 32018037

Ghadirivasfi M, Nohesara S, Ahmadkhaniha H-R, et al: Hypomethylation of the serotonin receptor type-2A gene (HTR2A) at T102C polymorphic site in DNA derived from the saliva of patients with schizophrenia and bipolar disorder. Am J Med Genet B Neuropsychiatr Genet 156B(5):536–545, 2011 21598376

Han LKM, Aghajani M, Clark SL, et al: Epigenetic aging in major depressive disorder. Am J Psychiatry 175(8):774–782, 2018 29656664

Hobara T, Uchida S, Otsuki K, et al: Altered gene expression of histone deacetylases in mood disorder patients. J Psychiatr Res 44(5):263–270, 2010 19767015

Horvath S: DNA methylation age of human tissues and cell types. Genome Biol 14(10):R115, 2013 24138928

Horvath S, Mah V, Lu AT, et al: The cerebellum ages slowly according to the epigenetic clock. Aging (Albany NY) 7(5):294–306, 2015 26000617

Houtepen LC, van Bergen AH, Vinkers CH, et al: DNA methylation signatures of mood stabilizers and antipsychotics in bipolar disorder. Epigenomics 8(2):197–208, 2016 26792232

Iga J, Ueno S, Yamauchi K, et al: Altered HDAC5 and CREB mRNA expressions in the peripheral leukocytes of major depression. Prog Neuropsychopharmacol Biol Psychiatry 31(3):628–632, 2007 17258370

Januar V, Ancelin M-L, Ritchie K, et al: BDNF promoter methylation and genetic variation in late-life depression. Transl Psychiatry 5:e619, 2015 26285129

Kaminsky Z, Jones I, Verma R, et al: DNA methylation and expression of KCNQ3 in bipolar disorder. Bipolar Disord 17(2):150–159, 2015 25041603

Kang H-J, Bae K-Y, Kim S-W, et al: Longitudinal associations between glucocorticoid receptor methylation and late-life depression. Prog Neuropsychopharmacol Biol Psychiatry 84(Pt A):56–62, 2018 29432878

Kuan P-F, Waszczuk MA, Kotov R, et al: An epigenome-wide DNA methylation study of PTSD and depression in World Trade Center responders. Transl Psychiatry 7(6):e1158, 2017 28654093

Kuratomi G, Iwamoto K, Bundo M, et al: Aberrant DNA methylation associated with bipolar disorder identified from discordant monozygotic twins. Mol Psychiatry 13(4):429–441, 2008 17471289

Lam D, Ancelin M-L, Ritchie K, et al: DNA methylation and genetic variation of the angiotensin converting enzyme (ACE) in depression. Psychoneuroendocrinology 88:1–8, 2018 29132028

Lema C, Cunningham MJ: MicroRNAs and their implications in toxicological research. Toxicol Lett 198(2):100–105, 2010 20599482

Li S, Yang Q, Hou Y, et al: Hypomethylation of LINE-1 elements in schizophrenia and bipolar disorder. J Psychiatr Res 107:68–72, 2018 30326341

Li Y-J, Xu M, Gao Z-H, et al: Alterations of serum levels of BDNF-related miRNAs in patients with depression. PLoS One 8(5):e63648, 2013 23704927

Lim CH, Zainal NZ, Kanagasundram S, et al: Preliminary examination of microRNA expression profiling in bipolar disorder I patients during antipsychotic treatment. Am J Med Genet B Neuropsychiatr Genet 171(6):867–874, 2016 27177356

Liu L, Li Y, Tollefsbol TO: Gene-environment interactions and epigenetic basis of human diseases. Curr Issues Mol Biol 10(1-2):25–36, 2008 18525104

Lopez JP, Lim R, Cruceanu C, et al: miR-1202 is a primate-specific and brain-enriched microRNA involved in major depression and antidepressant treatment. Nat Med 20(7):764–768, 2014 24908571

McGowan PO, Sasaki A, D'Alessio AC, et al: Epigenetic regulation of the glucocorticoid receptor in human brain associates with childhood abuse. Nat Neurosci 12(3):342–348, 2009 19234457

McKinney BC, Lin C-W, Rahman T, et al: DNA methylation in the human frontal cortex reveals a putative mechanism for age-by-disease interactions. Transl Psychiatry 9(1):39, 2019 30696804

Melas PA, Wei Y, Wong CCY, et al: Genetic and epigenetic associations of MAOA and NR3C1 with depression and childhood adversities. Int J Neuropsychopharmacol 16(7):1513–1528, 2013 23449091

Meller VH, Joshi SS, Deshpande N: Modulation of chromatin by noncoding RNA. Annu Rev Genet 49:673–695, 2015 26631517

Moreau MP, Bruse SE, David-Rus R, et al: Altered microRNA expression profiles in postmortem brain samples from individuals with schizophrenia and bipolar disorder. Biol Psychiatry 69(2):188–193, 2011 21183010

Murata Y, Ikegame T, Koike S, et al: Global DNA hypomethylation and its correlation to the betaine level in peripheral blood of patients with schizophrenia. Prog Neuropsychopharmacol Biol Psychiatry 99:109855, 2020 31911076

Na K-S, Chang HS, Won E, et al: Association between glucocorticoid receptor methylation and hippocampal subfields in major depressive disorder. PLoS One 9(1):e85425, 2014 24465557

Na K-S, Won E, Kang J, et al: Brain-derived neurotrophic factor promoter methylation and cortical thickness in recurrent major depressive disorder. Sci Rep 6(1):21089, 2016 26876488

Nicolini C, Fahnestock M: The valproic acid-induced rodent model of autism. Exp Neurol 299(Pt A):217–227, 2018 28472621

Nohesara S, Ghadirivasfi M, Mostafavi S, et al: DNA hypomethylation of MB-COMT promoter in the DNA derived from saliva in schizophrenia and bipolar disorder. J Psychiatr Res 45(11):1432–1438, 2011 21820670

Numata S, Ishii K, Tajima A, et al: Blood diagnostic biomarkers for major depressive disorder using multiplex DNA methylation profiles: discovery and validation. Epigenetics 10(2):135–141, 2015 25587773

Oh G, Wang S-C, Pal M, et al: DNA modification study of major depressive disorder: beyond locus-by-locus comparisons. Biol Psychiatry 77(3):246–255, 2015 25108803

Peña CJ, Nestler EJ: Progress in epigenetics of depression, in Epigenetics and Psychiatric Disease (Progress in Molecular Biology and Translational Science, Vol 157). Edited by Grayson DR. Cambridge, MA, Academic Press, 2018, pp 41–66

Peng H, Zhu Y, Strachan E, et al: Childhood trauma, DNA methylation of stress-related genes, and depression: findings from two monozygotic twin studies. Psychosom Med 80(7):599–608, 2018 29781947

Quach A, Levine ME, Tanaka T, et al: Epigenetic clock analysis of diet, exercise, education, and lifestyle factors. Aging (Albany NY) 9(2):419–446, 2017 28198702

Rao JS, Keleshian VL, Klein S, et al: Epigenetic modifications in frontal cortex from Alzheimer's disease and bipolar disorder patients. Transl Psychiatry 2:e132, 2012 22760556

Sapolsky RM, Meaney MJ, McEwen BS: The development of the glucocorticoid receptor system in the rat limbic brain, III: negative-feedback regulation. Brain Res 350(1–2):169–173, 1985 3986611

Sato F, Tsuchiya S, Meltzer SJ, et al: MicroRNAs and epigenetics. FEBS J 278(10):1598–1609, 2011 21395977

Schroeder FA, Lin CL, Crusio WE, et al: Antidepressant-like effects of the histone deacetylase inhibitor, sodium butyrate, in the mouse. Biol Psychiatry 62(1):55–64, 2007 16945350

Sharma RP, Rosen C, Kartan S, et al: Valproic acid and chromatin remodeling in schizophrenia and bipolar disorder: preliminary results from a clinical population. Schizophr Res 88(1–3):227–231, 2006 16996718

Song Y, Miyaki K, Suzuki T, et al: Altered DNA methylation status of human brain derived neurotrophic factor gene could be useful as biomarker of depression. Am J Med Genet B Neuropsychiatr Genet 165B(4):357–364, 2014 24801253

Story Jovanova O, Nedeljkovic I, Spieler D, et al: DNA methylation signatures of depressive symptoms in middle-aged and elderly persons: meta-analysis of multiethnic epigenome-wide studies. JAMA Psychiatry 75(9):949–959, 2018 29998287

Sugawara H, Iwamoto K, Bundo M, et al: Hypermethylation of serotonin transporter gene in bipolar disorder detected by epigenome analysis of discordant monozygotic twins. Transl Psychiatry 1(7):e24, 2011 22832526

Sugawara H, Murata Y, Ikegame T, et al: DNA methylation analyses of the candidate genes identified by a methylome-wide association study revealed common epigenetic alterations in schizophrenia and bipolar disorder. Psychiatry Clin Neurosci 72(4):245–254, 2018 29430824

Tadić A, Müller-Engling L, Schlicht KF, et al: Methylation of the promoter of brain-derived neurotrophic factor exon IV and antidepressant response in major depression. Mol Psychiatry 19(3):281–283, 2014 23670489

Tikellis C, Thomas MC: Angiotensin-converting enzyme 2 (ACE2) is a key modulator of the renin angiotensin system in health and disease. Int J Pept 2012:256294, 2012 22536270

Tozzi L, Farrell C, Booij L, et al: Epigenetic changes of FKBP5 as a link connecting genetic and environmental risk factors with structural and functional brain changes in major depression. Neuropsychopharmacology 43(5):1138–1145, 2018 29182159

Uddin M, Koenen KC, Aiello AE, et al: Epigenetic and inflammatory marker profiles associated with depression in a community-based epidemiologic sample. Psychol Med 41(5):997–1007, 2011 20836906

Vialou V, Feng J, Robison AJ, et al: Epigenetic mechanisms of depression and antidepressant action. Annu Rev Pharmacol Toxicol 53:59–87, 2013 23020296

Wolf EJ, Maniates H, Nugent N, et al: Traumatic stress and accelerated DNA methylation age: a meta-analysis. Psychoneuroendocrinology 92:123–134, 2018 29452766

Yuan H, Mischoulon D, Fava M, et al: Circulating microRNAs as biomarkers for depression: many candidates, few finalists. J Affect Disord 233:68–78, 2018 28673667

Zhao J, Goldberg J, Bremner JD, et al: Association between promoter methylation of serotonin transporter gene and depressive symptoms: a monozygotic twin study. Psychosom Med 75(6):523–529, 2013 23766378

PART IV

Somatic Interventions for Mood Disorders

CHAPTER 14

Tricyclics, Tetracyclics, and Monoamine Oxidase Inhibitors

Matthew Macaluso, D.O., DFAPA

Like many established treatments in psychiatry, monoamine oxidase inhibitors (MAOIs) and tricyclic antidepressants (TCAs) were serendipitously discovered. MAOIs were discovered after World War II when compounds with a hydrazine base were developed (isocarboxazid) from excess rocket fuel and used to treat tuberculosis and, later, depression. Iproniazid, which was developed for tuberculosis in the 1950s, has known MAOI properties and resulted in improved mood for patients being treated for tuberculosis. Although hepatotoxicity limited iproniazid's use as an antidepressant, the development of other MAOIs led to their widespread use in the 1950s through the 1970s (Hillhouse and Porter 2015).

As with MAOIs, TCAs were serendipitously discovered in the late 1950s in efforts to produce more effective antipsychotic drugs. TCAs were created from chlorpromazine by substituting sulfur for an ethylene bridge and modifying the phenothiazine ring. These modifications led to the development of imipramine, the first TCA. The antidepressant properties of imipramine were discovered by the Swiss psychiatrist Kuhn (1958), who was studying imipramine as an antipsychotic. Kuhn observed that imipramine did not have effects on psychosis but instead was useful in treating depression.

Prior to the discovery of these drugs, the major treatments for depression included psychotherapy, psychoanalysis, hospitalization, sleep deprivation, or even psychosurgery in severe cases. The discovery of TCAs and MAOIs changed how the treatment of depression was conceptualized because effective medications were now available. During the heyday of the TCAs and MAOIs, depression was characterized as melancholic or nonmelancholic, a designation that influenced the choice of antidepressant. In addition, consideration was given to whether the patient's depression would respond to serotonergic versus noradrenergic antidepressants.

TCAs and MAOIs seemed to increase synaptic concentrations of serotonin and catecholamines. Therefore, developing other drugs that worked in a similar fashion was a goal in the 1960s and beyond. This led to the development of additional TCAs, MAOIs, and tetracyclic antidepressants, and eventually to the development of selective serotonin reuptake inhibitors (SSRIs) and serotonin-norepinephrine reuptake inhibitors (SNRIs). In the 1970s, tetracyclic antidepressants were developed from TCAs. Whereas TCAs were three-ringed compounds, tetracyclics were four-ringed compounds. When SSRIs and SNRIs were developed in the 1980s and 1990s, they represented a safer and better-tolerated alternative to TCAs, tetracyclics, and MAOIs.

The goal of this chapter is to review the classification, efficacy, safety, and tolerability of TCAs, tetracyclics, and MAOIs.

Classification, Safety, and Tolerability

Monoamine Oxidase Inhibitors

MAOIs have historically been classified based on their selectivity for specific isoforms of monoamine oxidase (MAO). For example, MAOIs are classified by their selectivity for the MAO-A versus the MAO-B receptor, with some MAOIs having activity at both receptors. MAO-A receptors deaminate epinephrine, norepinephrine, and serotonin, whereas MAO-B is involved in the catalyzation of benzylamine and β-phenylethylamine. Dopamine and tyramine are catalyzed through both MAO-A and MAO-B.

In addition to classification based on activity at MAO-A or MAO-B receptors, MAOIs are often subdivided into groups based on the reversibility or irreversibility of their inhibitory effects at specific MAO receptors. MAOIs with selective MAO-A activity seem to have antidepressant properties similar to those of MAOIs that have activity on both MAO-A and MAO-B receptors. Nonselective MAO-A/MAO-B inhibitors include isocarboxazid and phenelzine. Selective MAO-A inhibitors include moclobemide (as well as other agents not commonly used in clinical practice). Selective MAO-B inhibitors include selegiline and rasagiline, with the latter primarily used in Parkinson's disease (Table 14–1).

Use of MAOIs requires patients to maintain a special diet in which they avoid foods high in tyramine (e.g., certain cheeses, wine, beer, and cured meats) (Shulman and Walker 1999). Consuming tyramine leads to elevated levels of norepinephrine that cannot be effectively catalyzed because the MAOI blocks MAO, which breaks down tyramine. This can lead to elevated blood pressure, hypertensive crisis, or other serious side effects, including intracranial bleeding and death.

Individuals who are not taking MAOIs can tolerate high volumes of tyramine consumption, in the range of 40 mg or more per day. Individuals taking MAOIs, however, may experience a hypertensive crisis at tyramine levels as low as 8 mg/day (Stahl and Felker 2008). Therefore, patients who are prescribed MAOIs need to be educated on consuming a low-tyramine diet (Sathyanarayana Rao and Yeragani 2009). Revised dietary restrictions for patients taking MAOIs were published in 1999 because many foods that were previously considered to contain high amounts of tyramine (e.g., certain recipes of pizza) are now considered safe (Shulman and Walker 1999). In addition, use of the selegiline transdermal patch carries fewer dietary constraints in compari-

TABLE 14–1. Monoamine oxidase inhibitor (MAOI) classes, including FDA-approved dosage ranges

Nonselective MAO-A/MAO-B inhibitors (irreversible)	Selective MAO-A inhibitors	Selective MAO-B inhibitors (irreversible)
Phenelzine (15–30 mg every 8 hours to start; maintenance 15 mg/day)	Clorgyline (irreversible—never marketed)	Selegiline (6 mg/24 hours–12 mg/24 hours transdermal patch)
Tranylcypromine (15 mg twice daily; not to exceed 60 mg/day)	Moclobemide (reversible—300–600 mg/day in divided doses)	Pargyline (discontinued)

son with oral MAOIs, with restrictions required for high, but not low, dosages of selegiline, as noted in the package insert (Merck 2006):

> In its entirety, the data for [selegiline transdermal] 6 mg/24 hours support the recommendation that a modified diet is not required at this dose. Due to the more limited data available for [selegiline transdermal] 9 mg/24 hours and 12 mg/24 hours, patients receiving these doses should follow Dietary Modifications Required for Patients Taking [selegiline transdermal] 9 mg/24 hours and 12 mg/24 hours.

In addition to dietary restrictions, individuals require a washout period of proserotonergic drugs before starting MAOIs. This washout period is based on the half-life of the drug. Therefore, with the exception of fluoxetine, individuals switching from SSRIs to MAOIs require a 2-week washout of the SSRI before starting an MAOI. Fluoxetine, because of its longer half-life, requires a washout of 5 weeks before starting an MAOI. Patients taking MAOIs should avoid over-the-counter decongestants, cold medications containing dextromethorphan, certain weight-loss medications, and other drugs that have serotonergic effects or intensify the drug's sympathomimetic effects. A washout of other serotonergic drugs should be considered before starting MAOIs and should be based on the half-life of the proserotonergic medication. Conway et al. (2015) argued that MAOIs can be initiated rapidly and without (or with only minimal) washout under confinement or inpatient conditions.

Additional considerations for prescribers of MAOIs include the more common adverse effects of orthostatic hypotension, weight gain, sexual dysfunction, and insomnia, which are not unique to MAOIs and occur with other antidepressants that work on biogenic amine neurotransmitters. Management of these more common adverse effects associated with MAOIs can include lowering the dosage or discontinuing the drug in cases where the effect is bothersome or more serious for the patient. Alternatively, watchful waiting may be an appropriate management strategy in certain situations in which the adverse effect is less bothersome or serious, because in some cases the effects may resolve with time.

Tricyclic Antidepressants

TCAs historically were classified based on their chemical structure (i.e., primary vs. secondary amine). However, in modern psychopharmacology, that historical classifi-

in treating atypical depression. In addition, Søgaard et al. (1999) demonstrated sertraline to be more effective than moclobemide in treating atypical depression.

More recently, the STAR*D (Sequenced Treatment Alternatives to Relieve Depression) study compared tranylcypromine (up to 60 mg/day) with the combination of mirtazapine (up to 45 mg/day) and venlafaxine (up to 300 mg/day) (Rush et al. 2006). Participants in STAR*D who were assigned to tranylcypromine or to the mirtazapine/venlafaxine combination had failed to respond to three sequential trials of antidepressants. Remission rates based on 17-item Hamilton Rating Scale for Depression (HAM-D17) scores were modest for both groups: 7% for tranylcypromine versus 14% for the venlafaxine/mirtazapine combination. The average responder to tranylcypromine took approximately 8.6 weeks to develop a response, compared with 8.1 weeks for responders to the combination treatment. Response and remission rates seemed limited by adverse effects in both groups (Rush and Jain 2019).

Tricyclic Antidepressants

For TCAs, much has been written correlating drug level to therapeutic response, safety, and tolerability (Burke and Preskorn 2004; Preskorn 1986; Preskorn et al. 1988, 1989). For example, with imipramine, clinical response is better when combined plasma levels of imipramine and its metabolite desipramine exceed 150 ng/mL than when combined levels are lower. However, combined levels of imipramine and desipramine in excess of 250 ng/mL are not associated with higher response rates but instead result in more adverse effects. Nortriptyline, on the other hand, has a curvilinear dose-response relationship in which optimal response occurs in the midrange of blood levels (50–150 ng/mL) and not at the high or low range. With amitriptyline, most patients demonstrate optimal response when combined serum levels of amitriptyline and its active metabolite nortriptyline are between 80 and 200 ng/mL; however, amitriptyline demonstrates significant cardiac toxicity when combined plasma levels of amitriptyline and nortriptyline exceed 500 ng/mL.

Monitoring of plasma TCA levels is also important for preventing adverse effects. For example, in comparison with patients who are cytochrome P450 (CYP) 2D6 extensive metabolizers, those who are CYP2D6 poor metabolizers may develop plasma TCA levels fourfold higher or more (Macaluso and Preskorn 2011). Therefore, in individuals with CYP2D6 poor metabolizer status, standard dosages of a TCA can lead to toxic effects such as seizures or confusion.

Level 3 of STAR*D included the option to switch to nortriptyline, a TCA, or mirtazapine, a tetracyclic. Remission rates based on HAM-D17 data from STAR*D were 12% for the mirtazapine-treated group versus 20% for the nortriptyline-treated group (Fava et al. 2006). Remission rates based on data from the 16-item Quick Inventory of Depressive Symptomatology Self-Report were 8% for the mirtazapine group and 12% for the nortriptyline group (Fava et al. 2006). However, none of these outcomes was statistically significant. For patients who achieved remission, the mean time to remission was 5.7 weeks for mirtazapine, compared with 6.3 weeks for nortriptyline.

Tetracyclic Antidepressants

Mirtazapine has a unique method of action. By blocking the presynaptic α_2 heteroreceptors, it enhances serotonergic and noradrenergic neurotransmission (de Boer and

Ruigt 1995; Sitsen and Zivkov 1995). This boosts postsynaptic levels of serotonin in addition to blocking postsynaptic serotonin (5-hydroxytryptamine [5-HT]) type 2A (5-HT_{2A}), type 2C (5-HT_{2C}), and type 3 (5-HT_3) receptors (Anttila and Leinonen 2001; Haddjeri et al. 1995). Mirtazapine's 5-HT_{2A} receptor blockade promotes sleep restoration with no sexual adverse effects (Preskorn 1999). Its 5-HT_{2C} receptor blockade contributes to the adverse effect of weight gain, whereas its 5-HT_3 receptor blockade contributes to the lack of gastrointestinal adverse effects. In addition, mirtazapine blocks histamine H_1 receptors, which contributes to its adverse effects of sedation and weight gain. Mirtazapine is also associated with dizziness and transient elevations in plasma lipids and liver function values.

Mirtazapine's approved dosage range is 15–45 mg once daily; however, some studies have utilized higher dosages, in the range of 60 mg/day, although this use is off-label (Merck 2012, 2017). Patients treated with mirtazapine for major depressive disorder in acute clinical trials showed statistically significant symptomatic improvement compared with subjects given placebo within the first 1–2 weeks of treatment (Alam et al. 2013; Lavergne et al. 2005). In addition, patients taking mirtazapine for major depressive disorder showed continued improvements in response rates at 40 weeks in long-term clinical trials.

Conclusion

Prior to the development of drugs with novel mechanisms of action, modern antidepressants acting on biogenic amine neurotransmitters evolved from MAOIs and TCAs, paving the way for newer and safer methods of treating depression. In modern psychiatry, MAOIs and TCAs have niche uses in treating refractory illness or specific subtypes of depression. Although the safety risks posed by these medications can be serious and life threatening, many can be mitigated through careful patient selection, appropriate clinical monitoring, and education of patients and families.

References

Alam A, Voronovich Z, Carley JA: A review of therapeutic uses of mirtazapine in psychiatric and medical conditions. Prim Care Companion CNS Disord 15(5):PCC.13r01525, 2013 24511451

American Psychiatric Association: Practice Guideline for the Treatment of Patients With Major Depressive Disorder, 3rd Edition. Washington, DC, American Psychiatric Association, 2010

Anttila SA, Leinonen EV: A review of the pharmacological and clinical profile of mirtazapine. CNS Drug Rev 7(3):249–264, 2001 11607047

Burke MJ, Preskorn SH: Therapeutic drug monitoring of antidepressants, in Antidepressants: Past Present and Future. Handbook of Experimental Pharmacology Vol. 157. Edited by Preskorn SH, Stanga CY, Feighner JP, Ross R. Berlin, Springer-Verlag, 2004, pp 87–114

Conway CR, Gebara MA, Walker MC, et al: Clinical characteristics and management of treatment-resistant depression. J Clin Psychiatry 76(11):1569–1570, 2015 26646033

de Boer T, Ruigt GSF: The selective alpha2-adrenoceptor antagonist mirtazapine (Org 3770) enhances noradrenergic and 5HT1A mediated serotonergic neurotransmission. CNS Drugs 4 (suppl 1):29–38, 1995

Fava M, Rush AJ, Wisniewski SR, et al: A comparison of mirtazapine and nortriptyline following two consecutive failed medication treatments for depressed outpatients: a STAR*D report. Am J Psychiatry 163(7):1161–1172, 2006 16816220

Haddjeri N, Blier P, de Montigny C: Noradrenergic modulation of central serotonergic neurotransmission: acute and long-term actions of mirtazapine. Int Clin Psychopharmacol 10 (suppl 4):11–17, 1995 8930005

Hillhouse TM, Porter JH: A brief history of the development of antidepressant drugs: from monoamines to glutamate. Exp Clin Psychopharmacol 23(1):1–21, 2015 25643025

Kuhn R: The treatment of depressive states with G 22355 (imipramine hydrochloride). Am J Psychiatry 115(5):459–464, 1958 13583250

Lavergne F, Berlin I, Gamma A, et al: Onset of improvement and response to mirtazapine in depression: a multicenter naturalistic study of 4771 patients. Neuropsychiatr Dis Treat 1(1):59–68, 2005 18568129

Macaluso M, Preskorn SH: CYP 2D6 PM status and antidepressant response to nortriptyline and venlafaxine: is it more than just drug metabolism? J Clin Psychopharmacol 31(2):143–145, 2011 21346604

Merck: EMSAM (selegiline transdermal system). Whitehouse Station, NJ, Merck & Co, February 2006. Available at: https://www.accessdata.fda.gov/drugsatfda_docs/label/2006/021708s000_021336s000lbl.pdf. Accessed November 12, 2020.

Merck: REMERON® (mirtazapine) tablets. Whitehouse Station, NJ, Merck & Co, 2012. Available at: https://www.accessdata.fda.gov/drugsatfda_docs/label/2007/020415s019,021208s010lbl.pdf. Accessed November 12, 2020.

Merck: Merck Medication Guide: Mirtazapine. Whitehouse Station, NJ, Merck & Co, 2017. Available at: https://www.organon.com/product/usa/pi_circulars/r/remeron/remeron_tablets_pi.pdf. Accessed November 12, 2020.

Pande AC, Birkett M, Fechner-Bates S, et al: Fluoxetine versus phenelzine in atypical depression. Biol Psychiatry 40(10):1017–1020, 1996 8915561

Preskorn SH: Tricyclic antidepressant plasma level monitoring: an improvement over the dose-response approach. J Clin Psychiatry 47 (1 suppl):24–30, 1986 2867088

Preskorn SH: Outpatient Management Of Depression: A Guide for the Primary Care Practitioner, 2nd Edition. Caddo, OK, Professional Communications Inc, 1999

Preskorn SH, Dorey RC, Jerkovich GS: Therapeutic drug monitoring of tricyclic antidepressants. Clin Chem 34(5):822–828, 1988 3131042

Preskorn SH, Jerkovich GS, Beber JH, et al: Therapeutic drug monitoring of tricyclic antidepressants: a standard of care issue. Psychopharmacol Bull 25(2):281–284, 1989 2690169

Quitkin F, Rifkin A, Klein DF: Monoamine oxidase inhibitors: a review of antidepressant effectiveness. Arch Gen Psychiatry 36(7):749–760, 1979 454092

Rush AJ, Jain SB: Clinical implications of the STAR*D trial. Handb Exp Pharmacol 250:51–99, 2019 30203327

Rush AJ, Trivedi MH, Wisniewski SR, et al: Acute and longer-term outcomes in depressed outpatients requiring one or several treatment steps: a STAR*D report. Am J Psychiatry 163(11):1905–1917, 2006 17074942

Sathyanarayana Rao TS, Yeragani VK: Hypertensive crisis and cheese. Indian J Psychiatry 51(1):65–66, 2009 19742203

Shulman KI, Walker SE: Refining the MAOI diet: tyramine content of pizzas and soy products. J Clin Psychiatry 60(3):191–193, 1999 10192596

Sitsen JM, Zivkov M: Mirtazapine: clinical profile. CNS Drugs 4 (suppl 1):39–48, 1995

Søgaard J, Lane R, Latimer P, et al: A 12-week study comparing moclobemide and sertraline in the treatment of outpatients with atypical depression. J Psychopharmacol 13(4):406–414, 1999 10667618

Stahl SM, Felker A: Monoamine oxidase inhibitors: a modern guide to an unrequited class of antidepressants. CNS Spectr 13(10):855–870, 2008 18955941

Thase ME, Trivedi MH, Rush AJ: MAOIs in the contemporary treatment of depression. Neuropsychopharmacology 12(3):185–219, 1995 7612154

CHAPTER 15

Selective Serotonin Reuptake Inhibitors and Related Antidepressants

Richard C. Shelton, M.D.

The introduction of the selective serotonin reuptake inhibitors (SSRIs) had an enormous impact on the practice of medicine in general and on the practice of psychiatry in particular. Prior to the introduction of fluoxetine in the U.S. market in late 1997, antidepressants were infrequently used in the primary care setting and, when used, were frequently used at subtherapeutic dosages. Since then, antidepressants have become among the most widely prescribed drugs worldwide, with a market representing billions of dollars per year. The SSRIs and later medications have changed the face of the treatment of depression. This chapter reviews antidepressant medications approved by the FDA since 1997.

Background and History

Tricyclic antidepressants (TCAs) and monoamine oxidase inhibitors (MAOIs) have a high side-effect burden, cardiotoxicity, risk in overdose, and drug interactions that limit their usefulness in practice. By the late 1960s, it was clear that newer treatments with improved risk and tolerability profiles were needed. Because both the MAOIs and TCAs appeared to work by enhancing monoaminergic synaptic transmission, including that of norepinephrine, serotonin, and, to a lesser degree, dopamine, investigators pursued the hypothesis that the therapeutic effects of these drugs resulted from increased levels of these neurotransmitters, culminating in the monoamine hypothesis of depression (Schildkraut 1965). Initially, this largely focused on noradrenergic mechanisms, but later work by investigators such as Arvid Carlsson, James Maas, and others began to shift the focus toward serotonin as an important target of antidepressant action (Nemeroff and Owens 2003). Pharmaceutical research in Europe and the U.S. focused on developing drugs that block the serotonin reuptake site, referred to as the serotonin transporter (SERT), without the concomitant receptor binding profile of the TCAs. This led to the synthesis of zimelidine, the first marketed SSRI, and fluoxetine, the first SSRI marketed in the United States (Fuller et al. 1991; Huitfeldt and Montgomery 1983; Montgomery et al. 1981a, 1981b)

Following the remarkable success of fluoxetine, various companies introduced compounds that were relatively potent and selective antagonists of SERT. The "modern" era of antidepressant treatment had begun in earnest. In parallel with this development, many companies continued to focus considerable efforts on the synthesis of drugs that were similar to TCAs in action but were not serotonin selective. Much of the development of antidepressants over the past 30 years or more has focused on the goal of developing "cleaned-up" TCAs—drugs that inhibit the reuptake of norepinephrine, serotonin, or both but have low affinity for other receptors. The result was a new generation of antidepressants, which includes the SSRIs, the selective norepinephrine reuptake inhibitors (NRIs), and the dual serotonin-norepinephrine reuptake inhibitors (SNRIs).

Monoamine Transporters

Most antidepressant compounds, both old and newer, act by the blocking the transporter proteins for serotonin, norepinephrine, or both. SERT and the norepinephrine transporter (NET) are chemically related structures with distinct genetic loci. They are part of a larger family of transporters powered by Na+/K+ ATPases. The function of a transporter is to remove the neurotransmitter from the synapse, thus terminating stimulation of the postsynaptic neuron. In addition, the transporter serves as a recycling agent, allowing the presynaptic cell to reuse the serotonin that it collects (Blakely et al. 1994; Qian et al. 1995).

Like other members of the transporter family, SERT is a glycoprotein complex embedded in a plasma membrane by 12 transmembrane domains. Its glycosylation plays an important role in protein folding and protecting against degradation (Blakely et al. 1994). These transporters are located on the axon terminals and cell bodies of serotonergic neurons. Each transporter contains binding sites for serotonin, sodium, chlorine, potassium, and pharmacological agents (e.g., SSRIs, cocaine, and amphetamines). To initiate serotonin reuptake, SERT binds extracellular serotonin, sodium, and chlorine. This induces a conformational change in SERT that moves these ions and serotonin into the cell, where they are released. Intracellular potassium then binds to the complex, another conformational change ensues, and the complex returns to its initial configuration. SSRIs inhibit SERT by binding to a site on the SERT protein at a location other than the active uptake site for serotonin (allosteric inhibition). Thus, SSRIs do not completely prevent the SERT from functioning because they do not prevent the binding of serotonin. However, therapeutic dosages of SSRIs decrease SERT functioning by 60%–80%.

NET is structurally and functionally very similar to SERT, and many antidepressants inhibit both of these transporters. In addition, NET has a moderate affinity for dopamine, and therefore antidepressants that act on NET enhance transmission of both norepinephrine and dopamine (Pacholczyk et al. 1991). Some brain regions, particularly the frontal cortex, have low levels of dopamine transporters, and NET is the principal mechanism for reuptake of dopamine in these areas (Morón et al. 2002). Thus, even highly selective NET inhibitors, such as atomoxetine (a medication used for ADHD), can enhance both norepinephrine and dopamine transmission. Finally, at least one antidepressant, sertraline, has a modest effect on the transporter for dopamine directly, although the clinical implications of this are unknown (Owens et al. 1997). Binding affinities for the NET and SERT (expressed as the inhibition constant [Ki]) are listed in Table 15–1.

Desensitization of specific serotonin and norepinephrine receptors, which occurs after reuptake blockade, has been postulated to be the principal mechanism of action of antidepressants (Sulser et al. 1978). Hyman and Nestler (1996) have suggested that this desensitization serves as a marker of adaptation rather than the mechanism through which therapeutic actions are mediated. Enhanced transsynaptic signaling by norepinephrine and serotonin leads to downstream effects of gene expression that may, ultimately, result in therapeutic effects. Thus, rather than being directly associated with the antidepressant effects, receptor desensitization could primarily be related to the amelioration of side effects.

Therapeutic Implications of Serotonin and Norepinephrine Reuptake Blockade

Antidepressants, including the SSRIs, SNRIs, and NRIs, are indicated for not only the treatment of depression but also various other psychiatric conditions, particularly anxiety disorders. Table 15–2 lists the antidepressants available in the United States, their trade names and dosage ranges, and their FDA-approved indications.

Over the past 30 years, data have emerged to suggest that mood is not a simple "good" versus "bad" or "high" versus "low" construct. Rather, several component features have emerged. For example, L.A. Clark and Watson (1991) conceptualized the mood-anxiety spectrum as composed of three dominant bimodal factors. These emerged from factor analytic studies of mood descriptors in large healthy control and symptomatic populations, and comprise "somatic anxiety," "positive affect," and "general distress" (also termed "negative affect") (L.A. Clark and Watson 1991; R.A. Clark et al. 1994; Watson et al. 1995a, 1995b). Somatic anxiety involves physiological arousal, with features such as tachycardia, tachypnea, tremor, diaphoresis, and other evidence of acute fear, and is found in panic attacks. *Positive affect* suggests a bimodal dimension with a positive emotional state involving enthusiasm, motivation, and optimism at one end and anhedonia, which is fairly specific to depression, at the other end. *General distress* refers to a range of negative emotions (e.g., sadness, anxiety, worry, rumination, tension) and general dissatisfaction and is common to both anxiety and mood disorders (Brown et al. 1998). Focusing on these components may contribute to misdiagnosis or multiple diagnostic assignments (i.e., "comorbidity").

TABLE 15–1. Pharmacodynamics and pharmacokinetics of selected antidepressants

Drug	Ki[a] (SERT)	Ki[a] (NET)	Ki(NET)/ Ki(SERT)	Protein binding	Half-life
Citalopram	8.9	30,285	3,403	80%	20 hours[1]
Desvenlafaxine	40	558[2]	14	30%	11 hours
Duloxetine	0.8[3]	7.5[3]	9	95%	12.5 hours[4]
Escitalopram	0.8	7,800	9,750	56%	27–32 hours
Fluoxetine	20	2,186	109	95%	4–6 days
Fluvoxamine	14	4,743	339	80%	15 hours[5]
Levomilnacipran	11.2	91[5]	8	22%	12 hours
Nefazodone	549	713	1.3	99%[6]	4–8 hours[7]
Paroxetine	0.83	328	395	95%	21 hours
Sertraline[b]	3.3	1,716	520	98%	26 hours
Venlafaxine[c]	102	1,644	16	27%	5–7 hours
Vilazodone	0.1	56[8]	560	98%	20–22 hours
Vortioxetine	1.6[9]	113	71	98%	7–11 hours

Note. NET=norepinephrine transporter; SERT=serotonin transporter.
[a]Uptake binding site binding affinity is expressed as the inhibition constant (Ki), which is an inverse scale (i.e., lower values are more potent).
[b]The half-life of the principal metabolite desmethylsertraline is 66 hours.
[c]*O*-desmethylvenlafaxine's half-life is 11 hours.

Sources. Adapted from Owens et al. 1997 and manufacturer prescribing information except as noted:
[1]Fredricson Overø 1982.
[2]Bridge et al. 2008.
[3]Bymaster et al. 2001.
[4]Sharma et al. 2000.
[5]Bruno et al. 2016.
[6]van Harten 1995.
[7]DeVane et al. 2002.
[8]Sahli et al. 2016.
[9]Bang-Andersen et al. 2011.

A question arises as to whether therapeutic response maps to any of these dimensions of mood. Enhancement of serotonin transmission appears to improve elements of somatic anxiety (e.g., panic, social phobia) and general distress (e.g., generalized anxiety disorder), which seem to be class effects and are not specific to a limited set of compounds (Shelton and Tomarken 2001). This would distinguish the difference between therapeutic *effect*, based on some underlying neurochemical mechanism of action, and therapeutic *indication*, based on submission of research data to the FDA or other regulatory agencies. By contrast, SERT inhibitors seem to produce a more mixed effect with regard to positive affect. Although some patients clearly experience a broad effect on mood symptoms with SSRIs, only about one-third experience remission in a typical 8- to 12-week therapeutic trial. Moreover, some patients describe a mood "flattening" effect with SSRIs. In fact, persisting symptoms in depression are often in the "positive" rather than in the "negative" affective domains.

TABLE 15–2. Antidepressants and related compounds approved for the treatment of depressive, anxiety, or pain disorders by the FDA (excluding tricyclics)

Drug	U.S. trade name	Dosage range (mg/day)	FDA-approved indications
Bupropion	Wellbutrin Wellbutrin SR Wellbutrin XL Zyban	 150–400 150–450	Major depressive disorder Smoking cessation (Zyban)
Citalopram	Celexa	20–60	Major depressive disorder
Duloxetine	Cymbalta	60–120	Major depressive disorder Generalized anxiety disorder Fibromyalgia Diabetic peripheral neuropathic pain Chronic musculoskeletal pain
Escitalopram	Lexapro	10–20	Major depressive disorder Generalized anxiety disorder[a]
Fluoxetine	Prozac Prozac Weekly Serafem	20–80 90–180	Depression Bulimia nervosa Obsessive-compulsive disorder Panic disorder Premenstrual dysphoric disorder (Serafem)
Fluvoxamine	Luvox	50–300	Obsessive-compulsive disorder (adults, children)[b]
Levomilnacipran	Fetzima	40–120	Major depressive disorder
Milnacipran	Savella	12.5–200	Fibromyalgia[b]
Mirtazapine	Remeron Remeron SolTab	15–45	Major depressive disorder
Nefazodone	Serzone	200–600	Major depressive disorder
Paroxetine Paroxetine extended release	Paxil Paxil CR	20–50 25–62.5	Major depressive disorder Generalized anxiety disorder Panic disorder PTSD Premenstrual dysphoric disorder Social anxiety disorder)
Sertraline	Zoloft	50–200	Major depressive disorder Obsessive-compulsive disorder Panic disorder PTSD Premenstrual dysphoric disorder Social anxiety disorder
Venlafaxine	Effexor Effexor XR	75–375 75–225	Depression Generalized anxiety disorder Social anxiety disorder Panic disorder

TABLE 15–2. Antidepressants and related compounds approved for the treatment of depressive, anxiety, or pain disorders by the FDA (excluding tricyclics) *(continued)*

Drug	U.S. trade name	Dosage range (mg/day)	FDA-approved indications
Vilazodone	Viibryd	10–40	Major depressive disorder
Vortioxetine	Trintellix	10–20	Major depressive disorder

Note. CR=controlled release; SR=sustained release; XL=extended release; XR=extended release.
[a]Social anxiety disorder, obsessive-compulsive disorder, panic disorder outside the United States.
[b]Major depressive disorder outside the United States.

By contrast, the effects of norepinephrine (including the indirect effects on dopaminergic mechanisms) appear to be significant mediators of arousal and activation. Antidepressants that act on catecholamines have been shown to have a beneficial effect in the positive affect domain. Bupropion, a drug acting predominantly via a catecholaminergic mechanism, has been shown to have a more robust effect in the positive affective than the general distress domain (Tomarken et al. 2004). Although the therapeutic specificity of antidepressant mechanisms of action remains somewhat controversial, at least some evidence indicates that serotonergic agents shade toward antianxiety effects, whereas catecholaminergic drugs shade toward reduction of anhedonia.

Selective Serotonin Reuptake Inhibitors

As a class of drugs, SSRIs share many characteristics. In addition to their specificity for SERT and relatively low affinity for other neurotransmitter receptors, they have a lower side-effect burden relative to TCAs and MAOIs, are relatively safe in overdose, and are readily absorbed from the gastrointestinal tract. Most circulate in a form that is highly bound to protein and is in equilibrium with the unbound, biologically active form. Metabolized in the liver, these antidepressants are broken down by hepatic microsomal enzymes and conjugated, usually with glucuronic acid, allowing clearance in the urine. Thus, hepatic or renal dysfunction reduces clearance of the drug. Despite these similarities, these drugs are unique in terms of their receptor affinity and pharmacokinetic properties.

Today, five SSRIs are approved by the FDA for treatment of depression (fluoxetine, sertraline, paroxetine, citalopram, and escitalopram), and another, fluvoxamine, is marketed for obsessive-compulsive disorder (OCD) but has been approved for depression in Europe and elsewhere. Table 15–2 lists the available SSRIs, their typical dosing ranges, and their FDA-approved indications.

Clinical Use

Newer antidepressants are safer and better tolerated than older medications; therefore, clinicians are more likely to prescribe them, and patients are more willing to take them. The popularity of the SSRIs has stemmed largely from their increased tolerability and not from an increase in drug efficacy (i.e., "response" or "remission"). Although overall outcomes of treatment may not have improved, SSRIs and later drugs appear to have increased the proportion of patients treated with antidepressant drugs, which is likely to have a favorable effect independent of the benefits of any single agent.

Increases in antidepressant tolerability have resulted in a substantial shift among the physicians treating depression. Whereas depression was once treated mainly by mental health professionals, nearly three-quarters of all patients seeking treatment for depression now visit a primary care physician (Montano 1994). Between 1987 and 1997, the rate of people seeking treatment increased from 0.73 to 2.33 per 100 people per year (Olfson et al. 2002), a roughly threefold increase. The percentage of individuals in treatment for depression who are given antidepressants has doubled, from 37.3% in 1987 to 74.5% in 1997. Use is increasing in children as well: between 1988 and 1994, use of antidepressants in children increased three- to fivefold (Zito 2002). Antidepressants have become among the most prescribed medications worldwide. In the United States, sertraline ranks at number 14, escitalopram at 22, fluoxetine at 23, and bupropion at 23 (Kane 2021).

Specific Medications

Fluoxetine

In late 1987, fluoxetine (Prozac) became the first SSRI approved for use in the United States. Once ingested, it is converted to its active metabolite, norfluoxetine. Both the parent compound and the metabolite are relatively selective for SERT: the Ki values for fluoxetine and norfluoxetine are 0.90 and 2.3 nMol, respectively, versus [^{3}H]citalopram in human transfected cells (SERT affinity), as opposed to 777 and 3,947 nMol versus [^{3}H]nisoxetine binding (NET affinity) (Owens et al. 1997). Typical fluoxetine dosing starts at 20 mg, taken once daily, and dosage can be increased in increments of 10–20 mg in a dosing range of up to 80 mg/day. Due to the relatively long half-lives of fluoxetine and norfluoxetine (4–6 days for fluoxetine, 7–15 days for norfluoxetine), a weekly dosing schedule and formulation (Prozac Weekly) have been approved, with a dosage of 90 mg taken once or twice per week. Fluoxetine's long half-life also makes it less likely than other SSRIs to produce a discontinuation syndrome in patients who stop treatment (Haddad 2001). Fluoxetine is very highly protein bound (98%) and is a potent inhibitor of cytochrome P450 (CYP) 2D6 and 2C19, and somewhat less so for 2B6 and 2C9 (Table 15–3).

Fluoxetine has been studied for a variety of conditions and is currently approved in the United States for depression, bulimia nervosa, OCD, panic disorder, and premenstrual dysphoric disorder (see Table 15–2). It remains the most commonly prescribed antidepressant in the United States (Kane 2021).

Sertraline

Sertraline (Zoloft), which was approved in 1992, has been among the most widely used antidepressants. Like fluoxetine, sertraline has been studied for a wide group of disorders and has been approved by the FDA for depression, OCD, panic disorder, PTSD, premenstrual dysphoric disorder, and social anxiety disorder (see Table 15–2). It is highly protein bound (see Table 15–1) and inhibits metabolism of other drugs via CYP2D6, CYP2B6, CYP2C, and CYP3A4 (see Table 15–3). The primary metabolic pathway for sertraline is CYP2B6.

TABLE 15–3. Metabolic pathways and relative inhibition of selected cytochrome P450 (CYP) enzymes by newer antidepressants

Drug	Primary metabolic pathway(s)	Secondary metabolic pathway(s)	CYP enzyme inhibited	Relative inhibition[a]
Bupropion	CYP2B6	CYP1A2, CYP2A6, CYP2C9, CYP3A4, CYP2E1, CYP2C19	CYP2D6	+
Citalopram/ Escitalopram	CYP2C19	CYP2D6, CYP3A4	CYP1A2 CYP2C	+ +
Duloxetine	CYP1A2, CYP2D6	—	CYP2D6[b]	++
Desvenlafaxine[c]	CYP3A4	—	None	–
Fluoxetine	CYP2D6	CYP2C19, CYP2D6, CYP3A4/5[d]	CYP2B6 CYP2C9 CYP2C19 CYP2D6	+ + +++ +++
Fluvoxamine[e]	Unknown	Unknown	CYP1A2 CYP2B6 CYP2D6 CYP2C9 CYP2C19 CYP2D6 CYP3A4	+++ + + ++ +++ + ++
Levomilnacipran / milnacipran	CYP3A4	—	None	–
Mirtazapine	CYP1A2, CYP2D6, CYP3A4	—	CYP2D6	+
Nefazodone	CYP3A4	CYP2D6[f]	CYP3A4	+++
Paroxetine	CYP2D6	—	CYP2B6 CYP2C9 CYP2C19 CYP2D6 CYP3A4	+++ + + +++ +
Sertraline	CYP2B6	—	CYP2D6 CYP2B6 CYP2C CYP3A4	++ ++ ++ ++
Venlafaxine	CYP2D6	—	None	–
Vilazodone	CYP3A4	—	None	–
Vortioxetine	CYP2D6	—	None	–

Note. —=no data available.
[a]Relative inhibition: –=minimal or zero; +=mild; ++=moderate; +++=strong.
[b]Skinner et al. 2003.
[c]Primary metabolism is via glucuronidation by UGT1A1, 1A3, 2B4, and 2B15.
[d]Secondary pathways contribute little to fluoxetine's metabolism unless CYP2D6 metabolism is reduced.
[e]van Harten 1995.
[f]Forms the psychoactive drug *meta*-chlorophenylpiperazine.
Source. Data from Nemeroff et al. 1996; Greenblatt et al. 1998; manufacturers' prescribing information.

A typical starting dosage is 50 mg/day (although lower dosages are sometimes used in anxiety disorders such as panic), and sertraline can be prescribed at dosages up to 200 mg/day. It is a very potent SERT inhibitor: sertraline and its primary metabolite desmethylsertraline potently block SERT, as measured by displacement of [^{3}H]citalopram (Ki=0.15 and 3.7 nMol, respectively) or [^{3}H]serotonin (Ki=3.3 and 187 nMol) (Owens et al. 1997). Both are weak norepinephrine reuptake inhibitors (Ki vs. [^{3}H]citalopram or [^{3}H]serotonin in the range of 85–328 nMol for sertraline and 811–2,365 nMol for desmethylsertraline).

Sertraline is sometimes touted as a dopamine reuptake inhibitor, although the binding affinity for the dopamine transporter is modest. Tatsumi et al. (1997) found the affinity for sertraline and desmethylsertraline to be K_D=25 and 129 nMol, respectively. However, this is much more potent than other antidepressant drugs (e.g., citalopram's K_D=28,100 nMol). To our knowledge, sertraline has not been tested via putative dopaminergic markers in humans (e.g., PET scanning), and its effect at the dopamine transporter in humans is unknown.

Paroxetine

Paroxetine (Paxil) was released soon after sertraline and was initially touted as a highly selective SERT inhibitor as a result of its high potency of SERT binding and its high ratio of serotonin-to-NET binding affinity (Boyer and Feighner 1992). Like other SSRIs, paroxetine has been widely studied, and it is approved for the treatment of depression, generalized anxiety disorder, panic disorder, PTSD, premenstrual dysphoric disorder, and social phobia (see Table 15–2). The usual dosage is 20 mg taken once daily, and this can be increased to 60 mg/day. It has a mild affinity to muscarinic receptors, leading some patients to experience anticholinergic side effects such as dry mouth and constipation (Owens et al. 1997). An enteric-coated controlled-release form of paroxetine (Paxil CR) is available and appears to be associated with somewhat lower rates of initial gastrointestinal side effects than the immediate-release version.

Paroxetine truly is a potent blocker of SERT: Ki=0.65 nMol ([^{3}H]citalopram displacement) or 0.83 nMol ([^{3}H]serotonin displacement) (Owens et al. 1997). However, although the ratio of SERT/NET inhibition is high, binding at the NET is not inconsequential: in vitro Ki=85 and 328 nMol versus [^{3}H]nisoxetine and [^{3}H]norepinephrine, respectively (Owens et al. 1997), which is mirrored by in vivo effects in rats (Owens et al. 2000). An important question, then, is whether this is reflected in human pharmacology.

Prior tests of NET blockade by paroxetine in humans, such as the tyramine pressor test, have been negative, although the dosage of paroxetine was low in those studies (20 mg/day). However, Gilmor et al. (2002) found that paroxetine inhibited norepinephrine uptake by 27% at an average serum concentration of 100 ng/mL and by 43% at 200 ng/mL, suggesting that paroxetine could be a meaningful norepinephrine reuptake inhibitor in humans, at least at higher dosages. However, the relationship between the in vitro effects measured in this study and in vivo effects in the brains of humans is unclear.

Paroxetine is highly protein bound (see Table 15–1) and inhibits a wide range of CYP enzymes, including potent inhibition of CYP2B6 and 2D6 and mild inhibition of CYP2C9, 2C19, and 3A4. It is therefore prone to significant drug-drug interactions. It is predominantly metabolized by CYP2D6.

Citalopram and Escitalopram

Citalopram (Celexa) and its s-enantiomer, s-citalopram (escitalopram, Lexapro), have been approved for depression in the United States. These drugs are potent and selective SERT inhibitors (Ki ~1–10 nMol) with negligible effects on the norepinephrine or dopamine transporters (Ki>3,000 nMol) (Owens et al. 1997). They also have very low binding affinity at other receptor sites (e.g., receptors for norepinephrine, serotonin, dopamine, histamine, or acetylcholine) (Baumann 1996). Citalopram is prescribed at a dosage of 20 mg/day, which can be increased to 60 mg/day or more. Escitalopram typically is dosed in a range of 10–30 mg/day. Only the s-enantiomer is the active form of the compound (Burke 2002); when citalopram is administered, only about 35% of the circulating plasma level in humans is in the escitalopram form (Rochat et al. 1995). Comparative clinical trials usually have calculated absolute doses of escitalopram at one-half the dose of citalopram (e.g., 10 mg vs. 20 mg) (Montgomery et al. 2001), which, therefore, may not be therapeutically equivalent.

Citalopram and escitalopram are substrates for CYP3A4, 2C19, and 2D6, although 2C19 predominates (Olesen and Linnet 1999; von Moltke et al. 1999). Neither citalopram nor the s-enantiomer substantially inhibits CYP metabolism, although modest inhibition of 1A2 and 2C have been reported (Greenblatt et al. 1998; Nemeroff et al. 1996). Escitalopram appears to have a somewhat lower plasma protein binding affinity (56%) in contrast to racemic citalopram (~80%) (DeVane 1998). This suggests that protein binding of the r-enantiomer is higher still, a potential therapeutic advantage for escitalopram when plasma protein displacement is of concern.

Fluvoxamine

Fluvoxamine (Luvox) is an SSRI approved in the United States only for the treatment of OCD, although it has been used as an antidepressant in Europe since 1984 (Rapaport et al. 1996). Placebo-controlled depression registration trials were conducted in the United States, but the findings were not sufficient to gain FDA approval (Ware 1997). Trials in OCD in both adults and children have suggested a robust effect (Goodman et al. 1997; Grados and Riddle 2001; Riddle et al. 2001).

The effects of fluvoxamine in depression, OCD, and other anxiety disorders are predictable based on the primary mechanism of action: the drug is a highly potent SERT inhibitor (Ki=1.6 nMol vs. [^{3}H]citalopram and 14 nMol vs. [^{3}H]serotonin) with minimal effects on NET (Ki=4,743 nMol) (Owens et al. 1997). Like other SSRIs, fluvoxamine inhibits various CYP enzymes, including 1A2, 2B6, 2D6, 2C19, 2C9, and 3A4 (see Table 15–3). It therefore is prone to many drug interactions (Table 15–4). Protein binding is relatively high at 80%, although this is lower than other SSRIs (see Table 15–1). It is metabolized into various relatively inactive compounds, primarily via oxidative deamination and demethylation. The half-life of the drug is about 15 hours initially, although this is increased with continued exposure as a result of autoinhibition of metabolism (van Harten 1995). Although the starting dosage usually is 50 mg/day, fluvoxamine tends to be effective in a dosage range of 150–200 mg/day.

Fluvoxamine is approved only for OCD in the United States, and a question is whether it should be used for this indication if other SSRIs (e.g., sertraline) have failed. Fluvoxamine is a moderately potent agonist at sigma-1 (σ_1) receptors (Ki=39 nM) (Hashimoto 2009). Sigma-1 receptors are orphan receptors, meaning that their natural endogenous ligands are unknown, although many amines and hormones bind to them (Fontanilla et al. 2009; Maurice and Su 2009). σ_1 Receptor agonists show antidepressant and anxiolytic effects (Hindmarch and Hashimoto 2010). Whether these σ_1 receptor agonist effects contribute to benefits in OCD is unknown.

Comparative Effectiveness

Drug responsiveness generally refers to a significant decrease in symptomatology, for example, as measured by a decrease of 50% or greater in score on a scale for depression, such as the Hamilton Rating Scale for Depression (HAM-D). In contrast, a patient is considered to be "in remission" if his or her level of symptoms is brought within the normal range, typically defined as a 17-item HAM-D score of 7 or less. Although response rather than remission has long been the primary measure of efficacy, many investigators are advocating the use of remission rates with the suggestion that remission is a better indicator for long-term outcome (Thase 2003). Generally speaking, rates of response do not vary significantly between antidepressant drugs (Kroenke et al. 2001). Most effective antidepressants produce rates of response in a typical 8- to 12-week clinical trial of 60%–75%. By contrast, remission rates in those same trials can be quite low, ranging from 30% to 50%. It is important not to consider these rates as somehow representing what would happen in clinical practice; trials are artificially truncated, and data usually are reported as last observation carried forward. Therefore, reports of remission may be valid for comparing effectiveness but may not reflect the realities of treatment.

However, some data indicate that SSRIs may induce remission at a rate that is less than that of alternative treatments, at least among certain subpopulations. Specifically, evidence suggests that TCA compounds may be more effective than SSRIs at treating individuals with the melancholic subtype of depression (Perry 1996). It has been speculated that the reason for this more favorable response characteristic is that TCAs generally block the reuptake of both norepinephrine and serotonin. The Danish University Antidepressant Group (1986, 1990) found that clomipramine, a potent norepinephrine and SERT inhibitor, produced a higher proportion of remission compared with either citalopram or paroxetine. In addition, a meta-analysis of registration trials with venlafaxine, a putative serotonin-norepinephrine reuptake inhibitor, suggested that a slightly higher (but statistically significant) proportion of patients achieve therapeutic remission with this drug in comparison with the SSRIs (Thase et al. 2001). Alternatively, some recent data suggest that the overall therapeutic effect of venlafaxine may not be greater than that of comparably dosed SSRIs (Montgomery et al. 2004). Therefore, whether SNRIs exert a greater effect than SSRIs or a heightened effect in a subgroup of depressed patients remains an open question.

The concept of "subgroup specificity" of response was initially supported by findings in the atypical subtype of depression, suggesting that individuals with this subtype preferentially responded to SSRIs. Atypical depression is characterized by so-called reverse vegetative features, including increased appetite and sleep along with heightened mood reactivity (see Chapter 35, "Atypical Depression, Dysthymia, and Cyclothymia"). The boundaries of this condition were described in the past in regard to differential responsiveness to treatment, specifically a tendency to preferentially respond to MAOIs relative to TCAs. Earlier open and small-scale controlled treatment research suggested that individuals with this subtype might be more likely to respond

TABLE 15–4. Representative medications metabolized by specific cytochrome P450 (CYP) enzymes

1A2			
Acetaminophen	Estradiol	Olanzapine	Theophylline
Amitriptyline	Fluvoxamine	Ondansetron	Tizanidine
Caffeine	Haloperidol	Phenacetin	Triamterene
Clomipramine	Imipramine	Propranolol	Verapamil
Clozapine	Mexiletine	Riluzole	S-warfarin
Cyclobenzaprine	Nabumetone	Ropivacaine	Zileuton
Duloxetine	Naproxen	Tacrin	Zolmitriptan
2B6			
Artemisinin	Ifosphamide	Methadone	Selegiline
Bupropion	Ketamine	Nevirapine	Sertraline
Cyclophosphamide	Meperidine	Propofol	Sorafenib
Efavirenz			
2C9			
Amitriptyline	Glipizide	Nateglinide	Tamoxifen
Celecoxib	Glyburide	Piroxicam	Tolbutamide
Diclofenac	Ibuprofen	Rosiglitazone	Torsemide
Fluoxetine	Irbesartan	S-naproxen	Valproic acid
Fluvastatin	Lornoxicam	S-warfarin	Verapamil
Glibenclamide	Losartan	Suprofen	Zakirlukast
Glimepiride	Meloxicam		
2C19			
Amitriptyline	Escitalopram	Nelfinavir	Proguanil
Carisoprodol	Esomeprazole	Nilutamide	Propranolol
Chloramphenicol	Hexobarbital	Omeprazole	R-mephobarbital
Citalopram	Imipramine	Pantoprazole	R-warfarin
Clomipramine	Indomethacin	Phenobarbitone	S-mephenytoin
Clopidogrel	Labetalol	Phenytoin	Teniposide
Cyclophosphamide	Lansoprazole	Primidone	Voriconazole
Diazepam	Moclobemide	Progesterone	

TABLE 15–4. Representative medications metabolized by specific cytochrome P450 (CYP) enzymes *(continued)*

2D6			
Alprenolol	Desipramine	Metoclopramide	Promethazine
Amitriptyline	Dexfenfluramine	Mexiletine	Propafenone
Amphetamine	Dextromethorphan	Minaprine	Propranolol
Aripiprazole	Donepezil	Nebivolol	Risperidone
Atomoxetine	Duloxetine	Nortriptyline	S-metoprolol
Bufuralol	Encainide	Ondansetron	Sparteine
Carvedilol	Flecainide	Oxycodone	Tamoxifen
Chlorpheniramine	Fluoxetine	Paroxetine	Thioridazine
Chlorpromazine	Fluvoxamine	Perhexiline	Timolol
Clomipramine	Haloperidol	Perphenazine	Tramadol
Clonidine	Imipramine	Phenacetin	Venlafaxine
Codeine	Lidocaine	Phenformin	Zuclopenthixol
Debrisoquine			

3A4,5,7			
Alfentanil	Dexamethasone	Lovastatin	Saquinavir
Alprazolam	Dextromethorphan	Methadone	Sildenafil
Amlodipine	Diazepam	Midazolam	Simvastatin
Aprepitant	Diltiazem	Nateglinide	Sirolimus
Aripiprazole	Docetaxel	Nelfinavir	Sorafenib
Astemizole	Domperidone	Nevirapine	Sunitinib
Atorvastatin	Eplerenone	Nifedipine	Tacrolimus
Boceprevir	Erythromycin	Nisoldipine	Telaprevir
Buspirone	Estradiol	Nitrendipine	Telithromycin
Cafergot	Felodipine	Ondansetron	Temsirolimus
Carbamazepine	Fentanyl	Paclitaxel	Terfenadine
Cerivastatin	Finasteride	Pimozide	Testosterone
Chlorpheniramine	Gleevec	Progesterone	Trazodone
Cilostazol	Haloperidol	Propranolol	Triazolam
Cisapride	HIV antivirals[a]	Quetiapine	Vemurafenib
Clarithromycin	Hydrocortisone	Quinidine	Verapamil
Cocaine	Indinavir	Quinine	Vincristine
Codeine	Irinotecan	Risperidone	Zaleplon
Cyclosporine	Lercanidipine	Romidepsin	Ziprasidone
Dapsone	Lidocaine	Salmeterol	Zolpidem

[a]HIV antivirals: indinavir, ritonavir, saquinavir, nelfinavir, nevirapine.

Source. Adapted from Indiana University Department of Medicine: "Drug Interactions Flockhart Table™." Available at: https://drug-interactions.medicine.iu.edu/MainTable.aspx. Accessed June 30, 2021.

to SSRIs than to TCAs. However, at least two subsequent controlled trials did not support this contention, and another report suggested that atypical features predicted earlier relapse in continuation and maintenance treatment after initial response.

In spite of this recent debate over the efficacy of SSRIs, these new antidepressants have clearly had a positive impact on patient care because they have made pharmacological treatment much more accessible to many patients with depression. Their relatively long half-lives (most are around 24 hours) have made once-daily dosing possible, a factor that promotes drug adherence.

Clinically Relevant Mechanisms of Action

When is an SSRI truly selective? Early in the evolution of SSRIs, serotonin selectivity was touted as a therapeutic advantage, playing off of the idea that the broader receptor binding profiles of TCAs produced considerable side effects; theoretically, then, selectivity would be expected to reduce the side-effect burden. However, given more recent data suggesting a modestly improved effect with SNRIs, several studies have tested the relative selectivity of antidepressant drugs. Most of the newer antidepressants are more potent serotonin than norepinephrine reuptake inhibitors, and determining when a drug has a dual versus single mechanism has been the focus of fierce debate. Much discussion has focused on the relative binding affinities of drugs for the SERT and NET in vitro (expressed as SERT/NET ratio), which is essentially a meaningless concept. The potency of a given drug at a site of action is the product of both binding affinity and concentration. Therefore, a drug with very low affinity but a high concentration in the brain may ultimately produce an equivalent effect to another drug with the opposite properties.

Paroxetine did not show evidence of a stronger effect on the tyramine pressor test as compared with amitriptyline (Hassan et al. 1985). Given the very high ratio of SERT/NET binding affinity, this finding has been taken as evidence of paroxetine's relative selectivity for the SERT. However, although paroxetine binds to the SERT much more potently, its affinity for the NET may not be trivial relative to other antidepressants. The in vitro binding affinity of [^{3}H]norepinephrine for the human NET is Ki=328 nMol, while that of venlafaxine is Ki=1,644 nMol. We have used the term "serotonin-selective dose" to describe dosages of antidepressants in which the serotonergic effects predominate over the noradrenergic effects—for example, paroxetine 20 mg/day, sertraline 50 mg/day, or venlafaxine 75 mg/day. However, based on relative affinity, certain compounds show changes in binding affinity (e.g., for NET) as the dosage is increased, although exactly where these effects occur can be obscure. Gilmor et al. (2002), as noted earlier, found that higher plasma levels of paroxetine produced moderate blockade of the NET; low concentrations of paroxetine produced relatively modest NET blockade (27%), but this effect increased somewhat at 200 ng/mL (43%), leading the authors to conclude that paroxetine at higher dosages and plasma concentrations could have a clinically meaningful noradrenergic effect. Again, the actual effect within the brain is unclear.

Related Side Effects

Certain side effects are common among SSRIs. These include nausea, vomiting, diarrhea, somnolence, fatigue, dizziness, tremor, insomnia, decreased libido, and erectile dysfunction. Most side effects dissipate within 2 weeks of starting the medication, except for sexual dysfunction, which can be more persistent.

Serotonin-Norepinephrine Reuptake Inhibitors

Venlafaxine and Desvenlafaxine

Venlafaxine (Effexor and Effexor XR) was introduced into the United States in 1994, and its primary metabolite, *O*-desmethylvenlafaxine (desvenlafaxine) (Pristiq), in 2008. Both are weak inhibitors of serotonin and norepinephrine reuptake (see Table 15–1) and very weak inhibitors of dopamine reuptake. Nonetheless, as noted earlier, in human studies venlafaxine shows significant effects in measurements of both SERT and NET blockade. This is due in part to the relatively high blood and cerebrospinal fluid levels of the parent compound and the primary metabolite desvenlafaxine and the very low protein binding of both. The low protein binding, and the fact that the drugs do not significantly affect CYP enzymes, suggests that drug-drug interactions would not typically be expected to occur (Ereshefsky and Dugan 2000). The primary metabolic pathway is CYP2D6 for venlafaxine and CYP3A4 for desvenlafaxine, although the latter is primarily eliminated via direct glucuronide conjugation mediated by uridine 5'-diphospho-glucuronosyltransferase (UGT) 1A1, 1A3, 2B4, and 2B15 enzymes (Fossom 2008).

Venlafaxine is approved in a dosing range of 75–225 mg/day for the extended-release form (Effexor XR) and 375 mg/day for the immediate-release form (Effexor) (see Table 15–2). Due to venlafaxine's short half-life, twice-daily dosing is required for the immediate-release form; however, the extended-release form and desvenlafaxine (which is available only in an extended-release form) can be dosed once a day. Desvenlafaxine is approved at a dosage range of 50–100 mg/day. Venlafaxine has been approved by the FDA for the treatment of both major depressive disorder (MDD) and generalized anxiety disorder (Gutierrez et al. 2003), and desvenlafaxine only for MDD. Montgomery et al. (2002) conducted a survival analysis with data from two longer-term studies of venlafaxine in MDD and found an overall better response and fewer dropouts at 150 mg/day relative to the 75 and the 37.5 mg/day dosages, indicating that higher dosages may be more effective (Montgomery et al. 2002).

As discussed, both venlafaxine and desvenlafaxine have short half-lives, and therefore, discontinuation reactions can be observed even after only brief interruptions (Haddad 2001). Like other sustained-release preparations (e.g., Paxil CR), venlafaxine XR and desvenlafaxine extended-release are not less prone to inducing such reactions. Therefore, patients should be warned about interruptions in dosing. Venlafaxine and desvenlafaxine are also associated with mild elevations in blood pressure; the immediate-release form of venlafaxine at higher dosages is more liable in this regard. It should be emphasized that these are not severe hypertensive events as seen with MAOIs, and hypertensive responses are not more common in patients with a history of hypertension. However, monitoring blood pressure is recommended (Feighner 1995). Other common side effects associated with venlafaxine and desvenlafaxine include nausea, somnolence, dry mouth, constipation, sweating, decreased libido, and erectile dysfunction.

Duloxetine

Duloxetine (Cymbalta) is another dual reuptake inhibitor approved for marketing for MDD in the United States. Dosing in clinical trials has ranged up to 40 mg twice per day, and the drug has shown good tolerability (Nemeroff et al. 2002; Schatzberg 2003; Sharma et al. 2000). In contrast to venlafaxine, this drug appears to induce low rates of spontaneous hypertension (<2%) (Schatzberg 2003).

Because mild hypertensive reactions occur with other norepinephrine reuptake inhibitors (e.g., TCAs, venlafaxine), the question arises of whether duloxetine causes a clinically meaningful blockade of norepinephrine reuptake. Duloxetine binds to SERT and NET at Ki=0.8 and 7.5 nMol, respectively, yielding a SERT/NET ratio of 9 (as opposed to 16 for venlafaxine [Owens et al. 1997]) (see Table 15–1) (Bymaster et al. 2001).

Work by Turcotte et al. (2001) and Chalon et al. (2003) called into question the in vivo potency of duloxetine in blocking norepinephrine reuptake. Both studies involved administering duloxetine to healthy volunteers and performing the tyramine pressor test as described earlier for venlafaxine. In both instances, duloxetine did not produce the expected increase in blood pressure induced by the administration of tyramine, in contrast to TCAs, although in the latter study it did increase whole-body norepinephrine turnover (an indirect measure of reuptake inhibition). Duloxetine showed evidence of SERT blockade, which is in contrast to both in vitro studies and in vivo studies in animals, which indicated potent norepinephrine reuptake inhibition. In addition, meta-analyses of clinical trials suggest that duloxetine was no more effective than SSRIs for MDD (Cipriani et al. 2009, 2012, 2016).

Additional support for duloxetine's norepinephrine reuptake inhibition comes from the considerable number of preclinical (Wang et al. 2015, 2016) and clinical (Citrome and Weiss-Citrome 2012; Pergolizzi et al. 2013) studies on its use in pain. Potent SNRIs such as TCAs and milnacipran improve peripheral pain (Häuser et al. 2012). These effects on pain are mediated through three mechanisms: serotonin and norepinephrine reuptake inhibition and sodium channel blockade. Serotonin and norepinephrine have inhibitory effects on sensory transmission in nociceptive fibers in the dorsal horn of the spinal cord (Micó et al. 2006). Duloxetine (Wang et al. 2010) and TCAs such as amitriptyline (Furgała et al. 2018) also block $Na_v1.3$, $Na_v1.7$, and $Na_v1.8$ voltage-gated sodium channels, which produces antinociceptive effects in preclinical models (Horishita et al. 2017) that may mediate some of the beneficial effects on pain. Duloxetine is approved in the United States for the treatment of fibromyalgia, diabetic neuropathic pain, and chronic musculoskeletal pain. In addition, duloxetine has been shown to be effective in reducing urinary stress incontinence in women, which also supports a meaningful norepinephrine reuptake inhibition effect (Moore 2004).

Common side effects with duloxetine include nausea, dry mouth, somnolence, constipation, decreased appetite, and sweating. The effects on sexual function were assessed in four clinical trials using the Arizona Sexual Experience Scale (ASEX) (Eli Lilly 2020). Overall, patients treated with duloxetine experienced more sexual dysfunction than did patients treated with placebo, as indicated by the ASEX total score. A sex-specific analysis showed that sexual dysfunction occurred only in males, who had more difficulty achieving orgasm with duloxetine compared with placebo. Females did not experience more sexual dysfunction on duloxetine than on placebo as measured by ASEX total score; in fact, women given duloxetine or placebo and men given placebo experienced a slight improvement in ASEX total score. Duloxetine and placebo were generally neutral on other aspects of sexual function, including sex drive and sexual arousal in both men and women and the ability to achieve an erection in men.

The primary metabolic pathways of duloxetine are via CYP1A2 and 2D6. It is highly protein bound and is a moderate inhibitor of CYP2D6. It therefore has a moderate potential for drug-drug interactions.

Milnacipran and Levomilnacipran

Milnacipran (Savella) and its levorotary enantiomer levomilnacipran (Fetzima) (Zadka et al. 2016) are highly potent SERT and NET inhibitors approved both in and outside of the United States for a range of conditions, including depression and pain. Milnacipran is approved outside of the United States for MDD, but it has never received FDA approval for this indication and is approved only for fibromyalgia. Levomilnacipran is only approved in the United States for MDD. The effects of SNRIs for pain syndromes are discussed further in the earlier section on duloxetine.

Milnacipran and levomilnacipran are more "balanced" SNRIs in that NET binding is higher relative to SERT binding than for other SNRIs. The relative SERT/NET ratios of SNRIs are as follows: venlafaxine, 30:1; desvenlafaxine, 14:1; duloxetine, 10:1; milnacipran, 1.6:1.0; and levomilnacipran, 1:2 (Sansone and Sansone 2014). In spite of the relatively high NET binding affinity, levomilnacipran produces only modest increases in blood pressure and pulse in the dosing range of 40–120 mg/day (Allergan 2019). Common side effects include nausea, vomiting, dizziness, sweating, insomnia, constipation, urinary hesitancy, tachycardia, and palpitations. Effects on sexual interest were assessed in at least one clinical trial with levomilnacipran (Gommoll et al. 2014), using the ASEX as described earlier with duloxetine. In this trial, no differences were found in ASEX total score between levomilnacipran and placebo in the overall groups for males and females separately. By contrast, erectile dysfunction in men was reported in clinical trials in 6%, 8%, and 10% of men given levomilnacipran 40, 80, or 120 mg/day, respectively, versus 2% in those given placebo (Allergan 2019). Rates of other sexual side effects in both women and men participating in clinical trials were low, but these trials may have underestimated the frequency. Milnacipran and levomilnacipran are metabolized by CYP3A4 and do not inhibit any CYP enzymes.

Other Antidepressants

Nefazodone

Nefazodone (Serzone) is a phenylpiperazine derivative that is structurally similar to trazodone but with an improved side-effect profile (Owens et al. 1997). It has low potency for the human SERT and NET (Ki=549 and 713 nMol, respectively) (Owens et al. 1997). By contrast, binding of nefazodone and its principal metabolite, hydroxynefazodone, to the serotonin (5-hydroxytryptamine [5-HT]) type 2A (5-HT_{2A}) receptor is considerably greater (ketanserin binding Ki=7.1 and 7.2 nMol, respectively) (Owens et al. 1997). Therefore, blockade of this receptor seems to be the basis of the therapeutic effect of nefazodone, much like trazodone. 5-HT_{2A} blockade shows antidepressant- and antianxiety-like effects in animal behavioral models. Nefazodone is a relatively potent norepinephrine α_1 receptor antagonist (Ki=5.5 nMol) (Owens et al. 1997) and a moderately potent histamine-1 blocker (Ki=30 nMol), which may account for some of the side effects associated with the drug, including orthostatic hypotension and sedation. The drug has a very short half-life (4–8 hours [DeVane et al. 2002]), requiring it to be taken at least twice per day. It is usually started at a dosage of 200 mg/day, which is typically advanced to the 300–600 mg/day range, divided into two doses. Rates of sexual dysfunction are relatively low.

There are some significant concerns associated with this drug. For example, it is a potent inhibitor of CYP3A4, an enzyme responsible for the metabolism of many drugs (see Table 15–3) (Nemeroff et al. 1996). In addition, it has been reported to induce severe hepatotoxicity resulting in liver failure. The rate of serious hepatotoxicity is low (~1/250,000–300,000 exposures [Sedky et al. 2012]), but the outcome is potentially catastrophic. Routine monitoring of hepatic function has not been established to be effective in preventing toxicity and is not required by the FDA, although early detection may improve outcome. Alternatively, counseling patients with regard to this adverse outcome and the symptoms of hepatic dysfunction (e.g., nausea, jaundice, anorexia, malaise) is essential. Furthermore, nefazodone should be avoided in people with baseline elevated transaminases, not because of an increased risk in these patients but because of difficulties in prospective monitoring (Sedky et al. 2012).

Nefazodone is metabolized by CYP3A4, with CYP2D6 being a minor secondary pathway. However, in the case of CYP3A4 inhibition, a higher proportion of metabolism is via CYP2D6. This is important because CYP2D6 metabolism forms *meta*-chlorophenylpiperazine, a psychoactive drug with anxiety-producing effects (Preskorn et al. 2012).

Vilazodone

Vilazodone (Viibryd) is a very potent SERT inhibitor (Ki=0.1 nMol) and a 5-HT_{1A} receptor partial agonist (half-maximal inhibitory concentration [IC_{50}]=0.2 nMol) (Hughes et al. 2005). It has low (although not trivial) affinity for the NET and the dopamine transporter (Ki=56 and 37 nMol, respectively) and extremely low binding to other receptors (Hughes et al. 2005). It is approved in the United States for the treatment of MDD. Partial-agonist actions at 5-HT_{1A} receptors are similar to those of buspirone; therefore, vilazodone is expected to have significant antianxiety and antidepressant effects. This is supported by studies in some (but not all) anxiety models (Treit et al. 2001). The clinical benefit in patients with generalized anxiety disorder was shown in three well-designed controlled trials with a total of 844 participants (Zareifopoulos and Dylja 2017). However, the development of vilazodone for this indication was suspended by the manufacturer. Nevertheless, vilazodone appears to be effective for anxiety symptoms in patients with MDD (Thase et al. 2014).

Comparative effectiveness against other antidepressants is unknown. One important outstanding question is whether vilazodone is more effective than simply combining an SSRI, such as escitalopram, with buspirone, both of which are generic and very inexpensive, unlike the branded vilazodone. Vilazodone has a higher affinity for 5-HT_{1A} receptors than buspirone (IC_{50}=0.2 vs. 24 nMol), but whether this translates into superior efficacy is unknown.

Side effects commonly associated with vilazodone include nausea, diarrhea, vomiting, dry mouth, dizziness, and insomnia. The FDA-approved product information includes warnings regarding acute pancreatitis and hyponatremia related to the syndrome of inappropriate antidiuretic hormone secretion (SIADH). However, the frequency of these more serious reactions is low. It is metabolized by CYP3A4 and does not inhibit CYP enzymes.

Vortioxetine

Vortioxetine (Trintellix) is approved for the treatment of MDD in the United States (Pae et al. 2015a). It is a complex and unique medication in that it is a potent SERT inhibitor (1.6 nMol), but it also has significant affinity for a number of serotonin receptors. It is a 5-HT_{1A} receptor agonist (Ki=15 nMol), a partial agonist at 5-HT_{1B} receptors, and an antagonist at 5-HT_{1D}, 5-HT_3, and 5-HT_7 receptors (Sanchez et al. 2015). Although the clinical implications of some of these binding effects are unknown, some actions can be predicted on the basis of both preclinical and clinical pharmacology. For example, actions at 5-HT_{1A} and 5-HT_3 receptors are expected to produce antianxiety effects, and this is supported by both animal studies (Mørk et al. 2012) and human clinical trials (Pae et al. 2015b). A recent meta-analysis of four randomized controlled trials in generalized anxiety disorder showed a significant, albeit modest, clinical effect (Pae et al. 2015b), although a second meta-analysis drew the opposite conclusion (Fu et al. 2016). It is not currently approved for the treatment of generalized anxiety disorder.

Both 5-HT_{1A} agonists and 5-HT_7 antagonists increase dopamine efflux in areas such as the frontal cortex and nucleus accumbens (Huang et al. 2012). Increases in both norepinephrine and dopamine have been shown with vortioxetine in the medial prefrontal cortex, nucleus accumbens, and hippocampus. These actions may improve attention and executive function. One well-done controlled trial showed a significantly greater effect of vortioxetine on the digit symbol substitution test (DSST) compared with placebo (Mahableshwarkar et al. 2015). Path analysis showed that vortioxetine had an effect on the DSST that was independent of its effect on depression. The DSST taps into a number of cognitive domains, including attention, memory, and executive function, and the clinical significance of improvement on this test is unknown. Other trials did not show a significant difference between vortioxetine and SSRIs on cognition (Baune et al. 2018b; Nierenberg et al. 2019; Vieta et al. 2018); however, a recent meta-analysis suggested that vortioxetine may have a greater effect than SSRIs, TCAs, and placebo on the DSST (Baune et al. 2018a).

Common side effects of vortioxetine include nausea, vomiting, diarrhea, constipation, dizziness, and sexual dysfunction. With the exception of nausea, these effects occur in less than 10% of patients in clinical trials, although, as noted earlier, sexual dysfunction may be underreported in clinical trials. Vortioxetine is a CYP2D6 substrate and does not inhibit CYP enzymes.

Reboxetine and Atomoxetine

Both reboxetine (Edronax, Vestra) (Brunello et al. 2002; Kasper et al. 2000) and atomoxetine (tomoxetine; Strattera) (Kratochvil et al. 2003) are potent and relatively selective norepinephrine reuptake inhibitors. Therefore, these drugs are similar in their therapeutic potential to TCAs such as desipramine. Although the effectiveness of reboxetine for MDD is supported by several studies, and it is available outside of the United States, FDA-regulated controlled registration trials were negative, and the drug was never approved (Page 2003). This may be the result of failed rather than negative trials—that is, caused by a relatively high placebo response rate. On the other hand, atomoxetine has received FDA approval in the United States for ADHD as a result of significant controlled trials. Atomoxetine has not been approved for depression; it was shown in at least one published Phase II clinical trial to be effective in depression (Chouinard et al. 1984), although subsequent depression trials have been negative. In addition, atomoxetine is not effective as an adjunct to SSRIs (Michelson et al. 2007), and it does not effectively improve depression in children with ADHD (Bangs et al. 2007).

Special Considerations

Serotonin Reuptake Inhibitor Discontinuation Syndrome

Abrupt termination of treatment with SERT inhibitors can result in a rapid onset of one or more characteristic symptoms now associated with the discontinuation syndrome: anxiety, crying, dizziness, headache, increased dreaming, insomnia, irritability, myoclonus, nausea (with occasional vomiting), paresthesias (including "electrical sensations"), and tremor. This phenomenon appears to be linked to three significant factors: SERT blockade, short half-life, and a relatively rapid decrease in dosage or termination of the medication. The anticholinergic effects of TCAs also have been touted as contributing to the problems associated with these drugs, especially in the face of symptoms that are more consistent with cholinergic rebound (including gastrointestinal hypermotility, movement disorders such as akathisia, and arrhythmias). However, this is a consistent property of SERT inhibitors, although half-life is key: long-half-life drugs such as fluoxetine seldom produce significant discontinuation syndrome, whereas short-half-life drugs such as paroxetine or venlafaxine very often do (Michelson et al. 2000; Rosenbaum et al. 1998).

Serotonin reuptake inhibitor discontinuation syndrome is not peculiar to the newer generation of agents, such as venlafaxine. In fact, the phenomenon has been reported with TCAs such as imipramine and clomipramine and with MAOIs (Lejoyeux and Adès 1997). The highest relative rates of discontinuation symptoms have been with TCAs (21.5%–100%) (Lejoyeux and Adès 1997), although this has not been confirmed in head-to-head comparisons. Prevention is the ideal approach to managing the syndrome. When patients are being treated with shorter-half-life agents, slow tapering typically prevents significant symptoms. Furthermore, patients on any serotonin reuptake inhibitor should be warned about the incidence of discontinuation symptoms after abrupt withdrawal. However, even with very slow tapering, some patients experience intolerable symptoms. Slowing the tapering process sometimes helps, but at times the substitution of another drug with a longer half-life is needed. Fluoxetine can be added to shorter-half-life medications, followed by tapering of the first medication and then by tapering of fluoxetine (Haddad 2001).

In utero exposure to antidepressants and subsequent postpartum discontinuation effects in infants also are of concern (Costei et al. 2002). One study showed an enhancement of perinatal complications, particularly respiratory distress, in infants born to mothers taking paroxetine at the time of delivery relative to infants exposed to paroxetine earlier in pregnancy but not at delivery (Costei et al. 2002). This advocates avoiding short-half-life SERT inhibitors late in pregnancy. Alternative strategies include discontinuation of the antidepressant well before delivery (although this risks the return of depression) or substitution of a longer-half-life drug early in pregnancy. Pregnancy issues should be considered when prescribing short-half-life drugs in women of reproductive potential.

Sexual Dysfunction

Sexual dysfunction is a side effect common to all SERT inhibitors; although these drugs have other chemical properties including α-adrenergic blockade and anticholinergic effects, the most consistent theme is the blockade of SERT. Sexual side effects were reported with serotonergic TCAs in the past. Common side effects of serotonin reuptake inhibitors include decreased libido, impairment in erection (in men) or labial engorgement (in women), and inhibition of orgasm. Therefore, patients taking these medications must be monitored carefully for persisting sexual side effects, because this class of adverse reactions contributes significantly to premature discontinuation. Reported rates of sexual dysfunction with serotonin reuptake inhibitors have varied widely, depending more on the ascertainment method than on the type of drug. Conservatively, about half of the patients treated with serotonin reuptake inhibitors experience significant dysfunction, with 15% or more having persistent symptoms (Ferguson 2001).

Caution needs to be exercised when evaluating sexual dysfunction associated with serotonin reuptake inhibitors. Decreased sex drive and arousal are common in depression; about half of patients with depression report significantly decreased sexual interest. Therefore, a baseline sexual history is an important part of information gathering in the evaluation of depression. Persistent sexual dysfunction may be a side effect of antidepressant therapy but may also be a residual symptom of depression, and, if so, should be addressed accordingly.

Management of sexual dysfunction can involve several different possible approaches. As noted, many individuals experience some improvement with time. However, it often is an intolerable side effect and should be managed aggressively to prevent premature termination of treatment. Decreasing the dosage or discontinuing the medication for a short period has been recommended, although this typically is ineffective and risks a return of depressive symptoms or discontinuation syndrome. One alternative is switching to a drug with fewer side effects: for example, switching from the serotonin reuptake inhibitor to bupropion, nefazodone, or mirtazapine has been reported to be effective. However, some patients experience a significant return of depressive symptoms on tapering of the serotonin reuptake inhibitor and therefore must be restarted on the original drug. Adding bupropion to the serotonin reuptake inhibitor is one management strategy; the addition of bupropion in the dosage range of 100–300 mg/day has been reported to be somewhat effective, although relatively few controlled clinical trial data are available (Safarinejad 2011).

Suicide Risk

In 1990, Teicher et al. (1990) reported on a series of six inpatients who, at baseline, had reported no suicidal ideation but developed intense suicidal preoccupation after initiating treatment with fluoxetine. According to the authors, this state persisted for periods of between 3 days and 3 months after discontinuation. This set off a firestorm of controversy about the potential of SSRIs to induce suicidal ideation in patients who did not previously have thoughts of self-harm. Furthermore, allegations arose that the risk of suicidal ideation with SSRIs has been downplayed by researchers due to economic interests that are the product of financial relationships between pharmaceutical companies and universities (Healy 2003).

Some epidemiological data suggest that SSRIs do, in fact, enhance suicidal ideation in certain patients. For example, Donovan et al. (2002) retrospectively evaluated 2,776 cases of deliberate self-harm that presented to the emergency department of the Derbyshire Royal Infirmary in the United Kingdom. The incidence of self-harm by drug was estimated from the number of prescriptions written for either a TCA or SSRI in the Southern Derbyshire district for the same time interval. Donovan and colleagues found a higher incidence of deliberate self-harm among the patients taking SSRIs than among those taking TCAs. The relative risk of overdose (setting imipramine at 1.0) was highest for fluoxetine, at 2.8, followed closely by flupentixol (an antipsychotic), at 2.6. The mean relative risk for SSRIs was 2.3, and for TCAs was 1.7. However, as the authors noted, the SSRI-related risk was skewed by the risk for fluoxetine; for example, the risk with sertraline was 1.4, and the risk with paroxetine was 1.9, whereas the risk for the TCAs clomipramine and lofepramine was 2.0 and 2.5, respectively. These kinds of data have led some to conclude that the risk of self-harm is increased with SSRIs, especially fluoxetine (Healy 2002). However, as the authors noted:

> Equally relevant, however, is the pragmatic consideration that prescribers are heeding advice to prescribe safer-in-overdose antidepressants to patients who are perceived to be at greater risk of [deliberate self harm]. This effectively "loads the dice" against antidepressants such as the SSRIs, so that this manifests as an apparent excess of self-harm behaviour in patients who had been prescribed these antidepressants. (Donovan et al. 2002, p. 556)

That is, people at higher risk of suicide are more likely to be prescribed medications that are safer in overdose.

Data from controlled clinical trials generally have not indicated that SSRIs enhance risk relative to non-SSRI antidepressants or placebo, with the exception of adolescents and young adults (discussed later). Khan et al. (2000) assessed the frequency of suicides and suicide attempts along with symptom reduction derived from adult clinical trial information for seven drugs in the FDA database: fluoxetine, sertraline, paroxetine, venlafaxine, nefazodone, mirtazapine, and bupropion. A total of 19,639 participants were included. The authors found no differences between the three groups compared collectively, or within any given drug dataset; however, fluoxetine information was not available for that analysis. Therefore, no comment could be made in regard to the suicide risk for fluoxetine per se, but this has been assessed by other studies. Beasley et al. (1991) conducted a meta-analysis of 17 controlled clinical trials comparing fluoxetine (n=1,765 exposures) with TCAs (n=731), placebo (n=569), or both. The pooled incidence of suicidal behavior did not differ between groups (suicidal acts: fluoxetine 0.3%, TCAs 0.4%, placebo 0.2%; suicidal ideation: fluoxetine 1.2%, TCAs 3.6%, placebo 2.5%). Together, these data make a compelling case for a lack of association between SSRIs and an increase in suicidal potential.

More recently, small differences in rates of suicidal ideation, attempts, or nonsuicidal self-injury from individual clinical trials have led the FDA and other regulatory authorities to issue warnings about the potential for certain SSRIs to enhance suicide risk in adolescents. The FDA issued an initial warning based on a meta-analysis of three unpublished controlled trials in depressed adolescents that failed to show differences between paroxetine and placebo (Wooltorton 2003). In these studies, suicidal thoughts, suicide attempts, and episodes of self-harm were more frequent among adolescents taking paroxetine (5.3% of 378) versus placebo (2.8% of 285). A similar result was demonstrated in studies of adolescents with social anxiety disorder (paroxetine 2.4% of 165 vs. 0% of 157). In this review, the author stated that "Paroxetine is contraindicated for patients under the age of 18...any pediatric patient currently taking paroxetine should be screened for suicidal thoughts, suicide attempts or episodes of self-harm" (Wooltorton 2003, p. 446).

Based on similar data, clinicians have been warned about the risk of suicidal behavior in adolescents treated with venlafaxine XR. This FDA warning came from an analysis of children and adolescents between the ages of 6 and 17 years treated in both open and controlled clinical trials. In a "Dear Healthcare Professional" letter, Wyeth, the manufacturer of venlafaxine, outlined adverse event information from trials in depression and generalized anxiety disorder conducted in children and adolescents. The company noted an excess of discontinuations for adverse events in three categories—hostility (venlafaxine 2% vs. placebo <1%), suicidal ideation (2% vs. 0%), and abnormal or changed behavior (1% vs. 0%)—and concluded: "Effexor and Effexor XR have not been and are not now recommended for use in pediatric patients" (Wyeth Pharmaceuticals 2003).

Subsequent, more comprehensive assessments of the FDA clinical trials databases indicated that the risk of suicidal ideation and self-injury (although not completed suicides) was highest in pediatric populations and progressively declined with age (McCain 2009). Setting the suicide rate of 25- to 30-year-old subjects as the comparator, the odds ratio for suicidality was highest among pediatric patients (OR 2.22) and lowest among subjects age 65 and older (OR 0.39) (McCain 2009).

Clinical trials databases are not the best for evaluating risk of increased suicidal potential, because patients with active suicidal ideation typically are excluded from outpatient trials and subsets of patients who may be at greater risk, such as those with borderline personality disorder, are routinely excluded as well. One of the better datasets for evaluating risks in adolescents comes from the Treatment of Adolescent Depression Study (TADS; Emslie et al. 2006), given that adolescents with suicidal ideation were not systematically excluded from participation. Adolescents with MDD were randomized to treatment with fluoxetine, cognitive-behavioral therapy (CBT), combined treatment, or placebo. Notably, in the TADS, as in the FDA-analyzed studies cited earlier, no increase in actual suicides was found. The rates of new-onset suicidal ideation were as follows: fluoxetine alone, 7.3%; CBT, 3.6%; combined treatment, 2.8%; and placebo, 2.7%. The rates of suicide attempts were as follows: fluoxetine alone, 1.8%; CBT, 1%; combined treatment, 1.9%; and placebo, 0%. Finally, the rates of all suicide-related events were as follows: fluoxetine alone, 9.2%; CBT, 4.5%; combined treatment, 4.7%; and placebo, 2.7%. These data certainly suggest that fluoxetine increases the frequency of suicidal ideation and attempts, although not that of completed suicide.

Two other interesting observations come from this study. First, combining fluoxetine with CBT reduces the rate of suicidal ideation, although not attempts. The observation of reduced suicidal ideation may be due to the fact that combined treatment was more effective than either monotherapy condition; the response rates were as follows: fluoxetine alone, 60.6%; CBT, 43.2%; combined treatment, 71.0%; and placebo, 34.8%. Second, CBT alone increased suicide-related events to a small degree, a finding that may mean that any effective treatment may increase the likelihood of suicide events in a small number of adolescents. The fact that all active treatments increased suicidal ideation and self-injury argues for heightened vigilance in depressed adolescent patients.

A key question, then, is why is there an apparent excess at all? The TADS is informative in determining possible mediators of the increased risk for suicidal ideation and behavior. Important side effects such as "mania spectrum," "agitation spectrum," and anxiety were increased in patients treated with fluoxetine. These symptoms suggest that the antidepressant may have been inducing a manic or mixed state that could have led to an increase in agitation, anxiety, irritability, hostility, and suicidal preoccupation. Second, antidepressants can induce anxiety and agitation in patients with depression even in the absence of a bipolar diathesis, but with a similar outcome. Furthermore, some medications such as paroxetine and venlafaxine have relatively short half-lives and are known to induce withdrawal reactions. Missing one or more doses could result in an abrupt return of depressive, anxious, and other symptoms, leading to suicidal ideation. These kinds of factors together could contribute to an excess of suicidal ideation, suicide attempts, or self-injury in the TADS and FDA datasets.

Olfson et al. (2003) evaluated the relationship between the changes in regional antidepressant medication treatment and suicide in adolescents from 1990 to 2000, using a large pharmacy database. They found that a 1% increase in frequency of prescription of antidepressant drugs resulted in a decrease in suicide frequency of 0.23 per 100,000. For the period of 1991–2001 in the United States, the suicide rate for children ages 10–14 years showed a decline of approximately 14%, whereas the rate for 15- to 19-year-olds showed a decline of 31.5% (Centers for Disease Control and Prevention 2004). The increase in frequency of antidepressant prescriptions over the same period suggested that these medications contributed to this decline. Similar results were shown in subsequent studies (Gibbons et al. 2005; Grunebaum et al. 2004; Ludwig and Marcotte 2005).

The FDA and other regulatory agencies required all antidepressants to have a "black box warning" about new-onset suicidal ideation or behavior starting in 2004. Following this change, the rates of suicide among adolescents began to increase after more than a decade of decline (Bridge et al. 2008). In the period after the black box warnings, the frequency of antidepressant medication prescriptions for adolescents declined (Busch and Barry 2009), but the frequency of diagnosis of depression among adolescents also declined (Adegbite-Adeniyi et al. 2012; Libby et al. 2007; Olfson et al. 2008). Although the frequency of prescribing antidepressants for adolescents has increased somewhat since that initial decline, the rate of suicide continues to increase, particularly among girls (Curtin et al. 2016).

Drug-Drug Interactions

Although the newer antidepressants are generally safe drugs, they do confer risks for serious drug-drug interactions under certain circumstances. Perhaps the most serious is the combination of SSRIs and MAOIs, which can lead to the development of a potentially fatal "serotonin syndrome." These drugs should never be taken in combination, and patients should not begin taking an MAOI for at least 2 weeks after discontinuing an SSRI (for fluoxetine the washout period should be 4 weeks or longer). Serotonin syndrome presents within 24 hours of initiating or increasing the dosage of a serotonin agent and results from overstimulation of 5-HT_{1A} and possibly 5-HT_2 receptors. It consists of a constellation of mental, autonomic, and neurological symptoms. The full-blown syndrome is diagnosed when a patient presents with at least four major symptoms or at least three major and two minor symptoms. Major symptoms include confusion, elevated mood, coma, fever, tremors, chills, and rigidity (among others), and minor symptoms include agitation, insomnia, tachycardia, tachypnea, and impaired coordination. Treatment always involves discontinuing the serotonergic agent and replacing fluids.

A second way in which drug-drug interactions can occur is through competitive protein binding. Antidepressants circulate in a state highly bound to proteins such as albumin, and other drugs that circulate in a highly bound state can displace the antidepressants, resulting in an increase in the fraction of the drug that is unbound. This may amplify the drug's effects, particularly its side effects (see Table 15–1). Most antidepressant medications are highly protein bound (>95%), with the exception of venlafaxine (27%), desvenlafaxine (30%), levomilnacipran (22%), and escitalopram (56%). Therefore, most antidepressants can displace drugs such as warfarin in plasma proteins.

Finally, a third risk for drug-drug interaction is that some medications inhibit CYP enzymes, the microsomal enzymes of the liver that metabolize many drugs before they are cleared from the body (see Tables 15–3 and 15–4). The antidepressants themselves are broken down by these enzymes, and some even inhibit their own metabolism. CYP2D6 is strongly inhibited by fluoxetine and paroxetine and weakly inhibited by sertraline and citalopram (Nemeroff et al. 1996). Drugs that are normally metabolized by this isoform include antipsychotics, antiseizure medication, β-blockers, and angiotensin-converting enzyme inhibitors. CYP3A4 is inhibited by nefazodone, norfluoxetine, and fluvoxamine, and thus these drugs can cause increased plasma levels of cyclosporine and other drugs metabolized by CYP3A4 (Nemeroff et al. 1996). Venlafaxine and mirtazapine may have lower potential for drug-drug interactions than other antidepressants.

Conclusion

The introduction of SSRIs and newer antidepressants has dramatically changed the treatment of depression over the past three decades. Earlier antidepressants such as the TCAs were effective but had significant side effects because they interacted with various neurotransmitter receptors. SSRIs rapidly became the most widely prescribed class of antidepressants—indeed, one of the most widely prescribed classes of drugs—and have been used for the treatment of depression in millions of people worldwide. Although questions remain about their comparative effectiveness, they continue to be widely used. These medications remain the mainstays of MDD treatment.

References

Adegbite-Adeniyi C, Gron B, Rowles BM, et al: An update on antidepressant use and suicidality in pediatric depression. Expert Opin Pharmacother 13(15):2119–2130, 2012 22984934

Allergan: Fetzima prescribing information. Madison, NJ, Allergan, October 2019. Available at: media.allergan.com/actavis/actavis/media/allergan-pdf-documents/product-prescribing/10092019-FETZIMA-v2_0USPI2220-v2_0MG2220-(clean).pdf. Accessed November 13, 2020.

Bang-Andersen B, Ruhland T, Jørgensen M, et al: Discovery of 1-[2-(2,4-dimethylphenylsulfanyl)phenyl]piperazine (Lu AA21004): a novel multimodal compound for the treatment of major depressive disorder. J Med Chem 54(9):3206–3221, 2011 21486038

Bangs ME, Emslie GJ, Spencer TJ, et al: Efficacy and safety of atomoxetine in adolescents with attention-deficit/hyperactivity disorder and major depression. J Child Adolesc Psychopharmacol 17(4):407–420, 2007 17822337

Baumann P: Pharmacokinetic-pharmacodynamic relationship of the selective serotonin reuptake inhibitors. Clin Pharmacokinet 31(6):444–469, 1996 8968657

Baune BT, Brignone M, Larsen KG: A network meta-analysis comparing effects of various antidepressant classes on the Digit Symbol Substitution Test (DSST) as a measure of cognitive dysfunction in patients with major depressive disorder. Int J Neuropsychopharmacol 21(2):97–107, 2018a 29053849

Baune BT, Sluth LB, Olsen CK: The effects of vortioxetine on cognitive performance in working patients with major depressive disorder: a short-term, randomized, double-blind, exploratory study. J Affect Disord 229:421–428, 2018b 29331703

Beasley CM Jr, Dornseif BE, Bosomworth JC, et al: Fluoxetine and suicide: a meta-analysis of controlled trials of treatment for depression. BMJ 303(6804):685–692, 1991 1833012

Blakely RD, De Felice LJ, Hartzell HC: Molecular physiology of norepinephrine and serotonin transporters. J Exp Biol 196:263–281, 1994 7823027

Boyer WF, Feighner JP: An overview of paroxetine. J Clin Psychiatry 53 (suppl):3–6, 1992 1531819

Bridge JA, Greenhouse JB, Weldon AH, et al: Suicide trends among youths aged 10 to 19 years in the United States, 1996–2005. JAMA 300(9):1025–1026, 2008 18768413

Brown TA, Chorpita BF, Barlow DH: Structural relationships among dimensions of the DSM-IV anxiety and mood disorders and dimensions of negative affect, positive affect, and autonomic arousal. J Abnorm Psychol 107(2):179–192, 1998 9604548

Brunello N, Mendlewicz J, Kasper S, et al: The role of noradrenaline and selective noradrenaline reuptake inhibition in depression. Eur Neuropsychopharmacol 12(5):461–475, 2002 12208564

Bruno A, Morabito P, Spina E, et al: The role of levomilnacipran in the management of major depressive disorder: a comprehensive review. Curr Neuropharmacol 14(2):191–199, 2016 26572745

Burke WJ: Escitalopram. Expert Opin Investig Drugs 11(10):1477–1486, 2002 12387707
Busch SHB, Barry CL: Pediatric antidepressant use after the black-box warning. Health Aff (Millwood) 28(3):724–733, 2009 19414881
Bymaster FP, Dreshfield-Ahmad LJ, Threlkeld PG, et al: Comparative affinity of duloxetine and venlafaxine for serotonin and norepinephrine transporters in vitro and in vivo, human serotonin receptor subtypes, and other neuronal receptors. Neuropsychopharmacology 25(6):871–880, 2001 11750180
Centers for Disease Control and Prevention: Suicide and attempted suicide—China, 1990–2002. MMWR Morb Mortal Wkly Rep 53(22):481–484, 2004 15190245
Chalon SA, Granier LA, Vandenhende FR, et al: Duloxetine increases serotonin and norepinephrine availability in healthy subjects: a double-blind, controlled study. Neuropsychopharmacology 28(9):1685–1693, 2003 12784100
Chouinard G, Annable L, Bradwejn J: An early phase II clinical trial of tomoxetine (LY139603) in the treatment of newly admitted depressed patients. Psychopharmacology (Berl) 83(1):126–128, 1984 6429697
Cipriani A, Furukawa TA, Salanti G, et al: Comparative efficacy and acceptability of 12 new-generation antidepressants: a multiple-treatments meta-analysis. Lancet 373(9665):746–758, 2009 19185342
Cipriani A, Koesters M, Furukawa TA, et al: Duloxetine versus other anti-depressive agents for depression. Cochrane Database Syst Rev 10:CD006533, 2012 23076926
Cipriani A, Zhou X, Del Giovane C, et al: Comparative efficacy and tolerability of antidepressants for major depressive disorder in children and adolescents: a network meta-analysis. Lancet 388(10047):881–890, 2016 27289172
Citrome L, Weiss-Citrome A: A systematic review of duloxetine for osteoarthritic pain: what is the number needed to treat, number needed to harm, and likelihood to be helped or harmed? Postgrad Med 124(1):83–93, 2012 22314118
Clark DA, Steer RA, Beck AT: Common and specific dimensions of self-reported anxiety and depression: implications for the cognitive and tripartite models. J Abnorm Psychol 103(4):645–654, 1994 7822565
Clark LA, Watson D: Tripartite model of anxiety and depression: psychometric evidence and taxonomic implications. J Abnorm Psychol 100(3):316–336, 1991 1918611
Costei AM, Kozer E, Ho T, et al: Perinatal outcome following third trimester exposure to paroxetine. Arch Pediatr Adolesc Med 156(11):1129–1132, 2002 12413342
Curtin SC, Warner M, Hedegaard H: Increase in suicide in the United States, 1999–2014. NCHS Data Brief (241):1–8, 2016 27111185
Danish University Antidepressant Group: Citalopram: clinical effect profile in comparison with clomipramine. A controlled multicenter study. Psychopharmacology (Berl) 90(1):131–138, 1986 2876451
Danish University Antidepressant Group: Paroxetine: a selective serotonin reuptake inhibitor showing better tolerance, but weaker antidepressant effect than clomipramine in a controlled multicenter study. J Affect Disord 18(4):289–299, 1990 2140382
DeVane CL: Differential pharmacology of newer antidepressants. J Clin Psychiatry 59 (suppl 20):85–93, 1998 9881541
DeVane CL, Grothe DR, Smith SL: Pharmacology of antidepressants: focus on nefazodone. J Clin Psychiatry 63 (1 suppl 1):10–17, 2002 11890560
Donovan S, Clayton A, Beeharry M, et al: Deliberate self-harm and antidepressant drugs. Investigation of a possible link. Br J Psychiatry 177:551–556, 2000 11102331
Eli Lilly: Cymbalta prescribing information. Indianapolis, IN, Eli Lilly, May 2020. Available at: pi.lilly.com/us/cymbalta-pi.pdf. Accessed November 16, 2020.
Emslie G, Kratochvil C, Vitiello B, et al: Treatment for Adolescents with Depression Study (TADS): safety results. J Am Acad Child Adolesc Psychiatry 45(12):1440–1455, 2006 17135989
Ereshefsky L, Dugan D: Review of the pharmacokinetics, pharmacogenetics, and drug interaction potential of antidepressants: focus on venlafaxine. Depress Anxiety 12 (suppl 1):30–44, 2000 11098412

Feighner JP: Cardiovascular safety in depressed patients: focus on venlafaxine. J Clin Psychiatry 56(12):574–579, 1995 8530334

Ferguson JM: The effects of antidepressants on sexual functioning in depressed patients: a review. J Clin Psychiatry 62 (suppl 3):22–34, 2001 11229450

Fontanilla D, Johannessen M, Hajipour AR, et al: The hallucinogen N,N-dimethyltryptamine (DMT) is an endogenous sigma-1 receptor regulator. Science 323(5916):934–937, 2009 19213917

Fossom LH: Review and Evaluation of Pharmacology/Toxicology Data: Desvenlafaxine. Silver Spring, MD, U.S. Food and Drug Administration, Center for Drug Evaluation and Research, 2008

Fredricson Overø K: Kinetics of citalopram in man; plasma levels in patients. Prog Neuropsychopharmacol Biol Psychiatry 6(3):311–318, 1982 6959195

Fu J, Peng L, Li X: The efficacy and safety of multiple doses of vortioxetine for generalized anxiety disorder: a meta-analysis. Neuropsychiatr Dis Treat 12:951–959, 2016 27143896

Fuller RW, Wong DT, Robertson DW: Fluoxetine, a selective inhibitor of serotonin uptake. Med Res Rev 11(1):17–34, 1991 1994152

Furgała A, Sałat R, Sałat K: Acute cold allodynia induced by oxaliplatin is attenuated by amitriptyline. Acta Neurobiol Exp (Warsz) 78(4):315–321, 2018 30624430

Gibbons RD, Hur K, Bhaumik DK, et al: The relationship between antidepressant medication use and rate of suicide. Arch Gen Psychiatry 62(2):165–172, 2005 15699293

Gilmor ML, Owens MJ, Nemeroff CB: Inhibition of norepinephrine uptake in patients with major depression treated with paroxetine. Am J Psychiatry 159(10):1702–1710, 2002 12359676

Gommoll CP, Greenberg WM, Chen C: A randomized, double-blind, placebo-controlled study of flexible doses of levomilnacipran ER (40–120mg/day) in patients with major depressive disorder. J Drug Assess 3(1):10–19, 2014 27536449

Goodman WK, Ward H, Kablinger A, et al: Fluvoxamine in the treatment of obsessive-compulsive disorder and related conditions. J Clin Psychiatry 58 (suppl 5):32–49, 1997 9184625

Grados MA, Riddle MA: Pharmacological treatment of childhood obsessive-compulsive disorder: from theory to practice. J Clin Child Psychol 30(1):67–79, 2001 11294079

Greenblatt DJ, von Moltke LL, Harmatz JS, Shader RI: Drug interactions with newer antidepressants: role of human cytochromes P450. J Clin Psychiatry 59 (suppl 15):19–27, 1998 9786307

Grunebaum MF, Ellis SP, Li S, et al: Antidepressants and suicide risk in the United States, 1985–1999. J Clin Psychiatry 65(11):1456–1462, 2004 15554756

Gutierrez MA, Stimmel GL, Aiso JY: Venlafaxine: a 2003 update. Clin Ther 25(8):2138–2154, 2003 14512125

Haddad PM: Antidepressant discontinuation syndromes. Drug Saf 24(3):183–197, 2001 11347722

Hashimoto K: Sigma-1 receptors and selective serotonin reuptake inhibitors: clinical implications of their relationship. Cent Nerv Syst Agents Med Chem 9(3):197–204, 2009 20021354

Hassan SM, Wainscott G, Turner P: A comparison of the effect of paroxetine and amitriptyline on the tyramine pressor response test. Br J Clin Pharmacol 19(5):705–706, 1985 3159408

Häuser W, Wolfe F, Tölle T, et al: The role of antidepressants in the management of fibromyalgia syndrome: a systematic review and meta-analysis. CNS Drugs 26(4):297–307, 2012 22452526

Healy D: SSRIs and deliberate self-harm. Br J Psychiatry 180:547–548, author reply 547–548, 2002 12042235

Healy D: In the grip of the python: conflicts at the university-industry interface. Sci Eng Ethics 9(1):59–71, 2003 12645230

Hindmarch I, Hashimoto K: Cognition and depression: the effects of fluvoxamine, a sigma-1 receptor agonist, reconsidered. Hum Psychopharmacol 25(3):193–200, 2010 20373470

Horishita T, Yanagihara N, Ueno S, et al: Antidepressants inhibit Nav1.3, Nav1.7, and Nav1.8 neuronal voltage-gated sodium channels more potently than Nav1.2 and Nav1.6 channels expressed in Xenopus oocytes. Naunyn Schmiedebergs Arch Pharmacol 390(12):1255–1270, 2017 28905186

Huang M, Horiguchi M, Felix AR, et al: 5-HT1A and 5-HT7 receptors contribute to lurasidone-induced dopamine efflux. Neuroreport 23(7):436–440, 2012 22415605

Hughes ZA, Starr KR, Langmead CJ, et al: Neurochemical evaluation of the novel 5-HT1A receptor partial agonist/serotonin reuptake inhibitor, vilazodone. Eur J Pharmacol 510(1–2):49–57, 2005 15740724

Huitfeldt B, Montgomery SA: Comparison between zimelidine and amitriptyline of efficacy and adverse symptoms—a combined analysis of four British clinical trials in depression. Acta Psychiatr Scand Suppl 308:55–69, 1983 6230896

Hyman SE, Nestler EJ: Initiation and adaptation: a paradigm for understanding psychotropic drug action. Am J Psychiatry 153(2):151–162, 1996 8561194

Kane SP: The Top 300 Drugs of 2021. Updated July 3, 2021. ClinCalc DrugStats Database, Version 21.2. Available at: https://clincalc.com/DrugStats/Top300Drugs.aspx. Accessed August 30, 2021.

Kasper S, el Giamal N, Hilger E: Reboxetine: the first selective noradrenaline re-uptake inhibitor. Expert Opin Pharmacother 1(4):771–782, 2000 11249515

Khan A, Warner HA, Brown WA: Symptom reduction and suicide risk in patients treated with placebo in antidepressant clinical trials: an analysis of the Food and Drug Administration database. Arch Gen Psychiatry 57(4):311–317, 2000 10768687

Kratochvil CJ, Vaughan BS, Harrington MJ, et al: Atomoxetine: a selective noradrenaline reuptake inhibitor for the treatment of attention-deficit/hyperactivity disorder. Expert Opin Pharmacother 4(7):1165–1174, 2003 12831341

Kroenke K, West SL, Swindle R, et al: Similar effectiveness of paroxetine, fluoxetine, and sertraline in primary care: a randomized trial. JAMA 286(23):2947–2955, 2001 11743835

Lejoyeux M, Adès J: Antidepressant discontinuation: a review of the literature. J Clin Psychiatry 58 (suppl 7):11–15, discussion 16, 1997 9219488

Libby AM, Brent DA, Morrato EH, et al: Decline in treatment of pediatric depression after FDA advisory on risk of suicidality with SSRIs. Am J Psychiatry 164(6):884–891, 2007 17541047

Ludwig J, Marcotte DE: Anti-depressants, suicide, and drug regulation. J Policy Anal Manage 24(2):249–272, 2005 15776534

Mahableshwarkar AR, Zajecka J, Jacobson W, et al: A randomized, placebo-controlled, active-reference, double-blind, flexible-dose study of the efficacy of vortioxetine on cognitive function in major depressive disorder. Neuropsychopharmacology 40(8):2025–2037, 2015 25687662

Maurice T, Su TP: The pharmacology of sigma-1 receptors. Pharmacol Ther 124(2):195–206, 2009 19619582

McCain JA: Antidepressants and suicide in adolescents and adults: a public health experiment with unintended consequences? Pharmacy & Therapeutics 34(7):355–378, 2009 20140100

Michelson D, Fava M, Amsterdam J, et al: Interruption of selective serotonin reuptake inhibitor treatment. Double-blind, placebo-controlled trial. Br J Psychiatry 176:363–368, 2000 10827885

Michelson D, Adler LA, Amsterdam JD, et al: Addition of atomoxetine for depression incompletely responsive to sertraline: a randomized, double-blind, placebo-controlled study. J Clin Psychiatry 68(4):582–587, 2007 17474814

Micó JA, Ardid D, Berrocoso E, et al: Antidepressants and pain. Trends Pharmacol Sci 27(7):348–354, 2006 16762426

Montano CB: Recognition and treatment of depression in a primary care setting. J Clin Psychiatry 55 (suppl):18–34, discussion 35–37, 1994 7814355

Montgomery SA, McAuley R, Rani SJ, et al: A double blind comparison of zimelidine and amitriptyline in endogenous depression. Acta Psychiatr Scand Suppl 290:314–327, 1981a 6452798

Montgomery SA, Rani SJ, McAuley R, et al: The antidepressant efficacy of zimelidine and maprotiline. Acta Psychiatr Scand Suppl 290:219–224, 1981b 6452792

Montgomery SA, Loft H, Sánchez C, et al: Escitalopram (S-enantiomer of citalopram): clinical efficacy and onset of action predicted from a rat model. Pharmacol Toxicol 88(5):282–286, 2001 11393591

Montgomery SA, Mahé V, Haudiquet V, et al: Effectiveness of venlafaxine, extended release formulation, in the short-term and long-term treatment of generalized anxiety disorder: results of a survival analysis. J Clin Psychopharmacol 22(6):561–567, 2002 12454555

Montgomery SA, Huusom AK, Bothmer J: A randomised study comparing escitalopram with venlafaxine XR in primary care patients with major depressive disorder. Neuropsychobiology 50(1):57–64, 2004 15179022

Moore K: Duloxetine: a new approach for treating stress urinary incontinence. Int J Gynaecol Obstet 86 (suppl 1):S53–S62, 2004 15302567

Mørk A, Pehrson A, Brennum LT, et al: Pharmacological effects of Lu AA21004: a novel multimodal compound for the treatment of major depressive disorder. J Pharmacol Exp Ther 340(3):666–675, 2012 22171087

Morón JA, Brockington A, Wise RA, et al: Dopamine uptake through the norepinephrine transporter in brain regions with low levels of the dopamine transporter: evidence from knockout mouse lines. J Neurosci 22(2):389–395, 2002 11784783

Nemeroff CB, Owens MJ: Neuropharmacology of paroxetine. Psychopharmacol Bull 37 (suppl 1):8–18, 2003 14566196

Nemeroff CB, DeVane CL, Pollock BG: Newer antidepressants and the cytochrome P450 system. Am J Psychiatry 153(3):311–320, 1996 8610817

Nemeroff CB, Schatzberg AF, Goldstein DJ, et al: Duloxetine for the treatment of major depressive disorder. Psychopharmacol Bull 36(4):106–132, 2002 12858150

Nierenberg AA, Loft H, Olsen CK: Treatment effects on residual cognitive symptoms among partially or fully remitted patients with major depressive disorder: a randomized, double-blinded, exploratory study with vortioxetine. J Affect Disord 250:35–42, 2019 30826492

Olesen OV, Linnet K: Studies on the stereoselective metabolism of citalopram by human liver microsomes and cDNA-expressed cytochrome P450 enzymes. Pharmacology 59(6):298–309, 1999 10575324

Olfson M, Marcus SC, Druss B, et al: National trends in the outpatient treatment of depression. JAMA 287(2):203–209, 2002 11779262

Olfson M, Shaffer D, Marcus SC, et al: Relationship between antidepressant medication treatment and suicide in adolescents. Arch Gen Psychiatry 60(10):978–982, 2003 14557142

Olfson M, Marcus SC, Druss BG: Effects of Food and Drug Administration warnings on antidepressant use in a national sample. Arch Gen Psychiatry 65(1):94–101, 2008 18180433

Owens MJ, Morgan WN, Plott SJ, et al: Neurotransmitter receptor and transporter binding profile of antidepressants and their metabolites. J Pharmacol Exp Ther 283(3):1305–1322, 1997 9400006

Owens MJ, Knight DL, Nemeroff CB: Paroxetine binding to the rat norepinephrine transporter in vivo. Biol Psychiatry 47(9):842–845, 2000 10812044

Pacholczyk T, Blakely RD, Amara SG: Expression cloning of a cocaine- and antidepressant-sensitive human noradrenaline transporter. Nature 350(6316):350–354, 1991 2008212

Pae CU, Wang SM, Han C, et al: Vortioxetine: a meta-analysis of 12 short-term, randomized, placebo-controlled clinical trials for the treatment of major depressive disorder. J Psychiatry Neurosci 40(3):174–186, 2015a 25350320

Pae CU, Wang SM, Han C, et al: Vortioxetine, a multimodal antidepressant for generalized anxiety disorder: a systematic review and meta-analysis. J Psychiatr Res 64:88–98, 2015b 25851751

Page ME: The promises and pitfalls of reboxetine. CNS Drug Rev 9(4):327–342, 2003 14647527

Pergolizzi JV Jr, Raffa RB, Taylor R Jr, et al: A review of duloxetine 60 mg once-daily dosing for the management of diabetic peripheral neuropathic pain, fibromyalgia, and chronic musculoskeletal pain due to chronic osteoarthritis pain and low back pain. Pain Pract 13(3):239–252, 2013 22716295

Perry PJ: Pharmacotherapy for major depression with melancholic features: relative efficacy of tricyclic versus selective serotonin reuptake inhibitor antidepressants. J Affect Disord 39(1):1–6, 1996 8835647

Preskorn SHS, Stanga CY, Feighner JP, Ross R (eds): Antidepressants: Past, Present, and Future (Handbook of Experimental Pharmacology, Vol 157). New York, Springer, 2012

Qian Y, Melikian HE, Rye DB, et al: Identification and characterization of antidepressant-sensitive serotonin transporter proteins using site-specific antibodies. J Neurosci 15(2):1261–1274, 1995 7869097

Rapaport M, Coccaro E, Sheline Y, et al: A comparison of fluvoxamine and fluoxetine in the treatment of major depression. J Clin Psychopharmacol 16(5):373–378, 1996 8889909
Riddle MA, Reeve EA, Yaryura-Tobias JA, et al: Fluvoxamine for children and adolescents with obsessive-compulsive disorder: a randomized, controlled, multicenter trial. J Am Acad Child Adolesc Psychiatry 40(2):222–229, 2001 11211371
Rochat B, Amey M, Baumann P: Analysis of enantiomers of citalopram and its demethylated metabolites in plasma of depressive patients using chiral reverse-phase liquid chromatography. Ther Drug Monit 17(3):273–279, 1995 7624924
Rosenbaum JF, Fava M, Hoog SL, et al: Selective serotonin reuptake inhibitor discontinuation syndrome: a randomized clinical trial. Biol Psychiatry 44(2):77–87, 1998 9646889
Safarinejad MR: Reversal of SSRI-induced female sexual dysfunction by adjunctive bupropion in menstruating women: a double-blind, placebo-controlled and randomized study. J Psychopharmacol 25(3):370–378, 2011 20080928
Sahli ZT, Banerjee P, Tarazi FI: The preclinical and clinical effects of vilazodone for the treatment of major depressive disorder. Expert Opin Drug Discov 11(5):515–523, 2016 26971593
Sanchez C, Asin KE, Artigas F: Vortioxetine, a novel antidepressant with multimodal activity: review of preclinical and clinical data. Pharmacol Ther 145:43–57, 2015 25016186
Sansone RA, Sansone LA: Serotonin norepinephrine reuptake inhibitors: a pharmacological comparison. Innov Clin Neurosci 11(3–4):37–42, 2014 24800132
Schatzberg AF: Efficacy and tolerability of duloxetine, a novel dual reuptake inhibitor, in the treatment of major depressive disorder. J Clin Psychiatry 64 (suppl 13):30–37, 2003 14552654
Schildkraut JJ: The catecholamine hypothesis of affective disorders: a review of supporting evidence. Am J Psychiatry 122(5):509–522, 1965 5319766
Sedky K, Nazir R, Joshi A, et al: Which psychotropic medications induce hepatotoxicity? Gen Hosp Psychiatry 34(1):53–61, 2012 22133982
Sharma A, Goldberg MJ, Cerimele BJ: Pharmacokinetics and safety of duloxetine, a dual-serotonin and norepinephrine reuptake inhibitor. J Clin Pharmacol 40(2):161–167, 2000 10664922
Shelton RC, Tomarken AJ: Can recovery from depression be achieved? Psychiatr Serv 52(11):1469–1478, 2001 11684742
Skinner MH, Kuan HY, Pan A, et al: Duloxetine is both an inhibitor and a substrate of cytochrome P4502D6 in healthy volunteers. Clin Pharmacol Ther 73(3):170–177, 2003 12621382
Sulser F, Vetulani J, Mobley PL: Mode of action of antidepressant drugs. Biochem Pharmacol 27(3):257–261, 1978 202286
Tatsumi M, Groshan K, Blakely RD, et al: Pharmacological profile of antidepressants and related compounds at human monoamine transporters. Eur J Pharmacol 340(2–3):249–258, 1997 9537821
Teicher MH, Glod C, Cole JO: Emergence of intense suicidal preoccupation during fluoxetine treatment. Am J Psychiatry 147(2):207–210, 1990 2301661
Thase ME: Effectiveness of antidepressants: comparative remission rates. J Clin Psychiatry 64 (suppl 2):3–7, 2003 12625792
Thase ME, Entsuah AR, Rudolph RL: Remission rates during treatment with venlafaxine or selective serotonin reuptake inhibitors. Br J Psychiatry 178:234–241, 2001 11230034
Thase ME, Chen D, Edwards J, et al: Efficacy of vilazodone on anxiety symptoms in patients with major depressive disorder. Int Clin Psychopharmacol 29(6):351–356, 2014 24978955
Tomarken AJ, Dichter GS, Freid C, et al: Assessing the effects of bupropion SR on mood dimensions of depression. J Affect Disord 78(3):235–241, 2004 15013248
Treit D, Degroot A, Kashluba S, et al: Systemic EMD 68843 injections reduce anxiety in the shock-probe, but not the plus-maze test. Eur J Pharmacol 414(2–3):245–248, 2001 11239925
Turcotte JE, Debonnel G, de Montigny C, et al: Assessment of the serotonin and norepinephrine reuptake blocking properties of duloxetine in healthy subjects. Neuropsychopharmacology 24(5):511–521, 2001 11282251
van Harten J: Overview of the pharmacokinetics of fluvoxamine. Clin Pharmacokinet 29 (suppl 1):1–9, 1995 8846617

Vieta E, Sluth LB, Olsen CK: The effects of vortioxetine on cognitive dysfunction in patients with inadequate response to current antidepressants in major depressive disorder: a short-term, randomized, double-blind, exploratory study versus escitalopram. J Affect Disord 227:803–809, 2018 29673132

von Moltke LL, Greenblatt DJ, Grassi JM, et al: Citalopram and desmethylcitalopram in vitro: human cytochromes mediating transformation, and cytochrome inhibitory effects. Biol Psychiatry 46(6):839–849, 1999 10494454

Wang CF, Russell G, Strichartz GR, et al: The local and systemic actions of duloxetine in allodynia and hyperalgesia using a rat skin incision pain model. Anesth Analg 121(2):532–544, 2015 26049779

Wang CF, Russell G, Wang SY, et al: R-duloxetine and N-methyl duloxetine as novel analgesics against experimental postincisional pain. Anesth Analg 122(3):719–729, 2016 26646348

Wang SY, Calderon J, Kuo Wang G: Block of neuronal Na+ channels by antidepressant duloxetine in a state-dependent manner. Anesthesiology 113(3):655–665, 2010 20693878

Ware MR: Fluvoxamine: a review of the controlled trials in depression. J Clin Psychiatry 58 (suppl 5):15–23, 1997 9184623

Watson D, Clark LA, Weber K, et al: Testing a tripartite model, II: exploring the symptom structure of anxiety and depression in student, adult, and patient samples. J Abnorm Psychol 104(1):15–25, 1995a 7897037

Watson D, Weber K, Assenheimer JS, et al: Testing a tripartite model, I: evaluating the convergent and discriminant validity of anxiety and depression symptom scales. J Abnorm Psychol 104(1):3–14, 1995b 7897050

Wooltorton E: Paroxetine (Paxil, Seroxat): increased risk of suicide in pediatric patients. CMAJ 169(5):446, 2003 12952810

Wyeth Pharmaceuticals: Dear Healthcare Professional Letter (Important Safety Information Regarding the Use of Effexor® (venlafaxine HCI) Tablets and Effexor® XR (venlafaxine HCI) Capsules in Children and Adolescents). August 22, 2003. Archived safety alert available at: https://www.healthycanadians.gc.ca/recall-alert-rappel-avis/hc-sc/2003/14212a-eng.php. Accessed August 3, 2021.

Zadka Ł, Dziwota E, Olajossy M: Levomilnacipran: a successor of milnacipran with a higher noradrenergic selectivity. Acta Pol Pharm 73(2):285–289, 2016 27180420

Zareifopoulos N, Dylja I: Efficacy and tolerability of vilazodone for the acute treatment of generalized anxiety disorder: a meta-analysis. Asian J Psychiatr 26:115–122, 2017 28483071

Zito JM: Five burning questions. J Dev Behav Pediatr 23 (1 suppl):S23–S30, 2002 11875287

CHAPTER 16

Lithium and Mood Stabilizers

Keming Gao, M.D., Ph.D.
Yuanhan Bai, M.D., M.S.
Joseph R. Calabrese, M.D.

Mood stabilizers are not only the cornerstone for the clinical management of bipolar disorder (Gao et al. 2015a) but also commonly recognized as possessing efficacy in the treatment of major depressive disorder (MDD) (Zhou et al. 2015). An ideal mood stabilizer would exhibit a broad spectrum of efficacy that covers all acute phases (depression, mania, and hypomania) and psychosis, prevents all abnormal mood variations of bipolar disorder, and does not aggravate or worsen any feature of the illness. However, all medications approved for bipolar disorder by the FDA have been based on the efficacy of a medication in the acute treatment of mania or bipolar depression or of a medication that prevents the relapse of any mood episodes (Gao et al. 2015a). Therefore, any medication approved for any phase of bipolar treatment can be considered a mood stabilizer. Accordingly, lithium, valproic acid/divalproex, lamotrigine, carbamazepine, and almost all atypical antipsychotics are mood stabilizers (Gao et al. 2015a).

While the evidence of efficacy of these drugs in bipolar disorder is strongly supported by large randomized, double-blind, placebo-controlled trials (DBPCTs), the evidence of efficacy in MDD is less convincing, although some atypical antipsychotics have been approved as adjunctive therapy to traditional antidepressants for treatment-resistant MDD (Aftab and Gao 2017). This chapter discusses use of lithium and anticonvulsant mood stabilizers, including valproic acid/divalproex, lamotrigine, and carbamazepine, in the treatment of mood disorders.

Lithium

Pharmacokinetics

Lithium negligibly binds to plasma protein and is eliminated almost exclusively via kidney. Of importance, age-related changes require careful consideration in the elderly. Elimination may be substantially increased or decreased by certain medications, such as certain diuretics and nonsteroidal anti-inflammatory drugs. Oral lithium is absorbed completely within 8 hours, and peak plasma levels are reached between 1 and 3 hours after ingestion. Absorption is not affected by the presence of food. Limited data suggest that brain/serum lithium concentration ratios vary widely and may positively correlate with age, weakly to moderately correlate with serum levels in the therapeutic range, and only significantly correlate with daily dosing for longer than 6 months. Higher brain/serum ratios were reported with single daily doses of lithium at bedtime than with twice-daily dosing.

Lithium in Acute Mania

The efficacy of lithium in the treatment of acute mania is supported by numerous DBPCTs. Lithium and valproic acid/divalproex are also commonly used for combination or adjunctive therapy with other medications for acute mania or bipolar depression. With a few exceptions, overall evidence supports that lithium monotherapy is as effective as other antimanic agents (Gao et al. 2015a), and combining lithium with an anticonvulsant mood stabilizer or an atypical antipsychotic is more effective than lithium alone. However, it has not been shown to be superior to placebo or divalproex in reducing manic symptoms in children and adolescents. In contrast, lithium appeared to be significantly less effective in reducing manic symptoms compared with risperidone (Duffy et al. 2018). A recent randomized, double-blind study of lithium versus divalproex in elderly patients with manic symptoms supported its use in the elderly with bipolar disorder. Both lithium and divalproex reduced manic symptoms significantly, but lithium was more effective than divalproex in patients with a Young Mania Rating Scale score greater than 30 points (Young et al. 2017).

Lithium in Acute Bipolar Depression

Early studies of lithium in bipolar depression were confounded by study designs and small sample sizes. In a bipolar depression study with quetiapine, lithium monotherapy was not significantly superior to placebo in reducing depressive symptoms regardless of lithium levels, but quetiapine monotherapy was (Gao et al. 2015a); however, lithium plus adjunctive personalized treatment was as effective as quetiapine plus adjunctive personalized treatment for bipolar depression (Nierenberg et al. 2016). Lithium reduced depression and anxiety symptoms as well as quetiapine did in patients with bipolar depression and different comorbidities (Gao et al. 2018). Lithium or divalproex plus lurasidone was indicated for bipolar depression. Although lithium and lamotrigine alone were not effective in reducing depressive symptoms, the two used in combination were significantly superior to lithium monotherapy. Lithium plus modafinil was also more efficacious in patients who had not responded to lithium monotherapy, but the results of adding armodafinil or antidepressant(s) to lithium or other mood stabilizers were inconsistent (Gao et al. 2015b). In some studies of bipolar II depression, lithium appeared significantly less effective than antidepressants for acute and long-term treatments (McElroy and Israel 2019).

Lithium in Maintenance Treatment of Bipolar Disorder

The efficacy of lithium monotherapy or adjunctive therapy was evaluated with modern study designs and DSM nomenclature during the development of divalproex, lamotrigine, olanzapine, and quetiapine for maintenance treatment of bipolar disorder (Gao et al. 2016). The overall impression was that lithium was as effective as other FDA-approved agents in preventing any mood relapse and more effective in preventing manic than depressive relapse. Lithium, along with quetiapine and lamotrigine, was the only medication superior to placebo in preventing depressive relapse, although lithium's magnitude was less than that of the other two medications (Gao et al. 2016). However, in a population-based study, lithium was more effective than valproic acid, olanzapine, and quetiapine (Hayes et al. 2016a), and in another study, lithium appeared to be superior to carbamazepine in preventing mood relapses (Peselow et al. 2016). Lithium and divalproex were similar in preventing mood relapses in patients with rapid-cycling bipolar disorder, but lithium plus divalproex was not significantly different from lithium alone in patients with comorbid substance use disorder (Gao et al. 2015a). In children and adolescents, data on lithium's long-term use were limited (Hafeman et al. 2020).

Lithium in Pregnancy and the Peripartum

Overall, there is a moderate level of agreement among international practice guidelines on the potential teratogenic effects of lithium, valproic acid, and carbamazepine (Graham et al. 2018). Valproic acid is not recommended during pregnancy, but no authoritative data support the discontinuation of lithium, lamotrigine, or carbamazepine during pregnancy (Scrandis 2017). Exposure to lithium or anticonvulsants, including valproic acid, lamotrigine, topiramate, and carbamazepine, in the first 20 weeks of pregnancy was not associated with an increased risk for ischemic placenta disease (Cohen et al. 2019). However, an increased risk for cardiac or major congenital malformations from uterine exposure to lithium was confirmed (Munk-Olsen et al. 2018; Patorno et al. 2017). Although children from ages 1 to 15 years who had lithium exposure *in utero* had normal development (Poels et al. 2018b), current data on the long-term effects of prenatal psychotropic exposure on child development are both limited and of poor quality (Haskey and Galbally 2017).

Lithium use during pregnancy may have some benefits for mothers, including mood stabilization and relapse prevention (Poels et al. 2018a), but it increases the risk for major congenital malformations in their children. If a patient has to take lithium during pregnancy, a minimal effective dosage should be attempted. Levels should be monitored closely, and high-resolution ultrasound should be performed at week 20 (Poels et al. 2018a; Wesseloo et al. 2017b). Immediately restarting lithium after delivery is recommended for women who discontinue it during pregnancy. Because newborns with lithium exposure are likely to have complications, specialized hospitals with comprehensive care for mothers and newborns should be considered for delivery whenever possible.

Lithium in Major Depressive Disorder

DBPCTs of lithium as an adjunctive therapy to antidepressants have been small, of short duration, and mainly focused on tricyclic antidepressants. A network meta-analysis of 48 trials at different stages of treatment-resistant depression found that lithium, quetiapine, aripiprazole, and thyroid hormone adjunctive therapy to antidepressant(s) were significantly more effective than placebo (Zhou et al. 2015), but a remission rate of 15.9% with lithium augmentation in patients with stage 2 treatment-resistant depression in a Sequenced Treatment Alternatives to Relieve Depression (STAR*D) study (Nierenberg et al. 2006) suggests that the benefit with lithium augmentation is relatively small.

Lithium in Suicide Prevention

It has been reported that lithium possesses some degree of antisuicidal efficacy in adults and in children and adolescents, based on observational studies and randomized trials (Hafeman et al. 2020; Tondo and Baldessarini 2018). This antisuicidal effect appeared not to be solely related to lithium's mood-stabilizing properties, because nonresponders also had fewer suicide attempts while taking lithium (Sarai et al. 2018). A prospective 8-year study found that rates of suicidal behavior were significantly reduced during treatment with lithium but not with valproic acid (Song et al. 2017). Overall evidence suggests that the antisuicidal effects of lithium are long term.

Safety and Tolerability

In efficacy and effectiveness DBPCTs, lithium was relatively well tolerated, comparable with placebo or active comparators (Bai et al. 2019). Irreversible chronic kidney disease, nephrogenic diabetes insipidus, and hyperparathyroidism may be avoided if detected earlier. Patients taking atypical antipsychotics and lithium had significantly higher rates of urinary concentrating deficiency than those taking lithium alone. Both lithium and anticonvulsant mood stabilizers were associated with an increased risk of chronic kidney disease, but the use of lithium was not associated with an increased risk for end-stage renal disease (Kessing et al. 2015). No benefit was found for discontinuing lithium in patients with chronic kidney disease (Kessing et al. 2017).

The magnitude of risk from lithium-related reduction in glomerular filtration rate (GFR), chronic kidney disease, or end-stage renal disease has yet to be determined, although overall evidence suggests that the risk is small (Azab et al. 2015). Factors associated with a decline in GFR, in order of decreasing importance, were longer lithium treatment, lower lithium dosages, higher serum lithium levels, older age, and medical comorbidity, especially cardiovascular comorbidity (Aiff et al. 2019; Tondo et al. 2017). Lithium dosing more than once a day, lithium levels greater than or equal to 0.6 mEq/L, and use of first-generation antipsychotics were independently associated with an increased risk of renal dysfunction.

Clinical Applications

Lithium is recommended as a first-line medication for mania, bipolar depression, and maintenance treatment of bipolar disorder (Yatham et al. 2018). Patients with a mania-depression interval sequence, family history of bipolar disorder, shorter prelithium illness duration, later age at onset, and absence of rapid cycling or psychosis may respond better to lithium (Hui et al. 2019). For mania, lithium carbonate 300 mg three or four times daily, with a target blood level of 0.8–1.2 mEq/L, is reasonable; clinicians should obtain a trough plasma level on days 4 or 5 in healthy adults and watch for any signs of toxicity. For milder mania or hypomania, 300 mg twice a day and a lower target blood level (0.6–0.8 mEq/L) may sufficiently stabilize mood. For bipolar depression, lithium can be started at 300 mg/day for 3 days, and then raised to a dosage of 600 mg/day, with target lithium levels ranging from 0.6 mEq/L to 1.2 mEq/L, depending on the maintenance goal. For maintenance, a higher therapeutic level is more effective in preventing manic relapse, although lower levels of 0.6–0.8 mEq/L may be adequate for preventing depressive relapses. For the elderly, serum levels of 0.4–0.8 mEq/L for patients ages 60–79 years and 0.4–0.7 mmol/L for patients ages 80 years and older were recommended (Shulman et al. 2019). Therapeutic levels at 0.4–0.6 mEq/L may be acceptable for good responders with poor lithium tolerance (Nolen et al. 2019). However, subtherapeutic dosages of lithium (300–600 mg/day) had minimal benefits for improving acute depressive or manic symptoms (Nierenberg et al. 2013). No therapeutic levels have been established for MDD, although therapeutic levels for bipolar disorder were often used in previous studies. Because lithium appeared to have better tolerability in manic patients than in depressed patients (Gao et al. 2008), adjustment of the lithium dosage and titration speed may be necessary based on the phase of illness.

Tremor, headache, constipation, nausea, vomiting, upset stomach, sedation, fatigue, and dizziness are common acute side effects of lithium. Weight gain, thirst, and polyuria are also observed with long-term use. Gastrointestinal disturbances and tremor can be mitigated by slower dosing strategies. These adverse effects typically subside within 1–2 weeks. Worsening of any of these adverse effects or the emergence of bradycardia, syncope, confusion, or ataxic gait should prompt a check of the patient's lithium level to rule out lithium toxicity. The possibility of drug interactions must always be considered, particularly with thiazide diuretics, angiotensin converting enzyme inhibitors, nonsteroidal anti-inflammatory drugs, and other psychotropics. In addition, lithium caused small but significant impairment in immediate verbal learning and memory and creativity, as well as psychomotor performance, in patients receiving long-term treatment (Wingo et al. 2009). An increased risk for cataract with long-term lithium use was reported in a population-based study from Taiwan (Chu et al. 2018). Lithium does not appear to affect bone density.

General medical history, physical examination, complete blood count, comprehensive metabolic panel, thyroid function tests, and pregnancy tests for women of childbearing age are recommended before starting lithium. Routine electrocardiographic monitoring is not necessary, but for high-risk patients older than 60 years or patients with ischemic heart disease, hypertension, hyperlipidemia, diabetes, cigarette smoking, or a family history of cardiovascular disease, a baseline electrocardiogram and subsequent testing every 6–12 months may be necessary (Mehta and Vannozzi 2017). Creatinine, calcium, and thyroid-stimulating hormone (TSH) should be measured every 2–3 months for the first 6 months and then every 6–12 months thereafter (Gao et al. 2015a; Shine et al. 2015). For patients with an emerging lack of energy or worsening depression, TSH levels should be checked. For patients with GFR levels lower than 60, creatinine levels should be checked more frequently. Excessive fluid intake and frequent urination need 24-hour urine volume and osmolality testing and urinalysis.

Anticonvulsant Mood Stabilizers

Pharmacokinetics

Bioavailability of divalproex is close to 100%, and that of the extended-release form is close to 90%. Peak plasma concentrations are achieved within 3–5 hours, although the extended-release form may take up to 17 hours. Half-life is about 12–16 hours, and steady states are usually achieved within 3–4 days. Valproic acid/divalproex is metabolized almost entirely by the liver cytochrome P450 (CYP) 2D6 system. Coadministration with microsomal enzyme–inducing drugs, such as carbamazepine, will decrease plasma levels of valproic acid. Toxicity can occur when divalproex is given along with other highly protein-bound drugs. Valproic acid/divalproex inhibits lamotrigine metabolism by 50% when it is coadministered.

Oral lamotrigine is rapidly absorbed, with negligible first-pass metabolism. Peak concentrations are reached in approximately 2–4 hours, and its half-life is approximately 25 hours. Lamotrigine is approximately 55% protein bound. At steady-state concentrations, lamotrigine levels are linear within a dosage range of 100–700 mg/day; renal insufficiency and hepatic disease reduce its clearance. The rate of clearance increases during each trimester of pregnancy, reaching a peak of baseline clearance by gestational week 32. The dosage of lamotrigine should immediately be decreased by 20%–25% after delivery for women whose dosage was increased during pregnancy (Kemp et al. 2017).

Carbamazepine is 80% bioavailable, nearly 80% protein bound, and primarily metabolized via the CYP3A4 system. Half-life is between 35 and 40 hours, but this falls to 12–17 hours with repeated dosing. Oxcarbazepine is a keto analogue of carbamazepine and is 67% protein bound. Oxcarbazepine is a pro-drug for 10-monohydroxy derivative (MHD), which is 38% protein bound and has less hepatic microsomal enzyme induction and autoinduction. Overall, more than 96% of oxcarbazepine is excreted by the kidneys. The half-life of MHD is 8–10 hours, and peak serum concentrations are reached in 4–6 hours; half-life does not change appreciably with repeated dosing. The relationship between oxcarbazepine dosage and plasma concentration appears linear within 300–2,700 mg/day.

Anticonvulsant Mood Stabilizers in Acute Mania

Divalproex sodium was the first anticonvulsant approved for treatment of bipolar mania by the FDA (Gao et al. 2015a). Its antimanic effect was further verified during the development of olanzapine. Like lithium, valproic acid/divalproex was commonly used as an adjunctive therapy with atypical antipsychotics or other medications for mania. Valproic acid monotherapy was not found to be significantly superior to placebo in children ages 10–17 years or in adolescents with manic or mixed symptoms, but it was superior to placebo in children ages 3–7 years (Kowatch et al. 2015). Valproic acid appeared to be less effective than antipsychotics in children and adolescents with mania.

Two large well-designed DBPCTs of carbamazepine monotherapy in acute mania confirmed its efficacy in reducing manic symptoms from early small sample studies (Gao et al. 2015a). A Cochrane review found the quality of studies of oxcarbazepine in bipolar disorder to be poor. Oxcarbazepine was not significantly superior to placebo in reducing manic symptoms in children and adolescents with bipolar disorder.

Anticonvulsant Mood Stabilizers in Acute Bipolar Depression

A meta-analysis of divalproex in bipolar depression found that the efficacy for response was comparable with FDA-approved medications for bipolar depression (Gao et al. 2015a). Lamotrigine monotherapy was not superior to placebo in acute bipolar depression in most studies, but a meta-analysis of all DBPCTs found it to be superior to placebo for treatment response, and patients with higher baseline depression severity had more benefits (Gao et al. 2015a). Lamotrigine was similar in response and remission rates to olanzapine-fluoxetine combination, the first approved medication for bipolar depression, in bipolar I patients with an index episode of depression (Gao et al. 2015b). Lamotrigine adjunctive therapy with lithium and valproic acid in rapid-cycling bipolar disorder, with or without a current substance use disorder, was not significantly superior to placebo. There is limited evidence of lamotrigine use in pediatric and geriatric patients with bipolar disorder. Valproic acid and lamotrigine may have potential benefit for comorbid substance use disorder in patients with bipolar disorder (Coles et al. 2019).

Anticonvulsant Mood Stabilizers in Maintenance Treatment of Bipolar Disorder

Valproic acid/divalproex is commonly used as a maintenance therapy for bipolar disorder, although it was not approved by the FDA for this indication (Gao et al. 2015a, 2016). In contrast, lamotrigine was the second medication approved by the FDA for maintenance treatment of bipolar disorder. Both lamotrigine and lithium were shown to exhibit efficacy in protecting against an emerging mood episode compared with placebo in two 18-month DBPCTs (Gao et al. 2016). However, lamotrigine plus divalproex did not have significant advantage over lamotrigine alone in the maintenance treatment of patients with an index episode of bipolar depression (Bowden et al. 2012).

Similarly, lamotrigine or divalproex adjunctive to aripiprazole in patients with an index manic or mixed episode was not significantly different from lamotrigine or divalproex alone (Gao et al. 2016). In contrast, quetiapine plus lamotrigine was more effective than quetiapine alone in reducing depressive symptoms in bipolar patients with an index episode of depression (Geddes et al. 2016). For carbamazepine, monotherapy produced variable results (Gao et al. 2015a), but there was stronger evidence supporting its use in combination with other mood stabilizers for maintenance, particularly with lithium.

Anticonvulsant Mood Stabilizers in Pregnancy and Peripartum

Data from epilepsy studies have determined that early gestational exposure to valproic acid is associated with the highest risk (≈10%) of major congenital malformations among anticonvulsants, in a dose-dependent fashion (Andrade 2018). Valproic acid exposure is also significantly associated with cognitive developmental delay, autism, and psychomotor delay (Veroniki et al. 2017b), as well as low IQ (Bromley et al. 2014). Carbamazepine is consistently associated with a higher risk of major congenital malformations relative to unexposed control groups and certain other anticonvulsants. Oxcarbazepine monotherapy is associated with an increased risk for autism, and carbamazepine polytherapy is associated with psychomotor delay (Bromley et al. 2014). However, at conventional dosages, lamotrigine, levetiracetam, and oxcarbazepine, and possibly zonisamide and gabapentin, are associated with absolute major congenital malformation risks similar to those in the general population (Andrade 2018; Veroniki et al. 2017a). Nevertheless, a significantly increased risk for autism associated with exposure to lamotrigine monotherapy or lamotrigine plus valproic acid has been reported (Veroniki et al. 2017b).

Although lamotrigine and lithium did not exhibit significant differences in mood relapses or in the prevention of severe postpartum episodes (Wesseloo et al. 2017a), the choice of a drug during pregnancy is complicated and should depend on safety and efficacy. Data for lamotrigine appear to be more favorable than for other anticonvulsant mood stabilizers and lithium, but its long-term effect on development remains uncertain. Even if lamotrigine is indicated during pregnancy, a minimal effective dosage should be maintained, although no dose-dependent effect was observed with lamotrigine for major congenital malformations and IQ (Andrade 2018).

Anticonvulsant Mood Stabilizers in Major Depressive Disorder

Some evidence suggests that adjunctive valproic acid, as well as carbamazepine and lamotrigine, had beneficial effects for MDD. An RCT in treatment-resistant depression found that valproic acid augmentation to paroxetine was as effective as risperidone, buspirone, trazodone, or thyroid hormone augmentation, with the highest remission rate of 48.7% (Fang et al. 2011). For lamotrigine, three large DBPCTs in non-treatment-resistant depression did not find a significant difference from placebo. Similarly, lamotrigine adjunctive therapy to antidepressants in MDD also did not significantly differ from placebo (Solmi et al. 2016). A network meta-analysis did not find a significant difference between lamotrigine and placebo adjunctive therapy to antidepressants in MDD (Zhou et al. 2015). However, a more recent meta-analysis including all studies of lamotrigine in mood disorders found that, as a whole, lamotrigine was significantly superior to placebo in reducing depressive symptoms, but the results in subgroups were less robust (Solmi et al. 2016).

Anticonvulsant Mood Stabilizers in Suicide Prevention

Although the warning for suicidality from anticonvulsants was issued by the FDA in 2008 after the agency conducted a meta-analysis of 199 RCTs involving 11 anticonvulsants, a number of studies and reviews in patients with bipolar disorder found that anticonvulsants did not have an increased risk for self-harm, suicide attempt, or completed suicide compared with placebo or lithium (Chen et al. 2019; Hayes et al. 2016b; Song et al. 2017). Anticonvulsant mood stabilizers can even reduce patients' risk for suicide attempt compared with that for patients who did not receive any psychotropic medication, although the antisuicidal effect from anticonvulsant mood stabilizers might be weaker than that from lithium (Hafeman et al. 2020; Tondo and Baldessarini 2018).

Safety and Tolerability

Overall, valproic acid/divalproex, lamotrigine, carbamazepine, and oxcarbazepine were well tolerated in acute and maintenance treatment of bipolar disorder (Bai et al. 2019). Diarrhea, somnolence, nausea, vomiting, dizziness, dyspepsia, abdominal pain, headache, and increased appetite are common side effects of divalproex. Ataxia, vomiting, dry mouth, dyspepsia, constipation, dizziness, and somnolence are common side effects of carbamazepine. Dizziness, dry mouth, headache, and somnolence are reported with lamotrigine use. Adverse effects during initial therapy with divalproex, lamotrigine, or carbamazepine are usually mild, transient, and easily managed, but rare, serious, and life-threatening adverse effects can potentially occur, including agranulocytosis, aplastic anemia, and hyponatremia with carbamazepine; pancreatitis and hyperammonemia with valproic acid/divalproex; and hepatic failure with valproic acid/divalproex and carbamazepine.

Rashes with carbamazepine and lamotrigine are a major concern that can affect their use. In a recent systematic review of lamotrigine in 122 RCTs, 8.6% of patients with bipolar disorder developed skin reactions, and only 0.02% developed Stevens-Johnson syndrome or toxic epidermal necrolysis (Bloom and Amber 2017). However, risk of rash with lamotrigine was increased in children younger than 12 years with coadministration of valproic acid, or by exceeding the recommended initial dosage or rate of dosage escalation. Therefore, to minimize the risk of life-threatening rash, careful attention should be given to the starting dosage, the rate of titration, and the coadministration of other drugs, such as valproic acid, that can prolong the elimination of lamotrigine. Hepatic failure from valproic acid in children younger than 12 years was also reported.

Clinical Applications

Divalproex and lamotrigine were recommended as a first-line medication for acute mania and bipolar I depression, respectively. Both medications were also recommended as first-line medications for the maintenance treatment of bipolar disorder (Yatham et al. 2018). Before initiating valproic acid/divalproex, a general medical history with special attention to the hepatic or hematological system, a comprehensive metabolic panel, a complete blood count, and a pregnancy test in women of childbearing age should be obtained. For acute mania, divalproex oral loading with a dosage of 20–30 mg/kg/day is suggested over standard gradual titration schedules because of its faster antimanic effect. Divalproex 250 mg three times a day or 500 mg twice a day is recommended for patients with less severe mania or for elderly patients. Reduced dosage, slower titration, and use of a slow-release divalproex formulation may lessen some acute side effects.

No pretreatment laboratory monitoring is required before initiating lamotrigine, although a routine physical examination, basic baseline chemistries, and pregnancy tests are advisable. Any rash that cannot readily be explained by a known cause (e.g., contact dermatitis) should lead to immediate discontinuation of lamotrigine, and patients should notify their treating physician(s) prior to resuming therapy. In unclear or difficult cases, dermatological consultation should be obtained before restarting or rechallenging with lamotrigine. Rechallenging can be initiated in those who have non-life-threatening rashes after a careful risk and benefit assessment with a slower titration schedule. Flu-like symptoms, unexplained widespread skin pain, red or purple skin rashes, or blisters or mucous on the skin need emergency attention. To reduce the risk for severe rashes, standard titration schedules showed be followed. The presence of an enzyme-inducing drug, such as carbamazepine, requires doubling of the lamotrigine dosage, whereas coadministration of lamotrigine with valproic acid/divalproex requires a 50% reduction in the lamotrigine dosage. Coadministration of lamotrigine with estrogen-containing oral contraceptives may require an increase in the lamotrigine dose.

As with valproic acid/divalproex, a general medical history and physical examination, comprehensive metabolic panel, complete blood count, and pregnancy test in women of childbearing age should be performed before starting carbamazepine/oxcarbazepine. More frequent monitoring is indicated in elderly patients or any patient taking carbamazepine/oxcarbazepine who develops fever, easy bruising or bleeding, weakness, or infection. No clear target serum levels of carbamazepine for acute mania have been established, although a range of 6–12 μg/mL is recommended. Immediate-release carbamazepine therapy may be started at dosages of 200–600 mg/day, with incremental increases of 200 mg/day every 2–5 days up to 1,000 mg/day, followed by careful monitoring of blood levels, side effects, and clinical efficacy. The beaded extended-release form may be started at 400 mg/day and increased as tolerated up to 1,600 mg/day. Many factors can affect carbamazepine blood levels, including auto-induction metabolism and significant drug-to-drug interactions.

Conclusion

Lithium has a spectrum of efficacy and effectiveness in the acute and maintenance treatment of bipolar disorder. Valproic acid/divalproex and carbamazepine have also been shown to exhibit efficacy in acute mania, and lamotrigine in maintenance treatment of bipolar disorder. Overall, combinations of lithium with valproic acid/divalproex, carbamazepine, or atypical antipsychotics for mania and combinations of lithium and lamotrigine for bipolar depression are more effective than monotherapies. It is reasonable to use lithium or an anticonvulsant mood stabilizer(s) as adjunctive or combination therapy with other medications in patients with bipolar disorder or MDD who fail to respond to standard monotherapy treatments. Lithium and anticonvulsant mood stabilizers have different short- and long-term side effects. Regular monitoring may reduce the risk for lithium-related end-stage renal disease, valproic acid–related hepatitis, and other potential life-threatening side effects. To minimize the risk of serious life-threatening rash with lamotrigine, the recommended titration schedule should strictly be adhered to. Because most patients with a mood disorder, especially bipolar disorder, need long-term if not lifelong medication treatment, the long-term safety and side-effect burden should be seriously considered from the beginning.

References

Aftab A, Gao K: The preclinical discovery and development of brexpiprazole for the treatment of major depressive disorder. Expert Opin Drug Discov 12(10):1067–1081, 2017 28718334

Aiff H, Attman PO, Ramsauer B, et al: Cardiovascular comorbidity increases the risk for renal failure during prophylactic lithium treatment. J Affect Disord 243:416–420, 2019 30268957

Andrade C: Major congenital malformations associated with exposure to antiepileptic drugs during pregnancy. J Clin Psychiatry 79(4):18f12449, 2018 30153402

Azab AN, Shnaider A, Osher Y, et al: Lithium nephrotoxicity. Int J Bipolar Disord 3(1):13, 2015 26043842

Bai Y, Liu T, Xu A, et al: Comparison of common side effects from mood stabilizers and antipsychotics between pediatric and adult patients with bipolar disorder: a systematic review of randomized, double-blind, placebo-controlled trials. Expert Opin Drug Saf 18(8):703–717, 2019 31203678

Bloom R, Amber KT: Identifying the incidence of rash, Stevens-Johnson syndrome and toxic epidermal necrolysis in patients taking lamotrigine: a systematic review of 122 randomized controlled trials. An Bras Dermatol 92(1):139–141, 2017 28225977

Bowden CL, Singh V, Weisler R, et al: Lamotrigine vs. lamotrigine plus divalproex in randomized, placebo-controlled maintenance treatment for bipolar depression. Acta Psychiatr Scand 126(5):342–350, 2012 22708645

Bromley R, Weston J, Adab N, et al: Treatment for epilepsy in pregnancy: neurodevelopmental outcomes in the child. Cochrane Database Syst Rev 10(10):CD010236, 2014 25354543

Chen TY, Kamali M, Chu CS, et al: Divalproex and its effect on suicide risk in bipolar disorder: a systematic review and meta-analysis of multinational observational studies. J Affect Disord 245:812–818, 2019 30699864

Chu CS, Lin CH, Lan TH, et al: Associations between use of mood stabilizers and risk of cataract: a population-based nested case-control study. J Affect Disord 227:79–81, 2018 29053979

Cohen JM, Huybrechts KF, Patorno E, et al: Anticonvulsant mood stabilizer and lithium use and risk of adverse pregnancy outcomes. J Clin Psychiatry 80(4):18m12572, 2019 31237992

Coles AS, Sasiadek J, George TP: Pharmacotherapies for co-occurring substance use and bipolar disorders: a systematic review. Bipolar Disord 21(7):595–610, 2019 31077521

Duffy A, Heffer N, Goodday SM, et al: Efficacy and tolerability of lithium for the treatment of acute mania in children with bipolar disorder: a systematic review: a report from the ISBD-IGSLi joint task force on lithium treatment. Bipolar Disord 20(7):583–593, 2018 30221434

Fang Y, Yuan C, Xu Y, et al: A pilot study of the efficacy and safety of paroxetine augmented with risperidone, valproate, buspirone, trazodone, or thyroid hormone in adult Chinese patients with treatment-resistant major depression. J Clin Psychopharmacol 31(5):638–642, 2011 21869688

Gao K, Ganocy SJ, Gajwani P, et al: A review of sensitivity and tolerability of antipsychotics in patients with bipolar disorder or schizophrenia: focus on somnolence. J Clin Psychiatry 69(2):302–309, 2008 18211129

Gao K, Kemp DE, Wu R, Calabrese JR: Mood stabilizers, in Psychiatry, 4th Edition. Edited by Tasman A, Kay J, Lieberman JA, et al. Chichester, UK, Wiley-Blackwell, 2015a, pp 2129–2153

Gao K, Wu R, Grunze H, Calabrese JR: Pharmacological treatment of acute bipolar depression, in Bipolar Book: History, Neurobiology, and Treatment. Edited by Yildiz A, Ruiz P, Nemeroff C. New York, Oxford University Press, 2015b, pp 281–298

Gao K, Wu R, Calabrese JR: Pharmacological treatment of the maintenance phase of bipolar depression: efficacy and side effects, in Bipolar Depression: Molecular Neurobiology, Clinical Diagnosis, and Pharmacotherapy, 2nd Edition. Edited by Zarate CA, Manji HK. Cham, Switzerland, Springer International, 2016, pp 213–242

Gao K, Goto T, Yuan C, et al: A pilot study of the effectiveness of lithium versus quetiapine immediate release monotherapy in patients with bipolar spectrum disorders. J Clin Psychopharmacol 38(5):422–434, 2018 30102627

Geddes JR, Gardiner A, Rendell J, et al; CEQUEL Investigators and Collaborators: Comparative evaluation of quetiapine plus lamotrigine combination versus quetiapine monotherapy (and folic acid versus placebo) in bipolar depression (CEQUEL): a 2 × 2 factorial randomised trial. Lancet Psychiatry 3(1):31–39, 2016 26687300

Graham RK, Tavella G, Parker GB: Is there consensus across international evidence-based guidelines for the psychotropic drug management of bipolar disorder during the perinatal period? J Affect Disord 228:216–221, 2018 29274567

Hafeman DM, Rooks B, Merranko J, et al: Lithium versus other mood-stabilizing medications in a longitudinal study of youth diagnosed with bipolar disorder. J Am Acad Child Adolesc Psychiatry 59(10):1146–1155, 2020 31369795

Haskey C, Galbally M: Mood stabilizers in pregnancy and child developmental outcomes: a systematic review. Aust N Z J Psychiatry 51(11):1087–1097, 2017 28825316

Hayes JF, Marston L, Walters K, et al: Lithium vs. valproate vs. olanzapine vs. quetiapine as maintenance monotherapy for bipolar disorder: a population-based UK cohort study using electronic health records. World Psychiatry 15(1):53–58, 2016a 26833609

Hayes JF, Pitman A, Marston L, et al: Self-harm, unintentional injury, and suicide in bipolar disorder during maintenance mood stabilizer treatment: a UK population-based electronic health records study. JAMA Psychiatry 73(6):630–637, 2016b 27167638

Hui TP, Kandola A, Shen L, et al: A systematic review and meta-analysis of clinical predictors of lithium response in bipolar disorder. Acta Psychiatr Scand 140(2):94–115, 2019 31218667

Kemp DE, van der Loos M, Gao K, et al: Lamotrigine, in The American Psychiatric Association Publishing Textbook of Psychopharmacology, 5th Edition. Edited by Schatzberg AF, Nemeroff CB. Washington, DC, American Psychiatric Association Publishing, 2017, pp 1001–1016

Kessing LV, Gerds TA, Feldt-Rasmussen B, et al: Use of lithium and anticonvulsants and the rate of chronic kidney disease: a nationwide population-based study. JAMA Psychiatry 72(12):1182–1191, 2015 26535805

Kessing LV, Feldt-Rasmussen B, Andersen PK, et al: Continuation of lithium after a diagnosis of chronic kidney disease. Acta Psychiatr Scand 136(6):615–622, 2017 29049864

Kowatch RA, Scheffer RE, Monroe E, et al: Placebo-controlled trial of valproic acid versus risperidone in children 3–7 years of age with bipolar I disorder. J Child Adolesc Psychopharmacol 25(4):306–313, 2015 25978742

McElroy SL, Israel A: Antidepressant medications in bipolar II disorder, in Bipolar II Disorder: Recognition, Understanding, and Treatment. Edited by Swartz HA, Suppes T. Washington, DC, American Psychiatric Association Publishing, 2019, pp 183–201

Mehta N, Vannozzi R: Lithium-induced electrocardiographic changes: a complete review. Clin Cardiol 40(12):1363–1367, 2017 29247520

Munk-Olsen T, Liu X, Viktorin A, et al: Maternal and infant outcomes associated with lithium use in pregnancy: an international collaborative meta-analysis of six cohort studies. Lancet Psychiatry 5(8):644–652, 2018 29929874

Nierenberg AA, Fava M, Trivedi MH, et al: A comparison of lithium and T(3) augmentation following two failed medication treatments for depression: a STAR*D report. Am J Psychiatry 163(9):1519–1530; quiz 1665, 2006 16946176

Nierenberg AA, Friedman ES, Bowden CL, et al: Lithium treatment moderate-dose use study for bipolar disorder: a randomized comparative effectiveness trial of optimized personalized treatment with and without lithium. Am J Psychiatry 170(1):102–110, 2013 23288387

Nierenberg AA, McElroy SL, Friedman ES, et al: Bipolar CHOICE (Clinical Health Outcomes Initiative in Comparative Effectiveness): a pragmatic 6-month trial of lithium versus quetiapine for bipolar disorder. J Clin Psychiatry 77(1):90–99, 2016 26845264

Nolen WA, Licht RW, Young AH, et al: What is the optimal serum level for lithium in the maintenance treatment of bipolar disorder? A systematic review and recommendations from the ISBD/IGSLI Task Force on treatment with lithium. Bipolar Disord 21(5):394–409, 2019 31112628

Patorno E, Huybrechts KF, Hernandez-Diaz S: Lithium use in pregnancy and the risk of cardiac malformations. N Engl J Med 377(9):893–894, 2017 28854098

Peselow ED, Clevenger S, IsHak WW: Prophylactic efficacy of lithium, valproic acid, and carbamazepine in the maintenance phase of bipolar disorder: a naturalistic study. Int Clin Psychopharmacol 31(4):218–223, 2016 26523730

Poels EMP, Bijma HH, Galbally M, et al: Lithium during pregnancy and after delivery: a review. Int J Bipolar Disord 6(1):26, 2018a 30506447

Poels EMP, Schrijver L, Kamperman AM, et al: Long-term neurodevelopmental consequences of intrauterine exposure to lithium and antipsychotics: a systematic review and meta-analysis. Eur Child Adolesc Psychiatry 27(9):1209–1230, 2018b 29948232

Sarai SK, Mekala HM, Lippmann S: Lithium suicide prevention: a brief review and reminder. Innov Clin Neurosci 15(11–12):30–32, 2018 30834169

Scrandis DA: Bipolar disorder in pregnancy: a review of pregnancy outcomes. J Midwifery Womens Health 62(6):673–683, 2017 29083536

Shine B, McKnight RF, Leaver L, et al: Long-term effects of lithium on renal, thyroid, and parathyroid function: a retrospective analysis of laboratory data. Lancet 386(9992):461–468, 2015 26003379

Shulman KI, Almeida OP, Herrmann N, et al: Delphi survey of maintenance lithium treatment in older adults with bipolar disorder: an ISBD task force report. Bipolar Disord 21(2):117–123, 2019 30375703

Solmi M, Veronese N, Zaninotto L, et al: Lamotrigine compared to placebo and other agents with antidepressant activity in patients with unipolar and bipolar depression: a comprehensive meta-analysis of efficacy and safety outcomes in short-term trials. CNS Spectr 21(5):403–418, 2016 27686028

Song J, Sjölander A, Joas E, et al: Suicidal behavior during lithium and valproate treatment: a within-individual 8-year prospective study of 50,000 patients with bipolar disorder. Am J Psychiatry 174(8):795–802, 2017 28595491

Tondo L, Baldessarini RJ: Antisuicidal effects in mood disorders: are they unique to lithium? Pharmacopsychiatry 51(5):177–188, 2018 29672801

Tondo L, Abramowicz M, Alda M, et al: Long-term lithium treatment in bipolar disorder: effects on glomerular filtration rate and other metabolic parameters. Int J Bipolar Disord 5(1):27, 2017 28480485

Veroniki AA, Cogo E, Rios P, et al: Comparative safety of anti-epileptic drugs during pregnancy: a systematic review and network meta-analysis of congenital malformations and prenatal outcomes. BMC Med 15(1):95, 2017a 28472982

Veroniki AA, Rios P, Cogo E, et al: Comparative safety of antiepileptic drugs for neurological development in children exposed during pregnancy and breast feeding: a systematic review and network meta-analysis. BMJ Open 7(7):e017248, 2017b 28729328

Wesseloo R, Liu X, Clark CT, et al: Risk of postpartum episodes in women with bipolar disorder after lamotrigine or lithium use during pregnancy: a population-based cohort study. J Affect Disord 218:394–397, 2017a 28501739

Wesseloo R, Wierdsma AI, van Kamp IL, et al: Lithium dosing strategies during pregnancy and the postpartum period. Br J Psychiatry 211(1):31–36, 2017b 28673946

Wingo AP, Wingo TS, Harvey PD, Baldessarini RJ: Effects of lithium on cognitive performance: a meta-analysis. J Clin Psychiatry 70(11):1588–1597, 2009 19689922

Yatham LN, Kennedy SH, Parikh SV, et al: Canadian Network for Mood and Anxiety Treatments (CANMAT) and International Society for Bipolar Disorders (ISBD) 2018 guidelines for the management of patients with bipolar disorder. Bipolar Disord 20(2):97–170, 2018 29536616

Young RC, Mulsant BH, Sajatovic M, et al: GERI-BD: a randomized double-blind controlled trial of lithium and divalproex in the treatment of mania in older patients with bipolar disorder. Am J Psychiatry 174(11):1086–1093, 2017 29088928

Zhou X, Ravindran AV, Qin B, et al: Comparative efficacy, acceptability, and tolerability of augmentation agents in treatment-resistant depression: systematic review and network meta-analysis. J Clin Psychiatry 76(4):e487–e498, 2015 25919841

CHAPTER 17

Role of Antipsychotics in Mood Disorder Treatment

Ilang M. Guiroy, M.D.
Tyler Wright, M.D., M.P.H.
Brian W. Wu, M.D., Ph.D.
Henry A. Nasrallah, M.D.

As with many other discoveries in the history of psychopharmacology, the use of antipsychotic medications in mood disorders began with serendipity. The first antipsychotic agent, chlorpromazine, was initially introduced as an anesthetic (Nasrallah and Tandon 2017), but it soon became apparent that it controlled not only the delusions and hallucinations of schizophrenia but also those of mania. Other first-generation antipsychotics (FGAs), such as haloperidol, were later approved for use in mania (which is a psychotic disorder), and many of the second-generation antipsychotics (SGAs; i.e., atypical antipsychotics) were also approved by the FDA for the treatment of mania on the basis of efficacy findings in controlled clinical trials.

The use of antipsychotic drugs for the treatment of depression began with the use of FGAs for depression with delusions or psychosis. The first tricyclic antidepressant (TCA), imipramine, was another serendipitous discovery, found when the three-ring phenothiazine structure of chlorpromazine was being modified to create a new antipsychotic that turned out to help depression but not schizophrenia. Subsequently, another drug developed as an antidepressant, amoxapine, turned out to have antipsychotic properties. A popular combination for psychotic depression in the 1970s was a single pill containing a combination of the TCA amitriptyline (trade name Elavil) and the FGA perphenazine (Trilafon). This combination drug was called Triavil.

When the selective serotonin receptor inhibitors (SSRIs) were introduced in the late 1980s (fluoxetine) and 1990s (sertraline, paroxetine, citalopram), it soon became apparent that they increase prolactin levels, which implies that they reduce dopamine activity by increasing serotonin activity and can technically be considered to have a mild antipsychotic effect. Finally, several SGAs demonstrated antidepressant effects (apart from their antimanic effects), either as monotherapy for bipolar depression or as adjunctive therapy with antidepressants for patients with depression that had not fully responded to antidepressants (this topic is discussed later in chapter).

Finally, there are the interesting cases of ketamine and pimavanserin, both of which have been shown to have antidepressants effects. Ketamine is a psychogenic hallucinogen found to have rapid antidepressant effects in treatment-resistant and refractory depression. Pimavanserin, an inverse agonist of serotonin (5-hydroxytryptamine [5-HT]) type 2A (5-HT_{2A}) receptors (with no dopamine receptor–blocking effects whatsoever), was approved in 2016 by the FDA for treatment of delusions and hallucinations associated with Parkinson's disease. In a recent trial (Papakostas et al. 2020), pimavanserin demonstrated significant antidepressant effects when added to a partially effective antidepressant. Ketamine highlights the role of hyperactive *N*-methyl-D-aspartate (NMDA) glutamate receptors as a possible etiology of depression, whereas pimavanserin points to inverse agonism of 5-HT_{2A} receptors as a therapeutic mechanism for treating depression. Both are new insights into therapeutic strategies for depression and may shed additional light on the neurobiology of depression.

First-Generation Antipsychotics for Treatment of Mood Disorders

Mood disorders are highly prevalent and are a critical subgroup of psychiatric disorders. They include major depressive disorder (MDD), bipolar mania, and bipolar depression (Vieta and Sanchez-Moreno 2008). Lithium has long been a first-line therapy for the treatment of bipolar disorder (since the early 1970s), together with anticonvulsants such as carbamazepine (since the early 1980s) and valproate (since the early 1990s). The advent of antipsychotic agents in the early 1950s led to their use in all psychotic disorders, a group that included not only schizophrenia and schizoaffective disorder but also bipolar mania and psychotic depression. Beginning with chlorpromazine, a strong dopamine type 2 (D_2) receptor antagonist, the FGAs were soon being widely used to treat MDD with or without psychotic features, The SGAs were modeled after clozapine to have stronger 5-HT_{2A} antagonism in addition to dopamine receptor antagonism; they were introduced in the mid-1990s and became widely used for the treatment of bipolar disorder and MDD both as monotherapy and in combination with mood stabilizers or antidepressants.

Haloperidol, a butyrophenone derivative representing the first nonphenothiazine antipsychotic, was an FGA that became widely used in mood disorders. Its use in bipolar disorder was studied as early as the 1970s, but it was not until decades later that placebo-controlled trials took place (Vieta and Sanchez-Moreno 2008). Haloperidol was shown to be significantly more efficacious than placebo (both as monotherapy and in combination with lithium or valproate) for the treatment of mania (Cipriani et al. 2006). After the introduction of the SGAs, haloperidol was found to be as efficacious as the SGA olanzapine for bipolar mania. Haloperidol was associated with less weight gain but higher rates of extrapyramidal side effects (EPS). The olanzapine group had significant improvement in quality of life in several measures when compared with the haloperidol group (Tohen et al. 2003a).

The TCA amoxapine became a popular antidepressant in the United States in the 1980s because its response time was generally faster than that of other medications in its class (Ban 1979). However, in both human and animal studies, this TCA was found to have antipsychotic properties but also was associated with EPS and increased prolactin levels. It is believed that these effects are due to amoxapine's strong antidopaminergic effects (Lydiard and Gelenberg 1981).

Reduction of dopamine tone may be a mechanism shared by SSRIs and antipsychotics. One hypothesis about the etiology of SSRI-associated sexual side effects suggests that they are the result of hyperprolactinemia. Increased serotonin inhibits dopamine activity, which leads to the release of prolactin (Lyons et al. 2016), and increased serotonin in the brain can act upon neural dopamine receptors (Zhou et al. 2005). SSRI-associated sexual side effects can include decreased libido, arousal issues, and delayed or absent orgasm or ejaculation (Rosen et al. 1999); problems such as menstrual disturbances, impotence, and decreased fertility have also been reported and can motivate a patient to discontinue SSRI therapy (Lyons et al. 2016). Antipsychotics are also well known to cause sexual side effects secondary to blockade of D_2 receptors (Park et al. 2012).

The First Combination Therapy of an Antipsychotic and an Antidepressant

The combination of perphenazine, an FGA, with amitriptyline, a TCA (i.e., Etrafon or Triavil), was targeted toward patients with schizophrenia who also presented with depression as well as toward patients who presented with depression in addition to agitation or anxiety. It was believed that these two drugs had additive effects when used together and that this combination represented a "broad-spectrum psychotherapeutic agent" that would be effective for these diagnoses. In the 1960s, a series of small studies by Dorfman (1963), Kennedy and Miller (1963), and Smith (1963) had found this drug combination to be effective. One study (Smith e Incas 1965) found that recurrent depressions responded most rapidly. "Excellent" response was found in 23 of 36 patients (64%), whose diagnoses included severe disorders such as bipolar disorder, schizophrenia, and violent tantrums.

In a study that compared amitriptyline-perphenazine combination therapy with monotherapy of either drug in the treatment of patients with psychotic depression, 78% (14 of 18) of the patients assigned to the combination therapy were responders, in comparison with only 41% (7 of 17) of those assigned to amitriptyline alone and only 19% (3 of 16) of those assigned to perphenazine alone (Spiker et al. 1985).

However, as with other medications, this combination therapy should be used with caution in patients with bipolar depression because it can precipitate a switch into a manic or hypomanic state. A thorough patient history, including family and psychiatric history, should be taken, and caregivers for patients who are beginning this therapy should monitor them closely for behavioral changes or the onset of suicidality (Angst and Marneros 2001).

When Unipolar and Bipolar Disorder Were Treated With the Same Drugs

As far back as Ancient Greece, mania and depression have been seen as separate but related conditions (Angst and Marneros 2001). Kraepelin was the first psychiatrist to describe two different types of psychosis, which he labeled *dementia praecox* and *manic-depressive illness* (Trede et al. 2005). This classification was reflected in DSM-II (American Psychiatric Association 1968), which used classifications such as *recurrent mania, recurrent depression*, and *recurrent mania and depression*. However, beginning with DSM-III (American Psychiatric Association 1980), bipolar disorder (the new name for manic-depressive illness) and MDD were listed as two separate conditions, with bipolar disorder distinguished from MDD by the presence of mania. In their review of the differences between bipolar and unipolar depression, Cuellar et al. (2005) noted that the separation of the two disorders in DSM-III was guided by "increasing evidence support[ing] the biological etiology and more severe lifetime course" of bipolar disorder compared with MDD).

Distinguishing between MDD and bipolar disorder for diagnostic purposes can be difficult because depressive episodes can be a part of both disorders (Cuellar et al. 2005). The distinction made between bipolar and unipolar depression has been a guiding principle of research for many decades (Cuellar et al. 2005), and this distinction is important because optimal treatment depends on the accuracy of the diagnosis. Specifically, the use of antidepressant monotherapy for patients presenting with bipolar depression can lead to negative outcomes, including increased mood instability and easier triggering of a mood episode.

Second-Generation (Atypical) Antipsychotics for Treatment of Mood Disorders

Bipolar Depression

Olanzapine-Fluoxetine Combination

In the past, combination therapies (e.g., amitriptyline and perphenazine) were widely prescribed in psychiatry. However, serious side effects, including suicidality and tardive dyskinesia, led to their use falling out of favor in the 1980s. More recently, the FDA approved a combination of fluoxetine and olanzapine (trade name Symbyax) for the treatment of bipolar I depression (Shelton 2006). The combination of these two medications is believed to result in higher serotonin levels, which may help depressive symptoms (Shelton 2003). In patients with nonpsychotic, nonbipolar depression who had not responded to SSRI monotherapy, the olanzapine-fluoxetine combination (OFC) produced improvement in symptoms within 1 week of beginning treatment. This improvement persisted throughout the length of the trial (Shelton et al. 2001).

However, OFC has several side effects of concern (Shelton 2006). Olanzapine and other SGAs have been linked to metabolic dysregulation, including weight gain, hyperlipidemia, hyperglycemia, and diabetes mellitus (Newcomer 2005). To prevent these adverse cardiometabolic effects, a standard weight management program involving diet and exercise should be implemented at the start of therapy, with or without the use of appetite suppressants such as topiramate. Biometric data, such as weight and waist circumference, should also be carefully monitored (Shelton 2006).

Quetiapine

Quetiapine (trade name Seroquel) was developed in an attempt to create a drug similar to clozapine without the risk of agranulocytosis. It is a multireceptor antagonist that has low affinity for the D_2 receptor and high affinity for the 5-HT_{2A} receptor, consistent with other SGAs; it is also a strong antagonist at histamine (H_1) receptors, a property that explains its sedative effects. The effective dosage range used in placebo-controlled clinical trials was 150–750 mg/day. The maximum plasma concentration was observed after 1–2 hours, and the half-life was 7 hours. Quetiapine was found to be effective for monotherapy in the acute and maintenance treatment of bipolar disorder and to be significantly better than placebo (Nemeroff et al. 2002). Lithium and quetiapine produced similar rates of symptom improvement; however, quetiapine also caused significant weight gain, somnolence, and dry mouth. No significant EPS were noted in a 12-week study (Bowden et al. 2005). In the maintenance treatment of bipolar disorder, quetiapine taken as an adjunct to lithium or valproate is particularly effective in reducing both manic and depressive episodes (Lindström et al. 2017).

Quetiapine was the first SGA to be approved as monotherapy for bipolar depression, by virtue of the norepinephrine reuptake inhibition side effects of its active metabolite, norquetiapine. It was found to be equivalent to lithium in efficacy (Weisler et al. 2011). Later clinical trials showed that quetiapine's efficacy for unipolar depression was similar to that of paroxetine, but because of its metabolic side effects, quetiapine was not approved for monotherapy of depression. However, FDA approved it for use as adjunctive therapy with an antidepressant for treatment-resistant depression (defined as inadequate response to one to three antidepressants).

Lurasidone

Lurasidone (trade name Latuda) received FDA approval for the treatment of acute depression associated with bipolar I disorder in adults (Bawa and Scarff 2015), either as monotherapy or as adjunctive treatment to either lithium or valproate (Loebel et al. 2014). The Program to Evaluate the Antidepressant Impact of Lurasidone (PREVAIL) was planned in 2009 by Sunovion (the manufacturer of lurasidone) to determine the effectiveness of the drug in the treatment of depression associated with bipolar I disorder. In this 6-week double-blind monotherapy study, patients were separated into three groups: lurasidone 20–60 mg/day, lurasidone 80–120 mg/day, or placebo. The primary efficacy parameter was a change from baseline in total Montgomery-Åsberg Depression Rating Scale (MADRS) score at week 6.

Based on this parameter, patients in the lurasidone-treated groups showed significantly greater improvement when compared with the placebo group (i.e., −15.4 for both lurasidone groups and −10.7 for placebo). Additionally, the response rates were higher in both lurasidone-treated groups versus the placebo group, with a number needed to treat (NNT) of 5 for both lurasidone groups. Remission rates were significantly higher for both lurasidone groups as well, with NNTs of 6 and 7 for the lower and higher dosages of lurasidone, respectively (McIntyre et al. 2013). The manufacturer determined that lurasidone significantly improved depressive symptoms in patients with bipolar depression at dosage ranges of 20–120 mg/day (Loebel et al. 2014). In addition, patients who received lurasidone showed significant improvements in scores on the Sheehan Disability Scale and a quality-of-life scale compared with patients who received placebo.

Treatment-Resistant Depression

Aripiprazole as Adjunctive Therapy

Aripiprazole (trade name Abilify; Otsuka American Pharmaceutical 2020) was the first partial agonist antipsychotic thought to stabilize the dopamine system by reducing dopamine activity when it is high and enhancing dopamine activity when it is low. Aripiprazole is an agonist of presynaptic dopamine autoreceptors, a postsynaptic partial agonist at the D_2 receptor, and a partial agonist at the 5-HT_{1A} receptor (Burris et al. 2002). Time to peak plasma concentration is 3–5 hours. Aripiprazole has a half-life of 75 hours, and the active metabolite's half-life is 94 hours (Kinghorn and McEvoy 2005). Among the antipsychotics, aripiprazole does not lengthen the QTc interval, does not cause hyperprolactinemia, is less frequently associated with EPS (although it has been associated with akathisia), and is less frequently associated with severe metabolic syndrome and weight gain.

Like quetiapine, aripiprazole is FDA approved as an adjunctive therapy for treatment-resistant MDD. However, in two FDA registration trials examining the efficacy of aripiprazole for bipolar depression, aripiprazole failed to outperform placebo. For bipolar I disorder maintenance therapy, aripiprazole used as an adjunct to lithium or valproic acid increased the time to relapse to depressive or manic episodes (Marcus et al. 2011). A small study showed that over 100 weeks, aripiprazole monotherapy was better than placebo in delaying time to manic relapse but not in delaying time to depressive relapse (Keck et al. 2007). Aripiprazole is particularly effective as an adjunct to SSRI therapy in treatment-resistant depression (Papakostas et al. 2005). In a randomized, placebo-controlled study of older adults (age >60 years) with treatment-resistant depression, 44% of patients who received aripiprazole augmentation of their antidepressant treatment (i.e., venlafaxine extended release) achieved and sustained remission (vs. 29% of those who received placebo) (Lenze et al. 2015). A secondary analysis of MADRS scores on specific items found that the presence of sleep disturbance and the absence of anhedonia were predictive of symptom remission in response to aripiprazole augmentation (Gebara et al. 2018).

Brexpiprazole as Adjunctive Therapy

Brexpiprazole (trade name Rexulti) displays partial agonism at the 5-HT_{1A} and D_2 receptors and antagonism at the 5-HT_{2A} receptor and the norepinephrine α_{1B} and α_{2c} receptors, and it shows moderate affinity for H_1 receptors. In 2015, brexpiprazole received FDA approval for adjunctive use in treatment-resistant MDD. In a double-blind randomized controlled trial, Thase et al. (2015) found that symptom reductions with brexpiprazole were clinically and statistically significantly greater than those with placebo.

Cariprazine as Monotherapy and Adjunctive Therapy

Durgam et al. (2016a) conducted a randomized, double-blind, placebo-controlled study to examine the effectiveness of cariprazine as an adjunct to antidepressant treatment in patients with treatment-resistant depression. In the study, patients continued their antidepressant treatment and were randomly assigned (1:1:1) to receive adjunctive cariprazine 1–2 mg/day, cariprazine 2.0–4.5 mg/day, or placebo and were monitored for 8 weeks. The primary and secondary efficacy parameters were change from baseline to week 8 in MADRS and Sheehan Disability Scale scores, respectively. On the basis of the MADRS total score, cariprazine at 2.0–4.5 mg/day was found to be superior to placebo.

Durgam et al. (2016b) also conducted an 8-week randomized, double-blind, placebo-controlled study in patients with bipolar I depression who were currently experiencing a major depressive episode. Patients were placed into either the placebo group or one of three fixed-dosage cariprazine groups (0.75 mg/day, 1.5 mg/day, or 3 mg/day). The primary and secondary outcomes in this study were scores from the MADRS and the Clinical Global Impressions–Severity scale, respectively, at 6 weeks. Only the cariprazine 1.5 mg/day group showed statistically significant improvement on every efficacy measure. The cariprazine 3 mg/day group showed some efficacy, but it was not statistically significant compared with the placebo group.

Bipolar Mania

Ziprasidone

Ziprasidone (trade name Geodon) was the fifth SGA to be developed. It is an antagonist at the $5\text{-}HT_{2A}$ and D_2 receptors. The time to maximum plasma concentration is 3–7 hours. The half-life is 4–7 hours if the drug taken with food; ziprasidone is best absorbed when taken with a meal. In comparison with other SGAs, ziprasidone is less likely to cause metabolic syndrome or hyperprolactinemia (Caley and Cooper 2002) but is more likely to cause QTc prolongation (Mandrioli et al. 2015). Although approval of ziprasidone was initially delayed due to concerns that QTc prolongation would increase risk for arrhythmias and torsades de pointes, postmarketing studies have not shown an increase in nonsuicidal mortality in real-world use of ziprasidone compared with olanzapine (Camm et al. 2012). Ziprasidone was approved for bipolar mania but was not superior to placebo as a monotherapy treatment for bipolar I depression or as an adjunctive therapy for treatment-resistant MDD (Patkar et al. 2015). Ziprasidone's nonsuperiority to placebo was replicated in multiple studies, including those examining ziprasidone as an adjunct to lithium or divalproex in patients with acute mania (Sachs et al. 2012).

Olanzapine

Olanzapine (trade name Zyprexa) was the first SGA to receive approval as monotherapy for bipolar mania. A randomized controlled trial found olanzapine monotherapy (5–20 mg/day) to have a faster onset of symptom reduction than divalproex (14 days vs. 62 days) for acute mania (Tohen et al. 2003b). However, over 47 weeks, no significant differences were found between the two agents in symptomatic mania remission and relapse rates. Tolerability was generally better for divalproex than for olanzapine.

Asenapine: A Sublingual Antipsychotic

The development of asenapine (trade name Saphris) was almost derailed by its poor bioavailability and extensive hepatic-gastrointestinal metabolism. Thus, it became the first sublingual SGA and is absorbed via the oral mucosa. On the basis of successful controlled clinical trials, asenapine received FDA approval for both schizophrenia and mania, but not for depression. It is an antagonist at D_2 and 5-HT_{2A} receptors. In addition, it exhibits a high affinity for multiple serotonin, dopamine, α-adrenergic, and histamine receptors. The peak plasma concentration is 30–90 minutes, and the half-life is 24 hours (Citrome 2014). When used for bipolar maintenance, asenapine monotherapy was found to be superior to placebo in delaying relapse to manic and depressive episodes (NNT=5). Side effects include somnolence, akathisia, and sedation (Szegedi et al. 2018). Patients receiving asenapine experienced greater symptom remission of acute mania (NNT=22) in comparison with placebo-treated patients, but not in comparison with olanzapine-treated patients (NNT=12) (McIntyre et al. 2010).

Role of Long-Acting Injectables in Mood Disorder Treatment

Long-Acting Risperidone

Quiroz et al. (2010) performed the largest published randomized controlled trial to date studying the effectiveness of injectable long-acting risperidone (LAR) as maintenance monotherapy for bipolar disorder. Patients with a history of more manic episodes than depressed episodes who were either currently stable or in a manic or mixed state were randomly assigned to continue the same dosage of LAR or to switch to placebo. They were then followed for 26 weeks, with a primary endpoint of time to relapse to any mood episode (depressive, manic, hypomanic, or mixed). Among patients assigned to receive LAR, 29% relapsed, compared with 57% of patients assigned to receive placebo. LAR therapy was superior to placebo in delaying time to relapse to any mood episode, regardless of whether patients were acutely manic or stable on risperidone, other antipsychotics, or mood stabilizers at enrollment.

Aripiprazole Once-Monthly Injections

The efficacy of oral aripiprazole in bipolar I disorder as both monotherapy and adjunctive therapy in both acute and maintenance treatment of bipolar mania has already been established in randomized controlled studies, and it has received FDA approval for the treatment of manic or mixed episodes associated with bipolar I disorder. Research on the use of long-acting injectables in the treatment of bipolar I disorder is limited. Some studies have examined the effectiveness of aripiprazole once-monthly 400-mg (AOM 400) injections in the treatment of bipolar I disorder in the maintenance phase. In a double-blind, randomized, placebo-controlled, multicenter withdrawal study, patients (N=133) were transitioned to and stabilized on oral aripiprazole monotherapy and then transitioned to AOM 400 injections every 4 weeks (Calabrese et al. 2017). After 8 weeks on AOM 400, patients who met stability criteria were randomly assigned (in a one-to-one ratio) to the maintenance phase, consisting of 52 weeks of double-blind treatment with either AOM 400 or placebo. The primary efficacy endpoint was time from randomization to recurrence of any mood episode. After 1 year, the time to recurrence of any mood episode was reduced by approximately one-half among patients receiving AOM 400 compared with those receiving placebo; 26.5% of patients in the AOM 400 group experienced a mood episode recurrence, compared with 51.1% of patients in the placebo group.

Pimavanserin: Beyond Parkinson's Disease

Pimavanserin is a newer antipsychotic that was approved for the treatment of hallucinations and delusions associated with Parkinson's disease psychosis due to its unique absence of any dopamine blockade and its action as an inverse agonist at the 5-HT_{2A} and 5-HT_{2C} receptors (Acadia Pharmaceuticals 2016). It does not worsen the motor symptoms of Parkinson's disease like dopamine antagonists do. Clinical trials examining the effectiveness of pimavanserin as an adjunctive therapy for treatment-resistant MDD are currently under way. Recently, Acadia Pharmaceuticals (2019) completed the Phase II CLARITY study, a 10-week randomized, double-blind, placebo-controlled multicenter study that evaluated the efficacy, safety, and tolerability of pimavanserin administered as an adjunctive treatment to patients with MDD who had an inadequate response to an SSRI or a serotonin-norepinephrine reuptake inhibitor (SNRI). The researchers found significant reductions in scores on the 17-item Hamilton Depression Rating Scale (the primary outcome measure) among patients given pimavanserin compared with those given placebo. These encouraging results led to initiation of the Phase III CLARITY program to continue to evaluate pimavanserin as an adjunctive therapy for patients who are already taking a stable dosage of an SSRI or SNRI but are having an inadequate response (Fava et al. 2019).

Conclusion

Antipsychotic medications, both first- and second-generation agents, have been widely used for mood disorders, sometimes off-label but more recently (with SGAs) for FDA-approved indications based on findings from controlled clinical trials. Antipsychotics have been demonstrated to be quite useful for unipolar depression (MDD) both as monotherapy and in combination with antidepressants, especially for patients with treatment-resistant illness. On the other hand, bipolar depression, which for decades has been treated with the traditional antidepressants approved for unipolar depression (MDD), now has three SGA medications approved by the FDA (quetiapine in 2005, lurasidone in 2013, and cariprazine in 2019) for use either as monotherapy or as an adjunct to treatment with a mood stabilizer (lithium or valproate). The manic phase of bipolar disorder has been successfully treated since the 1950s with the FGAs and since 2003 with various SGAs. The exact mechanisms by which antipsychotic drugs exert their antidepressant effects remain unknown, but recent reports of the antidepressant efficacy of the first nondopaminergic antipsychotic drug, pimavanserin, which is an inverse agonist of serotonin 5-HT_{2A}, suggest that the 5-HT_{2A} antagonism of the SGAs (in addition to their dopamine antagonism) may play a role in their antidepressant effects. Further research into the role of antipsychotic drugs in treating mood disorders is warranted.

References

Acadia Pharmaceuticals: Nuplazid [package insert]. San Diego, CA, Acadia Pharmaceuticals, Inc, 2016

Acadia Pharmaceuticals: Acadia Pharmaceuticals to present phase 2 CLARITY results for pimavanserin as an adjunctive treatment in major depressive disorder at the 2019 American Psychiatric Association Annual Meeting. BioSpace, May 18, 2019. Available at: https://www.biospace.com/article/releases/acadia-pharmaceuticals-to-present-phase-2-clarity-results-for-pimavanserin-as-an-adjunctive-treatment-in-major-depressive-disorder-at-the-2019-american-psychiatric-association-annual-meeting/. Accessed July 27, 2019.

American Psychiatric Association: Diagnostic and Statistical Manual of Mental Disorders, 2nd Edition. Washington, DC, American Psychiatric Association, 1968

American Psychiatric Association: Diagnostic and Statistical Manual of Mental Disorders, 3rd Edition. Washington, DC, American Psychiatric Association, 1980

Angst J, Marneros A: Bipolarity from ancient to modern times: conception, birth and rebirth. J Affect Disord 67(1–3):3–19, 2001 11869749

Ban TA: Amoxapine and viloxazine: review of the literature with special reference to clinical studies. Psychopharmacol Bull 15(3):22–25, 1979 386404

Bawa R, Scarff JR: Lurasidone: a new treatment option for bipolar depression—a review. Innov Clin Neurosci 12(1–2):21–23, 2015 25852975

Bowden CL, Grunze H, Mullen J, et al: A randomized, double-blind, placebo-controlled efficacy and safety study of quetiapine or lithium as monotherapy for mania in bipolar disorder. J Clin Psychiatry 66(1):111–121, 2005 15669897

Burris KD, Molski TF, Xu C, et al: Aripiprazole, a novel antipsychotic, is a high-affinity partial agonist at human dopamine D2 receptors. J Pharmacol Exp Ther 302(1):381–389, 2002 12065741

Calabrese JR, Sanchez R, Jin N, et al: Efficacy and safety of aripiprazole once-monthly in the maintenance treatment of bipolar I disorder: a double-blind, placebo-controlled, 52-week randomized withdrawal study. J Clin Psychiatry 78(3):324–331, 2017 28146613

Caley CF, Cooper CK: Ziprasidone: the fifth atypical antipsychotic. Ann Pharmacother 36(5):839–851, 2002 11978164

Camm AJ, Karayal ON, Meltzer H, et al: Ziprasidone and the corrected QT interval: a comprehensive summary of clinical data. CNS Drugs 26(4):351–365, 2012 22452529

Cipriani A, Rendell JM, Geddes JR: Haloperidol alone or in combination for acute mania. Cochrane Database Syst Rev (3):CD004362, 2006 16856043

Citrome L: Asenapine review, part I: chemistry, receptor affinity profile, pharmacokinetics and metabolism. Expert Opin Drug Metab Toxicol 10(6):893–903, 2014 24793403

Cuellar AK, Johnson SL, Winters R: Distinctions between bipolar and unipolar depression. Clin Psychol Rev 25(3):307–339, 2005 15792852

Dorfman W: The use of protriptyline (MK-240) as an antidepressant; a preliminary report. Am J Psychiatry 120(6):594–595, 1963 14086441

Durgam S, Earley W, Guo H, et al: Efficacy and safety of adjunctive cariprazine in inadequate responders to antidepressants: a randomized, double-blind, placebo-controlled study in adult patients with major depressive disorder. J Clin Psychiatry 77(3):371–378, 2016a 27046309

Durgam S, Earley W, Lipschitz A, et al: An 8-week randomized, double-blind, placebo-controlled evaluation of the safety and efficacy of cariprazine in patients with bipolar I depression. Am J Psychiatry 173(3):271–281, 2016b 26541814

Fava M, Dirks B, Freeman MP, et al: A phase 2, randomized, double-blind, placebo-controlled study of adjunctive pimavanserin in patients with major depressive disorder and an inadequate response to therapy (CLARITY). J Clin Psychiatry 80(6):19m12928, 2019 31556975

Gebara MA, DiNapoli EA, Kasckow J, et al: Specific depressive symptoms predict remission to aripiprazole augmentation in late-life treatment resistant depression. Int J Geriatr Psychiatry 33(2):e330–e335, 2018 28975710

Keck PE Jr, Calabrese JR, McIntyre RS, et al: Aripiprazole monotherapy for maintenance therapy in bipolar I disorder: a 100-week, double-blind study versus placebo. J Clin Psychiatry 68(10):1480–1491, 2007 17960961

Kennedy RE, Miller JJ: Amitriptyline-perphenazine in the treatment of schizophrenia. Am J Psychiatry 119(11):1092–1093, 1963 14031956

Keshavan MS, Lawler AN, Nasrallah HA, et al: New drug developments in psychosis: challenges, opportunities and strategies. Prog Neurobiol 152:3–20, 2017 27519538

Kinghorn WA, McEvoy JP: Aripiprazole: pharmacology, efficacy, safety and tolerability. Expert Rev Neurother 5(3):297–307, 2005 15938662

Lenze EJ, Mulsant BH, Blumberger DM, et al: Efficacy, safety, and tolerability of augmentation pharmacotherapy with aripiprazole for treatment-resistant depression in late life: a randomised, double-blind, placebo-controlled trial. Lancet 386(10011):2404–2412, 2015 26423182

Lindström L, Lindström E, Nilsson M, et al: Maintenance therapy with second generation antipsychotics for bipolar disorder—a systematic review and meta-analysis. J Affect Disord 213:138–150, 2017 28222360

Loebel A, Cucchiaro J, Silva R, et al: Lurasidone monotherapy in the treatment of bipolar I depression: a randomized, double-blind, placebo-controlled study. Am J Psychiatry 171(2):160–168, 2014 24170180

Lydiard RB, Gelenberg AJ: Amoxapine—an antidepressant with some neuroleptic properties? A review of its chemistry, animal pharmacology and toxicology, human pharmacology, and clinical efficacy. Pharmacotherapy 1(3):163–178, 1981 6152816

Lyons DJ, Ammari R, Hellysaz A, et al: Serotonin and antidepressant SSRIs inhibit rat neuroendocrine dopamine neurons: parallel actions in the lactotrophic axis. J Neurosci 36(28):7392–7406, 2016 27413150

Mandrioli R, Protti M, Mercolini L: Evaluation of the pharmacokinetics, safety and clinical efficacy of ziprasidone for the treatment of schizophrenia and bipolar disorder. Expert Opin Drug Metab Toxicol 11(1):149–174, 2015 25483358

Marcus R, Khan A, Rollin L, et al: Efficacy of aripiprazole adjunctive to lithium or valproate in the long-term treatment of patients with bipolar I disorder with an inadequate response to lithium or valproate monotherapy: a multicenter, double-blind, randomized study. Bipolar Disord 13(2):133–144, 2011 21443567

McIntyre RS, Cohen M, Zhao J, et al: Asenapine in the treatment of acute mania in bipolar I disorder: a randomized, double-blind, placebo-controlled trial. J Affect Disord 122(1–2):27–38, 2010 20096936

McIntyre RS, Cha DS, Kim RD, et al: A review of FDA-approved treatment options in bipolar depression. CNS Spectr 18 (suppl 1):4–20, quiz 21, 2013 24237641

Nasrallah HA, Tandon R: Classic antipsychotic medications, in Essentials of Clinical Psychopharmacology, 4th Edition. Edited by Schatzberg AF, Nemeroff CB. Washington, DC, American Psychiatric Publishing, 2017, pp 603–621

Nemeroff CB, Kinkead B, Goldstein J: Quetiapine: preclinical studies, pharmacokinetics, drug interactions, and dosing. J Clin Psychiatry 63 (suppl 13):5–11, 2002 12562141

Newcomer JW: Second-generation (atypical) antipsychotics and metabolic effects: a comprehensive literature review. CNS Drugs 19 (1 suppl 1):1–93, 2005 15998156

Otsuka American Pharmaceutical: Abilify prescribing information. June 2020. Available at: https://www.otsuka-us.com/sites/g/files/qhldwo3916/files/media/static/Abilify-M-PI.pdf. Accessed November 17, 2020.

Papakostas GI, Petersen TJ, Kinrys G, et al: Aripiprazole augmentation of selective serotonin reuptake inhibitors for treatment-resistant major depressive disorder. J Clin Psychiatry 66(10):1326–1330, 2005 16259548

Papakostas GI, Fava M, Freeman MP, et al: Effect of pimavanserin on anxious depression in patients with major depression and an inadequate response to previous therapy: secondary analysis of the clarity study. Int Clin Psychopharmacol 35(6):313–321, 2020 32804742

Park YW, Kim Y, Lee JH: Antipsychotic-induced sexual dysfunction and its management. World J Mens Health 30(3):153–159, 2012 23596605

Patkar AA, Pae CU, Vöhringer PA, et al: A 13-week, randomized double-blind, placebo-controlled, cross-over trial of ziprasidone in bipolar spectrum disorder. J Clin Psychopharmacol 35(3):319–323, 2015 25882763

Quiroz JA, Yatham LN, Palumbo JM, et al: Risperidone long-acting injectable monotherapy in the maintenance treatment of bipolar I disorder. Biol Psychiatry 68(2):156–162, 2010 20227682

Rosen RC, Lane RM, Menza M: Effects of SSRIs on sexual function: a critical review. J Clin Psychopharmacol 19(1):67–85, 1999 9934946

Sachs GS, Vanderburg DG, Karayal ON, et al: Adjunctive oral ziprasidone in patients with acute mania treated with lithium or divalproex, part 1: results of a randomized, double-blind, placebo-controlled trial. J Clin Psychiatry 73(11):1412–1419, 2012 23218157

Shelton RC: The combination of olanzapine and fluoxetine in mood disorders. Expert Opin Pharmacother 4(7):1175–1183, 2003 12831342

Shelton RC: The return of fixed combinations in psychiatry: fluoxetine and olanzapine combination. Ther Clin Risk Manag 2(2):187–192, 2006 18360592

Shelton RC, Tollefson GD, Tohen M, et al: A novel augmentation strategy for treating resistant major depression. Am J Psychiatry 158(1):131–134, 2001 11136647

Smith ME: Perphenazine and amitriptyline as adjuncts to psychotherapy. Am J Psychiatry 120(1):76–77, 1963 13989519

Smith e Incas J: Combined amitriptyline and perphenazine (Etrafon) in the treatment of severe emotional disorders. J Natl Med Assoc 57(4):284–286, 1965 5864895

Spiker DG, Weiss JC, Dealy RS, et al: The pharmacological treatment of delusional depression. Am J Psychiatry 142(4):430–436, 1985 3883815

Szegedi A, Durgam S, Mackle M, et al: Randomized, double-blind, placebo-controlled trial of asenapine maintenance therapy in adults with an acute manic or mixed episode associated with bipolar I disorder. Am J Psychiatry 175(1):71–79, 2018 28946761

Thase ME, Youakim JM, Skuban A, et al: Efficacy and safety of adjunctive brexpiprazole 2 mg in major depressive disorder: a phase 3, randomized, placebo-controlled study in patients with inadequate response to antidepressants. J Clin Psychiatry 76(9):1224–1231, 2015 26301701

Tohen M, Goldberg JF, Gonzalez-Pinto Arrillaga AM, et al: A 12-week, double-blind comparison of olanzapine vs haloperidol in the treatment of acute mania. Arch Gen Psychiatry 60(12):1218–1226, 2003a 14662554

Tohen M, Ketter TA, Zarate CA, et al: Olanzapine versus divalproex sodium for the treatment of acute mania and maintenance of remission: a 47-week study. Am J Psychiatry 160(7):1263–1271, 2003b 12832240

Trede K, Salvatore P, Baethge C, et al: Manic-depressive illness: evolution in Kraepelin's Textbook, 1883–1926. Harv Rev Psychiatry 13(3):155–178, 2005 16020028

Vieta E, Sanchez-Moreno J: Acute and long-term treatment of mania. Dialogues Clin Neurosci 10(2):165–179, 2008 18689287

Weisler RH, Nolen WA, Neijber A, et al: Continuation of quetiapine versus switching to placebo or lithium for maintenance treatment of bipolar I disorder (Trial 144: a randomized controlled study). J Clin Psychiatry 72(11):1452–1464, 2011 22054050

Zhou FM, Liang Y, Salas R, et al: Corelease of dopamine and serotonin from striatal dopamine terminals. Neuron 46(1):65–74, 2005 15820694

CHAPTER 18

Electroconvulsive Therapy

William McDonald, M.D.

Electroconvulsive therapy (ECT) has been referred to as the "gold standard" in the treatment of mood disorders (Kellner et al. 2012). ECT is the penultimate treatment in algorithmic strategies for patients whose depression is most resistant (Conway et al. 2017; Thase and Rush 1997), and failure to respond to a course of ECT is considered as confirmation that a patient has treatment-resistant depression (TRD) (Fink 2001). However, some have argued that ECT should be used earlier in the TRD algorithm, given the negative effects of chronic depression on quality of life, morbidity, and mortality, associated specifically with completed suicide (Beale and Kellner 2000). A study of the cost-effectiveness of ECT found that it significantly reduced patient time in depression, especially when offered early in the treatment course (Ross et al. 2018). The economic advantages were most apparent when ECT was initiated after only two antidepressant failures, in line with a widely accepted algorithm for when to consider ECT (Conway et al. 2017).

Psychotherapy and pharmacological trials may take weeks or months to be effective in TRD. In the Sequenced Treatment Alternatives to Relieve Depression (STAR*D) trial funded by the National Institute of Mental Health, researchers tested an evidence-based treatment algorithm and found that after two unsuccessful trials of antidepressant medication, the patient's chance of remission was as low as 15%, and the rate of relapse if they did respond was as high as 65% (Rush et al. 2019). Patients in populations with treatment-resistant illness who are administered ECT generally have remission rates of 60%–80% (O'Connor et al. 2001), with a relapse rate of less than 50% when they are maintained on a standardized maintenance pharmacotherapy regimen in the 6 months following a successful acute course of ECT (Sackeim et al. 2001). Furthermore, ECT has been shown to be effective in rapidly decreasing suicidal ideation (Kellner et al. 2005), with remission rates as high as 95% in patients with psychotic depression (Petrides et al. 2001).

Despite the clinical efficacy of ECT, the rate of U.S. hospitals providing it actually decreased significantly in the period from 1993 to 2009, dropping from 14.8% to 10.6%

(Case et al. 2013). A meta-analysis of 18 studies from 12 countries suggested a decline in the use of ECT in the period from 1973 to 2013, with significant variation among countries (Lesage et al. 2016). Some countries including China and The Netherlands have seen a rise in the use of ECT, whereas Canada (Rapoport et al. 2006) and Denmark (Munk-Olsen et al. 2006) have seen use remain stable. South London, England (Lambe et al. 2014), and Sydney, Australia (Plakiotis et al. 2012), have seen a decline.

Several potential reasons for the discrepancy in the efficacy and utilization of ECT, which are interrelated, include the availability of the treatment, the stigma associated with ECT, and concerns regarding side effects. The rates of use are directly related to the availability of the treatment and number of psychiatrists in the community and are indirectly related to state regulations restricting the use of ECT (Hermann et al. 1995). The availability of the treatment in the community is a product of both the attitudes of providers and patients toward the treatment and its associated costs.

There is no doubt that ECT has been unfairly stigmatized in the media and on the internet (Griffiths and O'Neill-Kerr 2019; Matthews et al. 2016; Sienaert 2016). Consider the impact of *One Flew Over the Cuckoo's Nest* on the perception of ECT (Hilton 2007). Researchers have found an indirect relationship between stigmatizing attitudes toward ECT and individuals' personal and factual knowledge related to the treatment (Kring et al. 2018). Patient family members (Elias et al. 2019), psychologists, nurses, social workers (Janicak et al. 1985), and medical students (Trenton and Pelchat 2016) reported a more positive view of ECT that was directly related to their familiarity with the procedure. Whether ECT is recommended is also related to the psychiatrist's view of the procedure (Latey and Fahy 1985). Providing full informed consent to patients and education to families and caregivers can mitigate unfounded concerns about the procedure and allow patients to make an informed decision regarding their treatment (Sackeim et al. 1995).

The costs associated with ECT can also be a barrier to its availability. ECT is increasingly being administered in treatment settings with anesthesia providers and advanced medical equipment monitoring the patient during and after the treatment. As a result, ECT is one of the safest procedures performed under general anesthesia, with a mortality rate of 1 death in 73,440 in a Veterans Affairs study (0.001%) (Watts et al. 2011) and 0.002% in a study that included 32 countries with 766,180 total treatments (Tørring et al. 2017). The increased costs associated with these medical advances may be a barrier for some patients, although the overall cost savings of ECT and improvement in areas such as patient quality of life are clear (Giacobbe et al. 2018; McCall et al. 2006; McDonald et al. 1998; Ross et al. 2018; Steffens et al. 1995).

Given the advantages of ECT in treating the most refractory mood disorders, ECT research has been focused on improving its safety while maintaining its efficacy. This research has resulted in several important modifications in the administration of ECT, including identifying patient characteristics associated with response to ECT, personalizing the treatment parameters based on the identified seizure threshold, using alternative electrode placements, and employing strategies to prevent or minimize relapse.

This review focuses on the evidence for identifying the "ideal patient" for ECT and on maximizing the efficacy of ECT in the treatment of mood disorders. A number of neuromodulation treatments can also be effective in TRD (e.g., repetitive transcranial magnetic stimulation [rTMS], transcranial direct current stimulation [tDCS], vagal nerve stimulation [VNS], deep brain stimulation [DBS]); data are limited on which treatment would be most appropriate for the individual patient. Understanding where ECT fits in the treatment of patients with mood disorders can help personalize treatment.

Identifying Patients Most Likely to Benefit

Clinical Markers of Response

An algorithm that determines which patients should be considered for ECT should weigh the relative risks and benefits of ECT compared with those of alternative treatments for major depressive disorder. Should the patient receive another course of antidepressants, a trial of rTMS, off-label ketamine infusions or nasal esketamine insufflation therapy, VNS, or investigational treatments such as DBS? In fact, relatively few data comparing the efficacy of these treatments are available. ECT is often used to provide evidence of treatment resistance (e.g., early investigational trials of VNS and DBS), or alternative treatments are used instead of ECT in patients concerned about the cognitive side effects of the treatment (e.g., esketamine and rTMS). Understanding the ideal patient for this treatment based on the patient's clinical characteristics is an important role of the practitioner prescribing a course of ECT to an individual patient for TRD.

When determining which patients are most appropriate for ECT, several patient clinical characteristics associated with an acute response to ECT should be considered. Response to ECT has been associated with increased age and a diagnosis of psychotic depression (Dombrovski et al. 2005; Haq et al. 2015; van Diermen et al. 2018). Additional predictors of response include psychomotor retardation and increased depression severity (Haq et al. 2015; Heijnen et al. 2019; van Diermen et al. 2018). Negative predictors include a diagnosis of comorbid personality disorder (specifically borderline personality disorder), alcohol or substance use disorder, or dysthymia; increased duration of a depressive episode; and a history of medication treatment resistance (Dombrovski et al. 2005; Fesko et al. 2004; Gálvez et al. 2013; Haq et al. 2015; Heijnen et al. 2010; Medda et al. 2014a; Moss and Vaidya 2014; Nordenskjöld et al. 2012; Rasmussen 2015).

One important clinical marker is the rate of remission in patients with unipolar depression versus patients with bipolar depression receiving an acute course of ECT. Bipolar depression is an understudied area in mood disorders, which is unfortunate given the relatively poor response to treatment for bipolar depression and the risks for worsening the course of bipolar illness with adjunctive antidepressants (Cheniaux and Nardi 2019). In a meta-analysis of patients receiving ECT who had a diagnosis of either unipolar or bipolar depression, the overall remission rates in both groups were equivalent: 50.9% and 53.2%, respectively (Dierckx et al. 2012). A more recent meta-analysis found similar results, with remission rates of 52.3% in both unipolar and bipolar depression, although a statistically higher rate of response and speed of response were found in the patients with bipolar depression (Bahji et al. 2019). Manic symptoms during a depressive episode (as measured by the Young Mania Rating Scale) in patients with unipolar or bipolar depression have been shown to have a decreased response to ECT (Perugi et al. 2012).

Biological Markers of Response

Biological markers, including genetic and physiological assessments, are potentially important in determining an individual's response to ECT. Researchers have correlated baseline neuroimaging findings, including decreased hippocampal volume, increased amygdala volume, and connectivity between prefrontal and default mode networks, with a positive response to ECT. Negative predictors of response include deep white matter hyperintensities and medial temporal atrophy (Levy et al. 2019; van Waarde et al. 2015). Machine learning models have also been used to determine neuroimaging biomarkers for response and have found a positive association between pretreatment subgenual cingulate volume and ECT response (Redlich et al. 2016).

Yao et al. (2019) recently reviewed laboratory and physiological markers associated with response to ECT. As they pointed out, much of the data are preclinical data in laboratory animals. The human data are preliminary, but some evidence has shown that polymorphisms of the glutamate receptor ionotropic kainate–4 gene (*GRIK4*) may predict response/nonresponse to ECT (Minelli et al. 2016). There is also preliminary evidence that genes involved in dopamine metabolism (catechol-*O*-methyltransferase [*COMT*]) and neurotransmitters associated with depression (tryptophan hydrolase, serotonin and norepinephrine transporters) are associated with response to ECT in depressed patients (Benson-Martin et al. 2016). Yao et al. (2019) also described very preliminary data in a small study ($N=11$) that associated the methylation rate of the brain-derived neurotrophic factor gene (*BDNF*) with remission in ECT (Kleimann et al. 2015).

Electroencephalographic and polysomnographic results and abnormalities in the hypothalamic-pituitary-adrenal (HPA) axis are also physiological markers of response to ECT (Yao et al. 2019). Most of these findings suffer from problems with specificity and sensitivity that make them difficult to use in prescribing ECT clinically, but they do provide insights into the mechanisms by which ECT exerts its therapeutic effect. The first electroencephalographic findings were from Max Fink (1979), who demonstrated that delta-wave or slow electroencephalographic rhythms during the ECT-induced seizure were necessary for clinical improvement. More recent findings support the use of electroencephalography in predicting response to ECT. Twenty-one-channel resting electroencephalography findings showed greater baseline anterior delta coherence (hypothesized to show intact neural circuitry, which could allow for better seizure propagation) (Scangos et al. 2019), ictal spectral amplitude and coherence, shorter latency until slow-wave onset (Krystal et al. 1995), and postictal electroencephalographic seizure suppression (Jagadisha et al. 2003; Scangos et al. 2019). However, some studies have found that electroencephalographic seizure expression is not related to ECT response (Nobler et al. 2000). Another line of reasoning is that the postictal response (e.g., reduced blood flow in the frontal regions and increased postictal slow-wave activities) is correlated with clinical response. These researchers hypothesize that the response to ECT is linked to activation of inhibitory GABA mechanisms (Sackeim 1994).

Sleep parameters have also been investigated as predictors of response. ECT is associated with an increase in the quality of sleep indices. Patients who achieved stable remission over time demonstrated significant increases in slow-wave sleep and rapid eye movement (REM) sleep duration and significant decreases in REM density compared with patients who did not experience symptom remission (Göder et al. 2016). In this same study, a higher density of the first REM sleep period was significantly associated with better ECT outcome. Grunhaus et al. (1994) found that patients who had a significantly shorter REM latency after a successful course of ECT were more likely to relapse in the 6 months following treatment.

The HPA axis is often investigated using the dexamethasone suppression test, and nonsuppression of cortisol by dexamethasone is evidence of the overactivity of the HPA axis in depression (Carroll 1982; Keller et al. 2017). Higher pretreatment levels of post-dexamethasone cortisol have been correlated with a positive response to ECT (Vukadin et al. 2011; Watts and Groft 2010). A small study found that five of six patients who went from nonsuppressors to suppressors of cortisol had a positive response to ECT, and the one patient who did not convert was a nonresponder (Albala et al. 1981). However, in a study of 42 patients, dexamethasone suppression test results did not predict who would remain in remission at 6-month follow-up, and, in fact, patients who had converted from nonsuppressors to suppressors were less likely to maintain remission at 6 months (Coryell and Zimmerman 1983).

Another potential marker is inflammation at baseline, including elevated levels of interleukin-6 (IL-6) (Kruse et al. 2018) and C-reactive protein (CRP) (Carlier et al. 2019), which have also been associated with a positive response to antidepressant medications. In one study, higher levels of IL-6 at baseline, and not other markers of inflammation (e.g., CRP), were found in women who responded to ECT (Kruse et al. 2018). Decreasing levels of IL-6 during treatment were associated with a positive ECT response (Järventausta et al. 2017). A review of inflammatory markers and ECT response found that ECT treatments were associated with an inflammatory response after a session and that the treatments could produce a longer-term reduction in cortisol levels, tumor necrosis factor α, and IL-6 (Yrondi et al. 2018).

ECT in Special Populations

ECT has been shown to be safe and effective during pregnancy for comorbid mood disorders (Ward et al. 2018). In this review, there was no evidence that ECT increased the risk of premature contractions, preterm labor, miscarriages, or congenital abnormalities (Ward et al. 2018). Another review of nine publications on ECT in pregnancy reported complications, including fetal arrhythmia, fetal bradycardia, premature birth, developmental delay, abdominal pain, uterine contraction, vaginal bleeding, placental abruption, and threatened abortion (Coshal et al. 2019); however, the authors concluded that, overall, ECT was relatively safe in pregnancy. These reviews and others (Anderson and Reti 2009; Calaway et al. 2016; Pompili et al. 2014; Saatcioglu and Tomruk 2011; Spodniaková et al. 2015) outline the importance of weighing the risks to the mother and fetus from a severe affective episode against the risks and efficacy of ECT in mood disorders. Some researchers have concluded that ECT should be used only as a last resort during pregnancy (Leiknes et al. 2015).

ECT has been shown to be both safe and effective in children and adolescents with intractable mood disorders (Benson and Seiner 2019; Cohen et al. 1997; Grover et al. 2013; Lima et al. 2013; Puffer et al. 2016; Shoirah and Hamoda 2011; Wachtel et al. 2011; Zhand et al. 2015). A negative predictor of response in adolescent females was nonsuicidal self-injury (Rootes-Murdy et al. 2019), a syndrome often associated with borderline personality disorder. This finding is congruent with the decreased response rate in adults with borderline personality disorder (Rasmussen 2015).

Safety and Efficacy in the Treatment of Mania

In a prospective study of more than 4,400 U.S. hospitals and 14,000 inpatients diagnosed with mania secondary to bipolar disorder, 18% of patients were treated with ECT and had significantly shorter lengths of stays and lower health care costs (Patel et al. 2019). In a comprehensive review of 589 patients with acute mania, Mukherjee et al. (1994) reported that ECT was an effective treatment, with more than 80% of patients remitting or showing marked clinical improvement. As with depression, patients in manic states that are more resistant to medication treatment have a lower response to ECT (Mukherjee et al. 1994). Positive clinical predictors of response to ECT include features of anxiety, depressed mood, and agitation as opposed to psychosis with or without mixed manic symptoms (Perugi et al. 2013).

Given the known destabilizing effect of antidepressants on bipolar states (Nivoli et al. 2012), some researchers have supported ECT as the perfect mood stabilizer for both the manic and depressive states of bipolar disorder (Medda et al. 2014b). Yet, as concluded in a review published in 2012 on an algorithm for the treatment of hypomania and mania, the data on ECT may be more "experience-based than evidence-based" (Nivoli et al. 2012).

It is unclear which electrode placement is most efficacious in bipolar mania. In a randomized study of 36 patients, bifrontal placement was as effective as bitemporal placement in the treatment of acute mania, with fewer cognitive side effects (Hiremani et al. 2008). There are also limited data comparing right unilateral ECT with bilateral ECT.

Bipolar patients with mixed states have a positive response to ECT (Gruber et al. 2000; Medda et al. 2010; Valentí et al. 2008; Vieta 2005); in one study, bipolar patients with mixed symptoms had a more rapid response and a greater decrease in suicidal ideation than bipolar patients in a depressive episode (Ciapparelli et al. 2001). ECT has also been shown to be effective in delirious mania, defined as the rapid onset of delirium, psychosis, mania, and often catatonic symptoms that may be present in up to 15% of patients with acute mania (Jacobowski et al. 2013). ECT is effective in patients with mania who are pregnant; it may have the advantage of decreasing the risks to both the mother and fetus due to the morbidity of a prolonged manic episode without the potential teratogenicity of anticonvulsants (Khan et al. 2016; Spodniaková et al. 2015). ECT is also effective in children and adolescents with bipolar disorder, having been used effectively in patients with mania in this population (Hill et al. 1997; Shoirah and Hamoda 2011).

Safety and Efficacy in the Treatment of Catatonia

Catatonic syndromes are present in approximately 10% of acutely ill psychiatric patients, and mood disorders are the most common cause of catatonia (Taylor and Fink 2003). ECT is very effective in the treatment of catatonia related to a mood disorder, particularly when benzodiazepines are ineffective (Kellner et al. 2020; Luchini et al. 2015; Medda et al. 2015; Unal et al. 2017). ECT is also effective in children with catatonia (Dhossche and Withane 2019; Grover et al. 2013; Jacob et al. 2014; Puffer et al. 2016; Raffin et al. 2015; Wachtel et al. 2011).

Maximizing Efficacy

Research on the treatment of mood disorders since the 1990s has focused on improving the safety of ECT while maintaining efficacy. ECT is a very effective treatment for mood disorders; however, its efficacy depends on use of modern evidence-based methodology, as described in the following subsection.

Maximizing the Efficacy of ECT While Minimizing Side Effects

Clinicians or researchers agree that ECT is one of the most efficacious treatments for mood disorders. The debate is really around its risks, which are primarily related to cardiovascular and cognitive side effects, versus its benefits. Many of the advancements in ECT have centered on maintaining its efficacy while decreasing its potential risks. Cardiovascular side effects are primarily due to the adrenergic surge from the induced seizure, which has been compared to a cardiac stress test. The patient's heart rate can accelerate from a base rate of 70 beats per minute to 130 beats per minute in a matter of seconds. This risk has been mitigated by carefully prescreening patients, ensuring that anesthesia providers are included on the ECT team, and using cardiovascular medications (e.g., β-blockers and calcium channel blockers) during the treatment. The risk is higher in patients with preexisting cardiac conditions, including hypertension, coronary artery disease, and arrhythmias (Andrade et al. 2016). However, overall, the rates of cardiovascular side effects are low, and concerns mainly apply to high-risk individuals, who can be managed with prophylactic cardiac medications during ECT (McDonald et al. 2017).

Cognitive side effects of ECT continue to be a significant concern for patients and a major focus of research, which has investigated both decreasing the energy required to initiate the seizure and using alternative electrode placements that do not directly stimulate areas related to memory and cognition. The development of the brief-pulse bidirectional square-wave ECT device in the mid-1980s was arguably one of the most important developments in ECT technology to date (Nilsen et al. 1986). The brief-pulse device is more efficient in inducing seizures than the original sine-wave device, which allows practitioners to deliver a stimulus using less energy and has resulted in a significant decrease in ECT-associated cognitive side effects. In one study comparing the sine-wave and brief-pulse devices in a community setting, patients treated with the sine-wave machines had a significant slowing in reaction time both immediately and 6 months after the index course of ECT compared with the brief-pulse group (Sackeim et al. 2007).

Another area of investigation is electrode placement, with the hypothesis that the point of stimulation is related to the degree of cognitive side effects. The original electrode placement was a bitemporal placement, in which electrodes are placed above the temples, 3 cm above a line intersecting the outer canthus of the eye and the tragus of the ear. This places the stimulus over the temporal lobes, potentially stimulating subcortical structures associated with cognition, including the amygdala and hippocampus. An alternative placement is the d'Elia placement, in which the electrodes are positioned over the right temple and 2 cm lateral to the vertex, thereby avoiding direct stimulation of cognitive areas associated with language in the dominant (left) hemisphere (d'Elia and Raotma 1975). Early studies showed that this placement, referred to as right unilateral ECT, had fewer cognitive side effects than bitemporal ECT (Sackeim et al. 2007). This strategy was refined with the bifrontal placement of electrodes over the frontal lobes (Letemendia et al. 1993).

The safety of ECT was further improved in the 1990s by advances in the understanding of the relationship between the seizure threshold and the efficacy of ECT. Again, this progress was rooted in improved knowledge regarding how the amount of energy used to create a seizure affected the seizure's impact on patient cognition. Through a series of studies, Harold Sackeim and his colleagues demonstrated that the efficacy of ECT was dependent on the magnitude of the electrical stimulus relative to the seizure threshold (McCall et al. 2000; Sackeim et al. 1993, 2000). These studies determined the stimulus threshold for each patient by using increasing stimulus doses to identify the minimal amount of energy needed to initiate a seizure. The studies by these researchers demonstrated that right unilateral electrode placement was effective only at 6 times the seizure threshold or higher and that bitemporal placement was most effective at 1.5–2.5 times the threshold. A pivotal study by the Consortium on Research in ECT (CORE) group led by Charles Kellner compared right unilateral ECT at 6 times the seizure threshold with bitemporal and bifrontal ECT at 1.5 times the threshold; the group demonstrated that all three electrode placements had equivalent efficacy and cognitive side effects (Kellner et al. 2010). This study confirmed that electrode placement and the seizure threshold were important for both determining the ideal parameters of and personalizing ECT treatment.

A recent development has been in the manipulation of one parameter of the ECT stimulus—the pulse width. The ECT stimulus is a pulse of energy composed of a pulse width (milliseconds), frequency (stimulations per second), and length (measured in seconds). The chronaxie is the amount of energy needed to depolarize a neuron; the most efficient pulse would use less energy to depolarize the neuron and potentially have fewer cognitive side effects. An early test of this hypothesis demonstrated that very short pulse widths, or ultrabrief pulse widths (<0.5 milliseconds), were as effective as longer pulse widths in treating depression and were associated with fewer cognitive side effects (Sackeim et al. 2008). The CORE group assessed the efficacy of ultrabrief right unilateral ECT in a vulnerable patient population—older patients with major depressive disorder—in their multisite Prolonging Remission in Depressed Elderly (PRIDE) study (Kellner et al. 2016a, 2016b; Lisanby et al. 2020). They evaluated the safety and efficacy of this approach in 240 elderly adults (age ≥60 years). In phase 1 of the study, 61.7% of patients remitted (and 70% responded); 10% did not remit and the other 28.3% dropped out. Overall, the changes in cognitive function were mild and the treatments were well tolerated.

Using evidence-based techniques to administer ECT can improve the safety of treating patients with mood disorders. Cognition needs to be monitored carefully because patients can have both anterograde and retrograde memory problems. Tools have been developed for bedside testing to monitor cognition; one recent scale is the Electroconvulsive Therapy Cognitive Assessment (Hermida et al. 2020), which is a

30-point scale that assesses multiple areas potentially affected by ECT, including attention and concentration as well as anterograde and retrograde memory functions. Like the Mini-Mental State Examination and Montreal Cognitive Assessment scales, this assessment can be done at the patient's bedside by a nurse, but unlike these older scales, it also includes assessment of retrograde memory.

Minimizing Relapse

Most clinicians and researchers in the field of mood disorders recognize that it is important to develop treatments that not only treat the acute episode but also manage relapse, particularly in the 6 months following the index episode. Patients with chronic depression and multiple treatment failures are more likely to relapse, and maintaining euthymia is often a central goal of treatment. The relapse rates in the year following a successful course of ECT are approximately 50%, with most patients relapsing within 6 months (Jelovac et al. 2013). The rates are higher among patients with psychotic depression and "double depression" (major depressive disorder and dysthymia) (Bourgon and Kellner 2000) and patients whose illness failed to respond to multiple antidepressant trials prior to their successful index session of ECT (Sackeim et al. 1990).

One strategy to manage relapse is to use a protocolized pharmacotherapy regimen with novel antidepressant strategies. Most patients whose illness is considered medication resistant have primarily failed to respond to selective serotonin reuptake inhibitors (SSRIs) and serotonin-norepinephrine reuptake inhibitors (SNRIs). The tricyclic antidepressants (TCAs) and monoamine oxidase inhibitors (MAOIs) are more difficult to use because of to their side-effect profiles and issues with patient compliance. Yet TCAs have been shown to be the most effective antidepressants in preventing relapse after ECT (Jelovac et al. 2013). Lithium has also been shown to be an excellent augmenting agent with proven efficacy in relapse prevention (Brus et al. 2019), although practitioners may be reluctant to use lithium for maintenance therapy (Atiku et al. 2015).

For most patients, the combination of a TCA with lithium would be a novel treatment. An early study showed that the relapse rate in the 6 months following a successful course of ECT was significantly reduced when the patient was maintained on a combination of lithium and nortriptyline compared with nortriptyline alone or placebo, with relapse rates of 39%, 60%, and 84%, respectively (Tew et al. 2007). In a randomized controlled trial, the CORE group compared continuation pharmacology using nortriptyline and lithium with continuation ECT in 201 patients who had remitted with an acute course of bilateral ECT (Kellner et al. 2006). Approximately half the patients in each group relapsed, and continuation ECT and pharmacotherapy were equivalent in terms of preventing relapse. Continuation ECT was well tolerated, with mild and transient cognitive side effects. A later analysis showed an association of higher relapse rates with increasing medication resistance prior to ECT (Rasmussen et al. 2009).

Phase 2 of the PRIDE study examined continuation ECT after a successful course of ultrabrief right unilateral ECT and showed that tapering ECT helped prevent relapse (Kellner et al. 2016a). This study also showed that a combination of venlafaxine and lithium with ECT was more effective in preventing relapse than venlafaxine and lithium alone. In clinical practice, the combination of pharmacotherapy and continuation ECT is the most common approach and appears to also be the most effective (Youssef and McCall 2014). Given the high risk of relapse, a maintenance strategy that includes tapering ECT after an acute course and starting a novel medication trial, which could include a combination of lithium and a TCA or perhaps an SNRI, would be the most appropriate. For patients who relapse in the 6 months following their acute course, continuation ECT combined with antidepressant medication should be considered.

Innovations in Neuromodulation and ECT

The focus of research has been to maintain the efficacy of ECT while minimizing its cognitive and other side effects. As discussed, previous innovations have included changes in the configuration of the pulse width and placement of the electrodes, as well as limiting the amount of energy used to create the seizure to ensure a therapeutic seizure while limiting side effects. The research in novel neuromodulation devices has focused on using subconvulsive seizures and limiting the convulsive seizures to areas related to mood and away from neurological structures associated with memory and cognition (e.g., hippocampus and amygdala).

rTMS and VNS use FDA-approved neuromodulation devices that have targeted depression using subconvulsive stimuli. rTMS administers a series of magnetic stimulations, usually over the left or right dorsolateral prefrontal cortex, to stimulate or depress firing of the underlying neurons. It has been shown to be effective in the treatment of major depressive disorder (George et al. 2010; O'Reardon et al. 2007). Similar to ECT, rTMS is less effective in patients whose illness has failed to respond to multiple antidepressant trials and who have chronic depression (Garnaat et al. 2019). ECT has an advantage over rTMS in the most severely ill and psychotic patients because those treated with ECT can begin to show improvement in a few days to a few weeks, whereas those given rTMS may need to wait 4–6 weeks to experience the full benefit. ECT has also been shown to be effective in stimulating subcortical areas known to be involved in depression (e.g., subcortical cingulate), while rTMS stimulates primarily cortical tissue and has only an indirect effect on subcortical areas known to be central to mood disorders. However, recent advances in rTMS technology (see Chapter 19, "Transcranial Magnetic Stimulation") have addressed many of these potential deficiencies and include research into shortening the treatment time from weeks to days, targeting more subcortical areas, and improving efficacy in severely depressed patients (McDonald and van Rooij 2019). Continued research in this area will be important; rTMS has distinct advantages over ECT because it has essentially no cognitive or cardiovascular side effects and no need for anesthesia. Some have described rTMS and ECT as complementary and not competitive alternatives for patients with depression, with ECT being clearly more effective in specific populations (e.g., psychotic depression) but the two modalities having considerable overlap in the treatment of other depressed populations (Fitzgerald 2004).

tDCS uses a low-intensity neuromodulation device that is currently in clinical trials. This device uses a positively charged anode electrode and negatively charged cathode electrode positioned on the scalp to excite or inhibit, respectively, cortical neurons underlying membrane potentials. tDCS is very safe and has the potential to be adapted for use by patients in their homes. Early trials have shown positive results in the treatment of depression, although the results have been relatively modest and show less effectiveness in TRD (Jog et al. 2019).

VNS delivers a subconvulsive stimulus and requires a surgical procedure to attach the device to the vagal nerve. VNS can also take months to be effective, and its clinical application has been slowed by the cost and the fact that the Centers for Medicare and Medicaid Services (CMS) and most insurance carriers have not approved payment for the procedure. However, VNS has been shown to be effective in patients with highly treatment-resistant illness (i.e., failure of eight or more antidepressant medications and nonresponse to ECT) and can produce a durable response over years (Aaronson et al. 2017). CMS is currently funding a study to reevaluate the safety and efficacy of VNS that, if positive, could open the way to increased coverage for this treatment. VNS is discussed in more detail in Chapter 20 ("Vagus Nerve Stimulation and Deep Brain Stimulation").

One of the most innovative and targeted research approaches to subconvulsive stimuli is DBS. DBS is both subconvulsive and targeted to a few millimeters of tissue. Early studies found that DBS was effective in patients whose illness was nonresponsive to ECT and in those with chronic depression (Bergfeld et al. 2016; Holtzheimer et al. 2012). The efficacy of DBS in large clinical trials has been mixed. Different groups are using different targets and different stimulus parameters with variable results, so more research is needed before DBS can be used clinically. The specificity of DBS, which can target specific white matter bundles in individuals with severe TRD, can provide perhaps the most personalized approach to therapy for chronic depression that is resistant to other treatments, including ECT (Conroy and Holtzheimer 2019).

A second approach has been to use a convulsive stimulus but to focus the stimulus away from cognitive areas and on neuroanatomical areas associated with depression. Two investigational devices include magnetic stimulation therapy (MST) and focal electrically administered seizure therapy (FEAST). MST relies on the principle that magnetic fields can be used to apply a more focal seizure than an electrical stimulus applied to the scalp because these fields pass unimpeded though the skull to stimulate a more defined brain area (Deng et al. 2011). The result is more focal stimulation of the cortex and decreased stimulation of areas in the temporal lobes involved in cognitive processing and memory. Although anesthesia is still required for MST (because the stimulus results in a generalized seizure), preliminary studies have shown it is as effective as ECT but with fewer cognitive side effects (Fitzgerald et al. 2013). Notably, some of the earlier studies have included patients with bipolar depression and psychotic depression, although no definitive conclusions can be drawn about the efficacy of MST in these disorders because the studies are preliminary (Kallioniemi et al. 2019). MST has also been shown to be effective in alleviating suicidal ideation (Sun et al. 2016).

FEAST uses ECT technology to initiate a seizure in the prefrontal cortex prior to generalization of the seizure. The FEAST stimulus is unidirectional and uses novel electrodes and placement that result in increased focality and a more efficient seizure induction (Sahlem et al. 2016; Spellman et al. 2009). The preliminary research, as well as preclinical studies in primates, has demonstrated that FEAST can induce an antidepressant response with a relatively short time to reorientation (Nahas et al. 2013;

Sahlem et al. 2016) and shows a more focal onset of seizure activity in the prefrontal cortex (Chahine et al. 2014).

There are other advanced investigational technologies using neuromodulation procedures that potentially could offer treatment for patients with the most resistant illness; these include closed-loop/adaptive DBS, optogenetics, magnetogenetics, and high- and low-intensity focused ultrasound (Kilian et al. 2019). Continued refinement of these procedures and determination of which patients will be most likely to benefit are important areas of research (McDonald 2019).

Conclusion

ECT is safe and effective in the treatment of TRD, with remission rates ranging from 60% to 80% and half of the patients remaining well over the following 6 months, when the potential for relapse is highest. Technical modifications to improve the safety and tolerability of ECT have included development of individualized dosing strategies, use of electrode placements that minimize direct stimulation of cognitively sensitive neuroanatomical areas, and adjustment of the stimulus parameters. From a medical perspective, these refinements have significantly improved the safety of ECT while maintaining its efficacy in the treatment of affective disorders. Unfortunately, the public perception of ECT continues to lag the research, although many studies show that patients receiving ECT and their families rate the experience favorably (Brown et al. 2018) and that perception is understandably related to the treatment practices of the ECT staff (Chakrabarti et al. 2010; Knight et al. 2017).

There are two clinical areas in which ECT clearly has an advantage over other FDA-approved neuromodulation devices: speed of response and rate of remission in the most severe psychiatric syndromes, including psychotic depression and catatonia. Two other FDA-approved treatments, rTMS and VNS, offer alternatives for some patients, and it is important to identify which populations will benefit from these treatments. Investigational therapies using neuromodulation are providing new treatment options for patients with severe depression who do not respond to ECT.

References

Aaronson ST, Sears P, Ruvuna F, et al: A 5-year observational study of patients with treatment-resistant depression treated with vagus nerve stimulation or treatment as usual: comparison of response, remission, and suicidality. Am J Psychiatry 174(7):640–648, 2017 28359201

Albala AA, Greden JF, Tarika J, et al: Changes in serial dexamethasone suppression tests among unipolar depressive receiving electroconvulsive treatment. Biol Psychiatry 16(6):551–560, 1981 7260217

Anderson EL, Reti IM: ECT in pregnancy: a review of the literature from 1941 to 2007. Psychosom Med 71(2):235–242, 2009 19073751

Andrade C, Arumugham SS, Thirthalli J: Adverse effects of electroconvulsive therapy. Psychiatr Clin North Am 39(3):513–530, 2016 27514303

Atiku L, Gorst-Unsworth C, Khan BU, et al: Improving relapse prevention after successful electroconvulsive therapy for patients with severe depression: completed audit cycle involving 102 full electroconvulsive therapy courses in West Sussex, United kingdom. J ECT 31(1):34–36, 2015 25029538

Bahji A, Hawken ER, Sepehry AA, et al: ECT beyond unipolar major depression: systematic review and meta-analysis of electroconvulsive therapy in bipolar depression. Acta Psychiatr Scand 139(3):214–226, 2019 30506992
Beale MD, Kellner CH: ECT in treatment algorithms: no need to save the best for last. J ECT 16(1):1–2, 2000 10735326
Benson NM, Seiner SJ: Electroconvulsive therapy in children and adolescents: clinical indications and special considerations. Harv Rev Psychiatry 27(6):354–358, 2019 31714466
Benson-Martin JJ, Stein DJ, Baldwin DS, et al: Genetic mechanisms of electroconvulsive therapy response in depression. Hum Psychopharmacol 31(3):247–251, 2016 27062668
Bergfeld IO, Mantione M, Hoogendoorn ML, et al: Deep brain stimulation of the ventral anterior limb of the internal capsule for treatment-resistant depression: a randomized clinical trial. JAMA Psychiatry 73(5):456–464, 2016 27049915
Bourgon LN, Kellner CH: Relapse of depression after ECT: a review. J ECT 16(1):19–31, 2000 10735328
Brown SK, Nowlin RB, Sartorelli R, et al: Patient experience of electroconvulsive therapy: a retrospective review of clinical outcomes and satisfaction. J ECT 34(4):240–246, 2018 29613943
Brus O, Cao Y, Hammar Å, et al: Lithium for suicide and readmission prevention after electroconvulsive therapy for unipolar depression: population-based register study. BJPsych Open 5(3):e46, 2019 31189487
Calaway K, Coshal S, Jones K, et al: A systematic review of the safety of electroconvulsive therapy use during the first trimester of pregnancy. J ECT 32(4):230–235, 2016 27327556
Carlier A, Berkhof JG, Rozing M, et al: Inflammation and remission in older patients with depression treated with electroconvulsive therapy; findings from the MODECT study. J Affect Disord 256:509–516, 2019 31279250
Carroll BJ: The dexamethasone suppression test for melancholia. Br J Psychiatry 140:292–304, 1982 7093598
Case BG, Bertollo DN, Laska EM, et al: Declining use of electroconvulsive therapy in United States general hospitals. Biol Psychiatry 73(2):119–126, 2013 23059049
Chahine G, Short B, Spicer K, et al: Regional cerebral blood flow changes associated with focal electrically administered seizure therapy (FEAST). Brain Stimul 7(3):483–485, 2014 24795198
Chakrabarti S, Grover S, Rajagopal R: Perceptions and awareness of electroconvulsive therapy among patients and their families: a review of the research from developing countries. J ECT 26(4):317–322, 2010 21155155
Cheniaux E, Nardi AE: Evaluating the efficacy and safety of antidepressants in patients with bipolar disorder. Expert Opin Drug Saf 18(10):893–913, 2019 31364895
Ciapparelli A, Dell'Osso L, Tundo A, et al: Electroconvulsive therapy in medication-nonresponsive patients with mixed mania and bipolar depression. J Clin Psychiatry 62(7):552–555, 2001 11488367
Cohen D, Paillère-Martinot ML, Basquin M: Use of electroconvulsive therapy in adolescents. Convuls Ther 13(1):25–31, 1997 9152585
Conroy SK, Holtzheimer PE: Deep brain stimulation for treatment-resistant depression: predicting response and optimizing treatment. Pers Med Psychiatry 17:43–45, 2019
Conway CR, George MS, Sackeim HA: Toward an evidence-based, operational definition of treatment-resistant depression: when enough is enough. JAMA Psychiatry 74(1):9–10, 2017 27784055
Coryell W, Zimmerman M: The dexamethasone suppression test and ECT outcome: a six-month follow-up. Biol Psychiatry 18(1):21–27, 1983 6830923
Coshal S, Jones K, Coverdale J, et al: An overview of reviews on the safety of electroconvulsive therapy administered during pregnancy. J Psychiatr Pract 25(1):2–6, 2019 30633726
d'Elia G, Raotma H: Is unilateral ECT less effective than bilateral ECT? Br J Psychiatry 126:83–89, 1975 1092400
Deng ZD, Lisanby SH, Peterchev AV: Electric field strength and focality in electroconvulsive therapy and magnetic seizure therapy: a finite element simulation study. J Neural Eng 8(1):016007, 2011 21248385

Dhossche DM, Withane N: Electroconvulsive therapy for catatonia in children and adolescents. Child Adolesc Psychiatr Clin N Am 28(1):111–120, 2019 30389071
Dierckx B, Heijnen WT, van den Broek WW, et al: Efficacy of electroconvulsive therapy in bipolar versus unipolar major depression: a meta-analysis. Bipolar Disord 14(2):146–150, 2012 22420590
Dombrovski AY, Mulsant BH, Haskett RF, et al: Predictors of remission after electroconvulsive therapy in unipolar major depression. J Clin Psychiatry 66(8):1043–1049, 2005 16086621
Elias A, Ang A, Schneider A, George K: Family presence during electroconvulsive therapy. J ECT 35(2):91–94, 2019 30531395
Feske U, Mulsant BH, Pilkonis PA, et al: Clinical outcome of ECT in patients with major depression and comorbid borderline personality disorder. Am J Psychiatry 161(11):2073–2080, 2004 15514409
Fink M: Convulsive Therapy: Theory and Practice. New York, Raven Press, 1979
Fink M: Convulsive therapy: a review of the first 55 years. J Affect Disord 63(1–3):1–15, 2001 11246075
Fitzgerald P: Repetitive transcranial magnetic stimulation and electroconvulsive therapy: complementary or competitive therapeutic options in depression? Australas Psychiatry 12(3):234–238, 2004 15715781
Fitzgerald PB, Hoy KE, Herring SE, et al: Pilot study of the clinical and cognitive effects of high-frequency magnetic seizure therapy in major depressive disorder. Depress Anxiety 30(2):129–136, 2013 23080404
Gálvez V, Loo CK, Alonzo A, et al: Do benzodiazepines moderate the effectiveness of bitemporal electroconvulsive therapy in major depression? J Affect Disord 150(2):686–690, 2013 23668903
Garnaat SL, Fukuda AM, Yuan S, et al: Identification of clinical features and biomarkers that may inform a personalized approach to rTMS for depression. Pers Med Psychiatry 17:4–16, 2019
George MS, Lisanby SH, Avery D, et al: Daily left prefrontal transcranial magnetic stimulation therapy for major depressive disorder: a sham-controlled randomized trial. Arch Gen Psychiatry 67(5):507–516, 2010 20439832
Giacobbe P, Rakita U, Penner-Goeke K, et al: Improvements in health-related quality of life with electroconvulsive therapy: a meta-analysis. J ECT 34(2):87–94, 2018 29461332
Göder R, Hinrichsen I, Seeck-Hirschner M, et al: Sleep at baseline and after electroconvulsive therapy in patients with major depression. Psychiatry Res 246:683–687, 2016 27825788
Griffiths C, O'Neill-Kerr A: Patients', carers', and the public's perspectives on electroconvulsive therapy. Front Psychiatry 10:304, 2019 31133895
Grover S, Malhotra S, Varma S, et al: Electroconvulsive therapy in adolescents: a retrospective study from north India. J ECT 29(2):122–126, 2013 23296394
Gruber NP, Dilsaver SC, Shoaib AM, et al: ECT in mixed affective states: a case series. J ECT 16(2):183–188, 2000 10868328
Grunhaus L, Shipley JE, Eiser A, et al: Shortened REM latency postECT is associated with rapid recurrence of depressive symptomatology. Biol Psychiatry 36(4):214–222, 1994 7986885
Haq AU, Sitzmann AF, Goldman ML, et al: Response of depression to electroconvulsive therapy: a meta-analysis of clinical predictors. J Clin Psychiatry 76(10):1374–1384, 2015 26528644
Heijnen WT, Birkenhäger TK, Wierdsma AI, et al: Antidepressant pharmacotherapy failure and response to subsequent electroconvulsive therapy: a meta-analysis. J Clin Psychopharmacol 30(5):616–619, 2010 20814336
Heijnen WT, Kamperman AM, Tjokrodipo LD, et al: Influence of age on ECT efficacy in depression and the mediating role of psychomotor retardation and psychotic features. J Psychiatr Res 109:41–47, 2019 30472527
Hermann RC, Dorwart RA, Hoover CW, et al: Variation in ECT use in the United States. Am J Psychiatry 152(6):869–875, 1995 7755116
Hermida AP, Goldstein FC, Loring DW, et al: ElectroConvulsive therapy cognitive assessment (ECCA) tool: a new instrument to monitor cognitive function in patients undergoing ECT. J Affect Disord 269:36–42, 2020 32217341

Hill MA, Courvoisie H, Dawkins K, et al: ECT for the treatment of intractable mania in two prepubertal male children. Convuls Ther 13(2):74–82, 1997 9253527
Hilton C: An exploration of the patient's experience of electro-convulsive therapy in mid-twentieth century creative literature: a historical study with implications for practice today. J Affect Disord 97(1–3):5–12, 2007 16887198
Hiremani RM, Thirthalli J, Tharayil BS, et al: Double-blind randomized controlled study comparing short-term efficacy of bifrontal and bitemporal electroconvulsive therapy in acute mania. Bipolar Disord 10(6):701–707, 2008 18837864
Holtzheimer PE, Kelley ME, Gross RE, et al: Subcallosal cingulate deep brain stimulation for treatment-resistant unipolar and bipolar depression. Arch Gen Psychiatry 69(2):150–158, 2012 22213770
Jacob P, Gogi PK, Srinath S, et al: Review of electroconvulsive therapy practice from a tertiary Child and Adolescent Psychiatry Centre. Asian J Psychiatr 12:95–99, 2014 25440568
Jacobowski NL, Heckers S, Bobo WV: Delirious mania: detection, diagnosis, and clinical management in the acute setting. J Psychiatr Pract 19(1):15–28, 2013 23334676
Jagadisha GB, Gangadhar B, Janakiramiah N, et al: Post-seizure EEG fractal dimension and spectral power predict antidepressant response to unilateral ECT. Indian J Psychiatry 45(1):16–20, 2003 21206807
Janicak PG, Mask J, Trimakas KA, et al: ECT: an assessment of mental health professionals' knowledge and attitudes. J Clin Psychiatry 46(7):262–266, 1985 4008449
Järventausta K, Sorri A, Kampman O, et al: Changes in interleukin-6 levels during electroconvulsive therapy may reflect the therapeutic response in major depression. Acta Psychiatr Scand 135(1):87–92, 2017 27858966
Jelovac A, Kolshus E, McLoughlin DM: Relapse following successful electroconvulsive therapy for major depression: a meta-analysis. Neuropsychopharmacology 38(12):2467–2474, 2013 23774532
Jog MV, Wang DJJ, Narr KL: A review of transcranial direct current stimulation (tDCS) for the individualized treatment of depressive symptoms. Pers Med Psychiatry 17–18:17–22, 2019 31938757
Kallioniemi E, McClintock SM, Deng ZD, et al: Magnetic seizure therapy: towards personalized seizure therapy for major depression. Pers Med Psychiatry 17–18:37–42, 2019 32832741
Keller J, Gomez R, Williams G, et al: HPA axis in major depression: cortisol, clinical symptomatology and genetic variation predict cognition. Mol Psychiatry 22(4):527–536, 2017 27528460
Kellner CH, Fink M, Knapp R, et al: Relief of expressed suicidal intent by ECT: a consortium for research in ECT study. Am J Psychiatry 162(5):977–982, 2005 15863801
Kellner CH, Knapp RG, Petrides G, et al: Continuation electroconvulsive therapy vs pharmacotherapy for relapse prevention in major depression: a multisite study from the Consortium for Research in Electroconvulsive Therapy (CORE). Arch Gen Psychiatry 63(12):1337–1344, 2006 17146008
Kellner CH, Knapp R, Husain MM, et al: Bifrontal, bitemporal and right unilateral electrode placement in ECT: randomised trial. Br J Psychiatry 196(3):226–234, 2010 20194546
Kellner CH, Greenberg RM, Murrough JW, et al: ECT in treatment-resistant depression. Am J Psychiatry 169(12):1238–1244, 2012 23212054
Kellner CH, Husain MM, Knapp RG, et al: A novel strategy for continuation ECT in geriatric depression: phase 2 of the PRIDE study. Am J Psychiatry 173(11):1110–1118, 2016a 27418381
Kellner CH, Husain MM, Knapp RG, et al: Right unilateral ultrabrief pulse ECT in geriatric depression: phase 1 of the PRIDE study. Am J Psychiatry 173(11):1101–1109, 2016b 27418379
Kellner CH, Obbels J, Sienaert P: When to consider electroconvulsive therapy (ECT). Acta Psychiatr Scand 141(4):304–315, 2020 31774547
Khan SJ, Fersh ME, Ernst C, et al: Bipolar disorder in pregnancy and postpartum: principles of management. Curr Psychiatry Rep 18(2):13, 2016 26781551
Kilian H, Meyer D, Schlaepfer TE: Putative novel neuromodulatory treatments for affective disorders—what might emerge? Pers Med Psychiatry 17:46–50, 2019

Kleimann A, Kotsiari A, Sperling W, et al: BDNF serum levels and promoter methylation of BDNF exon I, IV and VI in depressed patients receiving electroconvulsive therapy. J Neural Transm (Vienna) 122(6):925–928, 2015 25387785

Knight F, Ridge D, McShane R, et al: Care, control, and the electroconvulsive therapy ritual: making sense of polarized patient narratives. Qual Health Res 27(11):1675–1685, 2017 28799472

Kring IS, Bergholt MD, Midtgaard J: The perspectives of former recipients and experts on stigmatization related to electroconvulsive therapy in Denmark: a focus group study. J Psychiatr Ment Health Nurs 25(5–6):358–367, 2018 29758121

Kruse JL, Congdon E, Olmstead R, et al: Inflammation and improvement of depression following electroconvulsive therapy in treatment-resistant depression. J Clin Psychiatry 79(2):17m11597, 2018 29489077

Krystal AD, Weiner RD, Coffey CE: The ictal EEG as a marker of adequate stimulus intensity with unilateral ECT. J Neuropsychiatry Clin Neurosci 7(3):295–303, 1995 7580187

Lambe S, Mogg A, Eranti S, et al: Trends in use of electroconvulsive therapy in South London from 1949 to 2006. J ECT 30(4):309–314, 2014 24625707

Latey RH, Fahy TJ: Electroconvulsive therapy in the Republic of Ireland 1982: a summary of findings. Br J Psychiatry 147:438–439, 1985 4075035

Leiknes KA, Cooke MJ, Jarosch-von Schweder L, et al: Electroconvulsive therapy during pregnancy: a systematic review of case studies. Arch Women Ment Health 18(1):1–39, 2015 24271084

Lesage A, Lemasson M, Medina K, et al: The prevalence of electroconvulsive therapy use since 1973: a meta-analysis. J ECT 32(4):236–242, 2016 27227401

Letemendia FJ, Delva NJ, Rodenburg M, et al: Therapeutic advantage of bifrontal electrode placement in ECT. Psychol Med 23(2):349–360, 1993 8332652

Levy A, Taib S, Arbus C, et al: Neuroimaging biomarkers at baseline predict electroconvulsive therapy overall clinical response in depression: a systematic review. J ECT 35(2):77–83, 2019 30628993

Lima NN, Nascimento VB, Peixoto JA, et al: Electroconvulsive therapy use in adolescents: a systematic review. Ann Gen Psychiatry 12(1):17, 2013 23718899

Lisanby SH, McClintock SM, Alexopoulos G, et al: Neurocognitive effects of combined electroconvulsive therapy (ECT) and venlafaxine in geriatric depression: phase 1 of the PRIDE study. Am J Geriatr Psychiatry 28(3):304–316, 2020 31706638

Luchini F, Medda P, Mariani MG, et al: Electroconvulsive therapy in catatonic patients: efficacy and predictors of response. World J Psychiatry 5(2):182–192, 2015 26110120

Matthews AM, Rosenquist PB, McCall WV: Representations of ECT in English-language film and television in the new millennium. J ECT 32(3):187–191, 2016 27008331

McCall WV, Reboussin DM, Weiner RD, et al: Titrated moderately suprathreshold vs fixed high-dose right unilateral electroconvulsive therapy: acute antidepressant and cognitive effects (see comments). Arch Gen Psychiatry 57(5):438–444, 2000 10807483

McCall WV, Prudic J, Olfson M, et al: Health-related quality of life following ECT in a large community sample. J Affect Disord 90(2–3):269–274, 2006 16412519

McDonald WM: Are modern neuromodulation therapies too precise? Pers Med Psychiatry 17:1–3, 2019

McDonald WM, van Rooij SJH: Targeting PTSD. Am J Psychiatry 176(11):894–896, 2019 31672041

McDonald WM, Phillips V, Figielo GS, et al: Cost-effective maintenance treatment of resistant geriatric depression. Psychiatric Annals 28:47–52, 1998

McDonald WM, Meeks TW, Carpenter LL, et al: Electroconvulsive therapy and other neuromodulation therapies, in The American Psychiatric Publishing Textbook of Psychopharmacology, 5th Edition. Edited by Schatzberg AF, Nemeroff CB. Washington, DC, American Psychiatric Press, 2017, pp 861–899

Medda P, Perugi G, Zanello S, et al: Comparative response to electroconvulsive therapy in medication-resistant bipolar I patients with depression and mixed state. J ECT 26(2):82–86, 2010 19710623

Medda P, Mauri M, Toni C, et al: Predictors of remission in 208 drug-resistant depressive patients treated with electroconvulsive therapy. J ECT 30(4):292–297, 2014a 24625706
Medda P, Toni C, Perugi G, et al: The mood-stabilizing effects of electroconvulsive therapy. J ECT 30(4):275–282, 2014b 25010031
Medda P, Toni C, Luchini F, et al: Catatonia in 26 patients with bipolar disorder: clinical features and response to electroconvulsive therapy. Bipolar Disord 17(8):892–901, 2015 26643014
Minelli A, Congiu C, Ventriglia M, et al: Influence of GRIK4 genetic variants on the electroconvulsive therapy response. Neurosci Lett 626:94–98, 2016 27222927
Moss L, Vaidya N: Does comorbid alcohol and substance abuse affect electroconvulsive therapy outcome in the treatment of mood disorders? J ECT 30(1):22–25, 2014 23859979
Mukherjee S, Sackeim HA, Schnur DB: Electroconvulsive therapy of acute manic episodes: a review of 50 years' experience. Am J Psychiatry 151(2):169–176, 1994 8296883
Munk-Olsen T, Laursen TM, Videbech P, et al: Electroconvulsive therapy: predictors and trends in utilization from 1976 to 2000. J ECT 22(2):127–132, 2006 16801829
Nahas Z, Short B, Burns C, et al: A feasibility study of a new method for electrically producing seizures in man: focal electrically administered seizure therapy (FEAST). Brain Stimul 6(3):403–408, 2013 23518262
Nilsen SM, Willis KW, Pettinati HM: Initial impression of two new brief-pulse electroconvulsive therapy machines. Convuls Ther 2(1):43–54, 1986 11940844
Nivoli AM, Murru A, Goikolea JM, et al: New treatment guidelines for acute bipolar mania: a critical review. J Affect Disord 140(2):125–141, 2012 22100133
Nobler MS, Luber B, Moeller JR, et al: Quantitative EEG during seizures induced by electroconvulsive therapy: relations to treatment modality and clinical features, I: global analyses. J ECT 16(3):211–228, 2000 11005043
Nordenskjöld A, von Knorring L, Engström I: Predictors of the short-term responder rate of electroconvulsive therapy in depressive disorders—a population based study. BMC Psychiatry 12:115, 2012 22900754
O'Connor MK, Knapp R, Husain M, et al: The influence of age on the response of major depression to electroconvulsive therapy: a C.O.R.E. report. Am J Geriatr Psychiatry 9(4):382–390, 2001 11739064
O'Reardon JP, Solvason HB, Janicak PG, et al: Efficacy and safety of transcranial magnetic stimulation in the acute treatment of major depression: a multisite randomized controlled trial. Biol Psychiatry 62(11):1208–1216, 2007 17573044
Patel RS, Jain SB, Youssef NA: Electroconvulsive treatment utilization for the inpatient management of severe manic episodes of bipolar disorder. J ECT 35(3):195–200, 2019 30870263
Perugi G, Medda P, Zanello S, et al: Episode length and mixed features as predictors of ECT nonresponse in patients with medication-resistant major depression. Brain Stimul 5(1):18–24, 2012 22037132
Perugi G, Medda P, Reis J, et al: Clinical subtypes of severe bipolar mixed states. J Affect Disord 151(3):1076–1082, 2013 24074482
Petrides G, Fink M, Husain MM, et al: ECT remission rates in psychotic versus nonpsychotic depressed patients: a report from CORE. J ECT 17(4):244–253, 2001 11731725
Plakiotis C, George K, O'Connor DW: Has electroconvulsive therapy use remained stable over time? A decade of electroconvulsive therapy service provision in Victoria, Australia. Aust N Z J Psychiatry 46(6):522–531, 2012 22375067
Pompili M, Dominici G, Giordano G, et al: Electroconvulsive treatment during pregnancy: a systematic review. Expert Rev Neurother 14(12):1377–1390, 2014 25346216
Puffer CC, Wall CA, Huxsahl JE, et al: A 20 year practice review of electroconvulsive therapy for adolescents. J Child Adolesc Psychopharmacol 26(7):632–636, 2016 26784386
Raffin M, Zugaj-Bensaou L, Bodeau N, et al: Treatment use in a prospective naturalistic cohort of children and adolescents with catatonia. Eur Child Adolesc Psychiatry 24(4):441–449, 2015 25159089
Rapoport MJ, Mamdani M, Herrmann N: Electroconvulsive therapy in older adults: 13-year trends. Can J Psychiatry 51(9):616–619, 2006 17007229

Rasmussen KG: Do patients with personality disorders respond differentially to electroconvulsive therapy? A review of the literature and consideration of conceptual issues. J ECT 31(1):6–12, 2015 25054362

Rasmussen KG, Mueller M, Rummans TA, et al: Is baseline medication resistance associated with potential for relapse after successful remission of a depressive episode with ECT? Data from the Consortium for Research on Electroconvulsive Therapy (CORE). J Clin Psychiatry 70(2):232–237, 2009 19192459

Redlich R, Opel N, Grotegerd D, et al: Prediction of individual response to electroconvulsive therapy via machine learning on structural magnetic resonance imaging data. JAMA Psychiatry 73(6):557–564, 2016 27145449

Rootes-Murdy K, Carlucci M, Tibbs M, et al: Non-suicidal self-injury and electroconvulsive therapy: outcomes in adolescent and young adult populations. J Affect Disord 250:94–98, 2019 30844603

Ross EL, Zivin K, Maixner DF: Cost-effectiveness of electroconvulsive therapy vs pharmacotherapy/psychotherapy for treatment-resistant depression in the United States. JAMA Psychiatry 75(7):713–722, 2018 29800956

Rush AJ, Aaronson ST, Demyttenaere K: Difficult-to-treat depression: a clinical and research roadmap for when remission is elusive. Aust N Z J Psychiatry 53(2):109–118, 2019 30378447

Saatcioglu O, Tomruk NB: The use of electroconvulsive therapy in pregnancy: a review. Isr J Psychiatry Relat Sci 48(1):6–11, 2011 21572236

Sackeim HA: Central issues regarding the mechanisms of action of electroconvulsive therapy: directions for future research. Psychopharmacol Bull 30(3):281–308, 1994 7878177

Sackeim HA, Prudic J, Devanand DP, et al: The impact of medication resistance and continuation pharmacotherapy on relapse following response to electroconvulsive therapy in major depression. J Clin Psychopharmacol 10(2):96–104, 1990 2341598

Sackeim HA, Prudic J, Devanand DP, et al: Effects of stimulus intensity and electrode placement on the efficacy and cognitive effects of electroconvulsive therapy (see comments). N Engl J Med 328(12):839–846, 1993 8441428

Sackeim HA, Devanand DP, Nobler M: Electroconvulsive therapy, in Psychopharmacology: The Fourth Generation of Progress. Edited by Bllom FE, Kupfer DJ. New York, Raven, 1995, pp 1123–1142

Sackeim HA, Prudic J, Devanand DP, et al: A prospective, randomized, double-blind comparison of bilateral and right unilateral electroconvulsive therapy at different stimulus intensities (see comments). Arch Gen Psychiatry 57(5):425–434, 2000 10807482

Sackeim HA, Haskett RF, Mulsant BH, et al: Continuation pharmacotherapy in the prevention of relapse following electroconvulsive therapy: a randomized controlled trial (see comments). JAMA 285(10):1299–1307, 2001 11255384

Sackeim HA, Prudic J, Fuller R, et al: The cognitive effects of electroconvulsive therapy in community settings. Neuropsychopharmacology 32(1):244–254, 2007 16936712

Sackeim HA, Prudic J, Nobler MS, et al: Effects of pulse width and electrode placement on the efficacy and cognitive effects of electroconvulsive therapy. Brain Stimul 1(2):71–83, 2008 19756236

Sahlem GL, Short EB, Kerns S, et al: Expanded safety and efficacy data for a new method of performing electroconvulsive therapy: focal electrically administered seizure therapy. J ECT 32(3):197–203, 2016 27379790

Scangos KW, Weiner RD, Coffey EC, et al: An electrophysiological biomarker that may predict treatment response to ECT. J ECT 35(2):95–102, 2019 30531398

Shoirah H, Hamoda HM: Electroconvulsive therapy in children and adolescents. Expert Rev Neurother 11(1):127–137, 2011 21158560

Sienaert P: Based on a true story? The portrayal of ECT in international movies and television programs. Brain Stimul 9(6):882–891, 2016 27522170

Spellman T, Peterchev AV, Lisanby SH: Focal electrically administered seizure therapy: a novel form of ECT illustrates the roles of current directionality, polarity, and electrode configuration in seizure induction. Neuropsychopharmacology 34(8):2002–2010, 2009 19225453

Spodniaková B, Halmo M, Nosáľová P: Electroconvulsive therapy in pregnancy—a review. J Obstet Gynaecol 35(7):659–662, 2015 25526509
Steffens DC, Krystal AD, Sibert TE, et al: Cost effectiveness of maintenance ECT. Convuls Ther 11(4):283–284, 1995 8919583
Sun Y, Farzan F, Mulsant BH, et al: Indicators for remission of suicidal ideation following magnetic seizure therapy in patients with treatment-resistant depression. JAMA Psychiatry 73(4):337–345, 2016 26981889
Taylor MA, Fink M: Catatonia in psychiatric classification: a home of its own. Am J Psychiatry 160(7):1233–1241, 2003 12832234
Tew JD Jr, Mulsant BH, Haskett RF, et al: Relapse during continuation pharmacotherapy after acute response to ECT: a comparison of usual care versus protocolized treatment. Ann Clin Psychiatry 19(1):1–4, 2007 17453654
Thase ME, Rush AJ: When at first you don't succeed: sequential strategies for antidepressant nonresponders. J Clin Psychiatry 58 (suppl 13):23–29, 1997 9402916
Tørring N, Sanghani SN, Petrides G, et al: The mortality rate of electroconvulsive therapy: a systematic review and pooled analysis. Acta Psychiatr Scand 135(5):388–397, 2017 28332236
Trenton A, Pelchat R: Medical students' perceptions of electroconvulsive therapy: the impact of direct exposure. J ECT 32(1):20–22, 2016 26075694
Unal A, Altindag A, Demir B, Aksoy I: The use of lorazepam and electroconvulsive therapy in the treatment of catatonia: treatment characteristics and outcomes in 60 patients. J ECT 33(4):290–293, 2017 28640169
Valentí M, Benabarre A, García-Amador M, et al: Electroconvulsive therapy in the treatment of mixed states in bipolar disorder. Eur Psychiatry 23(1):53–56, 2008 18191551
van Diermen L, van den Ameele S, Kamperman AM, et al: Prediction of electroconvulsive therapy response and remission in major depression: meta-analysis. Br J Psychiatry 212(2):71–80, 2018 29436330
van Waarde JA, Scholte HS, van Oudheusden LJ, et al: A functional MRI marker may predict the outcome of electroconvulsive therapy in severe and treatment-resistant depression. Mol Psychiatry 20(5):609–614, 2015 25092248
Vieta E: Bipolar mixed states and their treatment. Expert Rev Neurother 5(1):63–68, 2005 15853475
Vukadin M, Birkenhäger TK, Wierdsma AI, et al: Post-dexamethasone cortisol as a predictor for the efficacy of electroconvulsive therapy in depressed inpatients. J Psychiatr Res 45(9):1165–1169, 2011 21481419
Wachtel LE, Dhossche DM, Kellner CH: When is electroconvulsive therapy appropriate for children and adolescents? Med Hypotheses 76(3):395–399, 2011 21129852
Ward HB, Fromson JA, Cooper JJ, et al: Recommendations for the use of ECT in pregnancy: literature review and proposed clinical protocol. Arch Women Ment Health 21(6):715–722, 2018 29796968
Watts BV, Groft A: Retrospective evaluation of the dexamethasone suppression test as a predictor of response to electroconvulsive therapy in patients with comorbid major depressive disorder and posttraumatic stress disorder. J ECT 26(3):213–217, 2010 20386115
Watts BV, Groft A, Bagian JP, et al: An examination of mortality and other adverse events related to electroconvulsive therapy using a national adverse event report system. J ECT 27(2):105–108, 2011 20966769
Yao Z, McCall WV, Essali N, et al: Precision ECT for major depressive disorder: a review of clinical factors, laboratory, and physiologic biomarkers as predictors of response and remission. Pers Med Psychiatry 17:23–31, 2019
Youssef NA, McCall WV: Relapse prevention after index electroconvulsive therapy in treatment-resistant depression. Ann Clin Psychiatry 26(4):288–296, 2014 25401716
Yrondi A, Sporer M, Péran P, et al: Electroconvulsive therapy, depression, the immune system and inflammation: a systematic review. Brain Stimul 11(1):29–51, 2018 29111078
Zhand N, Courtney DB, Flament MF: Use of electroconvulsive therapy in adolescents with treatment-resistant depressive disorders: a case series. J ECT 31(4):238–245, 2015 25830809

CHAPTER 19

Transcranial Magnetic Stimulation

Andrew M. Fukuda, M.D., Ph.D.
Brian C. Kavanaugh, Psy.D.
Shiwen Yuan, M.D.
Linda L. Carpenter, M.D.

As is evident throughout this textbook, major depressive disorder (MDD) is a debilitating and widespread illness, with 19.4 million adults (18 years or older) in 2019 having at least one major depressive episode in the United States alone, according to the National Institute of Mental Health (NIMH; Substance Abuse and Mental Health Services Administration 2020). Although pharmacotherapy is successfully able to treat many, a substantial portion of those with MDD have limited responses to medications or develop intolerable side effects, so alternative treatment options are necessary.

Transcranial magnetic stimulation (TMS) is a noninvasive method for therapeutic modulation of brain activity. Although it has been increasingly used since 1985 (Barker and Cain 1985; Barker et al. 1985) as a research tool to elucidate certain aspects of brain function, TMS has been further developed and clinically utilized for treating patients with pharmacoresistant forms of MDD. Since the FDA cleared the first TMS device (Neuronetics, Malvern, Pennsylvania; 510[k] number: K083538) to treat MDD in 2008, multiple other devices have received regulatory approval for that same therapeutic indication. In 2018, a TMS device received the first FDA clearance for treatment of patients with obsessive-compulsive disorder (OCD), and a portable TMS device was FDA-cleared for treatment of migraine in 2013. Clinical research continues to explore the potential for TMS to treat a broad array of neuropsychiatric disorders and symptoms related to behavioral health, addiction, and overall wellness. However, the focus of this chapter is the use of TMS for MDD.

What Is Transcranial Magnetic Stimulation Therapy?

Application of TMS requires the delivery of a pulsed magnetic field from a TMS "coil" placed on the patient's head. The coil contains multiple windings of copper wire (or other material that conducts electricity) covered by a hard case and a cooling mechanism of some sort; electricity traveling through the coil in a fluctuating manner generates an electromagnetic field that is emitted from the coil and passes through skin, bone, and other cranial tissues without impedance, subsequently exerting its effects on the targeted regions of superficial cortex several centimeters below the surface. Consistent with Faraday's law of electromagnetic induction, pulsed magnetic fields from the TMS coil induce an electrical current in a perpendicular plane in the underlying tissues, which translates to the firing of neuronal action potentials when the intensity is at a certain threshold.

TMS coils can be constructed with internal windings in various shapes and sizes; most TMS therapy devices use a simple figure-eight-shaped coil, but one manufacturer has a system that uses larger and more complex coil geometries (known as Hesed or H-coils). Figure-eight coils deliver a stimulation that is fairly focal, whereas H-coils activate a broader area of cortex. In stationary TMS device systems such as those approved for MDD, one or more components provide electricity to the coil from a standard power source, and an integrated computer allows the clinician to select parameters for the desired protocol. Some systems include, or are capable of integration with, additional components to enhance their functionality, such as a robotic arm to hold the coil on the patient's head, gauges marking coordinates in multiple planes for frameless stereotaxis, or tracking tools and software to guide placement of the coil to a specific area on the patient's scalp (or MRI-guided navigation to stimulate a specific target in the patient's brain).

Standard commercial TMS devices emit magnetic pulses with a strength similar to that of a standard MRI scanner to patients who are awake and in a seated or reclined position. With each pulse, the person receiving TMS experiences a mild percussive sensation on the head underneath the coil, but this is generally well tolerated, and patients accommodate to it after several sessions (Borckardt et al. 2013). No anesthesia or sedation is required, and patients drive themselves to and from their daily outpatient treatment sessions. Immediate physiological after-effects of a single TMS application last about 30 minutes, but a series of repeated sessions (typically 20–30 over 4–6 weeks) is needed to produce enduring resolution of MDD symptoms.

Clinicians may choose from several parameters for delivering TMS therapy. Some of these parameters relate to the targeted brain region; for MDD, the target is most often the left dorsolateral prefrontal cortex (DLPFC), but evidence also exists for treatment over the right DLPFC or midline areas of the prefrontal cortex (PFC). Other parameters describe the characteristics of the magnetic energy itself—that is, relative intensity (strength of the magnetic field), frequency (number of magnetic pulses delivered per second [Hz]), pulse pattern (e.g., standard "trains" of pulses at 10 Hz vs. very rapid "bursts" or pulses delivered at a 5-Hz "carrier frequency"), and duration of the "rest" times between the strings of TMS pulses. Additional clinically relevant treatment parameters relate to how many total pulses a patient is given in a single session, how often the treatment sessions occur (typically once daily, 5 days per week), and how many treatment weeks compose a standard course of acute therapy for the disorder (typically 4–6 weeks, followed by additional treatments in a taper schedule).

Motor Threshold Procedure

One of the personalized-medicine features of TMS therapy relates to the fact that the intensity of stimulation is individually customized and calibrated against each patient's unique level of cortical excitability. A standard procedure done on the first day of a course of treatment involves finding the exact location on the patient's scalp that corresponds with the underlying spot in that patient's primary motor cortex where stimulation with a single TMS pulse generates the most robust response. With the correct placement, neurons connect, via corticospinal tracts and peripheral nerves, to produce a motor-evoked potential (identified as a visible "twitch" or alternatively by the peak amplitude of an evoked potential as measured by electromyogram) in the muscles of the fingers on the contralateral hand. This location on the scalp, along with the minimum intensity of magnetic energy required to elicit the contralateral muscle response, together define the "motor threshold" (MT).

Finding the MT location and determining the MT level are the first steps in delivery of TMS; application of TMS therapy sessions without this step could adversely impact both safety and efficacy because other treatment parameters are calibrated relative to a patient's MT. Data suggest no significant difference exists between MT levels determined by electromyogram and those determined by visual observation of a muscle twitch (Badran et al. 2019), so most clinical TMS devices rely on the latter method. MT level is the basis for knowing what *intensity of stimulation* is likely to modulate the activity of cortical neurons in a patient's brain. The FDA-cleared MDD treatment protocols involve delivery of TMS at 120% intensity relative to the MT level. This means that the intensity of all magnetic pulses targeting the PFC during a treatment session is 20% higher than the minimal (threshold) intensity needed for a single pulse to activate specific neurons in the patient's motor cortex as determined during the MT procedure on the first day.

The functional MT location on a patient's scalp is also a parameter that may subsequently guide *placement* of the coil on another area of the scalp for treatment of depression. The MT location (defined as the motor cortex location that optimally activated the contralateral thumb muscle or proximal hand muscles) is used by many to navigate the TMS coil to a scalp location (5–6 cm anteriorly in a parasagittal line) over the DLPFC for therapeutic stimulation. Although this method for finding the scalp target for delivery of stimulation to the left DLPFC was employed in all MDD regulatory trials, research has subsequently shown that fixed measurements from the MT location are not consistently reliable for targeting that brain region (Herwig et al. 2001).

Use in Pharmacoresistant Major Depressive Disorder

At present, FDA-cleared TMS devices for MDD are specifically indicated for use in patients whose illness has failed to respond to at least one antidepressant medication trial during the current depressive episode (hereafter referred to as treatment-resistant depression, or TRD). The first FDA clearance (in 2008) for a TMS device (with figure-eight coil) followed a series of regulatory trials by Neuronetics. Results of a large regulatory trial using an H-coil TMS device by BrainsWay (Jerusalem, Israel) generated the second FDA clearance for MDD in 2013. Since then, other device manufacturers have sought and achieved FDA clearance to market their TMS devices in the United States without conducting any new regulatory clinical trials; these approvals have been based on demonstration of technical equivalence to the Neuronetics device—that is, having similar figure-eight coils and stimulation features.

The TMS parameters and protocols for TRD used in the two major industry-sponsored sham-controlled regulatory trials (Neuronetics and BrainsWay) consisted of high-frequency (10 Hz and 18 Hz, respectively) pulses administered in short trains (4 and 2 seconds, respectively) at an intensity that was 120% of the patient's MT, interspersed with rest periods without any stimulation (20 and 26 seconds, respectively). The targeted area of the brain was the left DLPFC, although the broad area covered by the H-coils also delivered some stimulation to the right DLPFC. Treatment sessions were given 5 days per week for 4–6 weeks. Because large samples were used to demonstrate efficacy and safety in randomized, sham-controlled trials that employed rigorous and standardized methods across multiple study sites, these parameters define the "doses" of TMS that are considered to have the strongest evidence base for clinical care.

Numerous other TMS clinical trials investigating different parameters or approaches to TMS therapy have also been published, both before and after the two seminal FDA approvals. Several studies employing alternate designs (e.g., prospective open-label trials, randomized noninferiority trials, naturalistic treatment studies, and meta-analyses of pooled data from multiple smaller studies) provide varying degrees of compelling evidence that it is also safe and efficacious to administer TMS using various different stimulation parameters. Some of these have resulted in revision or extension of the original FDA-approved "labels" and now appear in the official "indication for use" documents associated with individual TMS devices. Results from several key investigations shaping the current evidence base for TMS to treat MDD are summarized in the discussion that follows.

Acute Efficacy

Three double-blinded randomized controlled trials (RCTs) comparing outcomes in groups receiving either active or sham treatments played pivotal roles in the establishment of TMS as an effective acute therapy for MDD. O'Reardon et al. (2007) reported acute-phase results of the Neuronetics-sponsored RCT that took place at 23 international sites (in the United States, Canada, and Australia) and included 301 medication-free patients. Both response and remission rates were significantly higher in the active group (24% response and 17% remission, respectively) compared with the sham-treatment group (15% response and 8% remission, respectively) after 6 weeks of treatment (30 sessions).

Results of a subsequent RCT funded by NIMH and without industry sponsorship was published in 2010 by George et al. (2010). Neuronetics' TMS devices (which have figure-eight-shaped coils) were donated to four university study sites where treatments were delivered using the same stimulation parameters reported by O'Reardon et al. (2007) during the blinded acute phase (n=190). Unique features of this study included a variable-length blinded phase (continuation beyond 3 weeks was contingent on threshold clinical improvement) and brain MRI evaluation to determine whether the position of the coil should be advanced anteriorly by another 1 cm (beyond the spot found, 5 cm anterior to the MT location) to target the left DLPFC. Activation of face and scalp muscles with small electrodes during stimulation trains was a method used to make the sham TMS feel more like active TMS and thus optimize the blinding. The response rate was 15% and remission rate 14% for the group treated with active TMS, whereas only 5% of sham-treated patient outcomes achieved both response and remission. The odds for remitting with active stimulation were 4.2 times greater than for remitting with sham (George et al. 2010).

A third clinical trial of marked importance in establishing TMS clinical efficacy for MDD was the pivotal RCT sponsored by BrainsWay (Levkovitz et al. 2015) using H-coil devices targeting the bilateral (predominantly left, but also right) DLPFCs in 212 patients with TRD at 20 different study sites across four countries. After 4 weeks (20 sessions), all participants transitioned to a schedule of two sessions per week for another 12 weeks, during which they received the same (blinded) active or sham stimulation. Acute-phase response and remission rates at week 5 (after 22 sessions) were significantly higher in the active group (37% and 30%, respectively) than for sham-treated subjects (28% and 16%, respectively). These results supported FDA clearance of the BrainsWay H-coil TMS device for TRD.

Following FDA clearance of the Neuronetics device and its early uptake by clinical practices, a large multisite naturalistic treatment study confirmed similar efficacy for patients with MDD who were treated outside of research protocols with the device (Carpenter et al. 2012). This study reflected "real-life" TMS clinical practice, where most patients are taking one or more antidepressant or other psychotropic medications at the time of referral and remain on concurrent medication during the TMS treatment course. Outcomes for 307 patients (whose treatment costs were supported by their health insurance or through self-pay) across 42 clinics demonstrated that about half (42%–58%, depending on which scale is used) of patients were responders (defined by at least 50% improvement from baseline) and approximately one-third reached the threshold scores for remission (27%–37% across three measures). These findings were largely consistent with other open-label data, such as the crossover phase in the Neuronetics regulatory trial (Avery et al. 2008).

Despite the apparent consistency of positive results across regulatory RCTs and naturalistic and open trials, a recent RCT investigating TMS in 164 U.S. veterans with TRD failed to demonstrate statistical superiority of active stimulation over sham TMS. Following 20–30 sessions (4–6 weeks) of blinded 10-Hz TMS sessions delivered by a figure-eight coil device, remission was achieved by 41% of those randomized to the active group and 37% randomized to the sham group (Yesavage et al. 2018). Comorbid PTSD emerged as a slight moderator of inferior outcomes, but the authors speculated that a high sham response rate in this study was likely attributable to the frequent contact veteran participants had with study personnel and other clinicians who not only monitored their participation in the trial's procedures but also enforced adherence to concurrent psychiatric medications.

The optimal number of TMS sessions or weeks of treatment was not known at the time each regulatory trial commenced, so several studies planned phases to evaluate whether additional TMS treatments (after the fixed number delivered in a blinded acute phase) would bring more patients to the point of response or remission. An open-label extension trial enrolled 77 participants who had not responded to 6 weeks of active TMS in the blinded trial and continued to provide daily (five per week) sessions for up to 6 additional weeks (Avery et al. 2008). Of these patients who had their acute course extended beyond 30 sessions, 32% went on to achieve response and 15% remission with the additional treatments.

An open-label follow-up phase after completion of 3–6 weeks in the blinded phase in the NIMH-funded trial allowed patients to receive additional 10-Hz sessions (over the same left DLPFC target) or several weeks of additional 1-Hz treatments above the *right* DLPFC (McDonald et al. 2011). The final remission rate climbed to 30% after that open phase, again suggesting that optimal outcomes for many patients will require extension of an acute course beyond 3–6 weeks. Data from the continuation phase of the BrainsWay pivotal trial also underscored this point: 61% of nonresponders following 4 weeks (20 sessions) of active TMS were "converted" to responders with 4 more weeks of active treatment delivered on a schedule of two sessions per week (Yip et al. 2017). The "take-home message" from these studies encourages patients and providers to continue with an extension of the acute TMS course when a trajectory of improvement is seen but remission is not achieved at the end of 4–6 weeks.

Maintenance and Retreatment

Although the durability of the positive effect following an acute course of TMS therapy is considered quite good overall, outcomes do vary, and no treatment modality to date offers a permanent cure for MDD. A prospective study followed 99 patients who had significant clinical benefit from their acute course of TMS and were maintained on one antidepressant medication after stopping stimulation (Janicak et al. 2010). Although 38% met criteria for some symptom worsening during the 6-month follow-up period, most improved when TMS was reintroduced, and only 10% of patients relapsed into a new major depressive episode. Naturalistic data from 257 TMS patients followed for 1 year showed that 63% of those who initially responded to TMS maintained their clinically improved state, but 36% of the group had received additional TMS sessions to maintain that status (Dunner et al. 2014). Several studies have shown that those who respond to or remit with their initial course of TMS are likely to respond or remit again when they undergo another acute treatment series initiated at the time of depression relapse (Fitzgerald et al. 2006a; Fukuda et al. 2019; Kelly et al. 2017).

Several approaches to maintenance TMS treatment have been prospectively investigated to prolong the time until subsequent depressive symptom relapse or episode recurrence (Fitzgerald et al. 2016; Haesebaert et al. 2018; Philip et al. 2016a; Wang et al. 2017), including regular or taper treatment schedules, intermittent "clusters" of maintenance TMS treatments, and symptom-triggered thresholds for repeat treatment series. No consensus has yet been found as to the best schedule or strategy for using TMS after finishing an initial acute series; it may be that individually customized scheduling is needed for each patient because some will remain well for a relatively long period of time and others will experience symptom relapse within days or weeks after their final acute-phase treatment series. Emerging evidence suggests that several different maintenance TMS practices are useful for preventing relapse, but more prospective controlled studies are needed to shape formal guidelines for the field.

Safety and Clinical Considerations

A meta-analysis of 29 RCTs of TMS (Berlim et al. 2014) reported dropout rates ranging from 0% to 17.6%, with the exception of one study in which a 45.5% discontinuation rate was seen in a group assigned to unilateral TMS (Blumberger et al. 2012); the events reported for that group were not judged to be side effects from stimulation, per se, or safety issues directly related to TMS. No difference was found between the overall dropout rates for high-frequency TMS treatment (7.5%) and sham treatment (7.6%), suggesting good overall tolerability of treatment with figure-eight coil devices. A meta-analysis of 19 studies comparing antidepressant effects between TMS delivered with H-coils and that with figure-eight coils found comparable treatment outcomes, although dropout rates were somewhat higher in H-coil trials (Gellersen and Kedzior 2019). Theta-burst stimulation (TBS), described in detail later, has shown a comparable safety profile to conventional TMS pattern protocols (Blumberger et al. 2018; Rachid 2017) when delivered with figure-eight coils; serious adverse effects, including seizures, were rare when TBS was delivered over the DLPFC.

Published reports (e.g., Ontario Health [Quality] 2021) and clinical experience have identified adverse effects attributable to TMS; these are typically mild to moderate in severity and transient. Headache (4.5%–60%) can be common, both during and after TMS application, in the early weeks of a course of treatment. A higher MT level (and hence, a greater magnetic pulse intensity and a stronger sensation of percussion on the scalp) is related to a more intense headache. Headache associated with TMS typically resolves with habituation or from the direct analgesic effect of the stimulation (Taylor et al. 2012). Notably, TMS does not increase the risk of migraine in a healthy population or in patients with a history of migraine; on the contrary, single-pulse TMS has been proven to be effective in treating acute migraine (Lipton et al. 2010). Scalp discomfort (4.5%–33% in most clinical trials, 78.9% in one particular trial [Loo et al. 2007]) is also common and may incorporate twitching or superficial muscle movements at or near the location of the TMS delivery site, occasionally extending to facial areas including the ipsilateral eye, ear, nose, or jaw. Nausea and other types of gastrointestinal discomfort have been reported in conjunction with rTMS (5%–22%), although in these studies, a similar rate of nausea and gastrointestinal discomfort was reported in conjunction with sham treatment as well (0%–22%) (Ontario Health [Quality] 2021); however, it is unclear whether events reported in this category are secondary to head pain, anxiety, presyncope, or concurrent medications.

Induction of hypomania has occurred during delivery of high-frequency protocols and is often preceded by treatment-emergent irritability or agitation (Dolberg et al. 2001). Damage to auditory acuity is a risk associated with some coil models when the intensity is set to relatively high settings and the delivery of pulse trains from the coil emits a loud clicking sound; however, this risk is avoided when ear protection (at least 30 dB noise reduction) is worn (U.S. Food and Drug Administration 2011). Skin burn from overheating of TMS coils is a theoretical risk; this is now prevented by FDA regulations that require all coils to have sensors that interrupt stimulation when the coil reaches a preset temperature limit. No evidence has been found of pathological changes in brain tissue resulting from TMS delivered within the established safety ranges (Mutz et al. 2019; Rossi et al. 2009; Wassermann 1998), but unknown risks remain for protocols that utilize stimulation parameters outside evidence-based data.

A vasovagal response associated with anxiety, pain, hypoglycemia, or dehydration may occur in the form of syncope during or after TMS (Wassermann 1998) and should be differentiated from a TMS-induced seizure. Often similar in appearance to seizure, syncope can happen during or after TMS applications and mimics seizure on the basis of diminished consciousness and limb movements (Rossi et al. 2009). Syncope is typically preceded by pallor, dizziness, weakness, visual field changes, and autonomic changes, and it usually resolves rapidly without the classic postictal confusion that occurs following seizures. Induction of seizure during TMS is a rare side effect estimated in 2012 to have a risk of 0.003% per treatment for figure-eight coils (Carpenter et al. 2012); since then, millions of treatments have been delivered safely, and the current seizure risk is likely much lower. A 2018 seizure estimate for TMS delivered by H-coils (which might be expected to carry greater seizure risk based on their large windings and relatively greater volume of current induction in the cortex) was less than 0.001% (Tendler et al. 2018). To date, TMS-associated seizure almost exclusively has occurred in patients with preexisting risks, including heavy alcohol use or withdrawal or concurrent use of seizure threshold–lowering medications (Rossi et al. 2009). The seizure tends to be tonic-clonic when it does occur, due to the direct stimulation of the motor cortex or adjacent areas spreading neuronal excitation. Constant observation of patients during TMS application allows for monitoring of signs (e.g., movement of contralateral hands or limbs during stimulation trains) that might herald the onset of a TMS-induced seizure.

A 2018 consensus report recommended elements of pre-TMS evaluation and informed consent that are crucial to ensure safe treatment (McClintock et al. 2018). A comprehensive review of the patient's medical, surgical, and psychiatric history determines indications for and potential risks and benefits of TMS therapy. Such an evaluation should particularly assess seizure risks and employ screening tools such as the TMS Adult Safety Screen (Keel et al. 2001) to facilitate quantification of risk factors. Accurate localization of the MT site optimizes stimulation amplitude, thus avoiding falsely high pulse intensity for treatment and minimizing side effects. Contraindications to TMS include ferromagnetic metal objects (e.g., medical implants, pacemakers, fragments, nonremovable piercings) in the head and neck areas close to the coil due to risk of heating or to movement of those objects causing damage to the surrounding tissues. Metal objects below the head and neck regions are generally considered safe due to rapid dissipation of the magnetic strength with distance (Deng et al. 2013).

Patients should be hemodynamically stable and comfortably seated in the TMS treatment chair, with sufficient support of their spine and adequate ear protection. Once the treatment session begins, they should be closely monitored. Providers should inspect the patient's contralateral hand for twitching or involuntary movements during a TMS session as a sign of excitation spread to the motor area, to determine the need to abort a treatment session or to make parameter adjustments to decrease risk of possible seizure. Evaluation of changes in sleep and mood, including emergence of irritability or agitation, should be conducted prior to each TMS application. For headaches or scalp discomfort, over-the-counter analgesics can be taken orally or used topically before or after a TMS session to effectively control the symptoms (Trevino et al. 2011). Reducing the intensity of TMS pulses also enhances tolerability, although evidence is limited for antidepressant effects when stimulation intensity is consistently delivered below 110% MT.

Outside of the indicated populations, the safe therapeutic use and clinical benefit of TMS have been suggested in preliminary studies of adolescents with depression (Donaldson et al. 2014; Wall et al. 2011), women with perinatal depression (Kim et al. 2011), and patients with geriatric depression (Sabesan et al. 2015), bipolar disorder depression (Yatham et al. 2018), or PTSD comorbid with MDD (Philip et al. 2016b).

Cost-Effectiveness

The cost of a standard outpatient acute TMS series (20–40 sessions) to treat MDD ranges from about $8,000 to $20,000 and remains less costly than a standard course of electroconvulsive therapy. Analyses have shown that TMS is cost-effective for TRD (Nguyen and Gordon 2015; Simpson et al. 2009) and non-treatment-resistant depression (Voigt et al. 2017).

Alternative Protocols for Major Depressive Disorder

When designing the first therapeutic TMS protocols for MDD, researchers selected high-frequency (5–25 Hz) stimulation targeting the left DLPFC on the basis of previously published imagining results showing that depressed patients showed decreased activity in that region, hyperactivity of the right DLPFC (George et al. 1994), and lateralized cognitive function abnormalities (Grimm et al. 2008) relative to healthy control subjects. Early TMS experiments identified opposite neuromodulatory effects of high- versus low-frequency TMS on excitability of cortical neurons in the motor cortex (Pascual-Leone et al. 1994), and high-frequency stimulation to the left DLPFC was hypothesized to reduce MDD symptoms by addressing a regional deficit in that hemisphere (George et al. 1995). Other parameters and cortical TMS targets have also been investigated for MDD; notable among them are protocols that deliver low-frequency (1 Hz) TMS to the right DLPFC (Berlim et al. 2013a), which was hypothesized to dampen excessive activity in the right hemisphere and was found to be better tolerated than high-frequency stimulation (Feinsod et al. 1998). Subsequent studies evaluated the potential utility of combining both high-frequency TMS on the left side and low-frequency on the right side with sequential-bilateral stimulation protocols (Berlim et al. 2013b; Fitzgerald et al. 2006b). Efficacy of all three protocols (high-frequency on left, low-frequency on right, and sequential bilateral) is superior to sham stimulation, and they appear to produce similar response rates (Berlim et al. 2013a; Chen et al. 2013, 2014).

"Accelerated" TMS protocols have applied multiple sessions per day to hasten the antidepressant effect (Sonmez et al. 2019); pilot studies have shown rates of success comparable with those of standard, once-daily session approaches, but prospective data showing superiority of accelerated TMS schedules are currently lacking. TMS treatments on a once-daily schedule (typically five per week on weekdays) define the standard of care at present.

TBS is a type of TMS pulse pattern originally inspired by observations of neuronal firing during rodent exploration behaviors in preclinical studies. Complex spike patterns were modeled by "bursts" of TMS pulses applied at a high frequency (50 Hz, or within the gamma frequency band of 30–60 Hz) and repeated approximately every 20 ms (5 Hz, mimicking the endogenous theta band rhythm). Theta-burst-patterned transcranial stimulation was adapted to human protocols, where it was found to promote superior brain plasticity compared with conventional TMS pulses (Suppa et al. 2016).

Experiments using intermittent TBS delivered at subthreshold intensity (i.e., 80% MT) were successful for inducing an *excitatory effect* on neurons when delivered in protocols containing short (2-second) trains of bursts following 10 seconds of rest (Huang et al. 2005). Continuous TBS protocols with an 80% MT intensity were likewise found to induce an *inhibitory effect* on the motor cortex when administered as a single, uninterrupted train of magnetic bursts (Di Lazzaro et al. 2011). Superior neuronal plasticity effects produced by TBS, compared with conventional TMS, eventually led to clinical investigations wherein TBS protocols were investigated as an alternative to conventional TMS therapy for the treatment of MDD. Several pilot studies investigating intermittent TBS over the left DLPFC for MDD demonstrated efficacy that was superior to sham (see the meta-analysis by Berlim et al. 2017), raising the exciting possibility that efficacy equivalent to that of the 37-minute standard session could be achieved with a TMS protocol duration of less than 4 minutes.

Ultimately, a large, randomized noninferiority trial was conducted at three Canadian sites in an open-label study comparing the outcomes of 4–6 weeks of standard 10-Hz stimulation with an intermittent TBS protocol using the Magventure figure-eight coil device. This study enrolled and randomly assigned 414 patients with MDD who were on stable concurrent antidepressants and other psychotropic medications (Blumberger et al. 2018). Unlike prior studies, the intermittent TBS was delivered at 120% MT in this trial, resulting in patient-rated pain ratings that were significantly higher than those for the 10-Hz stimulation condition. However, antidepressant efficacy was equivalent between intermittent TBS (which provided a therapeutic dose in 3 minutes) and 10-Hz stimulation (in which each session lasts 37.5 minutes), and the dropout rate did not differ between the two protocols. These results supported FDA clearance of intermittent TBS parameters for the Magventure device and several other devices that have established technical equivalence since then.

Several TMS devices now have FDA clearance for MDD treatment, and all are capable of delivering multiple different stimulation protocols. Although the original high-frequency left-sided protocols are currently the most commonly utilized as a result of strong evidence from multiple published RCTs, ongoing research into alternatives will continue to advance the field and define future standards.

Potential Mechanisms of Therapeutic Action

Multiple lines of research inform our understanding of how TMS works to relieve depression. Application of TMS transiently entrains cortical oscillatory rhythms (Brignani et al. 2008; Johnson et al. 2010) and subsequently modulates oscillatory rhythms (Ding et al. 2014; Fuggetta and Noh 2003) as measured by electroencephalogram. Interleaved imaging with TMS applied to the PFC shows it immediately induces activation in subcortical limbic regions directly beneath the coil (Li et al. 2004). Other studies have demonstrated the TMS-associated production of brain-derived neurotrophic factor (BDNF) and cellular proliferation in the hippocampus (Wang et al. 2014), as well as posttreatment increases in gray matter volume (Lan et al. 2016). This aligns with a study by Oliveira-Maia et al. (2017) suggesting that a pretreatment measure of brain plasticity in the motor cortex can predict who will respond clinically to TMS over the left DLPFC.

Neural network dysfunction has been hypothesized to be associated with MDD. A meta-analysis of resting-state functional MRI (fMRI) data showed specific abnormalities in brain connectivity in MDD (Kaiser et al. 2015), particularly hypoconnectivity with the frontoparietal network (FPN), whose key function is cognitive control or "top-down" regulation. Hypoconnectivity between the FPN and dorsal attention network (involved in externally oriented attention) is another prominent finding, along with hyperconnectivity within the default mode network (DMN; involved in internally oriented attention) and hyperconnectivity between the FPN and DMN. Similar regional deficits have been identified in structural imaging studies, such as increased cortical thickness in DMN structures and decreased cortical thickness in frontal and temporal regions (Li et al. 2020).

In recent years, a number of studies have obtained functional MRI or electroencephalographic data before and after a clinical course of TMS for MDD to identify neurobiological markers or mechanisms of its antidepressant effects. A universal mechanism for the therapeutic action in MDD has yet to be identified, perhaps in part due to the significant methodological variability of published studies, including various statistical/data analyses (e.g., regions vs. networks; positive vs. negative or anticorrelations), various modalities of brain assessment, a range of TMS parameters, and diverse stimulation targets. An emerging pattern of neuroimaging findings has been described in published reviews (Anderson et al. 2016; Philip et al. 2018; Taib et al. 2018).

With regard to regional changes observed following a standard course of TMS therapy, a review by Taib et al. (2018) identified alterations in a range of frontotemporoparietal and subcortical brain regions: the subgenual anterior cingulate cortex, perigenual anterior cingulate cortex, superior medial frontal gyrus, DLPFC, dorsomedial PFC, bilateral middle frontal gyri, left precuneus, hippocampus, thalami, putamen, parietal lobes, insula, right orbitofrontal cortex, and middle temporal cortex. With regard to network-specific findings, changes in the DMN, including activity increases and its connectivity to other networks, have been one of the most consistent findings; alterations in the FPN and salience network have also been noted (Anderson et al. 2016; Philip et al. 2018). Researchers have at times noted a surprising lack of findings in the FPN, given that the left DLPFC is a common site of TMS application and is also a hub of that network (Philip et al. 2018).

Additional work has sought to identify specific neurobiological predictors of clinical response to TMS, particularly within the context of the significant clinical heterogeneity found in MDD. One large-scale functional MRI study identified four neurophysiological "biotypes" of depression based on distinct patterns of dysfunctional connectivity (Drysdale et al. 2017). Although 82.5% of patients with "biotype 1" experienced (>25%) symptom improvement after TMS, only 61% with biotype 2 improved, and less than 30% of patients characterized by biotype 3 or 4 improved. Clinical symptoms did not predict treatment response, but the authors found that patterns of connectivity between the dorsomedial PFC (stimulation site) and the left amygdala, left DLPFC, bilateral orbitofrontal cortex, and posterior cingulate cortex did predict outcome with 78.3% accuracy.

Of particular relevance to TMS, Padmanabhan et al. (2019) investigated whether the location of the brain lesion in patients who had had a stroke was associated with the presence of poststroke depression. Although no single region uniformly led to depression, all lesions that did lead to depression mapped onto the left DLPFC–related brain circuit, highlighting the potential importance of the left DLPFC as a target for TMS administration and its relevance to subsequent clinical response. In a related study by Weigand et al. (2018), connectivity from the stimulation target (location under the TMS coil) to the subgenual cingulate region was examined as a function of clinical TMS outcome. Stimulation sites that were more anterolateral and those that were negatively correlated with the subgenual cingulate were both associated with a better TMS treatment response, but only the subgenual cingulate correlation persisted as a significant predictor in a replication cohort. Notably, the subgenual cingulate correlation predicted improvement in cognitive and affective symptoms of MDD but not somatic symptoms.

Conclusion

TMS therapy was first introduced into psychiatric practice following the 2008 FDA clearance of the first device to treat MDD. Since then, it has become a standard of care for TRD, with numerous clinical studies confirming its efficacy and safety. The field has evolved with regard to our understanding of TMS's effects and mechanisms, and recent exciting work suggests further potential for optimizing TMS outcomes with the discovery of new biomarkers and application of a personalized medicine approach. TMS therapy has not replaced electroconvulsive therapy but, rather, offers another option for adult outpatients with MDD who are not benefiting from standard antidepressant interventions such as pharmacotherapy and psychotherapy.

References

Anderson RJ, Hoy KE, Daskalakis ZJ, et al: Repetitive transcranial magnetic stimulation for treatment resistant depression: re-establishing connections. Clin Neurophysiol 127(11):3394–3405, 2016 27672727

Avery DH, Isenberg KE, Sampson SM, et al: Transcranial magnetic stimulation in the acute treatment of major depressive disorder: clinical response in an open-label extension trial. J Clin Psychiatry 69(3):441–451, 2008 18294022

Badran BW, Ly M, DeVries WH, et al: Are EMG and visual observation comparable in determining resting motor threshold? A reexamination after twenty years. Brain Stimul 12(2):364–366, 2019 30448078

Barker AT, Cain MW: The claimed vasodilatory effect of a commercial permanent magnet foil: results of a double-blind trial. Clin Phys Physiol Meas 6(3):261–263, 1985 4042555

Barker AT, Jalinous R, Freeston IL: Non-invasive magnetic stimulation of human motor cortex. Lancet 1(8437):1106–1107, 1985 2860322

Berlim MT, Van den Eynde F, Daskalakis ZJ: Clinically meaningful efficacy and acceptability of low-frequency repetitive transcranial magnetic stimulation (rTMS) for treating primary major depression: a meta-analysis of randomized, double-blind and sham-controlled trials. Neuropsychopharmacology 38(4):543–551, 2013a 23249815

Berlim MT, Van den Eynde F, Daskalakis ZJ: High-frequency repetitive transcranial magnetic stimulation accelerates and enhances the clinical response to antidepressants in major depression: a meta-analysis of randomized, double-blind, and sham-controlled trials. J Clin Psychiatry 74(2):e122–e129, 2013b 23473357

Berlim MT, van den Eynde F, Tovar-Perdomo S, et al: Response, remission and drop-out rates following high-frequency repetitive transcranial magnetic stimulation (rTMS) for treating major depression: a systematic review and meta-analysis of randomized, double-blind and sham-controlled trials. Psychol Med 44(2):225–239, 2014 23507264

Berlim MT, McGirr A, Rodrigues Dos Santos N, et al: Efficacy of theta burst stimulation (TBS) for major depression: an exploratory meta-analysis of randomized and sham-controlled trials. J Psychiatr Res 90:102–109, 2017 28254709

Blumberger DM, Mulsant BH, Fitzgerald PB, et al: A randomized double-blind sham-controlled comparison of unilateral and bilateral repetitive transcranial magnetic stimulation for treatment-resistant major depression. World J Biol Psychiatry 13(6):423–435, 2012 21736507

Blumberger DM, Vila-Rodriguez F, Thorpe KE, et al: Effectiveness of theta burst versus high-frequency repetitive transcranial magnetic stimulation in patients with depression (THREE-D): a randomised non-inferiority trial. Lancet 391(10131):1683–1692, 2018 29726344

Borckardt JJ, Nahas ZH, Teal J, et al: The painfulness of active, but not sham, transcranial magnetic stimulation decreases rapidly over time: results from the double-blind phase of the OPT-TMS trial. Brain Stimul 6(6):925–928, 2013 23769413

Brignani D, Manganotti P, Rossini PM, et al: Modulation of cortical oscillatory activity during transcranial magnetic stimulation. Hum Brain Mapp 29(5):603–612, 2008 17557296

Carpenter LL, Janicak PG, Aaronson ST, et al: Transcranial magnetic stimulation (TMS) for major depression: a multisite, naturalistic, observational study of acute treatment outcomes in clinical practice. Depress Anxiety 29(7):587–596, 2012 22689344

Chen J, Zhou C, Wu B, et al: Left versus right repetitive transcranial magnetic stimulation in treating major depression: a meta-analysis of randomised controlled trials. Psychiatry Res 210(3):1260–1264, 2013 24113125

Chen JJ, Liu Z, Zhu D, et al: Bilateral vs. unilateral repetitive transcranial magnetic stimulation in treating major depression: a meta-analysis of randomized controlled trials. Psychiatry Res 219(1):51–57, 2014 24889845

Deng ZD, Lisanby SH, Peterchev AV: Electric field depth-focality tradeoff in transcranial magnetic stimulation: simulation comparison of 50 coil designs. Brain Stimul 6(1):1–13, 2013 22483681

Di Lazzaro V, Dileone M, Pilato F, et al: Modulation of motor cortex neuronal networks by rTMS: comparison of local and remote effects of six different protocols of stimulation. J Neurophysiol 105(5):2150–2156, 2011 21346213

Ding L, Shou G, Yuan H, et al: Lasting modulation effects of rTMS on neural activity and connectivity as revealed by resting-state EEG. IEEE Trans Biomed Eng 61(7):2070–2080, 2014 24686227

Dolberg OT, Schreiber S, Grunhaus L: Transcranial magnetic stimulation-induced switch into mania: a report of two cases. Biol Psychiatry 49(5):468–470, 2001 11274660

Donaldson AE, Gordon MS, Melvin GA, et al: Addressing the needs of adolescents with treatment resistant depressive disorders: a systematic review of rTMS. Brain Stimul 7(1):7–12, 2014 24527502

Drysdale AT, Grosenick L, Downar J, et al: Resting-state connectivity biomarkers define neurophysiological subtypes of depression. Nat Med 23(1):28–38, 2017 27918562

Dunner DL, Aaronson ST, Sackeim HA, et al: A multisite, naturalistic, observational study of transcranial magnetic stimulation for patients with pharmacoresistant major depressive disorder: durability of benefit over a 1-year follow-up period. J Clin Psychiatry 75(12):1394–1401, 2014 25271871

Feinsod M, Kreinin B, Chistyakov A, et al: Preliminary evidence for a beneficial effect of low-frequency, repetitive transcranial magnetic stimulation in patients with major depression and schizophrenia. Depress Anxiety 7(2):65–68, 1998 9614593

Fitzgerald PB, Benitez J, de Castella AR, et al: Naturalistic study of the use of transcranial magnetic stimulation in the treatment of depressive relapse. Aust N Z J Psychiatry 40(9):764–768, 2006a 16911751

Fitzgerald PB, Benitez J, de Castella A, et al: A randomized, controlled trial of sequential bilateral repetitive transcranial magnetic stimulation for treatment-resistant depression. Am J Psychiatry 163(1):88–94, 2006b 16390894

Fitzgerald PB, Hoy KE, Anderson RJ, et al: A study of the pattern of response to rTMS treatment in depression. Depress Anxiety 33(8):746–753, 2016 27059158

Fuggetta G, Noh NA: A neurophysiological insight into the potential link between transcranial magnetic stimulation, thalamocortical dysrhythmia and neuropsychiatric disorders. Exp Neurol 245:87–95, 2013 23063603

Fukuda AM, Tirrell E, Gobin AP, et al: Repetitive transcranial magnetic stimulation for depression relapse or recurrence: naturalistic retreatment series outcomes. Brain Stimul 12(5):1328–1329, 2019 31266723

Gellersen HM, Kedzior KK: Antidepressant outcomes of high-frequency repetitive transcranial magnetic stimulation (rTMS) with F8-coil and deep transcranial magnetic stimulation (DTMS) with H1-coil in major depression: a systematic review and meta-analysis. BMC Psychiatry 19(1):139, 2019 31064328

George MS, Ketter TS, Post RM: Prefrontal cortex dysfunction in clinical depression. Depression 2(2):59–72, 1994

George MS, Wassermann EM, Williams WA, et al: Daily repetitive transcranial magnetic stimulation (rTMS) improves mood in depression. Neuroreport 6(14):1853–1856, 1995 8547583

George MS, Lisanby SH, Avery D, et al: Daily left prefrontal transcranial magnetic stimulation therapy for major depressive disorder: a sham-controlled randomized trial. Arch Gen Psychiatry 67(5):507–516, 2010 20439832

Grimm S, Beck J, Schuepbach D, et al: Imbalance between left and right dorsolateral prefrontal cortex in major depression is linked to negative emotional judgment: an fMRI study in severe major depressive disorder. Biol Psychiatry 63(4):369–376, 2008 17888408

Haesebaert F, Moirand R, Schott-Pethelaz AM, et al: Usefulness of repetitive transcranial magnetic stimulation as a maintenance treatment in patients with major depression. World J Biol Psychiatry 19(1):74–78, 2018 27807990

Herwig U, Padberg F, Unger J, et al: Transcranial magnetic stimulation in therapy studies: examination of the reliability of "standard" coil positioning by neuronavigation. Biol Psychiatry 50(1):58–61, 2001 11457424

Huang YZ, Edwards MJ, Rounis E, et al: Theta burst stimulation of the human motor cortex. Neuron 45(2):201–206, 2005 15664172

Janicak PG, Nahas Z, Lisanby SH, et al: Durability of clinical benefit with transcranial magnetic stimulation (TMS) in the treatment of pharmacoresistant major depression: assessment of relapse during a 6-month, multisite, open-label study. Brain Stimul 3(4):187–199, 2010 20965447

Johnson JS, Hamidi M, Postle BR: Using EEG to explore how rTMS produces its effects on behavior. Brain Topogr 22(4):281–293, 2010 19915972

Kaiser RH, Andrews-Hanna JR, Wager TD, et al: Large-scale network dysfunction in major depressive disorder: a meta-analysis of resting-state functional connectivity. JAMA Psychiatry 72(6):603–611, 2015 25785575

Keel JC, Smith MJ, Wassermann EM: A safety screening questionnaire for transcranial magnetic stimulation. Clin Neurophysiol 112(4):720, 2001 11332408

Kelly MS, Oliveira-Maia AJ, Bernstein M, et al: Initial response to transcranial magnetic stimulation treatment for depression predicts subsequent response. J Neuropsychiatry Clin Neurosci 29(2):179–182, 2017 27899052

Kim DR, Epperson N, Paré E, et al: An open label pilot study of transcranial magnetic stimulation for pregnant women with major depressive disorder. J Womens Health (Larchmt) 20(2):255–261, 2011 21314450

Lan MJ, Chhetry BT, Liston C, et al: Transcranial magnetic stimulation of left dorsolateral prefrontal cortex induces brain morphological changes in regions associated with a treatment resistant major depressive episode: an exploratory analysis. Brain Stimul 9(4):577–583, 2016 27017072

Levkovitz Y, Isserles M, Padberg F, et al: Efficacy and safety of deep transcranial magnetic stimulation for major depression: a prospective multicenter randomized controlled trial. World Psychiatry 14(1):64–73, 2015 25655160

Li Q, Zhao Y, Chen Z, et al: Meta-analysis of cortical thickness abnormalities in medication-free patients with major depressive disorder. Neuropsychopharmacology 45(4):703–712, 2020 31694045

Li X, Tenebäck CC, Nahas Z, et al: Interleaved transcranial magnetic stimulation/functional MRI confirms that lamotrigine inhibits cortical excitability in healthy young men. Neuropsychopharmacology 29(7):1395–1407, 2004 15100699

Lipton RB, Dodick DW, Silberstein SD, et al: Single-pulse transcranial magnetic stimulation for acute treatment of migraine with aura: a randomised, double-blind, parallel-group, sham-controlled trial. Lancet Neurol 9(4):373–380, 2010 20206581

Loo CK, Mitchell PB, McFarquhar TF, et al: A sham-controlled trial of the efficacy and safety of twice-daily rTMS in major depression. Psychol Med 37(3):341–349, 2007 17176505

McClintock SM, Reti IM, Carpenter LL, et al: Consensus recommendations for the clinical application of repetitive transcranial magnetic stimulation (rTMS) in the treatment of depression. J Clin Psychiatry 79(1):16cs10905, 2018 28541649

McDonald WM, Durkalski V, Ball ER, et al: Improving the antidepressant efficacy of transcranial magnetic stimulation: maximizing the number of stimulations and treatment location in treatment-resistant depression. Depress Anxiety 28(11):973–980, 2011 21898711

Mutz J, Vipulananthan V, Carter B, et al: Comparative efficacy and acceptability of non-surgical brain stimulation for the acute treatment of major depressive episodes in adults: systematic review and network meta-analysis. BMJ 364:l1079, 2019 30917990

Nguyen KH, Gordon LG: Cost-effectiveness of repetitive transcranial magnetic stimulation versus antidepressant therapy for treatment-resistant depression. Value Health 18(5):597–604, 2015 26297087

Oliveira-Maia AJ, Press D, Pascual-Leone A: Modulation of motor cortex excitability predicts antidepressant response to prefrontal cortex repetitive transcranial magnetic stimulation. Brain Stimul 10(4):787–794, 2017 28438543

Ontario Health (Quality): Repetitive transcranial magnetic stimulation for people with treatment-resistant depression: a health technology assessment. Ont Health Technol Assess Ser 21(4):1–232, 2021 34055112

O'Reardon JP, Solvason HB, Janicak PG, et al: Efficacy and safety of transcranial magnetic stimulation in the acute treatment of major depression: a multisite randomized controlled trial. Biol Psychiatry 62(11):1208–1216, 2007 17573044

Padmanabhan JL, Cooke D, Joutsa J, et al: A human depression circuit derived from focal brain lesions. Biol Psychiatry 86(10):749–758, 2019 31561861

Pascual-Leone A, Valls-Solé J, Wassermann EM, et al: Responses to rapid-rate transcranial magnetic stimulation of the human motor cortex. Brain 117(Pt 4):847–858, 1994 7922470

et al. 2008; Nemeroff et al. 2006). Additionally, patients who responded to ECT previously had a higher cumulative VNS response rate than those who did not respond to ECT, supporting the idea of ECT response as predictor for VNS response (Aaronson et al. 2017). However, VNS appears to be more efficient in patients with low to moderate but not extreme antidepressant resistance, and patients who had never received ECT were 3.9 times more likely to respond to VNS (Daban et al. 2008).

Overall, predictors of response have not been well examined. Yet one of the first symptoms to be ameliorated following onset of VNS concerns sleep disturbances. Improvement of sleep architecture may be predictive of an antidepressant effect and should be investigated in detail in future studies (Armitage et al. 2003).

In conclusion, the first studies may have been underdosed, considering the current recommendations of stimulation intensities greater than 1 mA (Daban et al. 2008), and RCTs with a double-blind, sham-controlled design are difficult to create due to common adverse events associated with VNS—mainly voice alterations and increased cough (Martin and Martín-Sánchez 2012; Schlaepfer et al. 2008b). Long-term naturalistic observational studies are urgently needed for a better evaluation of the antidepressant efficacy of VNS. Also, it is questionable that VNS has not found an uptake in general treatment and that reimbursement for the psychiatric use of VNS is lacking. The current RESTORE-LIFE study (ClinicalTrials.gov Identifier NCT03320304) may help address those questions.

Deep Brain Stimulation

DBS involves a permanent or intermittent electrical stimulation of a specific brain area. In a stereotactic surgical procedure, electrodes are implanted permanently in previously defined target areas. A transcutaneously programmable pulse generator, placed subcutaneously in the clavicular region, sends electric impulses to these electrodes (Figure 20–2). Typical parameter settings are frequencies between 90 Hz and 130 Hz, pulse widths of about 90 µs, and voltages between 4 V and 8 V (Schlaepfer and Bewernick 2013). Compared with ablative neurosurgical interventions, DBS is less invasive and mostly reversible, and its features are adjustable, allowing clinicians to maximize treatment benefit and minimize adverse events individually, as well as allowing sham-controlled hypothesis testing (Lozano et al. 2019; Schlaepfer et al. 2014).

History

Although the first attempts at electric brain stimulation and recording via intracerebral implantation of electrodes for psychiatric treatment purposes were made in the 1950s (Hariz et al. 2010), it was several decades later that a Grenoble group established modern DBS by introducing permanent electrical stimulation as an addition to thalamotomy for the treatment of extrapyramidal movement disorders in 1987 (Benabid et al. 1987). By 1994, the first patient with Parkinson's disease had been treated with DBS solely, resulting in an immense tremor reduction (Benabid et al. 1994). Since then, DBS has become a standard treatment for movement disorders, especially Parkinson's disease, and more than 150,000 patients have been treated with DBS (Medtronic 2017).

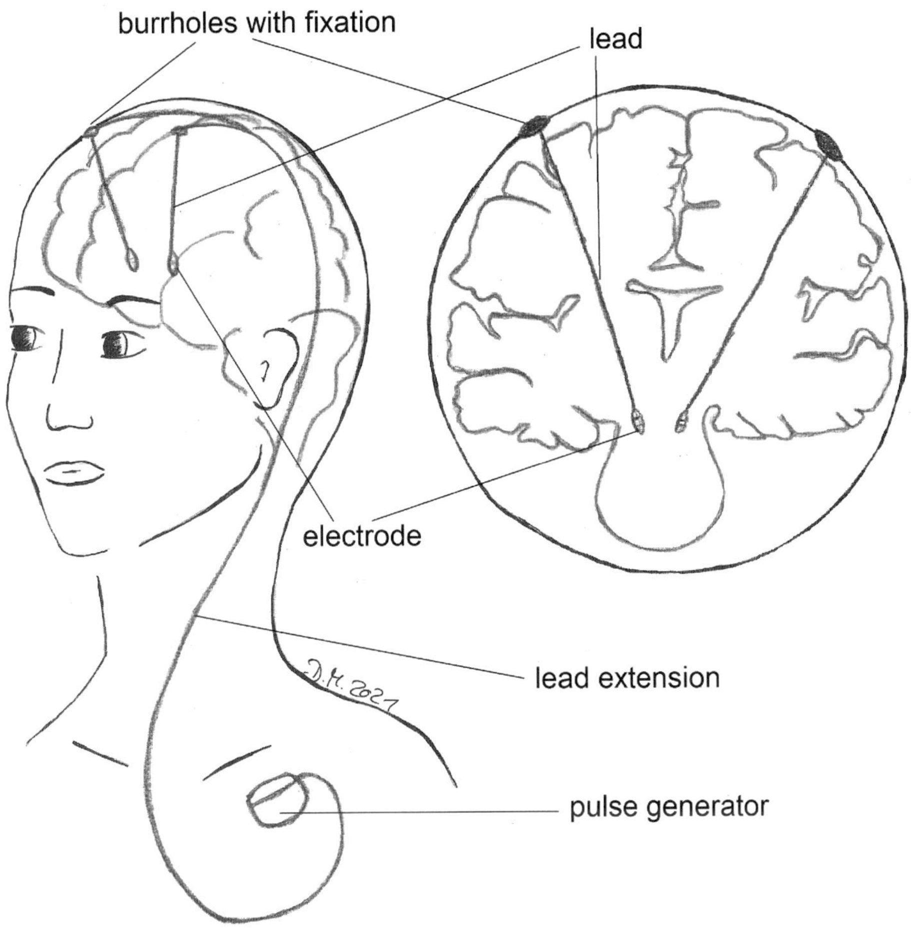

FIGURE 20–2. Schematic structure of a deep brain stimulation system.
To view this figure in color, see Plate 7 in Color Gallery in middle of book.
Source. Dora Meyer, 2021.

In Germany alone, about 800 new implantations have been counted annually since 2014, with a peak of about 1,000 in 2019 (Gemeinsamer-Bundesausschus 2021).

In 1999, DBS was successfully used for treatment of a psychiatric disorder, obsessive-compulsive disorder (OCD), for the first time (Nuttin et al. 1999). In an attempt to replace irreversible capsulotomy with DBS, the authors chose to stimulate the anterior limb of the internal capsule (ALIC), a target that had been used for capsulotomy previously. Inspired by their promising results, several research groups followed and demonstrated that electrical stimulation of different brain targets is associated with a remarkable reduction of obsessive and compulsive symptoms (Borders et al. 2018). Besides the subthalamic nucleus and nucleus accumbens, which have been proven effective in RCTs (Denys et al. 2010; Mallet et al. 2008), the superolateral branch of the medial forebrain bundle seems to be a promising new target in DBS for OCD (Coenen et al. 2017; Meyer et al. 2019), although RCTs are still pending. DBS for treatment-resistant OCD is approved by the FDA according to the Humanitarian Device Exemption (U.S. Food and Drug Administration 2020).

Development

Since about the turn of the century, DBS has also been under investigation for the treatment of treatment-resistant depression (TRD). Although it is approved for OCD, DBS is not yet approved for TRD therapy by the FDA. As outlined in the introduction to this chapter, depression is now conceptualized as a complex brain disorder involving several key brain circuits. Therefore, various potential structures within these circuits are under investigation as DBS targets for TRD (Drobisz and Damborská 2019). The following targets have been studied most thoroughly (Döbrössy et al. 2021; Figure 20–3): subgenual cingulate gyrus (SCG), capsular targets (ALIC and ventral capsule/ventral striatum [VC/VS]), nucleus accumbens, and superolateral medial forebrain bundle (slMFB).

Subgenual Cingulate Gyrus

Converging findings from clinical, anatomical, neurochemical, and functional imaging studies of depression, as well as studies using induced sadness in healthy subjects, resulted in a neuroanatomical model that describes depression as a "failure of the coordinated interactions of a distributed network of limbic-cortical pathways" (Mayberg 1997, p. 471). The SCG (also area Cg25 or Brodmann area 25) is highlighted as a switching point in this network. The prominent position of the SCG led to the hypothesis that high-frequency electrical stimulation of this area could result in a decrease in depressive symptoms by decreasing SCG activity. The first positive results with open-label stimulation (Mayberg et al. 2005) promoted further research on the neuropathology and optimal stimulation target for treatment purposes.

Capsular Targets: Anterior Limb of the Internal Capsule and Ventral Capsule/Ventral Striatum

Unlike the SCG, the ALIC and VC/VS were chosen mainly based on clinical observations. Both targets form part of the striatum, which is involved in the cortico-striato-thalamo-cortical (CSTC) network, seen as highly relevant in the pathophysiology of OCD (Alexander et al. 1986; Karas et al. 2019). The VC/VS contains the ventral half of the ALIC and impinges inferiorly on the VS (Greenberg et al. 2006). Due to their extreme spatial and functional proximity, the ALIC and VC/VS are summarized as capsular targets. Ablative procedures in the CSTC network have led to improvements in OCD and in TRD in about 35%–70% of treated patients (Greenberg et al. 2003). In addition to ablative procedures, DBS applied to CSTC targets has also improved OCD symptoms (Alonso et al. 2015; Blomstedt et al. 2013). In two trials intending to treat treatment-resistant OCD using DBS applied to the capsular targets, not only was a decrease in OCD symptoms reported, but also a decrease in depressive symptoms (Greenberg et al. 2006; Nuttin et al. 2003). These observations, along with the antidepressant effects of ablative procedures, led to the first study on VC/VS stimulation in TRD (Malone et al. 2009).

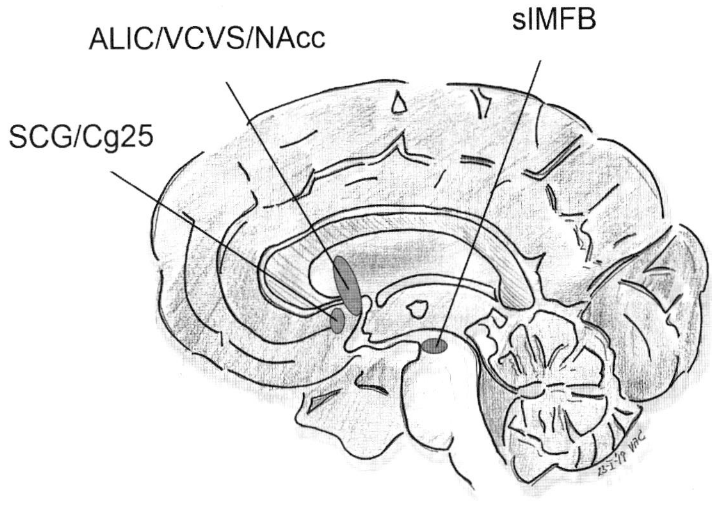

FIGURE 20–3. Experimental targets for deep brain stimulation in treatment-resistant depression.

To view this figure in color, see Plate 8 in Color Gallery in middle of book.

ALIC=anterior limb of the internal capsule; CG25=Brodmann area 25; NAcc=nucleus accumbens; SCG=subgenual cingulate gyrus; sIMFB=superolateral branch of the medial forebrain bundle; VCVS=ventral capsule/ventral striatum.

Source. Adapted from Figure 2 (Volker A. Coenen, 2019; p. 92) in Döbrössy M, Ramanathan C, Ashouri Vajari D, et al.: "Neuromodulation in Psychiatric Disorders: Experimental and Clinical Evidence for Reward and Motivation Network Deep Brain Stimulation: Focus on the Medial Forebrain Bundle." *European Journal of Neuroscience* 53(1):89–113, 2021. Available at: https://onlinelibrary.wiley.com/doi/10.1111/ejn.14975. Accessed October 26, 2021. Copyright © 2020, The Authors, used under the terms of the Creative Commons Attribution License.

Nucleus Accumbens

The nucleus accumbens forms part of the VS and is therefore located very close to the capsular stimulation targets. It is highly involved in processing reward and pleasure information: neuronal activity and dopamine release increase in the nucleus accumbens during expectation and experience of rewards (Adinoff 2004; Doyon et al. 2005; Schultz 2004), and increased VS activity is associated with induced euphoria (Aharon et al. 2001; Drevets et al. 2001; Knutson et al. 2001). A translational study found that long-term administration of an antidepressant could re-regulate activity of the nucleus accumbens in socially stressed mice (Berton et al. 2006). Based on these findings, it has been proposed that anhedonia—a key symptom of depression (American Psychiatric Association 2013)—represents a lack of reward-motivated behavior and is related to activity in the nucleus accumbens (Schlaepfer et al. 2008a). On a neuroanatomical level, the nucleus accumbens is interconnected with other brain areas involved in emotion processing, including the DBS target SCG, described earlier (Hamani et al. 2009; Vergani et al. 2016). It has therefore been concluded that stimulating the nucleus accumbens would result in modulation of other parts of emotion-related networks as well and would decrease anhedonia (Schlaepfer et al. 2008a).

Superolateral Branch of the Medial Forebrain Bundle

Similar to the nucleus accumbens, the medial forebrain bundle is highly associated with reward processing. It is located at the center of a distributed network that is considered the neural substrate of the reward circuitry and has been studied thoroughly in rodents (Wise 22005). This system—among others—is engaged in predicting and computing rewards, initiating exploration, and eliciting hedonic consummatory behavior (Carlezon and Chartoff 2007; Waraczynski 2006). Although well known in rodents, it was not until 2009 that the full structure of this network was visualized in humans (Coenen et al. 2009). Using diffusion tensor imaging, a procedure based on MRI analysis that allows imaging of fiber connections based on the anisotropy of the brain tissue, it has been shown that the human medial forebrain bundle originates in the ventral tegmental area and then splits into a lower and a superolateral branch.

The slMFB is of particular interest for DBS because of its neuroanatomical structure. The superolateral branch "shears out laterally, under-crosses the thalamus and ascends to the interior portion of the anterior limb of the internal capsule (ALIC)" (Coenen et al. 2011, p. 1974). The slMFB also accesses the ventral striatum and the nucleus accumbens directly, whereas direct connections with the white matter tracts surrounding the SCG are seen inconsistently (Coenen et al. 2011). This neuroanatomical description demonstrates the connecting position of the slMFB with the targets described earlier. In a diffusion tensor imaging study of healthy subjects, it was demonstrated that the historically most commonly chosen lesion targets for depression treatment are actually interconnected by fiber tracts that are mainly part of the slMFB (Schoene-Bake et al. 2010). In retrospect, this means that although these targets might have been selected for other reasons originally, the efficacy of the described DBS targets in TRD is best explained by their shared involvement in the reward system. Because the slMFB is a central connecting element in this system, it has been promoted as a stimulation target in itself (Coenen et al. 2011; Schlaepfer et al. 2014).

State of the Art

Table 20–A in the Appendix shows all published studies we know of that involved stimulation of the DBS targets described earlier for the treatment of TRD and included a response rate. The most commonly used clinician-rated instruments for assessing depression severity are the Hamilton Depression Rating Scale (HAM-D; Hamilton 1960) and the Montgomery-Åsberg Depression Rating Scale (MADRS; Montgomery and Åsberg 1979; Santor et al. 2006); different versions of the HAM-D may be used. Response is usually defined as greater than 50% improvement compared with baseline. In general, a substantial rate of response and even remission is achieved—especially in relation to the treatment-resistant illness in this population. Apparently, none of the targets presented seems to be substantially superior to the others. Due to the small number of RCTs, even a meta-analysis could not reliably determine a superior target (Kisely et al. 2018). Despite the generally high response rates, predominantly in open-label studies, response and remission rates vary substantially among studies and fluctuate over time. This is typical for studies with small sample sizes (Khan et al. 2018) and indicates that RCTs and meta-analyses are needed for a better estimation of the actual treatment efficacy. Although many study protocols set the end of study at 6 or 12 months (see Appendix Table 20–A), clinical long-term observations over many years have been reported in several publications. Thus, DBS for depression is a long-term treatment.

As mentioned, one of the great advantages of DBS over lesion procedures is that sham-controlled trials become feasible. Therefore, after some very promising open-label pilot trials and small controlled trials (see Appendix Table 20–A), two large, well-designed sham-controlled studies were started, with sample sizes determined on the basis of power analyses (Dougherty et al. 2015; Holtzheimer et al. 2017). Unfortunately, both studies were stopped after preliminary futility analyses did not find significant group differences in depressive symptoms between sham and active stimulation.

Nevertheless, instead of discarding DBS as treatment for TRD due to these preliminary findings, we should seek explanations for the failed trials of Dougherty et al. (2015 and Holtzheimer et al. (2017). First, these RCTs were highly underpowered. Their sample sizes (30 and 90, respectively) were much smaller than expected (208 and 201, respectively) and made them quite unlikely to yield statistically significant and replicable results (see Khan et al. 2018 for deeper insight into the problems of trial design in antidepressant treatment). The lack of a significant group difference does not necessarily point toward an ineffective treatment. Looking at the study design presented in Dougherty et al. (2015), one can argue that a treatment duration of 4 months before response assessment might be too brief in relation to the duration of illness in this severely ill and treatment-resistant population (Schlaepfer 2015). Furthermore, the time period for individual parameter adjustment was limited to a few days only, which seems much too short for this complex intervention. On the other hand, parameter adjustment in the study by Holtzheimer et al. (2017) followed a plan that might have been too strict. Reaching a stable response can take time (Bergfeld et al. 2016), a factor that should be considered in future trial designs (Mayberg et al. 2016).

Beyond these issues, it is also questionable whether the commonly used outcome parameters—the HAM-D and the MADRS—are sensitive enough for the assessment of symptom changes in severe depression. The chronically severe depression in the study population might result in ceiling effects. Therefore, DBS-specific measures of severe depression are urgently needed (Schlaepfer 2015). Furthermore, the HAM-D and MADRS are multidimensional measures that try to assess the whole depression syndrome. Efficacy analyses usually focus on the sum score. Unfortunately, similar sum scores can be achieved by a great number of unique symptom combinations and thereby cover up the nuances of the present depression manifestation (Fried and Nesse 2015). At the same time, a sum score reduction does not give any information about which aspects of the illness actually did improve (Khan et al. 2018). To improve interpretability, it therefore makes sense to look at single symptoms and to find measurements that contain fewer dimensions (Fried and Nesse 2015).

Finally, the HAM-D and MADRS actually ask for the patient's depressive symptoms in the past week. Comparing depression severity at baseline and at an arbitrarily chosen follow-up time point can be influenced by many variables other than treatment and does not tell anything about the course of treatment response (Schlaepfer 2015). For assessment of the whole process from baseline to end of study, the area under the curve has been proposed (Bewernick et al. 2017b; Schlaepfer 2015); this measure is the product of time and depression severity and contains all measuring points and thereby gives information about stability of illness/response. Especially for studies with long-term follow-up, this seems to be a more meaningful outcome parameter than the mere comparison between two points in time. In October 2018, a new large-scale RCT on the treatment of TRD with DBS was started, taking into account the difficulties of the studies by Dougherty et al. (2015) and Holtzheimer et al. (2017). The stimulation target is the slMFB (clinical trial identifier NCT03653858). Although no results have been reported yet, this study might be a milestone for DBS in TRD.

DBS has been in use for a while now, yet the exact mode of action remains unclear. Different hypotheses on the electrochemical processes induced by DBS have been put forward, the most common ones being direct inhibition of neural activity, direct excitation of neural activity, informational lesion, and synaptic filtering. These concepts focus on the acute effects of DBS in movement disorders; for an explanation of these concepts and the current evidence, see Lozano et al. (2019). Currently under investigation are neuroplastic changes induced by DBS in rodent models of depression (Falowski et al. 2011; Veerakumar et al. 2014).

Where does all this leave us? DBS is a promising treatment for depression with impressive results in open-label studies. Surprisingly, RCTs have not been as successful so far. This might be at least partially related to methodological difficulties that should be addressed in future studies. Further well-designed comparable studies on treatment efficacy that allow for meta-analysis are therefore urgently needed. At the same time, careful patient selection that considers individual risks is indispensable, because DBS is an invasive procedure that comes with certain risks (see the next section, "Safety"). Several targets are under investigation, and at this point we cannot determine which is the most effective—neither in general nor in the individual case. Generally, antidepressant effects may vary due to interactions of DBS target, parameter settings, and individual clinical characteristics (Dandekar et al. 2018). Deeper insight into this relationship could be a basis for personalized treatment, which is why clinical research should focus on single symptoms as well as on the whole syndrome. Ultimately, a better understanding of the mode of action of DBS is needed to improve target selection and parameter adjustment. So far, DBS should only be considered as a treatment alternative once all approved and well-evaluated treatment procedures have been exhausted. If this requirement is fulfilled, DBS, administered by an expert team in the context of clinical studies, may offer a chance for significant illness improvement.

Safety

Like any other treatment, DBS is associated with side effects. These side effects can be surgery-, stimulation-, or device-related. Broad overviews of adverse events reported thus far in DBS for TRD are presented in reviews by Kisely et al. (2018) and Dandekar et al. (2018). The main surgery-associated side effects are wound infection, erosion, lead migration, device-related infection, and hemorrhage. These adverse effects may be permanent but are transient in most cases. The incidence rate of hemorrhage in functional neurosurgery (lesion procedures and DBS in general) is about 5.0% (Zrinzo et al. 2012).

Stimulation-related adverse effects such as hypomanic symptoms, disinhibition, restlessness, anxiety, sweating, or headaches are mostly transient (Kisely et al. 2018). Parameter adjustment is required if adverse effects are persistent or experienced as stressful (Schlaepfer et al. 2014). Suicide attempts and completed suicides have been reported as well (i.e., Bergfeld et al. 2016; Bewernick et al. 2010; Kennedy et al. 2011). Because prospective studies indicate an increased risk of suicide in patients with TRD (Oquendo et al. 2006), this should be expected and demonstrates the necessity of close psychiatric supervision during studies and follow-up.

Symptom aggravation due to unintended (i.e., battery depletion) or planned (i.e., blinded stimulation) stimulation discontinuation has been reported (i.e., Bergfeld et al. 2016; Holtzheimer et al. 2012; Kilian et al. 2019). Although one study did not find clinical changes after a planned 48-hour stimulation discontinuation, metabolic changes become apparent after this short time period (Martin-Blanco et al. 2015). These findings support the hypothesis that continuous stimulation is essential for effective treatment.

Besides these general adverse events, different stimulation targets seem to be associated with specific side effects (see Dandekar et al. 2018). Due to small sample sizes and only partial data available from control groups, data on the efficacy and safety of DBS in TRD must be considered preliminary.

Ethical Considerations

Applying DBS for TRD should be and is discussed in light of ethical principles. Quite frequently, concerns regarding possible personality changes under DBS are voiced (Grant et al. 2014; Hildt 2006; Synofzik and Schlaepfer 2008). To address these concerns, it is necessary to reflect on what is meant by the term *personality*—a question that exceeds the scope of this chapter. In short, a quantitative analysis of personality traits before and after DBS for TRD did not reveal any changes (Bewernick et al. 2018). In qualitative analyses in DBS for Parkinson's disease and OCD, patients occasionally report feelings of strangeness or unfamiliarity with themselves (de Haan et al. 2015; Gilbert et al. 2017; Schüpbach et al. 2006). At the same time, effective treatment of psychiatric disorders can be conceptualized as purposefully changing aspects of an individual's personality (Synofzik and Schlaepfer 2008) and therefore leads to the question of whether a change in personality is inevitably undesirable (Grant et al. 2014; Synofzik and Schlaepfer 2008).

Regarding interpersonal relationships, poor social adjustment, especially in marital relationships and professional lives, has been reported after DBS for Parkinson's disease, despite the successful reduction of motor symptoms. This leads to the assumption that rapid improvement of a disabling condition might have a destabilizing effect (Baertschi et al. 2019; Schüpbach et al. 2006) that should be taken into account when informing patients about the potential risks and benefits of DBS and when defining outcome measures in studies on treatment efficacy, especially because very rapid improvement of depressive symptomatology has been observed in DBS for TRD (Schlaepfer et al. 2013). These considerations of DBS for psychiatric purposes are extended by a body of literature (i.e., Grant et al. 2014; Kuhn et al. 2009; Synofzik and Schlaepfer 2008) focused on the well-established principles of bioethical nonmaleficence, justice, and autonomy expounded by Beauchamp and Childress (2009). To ensure that these principles are not only discussed in general but also taken into account in every individual case and in planning clinical trials, guidelines for patient selection have been proposed (Nuttin et al. 2014).

Without question, DBS remains an invasive treatment and comes with certain risks. Thus, careful selection of patients and targets is important to ensure that patients receive the best treatment available. Regarding risk-benefit estimations, it is an advantage that surgery-related side effects are already well known due to the application of DBS in neurology (Kleiner-Fisman et al. 2006). Additionally, the side-effect risks of DBS must be balanced against the immense burden of disease (Mrazek et al. 2014) and the side effects of alternative treatments such as electroconvulsive therapy (Kolshus et al. 2017). As discussed earlier, depression is a complex syndrome. We should therefore aim for individualized patient care that takes into account the individual depression manifestation (Fried and Nesse 2015) and assesses the best-fitting DBS target. Ultimately, DBS pursues the same goal as all biological interventions for depression—reestablishing the balance of brain circuits involved in maintaining depression in general and TRD in particular.

References

Aaronson ST, Carpenter LL, Conway CR, et al: Vagus nerve stimulation therapy randomized to different amounts of electrical charge for treatment-resistant depression: acute and chronic effects. Brain Stimul 6(4):631–640, 2013 23122916

Aaronson ST, Sears P, Ruvuna F, et al: A 5-year observational study of patients with treatment-resistant depression treated with vagus nerve stimulation or treatment as usual: comparison of response, remission, and suicidality. Am J Psychiatry 174(7):640–648, 2017 28359201

Accolla EA, Aust S, Merkl A, et al: Deep brain stimulation of the posterior gyrus rectus region for treatment resistant depression. J Affect Disord 194:33–37, 2016 26802505

Adinoff B: Neurobiologic processes in drug reward and addiction. Harv Rev Psychiatry 12(6):305–320, 2004 15764467

Aharon I, Etcoff N, Ariely D, et al: Beautiful faces have variable reward value: fMRI and behavioral evidence. Neuron 32(3):537–551, 2001 11709163

Alexander GE, DeLong MR, Strick PL: Parallel organization of functionally segregated circuits linking basal ganglia and cortex. Annu Rev Neurosci 9(1):357–381, 1986 3085570

Alonso P, Cuadras D, Gabriëls L, et al: Deep brain stimulation for obsessive-compulsive disorder: a meta-analysis of treatment outcome and predictors of response. PLoS One 10(7):e0133591, 2015 26208305

American Psychiatric Association: Diagnostic and Statistical Manual of Mental Disorders, 5th Edition. Arlington, VA, American Psychiatric Association, 2013

Armitage R, Husain M, Hoffmann R, et al: The effects of vagus nerve stimulation on sleep EEG in depression: a preliminary report. J Psychosom Res 54(5):475–482, 2003 12726905

Baertschi M, Flores Alves Dos Santos J, Burkhard P, et al: The burden of normality as a model of psychosocial adjustment after deep brain stimulation for Parkinson's disease: a systematic investigation. Neuropsychology 33(2):178–194, 2019 30667249

Bajbouj M, Merkl A, Schlaepfer TE, et al: Two-year outcome of vagus nerve stimulation in treatment-resistant depression. J Clin Psychopharmacol 30(3):273–281, 2010 20473062

Beauchamp TL, Childress JF: Principles of Biomedical Ethics, 6th Edition. New York, Oxford University Press, 2009

Benabid AL, Pollak P, Louveau A, et al: Combined (thalamotomy and stimulation) stereotactic surgery of the VIM thalamic nucleus for bilateral Parkinson disease. Appl Neurophysiol 50(1–6):344–346, 1987 3329873

Benabid AL, Pollak P, Gross C, et al: Acute and long-term effects of subthalamic nucleus stimulation in Parkinson's disease. Stereotact Funct Neurosurg 62(1–4):76–84, 1994 7631092

Ben-Menachem E: Vagus-nerve stimulation for the treatment of epilepsy. Lancet Neurol 1(8):477–482, 2002 12849332

Ben-Menachem E, Mañon-Espaillat R, Ristanovic R, et al: Vagus nerve stimulation for treatment of partial seizures: 1. A controlled study of effect on seizures. Epilepsia 35(3):616–626, 1994 8026408

Bennabi D, Aouizerate B, El-Hage W, et al: Risk factors for treatment resistance in unipolar depression: a systematic review. J Affect Disord 171:137–141, 2015 25305428

Bergfeld IO, Mantione M, Hoogendoorn ML, et al: Deep brain stimulation of the ventral anterior limb of the internal capsule for treatment-resistant depression: a randomized clinical trial. JAMA Psychiatry 73(5):456–464, 2016 27049915

Berry SM, Broglio K, Bunker M, et al: A patient-level meta-analysis of studies evaluating vagus nerve stimulation therapy for treatment-resistant depression. Med Devices (Auckl) 6:17–35, 2013 23482508

Berton O, Nestler EJ: New approaches to antidepressant drug discovery: beyond monoamines. Nat Rev Neurosci 7(2):137–151, 2006 16429123

Berton O, McClung CA, DiLeone RJ, et al: Essential role of BDNF in the mesolimbic dopamine pathway in social defeat stress. Science 311(5762):864–868, 2006 16469931

Bewernick BH, Hurlemann R, Matusch A, et al: Nucleus accumbens deep brain stimulation decreases ratings of depression and anxiety in treatment-resistant depression. Biol Psychiatry 67(2):110–116, 2010 19914605

Bewernick BH, Kayser S, Sturm V, et al: Long-term effects of nucleus accumbens deep brain stimulation in treatment-resistant depression: evidence for sustained efficacy. Neuropsychopharmacology 37(9):1975–1985, 2012 22473055

Bewernick BH, Kayser S, Gippert SM, et al: Acute antidepressant effects of deep brain stimulation—review and data from slMFB-stimulation. Personalized Medicine in Psychiatry 3:1–7, 2017a. Available at: https://www.personalizedmedpsych.com/article/S2468-1717(17)30003-0/fulltext. Accessed October 26, 2021.

Bewernick BH, Kayser S, Gippert SM, et al: Deep brain stimulation to the medial forebrain bundle for depression—long-term outcomes and a novel data analysis strategy. Brain Stimul 10(3):664–671, 2017b 28259544

Bewernick BH, Kilian HM, Schmidt K, et al: Deep brain stimulation of the supero-lateral branch of the medial forebrain bundle does not lead to changes in personality in patients suffering from severe depression. Psychol Med 48(16):2684–2692, 2018 29493478

Blomstedt P, Sjöberg RL, Hansson M, et al: Deep brain stimulation in the treatment of obsessive-compulsive disorder. World Neurosurg 80(6):e245–e253, 2013 23044000

Borders C, Hsu F, Sweidan AJ, et al: Deep brain stimulation for obsessive compulsive disorder: a review of results by anatomical target. Ment Illn 10(2):7900, 2018 30542526

Carlezon WA Jr, Chartoff EH: Intracranial self-stimulation (ICSS) in rodents to study the neurobiology of motivation. Nat Protoc 2(11):2987–2995, 2007 18007634

Cepeda MS, Reps J, Fife D, et al: Finding treatment-resistant depression in real-world data: how a data-driven approach compares with expert-based heuristics. Depress Anxiety 35(3):220–228, 2018 29244906

Coenen VA, Honey CR, Hurwitz T, et al: Medial forebrain bundle stimulation as a pathophysiological mechanism for hypomania in subthalamic nucleus deep brain stimulation for Parkinson's disease. Neurosurgery 64(6):1106–1114, discussion 1114–1115, 2009 19487890

Coenen VA, Schlaepfer TE, Maedler B, et al: Cross-species affective functions of the medial forebrain bundle-implications for the treatment of affective pain and depression in humans. Neurosci Biobehav Rev 35(9):1971–1981, 2011 21184778

Coenen VA, Schlaepfer TE, Goll P, et al: The medial forebrain bundle as a target for deep brain stimulation for obsessive-compulsive disorder. CNS Spectr 22(3):282–289, 2017 27268576

Coenen VA, Bewernick BH, Kayser S, et al: Superolateral medial forebrain bundle deep brain stimulation in major depression: a gateway trial. Neuropsychopharmacology 44(7):1224–1232, 2019 30867553

Conway CR, Sheline YI, Chibnall JT, et al: Cerebral blood flow changes during vagus nerve stimulation for depression. Psychiatry Res 146(2):179–184, 2006 16510266

Conway CR, Sheline YI, Chibnall JT, et al: Brain blood-flow change with acute vagus nerve stimulation in treatment-refractory major depressive disorder. Brain Stimul 5(2):163–171, 2012 22037127

Conway CR, Chibnall JT, Gebara MA, et al: Association of cerebral metabolic activity changes with vagus nerve stimulation antidepressant response in treatment-resistant depression. Brain Stimul 6(5):788–797, 2013 23485649

Daban C, Martinez-Aran A, Cruz N, et al: Safety and efficacy of vagus nerve stimulation in treatment-resistant depression. A systematic review. J Affect Disord 110(1–2):1–15, 2008 18374988

Dandekar MP, Fenoy AJ, Carvalho AF, et al: Deep brain stimulation for treatment-resistant depression: an integrative review of preclinical and clinical findings and translational implications. Mol Psychiatry 23(5):1094–1112, 2018 29483673

Davidson B, Giacobbe P, Mithani K, et al: Lack of clinical response to deep brain stimulation of the medial forebrain bundle in depression. Brain Stimul 13(5):1268–1270, 2020 32540453

de Haan S, Rietveld E, Stokhof M, et al: Effects of deep brain stimulation on the lived experience of obsessive-compulsive disorder patients: In-depth interviews with 18 patients. PLoS One 10(8):e0135524, 2015 26312488

Denys D, Mantione M, Figee M, et al: Deep brain stimulation of the nucleus accumbens for treatment-refractory obsessive-compulsive disorder. Arch Gen Psychiatry 67(10):1061–1068, 2010 20921122

Döbrössy M, Ramanathan C, Ashouri Vajari D, et al: Neuromodulation in psychiatric disorders: experimental and clinical evidence for reward and motivation network deep brain stimulation: focus on the medial forebrain bundle. European Journal of Neuroscience 53(1):89–113, 2021. Available at: https://onlinelibrary.wiley.com/doi/10.1111/ejn.14975. Accessed October 26, 2021.

Dougherty DD, Rezai AR, Carpenter LL, et al: A randomized sham-controlled trial of deep brain stimulation of the ventral capsule/ventral striatum for chronic treatment-resistant depression. Biol Psychiatry 78(4):240–248, 2015 25726497

Doyon WM, Anders SK, Ramachandra VS, et al: Effect of operant self-administration of 10% ethanol plus 10% sucrose on dopamine and ethanol concentrations in the nucleus accumbens. J Neurochem 93(6):1469–1481, 2005 15935063

Drevets WC, Gautier C, Price JC, et al: Amphetamine-induced dopamine release in human ventral striatum correlates with euphoria. Biol Psychiatry 49(2):81–96, 2001 11164755

Drobisz D, Damborská A: Deep brain stimulation targets for treating depression. Behav Brain Res 359:266–273, 2019 30414974

Dunlop BW, Rajendra JK, Craighead WE, et al: Functional connectivity of the subcallosal cingulate cortex and differential outcomes to treatment with cognitive-behavioral therapy or antidepressant medication for major depressive disorder. Am J Psychiatry 174(6):533–545, 2017 28335622

Dunner DL, Rush AJ, Russell JM, et al: Prospective, long-term, multicenter study of the naturalistic outcomes of patients with treatment-resistant depression. J Clin Psychiatry 67(5):688–695, 2006 16841617

Eitan R, Fontaine D, Benoît M, et al: One year double blind study of high vs low frequency subcallosal cingulate stimulation for depression. J Psychiatr Res 96:124–134, 2018 29032294

Elger G, Hoppe C, Falkai P, et al: Vagus nerve stimulation is associated with mood improvements in epilepsy patients. Epilepsy Res 42(2–3):203–210, 2000 11074193

Englot DJ, Chang EF, Auguste KI: Vagus nerve stimulation for epilepsy: a meta-analysis of efficacy and predictors of response. J Neurosurg 115(6):1248–1255, 2011 21838505

Falowski SM, Sharan A, Reyes BA, et al: An evaluation of neuroplasticity and behavior after deep brain stimulation of the nucleus accumbens in an animal model of depression. Neurosurgery 69(6):1281–1290, 2011 21566538

Famm K, Litt B, Tracey KJ, et al: Drug discovery: a jump-start for electroceuticals. Nature 496(7444):159–161, 2013 23579662

Fenoy AJ, Schulz P, Selvaraj S, et al: Deep brain stimulation of the medial forebrain bundle: distinctive responses in resistant depression. J Affect Disord 203:143–151, 2016 27288959

Fenoy AJ, Schulz PE, Selvaraj S, et al: A longitudinal study on deep brain stimulation of the medial forebrain bundle for treatment-resistant depression. Transl Psychiatry 8(1):111, 2018 29867109

Fife D, Feng Y, Wang MY-H, et al: Epidemiology of pharmaceutically treated depression and treatment resistant depression in Taiwan. Psychiatry Res 252:277–283, 2017 28288438

Fried EI, Nesse RM: Depression sum-scores don't add up: why analyzing specific depression symptoms is essential. BMC Med 13(1):72, 2015 25879936

Galluccio L, Palazzo S, Santagati GE: Modeling signal propagation in nanomachine-to-neuron communications. Nano Communication Networks 2(4):213–222, 2011. Available at: https://www.sciencedirect.com/science/article/abs/pii/S1878778911000548?via%3Dihub. Accessed October 26, 2021.

Gemeinsamer-Bundesausschus: Qualitätsberichte der Krankenhäuser im XML-Format. 2014–2019. 2021. Available at: https://www.g-ba.de/themen/qualitaetssicherung/datenerhebung-zur-qualitaetssicherung/datenerhebung-qualitaetsbericht/. Accessed October 2021.

George MS, Rush AJ, Marangell LB, et al: A one-year comparison of vagus nerve stimulation with treatment as usual for treatment-resistant depression. Biol Psychiatry 58(5):364–373, 2005 16139582

Gilbert F, Goddard E, Viaña JNM, et al: I miss being me: phenomenological effects of deep brain stimulation. AJOB Neurosci 8(2):96–109, 2017

Grant RA, Halpern CH, Baltuch GH, et al: Ethical considerations in deep brain stimulation for psychiatric illness. J Clin Neurosci 21(1):1–5, 2014 24055023

Greenberg BD, Price LH, Rauch SL, et al: Neurosurgery for intractable obsessive-compulsive disorder and depression: critical issues. Neurosurg Clin N Am 14(2):199–212, 2003 12856488

Greenberg BD, Malone DA, Friehs GM, et al: Three-year outcomes in deep brain stimulation for highly resistant obsessive-compulsive disorder. Neuropsychopharmacology 31(11):2384–2393, 2006 16855529

Hamani C, Mayberg H, Snyder B, et al: Deep brain stimulation of the subcallosal cingulate gyrus for depression: anatomical location of active contacts in clinical responders and a suggested guideline for targeting. J Neurosurg 111(6):1209–1215, 2009 19480538

Hamilton M: A rating scale for depression. J Neurol Neurosurg Psychiatry 23(1):56–62, 1960 14399272

Handforth A, DeGiorgio CM, Schachter SC, et al: Vagus nerve stimulation therapy for partial-onset seizures: a randomized active-control trial. Neurology 51(1):48–55, 1998 9674777

Harden CL, Pulver MC, Ravdin LD, et al: A pilot study of mood in epilepsy patients treated with vagus nerve stimulation. Epilepsy Behav 1(2):93–99, 2000 12609137

Hariz MI, Blomstedt P, Zrinzo L: Deep brain stimulation between 1947 and 1987: the untold story. Neurosurg Focus 29(2):E1, 2010 20672911

Henry TR: Therapeutic mechanisms of vagus nerve stimulation. Neurology 59 (6 suppl 4):S3–S14, 2002 12270962

Henry TR, Bakay RA, Pennell PB, et al: Brain blood-flow alterations induced by therapeutic vagus nerve stimulation in partial epilepsy, II: prolonged effects at high and low levels of stimulation. Epilepsia 45(9):1064–1070, 2004 15329071

Hildt E: Electrodes in the brain: some anthropological and ethical aspects of deep brain stimulation. The International Review of Information Ethics 5(9):33–39, 2006. Available at: https://informationethics.ca/index.php/irie/article/view/193. Accessed October 26, 2021.

Hodgkin AL, Huxley AF: A quantitative description of membrane current and its application to conduction and excitation in nerve. J Physiol 117(4):500–544, 1952 1299123

Holtzheimer PE, Kelley ME, Gross RE, et al: Subcallosal cingulate deep brain stimulation for treatment-resistant unipolar and bipolar depression. Arch Gen Psychiatry 69(2):150–158, 2012 22213770

Holtzheimer PE, Husain MM, Lisanby SH, et al: Subcallosal cingulate deep brain stimulation for treatment-resistant depression: a multisite, randomised, sham-controlled trial. Lancet Psychiatry 4(11):839–849, 2017 28988904

Karas PJ, Lee S, Jimenez-Shahed J, et al: Deep brain stimulation for obsessive compulsive disorder: evolution of surgical stimulation target parallels changing model of dysfunctional brain circuits. Front Neurosci 12:998, 2019 30670945

Kennedy SH, Giacobbe P, Rizvi SJ, et al: Deep brain stimulation for treatment-resistant depression: follow-up after 3 to 6 years. Am J Psychiatry 168(5):502–510, 2011 21285143

Khan A, Mar KF, Brown WA: The conundrum of depression clinical trials: one size does not fit all. Int Clin Psychopharmacol 33(5):239–248, 2018 29939890

Kilian HM, Meyer DM, Bewernick BH, et al: Discontinuation of superolateral medial forebrain bundle deep brain stimulation for treatment-resistant depression leads to critical relapse. Biol Psychiatry 85(6):e23–e24, 2019 30253883

Kisely S, Li A, Warren N, Siskind D: A systematic review and meta-analysis of deep brain stimulation for depression. Depress Anxiety 35(5):468–480, 2018 29697875

Kleiner-Fisman G, Herzog J, Fisman DN, et al: Subthalamic nucleus deep brain stimulation: summary and meta-analysis of outcomes. Mov Disord 21 (suppl 14):S290–S304, 2006 16892449

Knutson B, Adams CM, Fong GW, Hommer D: Anticipation of increasing monetary reward selectively recruits nucleus accumbens. J Neurosci 21(16):RC159–RC159, 2001 11459880

Kolshus E, Jelovac A, McLoughlin DM: Bitemporal v. high-dose right unilateral electroconvulsive therapy for depression: a systematic review and meta-analysis of randomized controlled trials. Psychol Med 47(3):518–530, 2017 27780482

Kosel M, Brockmann H, Frick C, et al: Chronic vagus nerve stimulation for treatment-resistant depression increases regional cerebral blood flow in the dorsolateral prefrontal cortex. Psychiatry Res 191(3):153–159, 2011 21306877

Krishnan V, Nestler EJ: The molecular neurobiology of depression. Nature 455(7215):894–902, 2008 18923511

Kuhn J, Gaebel W, Klosterkoetter J, et al: Deep brain stimulation as a new therapeutic approach in therapy-resistant mental disorders: ethical aspects of investigational treatment. Eur Arch Psychiatry Clin Neurosci 259 (2 suppl 2):S135–S141, 2009 19876671

LivaNova: VNS Therapy System: Depression Physician's Manual, May 2020, U.S. Version. Available at: https://vnstherapy.info/. Accessed September 9, 2021.

Lomarev M, Denslow S, Nahas Z, et al: Vagus nerve stimulation (VNS) synchronized BOLD fMRI suggests that VNS in depressed adults has frequency/dose dependent effects. J Psychiatr Res 36(4):219–227, 2002 12191626

Lozano AM, Mayberg HS, Giacobbe P, et al: Subcallosal cingulate gyrus deep brain stimulation for treatment-resistant depression. Biol Psychiatry 64(6):461–467, 2008 18639234

Lozano AM, Giacobbe P, Hamani C, et al: A multicenter pilot study of subcallosal cingulate area deep brain stimulation for treatment-resistant depression. J Neurosurg 116(2):315–322, 2012 22098195

Lozano AM, Lipsman N, Bergman H, et al: Deep brain stimulation: current challenges and future directions. Nat Rev Neurol 15(3):148–160, 2019 30683913

Mahlich J, Tsukazawa S, Wiegand F: Estimating prevalence and healthcare utilization for treatment-resistant depression in Japan: a retrospective claims database study. Drugs Real World Outcomes 5(1):35–43, 2018 29185233

Mallet L, Polosan M, Jaafari N, et al: Subthalamic nucleus stimulation in severe obsessive-compulsive disorder. N Engl J Med 359(20):2121–2134, 2008 19005196

Malone DA Jr: Use of deep brain stimulation in treatment-resistant depression. Cleve Clin J Med 77 (suppl 3):S77–S80, 2010 20622083

Malone DA Jr, Dougherty DD, Rezai AR, et al: Deep brain stimulation of the ventral capsule/ventral striatum for treatment-resistant depression. Biol Psychiatry 65(4):267–275, 2009 18842257

Martin JL, Martín-Sánchez E: Systematic review and meta-analysis of vagus nerve stimulation in the treatment of depression: variable results based on study designs. Eur Psychiatry 27(3):147–155, 2012 22137776

Martín-Blanco A, Serra-Blasco M, Pérez-Egea R, et al: Immediate cerebral metabolic changes induced by discontinuation of deep brain stimulation of subcallosal cingulate gyrus in treatment-resistant depression. J Affect Disord 173:159–162, 2015 25462411

Mayberg HS: Limbic-cortical dysregulation: a proposed model of depression. J Neuropsychiatry Clin Neurosci 9(3):471–481, 1997 9276848

Mayberg HS, Lozano AM, Voon V, et al: Deep brain stimulation for treatment-resistant depression. Neuron 45(5):651–660, 2005 15748841

Mayberg HS, Riva-Posse P, Crowell AL: Deep brain stimulation for depression: keeping an eye on a moving target. JAMA Psychiatry 73(5):439–440, 2016 27049731

McGrath CL, Kelley ME, Dunlop BW, et al: Pretreatment brain states identify likely nonresponse to standard treatments for depression. Biol Psychiatry 76(7):527–535, 2014 24462230

Medtronic: Medtronic SureTune(TM)3 receives Health Canada license for deep brain stimulation therapy. June 6, 2017. Available at: https://www.medtronic.com/ca-en/about/news/surretune3_dbs.html. Accessed November 18, 2020.

Merkl A, Schneider GH, Schönecker T, et al: Antidepressant effects after short-term and chronic stimulation of the subgenual cingulate gyrus in treatment-resistant depression. Exp Neurol 249:160–168, 2013 24012926

Merkl A, Aust S, Schneider GH, et al: Deep brain stimulation of the subcallosal cingulate gyrus in patients with treatment-resistant depression: a double-blinded randomized controlled study and long-term follow-up in eight patients. J Affect Disord 227:521–529, 2018 29161674

Meyer D, Kilian H, Spanier S, et al: Rapid improvement of OCD symptoms and antidepressant response to deep brain stimulation of the superolateral medial forebrain bundle in OCD—a case series (W155; pp 468–469), in Abstracts Collection: ACNP 58th Annual Meeting: Poster Session III. Neuropsychopharmacology 44 (suppl 1):385–538, 2019. Available at: https://www.nature.com/articles/s41386-019-0547-9.pdf. Accessed October 26, 2021.

Millet B, Jaafari N, Polosan M, et al: Limbic versus cognitive target for deep brain stimulation in treatment-resistant depression: accumbens more promising than caudate. Eur Neuropsychopharmacol 24(8):1229–1239, 2014 24950819

Montgomery SA, Åsberg M: A new depression scale designed to be sensitive to change. Br J Psychiatry 134(4):382–389, 1979 444788

Mrazek DA, Hornberger JC, Altar CA, et al: A review of the clinical, economic, and societal burden of treatment-resistant depression: 1996–2013. Psychiatr Serv 65(8):977–987, 2014 24789696

Mu Q, Bohning DE, Nahas Z, et al: Acute vagus nerve stimulation using different pulse widths produces varying brain effects. Biol Psychiatry 55(8):816–825, 2004 15050863

Nahas Z, Marangell LB, Husain MM, et al: Two-year outcome of vagus nerve stimulation (VNS) for treatment of major depressive episodes. J Clin Psychiatry 66(9):1097–1104, 2005 16187765

Nahas Z, Teneback C, Chae J H, et al: Serial vagus nerve stimulation functional MRI in treatment resistant depression. Neuropsychopharmacology 32(8):1649–1660, 2007 17203016

Nemeroff CB, Mayberg HS, Krahl SE, et al: VNS therapy in treatment-resistant depression: clinical evidence and putative neurobiological mechanisms. Neuropsychopharmacology 31(7):1345–1355, 2006 16641939

Nuttin B, Cosyns P, Demeulemeester H, et al: Electrical stimulation in anterior limbs of internal capsules in patients with obsessive-compulsive disorder. Lancet 354(9189):1526, 1999 10551504

Nuttin BJ, Gabriëls LA, Cosyns PR, et al: Long-term electrical capsular stimulation in patients with obsessive-compulsive disorder. Neurosurgery 52(6):1263–1272, discussion 1272–1274, 2003 12762871

Nuttin B, Wu H, Mayberg H, et al: Consensus on guidelines for stereotactic neurosurgery for psychiatric disorders. J Neurol Neurosurg Psychiatry 85(9):1003–1008, 2014 24444853

Oquendo MA, Currier D, Mann JJ: Prospective studies of suicidal behavior in major depressive and bipolar disorders: what is the evidence for predictive risk factors? Acta Psychiatr Scand 114(3):151–158, 2006 16889585

Pardo JV, Sheikh SA, Schwindt GC, et al: Chronic vagus nerve stimulation for treatment-resistant depression decreases resting ventromedial prefrontal glucose metabolism. Neuroimage 42(2):879–889, 2008 18595737

Perez-Caballero L, Pérez-Egea R, Romero-Grimaldi C, et al: Early responses to deep brain stimulation in depression are modulated by anti-inflammatory drugs. Mol Psychiatry 19(5):607–614, 2014 23711979

Puigdemont D, Pérez-Egea R, Portella MJ, et al: Deep brain stimulation of the subcallosal cingulate gyrus: further evidence in treatment-resistant major depression. Int J Neuropsychopharmacol 15(1):121–133, 2012 21777510

Ramasubbu R, Anderson S, Haffenden A, et al: Double-blind optimization of subcallosal cingulate deep brain stimulation for treatment-resistant depression: a pilot study. J Psychiatry Neurosci 38(5):325–332, 2013 23527884

Raymaekers S, Luyten L, Bervoets C, et al: Deep brain stimulation for treatment-resistant major depressive disorder: a comparison of two targets and long-term follow-up. Transl Psychiatry 7(10):e1251, 2017 29087373

Riva-Posse P, Choi KS, Holtzheimer PE, et al: A connectomic approach for subcallosal cingulate deep brain stimulation surgery: prospective targeting in treatment-resistant depression. Mol Psychiatry 23(4):843–849, 2018 28397839

Rush AJ, George MS, Sackeim HA, et al: Vagus nerve stimulation (VNS) for treatment-resistant depressions: a multicenter study. Biol Psychiatry 47(4):276–286, 2000 10686262

Rush AJ, Marangell LB, Sackeim HA, et al: Vagus nerve stimulation for treatment-resistant depression: a randomized, controlled acute phase trial. Biol Psychiatry 58(5):347–354, 2005 16139580

Rush AJ, Trivedi MH, Wisniewski SR, et al: Acute and longer-term outcomes in depressed outpatients requiring one or several treatment steps: a STAR*D report. Am J Psychiatry 163(11):1905–1917, 2006 17074942

Sackeim HA, Rush AJ, George MS, et al: Vagus nerve stimulation (VNS) for treatment-resistant depression: efficacy, side effects, and predictors of outcome. Neuropsychopharmacology 25(5):713–728, 2001 11682255

Sackeim HA, Brannan SK, Rush AJ, et al: Durability of antidepressant response to vagus nerve stimulation (VNS). Int J Neuropsychopharmacol 10(6):817–826, 2007 17288644

Santor DA, Gregus M, Welch A: Eight decades of measurement in depression. Measurement: Interdisciplinary Research and Perspectives 4(3):135–155, 2006. Available at: https://www.tandfonline.com/doi/abs/10.1207/s15366359mea0403_1. Accessed October 26, 2021.

Schlaepfer TE: Deep brain stimulation for major depression—steps on a long and winding road. Biol Psychiatry 78(4):218–219, 2015 26195174

Schlaepfer TE, Bewernick BH: Ethische bewertung der methoden psychiatrischer neuromodulation, in Ethik Psychiatrischer Forschung. Edited by Helmchen H. Berlin, Germany, Springer Berlin Heidelberg, 2013, pp 133–152

Schlaepfer TE, Cohen MX, Frick C, et al: Deep brain stimulation to reward circuitry alleviates anhedonia in refractory major depression. Neuropsychopharmacology 33(2):368–377, 2008a 17429407

Schlaepfer TE, Frick C, Zobel A, et al: Vagus nerve stimulation for depression: efficacy and safety in a European study. Psychol Med 38(5):651–661, 2008b 18177525

Schlaepfer TE, Bewernick BH, Kayser S, et al: Rapid effects of deep brain stimulation for treatment-resistant major depression. Biol Psychiatry 73(12):1204–1212, 2013 23562618

Schlaepfer TE, Bewernick BH, Kayser S, et al: Deep brain stimulation of the human reward system for major depression—rationale, outcomes and outlook. Neuropsychopharmacology 39(6):1303–1314, 2014 24513970

Schlaepfer TE, Meyer-Lindenberg A, Synofzik M, et al: Invasive brain stimulation in the treatment of psychiatric illness. Dtsch Arztebl Int 118(3):31–36, 2021 33759753

Schoene-Bake J-C, Parpaley Y, Weber B, et al: Tractographic analysis of historical lesion surgery for depression. Neuropsychopharmacology 35(13):2553–2563, 2010 20736994

Schultz W: Neural coding of basic reward terms of animal learning theory, game theory, microeconomics and behavioural ecology. Curr Opin Neurobiol 14(2):139–147, 2004 15082317

Schüpbach M, Gargiulo M, Welter ML, et al: Neurosurgery in Parkinson disease: a distressed mind in a repaired body? Neurology 66(12):1811–1816, 2006 16801642

Synofzik M, Schlaepfer TE: Stimulating personality: ethical criteria for deep brain stimulation in psychiatric patients and for enhancement purposes. Biotechnol J 3(12):1511–1520, 2008 19072907

U.S. Food and Drug Administration: Humanitarian device exemption (HDE). November 16, 2020. Available at: www.accessdata.fda.gov/scripts/cdrh/cfdocs/cfhde/hde.cfm?id=H050003. Accessed November 18, 2020.

Veerakumar A, Challis C, Gupta P, et al: Antidepressant-like effects of cortical deep brain stimulation coincide with pro-neuroplastic adaptations of serotonin systems. Biol Psychiatry 76(3):203–212, 2014 24503468

Vergani F, Martino J, Morris C, et al: Anatomic connections of the subgenual cingulate region. Neurosurgery 79(3):465–472, 2016 27327267

Waraczynski MA: The central extended amygdala network as a proposed circuit underlying reward valuation. Neurosci Biobehav Rev 30(4):472–496, 2006 16243397

Wise RA: Forebrain substrates of reward and motivation. J Comp Neurol 493(1):115–121, 2005 16254990

Zobel A, Joe A, Freymann N, et al: Changes in regional cerebral blood flow by therapeutic vagus nerve stimulation in depression: an exploratory approach. Psychiatry Res 139(3):165–179, 2005 16043331

Zrinzo L, Foltynie T, Limousin P, et al: Reducing hemorrhagic complications in functional neurosurgery: a large case series and systematic literature review. J Neurosurg 116(1):84–94, 2012 21905798

APPENDIX TABLE 20–A. Findings from published studies of deep brain stimulation (DBS) targets for treatment-resistant depression

Target and reference	*N*	End of study	Maximum follow-up reported	Response		Remission		Sample	Comment on study design
				Definition	Rate (%)	Definition	Rate (%)		
Subgenual cingulate gyrus/Cg 25									
Eitan et al. 2018	9	13 months	13 months	≥40% reduction in MADRS score	Time point NA: 44.4	NA	NA	—	High- vs. low-frequency stimulation
Merkl et al. 2018	8	24 months	28 months to 4 years	≥50% reduction in HAMD-24 score	6 months: 37.5 12 months: 43 24 months: 33 28 months: 33	HAMD-24 score ≤10	6 months: 12.5 12 months: 14.2 24 months: 33.3 28 months: 33.3	Overlap with sample described in Merkl et al. 2013	4 weeks blinded sham or active stimulation
Riva-Posse et al. 2018	11	12 months	12 months	≥50% reduction in HAMD-17 score	6 months: 72.7 12 months: 81.8	HAMD-17 score ≤7	6 months: 45.4 12 months: 54.5	—	Pilot study on the utility of a prospective connectomic approach for surgery

APPENDIX TABLE 20–A. Findings from published studies of deep brain stimulation (DBS) targets for treatment-resistant depression *(continued)*

Target and reference	*N*	End of study	Maximum follow-up reported	Response		Remission		Sample	Comment on study design
				Definition	Rate (%)	Definition	Rate (%)		
Holtzheimer et al. 2017	90	12 months	24 months	≥40% reduction in MADRS score	6 months: 20 (stimulation group) 17 (control group) 12 months: 30 (stimulation group) 27 (control group) 18 months: 51 (of all patients) 24 months: 48 (of all patients)	MADRS score ≤10	6 months: 10 (stimulation group) 7 (control group) 12 months: 18 (stimulation group) 7 (control group) 18 months: 17 (of all patients) 24 months: 25 (of all patients)	—	6-month blinded sham/active stimulation study stopped after futility analysis
Accolla et al. 2016	5	NA	6 months	≥50% reduction in HAMD-24 and BDI scores	6 months: 20	NA	NA	Overlap with sample described in Merkl et al. 2013	Double-blind selection of best contact pair for stimulation, including 24-hour sham
Perez-Caballero et al. 2014	8	NA	1 month	≥50% reduction in HAMD-17 score	1 month: 37.5	HAMD-17 score ≤8	1 month: 25	Subsample of Puigdemont et al. 2012	Retrospective analysis of influence of analgesic/anti-inflammatory drugs

APPENDIX TABLE 20–A. Findings from published studies of deep brain stimulation (DBS) targets for treatment-resistant depression *(continued)*

Target and reference	*N*	End of study	Maximum follow-up reported	Response		Remission		Sample	Comment on study design
				Definition	Rate (%)	Definition	Rate (%)		
Subgenual cingulate gyrus/Cg 25 *(continued)*									
Ramasubbu et al. 2013	4	9 months	9 months	≥50% reduction in HAMD-17 score	3.5 months: 25 9 months: 50	NA	NA	—	12-week double-blind optimization phase, including 2 weeks of sham
Merkl et al. 2013	6	6 months	6–9 months	≥50% reduction in HAMD-24 score	6 months: 33.3	HAMD-24 score <10	6 months: 33.3	—	Double-blind, high-intensity stimulation for 5 days, followed by open-label study
Lozano et al. 2012	21	12 months	12 months	≥50% reduction in HAMD-17 score	1 month: 57 6 months: 48 12 months: 29	NA	NA	—	Multicenter pilot study
Puigdemont et al. 2012	8	12 months	12 months	≥50% reduction in HAMD-17 score	1 week: 87.5 1 month: 37.5 6 months: 87.5 12 months: 62.5%	HAMD-17 score ≤7	1 week: 50 1 month: NA 6 months: 37.5 12 months: 50	—	Preliminary findings of pre-randomization phase of an RCT

APPENDIX TABLE 20–A. Findings from published studies of deep brain stimulation (DBS) targets for treatment-resistant depression *(continued)*

Target and reference	*N*	End of study	Maximum follow-up reported	Response		Remission		Sample	Comment on study design
				Definition	Rate (%)	Definition	Rate (%)		
Holtzheimer et al. 2012	17	6 months	24 months	≥50% reduction in HAMD -17 score	6 months: 41 12 months: 36 24 months: 92	HAMD-17 score ≤7	6 months: 18 12 months: 36 24 months: 58	—	Single-blind discontinuation phase (after 4 weeks of single-blind sham and 24 weeks of active stimulation) was stopped after 3 patients relapsed
Kennedy et al. 2011	20	NA	6 years	≥50% reduction in HAMD -17 score	1 year: 62.5 2 years: 46.2 3 years: 75 Last follow-up: 64.3	HAMD-17 score ≤7	1 year: 18.8 2 years: 15.4 3 years: 50 Last follow-up: 42.9	Same sample as described in Lozano et al. 2008	Long-term follow-up
Lozano et al. 2008	20	12 months	12 months	≥50% reduction in HAMD-17 score	1 month: 35 6 months: 60 12 months: 55	HAMD-17 score ≤7	1 month: 10 6 months: 35 12 months: 35	Extended sample of Mayberg et al. 2005	Blinded stimulation during the immediate postoperative period
Mayberg et al. 2005	6	6 months	6 months	≥50% reduction in HAMD-17 score	1 month: 33.3 2 months: 83.3 6 months: 66.6	HAMD-17 score ≤8	1 month: 0 2 months: 0 6 months: 33.3	—	Blinded stimulation during the immediate postoperative period

APPENDIX TABLE 20–A. Findings from published studies of deep brain stimulation (DBS) targets for treatment-resistant depression *(continued)*

Target and reference	*N*	End of study	Maximum follow-up reported	Response		Remission		Sample	Comment on study design
				Definition	Rate (%)	Definition	Rate (%)		
Ventral capsule/Ventral striatum									
Dougherty et al. 2015	30	12 months plus long-term follow-up	24 months	≥50% reduction in MADRS score	4 months: 20 (stimulation group) 14.3 (control group) 12 months: 20 (of all patients) 24 months: 23.3 (of all patients)	MADRS score ≤10	12 months: 13 (of all patients) 24 months: 20 (of all patients)	—	Randomized controlled blinded phase for 4 months, followed by open-label stimulation
Malone 2010	17	NA	14–67 months	≥50% reduction in MADRS score	3 months: 53 6 months: 47 12 months: 53 Last follow-up: 71	MADRS score ≤11	3 months: 35 6 months: 29 12 months: 41 Last follow-up: 35	Slightly extended sample (+2 patients) of Malone et al. 2009	Multicenter pilot study
Malone et al. 2009	15	NA	6–51 months	≥50% reduction in HAMD-24 score	3 months: 46.7 6 months: 40 Last follow-up: 53.3	HAMD-24 score ≤10	3 months: 20 6 months: 20 Last follow-up: 40	—	Multicenter pilot study

APPENDIX TABLE 20–A. Findings from published studies of deep brain stimulation (DBS) targets for treatment-resistant depression *(continued)*

Target and reference	*N*	End of study	Maximum follow-up reported	Response		Remission		Sample	Comment on study design
				Definition	Rate (%)	Definition	Rate (%)		
Anterior limb of the internal capsule									
Raymaekers et al. 2017	7	NA	36–97 months	≥50% reduction in HAMD-17 score	3 years: 71.4 Last follow-up: 71.4	HAMD-17 score ≤7	3 years: 28.6 Last follow-up: 28.6	—	Double-blind crossover; stimulation target was varied systematically between ALIC, BNST, and ITP
Bergfeld et al. 2016	25	Maximum of 64 weeks	NA	≥50% reduction in HAMD-17 score	~12 months: 40	HAMD-17 score ≤7	~12 months: 20	—	Open-label stimulation for maximum of 1 year until response stable for ≥4 weeks, followed by 2×6 weeks blinded crossover sham/active stimulation

APPENDIX TABLE 20–A. Findings from published studies of deep brain stimulation (DBS) targets for treatment-resistant depression *(continued)*

Target and reference	*N*	End of study	Maximum follow-up reported	Response		Remission		Sample	Comment on study design
				Definition	Rate (%)	Definition	Rate (%)		
Nucleus accumbens									
Millet et al. 2014	6 included, 4 implanted	15 months	15 months	≥50% reduction in HAMD-17 score	5 months: 0 9 months: 0 15 months: 50	HAMD-17 score ≤7	5 months: 0 9 months: 0 15 months: 25	—	Crossover to caudate stimulation at 5 months (until month 9) in case of nonresponse to nucleus accumbens stimulation; multicenter pilot study
Bewernick et al. 2012	11	12 months	12 months to 4 years	≥50% reduction in HAMD-28 score	12 months: 45.5 Last follow-up: 45.5	HAMD-28 score ≤10	12 months: 9 Last follow-up: 9	Slightly extended sample (+ 1 patient) of Bewernick et al. 2010	Long-term follow-up
Bewernick et al. 2010	10	12 months	12 months	≥50% reduction in HAMD-28 score	12 months: 50	HAMD-28 score ≤10	Time point NA: 30	—	Pilot study

APPENDIX TABLE 20–A. Findings from published studies of deep brain stimulation (DBS) targets for treatment-resistant depression *(continued)*

Target and reference	*N*	End of study	Maximum follow-up reported	Response		Remission		Sample	Comment on study design
				Definition	Rate (%)	Definition	Rate (%)		
Superolateral branch of the medial forebrain bundle									
Davidson et al. 2020	2	6 months	8 months	≥50% reduction in HAMD-17 score	Any time point: 0	NA	NA	—	6 months of open-label stimulation followed by 2×2 weeks of double-blind OFF/ON
Coenen et al. 2019	16	12 months	12 months	≥50% reduction in MADRS score	12 months: 100 (of all patients)	MADRS score ≤10	12 months: 50 (of all patients)	—	Blinded stimulation for 8 weeks; staggered onset
Fenoy et al. 2018	6	12 months	12 months	≥50% reduction in MADRS score	12 months: 66.7	HAM-D score <7	12 months: 66.7	Slightly extended sample (+2 patients) of Fenoy et al. 2016	Long-term follow-up
Bewernick et al. 2017b	8	12 months	4 years	≥50% reduction in MADRS score	12 months: 75 Last follow-up: 87.5 (area under the curve)	MADRS score <10	12 months: 50	Slightly extended sample (+1 patient) of Schlaepfer et al. 2013	Long-term follow-up

Appendix Table 20–A. Findings from published studies of deep brain stimulation (DBS) targets for treatment-resistant depression *(continued)*

Target and reference	*N*	End of study	Maximum follow-up reported	Response		Remission		Sample	Comment on study design
				Definition	Rate (%)	Definition	Rate (%)		
Superolateral branch of the medial forebrain bundle *(continued)*									
Fenoy et al. 2016	4	12 months	6 months	≥50% reduction in MADRS score	1 week: 75 6 months: 50	NA	NA	—	Single-blind sham stimulation for 4 weeks; interim report
Schlaepfer et al. 2013	7	3 months	3–8 months	≥50% reduction in MADRS score	1 week: 57.1 3 months: 85.7 Last follow-up: 85.7	MADRS score <10	1 week: 42.9 3 months: 57.1 Last follow-up: 57.1	—	Pilot study

Single case studies are not reported.

ALIC =anterior limb of the internal capsule; BDI=Beck Depression Inventory; BNST=bed nucleus of the stria terminalis; HAM-D=Hamilton Rating Scale for Depression (HAMD-17, HAMD-24, and HAMD-28=17-item, 24-item, and 28-item HAM-D, respectively); ITP=inferior thalamic peduncle; MADRS=Montgomery-Åsberg Depression Rating Scale; NA=not available; RCT=randomized controlled trial.

Source. Adapted from eTable (https://www.ncbi.nlm.nih.gov/pmc/articles/PMC8129059/table/T2/) in Schlaepfer TE, Meyer-Lindenberg A, Synofzik M, et al.: "Invasive Brain Stimulation in the Treatment of Psychiatric Illness—Proposed Indications and Approaches." *Deutsches Ärzteblatt International* 118(3):31–36, 2021. Available at: https://www.ncbi.nlm.nih.gov/pmc/articles/PMC8129059/. Accessed January 7, 2022.
Table data based on reviews by Dandekar et al. 2018, Drobisz and Damborská 2019, and Kisely et al. 2018 with updates.

CHAPTER 21

Other Antidepressants

Bupropion, Mirtazapine, and Trazodone

Charles DeBattista, M.D.

Bupropion, mirtazapine, and trazodone represent pharmacologically unique antidepressants that do not fit neatly into other common antidepressant classes, such as the selective serotonin reuptake inhibitors (SSRIs), serotonin-norepinephrine reuptake inhibitors (SNRIs), tricyclic antidepressants (TCAs), and monoamine oxidase inhibitors (MAOIs). Each of these three drugs has found important clinical niches in the treatment of depression, whether used as monotherapies or as adjunctive agents in combination with other antidepressants. Bupropion and mirtazapine are commonly co-prescribed with SSRIs and SNRIs to augment antidepressant response, while trazodone has become among the more common agents prescribed for insomnia. The unique pharmacology of these drugs also makes them among the least likely antidepressants to be associated with sexual side effect. Although trazodone, mirtazapine, and bupropion have been available for decades, they remain important and widely prescribed agents in the treatment of depression.

Bupropion

Bupropion became of interest to medicinal chemists in the 1960s, when it was found to have antidepressant properties in screening tests but did not appear to have some of the downsides of the TCAs and the MAOIs. Bupropion has been available to clinicians in the United States since 1986, but its mechanism of action is still not completely understood. Among its distinct properties relative to most currently available antidepressants is that bupropion does not have serotonergic properties. It is not a significant inhibitor of the serotonin (5-hydroxytryptamine [5-HT]) transporter and does not act on serotonin type 2 (5-HT_2) or type 1A (5-HT_{1A}) receptors (Costa et al.

2019; Foley et al. 2006). This lack of serotonergic effects contributes to bupropion's low proclivity for causing sexual side effects (Pereira et al. 2014).

Bupropion's primary mechanism of action appears to be on the norepinephrine system (Khan et al. 2016), where it reduces the excretion of norepinephrine and its metabolites. Its active metabolites, including hydroxybupropion and erythrobupropion, inhibit the norepinephrine transporter, although less potently than most TCAs and SNRIs (Costa et al. 2019). Bupropion does appear to downregulate β-adrenergic receptors in the locus coeruleus, and chronic administration of bupropion is known to modestly inhibit tyrosine hydroxylase activity.

Although often characterized as a dopaminergic drug, bupropion's dopamine properties are less evident than its noradrenergic effects. For example, animal studies have reported that it increases dopamine concentrations in the nucleus accumbens and mildly inhibits dopamine reuptake, but human studies have been less consistent. Human PET studies have not demonstrated a significant effect of bupropion on the dopamine transporter (Meyer et al. 2002). In addition, the major metabolite of dopamine, homovanillic acid, does not appear to be significantly affected by bupropion administration (Goodnick et al. 1998).

Because if its noradrenergic and perhaps some dopaminergic effects, bupropion is an activating antidepressant commonly prescribed for patients with major depressive disorder (MDD) whose depression is characterized by fatigue, hyperphagia, and hypersomnia rather than patients with significant insomnia, anxiety, and anorexia (Jefferson 2008; Patel et al. 2016). Bupropion is also among the more common augmentation strategies used by clinicians to improve the antidepressant effect of SSRIs, SNRIs, and other antidepressants. Despite the popularity of bupropion augmentation, few placebo-controlled trials have ever been completed with this strategy. However, bupropion augmentation has been examined in several large, randomized comparative efficacy studies, including the Sequenced Treatment Alternatives to Relieve Depression (STAR*D; Trivedi et al. 2006) and the Veterans Affairs Augmentation and Switching Treatments for Improving Depression Outcomes (VAST-D; Mohamed et al. 2017). In general, these studies have concluded that bupropion is about as useful as other augmenting agents, such as buspirone and aripiprazole, but not superior to them. Some open-label studies have suggested that adding bupropion to a serotonergic antidepressant can mitigate antidepressant-induced sexual side effects, but controlled studies have not been conclusive in this regard.

Bupropion is the only antidepressant with a specific indication for prevention of depressive episodes associated with seasonal affective disorder (SAD). Three registration trials with a total of 1,100 patients with SAD who were treated with bupropion extended-release demonstrated that an average dosage of 300 mg/day started in the fall was significantly more effective than placebo in preventing the recurrence of depression (Niemegeers et al. 2013). Subsequent analyses have shown that bupropion has a number needed to treat of 5 for preventing recurrences of depression in patients with SAD who have frequent recurrences.

In addition to the treatment of depression, bupropion has been FDA approved for two other indications. One indication is in the aid of smoking cessation. Registration trials and subsequent studies indicate that patients with nicotine dependence who were treated with 150–300 mg/day were more likely to abstain from smoking than those treated with placebo (Goldstein 1998; Jorenby 2002). The other approved indication is weight loss when used in a combination pill with naltrexone. Overweight or obese subjects who took the combination of bupropion and naltrexone for up to 56 weeks lost an average of 5% of their body weight, compared with approximately 3% of those given placebo (Greig and Keating 2015; Onakpoya et al. 2020). Off-label uses of bupropion for which there is some empirical support include the treatment of ADHD, persistent depressive disorder (dysthymia), and bipolar depression (in combination with a mood stabilizer). Unlike most antidepressants, bupropion has not consistently demonstrated benefit in the treatment of anxiety disorders, although some small positive studies in the treatment of social anxiety disorder have been reported.

Because bupropion is primarily metabolized via the cytochrome P450 (CYP) 2B6 isoenzyme, which is not involved in the metabolism of most medications, the risk of pharmacokinetic drug interactions is relatively small (Costa et al. 2019; Jefferson et al. 2005). Bupropion is a mild to moderate inhibitor of CYP2D6 and may interfere with the metabolism of substrates of this enzyme, although such interactions are rarely clinically significant. The most significant drug interaction may be with an MAOI, which may increase the risk of a hypertensive crisis (although not a serotonin syndrome). Drugs that lower the seizure threshold might also further increase the risk of seizure associated with bupropion.

Bupropion has a favorable side-effect profile in comparison with many other antidepressants (Saiz Ruiz et al. 2011). Because of its lack of serotonergic activity, it is less likely to be associated with sexual side effects. It does not induce orthostatic hypotension, and weight gain is uncommon. No significant anticholinergic side effects are associated with bupropion; dry mouth does occur but is thought to be related to the noradrenergic properties of the drug. The primary side effects are those associated with CNS activation. Bupropion is associated with worsening insomnia and should not be taken close to bedtime. It is not anxiolytic, and some anxious patients report an increase in anxiety and agitation with the drug. Likewise, bupropion can increase irritability in some patients. Increases in blood pressure and heart rate can occur. About 21% of patients in the MDD trials experienced some tremor with bupropion, which was about three times the rate of tremor seen in patients given placebo.

The most serious adverse event associated with bupropion is seizure (Davidson 1989), which is primarily associated with the immediate-release formulation. Seizure incidence is estimated at approximately 0.4% (4/1,000) for dosages less than or equal to 450 mg/day, with risk increasing substantially for dosages greater than 450 mg/day (i.e., up to 4.0% [4/100]). The seizure risk for the sustained- and extended-release formulations has been estimated at 0.1% (1/1,000), which is similar to the risk associated with other antidepressants.

Mirtazapine

Mirtazapine was synthesized in 1989 and approved in the United States in 1996 for the treatment of MDD. Mirtazapine is pharmacologically unique because it is not a monoamine reuptake inhibitor but has some noradrenergic and serotonergic receptor effects (Nutt 1997). For example, it is a presynaptic α_2 receptor antagonist that results in the presynaptic release of norepinephrine. The increase in norepinephrine in the synapse concurrently result in an increase in serotonergic neurotransmission via stimulation of α_1 receptors on serotonin neuron cell bodies. However, mirtazapine does not block α_2 receptors and is not associated with inducing hypotension. Mirtazapine is also an antagonist of the serotonin 5-HT_2 and 5-HT_3 receptors, as well as the histamine H_1 receptor.

In clinical trials, mirtazapine appears to be effective for both outpatients with milder depression and more severely ill inpatients with MDD. Early efficacy trials in MDD concluded that mirtazapine was as effective as the TCAs doxepin and amitriptyline (Mathur et al. 2002; Montgomery et al. 1998). In addition, mirtazapine appears in clinical trials to be as effective as various SSRIs, including paroxetine, fluoxetine, and citalopram (Thompson 1999). In some of these trials, mirtazapine had more rapid anxiolytic and antidepressant properties (Fawcett and Barkin 1998).

Mirtazapine has been used to treat common subtypes of depression. Some studies suggest that it is both effective and well tolerated in patients with geriatric depression (Bradley et al. 2016; Holland and Bhogle 2013). Side effects that can be problematic in some patients, including sedation and weight gain, may be desirable in some geriatric patients. In addition, studies have shown efficacy in the treatment of other subtypes of depression, including brief recurrent, atypical, and seasonal depression (Stahl et al. 1997).

In addition to its use in the monotherapy of depression, mirtazapine is frequently combined with other antidepressants to augment response. In the STAR*D trial, the combination of mirtazapine and venlafaxine was as effective as switching to an MAOI, tranylcypromine, and better tolerated in the treatment of patients with MDD whose illness had failed to respond to three consecutive antidepressant treatments (Trivedi et al. 2006). Still, only 13% of the subjects treated with a combination of venlafaxine and mirtazapine achieved a remission-level response in the STAR*D trial. Most but not all studies have found that adding 15–30 mg/day of mirtazapine to an SSRI or SNRI is effective in augmenting antidepressant response. However, the largest randomized controlled trial (RCT) conducted to date (Kessler et al. 2018) examined the efficacy of adding mirtazapine or placebo to SSRI or SNRI treatment in 480 primary care patients with MDD whose illness had not responded to monotherapy. No statistical advantage was found for adding mirtazapine over adding placebo. Likewise, the Combining Medications to Enhance Depression Outcomes trial (Rush et al. 2011), which examined the efficacy of combining mirtazapine with venlafaxine at the onset of MDD treatment, found no advantage over monotherapy in achieving response or remission.

Although mirtazapine is approved only for the treatment of MDD, there is reason to believe that the drug is beneficial in the treatment of some anxiety disorders (Gambi et al. 2005; Leinonen et al. 1999; Muehlbacher et al. 2005). Small and open-label studies have suggested some benefit for monotherapy with mirtazapine or for its use as an adjunctive agent in the treatment of social anxiety disorder, generalized anxiety disorder, and PTSD (Gambi et al. 2005; Muehlbacher et al. 2005; Ribeiro et al. 2001; Schneier et al. 2015). Among the most common uses of mirtazapine beyond the treatment of MDD is in the treatment of insomnia. Along with trazodone and quetiapine, mirtazapine is frequently used as a non-habit-forming strategy for the treatment of insomnia. Low dosages of mirtazapine (7.5 mg/day) were found to be as effective as 50 mg/day of quetiapine in a controlled trial of 19 healthy men with transient insomnia (Karsten et al. 2017), and mirtazapine increased total sleep time by 30 minutes and reduced awakenings by 40%. Studies of mirtazapine in the treatment of insomnia in patients with MDD, as well as in those with cancer, have indicated efficacy in improving sleep (Economos et al. 2020; Theobald et al. 2002).

Nonpsychiatric uses of mirtazapine include the treatment of pain syndromes and nausea. Mirtazapine, as a mixed serotonergic/adrenergic agent, has shown benefit in the treatment of pain disorders such as fibromyalgia. Several small, open-label and controlled studies have found it to be effective in the treatment of fibromyalgia with and without concomitant depression (Ottman et al. 2018; Welsch et al. 2018). Its 5-HT_3 receptor antagonist effects have found a role in the treatment of nausea and reduced appetite in patients with cancer, as well as in the pre- and postoperative management of nausea and anxiety in surgery patients (Chang et al. 2010; Kim et al. 2008).

The primary drug interactions with mirtazapine are pharmacodynamic rather pharmacokinetic. Although mirtazapine is partially metabolized via CYP2D6 and CYP3A4, potent inhibitors of these isoenzymes, such as paroxetine and ketoconazole, have modest and clinically insignificant effects on mirtazapine blood levels (Jaquenoud Sirot et al. 2012; Sitsen et al. 2001). On the other hand, the sedating effects of mirtazapine can be enhanced by the concomitant administration of CNS depressants, including alcohol, benzodiazepines, and most hypnotic drugs. Its α_2 effects have been associated with inducing a hypertensive crisis when used in combination with an MAOI (Ubogu and Katirji 2003). Thus, mirtazapine should be stopped at least 2 weeks before MAOI treatment begins.

The most common side effects of mirtazapine in MDD studies have been sedation/somnolence, dry mouth, and weight gain (Nutt 2002; Watanabe et al. 2010). More than half of patients taking mirtazapine experience somnolence, so it is generally taken at night. A counterintuitive effect is that lower dosages may be associated with more sedation than higher dosages. At a dosage of less than 15 mg/day, mirtazapine's antihistamine effects predominate over its noradrenergic and serotonergic actions (Shuman et al. 2019). Thus, patients experience more sedation at 7.5 mg/day than at 30 mg/day. On the other hand, most patients do not find 30 mg/day any more sedating than 15 mg/day. Many patients with MDD find the sedating effects to be useful in treating insomnia; however, few find the other major side effect, weight gain, to be as useful. The exceptions are patients who have lost weight secondary to their MDD, patients with a low BMI at baseline, and some geriatric patients. As mentioned, patients with cancer have sometimes benefited from the antinausea and appetite-increasing effects associated with mirtazapine. In MDD studies, mirtazapine was associated with a greater than 7% increase in body weight in approximately 7.5% of patients, and at least 20% of patients gained weight on the drug (PDR Staff 2017).

Mirtazapine is known to increase cholesterol and triglyceride levels in some patients. In premarketing studies, 15% of patients had an increase of more than 20% in cholesterol levels, and about 6% of patients had a significant increase in triglyceride levels (PDR Staff 2017). Statin agents appear to be effective in treating mirtazapine-associated increases in cholesterol and triglycerides. Postural hypotension is seen in about 7% of patients taking mirtazapine. This risk is higher in older patients and those taking antihypertensives but rarely is a basis for discontinuing the drug.

In contrast to most antidepressants, sexual side effects are not common with mirtazapine (Clayton et al. 2014). In fact, many patients who have antidepressant-induced sexual side effects have a resolution of these side effects when switched to mirtazapine.

Trazodone

Trazodone was the first alternative to the TCAs and MAOIs that was a serotonin-specific antidepressant. Introduced in the United States in 1981, it was considered a safer alternative to the older agents and was very popular among clinicians until other safe and easy-to-use agents, such as the SSRIs, became available later in the 1980s.

Trazodone is a postsynaptic 5-HT_{2A} and 5-HT_{2C} antagonist (Haria et al. 1994). The 5-HT_2 receptor interacts with the other receptors in the serotonin family, including the 5-HT_{1A} receptor, which appears to be important in the pathophysiology of both anxiety and depression. In addition, trazodone is a modest serotonin transporter inhibitor and an α_1-adrenergic receptor antagonist. It also inhibits the H_1 receptor, which contributes to its sedating properties.

The only FDA indication for trazodone is in the treatment of MDD. Many clinicians regard it as a less efficacious antidepressant than the TCAs or other antidepressants, particularly in patients with more serious depression. However, reviews of comparison studies have generally not found a significant difference in efficacy between trazodone and the TCAs or other antidepressants (Patten 1992; Yi et al. 2018). Many dozens of RCTs have been published since the 1970s demonstrating the efficacy of trazodone in the treatment of MDD. Early studies tended to employ more aggressive dosing, often reaching the target dosage of 300–600 mg/day in the first week. This rapid titration was often poorly tolerated because of the drug's sedative effects. Most but not all patients are able to tolerate a more gradual titration of the drug. Given the large number of other antidepressant choices that do not require a slow titration and are not as sedating, trazodone is used less commonly in the treatment of MDD now than it once was.

The most common off-label use of trazodone is in the treatment of insomnia. Trazodone, like mirtazapine, is a non-habit-forming alternative to traditional benzodiazepines and related hypnotic drugs. However, despite its popularity as a sleeping agent, very little research has been done on the utility of trazodone in the treatment of primary insomnia (Jaffer et al. 2017). Doses of 50–100 mg given 30 minutes before bedtime appear to reduce sleep latency and result in fewer awakenings. However, trazodone is also associated with small but significant worsening of daytime cognitive function, including verbal learning and short-term memory. It appears to be a useful adjunct in the treatment of insomnia associated with depression (Jindal 2009) and perhaps Alzheimer's disease (Camargos et al. 2014), but is less useful for primary insomnia and insomnia related to substance abuse.

Another off-label use of trazodone is in the treatment of anxiety disorders (Bossini et al. 2015; Charney et al. 1986; Rickels et al. 1993). Low-dosage trazodone has been compared with the TCAs and benzodiazepines in the treatment of generalized anxiety disorder. Small, mostly open-label studies have suggested benefit for the treatment of anxiety in patients with MDD, panic disorder, and phobic disorders. Trazodone has more recently found a place in veterinary medicine in the management of anxiety in pets (Gruen et al. 2014; Orlando et al. 2016).

The primary drug interactions of trazodone are pharmacodynamic. Its sedating effects can be exacerbated by coadministration of other sedating CNS depressants, such as benzodiazepines. Likewise, its α-adrenergic properties can exacerbate hypotension when it is coadministered with antihypertensives. When combined with anticoagulants such as warfarin, trazodone can increase bleeding times. Its use is generally contraindicated in combination with MAOIs because of the risk of serotonin syndrome.

Trazodone is a CYP3A4 substrate and so can interact with inducers and inhibitors of this isoenzyme (Haria et al. 1994). Thus, coadministration with CYP3A4 inhibitors such as indinavir or ketoconazole may increase trazodone blood levels and increase associated side effects. On the other hand, coadministration of trazodone with CYP3A4 inducers such as rifampin, carbamazepine, or phenytoin may render it less effective and require higher dosages. In turn, trazodone can increase the levels of phenytoin or digoxin, leading to toxicity associated with these drugs.

One of the metabolites of trazodone is *meta*-chlorophenylpiperazine, which is a hallucinogen and CYP2D6 substrate. Potent inhibitors of CYP2D6 such as fluoxetine and paroxetine have very rarely been associated with an increase in agitation, dysphoria, and hallucinations when combined with trazodone. The most common side effect of trazodone relative to placebo is sedation and somnolence (PDR Staff 2017). In clinical trials of trazodone, up to 40% of patients reported sedation or drowsiness, a rate that was two to four times the rate reported in the patients given placebo. As a result, most patients take trazodone primarily at night, although dosages greater than 100 mg/day are usually given in divided doses. Although sedation is the most commonly reported side effect, nausea was one of the most common reasons patients discontinued the drug in clinical trials. About 10% of patients reported nausea or vomiting in inpatient clinical trials with trazodone, compared with approximately 1% of placebo-treated patients. Among its more dangerous side effects, particularly in the elderly, is orthostatic hypotension; although the rate of hypotension is less than that seen with TCAs, trazodone's α_1-adrenergic receptor antagonism effect increases the risk of falls and syncope in older patients. The hypotension is dose related, and the risk is greater at higher dosages than at lower ones.

Trazodone, like mirtazapine and bupropion, is associated with lower rates of sexual dysfunction than most antidepressants (Clayton et al. 2014). That said, it does carry a risk of priapism that is not typical of other antidepressants. Priapism is mediated by the α_1-blocking properties of trazodone and is treated either by the direct injection of an α_1 agonist such as phenylephrine or, in some cases, by removal of excess blood in the penis via needle aspiration or surgery (Saenz de Tejada et al. 1991). The incidence of priapism is about 1/6,000, and the risk is higher among young males than older patients.

References

Bossini L, Coluccia A, Casolaro I, et al: Off-label trazodone prescription: evidence, benefits, and risks. Curr Pharm Des 21(23):3343–3351, 2015 26088119

Bradley B, Backus D, Gray E: Depression in the older adult: what should be considered? Ment Health Clin 6(5):222–228, 2016 29955474

Camargos EF, Louzada LL, Quintas JL, et al: Trazodone improves sleep parameters in Alzheimer disease patients: a randomized, double-blind, and placebo-controlled study. Am J Geriatr Psychiatry 22(12):1565–1574, 2014 24495406

Chang F-L, Ho S-T, Sheen MJ: Efficacy of mirtazapine in preventing intrathecal morphine-induced nausea and vomiting after orthopaedic surgery. Anaesthesia 65(12):1206–1211, 2010 21182602

Charney DS, Woods SW, Goodman WK, et al: Drug treatment of panic disorder: the comparative efficacy of imipramine, alprazolam, and trazodone. J Clin Psychiatry 47(12):580–586, 1986 3536889
Clayton AH, Croft HA, Handiwala L: Antidepressants and sexual dysfunction: mechanisms and clinical implications. Postgrad Med 126(2):91–99, 2014 24685972
Costa R, Oliveira NG, Dinis-Oliveira RJ: Pharmacokinetic and pharmacodynamic of bupropion: integrative overview of relevant clinical and forensic aspects. Drug Metab Rev 51(3):293–313, 2019 31124380
Davidson J: Seizures and bupropion: a review. J Clin Psychiatry 50(7):256–261, 1989 2500425
Economos G, Lovell N, Johnston A, et al: What is the evidence for mirtazapine in treating cancer-related symptomatology? A systematic review. Support Care Cancer 28(4):1597–1606, 2020 31858251
Fawcett J, Barkin RL: Review of the results from clinical studies on the efficacy, safety and tolerability of mirtazapine for the treatment of patients with major depression. J Affect Disord 51(3):267–285, 1998 10333982
Foley KF, DeSanty KP, Kast RE: Bupropion: pharmacology and therapeutic applications. Expert Rev Neurother 6(9):1249–1265, 2006 17009913
Gambi F, De Berardis D, Campanella D, et al: Mirtazapine treatment of generalized anxiety disorder: a fixed dose, open label study. J Psychopharmacol 19(5):483–487, 2005 16166185
Goldstein MG: Bupropion sustained release and smoking cessation. J Clin Psychiatry 59 (suppl 4):66–72, 1998 9554323
Goodnick PJ, Dominguez RA, DeVane CL, et al: Bupropion slow-release response in depression: diagnosis and biochemistry. Biol Psychiatry 44(7):629–632, 1998 9787888
Greig SL, Keating GM: Naltrexone ER/bupropion ER: a review in obesity management. Drugs 75(11):1269–1280, 2015 26105116
Gruen ME, Roe SC, Griffith E, et al: Use of trazodone to facilitate postsurgical confinement in dogs. J Am Vet Med Assoc 245(3):296–301, 2014 25029308
Haria M, Fitton A, McTavish D: Trazodone: a review of its pharmacology, therapeutic use in depression and therapeutic potential in other disorders. Drugs Aging 4(4):331–355, 1994 8019056
Holland J, Bhogle M: Sertraline and mirtazapine as geriatric antidepressants. Psychiatr Danub 25 (suppl 2):S286–S290, 2013 23995195
Jaffer KY, Chang T, Vanle B, et al: Trazodone for insomnia: a systematic review. Innov Clin Neurosci 14(7–8):24–34, 2017 29552421
Jaquenoud Sirot E, Harenberg S, Vandel P, et al: Multicenter study on the clinical effectiveness, pharmacokinetics, and pharmacogenetics of mirtazapine in depression. J Clin Psychopharmacol 32(5):622–629, 2012 22926595
Jefferson JW: Bupropion extended-release for depressive disorders. Expert Rev Neurother 8(5):715–722, 2008 18457528
Jefferson JW, Pradko JF, Muir KT: Bupropion for major depressive disorder: pharmacokinetic and formulation considerations. Clin Ther 27(11):1685–1695, 2005 16368442
Jindal RD: Insomnia in patients with depression: some pathophysiological and treatment considerations. CNS Drugs 23(4):309–329, 2009 19374460
Jorenby D: Clinical efficacy of bupropion in the management of smoking cessation. Drugs 62 (suppl 2):25–35, 2002 12109933
Karsten J, Hagenauw LA, Kamphuis J, et al: Low doses of mirtazapine or quetiapine for transient insomnia: a randomised, double-blind, cross-over, placebo-controlled trial. J Psychopharmacol 31(3):327–337, 2017 28093029
Kessler D, Burns A, Tallon D, et al: Combining mirtazapine with SSRIs or SNRIs for treatment-resistant depression: the MIR RCT. Health Technol Assess 22(63):1–136, 2018 30468145
Khan SR, Berendt RT, Ellison CD, et al: Bupropion hydrochloride. Profiles Drug Subst Excip Relat Methodol 41:1–30, 2016 26940167
Kim SW, Shin IS, Kim JM, et al: Effectiveness of mirtazapine for nausea and insomnia in cancer patients with depression. Psychiatry Clin Neurosci 62(1):75–83, 2008 18289144

Leinonen E, Skarstein J, Behnke K, et al: Efficacy and tolerability of mirtazapine versus citalopram: a double-blind, randomized study in patients with major depressive disorder. Int Clin Psychopharmacol 14(6):329–337, 1999 10565799
Mathur A, Chowdhary A, Jain M: A comparative study of the efficacy and safety of mirtazapine versus amitriptyline in the treatment of major depression. Indian J Psychiatry 44(3):260–265, 2002 21206581
Meyer JH, Goulding VS, Wilson AA, et al: Bupropion occupancy of the dopamine transporter is low during clinical treatment. Psychopharmacology (Berl) 163(1):102–105, 2002 12185406
Mohamed S, Johnson GR, Chen P, et al: Effect of antidepressant switching vs augmentation on remission among patients with major depressive disorder unresponsive to antidepressant treatment: the VAST-D randomized clinical trial. JAMA 318(2):132–145, 2017 28697253
Montgomery SA, Reimitz PE, Zivkov M: Mirtazapine versus amitriptyline in the long-term treatment of depression: a double-blind placebo-controlled study. Int Clin Psychopharmacol 13(2):63–73, 1998 9669186
Muehlbacher M, Nickel MK, Nickel C, et al: Mirtazapine treatment of social phobia in women: a randomized, double-blind, placebo-controlled study. J Clin Psychopharmacol 25(6):580–583, 2005 16282842
Niemegeers P, Dumont GJ, Patteet L, et al: Bupropion for the treatment of seasonal affective disorder. Expert Opin Drug Metab Toxicol 9(9):1229–1240, 2013 23705752
Nutt D: Mirtazapine: pharmacology in relation to adverse effects. Acta Psychiatr Scand Suppl 391:31–37, 1997 9265949
Nutt DJ: Tolerability and safety aspects of mirtazapine. Hum Psychopharmacol 17 (suppl 1):S37–S41, 2002 12404669
Onakpoya IJ, Lee JJ, Mahtani KR, et al: Naltrexone-bupropion (Mysimba) in management of obesity: a systematic review and meta-analysis of unpublished clinical study reports. Br J Clin Pharmacol 86(4):646–667, 2020 31918448
Orlando JM, Case BC, Thomson AE, et al: Use of oral trazodone for sedation in cats: a pilot study. J Feline Med Surg 18(6):476–482, 2016 26037387
Ottman AA, Warner CB, Brown JN: The role of mirtazapine in patients with fibromyalgia: a systematic review. Rheumatol Int 38(12):2217–2224, 2018 29860538
Patel K, Allen S, Haque MN, et al: Bupropion: a systematic review and meta-analysis of effectiveness as an antidepressant. Ther Adv Psychopharmacol 6(2):99–144, 2016 27141292
Patten SB: The comparative efficacy of trazodone and imipramine in the treatment of depression. CMAJ 146(7):1177–1182, 1992 1532532
Pereira VM, Arias-Carrión O, Machado S, et al: Bupropion in the depression-related sexual dysfunction: a systematic review. CNS Neurol Disord Drug Targets 13(6):1079–1088, 2014 24923342
PDR Staff: Physicians' Desk Reference, 71st Edition. Montvale, NJ, Medical Economics, 2017
Ribeiro L, Busnello JV, Kauer-Sant'Anna M, et al: Mirtazapine versus fluoxetine in the treatment of panic disorder. Braz J Med Biol Res 34(10):1303–1307, 2001 11593305
Rickels K, Downing R, Schweizer E, et al: Antidepressants for the treatment of generalized anxiety disorder. A placebo-controlled comparison of imipramine, trazodone, and diazepam. Arch Gen Psychiatry 50(11):884–895, 1993 8215814
Rush AJ, Trivedi MH, Stewart JW, et al: Combining medications to enhance depression outcomes (CO-MED): acute and long-term outcomes of a single-blind randomized study. Am J Psychiatry 168(7):689–701, 2011 21536692
Saenz de Tejada I, Ware JC, Blanco R, et al: Pathophysiology of prolonged penile erection associated with trazodone use. J Urol 145(1):60–64, 1991 1984101
Saiz Ruiz J, Gibert J, Gutiérrez Fraile M, et al: Bupropion: efficacy and safety in the treatment of depression. Actas Esp Psiquiatr 39 (suppl 1):1–25, 2011 22983817
Schneier FR, Campeas R, Carcamo J, et al: Combined mirtazapine and SSRI treatment of PTSD: a placebo-controlled trial. Depress Anxiety 32(8):570–579, 2015 26115513

Shuman M, Chukwu A, Van Veldhuizen N, et al: Relationship between mirtazapine dose and incidence of adrenergic side effects: an exploratory analysis. Ment Health Clin 9(1):41–47, 2019 30627503

Sitsen J, Maris F, Timmer C: Drug-drug interaction studies with mirtazapine and carbamazepine in healthy male subjects. Eur J Drug Metab Pharmacokinet 26(1–2):109–121, 2001 11554425

Stahl S, Zivkov M, Reimitz PE, et al: Meta-analysis of randomized, double-blind, placebo-controlled, efficacy and safety studies of mirtazapine versus amitriptyline in major depression. Acta Psychiatr Scand 96 (suppl 391):22–30, 1997 9265948

Theobald DE, Kirsh KL, Holtsclaw E, et al: An open-label, crossover trial of mirtazapine (15 and 30 mg) in cancer patients with pain and other distressing symptoms. J Pain Symptom Manage 23(5):442–447, 2002 12007762

Thompson C: Mirtazapine versus selective serotonin reuptake inhibitors. J Clin Psychiatry 60 (suppl 17):18–22, discussion 46–48, 1999 10446737

Trivedi MH, Fava M, Wisniewski SR, et al: Medication augmentation after the failure of SSRIs for depression. N Engl J Med 354(12):1243–1252, 2006 16554526

Ubogu EE, Katirji B: Mirtazapine-induced serotonin syndrome. Clin Neuropharmacol 26(2):54–57, 2003 12671522

Watanabe N, Omori IM, Nakagawa A, et al: Safety reporting and adverse-event profile of mirtazapine described in randomized controlled trials in comparison with other classes of antidepressants in the acute-phase treatment of adults with depression: systematic review and meta-analysis. CNS Drugs 24(1):35–53, 2010 20030418

Welsch P, Bernardy K, Derry S, et al: Mirtazapine for fibromyalgia in adults. Cochrane Database Syst Rev 8(8):CD012708, 2018 30080242

Yi XY, Ni SF, Ghadami MR, et al: Trazodone for the treatment of insomnia: a meta-analysis of randomized placebo-controlled trials. Sleep Med 45:25–32, 2018 29680424

CHAPTER 22

Ketamine and Other Investigational Agents

Gerard Sanacora, M.D., Ph.D.
Brandon M. Kitay, M.D., Ph.D.

Over the past decade, depression has emerged as the leading cause of disability worldwide (Vigo et al. 2016, 2020). The significant morbidity and mortality associated with depression (Kessler et al. 2003) extend beyond its impact on individual productivity (Stewart et al. 2003) and cost the United States nearly $210 billion in 2010, with a substantial proportion attributable to indirect costs unrelated to treatment (Greenberg et al. 2015). While many factors contribute to the growing prevalence of depression, including practical, structural, and psychological barriers that limit access to timely and robust treatment (Thornicroft et al. 2017), there is also great concern regarding the inadequacy of our standard pharmacotherapies (Insel and Wang 2009). Antidepressant medications remain among the three most commonly prescribed therapeutic classes in the United States (Hales et al. 2019; Martin et al. 2019), yet one-third to nearly one-half of all patients diagnosed with major depressive disorder (MDD) will not adequately benefit from multiple, often successive, courses of antidepressant therapy (Gaynes et al. 2009; Nie et al. 2018; Rush et al. 2006). This fact underscores our need for novel antidepressant treatments, because patients with treatment-resistant depression (TRD)—defined as depression that does not to respond to at least two trials of an oral antidepressant at an effective dosage for an adequate duration (Sackeim 2001)—have low chances of achieving meaningful symptomatic relief with further trials of standard antidepressant therapies (Zisook et al. 2008). Because patients with TRD account for the greatest share of health care burden among patients with depressive disorders (Amos et al. 2018; Pilon et al. 2019), considerable research efforts have focused on developing antidepressants with this population in mind.

For the past 70 years, the general class of antidepressant medications comprised an array of orally administered agents with pharmacodynamic properties that nearly all converged on a common mechanism of action: modulation and/or enhancement of monoaminergic (e.g., serotonin, norepinephrine, dopamine) neurotransmission. Based on serendipitous discoveries made in the late 1950s (Perez-Caballero et al. 2019; Schildkraut 1965), the "monoaminergic deficiency hypothesis of depression" (Coppen et al. 1967) has remained the cornerstone of antidepressant design. However, the growing recognition that these medications bring limited benefit to many patients has cast doubt on their true efficacy (Ioannidis 2008). Furthermore, the discrepancy of several weeks between demonstrable neurophysiological changes in the brain and clinical benefits, along with marked variability in response (Cipriani et al. 2018), has further challenged our understanding of the mechanism of monoamine-targeting antidepressants and, by extension, the pathophysiological processes underlying depression (Harmer et al. 2017).

One of the most impactful and rapidly expanding lines of scientific inquiry over the past 30 years has been the study of amino acid neurotransmission (GABA and glutamate) and of the critical roles these systems play in neurophysiology and neuroplasticity. Dysregulation of glutamatergic neurotransmission is now implicated in the pathophysiology of multiple neuropsychiatric disorders ranging from amyotrophic lateral sclerosis to schizophrenia and from traumatic brain injury to obsessive-compulsive disorder (Javitt et al. 2011). The involvement of the glutamatergic system in regulating neuroplasticity, through effects on both synaptogenesis and dendritic pruning, points to a central role of the system in a diverse range of neurological processes, including adaptive brain function. The widespread distribution and ubiquitous nature of the system highlight the diverse range of neurological processes that are likely influenced by the system. For example, the critical role of the glutamatergic system in mediating the brain's response to stress has identified a critical link between psychosocial/environmental stress and the pathophysiology of mood and anxiety disorders in humans (Duman et al. 2019; Lener et al. 2017; Popoli et al. 2011).

This expanded understanding of the neurophysiological contributions of amino acid neurotransmitter systems and their disruption in both murine models of chronic stress and patients suffering from depression has driven exploration of the therapeutic potential of readily available pharmacological agents capable of targeting these systems (Wilkinson and Sanacora 2019). These efforts led to a wave of discovery culminating in the FDA approval of the first novel non-monoaminergic antidepressant medication, esketamine. The drug is believed to primarily target the glutamatergic neurotransmitter system, providing a rapid onset of antidepressant effects in previously treatment-nonresponsive depressed patients (U.S. Food and Drug Administration 2019). In this chapter we briefly describe the process of discovery, review the clinical data surrounding the efficacy and safety of the emerging treatments associated with the glutamatergic system, and reevaluate our understanding of the unique mechanisms of action associated with these novel treatments.

Path to the Discovery of Ketamine's Antidepressant Action

Like most journeys leading to novel discoveries, the path to the discovery of esketamine as a novel antidepressant was characterized by a series of serendipitous observations, scientific breakthroughs, blind alleys, red herrings, and unexpected connections to other branches of science and medicine. In chronological order, we would need to look back over 60 years to a serendipitous observation reported by George Crane in 1959 (Crane 1959). Much like the original discovery of iproniazid's antidepressant effects, leading to the development of the monoamine oxidase inhibitor (MAOI) class of antidepressants (Slattery et al. 2004), Crane published his observations of rapid improvements in mood, sleep, and appetite following the initiation of Seromycin (D-cycloserine) for the treatment of tuberculosis. Although this study predated any understanding of D-cycloserine's effects on the glutamatergic system, and even the understanding of glutamate's role as a neurotransmitter, later work has shown us that D-cycloserine acts as a partial agonist at the glycine site of the glutamatergic *N*-methyl-D-aspartate (NMDA) receptor, possibly providing the mechanism of the drug's observed antidepressant action (Thomas et al. 1988). Also predating the understanding of glutamate's role in neurotransmission and pathophysiology, a second study designed to explore ketamine's effect on the psychoanalytical construct of abreaction in 100 hospitalized Iranian patients diagnosed with a variety of psychiatric disorders showed, back in 1973, that a single dose of ketamine could produce rapid improvement in symptoms (Khorramzadeh and Lotfy 1973). These reports did not directly lead to further studies with NMDA receptor–targeting drugs, but in retrospect they are seen as providing supportive evidence of the receptor's ability to mediate rapid-onset antidepressant effects.

The first line of investigation that provided a direct link to the development and approval of esketamine as an antidepressant treatment was a series of studies from Phil Skolnick's laboratory at the National Institutes of Health (Pilc et al. 2013). These studies found evidence of NMDA receptor abnormalities associated with stress-induced rodent models of mood disorders and identified the NMDA receptor as a pharmacological target for antidepressant drug development in the early 1990s. Other work at the time demonstrated that tricyclic antidepressants—in addition to their effects on monoamine neurotransmission—also modified NMDA receptor binding and function, suggesting that the receptor may be involved in the downstream mechanisms of even the classic antidepressants (Reynolds and Miller 1988). In parallel, there was an increasing awareness of corticolimbic circuitry emerging at the time, and how it related to depressive symptoms. Given that these are largely glutamatergic and GABAergic circuits, it was reasoned that drugs targeting these systems may produce more direct antidepressant effects, not requiring the secondary changes in neurophysiology necessary for the monoaminergic drugs to produce their antidepressant effects (Krystal et al. 2019). This work provided the foundational evidence for the seminal proof-of-concept study by Berman et al. (2000) demonstrating the antidepressant potential of ketamine, a well-characterized NMDA receptor antagonist. Remarkably, the findings showed that a single infusion of ketamine produced a rapid onset of antidepressant effects capable of lasting for days after a single administration in a small group of eight patients in a randomized crossover study design. However, interest in developing ketamine as a novel, rapidly acting antidepressant therapy only gained sustained momentum nearly 6 years later following the replication and confirmation efforts by Zarate et al. (2006) at the National Institute of Mental Health. This early work not only spurred interest in ketamine and ketamine-like compounds but also can be credited with more broadly reigniting interest in antidepressant drug development that had waned through the end of the twentieth century.

Clinical Applications of Ketamine and Esketamine for Major Depressive Disorder

Since the 2006 report of subanesthetic ketamine producing rapid-acting antidepressant effects in subjects with MDD, there has been a relative explosion of studies and case series exploring the effects of ketamine and related drugs in the treatment of a variety of neuropsychiatric disorders. Here we will attempt to present a review of the data currently available, focusing on mood disorders and organized by drug. Because this chapter largely covers investigational agents, this section aims to provide the essential information required to evaluate their potential clinical efficacy and to expand our understanding of the pathophysiology of the disorders or guide the development of novel treatment strategies.

Ketamine

The majority of studies to date have focused on the efficacy of ketamine or esketamine for the treatment of depressive episodes in patients who have not had an adequate response to standard oral antidepressant medications. Many of the initial published reports simply confirmed the short-term effects of ketamine at the subanesthetic dose of 0.5 mg/kg over a period of 40 minutes (Table 22–1) (McGirr et al. 2015; Newport et al. 2015). However, there is now an increasing number of studies specifically addressing many of the important clinical questions related to optimal dosing, frequency of treatments, and longer-term management plans, as well as route of delivery (Caddy et al. 2014, 2015). Additionally, there have been several studies examining the efficacy and safety of several drugs with pharmacological properties similar to ketamine, including esketamine, the only one of the drugs in this discussion to have received approval by the FDA for treatment of a psychiatric disorder at this time.

Optimal Dose: Intravenous Ketamine

The original Berman et al. (2000) study of ketamine in the treatment of MDD used a dose of 0.5 mg/kg delivered intravenously over a period of 40 minutes. This dose was chosen not based on theoretical grounds intending to optimize antidepressant efficacy, but because it was the dose capable of producing marked acute effects on perception and cognition while still allowing the subject to remain awake enough to answer questions (Krystal et al. 2019). Although studies employing rodent models suggest the existence of an "inverted U"–shaped dose-response curve associated with the antidepressant efficacy of ketamine (Chowdhury et al. 2017; Li et al. 2010), there are remarkably few studies attempting to identify the optimal dose of ketamine to provide clinical benefit. The largest existing study investigating the effects of dose on clinical response examined only the short-term outcomes related to a single intravenous infusion (provided over 40 minutes) of ketamine at four different doses (0.1 mg/kg, 0.2 mg/kg, 0.5 mg/kg, and 1.0 mg/kg) or a midazolam control (active placebo) (Fava et al. 2020). Although this study was underpowered for definitive comparisons to be made, ketamine at all doses showed numerically greater reductions in depression severity compared with midazolam. The 0.5-mg/kg dose and the 1.0-mg/kg dose were superior to the comparator (midazolam) at day 1 and day 3 following in-

TABLE 22–1. Representative selection of randomized controlled trials of ketamine in subjects with major depressive disorder (MDD)

	Sample size	Design	Route,[a] schedule, dose	Depression rating scale[b]	Outcome
Berman et al. 2000	9	Double-blind, crossover	IV, single, saline vs. 0.5 mg/kg (40-minute infusion)	HAM-D (25-item)	Significant improvement at 2 hours through 72 hours
Zarate et al. 2006	18	Double-blind, crossover	IV, single, saline vs. 0.5 mg/kg (40-minute infusion)	HAM-D (21-item)	Significant improvement at 2 hours through 1 week
Sos et al. 2013	30	Double-blind, crossover	IV, single, saline vs. 0.54 mg/kg (30-minute infusion)	MADRS	Significant improvement at day 1 through day 7
Murrough et al. 2013a	73	Double-blind	IV, single, midazolam (active placebo) vs. 0.5 mg/kg (40-minute infusion)	MADRS	Significant improvement at day 1 posttreatment over placebo
Lapidus et al. 2014	20	Double-blind, crossover	IN, single, saline vs. 50 mg	MADRS	Significant improvement at 40 minutes through 48 hours
Hu et al. 2016	30	Double-blind	IV, single, saline+oral escitalopram vs. 0.5 mg/kg+oral escitalopram (40-minute infusion)	MADRS	Significant improvement at 2 hours through 2 weeks
Singh et al. 2016b	68	Double-blind	IV, multiple, saline vs. 0.5 mg/kg twice weekly or thrice weekly (40-minute infusions), up to 4 weeks	MADRS	Significant improvement as early as 3 days and through 15 days

[a]Route: IN=intranasal; IV=intravenous.
[b]Rating scales: HAM-D=Hamilton Depression Rating Scale (25- or 21-item); MADRS=Montgomery-Åsberg Depression Rating Scale.

fusion and showed evidence of a longer duration of action (Fava et al. 2020; Salloum et al. 2020). The clinical responses to the lower ketamine doses (0.1 and 0.2 mg/kg) were less consistent, and there was not strong evidence of a standard linear dose-response relationship. In retrospect, the original choice of 0.5 mg/kg may have been an extremely fortuitous decision. However, there remains a need for further investigation toward determining the optimal dosing of ketamine and identifying potential factors moderating dose response—for example, concomitant medications (Anand et al. 2000) that would impede or improve clinical efficacy.

Optimal Dosing Schedule: Intravenous Ketamine

The studies in the first wave of research exploring the antidepressant effects of ketamine were limited to single administrations of the drug. They demonstrated peak antidepressant benefits occurring within 24–72 hours of dosing, but then a gradual diminution of the beneficial effect in most patients over the following days and weeks (Caddy et al. 2015). A few early reports presenting evidence that the antidepressant effects could be sustained by providing six doses over 2 weeks (aan het Rot et al. 2010; Murrough et al. 2013b) were met with great interest, because they started to show the potential of using ketamine in the clinical management of patients. Although there are now several studies providing mostly consistent evidence of sustained clinical benefit with repeated ketamine dosing, there remain unanswered questions surrounding the frequency of dosing, the parameters for continuation and maintenance of ketamine therapy, and the safety of repeated administrations. One of the few studies specifically designed to evaluate how the frequency of ketamine administration could impact treatment of depression randomly assigned participants to either twice-weekly or thrice-weekly dosing with either 0.5 mg/kg ketamine or saline placebo. Although both dosing frequencies showed clear beneficial effects of ketamine over placebo, there was no evidence to suggest that thrice-weekly dosing was superior to twice-weekly dosing in producing and sustaining the antidepressant effect over the duration of the study (Singh et al. 2016b). These data represent the most thorough examination of the initial dosing frequency for ketamine in the treatment of MDD available to date and provided the rationale for the design of pivotal trials leading to the FDA approval of esketamine.

Longer-Term Treatment Planning

The strategy for longer-term treatment planning with ketamine remains largely underdeveloped at this time. Although there are now large-scale pivotal trials performed with extended use of intranasal esketamine that may afford an opportunity for extrapolation (see subsection "Esketamine" later in this chapter), there remains relatively little work published specifically exploring the optimization of intravenous ketamine treatment. Reports from several programs and a survey of many academic and private clinics providing intravenous ketamine treatment for MDD suggest that in many patients, the antidepressant benefit can be sustained with intermittent treatments (Phillips et al. 2020; Szymkowicz et al. 2013; Vande Voort et al. 2016; Wilkinson et al. 2017, 2018), but the optimal frequency of dosing to preserve benefits with repeated dosing has not clearly been determined. A survey of relatively early adopters of the treatment in 2017 suggested that the majority of patients were returning for treatment approximately every 2–5 weeks after completing an index course lasting a few weeks. This finding appears to be consistent with other, more recent reports and clinical practice. However, the data supporting this frequency remain of low quality, and there is variability in the reported frequency of administration that suggests there may be individual differences influencing the optimal dosing frequency.

Potential Risks of Ketamine Administration and Maintenance Treatment

The choice of whether to initiate ketamine in the treatment of a depressive episode and whether to continue with maintenance ketamine treatments should include careful consideration of potential risks to the patient. The concerns associated with the use of ketamine in treatment for depression can be captured in four general categories.

First, there are acute physiological and psychological risks associated with the administration of ketamine. Administration of ketamine can alter cardiovascular function, increasing heart rate and blood pressure. Although increases are generally limited in intensity and duration, they should be considered a potential risk for individuals with underlying cardiac or cerebrovascular conditions. Ketamine administered at the dose described as most effective in the treatment of depression can also have marked effects on cognition and perception that can be anxiogenic and dysphoria-inducing to some patients. Although these effects are quite transient, typically lasting only minutes to 1 hour after the infusion has stopped, they can be subjectively unpleasant to some patients and in rare cases may have a longer duration. The ability to manage these acute risks requires a unique set of clinical skills and monitoring capabilities that has limited the broader use of the treatment modality largely to specialty outpatient clinics and academic settings.

Second, there are potential longer-term physiological consequences of repeated ketamine administration. Neurological, urinary, and gastrointestinal pathology have all been associated with repeated ketamine use. Multiple preclinical studies have demonstrated neurotoxic effects related to the administration of ketamine and other NMDA receptor antagonists (Costa et al. 2020). Although most of these studies examined the effects of high doses of the drugs and administration during sensitive periods of development, there is evidence that even repeated subanesthetic doses of ketamine can cause neurotoxic effects, including behavioral changes and cellular abnormalities in the hippocampus of cynomolgus monkeys (Li et al. 2020) and rodents (Schobel et al. 2013). These studies, paired with evidence that ketamine use disorder is associated with several worrisome alterations within the CNS, including decreased gray matter, impaired cognition, and increased proneness to psychosis, provide strong cause for concern (Edward Roberts et al. 2014; Morgan et al. 2012, 2014).

Frequent use of ketamine can also contribute to a range of uropathies, including ulcerative cystitis, contracted bladder, ureteral stenosis, vesicoureteral reflux, impaired peristalsis function of the renal pelvis or ureter, and even chronic kidney failure. Although the exact mechanism underlying ketamine's toxic effect on the urinary system has not been completely elucidated, it is thought to involve direct toxicity to the urothelium and possibly neurogenic inflammation (Castellani et al. 2020). Similar toxic effects of heavy frequent ketamine misuse have also been reported within the gastrointestinal system, resulting in epigastric pain, recurrent vomiting, and gastrointestinal bleeding (S.Y.W. Liu et al. 2017).

Fortunately, there have been very few reports suggesting neurotoxicity in the form of persistently impaired cognition or increased psychotic episodes associated with the clinical use of ketamine to treat depression to date. Similarly, there has not been clear evidence of significant uropathy or gastrointestinal disorders associated with appropriate use of ketamine to treat mood disorders. However, we should be aware that the onset of these symptoms may require prolonged exposure (Li et al. 2019), and the absence of a coordinated data collection system for patients receiving ketamine treatments could make it difficult to reliably identify such cases if they are to develop.

Third, there is a possibility that treatment with ketamine could lead to future drug abuse and encourage drug diversion. Ketamine is known to have abuse liability and has been classified as a Schedule III controlled substance by the FDA since 1999. Recreational misuse of the drug has been reported since the early 1970s, but its popularity as a "club drug" grew in the 1980s, spreading to urban centers in several international locations (Sassano-Higgins et al. 2016). Although there are reports suggesting discontinuation symptoms and tolerance associated with chronic, frequent ketamine misuse, there is no clear evidence of a typical withdrawal syndrome following ketamine discontinuation. The Monitoring the Future study, assessing the prevalence of substance misuse in teenagers and young adults, has reported consistent rates of ketamine misuse since 2002 (Johnston et al. 2016), with an annual U.S. prevalence of ketamine in 2018 of 0.7%, 0.9%, and 0.9%, respectively, among 12th graders, college students, and young adults. In response to concerns of ketamine misuse internationally, the World Health Organization Expert Committee on Drug Dependence reviewed the latest evidence on the potential harm to health and dependence-producing properties of ketamine in 2016 (World Health Organization 2016). The committee decided to uphold its previous recommendations issued in 2006, 2012, and 2014 that ketamine should not be scheduled or controlled under the international drug control conventions, citing that illicit use of ketamine has been reported on a relatively small global scale for the past several decades, with dependence and overdose being rare. Further supporting this decision is the recognition that ketamine plays an essential role as a general anesthetic in low-resource countries and that further controlling ketamine may limit the potential for expanding research into its use in treating depression and other psychiatric disorders. It will be interesting to see how the increased use of ketamine for the treatment of mood disorders will impact the illicit use of ketamine moving forward.

Lastly, the unknown impact of long-term treatment with ketamine on brain function in general poses considerable challenges in determining the risks and benefits of chronic or maintenance ketamine therapy, especially for patients with TRD. As mentioned, the large majority of studies involving ketamine have focused on the short-term benefits of the treatment (those lasting days to weeks). There has been relatively little high-quality work demonstrating the effectiveness and safety of continued ketamine treatment. This lack of data on long-term treatment is compounded by concerns of drug dependency, either physiological or psychological, that have led some to wonder whether it may be difficult for patients to successfully taper and discontinue use of the drug over time. These concerns can only be addressed with rigorous longitudinal inquiries. Unfortunately, unless a concerted effort is made to collect, analyze, and disseminate this data, guidance on this issue may remain elusive for the foreseeable future.

Comparing Routes of Delivery

Oral delivery is especially appealing for its ease of use and accessibility; however, ketamine is subject to extensive first-pass metabolism resulting in relatively low bioavailability (Clements et al. 1982), and an oral formulation could increase the risk of misuse and diversion. Despite these concerns, there have been over a dozen case reports and small proof-of-concept studies exploring the possibility of oral dosing for the treatment of mood disorders (Rosenblat et al. 2019). Although the volume and quality of the relatively small number of studies to date do not afford us a firm evidence base, there is evidence to suggest the potential for clinical benefit and otherwise acceptable overall tolerability of oral dosing, albeit at a much longer time to onset and smaller magnitude of antidepressant effect compared with intravenous dosing (Rosenblat et al. 2019). Attempts have also been made to explore the potential for sublingual (Lara et al. 2013; Nguyen et al. 2015), subcutaneous, intramuscular (Loo et al. 2016), and intranasal (Lapidus et al. 2014) dosing in order to avoid the complications of intravenous dosing. Again, the quality, size, and number of these studies do not allow any meaningful conclusions to be drawn regarding the comparable efficacy and safety of the different routes of administration (Andrade 2017). Collectively, these studies all seem to suggest, similarly to the rodent studies, that the efficacy and side-effect profiles are closely tied to the peak plasma levels achieved. The relevance of other pharmacokinetic factors to the ultimate clinical utility of the treatment—such as time to maximal concentration, area under the curve, and plasma clearance rate—still needs to be determined.

Esketamine

Adequately addressing efficacy and safety issues with high-quality data is expensive. Costs have been the major factor impeding the collection of high-quality data with racemic ketamine. However, many of these concerns have been successfully addressed in pursuing the FDA approval of esketamine nasal spray (Spravato™) as augmentation to an oral antidepressant for patients with TRD (Bahr et al. 2019). Ketamine is a racemic mixture composed of equal amounts of left- and right-handed enantiomers (mirror images of the molecule that are nonsuperimposable and cannot be made identical by reorientation). Esketamine is the (*S*)-enantiomer isolate of the racemate, analogous to the left hand as arketamine, the (*R*)-enantiomer, is to the right hand. While the enantiomers are identical in atomic composition, the unique structural orientation of each enantiomer results in different pharmacological properties. Esketamine has a greater affinity for the NMDA glutamate receptor, thus allowing for a greater amount of NMDA receptor blockade with lower doses of the drug (White et al. 1980). This difference in NMDA receptor binding affinity is believed to account for varying effects of the two enantiomers on several physiological and psychological measures (Vollenweider et al. 1997). Practically, the greater potency of esketamine also affords greater flexibility in the route of delivery, as a clinically therapeutic concentration may be delivered in a reduced volume of vehicle.

Evidence for Antidepressant Action

On the basis of the original hypothesis that the proximal effects of ketamine on the NMDA receptor generated the cascade of events resulting in antidepressant effects, the decision was made to explore the antidepressant action of esketamine, given its greater NMDA receptor affinity (Table 22–2). A small Phase II study was completed in 2016 showing esketamine's antidepressant action when the drug was delivered intravenously over 40 minutes, a protocol similar to the one most commonly used for racemic ketamine (Singh et al. 2016a). The results of the relatively small proof-of-concept study were nearly identical to those reported previously with racemic ketamine, with marked improvements in depression ratings seen within 1 day. In this case, however, there was evidence to support equal efficacy of a lower (0.2 mg/kg) dose of esketamine over placebo. This suggestion of enhanced potency of esketamine over racemic ketamine further afforded the advantage of considering an alternative route of delivery of a more concentrated solution, and the decision was made to explore the possibility of delivering the medication intranasally, which would be more practical for outpatient physicians to administer. As noted previously, there was preliminary evidence to suggest intranasal delivery of racemic ketamine could produce antidepressant effects, but the magnitude of the response appeared to be reduced (Lapidus et al. 2014). This relatively reduced efficacy was thought to be related to the inability to achieve optimal plasma and ultimately brain concentrations using the intranasal route. These new data suggested that the alternative use of esketamine may sufficiently affect NMDA receptor function even when provided intranasally.

Intranasal Esketamine in Clinical Trials

A Phase II study of 67 adults with TRD examining the effects of three fixed doses of intranasal esketamine suggested the presence of sustained antidepressant effects for doses ranging from 28 to 84 mg administered twice weekly, with the appearance of an ascending dose-response relationship (Daly et al. 2018). This study was followed by a series of large Phase III clinical trials: two randomized, placebo-controlled trials involving 223 and 346 participants, respectively, using either fixed (Fedgchin et al. 2019) or flexible (Popova et al. 2019) dosing of 56 mg and 84 mg; a relapse-prevention randomized withdrawal study with 705 participants (Daly et al. 2019); and a long-term safety study of 802 TRD patients receiving up to 1 year of weekly or biweekly treatments (Wajs et al. 2020). In addition, a flexible-dose study with doses of esketamine ranging from 28 mg to 84 mg was conducted in 138 TRD patients age 65 years or older (Ochs-Ross et al. 2020).

The flexible-dosing study comparing the change in depression severity from baseline to day 28 between two groups of TRD patients treated with either esketamine plus a new oral antidepressant or placebo plus this antidepressant showed a greater improvement in the group receiving esketamine, with most of the separation between the groups occurring over the first 24 hours and being sustained for the duration of the study (Popova et al. 2019). At the end of the 4-week study, two-thirds of patients randomly assigned to receive esketamine were taking 84 mg, and a greater proportion of patients treated with esketamine plus the oral antidepressant demonstrated a response (69.3% vs. 52.0%) or had experienced a remission of symptoms (52.5% vs. 31.0%). The results of the fixed-dose study were less clear (Fedgchin et al. 2019), highlighting that not all Phase III esketamine studies met their designated primary outcome. Although both doses (56 mg and 84 mg) produced numerically greater changes in the Montgomery-Åsberg Depression Rating Scale measure of depression severity, as well as higher rates of response (54.1% and 53.1%) and remission (36.0% and 38.8%) compared with saline placebo (38.9% and 30.6%, respectively), the primary outcome measure comparing the new oral antidepressant plus esketamine versus the new oral antidepressant plus placebo did not meet the prespecified statistical significance criterion. In total, the two studies consistently demonstrated an increased ben-

TABLE 22–2. Representative selection of randomized controlled trials of esketamine in subjects with treatment-resistant major depressive disorder

	Sample (age range)	Design	Route,[a] schedule, dose	Outcome[b,c]
Singh et al. 2016a	30 (18–64 y)	Double-blind	IV Single 40-minute infusion; saline vs. esketamine 0.2 mg/kg vs. 0.5 mg/kg	Significant improvement at each dose tested at 2 hours through 7 days
Daly et al. 2018 (Phase II)	67 (20–64 y)	Double-blind, delayed start, placebo controlled with open-label extension	IN Fixed-dose phase (28 mg, 56 mg, or 84 mg): twice weekly × 2 weeks; saline (placebo) vs. esketamine 28 mg vs. 56 mg vs. 84 mg Open-label, flexible-dose phase (starting at 56 mg on day 15): twice weekly × 2 weeks, then weekly × 3 weeks, then biweekly through 9 weeks	Significant improvement compared with placebo after week 1, with an ascending dose-response curve; improvement sustained with reduced dosing frequency and repeated administration
Fedgchin et al. 2019 (Phase III)	223 (18–64 y)	Double-blind, parallel-group, placebo controlled	IN Fixed dose (56 mg or 84 mg), twice weekly × 4 weeks; saline (placebo) vs. esketamine 56 mg vs. 84 mg	Response rate, day 28: placebo = 39%; 56 mg = 54% (P=0.027 vs. placebo); 84 mg = 53% (P=0.088 vs. placebo)
Popova et al. 2019 (Phase III)	346 (18–64 y)	Double-blind, parallel-group, placebo controlled	IN Flexible dose; twice weekly × 4 weeks; saline (placebo) vs. esketamine 56 mg or 84 mg	Response rate, day 28: placebo = 52%; esketamine 56 mg or 84 mg = 69% (P=0.020 vs. placebo)

TABLE 22–2. Representative selection of randomized controlled trials of esketamine in subjects with treatment-resistant major depressive disorder *(continued)*

	Sample (age range)	Design	Route,[a] schedule, dose	Outcome[b,c]
Daly et al. 2019 (Phase III)	705 (18–64 y)	Double-blind, randomized withdrawal following stable response or remission at week 16	IN Flexible dose; twice weekly × 4 weeks, then weekly or biweekly to 12 weeks, then random assignment to placebo vs. esketamine continuation	Significant decrease in risk of relapse with esketamine continuation in stable responders (51% risk reduction, HR=0.49; 95% CI=0.29–0.84) and remitters (70% risk reduction, HR=0.30; 95% CI=0.16–0.55)
Wajs et al. 2020 (Phase III)	802 (≥18 y)	Open-label, long-term safety	IN Flexible dose (28 mg, 56 mg, or 84 mg) Induction phase: twice weekly × 4 weeks 48-week optimization/maintenance phase: weekly or biweekly for patients who were responders	Common treatment-emergent adverse events: dizziness (32.9%), dissociation (27.6%), nausea (25.1%), headache (24.9%)
Ochs-Ross et al. 2020 (Phase III)	138 (≥65 y)	Double-blind, parallel group, placebo controlled	IN Flexible dose; twice weekly × 4 weeks; saline (placebo) vs. esketamine 28 mg, 56 mg, or 84 mg	Response rate, week 4: placebo = 13%; esketamine 56 mg or 84 mg = 27% (*P*=0.058 vs. placebo)

[a]Route: IN=intranasal; IV=intravenous.
[b]Rating scale used in all studies: Montgomery-Åsberg Depression Rating Scale.
[c]Outcome: P=*P* value (difference from placebo); [HR]=hazard ratio; CI=confidence interval.

efit from the addition of esketamine to the initiation of a new oral antidepressant in TRD patients, with the separation between the two treatment conditions occurring within the first day and persisting, but not growing, over the remaining 4 weeks of the study. The short-term Phase III flexible esketamine dosing trial in patients age 65 years or older also did not meet its primary outcome, although esketamine also demonstrated a trend toward improvement over placebo when added to a new oral antidepressant (Ochs-Ross et al. 2020). While rates of treatment-emergent adverse events and tolerability in this older patient population were comparable to rates in studies with younger patients, the patients in this study remained at lower induction doses in earlier phases of the study, which may have resulted in a delay in separation of response from control. Sub-analyses from this study also suggested that treatment response in patients older than 75 years may be similar to that in patients from other esketamine trials encompassing a younger age groups and that patients older than 65 years may require longer overall periods of induction or acute-phase treatment to achieve benefits similar to those in younger cohorts. These issues remain open questions for further study with respect to esketamine.

The next important question addressed in this series of trials related to the safety of repeated dosing over an extended period and durability of the benefit with and without continued treatment. The long-term safety study was able to demonstrate persistent antidepressant effects lasting for up to a year with either ongoing weekly or every-other-week dosing in a large percentage of the patients responding to the initial 4-week index course (Wajs et al. 2020). However, the randomized withdrawal study provided evidence suggesting that in many cases patients may require ongoing treatments with esketamine in order to maintain the antidepressant response (Daly et al. 2019). The increase in relapse rate following discontinuation was notably higher in the patients who experienced a response (>50% improvement in symptom severity) but not remission, with 57.6% having a return of their depression after discontinuation of the esketamine over the course of the study. If esketamine treatment was maintained along with the oral antidepressant, slightly over one-fourth of the patients relapsed, whether they had achieved remission or not.

The long-term safety study (Wajs et al. 2020) also helped to address the major concern of adverse effects. Here, participants could receive esketamine dosed at flexible intervals between dosing sessions, either weekly or biweekly interchangeably, depending on 4-week interval symptom scores over the course of 1 year. As expected, there were several common transient treatment emergent adverse events, including dizziness, dissociation, nausea, and headache, all occurring in one-fourth to one-third of patients treated over that time period. Only about one-tenth of the patients discontinued esketamine because of these side effects. Seven percent of the participants experienced serious adverse events over the study duration, and two deaths were reported, but neither of the deaths was considered to be related to esketamine. It is important to note that no evidence of respiratory depression was found during the treatments.

To address concerns regarding long-term CNS and urinary system exposure to repeated dosing of the drug, cognitive performance and urinary symptoms were closely monitored. Cognitive performance generally either improved or remained stable relative to baseline assessments, and there were no reported cases of interstitial cystitis over the duration of the study. In general, treatment-emergent dissociative symptoms were transient, resolving within 90 minutes after the start dosing. However, the intensity of the transient adverse events, especially sedation and dissociation, in some individuals, and the remaining concerns for substance misuse and drug diversion, led the FDA to restrict distribution and use of the treatment under a Risk Evaluation and Mitigation Strategy that requires patients to administer the drug in the presence of a health care provider in an approved health care setting, with monitoring lasting at least 2 hours after initiating dosing (U.S. Food and Drug Administration 2020).

Other Investigational Glutamatergic Agents in the Pipeline

The unwanted side effects experienced with ketamine and esketamine, along with the restrictions on the accessibility of treatments requiring in-office administration, have prompted the search for other pharmacotherapies with similar mechanisms of action and abilities to produce rapid-onset antidepressant effects, but with improved safety profiles. Many of the novel drugs under investigation are pharmacologically quite similar to ketamine, either having direct effects on the NMDA receptor or targeting other components of glutamatergic or GABAergic neurotransmission. Other drugs target shared intracellular mechanisms with ketamine or produce physiological and/or psychological effects similar to those of ketamine.

Arketamine is the sister enantiomer of esketamine contained within the racemic mixture. Given that arketamine has a lower affinity for the NMDA receptor, reduced anesthetic properties, and fewer acute effects on cognition and perception (Vollenweider et al. 1997), it has not been the target of nearly as much research. However, many of these same properties make it an extremely interesting prospect clinically, if it retains some of the same antidepressant properties as the racemic mixture. Although there are several reports of the R-enantiomer having antidepressant-like properties in rodent studies (Yang et al. 2015), only one very small open-label clinical trial has been published to date suggesting it may possess rapid-onset antidepressant properties at doses producing minimal transient effects on arousal, cognition, and perception (Leal et al. 2021). Much attention was drawn to a report demonstrating that a metabolite of ketamine, (2R,6R)-hydroxynorketamine (HNK), exerts behavioral, electroencephalographic, electrophysiological, and cellular antidepressant-related actions, and is essential for ketamine to produce antidepressant effects in mice (Zanos et al. 2016). The finding that this metabolite appeared to have a very low affinity for the NMDA receptor raised questions about the true role of the NMDA receptor in ketamine's mechanism of action. However, conflicting studies in the rodent models (Shirayama and Hashimoto 2018) and two recent studies documenting a relationship between higher (2S,6S;2R,6R)-HNK concentrations and weaker antidepressant response in humans have made it challenging to interpret the contribution of these metabolites to the overall mechanism of antidepressant action (Farmer et al. 2020; Grunebaum et al. 2019).

Several pharmacological relatives of ketamine have also been investigated for potential antidepressant properties. Similar to ketamine, lanicemine (AR-R 15896AR, AZD-6765, BHV-5000) is a nonselective NMDA receptor antagonist with moderately high affinity for the receptor. With data suggesting rapid-onset antidepressant effects following a single infusion (Sanacora et al. 2014), the drug was advanced to Phase II randomized, placebo-controlled trials. The first of these studies, comparing fixed doses of 100 mg and 150 mg lanicemine with saline placebo in 152 participants, showed both doses of the drug to have superior antidepressant effects compared with placebo on a variety of measures (Sanacora et al. 2014). However, a second study of 300 participants randomly assigned to receive fixed doses of 50 mg or 100 mg, or placebo, did not show either of the doses to have antidepressant effects superior to those of placebo (Sanacora et al. 2017), leaving questions of whether the initial study resulted in a type I error or whether the high placebo response rate in the second study obscured any potential antidepressant efficacy.

Memantine, another nonselective NMDA receptor antagonist that has notable differences in receptor affinity, was also studied for antidepressant properties in a few small-scale clinical trials in mood disorders under various study designs. In general, these studies did not produce evidence to suggest a meaningful antidepressant response (Kishi et al. 2017).

Early in the search for ketamine-related compounds with possible antidepressant action, Traxoprodil (CP-101,606), an NR2B subunit–selective NMDA receptor antagonist, was studied in a novel proof-of-concept small clinical trial. Although the results suggested that the drug has antidepressant properties (Preskorn et al. 2008), the drug was not pursued, likely because of concerns about QTc prolongation (Machado-Vieira et al. 2017). Rislenemdaz (CERC-301, MK-0657), a second NR2B subunit–selective NMDA receptor antagonist that was delivered orally, was studied in Phase II studies that failed to show efficacy on the primary endpoint according to publications and press releases from the company (Ibrahim et al. 2012).

Dextromethorphan, the commonly used cough suppressant, is also known to have antagonist effects on the NMDA receptor in addition to activity at sigma$_1$ and mu opioid receptors, the serotonin transporter (5HTT), and calcium channels, and has been studied for antidepressant properties in a variety of forms. Retrospective case series suggested that dextromethorphan combined with the cytochrome P450 (CYP) 2D6 inhibitor quinidine to slow the rate of metabolism could benefit patients with refractory mood disorders (Kelly and Lieberman 2014; Nofziger et al. 2019). Several recent clinical trials examining the antidepressant efficacy of AXS-05, a combination of dextromethorphan and bupropion (an oral antidepressant that also acts as a CYP2D6 inhibitor), have been completed to date, with clinical trial results likely to be available in the coming years (Wilkinson and Sanacora 2019).

Other drugs attempting to target NMDA receptor function via interactions with the glycine binding regions of the receptor have also been examined. Rapastinel (GLYX-13), the most thoroughly studied at this time, has a unique course of drug development (Moskal et al. 2017). It was originally derived from studies aiming to create a monoclonal antibody that could be used to study synaptic plasticity by using material from newborn rat hippocampi as an immunogen. Further work led to the identification of a tetrapeptide component of the antibody, GLYX-13, that had activity on an NMDA receptor– and hippocampus-dependent test of associative learning and memory. Evidence showing GLYX-13 to override the effects of a competitive glycine site antagonist, 7-chlorokynurenic acid, suggested it was acting by modulating NMDA receptor function through interaction with the glycine binding site of the receptor. Initial preclinical work was very encouraging, with the drug demonstrating antidepressant-like effects and cellular changes consistent with those of ketamine in a variety of rodent models (R.J. Liu et al. 2017). Preliminary Phase II clinical trials further suggested clinical benefit in treating depression (Preskorn et al. 2015); however, three large Phase III clinical trials did not find the drug to have benefits superior to placebo in the treatment of depression (Tumolo 2019).

D-Serine, an endogenous amino acid neurotransmitter, is capable of modulating NMDA receptor activity by interacting with the glycine binding site on the receptor and producing an agonist-like action. As mentioned earlier, George Crane (1959) noted a rapid improvement in depressive symptoms when patients were treated with D-cycloserine, a closely related compound to D-serine, for tuberculosis in the late 1950s. More recently, there have been a series of preclinical studies showing that D-serine and D-cycloserine produce antidepressant effects in rodent models (MacKay et al. 2019). In parallel, there have been several small proof-of-concept studies suggesting that D-cycloserine may have beneficial effects in treating a number of psychiatric disorders, including MDD, especially when used in combination with other therapies. However, there are conflicting reports (Heresco-Levy et al. 2006, 2013; Schade and Paulus 2016). The interpretation of these studies is complicated by the fact that D-cycloserine can act as a partial agonist at the glycine site, making the dosage of the medication an extremely important variable in relation to drug effects. D-Cycloserine is now in clinical trials in the form of NRX-101 (D-cycloserine combined with lurasidone) for the maintenance of response in patients with bipolar depression with suicidal ideation who have responded to intravenous ketamine.

A third drug targeting the glycine site of the NMDA receptor was also recently evaluated for antidepressant activity. AV-101 (L-4-chlorokynurenine), the prodrug that is converted to 7-chlorokynurenic acid, which binds and modulates the glycine site of the NMDA receptor, had shown promising results in preclinical studies demonstrating antidepressant-like effects and cellular changes similar to those of ketamine in rodent models (Zanos et al. 2015). A small proof-of-concept study recently completed at the National Institute of Mental Health did not show evidence to support the drug's antidepressant effect in patients with depression, but it suggested that there may not have been sufficient conversion of the prodrug to 7-chlorokynurenic acid to effectively modulate activity of the receptor (Park et al. 2020).

Attempting to target the proposed downstream mechanisms involved in ketamine's antidepressant action, NV-5138, a small molecule that activates mTORC1 (mechanistic [mammalian] target of rapamycin complex 1) by binding to sestrin2, has been studied in rodent models and in early-phase clinical trials (Hasegawa et al. 2019; Kato et al. 2019). A single dose of NV-5138 produced rapid antidepressant actions in behavioral models of depression and increased the number and function of synapses as well as levels of synaptic proteins in the prefrontal cortex of rats. The Phase I studies were designed primarily to examine the safety, tolerability, and pharmacokinetics of the drug, but they also included a subset of patients with MDD. The results of these studies should be published in the near future and will provide information to suggest whether future clinical trials are warranted.

Moving even further downstream from what is believed to be ketamine's proximal mechanism of action, drugs targeting presynaptic glutamate release and postsynaptic activation of non-NMDA glutamate receptors are being evaluated for antidepressant properties. The extent of exploration for many of these drugs has been limited to preclinical investigations; however, several have been studied in early-phase clinical trials (Kadriu et al. 2019; Murrough et al. 2017; Wilkinson and Sanacora 2019).

Many of the drugs that failed to demonstrate clear efficacy in the clinical trials showed great promise in rodent models, and some even showed activation of purported mechanistic targets in human studies. It will be important for the future of translational antidepressant drug development to understand why these models presented incongruous results with the clinical trial data. For some, it may simply be the case that the drug under investigation did not adequately engage the appropriate target, as was suggested by the rodent models. For example, as noted above, AV-101 (L-4-chlorokynurenine) was developed as a prodrug to 7-chlorokynurenic acid, a well-characterized selective NMDA receptor glycine site antagonist that appeared highly effective in rodent models. However, the conversion to the active metabolite appears to be limited in humans, not allowing measurable concentrations of 7-chlorokynurenic acid to reach the central nervous system (Park et al. 2020). Similarly, rapastinel, another purported glycine site modulator, has an indirect effect on NMDA receptor ion channels as a functional modulator of the glycine site of the NMDA receptor in rodent models. Thus, the indirect effects may require several additional moderating factors and therefore reflect a greater chance of cross-species physiological variation.

Given these limitations, it is difficult to interpret how the negative clinical trials with those compounds inform us about the actual antidepressant potential of NMDA receptor modulation. The interpretation of the clinical trial data in relation to the underlying hypothesis of antidepressant mechanism of action is also complicated by the nuances and complexity of clinical trial designs. The early proof-of-concept studies with ketamine showed very large effect sizes that were obvious within hours of initial dosing. As the studies became more rigorous, with broader geographic distribution of patient samples and greater expectancy of drug effects, the magnitude of the effect size and speed of onset relative to the controlled arm of the studies may have been somewhat reduced. This reduction was readily observed within the ketamine and esketamine studies over time and was highlighted by the contrasting results of the two lanicemine studies (Sanacora et al. 2017). Altogether, this makes it very difficult to evaluate the potential of the entire class of drugs or the future likelihood of success for novel drugs with related mechanisms of action without understanding the finer details of each drug and study design.

Conclusion

The emergence of ketamine as a treatment for depression has changed the landscape of antidepressant drug development and expanded our understanding of the pathophysiology of mood disorders (Figure 22–1). It has proven that, contrary to long-held beliefs, antidepressant effects can be seen within hours of treatment onset and that it is possible to develop truly novel antidepressant drugs that do not have proximal effects on the monoaminergic system. It has also helped us reconceptualize our thinking about the mechanisms of antidepressant action. The fact that the antidepressant effect of ketamine is seen well beyond the presence of the active drug in the body suggests that treatment must initiate a cascade of physiological processes that ultimately

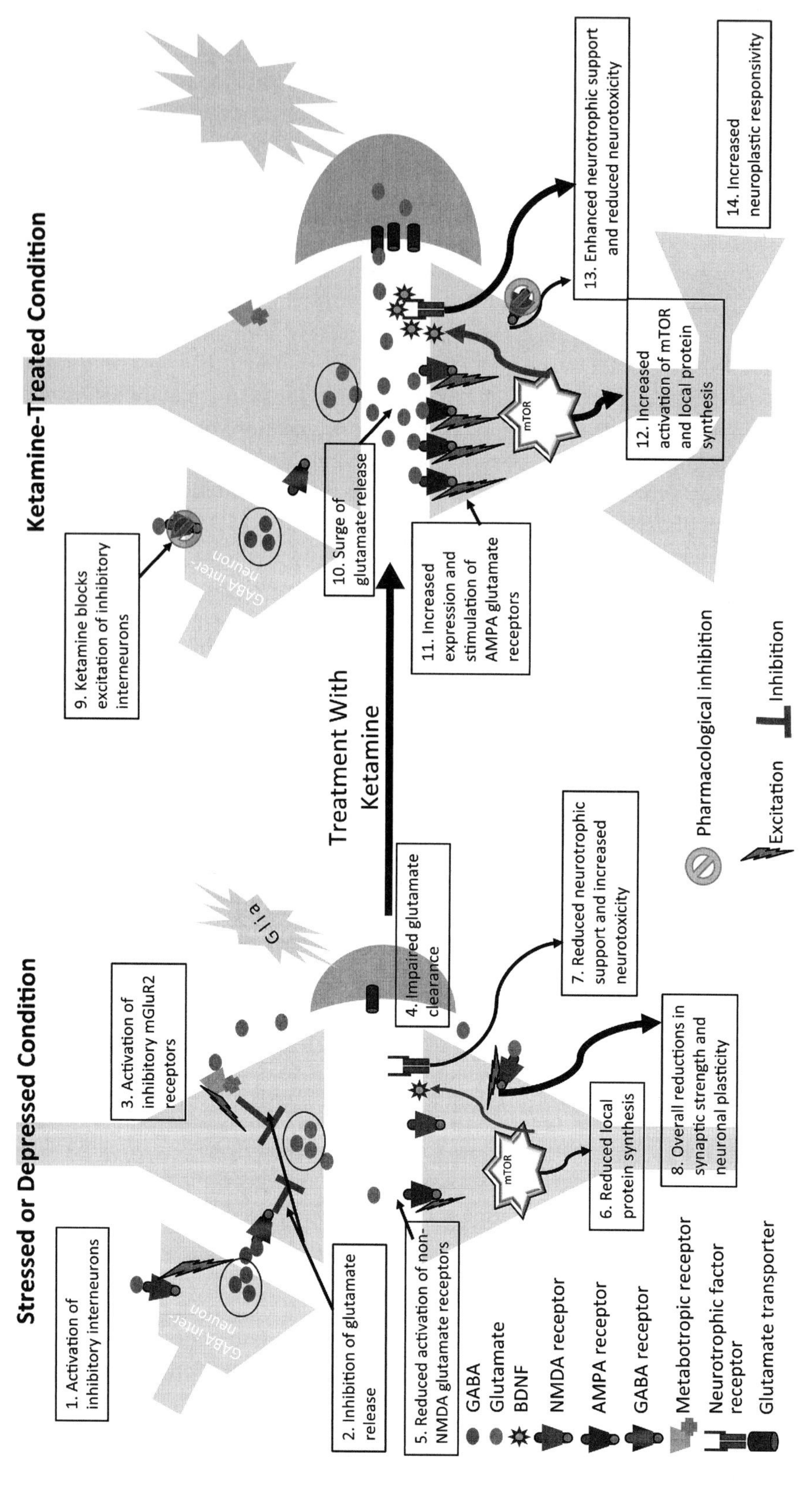

FIGURE 22–1. Proposed model depicting pathophysiological changes associated with mood disorders and ketamine's mechanism of antidepressant action.

To view this figure in color, see Plate 9 in Color Gallery in middle of book.

Stressed or Depressed Condition (under conditions of chronic stress and possibly reflecting pathophysiology of major depressive disorder)

1. Activation of inhibitory interneurons: Under usual conditions pyramidal glutamatergic neurons are under tonic inhibition by GABAergic interneurons that are themselves activated by glutamatergic inputs. ***2. Inhibition of glutamate release:*** The tonic inhibition limits release of glutamate into the synaptic cleft. ***3. Activation of inhibitory metabotropic glutamate (mGlu) receptors:*** Group II metabotropic glutamate receptors 2 and 3 (mGluR2/3) provide a second means of inhibiting glutamate release and are believed to serve as a sensor in a negative feedback loop, detecting increased levels of extrasynaptic glutamate and dampening any additional synaptic glutamate release. ***4. Impaired glutamate clearance:*** Under usual conditions, glutamate released into the synaptic cleft is rapidly cleared by excitatory amino acid transporters (EAATs). In most brain regions, glutamate clearance is predominantly accomplished through EAAT2, which is present on astroglial cells surrounding the synapse. Under conditions of chronic stress and possibly during depressive episodes, it is believed that the ability to clear glutamate is reduced, allowing for increased levels of extrasynaptic glutamate. ***5. Reduced activation of non–N-methyl-D-aspartate (NMDA) glutamate receptors:*** Reduced levels of synaptic glutamate release, and possibly elevated levels of extrasynaptic glutamate, are believed to decrease the number and activation of postsynaptic α-amino-3-hydroxy-5-methyl-4-isoxazolepropionic acid (AMPA) receptors. ***6. Reduced local protein synthesis:*** The mechanistic (mammalian) target of rapamycin (mTOR) is a kinase that regulates local protein synthesis in dendrites in a process mediating activity-dependent synaptic strengthening. Reductions in postsynaptic activation through AMPA receptors result in lower levels of mTOR activity, decreasing rates of local protein synthesis and synaptic strength. ***7. Reduced neurotrophic support and increased neurotoxicity:*** mTOR is believed to have a complex relationship with neurotrophic factors such as brain-derived neurotrophic factor (BDNF). There appears to be a positive feedback system in which increased mTOR activity results in increased expression of BDNF, and activation of the BDNF receptor tropomyosin receptor kinase B (TrkB) increases mTOR activity. Under conditions of chronic stress and possibly in depressive episodes, it is believed that BDNF expression and release are decreased in several critical brain regions. ***8. Overall reductions in synaptic strength and neuroplasticity:*** The effects of chronic stress result in decreased neurotrophic support and greater susceptibility of synaptic maintenance to the effects of potentially neurotoxic events, such as increased stimulation of extrasynaptic NMDA receptors. Ultimately, this results in a loss of synaptic strength and adaptive neuroplasticity and leads toward impaired neurotransmission and circuit function

Ketamine-Treated Condition

9. Ketamine blocks excitation of inhibitory interneurons: Several lines of evidence demonstrate the ability of ketamine to modulate glutamate release. One mechanism believed to mediate this effect is a selective inhibition of NMDA receptors on GABAergic interneurons. Inhibiting the inhibitory interneurons results in a release of the tonic inhibition. ***10. Surge of glutamate release:*** Whether through release of tonic inhibition or other mechanisms, there is good evidence demonstrating that a transient surge of glutamate release follows administration of subanesthetic doses of ketamine. ***11. Increased expression and stimulation of AMPA glutamate receptors:*** Increased levels of synaptic glutamate lead to activation of AMPA receptors in the postsynaptic membrane. There also appears to be an increased level of AMPA receptor expression and insertion following ketamine treatments that will likely amplify the effect. ***12. Increased activation of mTOR and local protein synthesis:*** Increased conductance through AMPA receptors stimulates intracellular messenger pathways, including that of the mTORC1 (mechanistic [mammalian] target of rapamycin complex 1) pathway, that promote translation of proteins necessary for neuronal plasticity. ***13. Enhanced neurotrophic support and reduced neurotoxicity:*** Neurotrophic factors such as BDNF are among the proteins that are increasingly expressed shortly following ketamine administration. The release of BDNF also appears to be stimulated by ketamine, and several studies suggest that this enhanced neurotrophic support is a necessary event in generating the ketamine-induced antidepressant-like effect in rodent models. Other studies suggest that blockade of extrasynaptic or specific subtypes of NMDA receptors further limits excitotoxic effects and promotes changes supporting neuronal plasticity. ***14. Increased neuroplastic responsivity:*** Combined, these actions are believed to increase synaptic plasticity, as reflected in synaptic strengthening, elevated levels of synaptogenesis, increased spine density, and ultimately changes in functional connectivity between brain regions involved in mood disorder pathophysiology.

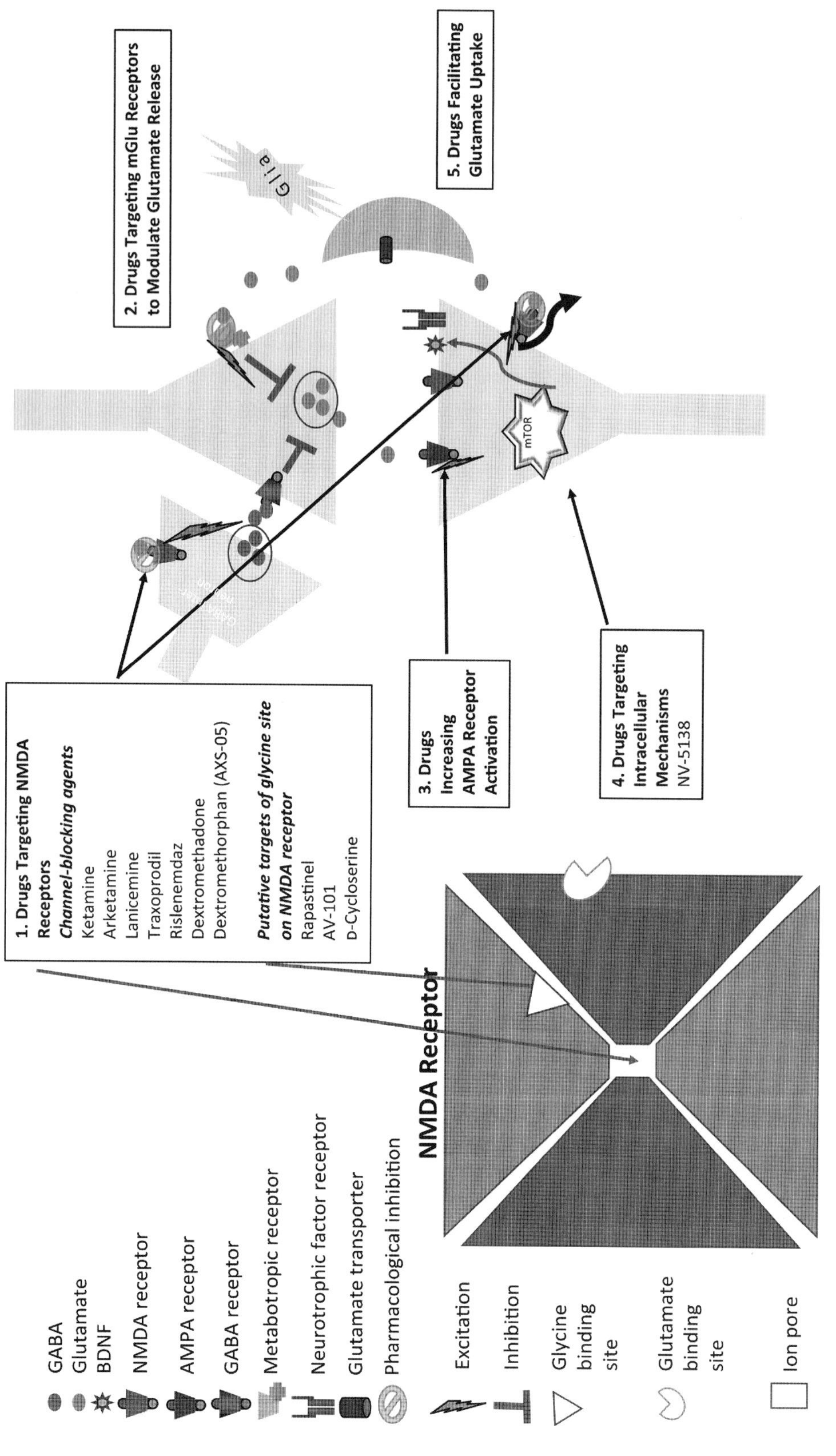

FIGURE 22–2. Novel drugs in development related to ketamine's proposed mechanism of action.

To view this figure in color, see Plate 10 in Color Gallery in middle of book.

1. Drugs targeting N-methyl-D-aspartate (NMDA) receptors: There are two major classifications of drugs currently in this category. The first class contains those drugs like ketamine that are primarily channel-blocking agents that interfere with the receptor's ion channel. These drugs can bind to selectively expressed subunits of the NMDA receptor or to sites common to all NMDA receptors. The second class contains drugs that are reported to act by modulating the binding or function of the glycine co-agonist site on the NMDA receptor. To varying degrees these drugs can indirectly modulate the ion transport through the receptor. These drugs are believed to produce their antidepressant effects by promoting enhanced presynaptic glutamate release and/or limiting neuronal toxicity. ***2. Drugs targeting metabotropic glutamate receptors 2 and 3 (mGluR2/3):*** mGluR2/3 activation serves to inhibit glutamate release and serves as a target to modulate glutamate release. On the basis of the proposed pathophysiological model presented above, arguments can be made for both inhibiting tonic glutamate release and transiently stimulating glutamate release, such as is believed to happen with ketamine treatment. Both positive and negative allosteric modulators of mGluR2/3 are being studied as treatment for mood disorders. ***3. Drugs stimulating α-amino-3-hydroxy-5-methyl-4-isoxazolepropionic acid (AMPA) receptor activation:*** These drugs can act either as more direct agonists of glutamate or as modulators of receptor function. To date there is preclinical evidence suggesting that drugs in this class possess antidepressant properties, but clinical confirmation is required. ***4. Drugs targeting intracellular mechanisms:*** Because preclinical evidence suggests that activation of the mechanistic (mammalian) target of the rapamycin complex 1 (mTORC1) pathway is critical to the mechanism of ketamine's action, there have been attempts to develop drugs that can more directly modulate the pathway downstream of the glutamatergic receptors. ***5. Drugs facilitating glutamate uptake:*** On the basis of evidence suggesting that glial cell abnormalities and impaired glutamate uptake are associated with the pathogenesis and pathophysiology of mood disorders, there have been attempts to identify and utilize drugs that can facilitate glutamate clearance in efforts to treat mood disorders. Rodent studies support this approach; however, the clinical studies for one potential agent, riluzole, have yielded inconsistent results at best. These equivocal findings may suggest that drugs that modulate glutamate uptake could have benefits prophylactically but may not be highly effective in treatment.

PART V

Psychotherapy of Mood Disorders

CHAPTER 23

Cognitive and Behavior Therapies for Depressive Disorders

W. Edward Craighead, Ph.D.

Evidence-based psychotherapies for the acute treatment of major depressive disorder (MDD) include Beck's eponymous cognitive-behavior therapy (CBT; Beck et al. 1979) and behavioral activation (BA; Jacobson et al. 2001), a contemporary form of behavior therapy. These therapies are short-term, educational, and fairly directive, typically comprising 16–20 sessions over 12–16 weeks. This chapter focuses on the description and clinical outcomes of BA and CBT, the most extensively evaluated of the efficacious psychotherapies. Notably, there are only minimal outcome data to support the choice of one over the other of these two therapies. Consequently, the decision regarding which of these therapies to implement is based on the therapist's competence, availability, and preference as well as the patient's treatment preference.

BA and CBT psychotherapies were derived from theoretical models and empirical psychopathological evidence regarding the etiology and maintenance of MDD. Behavior therapy (BT) was developed during the 1950s–1960s when mental health care professionals began applying empirically derived principles of learning theory to clinical intervention processes. BT and CBT (which began in earnest during the 1970s) are now mainstream models of psychosocial clinical interventions. Training in these conceptual models and their related interventions is a focus of most doctoral training programs in clinical psychology. Because the therapies are entirely compatible with biological models of contemporary psychiatry, training and clinical use of these therapies, along with interpersonal psychotherapy (IPT), are included in most psychiatry training programs.

BT derived from the conceptual framework of behaviorism, which may be traced to a variety of influences from around the world. In the United States, John B. Watson (1878–1958), who defined psychology as the "science of behavior," is most often credited with changing the focus of psychology from the study of the "mind" to the study of observable behaviors. Behaviorism became the primary conceptual framework underlying most basic psychological research from the 1920s through the 1970s.

Although occasional evaluations of a behavioral intervention were undertaken at earlier dates, extensive implementations and appraisals first emerged during the 1950s and 1960s (W.E. Craighead et al. 1995). The primary defining characteristic of BT was the application of principles of behaviorism to clinical phenomena as psychology moved from the basic science laboratories to informed clinical interventions. Two basic learning theory principles guided the development of BT: 1) principles of operant conditioning (first labeled behavior modification, now commonly called applied behavior analysis), championed by Skinner (1953) and his colleagues; and 2) principles of classical conditioning, applied (at least metaphorically) by Wolpe (1958) in his description of behavioral treatments for anxiety. Because anxiety was viewed as the core of "neuroses" within the then-prevailing psychodynamic model of psychopathology and treatment, BT initially focused on treatment of "anxiety" problems. Soon thereafter, clinical applications were developed for a variety of other disorders. The empirical evaluation of BT interventions, a fundamental hallmark, sustained BT and supported its efficacy for a wide range of clinical disorders (L.W. Craighead et al. 1994; Kazdin 1994).

During the 1970s, a confluence of factors resulted in a large proportion of behavior therapists shifting their focus to internal cognitive processes, producing the therapies now subsumed under the rubric of CBT. Like BT, CBT has not been monolithic; there are more than 20 different CBT approaches (Mahoney and Lyddon 1988), even when the so-called third-wave approaches of BT (e.g., mindfulness, dialectical behavior therapy; see Öst 2008) are omitted. CBT therapies emerged from three major developments. First, empirically oriented clinicians applied basic cognitive psychology constructs to the blossoming models and procedures of clinical intervention (e.g., Bandura's [1969] use of information processing in espousing his social learning theory). Second, the reformulation of behavioral self-control procedures as cognitive interventions influenced CBT (e.g., Meichenbaum 1977; Thoresen and Mahoney 1974). Finally, Ellis's (1962) and Beck's (1964, 1970) identification of cognitive therapies occurred in their clinical settings. Cognitive therapies, based on clinical experience rather than findings from basic psychology, rapidly lent themselves to empirical clinical trials. Ultimately, Beck and colleagues (e.g., Beck et al. 1979) combined BT and cognitive therapy into CBT.

BT and CBT share two cardinal assumptions: basic psychological research informs clinical models and procedures, and clinical scientists must evaluate the efficacy and effectiveness of interventions. Both BT and CBT (and IPT) are compatible with appropriate medication interventions in treating depression (W.E. Craighead and Dunlop 2014). The major difference between BT and CBT lies in the conceptualization of the psychopathology and the resulting specific intervention programs for various clinical disorders.

Individual Behavior Therapy

Several variants of BT were developed for the treatment of MDD; they all, however, shared the assumption that MDD results from avoidant coping strategies and decreases in behaviors that result in positive reinforcement. Consequently, behavior therapies for depression have focused on monitoring and increasing positive daily activities, decreasing negative life experiences, improving social and communication skills, and increasing adaptive behaviors such as assertiveness, as well as increasing adaptive behaviors resulting in response-contingent positive reinforcement.

Early Behavior Therapy

During the 1970s and early 1980s, Lewinsohn and his colleagues demonstrated that BT reduced aversive experiences and increased pleasant experiences—changes that resulted in decreased depression symptomatology (see summary in Lewinsohn and Gotlib 1995). Other investigators compared BT with the then-accepted antidepressant medication treatments. They found that BT was as effective as tricyclic antidepressants in reducing depression during a 12-week treatment period. During a 6-month follow-up, they found that acute BT treatment effects were maintained when patients were given essentially monthly booster sessions (Bellack et al. 1981, 1983; Hersen et al. 1984).

In 1979, McLean and Hakstian created an expanded BT by adding problem solving and Rehm's self-control (Rehm 1977) procedures. They completed a 10-week clinical trial comparing their expanded BT to relaxation therapy, insight-oriented psychotherapy, and amitriptyline. The expanded BT program was equal or superior to the other treatments. These outcomes were maintained at a 27-month follow-up, when individuals in the BT group were more socially active and productive than those in the other treatment conditions (McLean and Hakstian 1990).

In a consequential study, Keller et al. (2000) treated 681 adults with chronic MDD (MDD of at least 2 years' duration), current MDD superimposed on a preexisting dysthymic disorder ("double depression"), or recurrent MDD with incomplete remission between episodes and a total of at least 2 years' total duration of continuous illness. Patients were randomly assigned to receive 12 weeks of treatment with either an antidepressant (nefazodone), cognitive-behavioral analysis system of psychotherapy (CBASP), or the combination of CBASP and nefazodone. CBASP (McCullough et al. 2000) focuses on the consequences of the patient's behavior and the use of social problem solving to address interpersonal difficulties. Patients receiving nefazodone exhibited a more rapid reduction in symptoms during the first 4 weeks of treatment, but by the end of 12 weeks of treatment the outcomes were equivalent for the CBASP and nefazodone groups. Importantly, at the 12-week posttreatment assessment, the combination of CBASP and nefazodone was superior to either monotherapy intervention. Nemeroff et al. (2003), in a subsequent analysis of the study data, reported that CBASP (either alone or in combination with nefazodone) was an essential ingredient in the successful treatment of depressed patients who had experienced early life trauma.

Behavioral Activation

More recent iterations of BT for depression emanated from the work of Jacobson (for a review, see Dimidjian et al. [2011), who in a dismantling study of CBT, sought to identify its efficacious components for treating depression. Jacobson et al. (1996) evaluated the hypothesized mechanisms of change by randomly assigning depressed patients to one of the following three conditions: 1) the full CBT intervention (i.e., BA+automatic thoughts (AT)+schema work); 2) BA plus modification of distorted AT; or 3) BA alone. Like earlier BT, the BA treatment focused on decreasing avoidance (defined as a maladaptive coping strategy to avoid emotional stressors). To combat avoidance, BA included techniques such as monitoring daily activities, assessing pleasure in and mastery of activities, assigning increasingly difficult activities, imagining behaviors to be performed, discussing specific problems and identifying behavioral solutions to those problems, and intervening to ameliorate social skills deficits. Jacobson et al. (1996) found that BA alone and the full CBT treatment package were equally efficacious after the 20-session acute treatment trial and at 6-month follow-up. The treatment outcomes were maintained over a 2-year follow-up period—patients in all three treatments had equivalent rates of relapse, time to relapse, and number of symptom-free weeks (Gortner et al. 1998).

Jacobson and colleagues subsequently undertook a larger randomized trial comparing BA, CBT, paroxetine, and pill placebo. The placebo condition was maintained for 8 weeks. Paroxetine was found to be superior to placebo for the severely depressed patients; there were no differences between paroxetine and pill placebo for the more moderately depressed patients. At the end of the 16-week treatment, BA was equal in effectiveness to paroxetine among severely depressed patients, and both treatments were slightly superior to CBT (Dimidjian et al. 2006). A 2-year follow-up (Dobson et al. 2008) indicated that both BA and CBT were superior to paroxetine (even after being administered for 12 months) in maintaining the acute treatment effects. By illustrating the efficacy of BA across the MDD severity spectrum, these findings raised questions about the practice guidelines positing that only medication treatments are effective for severely depressed patients (American Psychiatric Association 2010).

Because of the *apparent* relative ease of conducting BA compared with CBT and IPT, there is widespread belief that BA can be more easily disseminated, a benefit that would be especially valuable to countries with limited mental health care services. This suggestion seems meritorious, given that Patel and colleagues have directed successful implementations of BA by less extensively trained local personnel in India (Patel et al. 2017, 2019). It should be noted, however, that the choice of 5–8 weekly sessions (instead of the typical 16 + weekly sessions) and the content of those 5–8 sessions remain unclear. Furthermore, the outcome measures included only brief self-report measures (e.g., the 9-item Patient Health Questionnaire [PHQ-9]; Kroenke et al. 2001) covering a relatively short period of time. Nevertheless, recent dissemination implementations in low- and middle-income countries show promise and are clearly needed.

Summary

Consistent findings support the efficacy of BT for MDD. Repeated meta-analyses have concluded that BA is at least as effective as CBT and antidepressant medications in treating MDD to remission (Cuijpers et al. 2007; Ekers et al. 2014; Huguet et al. 2018; Mazzucchelli et al. 2009). Nevertheless, for many years BT was overshadowed by outcome studies that focused on CBT and IPT as psychosocial interventions for MDD. However, given the relative efficacy, efficiency, and endurance of behavioral interventions and the recent results supporting the efficacy of CBASP and BA, it seems that this was an infelicitous turn of events. From a historical perspective, the lack of attention to BT was likely due to the unfortunate exclusion of BT from the influential Treatment of Depression Collaborative Research Program (TDCRP; Elkin et al. 1985) rather than the relative scientific merit and empirical outcomes of the then-extant comparative treatment studies.

Individual Cognitive-Behavior Therapy

As described earlier, CBT emerged as an amalgamation of three different developments: cognitive therapies per Ellis (1962) and Beck (1970, 1976); self-control and self-instructional training therapies (Mahoney 1974; Meichenbaum 1977); and the cognitive revolution in basic psychology theory and research that led to cognitively based interventions (Dember 1974). Early in the 1970s, there were several small studies utilizing some form of CBT, but it was Rush et al.'s (1977) extraordinarily important study that was largely responsible for the technique's inclusion in the TDCRP comparing CBT with IPT, pill placebo, and imipramine (Elkin et al. 1989). CBT rapidly became a viable treatment for MDD, at least partly because of its inclusion in the TDCRP and in Beck et al.'s (1979) manual written for that study.

Description

The typical CBT model (Figure 23–1) comprises three cognitive components: negative self-statements, cognitive errors, and underlying schemas or core beliefs. Within the model, MDD typically follows the occurrence of a life event; however, it is the combination of resulting automatic thoughts, information-processing deficits (cognitive errors), and enduring negative cognitive patterns (schemas/core beliefs) that leads to the development and maintenance of depression. CBT, consequently, focuses on assisting patients in changing their automatic statements, cognitive processes, and fundamental beliefs so they become more adaptive, positive, and internalized.

Automatic Thoughts

AT originate in response to a prompting event. One does not work to generate these thoughts, so they are labeled "automatic," as in springing up "naturally" and without effort. Beck et al.'s (1979) CBT manual noted that depressed individuals engage in negative AT or self-statements about themselves, the world, and the future (frequently referred to as the cognitive triad). Although depressed individuals can generally gain awareness of these thoughts, they typically are unaware of two things—their thoughts contain errors or distortions, and these AT serve to maintain or exacerbate negative mood. Depressed individuals do not view their AT as invalid (even when they are inaccurate), so their emotional responses to these AT are the same as if the AT were actually true.

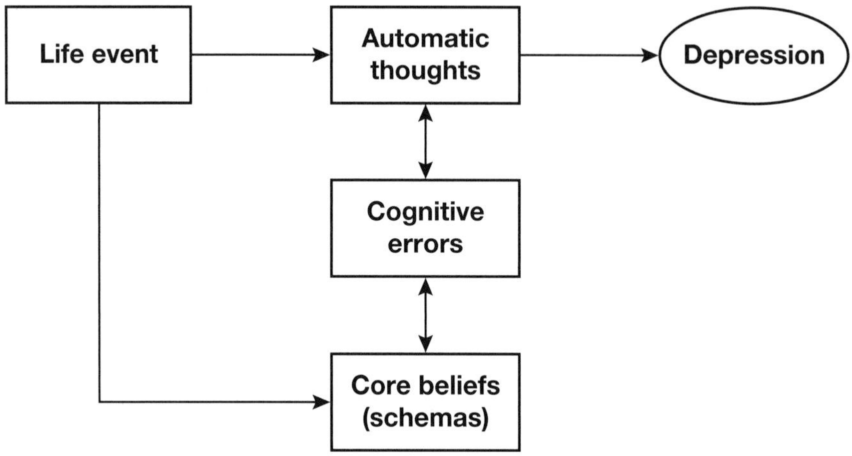

FIGURE 23–1. Cognitive model of depression.

Cognitive Distortions

As just described, the CBT model maintains that depressed thinking is negatively biased and automatic; additionally, and at a deeper level, depressed thought processes are also fraught and replete with cognitive distortions and processing errors. Cognitive distortions and errors may be activated by continuous negative self-statements, or they may surface from activation of the individual's underlying core beliefs or self-schemas. Cognitive distortions serve the role of processing errors that function, along with schemas, to screen out positive information or to process negative or neutral information in a negative manner.

Both A.T. Beck (1976) and J.S. Beck (1995) identified and described several examples of frequently occurring cognitive errors, including the following: 1) all-or-nothing thinking—viewing things in black-and-white terms rather than as existing on a continuum; 2) arbitrary inference—drawing negative conclusions in the absence of corroborating evidence; 3) overgeneralization—drawing conclusions that far exceed the bounds of the current situation; 4) selective abstraction—concentrating on one detail (typically negative) about a situation and ignoring others, thereby failing to see the whole picture; 5) magnification/minimization—magnifying the negative aspects of a person or situation and minimizing the positive aspects; 6) personalization—believing that external events happen because of one's own inherent inadequacy, weakness, or other flaw, thereby disregarding contradictory evidence; 7) emotional reasoning—thinking something must be true because of the strength of the feeling associated with the thought.

Core Beliefs (Schemas)

Beck (1976) postulated that depressed individuals utilize stable and negative cognitive patterns when interpreting information from their environments. These enduring patterns derive from fundamental beliefs—that is, depressed individuals' a priori assumptions about themselves. Beck and others (e.g., Young et al. 2003) refer to these fundamental beliefs as *schemas*. These depressogenic schemas become activated either directly by a major negative life event or indirectly through AT and cognitive processing errors about a life event. Sacco and Beck (1995) noted that the CBT theory of depression exemplifies a *diathesis-stress* model, wherein depressogenic core beliefs/schemas develop earlier in life (diathesis) and are latent until activated by negative life events (stress).

Process of CBT

A short-term (16–20 sessions over a period of 12–16 weeks), directive, and educational therapy, CBT attempts to change the depressed patient's negative view of the self, the world, and the future. The ultimate and essential goal of CBT is to correct the patient's long-standing pattern of faulty underlying core beliefs/schemas. Each session begins with the therapist, in collaboration with the patient, setting an "agenda" for the session. Over the course of treatment, CBT therapists consistently employ Socratic dialogue and freely use metaphors in discussing cognitive errors and correcting faulty beliefs.

Session 1 focuses on gathering the patient's history and achieving a correct diagnosis. During the second or third session (depending on the time necessary to complete history and diagnosis), the therapist presents the treatment rationale, designed to inform the client of the cognitive formulation and conceptualization of MDD as well as the upcoming processes of therapeutic sessions and change (Beck et al. 2001). Once the rationale is understood and accepted, early CBT sessions employ BT interventions. Various and controversial opinions exist regarding the purpose of the early behavioral interventions. Cognitively oriented CBT therapists maintain that the only purpose of behavioral strategies is to provide opportunities for monitoring behaviors and their associated thoughts and feelings; behavioral changes are not posited to be directly responsible for decreases in depression as BT therapists might view their impact (see Ilardi and Craighead 2006). During the third or fourth session, the therapist introduces self-monitoring techniques to help the patient gain an awareness of the relationship between AT and feelings. As the patient acquires a better understanding of this relationship, the therapist shifts to assisting the patient in developing alternative thoughts and identifying the resulting new feelings. Subsequently, patients are taught to perceive how their AT relate to their thought processes and logical errors, including the cognitive errors listed above. The middle sessions of CBT focus on identification of cognitive processing errors and mechanisms to correct the erroneous thought processes. Slightly over halfway through the therapy (typically sessions 9–10), the therapist introduces the concept of schemas, the beliefs underlying negative and positive thoughts and cognitive processes. Gradually, therapy focuses on changing these negative schemas (e.g., "I am worthless," "I am unlovable"), which are posited to play a central role in precipitating and maintaining major depressive episodes. Near the end of therapy (sessions 14–16), the focus shifts to termination and the use of cognitive strategies to prevent relapse or future recurrences of MDD.

CBT Outcome Data

CBT remains the most extensively evaluated and highly scrutinized psychosocial treatment for MDD. A number of early randomized controlled trials (RCTs) compared the relative effectiveness of CBT and tricyclic antidepressant medications (ADMs) (Elkin et al. 1989; Hollon et al. 1992; Rush et al. 1977; Simons et al. 1986). With the exception of the TDCRP (Elkin et al. 1989), all these studies found that CBT was as effective as tricyclic ADMs in alleviating MDD among outpatients. CBT compared favorably to ADMs when study physicians were free to prescribe the ADM of their choice (and free to switch medications during the treatment trial), provided that they prescribed at or above the established therapeutic dosages (Blackburn and Moore 1997). Additionally, CBT was as effective as the monoamine oxidase inhibitor phenelzine and was more effective than pill placebo in the treatment of atypical depression (Jarrett et al. 1999).

As noted earlier, the American Psychiatric Association published guidelines in 1993 (revised in 2010) stating that psychosocial interventions are not as appropriate as antidepressants for severely depressed individuals. At the time of that publication, CBT had not yet been compared with selective serotonin reuptake inhibitor (SSRI) ADMs. Additionally, unlike trials of ADMs, most studies demonstrating that CBT was an efficacious treatment for depression had not included pill-placebo control groups. Thus, considerable questions remained as to whether CBT could be considered equally as efficacious as ADMs with the same types of depressed subjects; moreover, one could not draw definitive conclusions about the relative efficacy of CBT compared with pill placebo (Klein 1996). As a result, various investigators in the early part of this century undertook studies with more severely depressed patients and compared CBT with SSRIs in pill-placebo controlled studies.

DeRubeis and colleagues (DeRubeis et al. 2005; Hollon et al. 2005) conducted perhaps the most illustrative and appropriately controlled acute treatment study that also included a long-term follow-up. They conducted an RCT (N=240 depressed patients) comparing CBT, paroxetine, and pill placebo. The paroxetine treatment arm included a flexible dosing strategy reflective of clinical practice with ADMs—that is, dosages could be increased up to 50 mg/day; patients who were unresponsive at 50 mg/day could have their treatment augmented with lithium or desipramine; and in cases in which paroxetine was intolerable, a switch could be made to another SSRI. For ethical reasons, the study was designed so that after 8 weeks of treatment, the "double blind" was broken and the pill-placebo condition was terminated. Data analyses conducted at that time showed that paroxetine was superior to pill placebo. Active treatments with paroxetine or CBT were continued for a total of 16 weeks. At the end of the 16-week acute treatment phase, participants who had responded to either treatment were continued in active treatment for 1 year. During the 1-year follow-up, one-half (randomly selected) of the paroxetine patients had their medication tapered to pill placebo, and the other half continued to receive the medication to which they had been responsive. CBT patients received three booster sessions, at least 1 month apart, during the 1-year follow up period. At the 1-year follow-up, all patients were terminated from treatment and followed naturalistically for an additional year.

The primary acute treatment finding was that ADMs and the CBT treatments were equally efficacious, with a categorical *response* rate of 58% for both treatments and *remission* rates of 46% for the ADM and 40% for CBT. The authors concluded, "It appears that cognitive therapy can be as effective as medications, even among more severely depressed outpatients, at least when provided by experienced cognitive therapists" (DeRubeis et al. 2005, p. 415). In the long-term follow-up phase of this study, CBT conferred greater maintenance of treatment gains among those who had responded to acute treatment (Hollon et al. 2005). Specifically, the relapse rate for the CBT condition was significantly lower than that of the patients who were successfully treated with ADM but then had the medication withdrawn at the end of 16 weeks (30.8% vs. 76.2% relapse), and CBT was as effective (30.8% relapse) as ADM for those who continued the ADM for a full year (47.2% relapse). This latter finding is particularly relevant for translating these results to real-world settings, because the typical period for which ADMs are *prescribed* is up to 1 year, but the average length of time that outpatients *take* prescribed ADMs is less than 16 weeks (Hirschfeld et al. 1997; Katon and Schulberg 1992; Keller et al. 1986). Moreover, fewer than 10% of outpatients with MDD complete an adequate course of ADM treatment (Venturini et al. 1999). Taken together, the findings reported by DeRubeis and Hollon and their colleagues suggest that CBT is at least as effective as an SSRI for moderate and severe depression, and that 16 weeks of treatment with CBT provides a sustained treatment effect for longer periods of time than does an ADM.

Comprehensive reviews of the relevant treatment literatures (David et al. 2018; DeRubeis et al. 2008) corroborate the conclusions reached in the preceding studies. Comparable effect sizes were reported for CBT and citalopram in the Sequenced Treatment Alternatives to Relieve Depression (STAR*D) study, the largest trial of antidepressants conducted to date (Trivedi et al. 2006). A series of meta-analyses have reached the same conclusions as the general clinical reviews; namely, both CBT and ADMs (most recently SSRIs) are equally effective for moderate and severe depression (see, e.g., Bortolotti et al. 2008; Cuijpers et al. 2016; Driessen et al. 2010). Finally, literature reviews and meta-analyses have reported that 1) the combination of CBT and ADMs is more effective than either monotherapy alone, but this may hold true only for *severely* depressed patients (Hollon et al. 2016); and 2) CBT and ADM combination treatment does not decrease the sustainable maintenance effects conferred by CBT for depression (e.g., W.E. Craighead and Dunlop 2014; Cuijpers et al. 2016). It should be noted, however, that all the reviewed treatment studies excluded inpatients and imminently suicidal outpatients.

Summary

Approximately 30%–35% of MDD patients who complete a course of CBT are largely asymptomatic and are considered "remitted." Another 30%–35% of CBT-treated patients have a 50% reduction in depressive symptoms and their symptoms no longer meet full criteria for MDD at posttreatment; these patients are typically referred to as "responders." Furthermore, among the studies reported herein, CBT appeared to confer some enduring prophylactic effects, with only 20%–30% of those successfully treated experiencing a relapse or recurrence during the first year following treatment. Indeed, 16 weeks (16–20 sessions) of CBT have consistently produced a 1-year follow-up success rate equal to that achieved by a full year of ADM treatment (Kennedy et al. 2018). Furthermore, CBT's maintenance effects are superior to short-term (16-week) ADM treatment (Cuijpers et al. 2016; Zhang et al. 2018).

Future Directions

Recent research has moved from comparisons of the relative effectiveness of CBT and other treatments to seeking knowledge regarding the moderators and mediators of treatments for MDD. Newer studies, consequently, focus on the identification of the

Hollon SD, Jarrett RB, Nierenberg AA, et al: Psychotherapy and medication in the treatment of adult and geriatric depression: which monotherapy or combined treatment? J Clin Psychiatry 66(4):455–468, 2005 15816788
Hollon SD, DeRubeis RJ, Fawcett J, et al: Effect of cognitive therapy with antidepressant medications vs antidepressants alone on the rate of recovery in major depressive disorder: a randomized clinical trial. JAMA Psychiatry 71(10):1157–1164, 2016 25142196
Huguet A, Miller A, Kisely S, et al: A systematic review and meta-analysis on the efficacy of Internet-delivered behavioral activation. J Affect Disord 235:27–38, 2018 29649708
Ilardi SS, Craighead WE: Rapid early response, cognitive modification, and nonspecific factors in cognitive behavior therapy for depression: a reply to Tang and DeRubies. Clin Psychol Sci Pract 6(3):295–299, 2006
Jacobson NS, Dobson KS, Truax PA, et al: A component analysis of cognitive-behavioral treatment for depression. J Consult Clin Psychol 64(2):295–304, 1996 8871414
Jacobson NS, Christopher RM, Sona D: Behavioral activation treatment for depression: returning to contextual roots. Clin Psychol Sci Pract 8(3):255–270, 2001
Jarrett RB, Schaffer M, McIntire D, et al: Treatment of atypical depression with cognitive therapy or phenelzine: a double-blind, placebo-controlled trial. Arch Gen Psychiatry 56(5):431–437, 1999 10232298
Katon W, Schulberg H: Epidemiology of depression in primary care. Gen Hosp Psychiatry 14(4):237–247, 1992 1505745
Kazdin AE: Methodology, design, and evaluation in psychotherapy research, in Handbook of Psychotherapy and Behavior Change. Edited by Bergin AE, Garfield SL. New York, Wiley, 1994, pp 19–71
Keller MB, Lavori PW, Coryell W, et al: Differential outcome of pure manic, mixed/cycling, and pure depressive episodes in patients with bipolar illness. JAMA 255(22):3138–3142, 1986 3702024
Keller MB, McCullough JP, Klein DN, et al: A comparison of nefazodone, the cognitive behavioral-analysis system of psychotherapy, and their combination for the treatment of chronic depression. N Engl J Med 342(20):1462–1470, 2000 10816183
Kennedy SM, Tonarely NA, Sherman JA, et al: Predictors of treatment outcome for the Unified Protocol for Transdiagnostic Treatment of Emotional Disorders in Children (UP-C). J Anxiety Disord 57:66–75, 2018 29776708
Klein DF: Preventing hung juries about therapy studies. J Consult Clin Psychol 64(1):81–87, 1996 8907087
Kroenke K, Spitzer RL, Williams JB: The PHQ-9: validity of a brief depression severity measure. J Gen Intern Med 16(9):606–613, 2001 11556941
Lewinsohn PM, Gotlib IH: Behavioral theory and treatment of depression, in Handbook of Depression, 2nd Edition. Edited by Beckham EE, Leber WR. New York, Guilford, 1995, pp 352–375
Mahoney MJ: Cognition and Behavior Modification. Cambridge, MA, Ballinger, 1974
Mahoney MJ, Lyddon WJ: Recent developments in cognitive approaches to counseling and psychotherapy. Couns Psychol 16(2):190–234, 1988
Mazzucchelli T, Kane R, Reese C: Behavioral activation treatments for depression in adults: a meta-analysis and review. Clin Psychol Sci Pract 16(4):383–411, 2009
McCullough ME, Pargament KI, Thoresen CE: The psychology of forgiveness: history, conceptual issues, and overview, in Forgiveness: Theory, Research, and Practice. Edited by McCullough ME, Pargament KI, Thoresen CE. New York, Guilford, 2000, pp 1–14
McLean PD, Hakstian AR: Clinical depression: comparative efficacy of outpatient treatments. J Consult Clin Psychol 47(5):818–836, 1979 389965
McLean PD, Hakstian AR: Relative endurance of unipolar depression treatment effects: longitudinal follow-up. J Consult Clin Psychol 58(4):482–488, 1990 2212186
Meichenbaum D: Cognitive-Behavior Modification: An Integrative Approach. New York, Plenum, 1977

Nemeroff CB, Heim CM, Thase ME, et al: Differential responses to psychotherapy versus pharmacotherapy in patients with chronic forms of major depression and childhood trauma. Proc Natl Acad Sci USA 100(24):14293–14296, 2003 14615578
Öst L-G: Efficacy of the third wave of behavioral therapies: a systematic review and meta-analysis. Behav Res Ther 46(3):296–321, 2008 18258216
Patel V, Weobong B, Weiss HA, et al: The Healthy Activity Program (HAP), a lay counsellor-delivered brief psychological treatment for severe depression, in primary care in India: a randomised controlled trial. Lancet 389(10065):176–185, 2017 27988143
Patel AR, Weobong B, Patel VH, et al: Psychological treatments for depression among women experiencing intimate partner violence: findings from a randomized controlled trial for behavioral activation in Goa, India. Arch Women Ment Health 22(6):779–789, 2019 31363925
Rehm LP: A self-control model of depression. Behav Ther 8(5):787–804, 1977
Rush AJ, Beck AT, Kovacs M, et al: Comparative efficacy of cognitive therapy and pharmacotherapy in the treatment of depressed outpatients. Cognit Ther Res 1(1):17–37, 1977
Sacco WP, Beck AT: Cognitive theory and therapy, in Handbook of Depression, 2nd Edition. Edited by Beckham EE, Leber WR. New York, Guilford, 1995, pp 329–351
Simons AD, Murphy GE, Levine JL, et al: Cognitive therapy and pharmacotherapy for depression. Sustained improvement over one year. Arch Gen Psychiatry 43(1):43–48, 1986 3942473
Skinner BF: Science and Human Behavior. New York, Macmillan, 1953
Thoresen CE, Mahoney MJ: Behavioral Self-Control. New York, Holt, Rinehart & Winston, 1974
Trivedi MH, Rush AJ, Wisniewski SR, et al: Evaluation of outcomes with citalopram for depression using measurement-based care in STAR*D: implications for clinical practice. Am J Psychiatry 163(1):28–40, 2006 16390886
Venturini F, Sung JCY, Nichol MB, et al: Utilization patterns of antidepressant medications in a patient population served by a primary care medical group. J Manag Care Pharm 5(3):243–249, 1999
Wolpe J: Psychotherapy by Reciprocal Inhibition. Redwood City, CA, Stanford University Press, 1958
Young JE, Klosko JS, Weishaar ME: Schema Therapy: A Practitioner's Guide. New York, Guilford, 2003
Zhang Z, Zhang L, Zhang G, et al: The effect of CBT and its modifications for relapse prevention in major depressive disorder: a systematic review and meta-analysis. BMC Psychiatry 18(1):50, 2018 29475431

CHAPTER 24

Interpersonal Psychotherapy for Depressive Disorders

John C. Markowitz, M.D.

Mood disorders are where interpersonal psychotherapy (IPT) began. In the 1970s, the late Gerald L. Klerman, M.D., Myrna M. Weissman, Ph.D., and colleagues were planning a randomized trial comparing pharmacotherapy and placebo for outpatients with major depressive disorder (MDD). Recognizing that many depressed patients received psychotherapy as part of their treatment, Klerman and Weissman decided to add psychotherapy to the study. Realizing that they had no gauge of what constituted typical psychotherapy in the community, these researchers decided to devise their own standardized treatment, which they hoped would not be too removed from community practice and which rely on interpersonal theory and, more particularly, on empirical research on interpersonal aspects of depression.

Klerman et al. (1984) developed a manual for this treatment and trained therapists to use it. The resultant psychotherapy worked as well as tricyclic antidepressant medication and better than control conditions, and the combination of this psychotherapy with pharmacotherapy had advantages over either modality alone (Klerman et al. 1974). Moreover, patients who received this interpersonally focused therapy developed new social skills over time, whereas patients who received medication alone did not. What became known as IPT has subsequently shown efficacy for MDD in repeated randomized controlled trials (RCTs) (Cuijpers et al. 2011) and for other subtypes of mood, and increasingly for nonmood, disorders as well (Cuijpers et al. 2016; Weissman et al. 2000). In this chapter I review basic aspects of IPT and its application to acute and chronic unipolar mood disorders.

History and Early Work

The history of IPT records a series of randomized clinical trials, beginning with trials in mood disorders. For many years, IPT paradoxically was very well researched but little practiced: it was almost purely a research intervention. Its research successes and recommendation by treatment guidelines (e.g., American Psychiatric Association 2010; Depression Guideline Panel 1993; Karasu et al. 1993), however, led to increasing interest and demand for training from clinicians. IPT has spread to different diagnoses, formats, and cultures. One of the relatively few empirically validated antidepressant psychotherapies, IPT has been tested in key studies such as the National Institute of Mental Health (NIMH) Treatment of Depression Collaborative Research Program (Elkin et al. 1985, 1989). The IPT manual (Weissman et al. 2018) has been translated into several languages, and this treatment has proved transportable to European, South American, and African, Australian, and Asian settings. Originally developed as an individual psychotherapy, IPT also shows promise in group, couples, and telether-apy formats.

Theoretical Model and Hypothesized Mechanisms

An eclectic treatment, IPT derives from several sources. One root is the interpersonal theory that arose in the United States after World War II. In contrast to the then-prevailing intrapsychically focused psychoanalytic thinking, psychiatrists such as Adolf Meyer, Harry Stack Sullivan (1953), Erich Fromm, and Frieda Fromm-Reichmann emphasized the status of humans as social beings and the effects of environment and current life events on psychopathology. Bowlby (1973, 1988) underscored the importance of attachment to primary caregivers as the basis for understanding affective responses to stress and to attachment in adult relationships. This theory provides a background for understanding IPT.

Research on psychosocial aspects of mood disorders confirmed the importance of life events as both precipitants and consequences of depression and indicated that social supports protect against depressive episodes (Brown and Harris 1978). Furthermore, research has connected the onset of mood disorders with life events such as the deaths of significant others (*complicated bereavement*), struggles with significant others (*role disputes*), and important life changes such as geographic moves, marriage or divorce, and beginning or ending jobs (*role transitions*) (Klerman et al. 1984). Negative life events are even more likely to follow the onset of depression than to precede it. Depressed patients withdraw socially, talk less to other people, and function less well in social and work settings. Regardless of whether a life event triggers a depressive episode, negative life events tend to follow its onset, confirming the patient's sense that life is spiraling downward and out of control.

IPT was developed as a simple, practical treatment by researchers. Its structure followed the logic of extant research on interpersonal aspects of depression. Patients are given the diagnosis of MDD according to standard diagnostic criteria (American Psychiatric Association 2013). Treatment focuses on problem areas defined as stressful triggers or consequences of depressive episodes: complicated bereavement following the death of a loved one, a struggle with a significant other, a major life change, or social isolation. The treatment does not demand a causal relation between mood event and life situation—the etiology of all psychiatric syndromes remains unknown and is surely multifaceted—but simply notes the association of the two. This connection between life situation and mood is one that many depressed patients forget; they guiltily blame themselves for their illness, its symptoms, and what is going wrong in their lives. IPT therapists encourage patients to see that by handling a situation well, they can make life go right and thereby improve their mood.

The mechanisms that make IPT efficacious are unknown. Research on IPT has been largely outcome research, designed to test whether the treatment works, rather than dismantling or process research to explore why it works; hence, more is known about appropriate target diagnoses for IPT than about its active ingredients. Nonetheless, IPT provides several likely helpful factors:

- The IPT therapist names the illness (e.g., MDD) and explicitly reassures the patient that what he or she is experiencing is a treatable illness and is not the patient's fault. This medical model gives the patient a temporary "sick role" (Parsons 1951) and shifts blame for symptoms from the overly guilty depressed patient to the syndrome.
- IPT helps the patient to understand connections between affects and actions in the interpersonal arena and to put them to effective use. This is a relatively simple and plausible central focus that even a depressed patient with concrete thinking and poor ability to concentrate can grasp.
- IPT focuses on building interpersonal skills such as self-assertion, effective expression of anger, and social risk-taking. Many depressed patients lack these important practical skills.
- The focus on understanding and confronting current interpersonal difficulties leads to "success experiences," that is, victorious interpersonal encounters (Frank 1971). These successes give the patient a greater sense of competence, agency, and control over his or her environment.
- IPT therapists assign no homework. This means that patients cannot fail to complete assignments, a frequent occurrence in other therapies that makes noncompliant patients feel like failures. Instead, the therapist primes the patient for encounters using role-play, then lets the time pressure of time-limited treatment push the patient toward eventual action.
- IPT focuses outside the office rather than on the therapeutic relationship. This has at least two positive consequences. First, therapists foster a positive therapeutic alliance; avoiding interpretations of the therapeutic relationship minimizes the risk of therapeutic ruptures (Safran and Muran 2000). Second, as termination approaches, patients can clearly see that they have done the hard work on, and hence deserve the credit for, their improved daily functioning and symptomatic gains.
- Therapeutic optimism, an important aspect of the IPT therapist's stance, is bolstered by research that IPT works.
- Preliminary recent research suggests that IPT may work through the repair of dysregulated affect and attachment (Milrod et al. 2020).

Conducting Interpersonal Psychotherapy

Techniques

IPT therapists define depression as a treatable *medical illness* that is not the patient's fault. This definition displaces burdensome blame from the patient to the illness. It also provides hope for improvement: an illness is far more treatable than a self-perceived intrinsic flaw. The IPT therapist uses DSM-5 (American Psychiatric Association 2013) to diagnose a mood disorder and a rating scale such as the Hamilton Rating Scale for Depression (HAM-D; Hamilton 1960) or the Beck Depression Inventory (BDI; Beck 1978) to assess and explain depressive symptoms. These instruments provide psychoeducation to help the patient to recognize that he or she is struggling with a common disorder with a predictable set of symptoms. The HAM-D and BDI have been used for decades, reinforcing that the problem is not a personal flaw but a long-recognized syndrome. The therapist gives the depressed patient the sick role (Parsons 1951), which excuses what the illness prevents him or her from doing, while still conferring responsibility to work in treatment to recover the lost healthy role. By solving an interpersonal problem—addressing complicated bereavement, a role dispute or transition, or an interpersonal deficit—the IPT patient can both improve his or her life situation and relieve symptoms of the depressive episode. This coupled formula, validated in repeated RCTs, can be offered with confidence and optimism.

IPT is an eclectic therapy that uses techniques seen in other treatment approaches yet can be clearly distinguished from other therapies by adherence ratings (Amole et al. 2017; Hill et al. 1992; Markowitz et al. 2000b). Its medical model of depressive illness mimics, and makes it highly compatible with, pharmacotherapy. Marital therapists find its approach to interpersonal issues familiar. IPT shares role-playing and a here-and-now focus with cognitive-behavioral therapy (CBT; Beck et al. 1979; Markowitz 2001). Akin to CBT as a time-limited, syndrome-targeted treatment, IPT is less structured, assigns no homework, and focuses on interpersonal problem areas and associated affect rather than automatic thoughts and core beliefs. Affect-focused, IPT overlaps with psychodynamic psychotherapies, and many early IPT research therapists came from psychodynamic backgrounds. Yet IPT also meaningfully differs from psychodynamic therapies in its focus on the present, not the past; its focus on real-life change rather than self-understanding; its medical model; and its avoidance of interpreting dreams and the transference (Markowitz et al. 1998b). No one technique or tactic makes IPT a unique and coherent approach; its overall strategies do.

Each of the four IPT interpersonal problem areas has discrete, if overlapping, goals for the therapist and patient to pursue. The therapist repeatedly helps the patient relate life events to mood and other symptoms. In each session after the first one, an *opening question* elicits an interval history of mood and events and focuses treatment on them. Other techniques include

- *Communication analysis*—the reconstruction and evaluation of recent affectively charged interpersonal encounters.
- *Exploration of the patient's wishes and options*—to pursue these in interpersonal situations.

- *Decision analysis*—to help the patient choose among options.
- *Role-playing*—to help patients rehearse tactics for real life.

IPT focuses on current interpersonal relationships in the patient's immediate social context. The IPT therapist attempts to intervene in symptom formation and social dysfunction associated with depression rather than aspects of personality. Personality is difficult to accurately assess during an episode of a major psychiatric disorder such as depression (Hirschfeld et al. 1983; Markowitz et al. 2015). IPT does help the patient build new social skills (Weissman et al. 1974, 1981), which may be as valuable as changing personality traits.

Phases of Treatment

As an acute treatment, IPT has three phases (Table 24–1) (Weissman et al. 2018). The *early phase*, lasting no more than three sessions, sets the stage for what follows. The therapist reviews symptoms, diagnoses depression by standard criteria (American Psychiatric Association 2013), and gives the patient the sick role. The psychiatric history includes an "interpersonal inventory," a careful cataloging of the patient's past and current social functioning and close relationships, including their patterns and mutual expectations. Initial sessions elucidate changes in relationships proximal to the onset of symptoms—for example, death of a loved one, children leaving home, worsening marital strife, or isolation from a confidant. The therapist looks for meaningful life events such as a career change or onset of a medical illness. This review provides a framework for understanding the social and interpersonal context of the depressive symptoms, and this framework becomes the basis of a treatment focus.

In clinical practice, the therapist assesses the need for medication on the basis of symptom severity, illness history and response to treatment, and patient preference. The therapist then educates the patient about the constellation of symptoms that define MDD, their psychosocial concomitants, and what the patient may expect from treatment. A formulation links the depressive syndrome to the patient's interpersonal situation (Markowitz and Swartz 2007), centered on one of four interpersonal problem areas: 1) grief, 2) interpersonal role disputes, 3) role transitions, or 4) interpersonal deficits (Table 24–2). With the patient's explicit acceptance of this formulation as the treatment focus, therapy enters the middle phase.

Any formulation perforce simplifies a patient's complex life story. Although many patients present with multiple interpersonal problems, the formulation isolates one or at most two salient problems related to the patient's mood disorder, either as precipitants or as consequences, and weaves them into an organizing fiction. More than two foci in a brief psychotherapy means no focus at all. Choice of focal problem area depends on clinical acumen, although research has shown that IPT therapists agree on the chosen areas (Markowitz et al. 2000a). Patients seem to find the foci credible.

In the *middle phase*, the IPT therapist pursues strategies appropriate to the focal interpersonal problem area (Weissman et al. 2018). To address grief (complicated bereavement after the death of a loved one), the therapist facilitates the catharsis of mourning and helps the patient to find new activities and relationships to compensate for the loss. For role disputes (conflicts with a spouse, other family member, boss, coworker, or friend), the therapist helps the patient to explore the relationship, the nature of the dis-

TABLE 24–1. Phases of interpersonal psychotherapy (IPT)

Early phase

Deal with the depression.

1. Review depressive symptoms.
2. Name the syndrome: formal diagnosis.
3. Provide psychoeducation about depression and its treatment.
4. Give the patient the "sick role."
5. Evaluate the need for medication.

Relate depression to interpersonal context: interpersonal inventory.

1. Determine the nature of interaction with significant persons.
2. Identify reciprocal expectations of the patient and significant others and whether these were fulfilled.
3. Discuss satisfying and unsatisfying aspects of relationships.
4. Detect recent changes in key relationships.
5. Determine changes the patient desires in his or her relationships.

Identify the major problem area.

1. Determine problem area related to current episode and set treatment goals.
2. Identify which relationship is related to the episode and what might change in it.

Explain IPT concepts and contract.

1. Outline the therapist's understanding of the problem: formulation.
2. Agree on treatment goals (focal problem area):
   a. *Brief* treatment (time limit)
   b. Target of improving depression (not character)
3. Describe IPT procedures: here-and-now focus, need to discuss important concerns, review of current interpersonal relationships, discussion of practical aspects of treatment.

Middle phase

Use specific strategies for treating grief, role disputes, role transitions, or interpersonal deficits.

Termination phase

Consolidate gains.

Foster independence.

Address guilt (and blame the therapy) if the patient's symptoms did not respond.

Review risk of relapse and recurrence.

Recontract for continuation or maintenance treatment if appropriate.

---

pute, whether it has reached an impasse, and available options to resolve it. If these options fail, the therapist and patient may conclude that the relationship has reached an impasse and consider ways to change the impasse or to end the relationship.

A role transition is a change in life status: beginning or ending a relationship or career, moving, being promoted, retiring, graduating, or receiving a diagnosis of a medical illness. The patient learns to manage the change by mourning the loss of the old role while recognizing positive and negative aspects of the new role he or she is assuming and taking steps to master it. The residual fourth IPT problem area, interpersonal deficits, comprises patients who lack all of the first three problem areas (i.e., have no recent life events). This least-defined focus, an anomalous non-life-event-

TABLE 24–2. Interpersonal psychotherapy problem areas

Problem area	Definition
Grief (complicated bereavement)	Death of a significant other
Role disputes	Struggle with a significant other
Role transitions	Life event that changes perceived social role
Interpersonal deficits	No life events; social isolation (used only if none of the above are appropriate)

based category for a life-event-based therapy, defines the patient as lacking the social skills to initiate or sustain relationships. Its goal is to help the patient develop new relationships and skills. Some patients who appear to fit this category may have DSM-IV (American Psychiatric Association 1994) dysthymic disorder, for which other IPT strategies have been developed (Markowitz 1998).

IPT sessions address current, here-and-now problems. Sessions open with the question "How have things been since we last met?" This orients the patient to recent interpersonal events and recent mood, which the therapist helps the patient to link. Therapists sympathize with patients' suffering and validate their emotions while taking an active, supportive, and hopeful stance to counter the depressed patient's pessimism. They elicit and emphasize the options for change in the patient's life, options that the depressive episode often has kept the patient from seeing or exploring fully. Understanding the situation does not suffice; therapists stress the need for patients to test these options to improve their lives and simultaneously treat their depressive episodes. Enacting a practical solution to the patient's focal interpersonal crisis within the envelope of the time-limited treatment is the implicit homework of IPT.

The *termination phase* of IPT, the last few sessions of acute treatment or last months of maintenance treatment, supports the patient's newly regained sense of competence by recognizing and consolidating therapeutic gains. The therapist enhances the patient's self-esteem and independence by underscoring that the patient's depressive episode has improved through the patient's interpersonal actions in changing a life situation. Moreover, the patient achieved this at a time when he or she had felt weakest. The therapist also helps the patient to anticipate triggers for and responses to depressive symptoms that might arise in the future. Relative to psychodynamic therapy, IPT deemphasizes termination: it is a graduation from successful treatment, a role transition that, like most, is bittersweet. The sadness of separation is distinguished from depressive feelings. If the patient has not improved, the therapist emphasizes that the treatment has failed, not the patient, and that alternative effective treatment options exist. Patients with multiple prior depressive episodes or significant residual symptoms who successfully complete acute treatment but remain at high risk for recurrence may contract for maintenance therapy as acute treatment draws to a close.

Indications and Contraindications

Research on psychotherapy outcome has lacked the resources available to pharmaceutical companies, whose products are accordingly better studied. Nonetheless, a series of RCTs comparing IPT with control conditions have defined the efficacy of IPT for patients with mood disorders. Indications for IPT thus have been determined not by random application but by RCTs. For some patient subgroups, IPT has been adapted in separate treatment manuals (e.g., Markowitz 1998; Mufson et al. 2011).

Still more interesting are comparative trials of IPT with CBT and medication, which have provided some data on differential therapeutics. No absolute contraindications exist for using IPT with nondelusional depressed outpatients, yet no treatment is ideal for all patients. Given a choice between two treatments of already established efficacy, the clinician must determine which factors may predict a better outcome for patients with a given diagnosis (Frances et al. 1984). The following section documents the efficacy of IPT for patients with unipolar, nondelusional mood disorders, first addressing acute and then chronic forms of depression (Table 24–3).

Acute Treatment of Major Depressive Disorder

IPT was first studied as an acute antidepressant treatment in a four-cell, 16-week randomized trial comparing IPT, amitriptyline, their combination, and a nonscheduled control treatment for 81 outpatients with MDD (DiMascio et al. 1979; Weissman et al. 1979). Amitriptyline worked more quickly, but IPT and amitriptyline did not significantly differ in symptom reduction at the end of treatment. Each reduced symptoms more efficaciously than did the control treatment, and combined amitriptyline-IPT was more efficacious than either active monotherapy. Not surprisingly, patients with psychotic depression who received IPT alone fared poorly. On naturalistic follow-up at 1 year, many patients had sustained improvement from the brief IPT intervention, and IPT patients had developed significantly better psychosocial functioning regardless of whether they had received medication. This effect on social function was not found for amitriptyline alone, nor had it been evident for IPT immediately after the 16-week trial (Weissman et al. 1981).

In the ambitious, multisite NIMH Treatment of Depression Collaborative Research Program (Elkin et al. 1989), investigators randomly assigned 250 outpatients with MDD to 16 weeks of IPT, CBT, or clinical management with either imipramine or pill placebo. Most subjects completed at least 15 weeks or 12 treatment sessions. More mildly depressed patients (defined as baseline 17-item HAM-D score <20) improved equally in all treatments. Among more severely depressed patients (HAM-D score ≥ 20), imipramine worked fastest and most consistently outperformed placebo. IPT was comparable to imipramine on several outcome measures, including HAM-D score, and superior to placebo for the more depressed patients. CBT was not superior to placebo among the more depressed patients.

Klein and Ross (1993) reanalyzed the NIMH Treatment of Depression Collaborative Research Program data with the Johnson-Neyman technique and found that medication outperformed the psychotherapies, which were superior to placebo, especially among more impaired patients. The authors found CBT inferior to IPT for patients with BDI scores greater than 30, a score demarcating the boundary between moderate and severe depression.

In a naturalistic follow-up study of Treatment of Depression Collaborative Research Program subjects at 18 months posttreatment, Shea et al. (1992) found no significant difference across treatments in recovery among patients whose symptoms

TABLE 24–3. Empirically based indications for interpersonal psychotherapy

Acute major depressive disorder
Geriatric patients
Adolescent patients
HIV-positive patients
Primary care patients
Antepartum and postpartum depressed women
Patients with marital disputes (conjoint therapy)
Recurrent major depressive disorder (maintenance prophylaxis)
Persistent depressive disorder (dysthymia)[a]
Bipolar disorder (adjunctive treatment)[a,b]
Interpersonal counseling for subsyndromal depression

[a]Preliminary results are encouraging.
[b]See Chapter 26 ("Psychotherapeutic Approaches to Bipolar Disorder") in this volume.

had remitted (i.e., those who had minimal or no symptoms after treatment and sustained this improvement during follow-up). Thirty percent of CBT, 26% of IPT, 20% of placebo, and 19% of imipramine subjects whose symptoms had acutely remitted remained in remission during that time span. Of the subjects whose symptoms had acutely remitted, relapse rates over the 18 months were 36% for CBT, 33% for IPT, 50% for imipramine (albeit medication had been stopped at 16 weeks), and 33% for placebo. The authors concluded that for many patients, 16 weeks of treatment was insufficient to achieve lasting recovery (Shea et al. 1992).

IPT works outside the United States as well. In a trial in the Hague, the Netherlands, Blom et al. (1996) first undertook a pilot trial and then completed a randomized trial of IPT, nefazodone, and their combination for 191 subjects with MDD (Blom et al. 2004). Results suggested that all three treatments had similar benefit. Subsequent trials have validated the efficacy of IPT for depression in many other countries (Weissman et al. 2018).

Depressed Geriatric Patients

IPT was first used with 30 depressed geriatric patients to enhance compliance in a 6-week pharmacotherapy trial and to enhance the pill placebo control group (Rothblum et al. 1982; Sholomskas et al. 1983). The investigators noted grief and role transitions as the modal treatment foci. They suggested modifications of IPT for older depressed patients, including a flexible duration of sessions, more practical advice and concrete support (e.g., arranging transportation, calling physicians), and increased recognition that major role changes may be impractical and detrimental (e.g., divorce at age 75 years). A 6-week trial comparing IPT with nortriptyline in depressed elderly patients showed some advantages for IPT, largely because of higher attrition in the medication group because of nortriptyline's side effects (Sloane et al. 1985).

Depressed Adolescents

Mufson et al. (1993) modified IPT to incorporate adolescent developmental issues. The researchers conducted an open feasibility and follow-up trial and then a controlled 12-week clinical trial comparing IPT for depressed adolescents (IPT-A) and clinical monitoring in 48 clinic-referred adolescents, ages 12–18, whose symptoms met DSM-III-R (American Psychiatric Association 1987) criteria for MDD. Patients were rated biweekly by a blinded independent evaluator to assess symptomatology, social functioning, and social problem-solving skills. Of the 48 patients, 32 (21 IPT-A, 11 control) completed the protocol.

Patients receiving IPT-A reported significantly greater improvement in depressive symptoms and social functioning, including functioning with friends and problem-solving skills. In the intent-to-treat sample, 75% of the IPT-A patients met the recovery criterion (HAM-D score ≤6), compared with 46% of the control subjects. The findings support the feasibility, patient acceptance, and efficacy of 12 weeks of IPT-A with acutely depressed adolescents in reducing depressive symptomatology and improving social functioning and interpersonal problem-solving skills (Mufson et al. 1999).

Mufson et al. (2004a) subsequently tested IPT-A in a large-scale effectiveness study in New York City school-based clinics; a 12-session course of IPT-A delivered by school counselors was compared with treatment as usual over 16 weeks. Adolescents with mood disorders who received IPT-A (N=63) again showed greater improvements than did those receiving usual treatment on independent, clinician, and self-report ratings of symptoms and social functioning. Thus, IPT-A has shown benefits in both efficacy and effectiveness trials. Mufson et al. (2004b) also have developed a group format for depressed adolescents, which might have economic benefits and take advantage of teenage peer support.

Rosselló and Bernal (1999) at the University of Puerto Rico compared IPT (n=22), CBT (n=25), and a wait-list control condition (n=24) in a 12-week RCT for adolescents (ages 13–18 years) whose symptoms met DSM-III-R criteria for MDD, dysthymia, or both. The investigators did not use Mufson and colleagues' IPT-A adaptation. Both IPT and CBT were more efficacious than the wait-list condition in reducing adolescents' self-rated depressive symptoms. IPT was more efficacious than CBT in increasing self-esteem and social adaptation. Effect sizes for improvement were 0.73 for IPT and 0.43 for CBT.

Mufson and colleagues have since adapted IPT-A as a group intervention, as a preventive intervention, and as an intervention for preadolescents (Weissman et al. 2018).

Depressed HIV-Positive Patients

Markowitz et al. (1992) modified IPT for depressed individuals with HIV (IPT-HIV) in the early years of the epidemic, when AIDS appeared to be an acute and lethal illness rather than the chronic disease it has now become. The adaptation emphasized common concerns among this population about illness and death, grief, and role transitions. A 16-week randomized trial in 101 subjects compared IPT-HIV, CBT, supportive psychotherapy, and imipramine plus supportive psychotherapy (Markowitz et al. 1998a). As with the subset of more severely depressed individuals in the Treatment of Depression Collaborative Research Program study (Elkin et al. 1989), all treatments were associated with symptom reduction, but IPT and imipramine plus supportive psychotherapy produced significantly greater symptomatic and functional improvement than CBT or supportive psychotherapy alone. Many patients reported improvement in neurovegetative symptoms that they had mistakenly attributed to HIV infection.

More recently, Heckman et al. (2017) successfully used telephone IPT to treat isolated rural patients with comorbid depression and HIV infection.

Depressed Primary Care Patients

Schulberg et al. (1996) compared IPT with pharmacotherapy for depressed primary care medical patients. The investigators integrated IPT into the primary care center. Not only did nurses take vital signs before sessions, but primary care patients received treatment for MDD without having to go to a "shrink": the mental health care came to them. If patients were medically hospitalized, attempts were made to continue IPT in the hospital.

Patients with MDD (N=276) were randomly assigned to receive IPT, nortriptyline, or their primary care physicians' usual care. IPT was given weekly for 16 weeks and then monthly for 4 months (Schulberg et al. 1996). Depressive symptoms declined more rapidly with either nortriptyline or IPT than with usual care. About 70% of those who completed the trial who had received nortriptyline or IPT, but only 20% of those who had received usual care, had recovered after 8 months. Subjects with a history of comorbid panic disorder had a poorer response across treatments than did those without a panic history (C. Brown et al. 1996), a finding subsequently corroborated by Frank et al. (2000).

Patients With Antepartum and Postpartum Depression

Pregnancy and nursing are key role transitions for women of childbearing age, who are prime candidates for depressive episodes (see Chapter 42, "Depression in Women," in this volume). Even though most antidepressant medications may carry little risk of teratogenesis and not all are detectable in breast milk, physicians are reluctant to prescribe medication, and patients are reluctant to accept it, during pregnancy and nursing. Thus, peripartum depression is an ideal target for IPT.

Spinelli (1997) at Columbia University tested IPT in women with antepartum depression. She added "complicated pregnancy" as a fifth interpersonal problem area. Timing and duration of sessions were adjusted in response to bed rest, delivery, obstetrical complications, and childcare. As with depressed HIV-positive and primary care patients, telephone sessions and hospital visits were sometimes necessary (Spinelli 1997). In a 16-week trial, Spinelli et al. (2016) found that IPT had greater efficacy than a control parenting education condition in treating women of generally low socioeconomic status with moderately severe depression.

O'Hara et al. (2000) compared IPT with a wait-list control condition in 120 women with postpartum depression in a 12-week trial with an 18-month follow-up. The research assessed both the symptom states of the postpartum mothers and their interactions with their infants (Stuart and O'Hara 1995). Of the IPT group, 38% met HAM-D and 44% met BDI remission criteria, compared with 14% on each measure for the control group. Sixty percent of IPT patients, in contrast to 16% of control subjects, reported more than a 50% reduction in BDI score. Mothers receiving IPT showed significantly improved social adjustment relative to the control group.

Klier et al. (2001) treated 17 women with postpartum depression in nine weekly 90-minute group IPT sessions followed by an hourlong individual termination session. Scores on the 21-item HAM-D declined from 19.7 to 8.0, suggesting the efficacy of this approach. In an exciting study of IPT as prevention, Zlotnick et al. (2001) treated 37 women at risk for postpartum depression with either four 60-minute sessions of an IPT-based group or usual care. Six of the 18 women in usual care developed depression by 3 months postpartum, compared with none of the 17 IPT group patients.

Depressed Patients With Marital Disputes (Conjoint IPT)

Stressful changes in relationships such as marital conflict, separation, and divorce can precipitate or complicate depressive episodes (Rounsaville et al. 1979). Treating marital role disputes in individual IPT often has the feel of unilateral couples therapy (Weissman et al. 2000), so extending IPT to a couples format was not difficult. Weissman and Klerman (1993) developed a manual for conjoint therapy for depressed patients with marital disputes (IPT-CM). IPT-CM includes the spouse in all sessions and focuses on the current marital dispute. Eighteen patients with MDD linked to onset or exacerbation of marital disputes were randomly assigned to 16 weeks of either individual IPT or IPT-CM. Patients showed similar reductions in depressive symptoms in both treatments, but patients receiving IPT-CM reported significantly better marital adjustment, marital affection, and sexual relationships (Foley et al. 1989). These pilot findings require replication with a larger sample and other control groups.

Maintenance Prophylaxis for Recurrent Major Depressive Disorder

A significant proportion of all depressions are chronic, and this chronicity may take two forms. First, most individuals who have a single episode of MDD have a greater than even chance of having a second lifetime episode; the more episodes one has, the greater the risk of subsequent episodes (Boland and Keller 2002). Patients with recurrent MDD require not only acute remission of symptoms but also prevention of relapse and recurrence. IPT is the first psychotherapy to have been tested as a maintenance treatment to prevent recurrence of depressive episodes. Second, many depressive episodes are chronic—either chronic MDD, milder but chronic DSM-IV dysthymic disorder, or so-called double depression (i.e., MDD superimposed on DSM-IV dysthymic disorder); DSM-5 has reclassified all of these under the rubric of "persistent depressive disorder (dysthymia)." Chronically depressed patients are still more hopeless and resigned than are acutely depressed patients, and the chronicity of their illness alters treatment strategies for their acute treatment.

IPT was first tested in an 8-month, six-cell trial (Klerman et al. 1974; Paykel et al. 1976). A study of this length today would be considered a continuation treatment because the concept of long-term maintenance antidepressant treatment has lengthened. Acutely depressed outpatient women (N=150) who had responded (with 50% or greater symptom reduction by interviewer rating) to a 4- to 6-week acute trial of amitriptyline were randomly assigned to 8 months of weekly IPT, amitriptyline, placebo alone, combined IPT-amitriptyline, combined IPT-placebo, or no treatment. Randomization to IPT or a low-contact psychotherapy condition occurred at entry into the continuation phase, whereas randomization to medication, placebo, or no treatment occurred at the end of the second month of continuation treatment. Maintenance pharmacotherapy was found to prevent relapse and symptom exacerbation, whereas IPT improved social functioning (Weissman et al. 1974). The effects of IPT on social functioning required 6–8 months to appear. Combined psychotherapy and pharmacotherapy produced the best outcomes.

Researchers in Pittsburgh, Pennsylvania, conducted two longer antidepressant maintenance trials of IPT (IPT-M). Frank et al. (1990, 1991) studied 128 outpatients with multiply and rapidly recurrent depression. Patients were given combined high-dosage (>200 mg/day) imipramine and weekly IPT until they responded; the high-dosage medication was continued while IPT was tapered to a monthly frequency during a 4-month continuation phase. Patients who remained in remission were then randomly assigned to 3 years of 1) ongoing high-dosage imipramine plus clinical management, 2) high-dosage imipramine plus monthly IPT, 3) monthly IPT alone, 4) monthly IPT plus placebo, or 5) placebo plus clinical management. High-dosage imipramine, with or without further IPT, proved most efficacious, protecting more than 80% of the patients over 3 years. Most placebo patients relapsed within the first few months. Once-monthly IPT, although less efficacious than medication, was statistically and clinically superior to the control condition in this high-risk patient population.

Reynolds et al. (1999) conducted a second 3-year maintenance study of geriatric patients with recurrent depression; they used IPT and nortriptyline in a design similar to that used in the Frank et al. (1990) study. The IPT manual was modified to allow more flexibility in the length of sessions, under the assumption that some elderly patients might have difficulty tolerating 50-minute sessions. The investigators found that geriatric patients needed to address early life relationships in psychotherapy, digressing from the here-and-now focus of IPT. Like Sholomskas et al. (1983), Reynolds and colleagues believed that therapists needed to help patients solve practical problems but acknowledged that some problems might not be resolvable, such as existential late-life issues or lifelong psychopathology (Rothblum et al. 1982). Elderly depressed patients whose sleep quality had normalized by the early continuation phase had an 80% chance of remaining well during the first year of maintenance treatment. Response rates were similar for patients who subsequently received either nortriptyline or IPT (Reynolds et al. 1999).

The acute treatment sample comprised 187 patients 60 years or older with recurrent MDD (Reynolds et al. 1999). These patients received combined IPT and nortriptyline. One hundred seven who had remission of symptoms and then achieved recovery after continuation therapy were randomly assigned to one of four 3-year maintenance conditions: 1) medication clinic with nortriptyline alone, with steady-state nortriptyline plasma levels maintained in a therapeutic window of 80–120 ng/mL; 2) medication clinic with placebo; 3) monthly maintenance IPT plus placebo; or 4) monthly maintenance IPT plus nortriptyline. Recurrence rates were 90% for placebo, 64% for IPT with placebo, 43% for nortriptyline alone, and 20% for combined treatment. Each monotherapy was statistically superior to placebo, whereas combined therapy showed superiority to IPT alone and a trend for superiority to nortriptyline alone. Patients in their 70s were more likely to have a recurrence, and to do so more quickly, than patients in their 60s. This study (Reynolds et al. 1999) corroborated the maintenance findings of Frank et al. (1990, 1991), with the difference that combined treatment showed advantages over pharmacotherapy alone for the geriatric population.

In both maintenance studies, the comparison of high-dosage tricyclic antidepressants with low-dose maintenance IPT is easy to misinterpret. No previous maintenance studies had ever used either such high dosages of medication or so low a dose of psychotherapy. Had the medication dosage been lowered comparably to the reduced psychotherapy dosage, recurrence in the medication groups might well have been greater;

had psychotherapy been more intensive, recurrence rates might have declined. Because there were no precedents for this research, the choice of a monthly dosing interval for maintenance IPT was reasonable and indeed showed some benefit. Several studies have since begun to test the effects of differing maintenance doses of psychotherapy.

These difficult, protracted studies have yielded exciting results. They showed that psychotherapy not only works acutely but also can continue working to ward off the return of a typically recurrent illness. These research trials also have contributed to the knowledge base on differential therapeutics by assessing potential moderators of outcome.

Persistent Depressive Disorder (Dysthymia)

Dysthymia is a syndrome, often of early onset, with high debility and comorbidity (see Chapter 35, "Atypical Depression, Dysthymia, and Cyclothymia," in this volume). Because dysthymic individuals often have been ill from an early age, they tend to accept their symptoms as part of themselves, an internal defect, and may not seek appropriate treatment. Early onset of symptoms impedes the development of social skills. Moreover, because these individuals often struggle through life without the evident crisis of a major depressive episode, people around them also may accept that they have nervous or melancholy characters and not press them to find treatment. Thus, many dysthymic individuals become patients late in the course of chronic illness and are resigned to their condition.

From an IPT perspective, dysthymic patients present an additional problem. As the description of IPT earlier in this chapter indicates, the IPT model connects recent life events with recent mood changes. This model nicely fits acute depression but makes less sense for the often decades-long cases of chronic depression. Accordingly, Markowitz (1998) modified IPT for DSM-IV dysthymic disorder (IPT-D), taking advantage of the patient's sense that the illness was part of his or her character. IPT-D encourages patients to reconceptualize what they consider their lifelong character flaws as ego-dystonic, chronic mood-dependent symptoms—as a chronic but treatable *state* rather than an immutable *trait*. Therapy itself is defined as an "iatrogenic role transition" from believing oneself flawed in personality to recognizing and treating the mood disorder. Markowitz (1994, 1998) openly treated 17 pilot subjects with 16 sessions of IPT-D: none worsened, and 11 subjects had remission of symptoms.

On the basis of these pilot results, investigators at Weill Medical College of Cornell University conducted a randomized trial comparing 16 weeks of IPT-D alone, sertraline plus clinical management, supportive psychotherapy, and combined IPT-D and sertraline for 86 patients with "pure" DSM-IV dysthymic disorder (i.e., no major depressive episode within the prior 6 months). Preliminary results in this underpowered trial found improvement across cells, with no statistically significant advantages for any condition, although post hoc analyses showed some advantages for the pharmacotherapy cells (Markowitz 2003). Other studies at Cornell University are comparing IPT with supportive psychotherapy for double depression and IPT plus Alcoholics Anonymous (AA) meetings with supportive psychotherapy plus AA meetings for chronically depressed patients with secondary alcohol abuse.

Browne et al. (2002) conducted one of the largest psychotherapy studies ever, treating 707 patients with DSM-IV (American Psychiatric Association 1994) dysthymic disorder. Most patients (68%) were women with a mean age in the early 40s. Half had early-onset (before age 21) dysthymic disorder, a third had current double depression, and two-thirds had a history of double depression. Patients were randomly assigned to receive sertraline (50–200 mg/day) alone, IPT alone, or combined IPT plus sertraline. The median dosage of sertraline was 100 mg/day in the sertraline-only group and 150 mg/day in the combined treatment cell. Treatment dosage in this community study was not fully balanced; IPT treatment (not adapted as described above) consisted of up to 12 (mean=10) 1-hour sessions over 6 months, whereas sertraline treatment usually endured for the 2 years of the study. Thus, the study compared acute psychotherapy with acute and maintenance pharmacotherapy.

Treatment outcome considered both symptoms and economics. Response was defined as a 40% or greater decrease on the Montgomery-Åsberg Depression Rating Scale (Montgomery and Åsberg 1979). (Many studies require a 50% decrement for response.) Of the 586 patients completing the 6-month acute phase, 60% of the sertraline-alone, 58% of the combined treatment, and 47% of the IPT-alone patients met response criteria. Sertraline, alone or combined with IPT, was significantly more efficacious than IPT alone. At the 2-year follow-up (N=525), IPT continued to lag in outcome, but both IPT groups had lower health and social services costs than did the sertraline-alone group, making the combination of IPT and sertraline most cost-effective. Concomitant IPT also decreased the likelihood of patients discontinuing their sertraline (Browne et al. 2002).

The first of these studies was underpowered. The second was large but included no control condition and a dosage imbalance between IPT and pharmacotherapy. The two trials did not provide definitive evidence of the utility of IPT for chronic and persistent depression but suggested that its benefits may be modest (Markowitz 2003).

Interpersonal Counseling for Subsyndromal Depression

Many primary care patients report psychiatric symptoms, but their symptoms do not meet full criteria for a psychiatric disorder. Their symptoms can be debilitating and, if ignored or misdiagnosed, may result in wasted use of medical procedures (Wells et al. 1989). Interpersonal counseling is a truncated form of IPT, designed for use by medical personnel without formal psychotherapy experience to treat distressed primary care patients whose symptoms do not meet full criteria for psychiatric syndromes. Interpersonal counseling was initially a one- to six-session intervention for nurse practitioners. The first session lasts up to 30 minutes; subsequent sessions are briefer.

The interpersonal counseling therapist assesses the patient's current functioning, recent life events, occupational and familial stressors, and changes in interpersonal relationships. Such events provide the context in which emotional and bodily symptoms presumably occur. Klerman et al. (1987) randomly assigned 128 primary care clinic patients who scored 6 or higher on the Goldberg General Health Questionnaire (GHQ) to receive either interpersonal counseling or usual care. Over an average of 3 months, interpersonal counseling subjects, often after receiving only one or two sessions, showed significantly greater symptom relief on the GHQ than did control subjects, especially mood improvement. Interpersonal counseling subjects subsequently used more mental health services, implying new awareness of their psychiatric symptomatology.

Mossey et al. (1996), noting that subsyndromal depressive symptoms delayed the recovery of hospitalized elderly patients, conducted a 10-session trial of interpersonal counseling for elderly hospitalized medical patients with minor depression. Patients were seen for hour-long sessions flexibly adjusted to the patient's medical status. Seventy-six hospitalized patients older than 60 years who had depressive symptoms on two consecutive assessments but whose symptoms did not meet full criteria for MDD were randomly assigned to receive either interpersonal counseling or usual care. Researchers also monitored a euthymic, untreated geriatric control group. Patients found interpersonal counseling feasible and tolerable. After 3 months, assessments showed nonsignificantly greater improvement on all outcome variables for interpersonal counseling relative to usual care, whereas control subjects showed a slight symptomatic worsening. Rehospitalization rates were virtually identical (11%–15%) for the interpersonal counseling and euthymic control groups and significantly less than those for the cohort in usual care (50%). Differences between interpersonal counseling and usual care groups reached statistical significance at 6 months on depressive symptom reduction and self-rated health but not physical or social functioning. The investigators thought that 10 sessions was insufficient for some patients and that maintenance interpersonal counseling might have been useful. Weissman et al. (2014) summarize the interpersonal counseling literature.

In a fascinating study in an area of Uganda ravaged by poverty, HIV, and depression, Bolton et al. (2003) used a dilute version of group IPT to treat depressed women. For lack of mental health professionals, treatment was conducted by local college graduates trained in what might be considered a form of interpersonal counseling. Researchers randomized assignment to either the interpersonal intervention or usual care by village rather than by depressed individual. Despite potential cultural differences, the interpersonal counseling group had a huge benefit relative to usual care, which was apparently minimal treatment. That the treatment had benefits for the village as a whole, even for villagers who had not participated in groups, is impressive. IPT proved transportable to this very different culture presumably because of its practical, present-focused emphasis on interpersonal relationships and problems, and because there was no need to teach what would have been an alien theory of cognition or unconscious drives, for example. This study sparked the application of interpersonal counseling for populations in other low-income countries.

Other Formats

Wilfley et al. (2000) have defined group IPT as a treatment format. Swartz et al. (2004) have tested IPT in a briefer, eight-session format for MDD with promising results. Weissman (1995) has developed a handbook of IPT for patients that includes psychoeducation and worksheets. Its utility has not been formally researched.

Differential Therapeutics

If two treatments have shown efficacy in treating depression, for which patients will one treatment likely yield a better outcome than the other? Outcome studies comparing such treatments are beginning to identify factors that moderate, or predict, treatment outcome (Table 24–4). The NIMH Treatment of Depression Collaborative Research Program, which compared IPT, CBT, and imipramine, suggested such moderating factors.

TABLE 24–4. Comparison of interpersonal psychotherapy (IPT) and cognitive-behavioral therapy (CBT)

Similarities

Common factors of psychotherapy

1. Sense of feeling understood (Relationship)
2. Framework for understanding (Rationale)
3. Hope and optimism (Remoralization)
4. Psychoeducation (Recognition)
5. Technique for getting better (Ritual)
6. Success experiences (Recovering control)

Common features of brief antidepressant psychotherapies

1. Manualized
2. Active
3. Time-limited (with comparable time courses)
4. Structured (CBT>IPT)
5. Here-and-now, current focus
6. Goals of self-assertion, mastery
7. Ultimate goal of new skills for prophylaxis
8. Can be combined with antidepressant medication

Technical similarities

1. Mobilizing patient to greater activity
2. Linking mood to activities and reactions to events, albeit with different emphases
3. Problem solving: "exploring options" vs. "empirical hypothesis testing"
4. Addressing "expectations" vs. "assumptions" about others
5. Role-playing

Differences

IPT: medical model

CBT: homework

Focus on affect (IPT) vs. thoughts→affect (CBT); hence, more external vs. more intrapsychic approach

Differential therapeutics of major depressive disorder: which works better for whom?

Predictor	IPT if predictor is...	CBT if predictor is...
Life events	Present	Absent
Social dysfunction (baseline)	Low	Very high (interpersonal deficits)
Symptom severity (baseline)	Higher	Lower
Personality traits	Obsessive	Avoidant

Sotsky et al. (1991) found that Treatment of Depression Collaborative Research Program depressed patients with low baseline levels of social dysfunction responded well to IPT, whereas those with severe social deficits (probably falling into the "interpersonal deficits" problem area) responded less well. In contrast, patients with greater symptom severity and difficulty in concentrating responded poorly to CBT. Initial greater severity of MDD and of impaired functioning predicted superior response to

Outcome Studies

Meta-analyses focused on short-term psychodynamic psychotherapy (usually consisting of 16–24 weekly sessions) have confirmed the efficacy of psychodynamic psychotherapy for the treatment of depression. A meta-analysis by Driessen et al. (2010) included 23 studies totaling 1,365 subjects. Short-term psychodynamic psychotherapy was found to be significantly more effective than control conditions, and the changes from pretreatment to posttreatment were large and maintained in follow-ups 1 year later. When short-term psychodynamic therapy was compared with other psychotherapies, no significant differences were found at 3-month or 12-month follow-ups. Those treatments that focused more on the supportive end of the continuum were equally as effective as those that were more expressive and focused.

Driessen et al. (2013) more recently compared the efficacy of psychodynamic psychotherapy with that of cognitive-behavioral therapy (CBT) in a randomized controlled trial involving 341 outpatients seeking treatment for MDD, making it the largest randomized controlled trial of dynamic psychotherapy conducted to date. Each group received 16 sessions of treatment. No statistically significant treatment differences were found for any of the outcome measures. The average posttreatment remission rate was 22.7%. The key finding was that psychodynamic psychotherapy was not inferior to CBT.

Cuijpers et al. (2008) conducted seven meta-analyses involving a total of 53 studies in which seven major types of psychotherapy for mild to moderate adult depression were directly compared with one another. Each major type of treatment had been examined in at least five randomized controlled trials, and psychodynamic psychotherapy was one of the treatments considered. The investigators found no evidence that any one of the treatments was more or less efficacious than another, with the exception of interpersonal therapy (somewhat more efficacious) and nondirective supportive treatment (somewhat less efficacious). They concluded that there were no large differences in efficacy among the major psychotherapies for mild to moderate depression.

A randomized controlled pilot investigation (Gibbons et al. 2012) found that short-term dynamic psychotherapy is effective for depression in a community mental health system. Forty treatment-seeking patients with moderate-to-severe depression were randomly assigned to receive twelve weeks of psychotherapy with either a community therapist trained in brief dynamic psychotherapy or a therapist providing treatment as usual (TAU). When the results were examined, it was determined that blind judges were able to discriminate the dynamic sessions from the TAU sessions on adherence to dynamic interventions. Moreover, although this pilot study did not have adequate statistical power to assess efficacy, moderate to large effect sizes for dynamic psychotherapy over TAU were noted: 50% of patients treated with dynamic therapy moved into a normative range on depressive symptoms compared with only 29% of patients treated with TAU.

This pilot study by Gibbons and colleagues was followed by a randomized clinical noninferiority trial in 2016 that directly compared cognitive therapy with dynamic therapy for treating MDD in a community mental health setting (Gibbons et al. 2016). The trial included 237 adults. The authors concluded that when intensive expert supervision is used in community mental health settings, dynamic therapy is not inferior to cognitive therapy on change in depression for the treatment of MDD.

The empirical data from randomized controlled trials focus on the less severe cases of depression, for which dynamic therapy has been shown to be efficacious. Much less is known about moderate to severe depression. A recently published pilot study (Fonagy et al. 2020) made an effort to evaluate the efficacy of treatment with more severely disturbed depressed patients. The 147 patients in the study were randomly assigned to receive one of three treatments: CBT, a control intervention, and dynamic interpersonal therapy (DIT). Sixteen sessions of treatment were delivered over a 5-month period. DIT is a psychodynamic treatment for depression that includes mentalization-based treatment. Patients whose symptoms meet criteria for MDD of a moderate to severe nature were assessed at baseline, 3 months, and 6 months using several measures. Patients who received DIT and those who received CBT showed equivalence on most outcomes. Moreover, they did better than patients who received the control intervention. The authors concluded that DIT was effective in a primary care setting at a comparable level to CBT, and was much more effective than a control condition. Further research is needed to clarify the role of DIT.

Despite the optimism for the efficacy of short-term treatment for depression, some concern has arisen. When short-term dynamic psychotherapy of 16 sessions or so is used for depression, a significant number of depressed patients do not respond adequately within this time frame. A randomized controlled trial investigating the effectiveness of long-term psychoanalytic psychotherapy (LTPP) compared that treatment approach with TAU for individuals diagnosed with treatment-resistant depression (Rost et al. 2019). Patients were rated over an 18-month treatment period and a 2-year follow-up. As expected, depressed patients with more maladaptive dependence and self-critical features did not benefit from LTPP or TAU. Patients with less maladaptive self-critical features benefited from both LTPP and TAU, while those with more maladaptive dependent features showed considerable gains from LTPP but not from TAU, with medium to large effect sizes. The authors concluded that clinicians need to modify and tailor treatment in accordance with the individual pretreatment personality features.

In this section on outcome studies, the reader will note that there are no controlled studies of bipolar depression using psychodynamic psychotherapy techniques. Bipolar illness is biologically driven to a great extent and does not tend to respond to psychodynamic techniques. Insight is generally absent in patients who are in the midst of a manic episode. However, having clarified this issue, clinicians treating bipolar patients can carefully note the connections between specific life events and relapse as part of the ongoing monitoring. Moreover, treaters can help their bipolar patients recognize the psychic discontinuity characteristic of the illness. In other words, the version of the self that appears during a manic episode may be viewed as entirely disconnected from the self in the euthymic phase. Clinicians can work with the patient to piece together the fragments of the self such that the patient has a more continuous narrative of his or her life (Gabbard 2014).

Implementing the Psychotherapy

The first step in psychotherapy of depression is establishing a therapeutic alliance. In a recent meta-analysis involving 200 research reports and more than 14,000 treatments, Flückiger et al. (2012) found that there is a robust correlation between the therapeutic alliance and positive outcome. The link is present regardless of whether disorder-specific manuals are used and regardless of the type of psychotherapy or the specificity of outcomes. Hence the therapist needs to make an effort to forge a positive alliance as the first order of business in psychotherapy of depression. Therapists should not judge or try to cheer up the patient as others do. They also should accept the notion that there are reasons to be depressed. Unlike others in the patient's family, they do not exhort the patient to snap out of it. A dynamic therapist will collaborate with the patient on a pursuit of possible factors that have contributed. The depressed individual has already heard others saying that there is no reason for depression, and the therapist must operate from the assumption that from the patient's vantage point, there *is* something to be depressed about. Empathy and active listening are far more important than interpreting or trying to talk the patient out of the demoralizing state.

As therapists listen to their patients tell their stories, they carefully evaluate the nature of stressors that may have triggered the depression. The therapist would want to know if the stressor involved loss and humiliation or if it reawakened early childhood losses or traumas. Meaning is an essential part of the psychodynamic exploration. Whatever the stressor was, the therapist wants to know about the meaning of that stressor to the patient. Is the triggering event reminiscent of other experiences of feelings or thoughts from the past? In many ways, the key to the establishment of a therapeutic alliance is for the therapist to pursue the "person" rather than trying to eradicate the "illness." Although it may sound counterintuitive, forming a bond with the patient and consistently trying to understand what is going on, with or without concurrent medication, may be the key to helping the patient.

Another approach that may serve to build a therapeutic alliance is a frank discussion about what psychotherapy is and what it is not. Therapists may also need to explain that much of mental life is unconscious and that problematic patterns in the patient's life are likely caused by factors that are not completely within the conscious awareness of the patient. The collaborative nature of therapy should also be spelled out (Gabbard 2017). A study by Goldman et al. (2013) found that psychodynamic therapists who are more collaborative in identifying specific goals and explicitly defining the focus of the treatment, as well as providing a clear rationale for their model, may facilitate a strong therapeutic alliance.

As the therapist continues to listen to the patient's story, questions about suicide can be gently introduced. If suicidal fantasies are present, the therapist wants to know what part of the patient or the patient's life is so horrific that suicide is the only answer. As the stressors are evaluated, a psychodynamic therapist listens closely to the themes that occur around relationship patterns and the rise and fall of the patient's self-esteem. Is the patient concerned about destructiveness or greed that may have harmed loved ones? Is the patient harboring a perfectionistic view of the self that seems out of reach? Has anger been turned inward, and is the patient tormented by a harsh superego or conscience that is constantly expecting more of the patient? Have there been significant losses recently that the patient feels are irreparable? What defense mechanisms seem to be prominent in the patient's efforts to manage the painful emotional state?

As the psychotherapist understands more about the patient, she may join the patient in trying to conceive new ways of living with different aspirations, perhaps not so idealized, and more realistic goals and objectives. Therapists must be patient and avoid rushing to tell patients what their goals should be. It is usually more useful to wait for the patient to articulate his or her goals so that they are "owned" by the patient. In the long run, it is best for the patient to struggle with the complex issues he is confronting as the therapist helps to articulate to the patient particular meanings that may be attached to his suffering.

While relational issues and interpersonal meaning are almost always connected to a depression, patients often do not want to discuss those interpersonal implications. They often prefer the notion that depression and suicidal wishes arise out of nowhere rather than seeing them as having emerged from significant relational conflicts. Even though some of the factors leading to the depression may be unconscious, careful attention to transference and countertransference developments may lead to further understanding about the patient's resistance to therapy or to change.

Common countertransference dilemmas occur in the psychotherapist of the depressed patient. These may include feelings of despair and hopelessness, anger that the patient does not get better more quickly, wishes to transfer the patient to another therapist, powerful rescue fantasies, and a host of other feelings that depend on the fit between therapist and patient. An impasse may arise between patient and therapist, and it is an opportunity for both therapist and patient to constructively collaborate on figuring out what is being recreated in the transference-countertransference.

Psychodynamic therapy is sometimes referred to as *expressive-supportive psychotherapy* (Gabbard 2017). On the expressive end of the continuum are comments that may be more challenging to the patient: interpretation of unconscious meanings, observations about aspects of the patient that are not in the patient's awareness, confrontations that are designed to make the patient aware of aspects of her character that may not be in her awareness, and clarifications that involve an effort to help the patient be clearer about what she may be trying to communicate. On the supportive end of the continuum are the following interventions: empathic validation of the patient's experience and feelings, psychoeducational interventions that are designed to inform the patient about aspects of depression or of the treatment literature, and advice and praise, both of which provide support to the patient who is highly self-critical and self-doubting. In a middle position, which is neither expressive nor supportive, one would find an intervention known as *encouragement to elaborate*. This type of comment may be as simple as "Tell me more about that" or "What comes to mind about that?" The goal is to help the patient describe a situation more fully. Throughout psychodynamic therapy, the therapist must adjust the interventions to the patient's capacity to tolerate them at a particular moment in the treatment. Hence the therapist moves back and forth along the continuum based on the patient's readiness to hear and contemplate what the therapist is saying.

Concerns about suicide must be repeatedly evaluated in the course of the therapy. Patients may wish to hide such feelings from the therapist, so an atmosphere must be created by the therapist such that suicidal ideas and wishes can be spoken about frankly with the therapist, who must not respond with dismay. Patients must be encouraged to articulate what they think that suicide would accomplish and how others might be affected by it.

A psychodynamic therapist must operate within a biopsychosocial perspective. While the therapist is trying to help a patient understand what depression is and what the patient's subjective experience reflects, he or she must also be thinking about which components of the depressive illness are more biological and require medication and which aspects are amenable to psychotherapy.

Psychotherapy today does not necessarily imply that the therapist and the patient are in the same room. Online apps, video conferencing platforms, texting, email, and phone therapy have dramatically changed the therapeutic playing field. Definitive research is not yet available, but practice is far ahead of empirically derived data on efficacy. Therapists are routinely receiving text messages from their patients, and these interactions frequently lead to more extended conversations via text. Phone therapy and videoconferencing therapy are also practiced in many situations where patient and therapist cannot be together for reasons of travel, relocation, or out-of-town business—or, as in the case of the COVID-19 pandemic, public health reasons. Most psychotherapists today view online communication with patients as virtually unavoidable (Gabbard 2019). Some of it, like appointment changes, may not be unprofessional or unethical, but breaches of confidentiality are always a risk with communications that are not in-person. Clinicians must be hypervigilant about how any remote communication is conducted.

References

Agid O, Shapira B, Zislin J, et al: Environment and vulnerability to major psychiatric illness: a case control study of early parental loss in major depression, bipolar disorder and schizophrenia. Mol Psychiatry 4(2):163–172, 1999 10208448

Arieti S: Psychotherapy of severe depression. Am J Psychiatry 134(8):864–868, 1977 879347

Bibring E: The mechanism of depression, in Affective Disorders: Psychoanalytic Contributions to Their Study. Edited by Greenacre P. New York, International Universities Press, 1953, pp 3–48

Bifulco A, Brown GW, Moran P, et al: Predicting depression in women: the role of past and present vulnerability. Psychol Med 28(1):39–50, 1998 9483682

Blatt SJ: Experiences of Depression: Theoretical, Clinical and Research Perspectives. Washington, DC, American Psychological Association, 2004

Busch FN, Rudden M, Shapiro T: Psychodynamic Treatment of Depression. Washington, DC, American Psychiatric Publishing, 2004

Cuijpers P, van Straten A, Andersson G, van Oppen P: Psychotherapy for depression in adults: a meta-analysis of comparative outcome studies. J Consult Clin Psychol 76(6):909–922, 2008 19045960

Driessen E, Cuijpers P, de Maat SCM, et al: The efficacy of short-term psychodynamic psychotherapy for depression: a meta-analysis. Clin Psychol Rev 30(1):25–36, 2010 19766369

Driessen E, Van HL, Don FJ, et al: The efficacy of cognitive-behavioral therapy and psychodynamic therapy in the outpatient treatment of major depression: a randomized clinical trial. Am J Psychiatry 170(9):1041–1050, 2013 24030613

Flückiger C, Del Re AC, Wampold BE, et al: How central is the alliance in psychotherapy? A multilevel longitudinal meta-analysis. J Couns Psychol 59(1):10–17, 2012 21988681

Fonagy P, Lemma A, Target M, et al: Dynamic interpersonal therapy for moderate to severe depression: a pilot randomized controlled and feasibility trial. Psychol Med 50(6):1010–1019, 2020 31084635

Freud F: Mourning and melancholia (1917), in The Standard Edition of the Complete Psychological Works of Sigmund Freud, Vol 14. Translated and edited by Strachey J. London, Hogarth Press, 1963, pp 237–260

Gabbard GO: Psychodynamic Psychiatry in Clinical Practice, 5th Edition. Arlington, VA, American Psychiatric Publishing, 2014

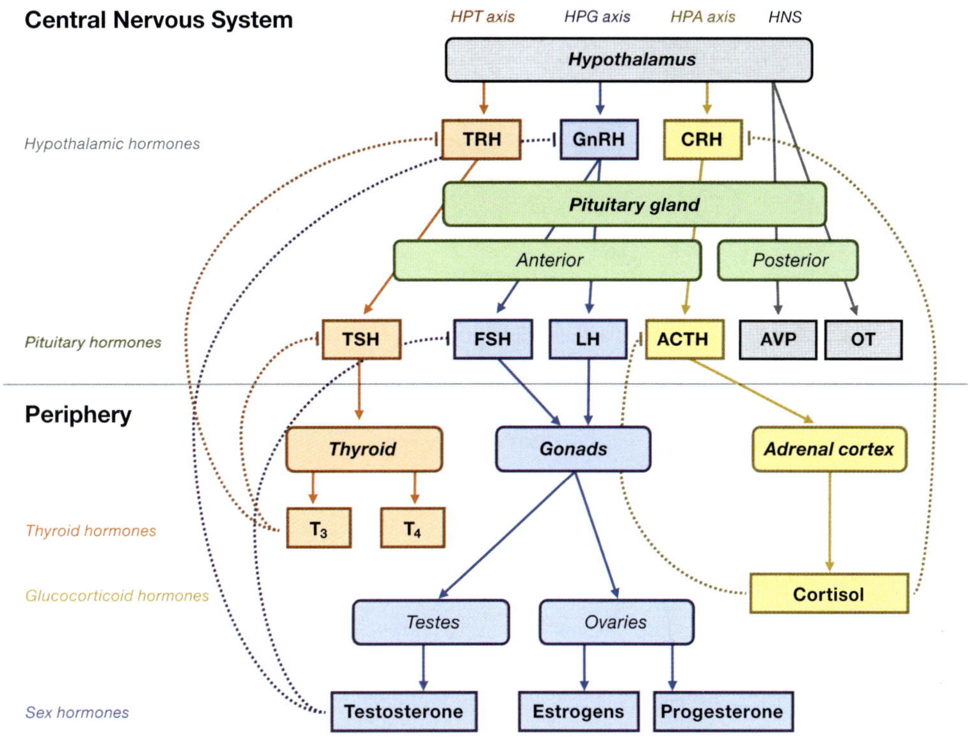

PLATE 1. Physiology of the neuroendocrine system.

Schematic representation of the four major components of the neuroendocrine system: the HPA, HPT, and HPG axes and the HNS. Hypothalamic neurons produce releasing hormones and HNS hormones. Releasing hormones act on the anterior pituitary gland, causing the release of stimulating hormones. HNS hormones are released from hypothalamic axons in the posterior pituitary, also called the neurohypophysis. The stimulating hormones produced in the pituitary gland then stimulate peripheral organs (thyroid, gonads, and adrenal cortex) to produce specific hormones, which in turn exert several biological functions (T_3, T_4; testosterone, progesterone, estrogens; and cortisol, respectively). These peripheral hormones also act backward within each axis, self-controlling their production via a negative feedback. The hypothalamic-pituitary-thyroid (HPT) axis is represented in *red*, the hypothalamic-pituitary-gonadal (HPG) axis in *blue*, the hypothalamic-pituitary-adrenal (HPA) axis in *yellow*, the hypothalamus and the hypothalamic-neurohypophysial system (HNS) in *black*, and the pituitary gland in *green*. *Arrows* indicate a stimulation, and *dotted lines* an inhibition. Hormone-producing organs are shown in *rounded boxes*, and hormonal products in *rectangles*.

ACTH=adrenocorticotropic hormone; AVP=arginine vasopressin; CRH=corticotropin-releasing hormone; FSH=follicle-stimulating hormone; GnRH=gonadotropin-releasing hormone; LH=luteinizing hormone; OT=oxytocin; T_3=triiodothyronine; T_4=thyroxine; TRH=thyrotropin-releasing hormone; TSH=thyroid-stimulating hormone.

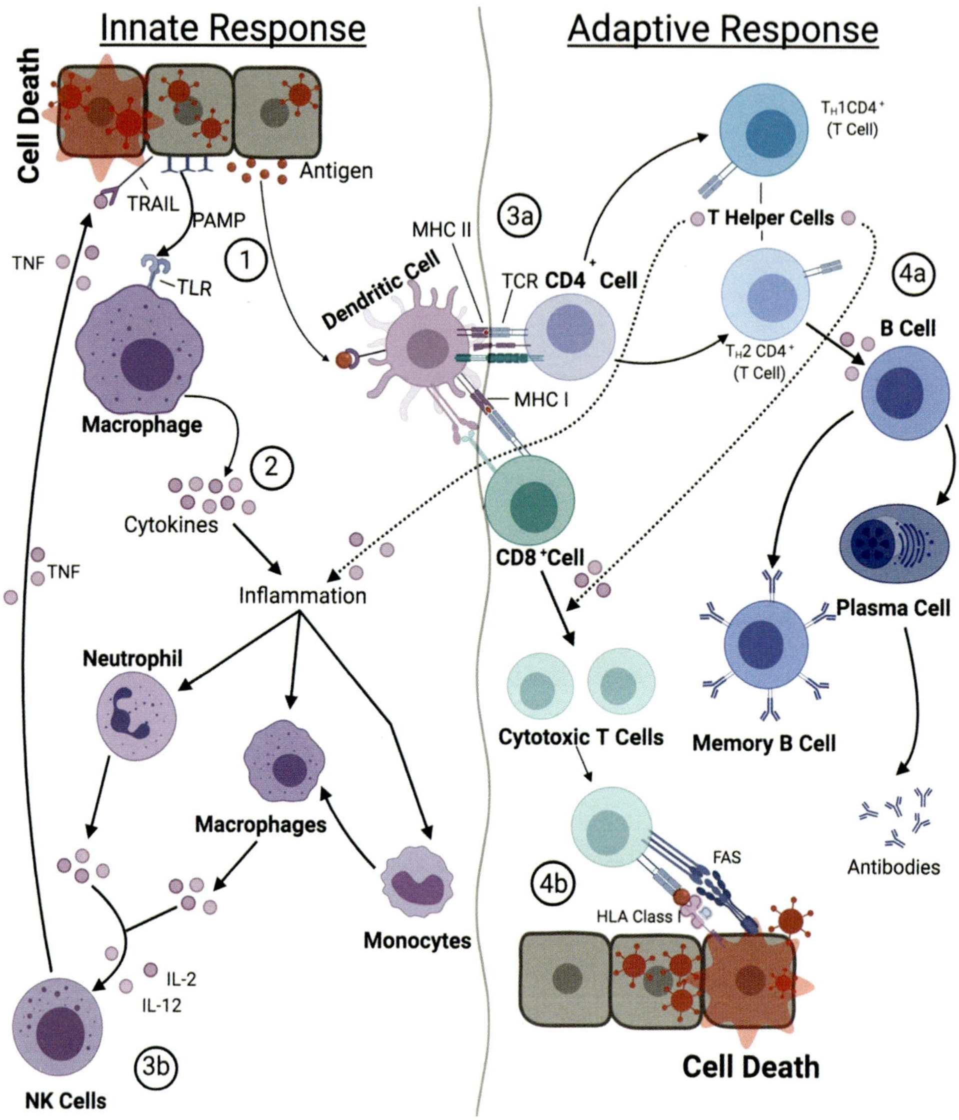

PLATE 2. Immune cells and their roles in the immune response.

(1) ***Immune recognition:*** A monocyte recognizes pathogen-associated molecular patterns (PAMPs) on an infected cell using a toll-like receptor (TLR). **(2)** ***Activation:*** Inflammatory cytokines are produced by cells at the site of infection, and this draws other innate immune cells. **(3a)** ***Antigen presentation:*** A dendritic cell presents fragments of pathogen to T cells, looking for a match. **(3b)** Meanwhile, innate immune cells such as natural killer (NK) cells and neutrophils directly and indirectly attack the infected cells, inducing apoptosis or cell death. **(4a)** B cells that can make antibodies effective against the pathogen mature into plasma cells for immediate production and memory cells to facilitate response if the same pathogen is encountered again. Mature lymphocytes will direct resolution of the response as it completes. **(4b)** Matching T cells mature into helper T cells and cytotoxic T cells that integrate the immune response and directly attack infected cells, respectively.

$CD8^+$ cell=a critical subpopulation of MHC class I restricted T cells; FAS=a type II membrane protein within the tumor necrosis family; HLA=human leukocyte antigen; IL=interleukin; MHC=major histocompatibility complex; TCR=T cell receptor; T_H1 $CD4^+$=a type of lymphocyte that helps coordinate the immune response by stimulating other immune cells; T_H2 $CD4^+$=a type of lymphocyte that helps coordinate the immune response by stimulating other immune cells; TNF=tumor necrosis factor; TRAIL=TNF-related apoptosis-inducing ligand.

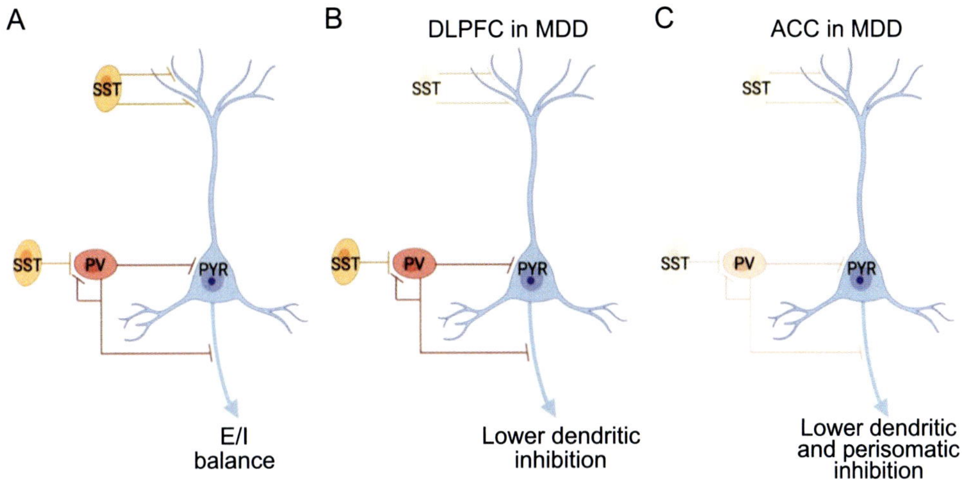

PLATE 3. Simplified diagram indicating neocortical microcircuitry and dysfunction in mood disorders.

(A) Canonical microcircuitry in unaffected comparison subjects with excitation/inhibition (E/I) balance. **(B)** In the dorsolateral prefrontal cortex (DLPFC) in subjects with major depressive disorder (MDD), lower expression of somatostatin (SST) (indicated by *lighter color*), but no change in parvalbumin (PV), was reported, suggesting lower levels of dendritic inhibition onto pyramidal cells (PYR). **(C)** In the anterior cingulate cortex (ACC) in MDD, lower levels of SST and lower PV (indicated by *lighter colors*) were reported, suggesting lower levels of dendritic and perisomatic inhibition onto pyramidal cells.
Created with BioRender.com.

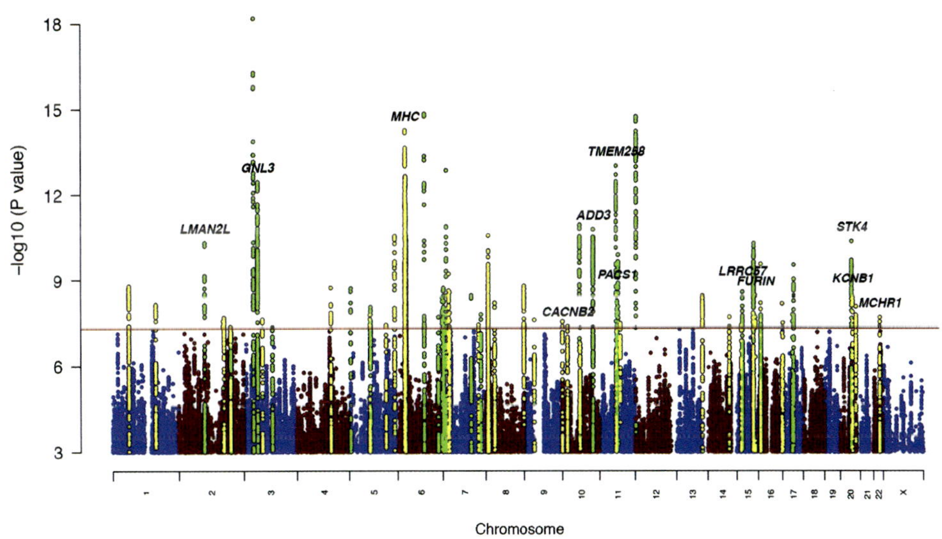

PLATE 4. Bipolar disorder genome-wide association study (GWAS) meta-analysis reveals many risk loci.

Manhattan plot for the primary GWAS meta-analysis of 41,917 bipolar disorder case subjects and 371,549 control subjects (Mullins et al. 2021). GWAS $-\log_{10}(P)$ values are plotted for all single-nucleotide polymorphisms (SNPs) across chromosomes 1–22. The *red line* shows the genome-wide significance threshold ($P<5\times10^{-8}$). SNPs in genome-wide significant loci are colored *green* for loci previously associated with bipolar disorder and *yellow* for novel associations from this study.

Source. Reprinted from Figure 1 in Mullins N, Forstner AJ, O'Connell KS, et al.: "Genome-Wide Association Study of More Than 40,000 Bipolar Disorder Cases Provides New Insights Into the Underlying Biology." *Nature Genetics* 53(6):817–829, 2021. PMCID: PMC8192451.

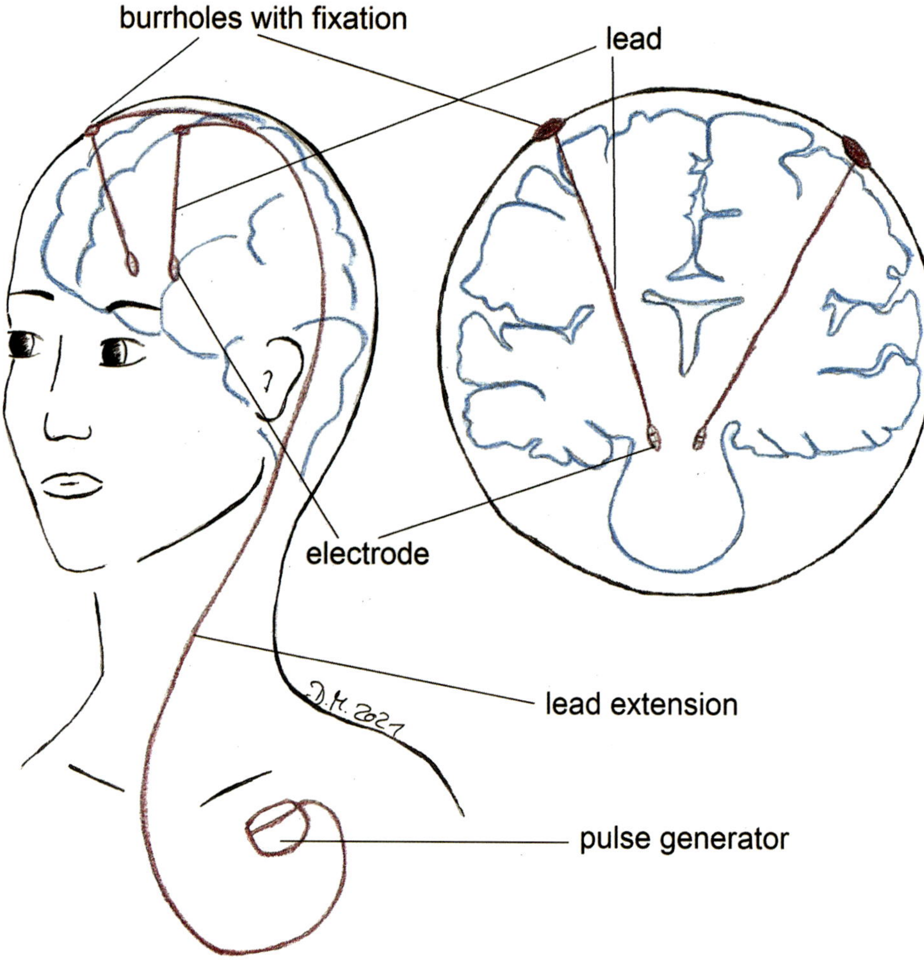

Plate 7. Schematic structure of a deep brain stimulation system.
Source. Dora Meyer, 2021.

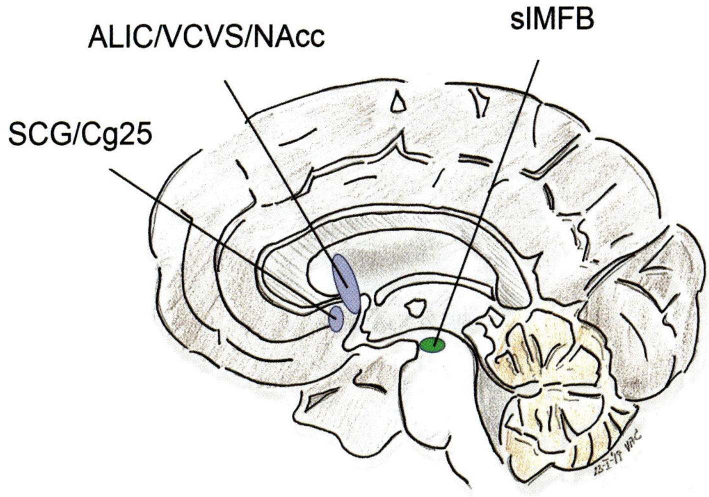

Plate 8. Experimental targets for deep brain stimulation in treatment-resistant depression.

ALIC=anterior limb of the internal capsule; CG25=Brodmann area 25; NAcc=nucleus accumbens; SCG= subgenual cingulate gyrus; slMFB=superolateral branch of the medial forebrain bundle; VCVS=ventral capsule/ventral striatum.

Source. Adapted from Figure 2 (Volker A. Coenen, 2019; p. 92) in Döbrössy M, Ramanathan C, Ashouri Vajari D, et al.: "Neuromodulation in Psychiatric Disorders: Experimental and Clinical Evidence for Reward and Motivation Network Deep Brain Stimulation: Focus on the Medial Forebrain Bundle." *European Journal of Neuroscience* 53(1):89–113, 2021. Available at: https://onlinelibrary.wiley.com/doi/10.1111/ejn.14975. Accessed October 26, 2021.

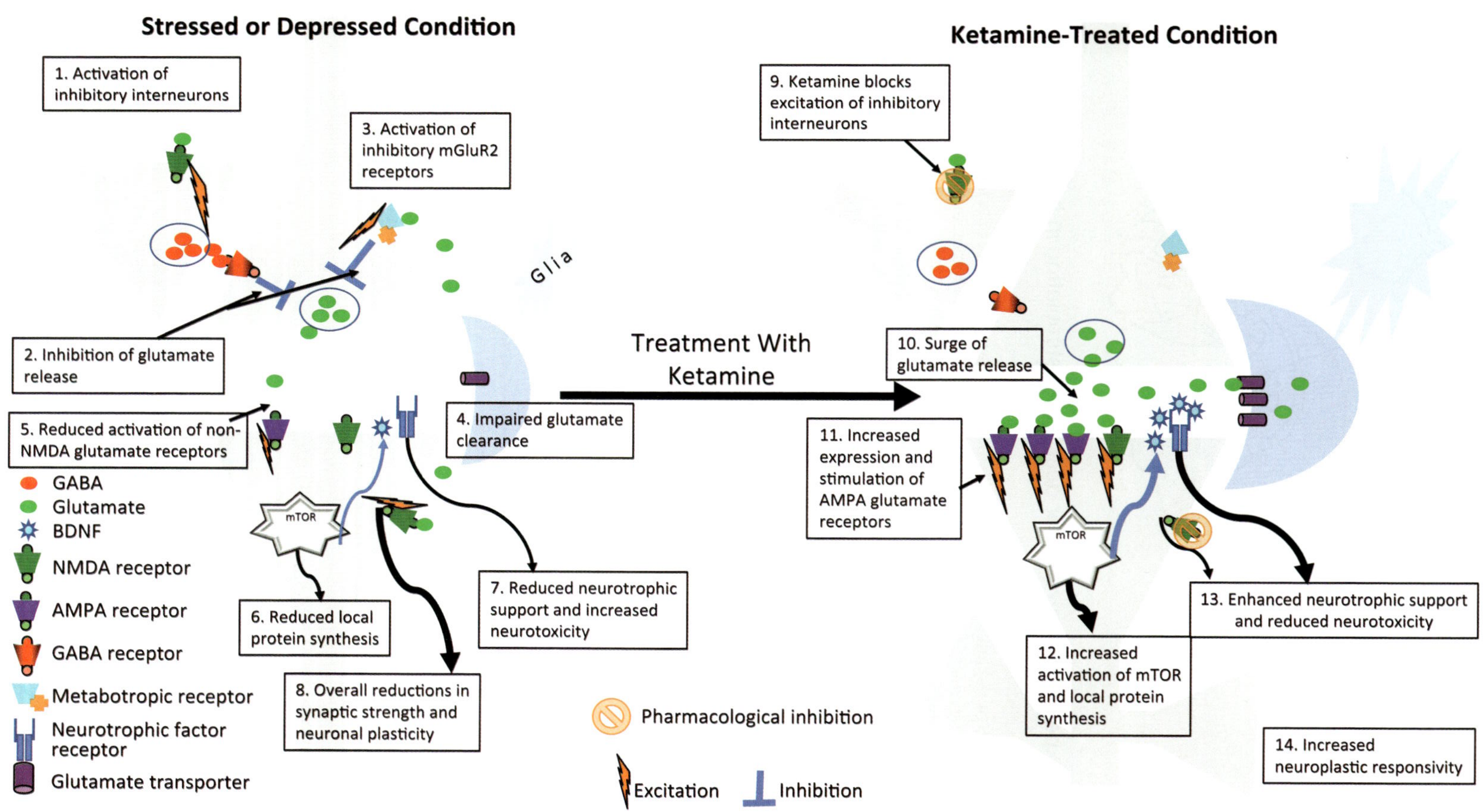
Stressed or Depressed Condition
Ketamine-Treated Condition
1. Activation of inhibitory interneurons
2. Inhibition of glutamate release
3. Activation of inhibitory mGluR2 receptors
4. Impaired glutamate clearance
5. Reduced activation of non-NMDA glutamate receptors
6. Reduced local protein synthesis
7. Reduced neurotrophic support and increased neurotoxicity
8. Overall reductions in synaptic strength and neuronal plasticity
Glia
mTOR
Treatment With Ketamine
9. Ketamine blocks excitation of inhibitory interneurons
10. Surge of glutamate release
11. Increased expression and stimulation of AMPA glutamate receptors
12. Increased activation of mTOR and local protein synthesis
13. Enhanced neurotrophic support and reduced neurotoxicity
14. Increased neuroplastic responsivity
GABA
Glutamate
BDNF
NMDA receptor
AMPA receptor
GABA receptor
Metabotropic receptor
Neurotrophic factor receptor
Glutamate transporter
Pharmacological inhibition
Excitation
Inhibition

PLATE 9. Proposed model depicting pathophysiological changes associated with mood disorders and ketamine's mechanism of antidepressant action.

Stressed or Depressed Condition (under conditions of chronic stress and possibly reflecting pathophysiology of major depressive disorder)

1. Activation of inhibitory interneurons: Under usual conditions pyramidal glutamatergic neurons are under tonic inhibition by GABAergic interneurons that are themselves activated by glutamatergic inputs. ***2. Inhibition of glutamate release:*** The tonic inhibition limits release of glutamate into the synaptic cleft. ***3. Activation of inhibitory metabotropic glutamate (mGlu) receptors:*** Group II metabotropic glutamate receptors 2 and 3 (mGluR2/3) provide a second means of inhibiting glutamate release and are believed to serve as a sensor in a negative feedback loop, detecting increased levels of extrasynaptic glutamate and dampening any additional synaptic glutamate release. ***4. Impaired glutamate clearance:*** Under usual conditions, glutamate released into the synaptic cleft is rapidly cleared by excitatory amino acid transporters (EAATs). In most brain regions, glutamate clearance is predominantly accomplished through EAAT2, which is present on astroglial cells surrounding the synapse. Under conditions of chronic stress and possibly during depressive episodes, it is believed that the ability to clear glutamate is reduced, allowing for increased levels of extrasynaptic glutamate. ***5. Reduced activation of non–N-methyl-D-aspartate (NMDA) glutamate receptors:*** Reduced levels of synaptic glutamate release, and possibly elevated levels of extrasynaptic glutamate, are believed to decrease the number and activation of postsynaptic α-amino-3-hydroxy-5-methyl-4-isoxazolepropionic acid (AMPA) receptors. ***6. Reduced local protein synthesis:*** The mechanistic (mammalian) target of rapamycin (mTOR) is a kinase that regulates local protein synthesis in dendrites in a process mediating activity-dependent synaptic strengthening. Reductions in postsynaptic activation through AMPA receptors result in lower levels of mTOR activity, decreasing rates of local protein synthesis and synaptic strength. ***7. Reduced neurotrophic support and increased neurotoxicity:*** mTOR is believed to have a complex relationship with neurotrophic factors such as brain-derived neurotrophic factor (BDNF). There appears to be a positive feedback system in which increased mTOR activity results in increased expression of BDNF, and activation of the BDNF receptor tropomyosin receptor kinase B (TrkB) increases mTOR activity. Under conditions of chronic stress and possibly in depressive episodes, it is believed that BDNF expression and release are decreased in several critical brain regions. ***8. Overall reductions in synaptic strength and neuroplasticity:*** The effects of chronic stress result in decreased neurotrophic support and greater susceptibility of synaptic maintenance to the effects of potentially neurotoxic events, such as increased stimulation of extrasynaptic NMDA receptors. Ultimately, this results in a loss of synaptic strength and adaptive neuroplasticity and leads toward impaired neurotransmission and circuit function.

Ketamine-Treated Condition

9. Ketamine blocks excitation of inhibitory interneurons: Several lines of evidence demonstrate the ability of ketamine to modulate glutamate release. One mechanism believed to mediate this effect is a selective inhibition of NMDA receptors on GABAergic interneurons. Inhibiting the inhibitory interneurons results in a release of the tonic inhibition. ***10. Surge of glutamate release:*** Whether through release of tonic inhibition or other mechanisms, there is good evidence demonstrating that a transient surge of glutamate release follows administration of subanesthetic doses of ketamine. ***11. Increased expression and stimulation of AMPA glutamate receptors:*** Increased levels of synaptic glutamate lead to activation of AMPA receptors in the postsynaptic membrane. There also appears to be an increased level of AMPA receptor expression and insertion following ketamine treatments that will likely amplify the effect. ***12. Increased activation of mTOR and local protein synthesis:*** Increased conductance through AMPA receptors stimulates intracellular messenger pathways, including that of the mTORC1 (mechanistic [mammalian] target of rapamycin complex 1) pathway, that promote translation of proteins necessary for neuronal plasticity. ***13. Enhanced neurotrophic support and reduced neurotoxicity:*** Neurotrophic factors such as BDNF are among the proteins that are increasingly expressed shortly following ketamine administration. The release of BDNF also appears to be stimulated by ketamine, and several studies suggest that this enhanced neurotrophic support is a necessary event in generating the ketamine-induced antidepressant-like effect in rodent models. Other studies suggest that blockade of extrasynaptic or specific subtypes of NMDA receptors further limits excitotoxic effects and promotes changes supporting neuronal plasticity. ***14. Increased neuroplastic responsivity:*** Combined, these actions are believed to increase synaptic plasticity, as reflected in synaptic strengthening, elevated levels of synaptogenesis, increased spine density, and ultimately changes in functional connectivity between brain regions involved in mood disorder pathophysiology.

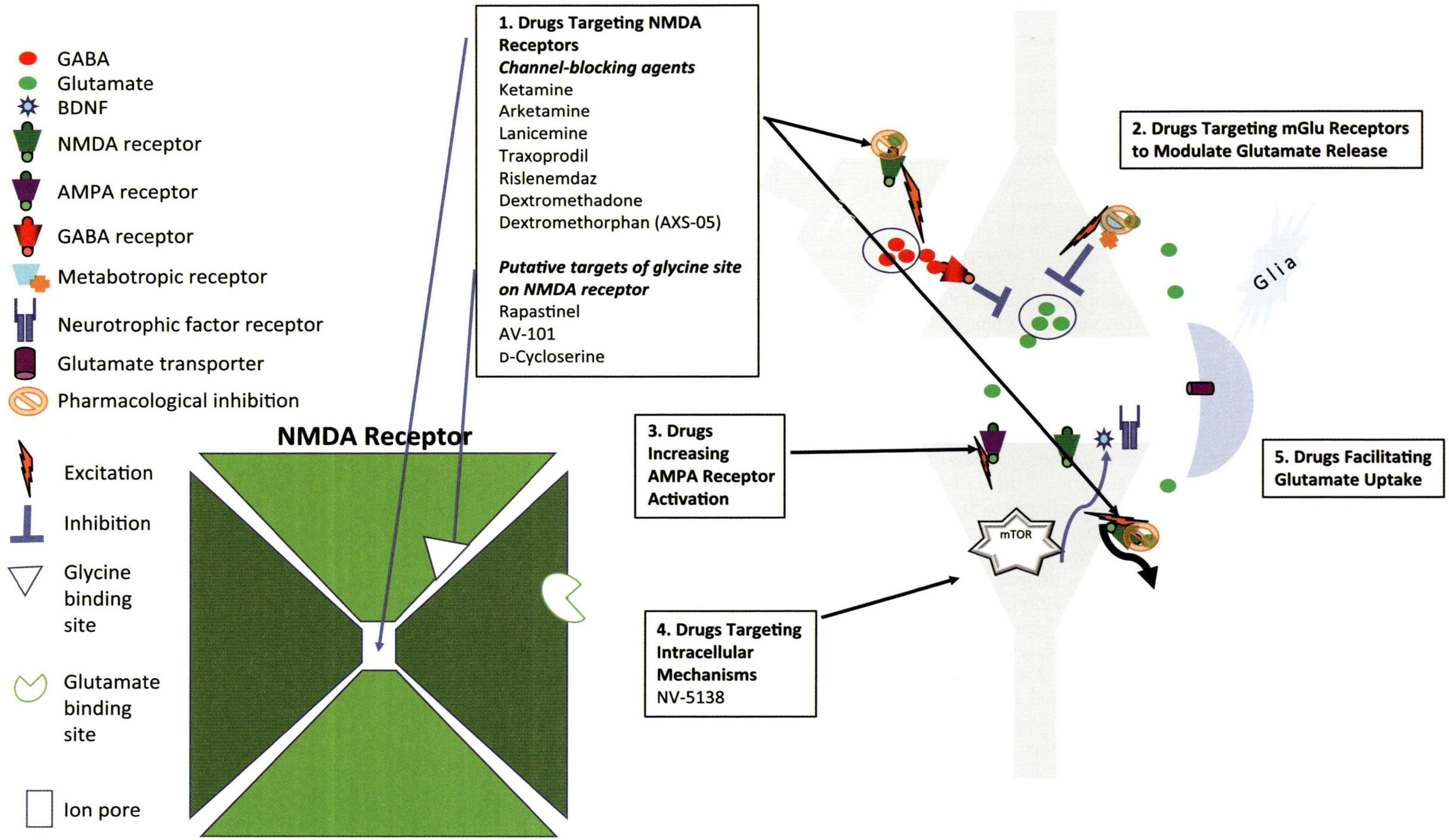

GABA
Glutamate
BDNF
NMDA receptor
AMPA receptor
GABA receptor
Metabotropic receptor
Neurotrophic factor receptor
Glutamate transporter
Pharmacological inhibition
Excitation
Inhibition
Glycine binding site
Glutamate binding site
Ion pore
NMDA Receptor
1. Drugs Targeting NMDA Receptors
Channel-blocking agents
Ketamine
Arketamine
Lanicemine
Traxoprodil
Rislenemdaz
Dextromethadone
Dextromethorphan (AXS-05)
Putative targets of glycine site on NMDA receptor
Rapastinel
AV-101
D-Cycloserine
2. Drugs Targeting mGlu Receptors to Modulate Glutamate Release
3. Drugs Increasing AMPA Receptor Activation
4. Drugs Targeting Intracellular Mechanisms
NV-5138
5. Drugs Facilitating Glutamate Uptake
Glia
mTOR

PLATE 10. Novel drugs in development related to ketamine's proposed mechanism of action.

1. Drugs targeting N-methyl-D-aspartate (NMDA) receptors: There are two major classifications of drugs currently in this category. The first class contains those drugs like ketamine that are primarily channel-blocking agents that interfere with the receptor's ion channel. These drugs can bind to selectively expressed subunits of the NMDA receptor or to sites common to all NMDA receptors. The second class contains drugs that are reported to act by modulating the binding or function of the glycine co-agonist site on the NMDA receptor. To varying degrees these drugs can indirectly modulate the ion transport through the receptor. These drugs are believed to produce their antidepressant effects by promoting enhanced presynaptic glutamate release and/or limiting neuronal toxicity. ***2. Drugs targeting metabotropic glutamate receptors 2 and 3 (mGluR2/3):*** mGluR2/3 activation serves to inhibit glutamate release and serves as a target to modulate glutamate release. On the basis of the proposed pathophysiological model presented above, arguments can be made for both inhibiting tonic glutamate release and transiently stimulating glutamate release, such as is believed to happen with ketamine treatment. Both positive and negative allosteric modulators of mGluR2/3 are being studied as treatment for mood disorders. ***3. Drugs stimulating α-amino-3-hydroxy-5-methyl-4-isoxazolepropionic acid (AMPA) receptor activation:*** These drugs can act either as more direct agonists of glutamate or as modulators of receptor function. To date there is preclinical evidence suggesting that drugs in this class possess antidepressant properties, but clinical confirmation is required. ***4. Drugs targeting intracellular mechanisms:*** Because preclinical evidence suggests that activation of the mechanistic (mammalian) target of the rapamycin complex 1 (mTORC1) pathway is critical to the mechanism of ketamine's action, there have been attempts to develop drugs that can more directly modulate the pathway downstream of the glutamatergic receptors. ***5. Drugs facilitating glutamate uptake:*** On the basis of evidence suggesting that glial cell abnormalities and impaired glutamate uptake are associated with the pathogenesis and pathophysiology of mood disorders, there have been attempts to identify and utilize drugs that can facilitate glutamate clearance in efforts to treat mood disorders. Rodent studies support this approach; however, the clinical studies for one potential agent, riluzole, have yielded inconsistent results at best. These equivocal findings may suggest that drugs that modulate glutamate uptake could have benefits prophylactically but may not be highly effective in treatment.

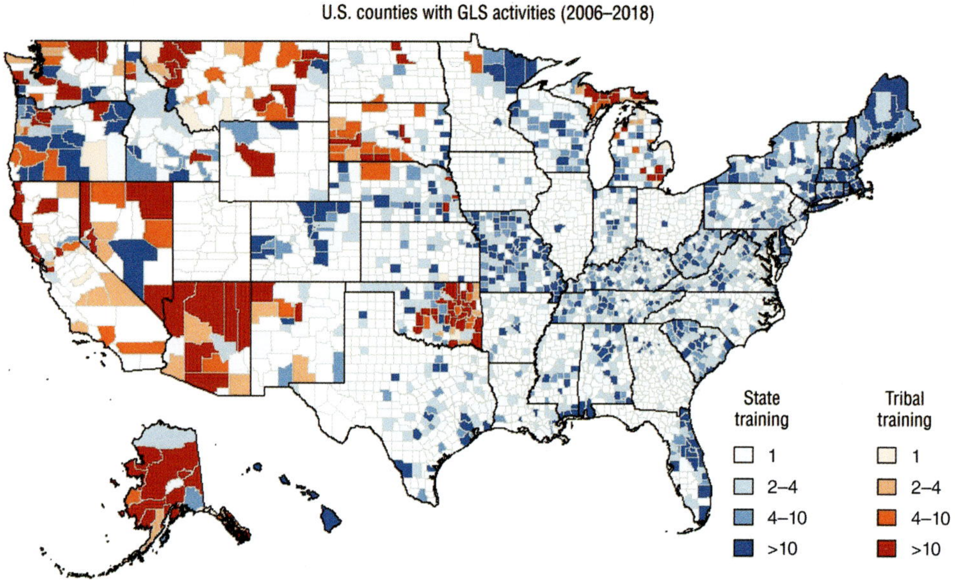

PLATE 11. **Locations and "densities" of Garrett Lee Smith Memorial Program (GLS) implementation: U.S. counties, 2006–2018.**

The GLS has been implemented in more than 1,500 U.S. counties (approximately 1,300 state and 200 tribal grantees).

Source. Reprinted from Slide 8 in Walrath C, Godoy Garraza L, Kuiper N: GLS Program Impact: The Evidence To Date. State & Tribal Plenary Presentation, March 20, 2018. Available at: https://www.sprc.org/system/files/private/event-training/STPlenary%20Christine%20Walrath-ST%20Plenary%20GLS%20ProgramImpact-March20-9am.pdf. Accessed November 30, 2020.

Gabbard GO: Long-Term Psychodynamic Psychotherapy: A Basic Text, 3rd Edition. Arlington, VA, American Psychiatric Association Publishing, 2017

Gabbard GO: Digital professionalism. Acad Psychiatry 43(3):259–263, 2019 30324397

Gibbons MBC, Thompson SM, Scott K, et al: Supportive-expressive dynamic psychotherapy in the community mental health system: a pilot effectiveness trial for the treatment of depression. Psychotherapy (Chic) 49(3):303–316, 2012 22962971

Gibbons MBC, Gallop R, Thompson D, et al: Comparative effectiveness of cognitive therapy and dynamic psychotherapy for major depressive disorder in a community mental health setting: a randomized clinical noninferiority trial. JAMA Psychiatry 73(9):904–911, 2016 27487573

Goldman RE, Hilsenroth MJ, Owen JJ, et al: Psychotherapy integration and alliance: use of cognitive-behavioral techniques within a short-term psychodynamic treatment model. Journal of Psychotherapy Integration 23:373–385, 2013. Available at: https://psycnet.apa.org/doiLanding?doi=10.1037%2Fa0034363. Accessed October 26, 2021.

Hammen CL: Stress and the course of unipolar and bipolar disorders, in Does Stress Cause Psychiatric Illness? Edited by Mazure CM. Washington, DC, American Psychiatric Press, 1995, pp 87–110

Heim C, Newport DJ, Heit S, et al: Pituitary-adrenal and autonomic responses to stress in women after sexual and physical abuse in childhood. JAMA 284(5):592–597, 2000 10918705

Jacobson E: Psychotic identification, in Depression: Comparative Studies of Normal, Neurotic, and Psychotic Conditions. Edited by Jacobson E. New York, International Universities Press, 1971, pp 242–263

Kendler KS, Kessler RC, Walters EE, et al: Stressful life events, genetic liability, and onset of an episode of major depression in women. Am J Psychiatry 152(6):833–842, 1995 7755111

Kendler KS, Karkowski LM, Prescott CA: Causal relationship between stressful life events and the onset of major depression. Am J Psychiatry 156(6):837–841, 1999 10360120

Kendler KS, Thornton LM, Prescott CA: Gender differences in the rates of exposure to stressful life events and sensitivity to their depressogenic effects. Am J Psychiatry 158(4):587–593, 2001 11282693

Kendler KS, Hettema JM, Butera F, et al: Life event dimensions of loss, humiliation, entrapment, and danger in the prediction of onsets of major depression and generalized anxiety. Arch Gen Psychiatry 60(8):789–796, 2003 12912762

Munjiza A, Kostic M, Pesic D, et al: Higher concentration of interleukin 6—A possible link between major depressive disorder and childhood abuse. Psychiatry Res 264:26–30, 2018 29626828

Nemeroff CB: The neurobiological consequences of child abuse (Distinguished Psychiatrist Lecture Series, Lecture 3). Presented at the 156th Annual Meeting of the American Psychiatric Association, San Francisco, CA, May 17–22, 2003

Rost F, Luyton P, Fearon P, et al: Personality and outcome in individuals with treatment-resistant depression—exploring differential treatment effects in the Tavistock Adult Depression Study (TADS). J Consult Clin Psychol 87(5):433–445, 2019 30998046

van Nierop M, Lecei A, Myin-Germeys I, et al: Stress reactivity links childhood trauma exposure to an admixture of depressive, anxiety, and psychosis symptoms. Psychiatry Res 260:451–457, 2018 29272730

CHAPTER 26

Psychotherapeutic Approaches to Bipolar Disorder

David J. Miklowitz, Ph.D.
Lisa A. O'Donnell, Ph.D.

Bipolar disorder is characterized by a relapse/remission course, with varying degrees of symptomatic and functional disability between episodes. Lithium, other mood stabilizers, and second-generation antipsychotics are usually recommended as first-line treatments for acute episodes of mania or depression. However, medication *alone* is often an insufficient strategy for managing the illness over the long term. Rates of recurrence are high even for individuals receiving medication (i.e., a recurrence rate of 41% at 1 year), with those younger than 18 years at greatest risk for recurrence (Gignac et al. 2015).

Increasingly, treatment guidelines for bipolar disorder are recommending a combination of medications and psychosocial treatments (Goodwin et al. 2016; Yatham et al. 2018). Adjunctive psychotherapies aim to reduce the impact of psychosocial stressors through increasing access to social supports; enhancing functioning in the areas of academic, school, and work performance; and enhancing quality of life despite limitations imposed by the illness. Consistent with many models of chronic disease management, treating bipolar disorder requires a biopsychosocial approach incorporating pharmacotherapy in the context of psychoeducation, illness management strategies, and skills training. This chapter reviews the current state of research evidence on the use of different forms of individual, group, and family therapy approaches in the treatment of bipolar disorder. Space constraints preclude a review of all existing open and randomized controlled trial (RCT) studies of each modality, but common themes observed across trials will be highlighted, along with recommendations for future research.

Individual Psychosocial Approaches

Interpersonal and Social Rhythm Therapy

Interpersonal psychotherapy (IPT) is based on the view that depression exists within the context of interpersonal stressors. These stressors typically occur in the areas of grief and loss, role transitions, interpersonal disputes, and social skills deficits. The social rhythm disruption theory proposes that among individuals with vulnerabilities to circadian disruption, life stressors that disrupt the regularity of daily and nightly routines can trigger mood episodes (Ehlers et al. 1988). Interpersonal and social rhythm therapy, or IPSRT, is a form of IPT specifically designed for individuals with bipolar disorder to assist them in regulating their sleep/wake cycles and other daily rhythms, managing interpersonal stressors, and preventing future depressive and manic episodes.

IPSRT is given in variable lengths and frequencies depending on the acute or long-term objectives of the program. The initial phases typically include assessment of the quality and number of the patient's relationships, identification of one or more interpersonal problem areas, psychoeducation about the link between daily routines and mood, and the recording of daily activities and sleep/wake cycles. The intermediate phase focuses on managing mood symptoms, regulating social and sleep/wake rhythms, and resolving key interpersonal problems. The preventive phase focuses on reinforcing regular social rhythms and working toward reducing the impact of interpersonal stressors in the future.

A 2-year clinical trial examined 175 acutely depressed, manic, or mixed-episode adults with bipolar I disorder who received pharmacotherapy and were randomly assigned to receive either IPSRT or intensive clinical management (ICM; psychoeducation, illness management strategies, general support) during an acute treatment phase (Frank et al. 2005). Then, after symptoms stabilized, patients were again randomized into a two-year maintenance phase of either IPSRT or ICM. Results found no differences between these four groups for time to remission. However, those in the acute IPSRT treatment arm had a longer time to recurrence, more time well, and better occupational functioning during the maintenance phase than those in the acute ICM condition. Moreover, the association between treatment with IPSRT and later recurrence was mediated by improvements in social rhythm stability during acute treatment.

In the only trial of psychotherapy given without concurrent medication, Swartz et al. (2018) allocated 92 acutely depressed adults with bipolar II disorder into one of two groups: IPSRT plus placebo or IPSRT plus quetiapine. In 12 weeks of treatment, the IPSRT plus quetiapine group improved faster in depression and hypomania scores compared with the IPSRT plus placebo group. Those receiving quetiapine were exposed to more severe side effects (including significantly greater weight gain) than those receiving IPSRT plus placebo. At a 5-year follow-up, both groups had similar symptom status.

In a study in New Zealand, 100 patients between the ages of 15 and 36 years (mean 26.6 years) with bipolar I disorder, bipolar II disorder, or bipolar disorder not otherwise specified (NOS) were randomly allocated to receive medication plus IPSRT or medication plus specialist supportive care (psychoeducation and supportive engagement) (Inder et al. 2015). Both treatments were administered in an average of 26–27 sessions over 18 months. The IPSRT included adaptations for adolescents with bipolar I or bipolar II disorder (Hlastala et al. 2010), such as age-relevant differences in sleep/wake cycles and areas of interpersonal conflict. The two treatment groups experienced similar reductions in depressive and manic symptoms and improvements in social functioning, with no group differences over 3 years in symptom severity or time to recurrence (Inder et al. 2017).

IPSRT was one of three psychotherapies found to hasten recovery in comparison with brief treatment in the Systematic Treatment Enhancement Program for Bipolar Disorder (STEP-BD) study (see discussion later in this chapter). Thus, the balance of evidence for IPSRT is positive, although the New Zealand study suggests that it may not outperform standard supportive care for younger patients. There are few data on moderators of response to IPSRT, such as whether patients who begin treatment with high social rhythm variability are more likely to benefit than those with minimal rhythm disruption.

Cognitive-Behavioral Therapy

Most psychotherapies referred to as "cognitive" assume that the meaning people attach to situations is the primary causal influence on their emotions and behaviors. Treatment of a recurrent mood disorder, then, involves identifying and challenging negativistic or distorted thinking and encouraging patients to consider alternative, healthier meanings to provocative situations. In extensions of cognitive-behavioral therapy (CBT) to bipolar disorder, the overly optimistic or grandiose thinking associated with hypomanic or manic episodes is addressed through cognitive restructuring, such as by encouraging patients to consider the risks as well as potential benefits of impulsive choices (Lam et al. 2003). Additionally, CBT attempts to reduce the withdrawal and avoidance associated with depression by increasing the patient's engagement with his or her environment (behavioral activation). More recent adaptations of CBT have also included exercise and healthy lifestyle management as ways of combating depressive mood states (Sylvia et al. 2019).

The average length of CBT for bipolar disorder is 20 individual sessions, including booster sessions, over a period of 6–9 months. Treatment typically starts with psychoeducation on topics such as medication adherence, stress management, and daily mood monitoring. Addressing automatic negative thoughts and core dysfunctional beliefs often makes up the body of treatment. For relapse prevention, CBT teaches patients to detect early warning signs of recurrence and implement prevention-oriented coping strategies.

Despite the large body of research supporting CBT as an effective treatment for major depressive disorder, evidence for its effectiveness in bipolar disorder is inconclusive. In the United Kingdom, Lam et al. (2003) randomly allocated 103 euthymic adults with bipolar I disorder to receive either cognitive therapy (CT) with medications and regular psychiatric follow-up or medications and psychiatric follow-up (usual care) only. Over 12 months, those receiving CT had fewer and shorter depressive episodes, fewer hospitalizations, and better social functioning than those in usual care. These results were maintained at the 30-month follow-up, although the effect on relapse reduction was significant only in the first 12 months (Lam et al. 2005).

Scott et al. (2006) conducted an RCT across five U.K. community mental health agencies, comparing pharmacotherapy alone with pharmacotherapy plus 22 sessions of individual CT over 18 months. The study (N=253) included acutely ill and remitted patients. There were no group differences in recurrence rates except for patients who had fewer than 12 lifetime episodes; these were less likely to experience a recurrence in CT plus pharmacotherapy than in pharmacotherapy alone. In turn, patients with more than 12 prior episodes were less likely to experience a recurrence in pharmacotherapy alone than in CT plus pharmacotherapy. This finding was interpreted as CT being more advantageous for individuals with a less recurrent form of bipolar disorder, or those earlier in the illness course.

Although CBT includes psychoeducation about bipolar disorder, there are group treatments that focus exclusively on psychoeducation (see section below) and do not contain all of the individual elements of CBT, such as cognitive restructuring. A large Canadian RCT with 204 adults with bipolar I or bipolar II disorder compared 20 sessions of individual CBT plus medications with 6 sessions of a brief group psychoeducation treatment plus medications. After 18 months, the brief group treatment was found to be just as effective as CBT in terms of symptom reduction and likelihood of relapse, and it could be delivered at a much lower cost (Parikh et al. 2012).

CBT contains many of the "nonspecific" features of supportive psychotherapy, such as empathy, support, and provision of illness-related information. Thus, the question arises as to whether the unique components of CBT account for its effects above and beyond its nonspecific components. In 76 euthymic adults with bipolar disorder, an RCT comparing 20 sessions of CBT with 20 sessions of supportive therapy found equivalent relapse rates over a 2-year follow-up (Meyer and Hautzinger 2012). Similar findings emerged from a pilot RCT of 32 depressed adults with bipolar I disorder that compared 18 sessions of CBT with 18 sessions of supportive therapy. Both groups showed similar improvements in depression and overall functioning, but neither group showed changes in manic symptoms (Deckersbach et al. 2018).

A U.K. study compared pharmacotherapy plus an 18-session recovery-focused CBT approach against pharmacotherapy alone in 67 euthymic adults with bipolar disorder (Jones et al. 2015). Compared with traditional CBT, recovery-focused CBT places a greater emphasis on working collaboratively with patients to address personal goals related to the disorder and its associated features. Over a 15-month follow-up, recovery-focused CBT was found to be associated with greater improvements in personal recovery and increased time to mood relapse compared with pharmacotherapy alone.

Overall, CBT appears to be an effective adjunct to pharmacotherapy for adults with bipolar disorder, although it is unclear whether it is any more effective than supportive therapy. Results from the Canadian trial indicate that group psychoeducation is a more cost-effective option. The effects of CBT appear to be more consistent for depressive symptoms than for manic symptoms.

Group Psychoeducation

Administering psychoeducation in a group format has many advantages, including reduced costs in settings where multiple patients need to learn the same set of coping skills. Patients report that groups are where they feel most understood and less stigmatized. In one of the first RCTs to examine group psychoeducation for individuals with bipolar disorder, Bauer et al. (2006) tested a "Life Goals Program" as part of a larger systematic care intervention. Patients in the trial (*N*=306) were randomly allocated to receive either "collaborative chronic care treatment" or treatment as usual (TAU). The collaborative chronic care treatment consisted of pharmacotherapy, a nurse care coordinator to help ensure medication adherence, and the Life Goals Program delivered in five weekly and then twice-monthly groups for up to 3 years. In addition to teaching relapse prevention strategies, the groups focused on the attainment of personalized life goals. Patients in the TAU condition received medication sessions and occasional psychotherapy, as per Veterans Affairs' usual care protocols. Over 3 years, patients receiving the collaborative chronic care intervention had 6.2 fewer weeks in mood episodes, as well as greater improvements in social and occupational functioning and quality of life, than patients receiving TAU. Contrary to the results for CBT, the effects were primarily on length of manic episodes; there were no differences between the conditions in the length of depressive episodes.

These results were largely replicated in a separate trial administered by the Group Health Cooperative organization of Washington State. Simon et al. (2006) randomly assigned 441 patients to a 2-year collaborative chronic care program or TAU (medication management visits). The probability of a new manic episode was significantly lower in the collaborative care group over 2 years, and these patients spent fewer weeks in manic episodes. There were no effects of collaborative care on depression severity or depressive recurrences.

The Barcelona trial, an influential study of group psychoeducation, compared 21 sessions of structured group psychoeducation with 21 sessions of unstructured supportive group therapy (standard care). Group psychoeducation according to the Barcelona model involves 90-minute patient groups run by two clinicians experienced in treating bipolar disorder (Colom et al. 2009). The goals are to educate the patients on the nature, causes, and treatment of bipolar disorder; the importance of monitoring one's moods; medication adherence; detection of prodromal symptoms of recurrence; and healthy lifestyle choices regarding sleep, diet, and substance use. The sessions usually include a 30- to 40-minute didactic presentation on one topic followed by an exercise and group discussion related to the topic.

All patients in the Barcelona trial (*N*=120) received standard pharmacotherapy, and all were in symptomatic remission at entry (Colom et al. 2003). Compared with those receiving standard care, those receiving group psychoeducation experienced fewer relapses and recurrences; increased time to relapse for depressed, hypomanic, manic, and mixed episodes; and lower rates of hospitalization. These findings were maintained for 5 years following the end of treatment (Colom et al. 2009). This study is important in suggesting not only that psychoeducation is effective in a group format but also that belonging to a group is not by itself sufficient; group treatment needs to be structured and oriented toward strategies for managing the illness.

A smaller 12-month RCT conducted in Brazil compared 16 sessions of the Barcelona group's psychoeducation program with 16 sessions of support and relaxation training for remitted bipolar I or bipolar II disorder patients (de Barros Pellegrinelli et al. 2013). Patients in the two groups did not differ in reductions in mood symptoms or improvements in psychosocial functioning over 12 months. Most of the patients had highly chronic depression (i.e., 10 or more episodes), suggesting that group treatment may be less effective among more chronic patients. Other differences from the Barcelona trial, such as the shorter treatment protocol (16 vs. 20 sessions) and the smaller sample size ($N=55$) and shorter follow-up, may have also affected these results.

In a study in Denmark, Kessing et al. (2014) randomly assigned 158 patients who had recently been discharged from the hospital with bipolar disorder (often only a single episode of mania) to either a 2-year intervention program at a specialized outpatient mood disorders clinic or standard psychiatric treatment in a different clinic. Patients in the specialty clinic began with acute treatment of depressive or manic symptoms involving three group psychoeducation sessions plus regular pharmacotherapy sessions for 6 months. Pharmacotherapy was delivered by trained physicians who followed international practice guidelines. When patients were fully or partially recovered from their index episode, they transitioned to maintenance group therapy consisting of 12 weekly group sessions, 3 booster sessions, and a 3- to 6-month discharge group focused on preparation for transfer to a community practitioner. Patients in the standard outpatient clinic condition received treatment in a local community mental health center or from a local psychiatrist or general practitioner, with pharmacological treatment based on the preferences of the physician rather than on treatment guidelines. These patients were not generally offered individual or group psychoeducation. All patients were followed for up to 6 years after discharge (average follow-up of 2.5 years).

The rates of rehospitalization among younger patients (ages 18–25; $n=29$) in the specialty service were lower than rates among patients in the standard treatment group, but these differences did not reach significance in the older patients ($n=129$), who composed the majority of the sample. Interestingly, the patients in the specialty service were more likely to be treated with (and were more adherent with) mood stabilizers and antipsychotics than patients in the standard care clinics, particularly those in the 18- to 25-year age group. Although many of the primary results did not reach conventional levels of significance, comparisons of effect sizes indicated that the more intensive specialty outpatient services, which focused on psychoeducation and evidence-based pharmacotherapy, were more effective in younger than in older patients.

Group psychoeducation appears to be a cost-effective approach for the long-term maintenance of bipolar disorder in euthymic adults. Further research is needed to determine whether younger patients who are early in the course of their disorder are better candidates for psychoeducation or CBT than older and more chronic and recurrent patients. The extent to which the effects of group psychoeducation are mediated by improved medication adherence is also worthy of investigation.

Family Interventions

In the late 1980s, evidence emerged that family attributes such as high expressed emotion (EE) in caregivers (i.e., high levels of criticism, hostility, or emotional overinvolvement) and negative interactional behaviors between patients and their parents/caregivers were associated with a more recurrent course of bipolar illness and poorer social functioning (Miklowitz et al. 1988; Priebe et al. 1989). High levels of EE have many causes among caregivers, but one appears to be their understanding of the illness: parents and spouses who are rated high in EE tend to attribute negative behaviors by the patient to internal and controllable causes (e.g., willfulness, personal choice), whereas parents and spouses rated low in EE are more likely to attribute these behaviors to less controllable factors, such as the presence of an illness (Hooley and Miklowitz 2018; Wendel et al. 2000).

Family-focused therapy (FFT) was developed to address family risk factors such as high EE (Miklowitz 2010). The objectives of FFT are to reduce family stress by 1) increasing family members' understanding of the illness, including how to recognize early warning signs of new episodes and how to intervene to help prevent relapse (psychoeducation); 2) enhancing constructive caregiver/patient communication through rehearsing skills such as active listening, making requests for changes in another person's behavior, and balancing positive and negative feedback (communication training); and 3) improving family problem-solving skills (identifying and defining problems, generating and evaluating solutions, implementing solutions) to enhance family and community functioning.

FFT is administered in the stabilization period following an acute manic or depressive episode. during which the focus is on assisting patients in returning to their preillness level of functioning. Typically, therapists meet with individual families (patient, parents or spouse, siblings) in weekly and then biweekly sessions that can extend to 6 or 9 months. Longer protocols (i.e., 21 sessions over 9 months) are recommended for patients who have fully syndromal manic and depressive episodes, whereas shorter protocols (12 sessions over 4 months) are recommended for children or adolescents in high-risk states (i.e., those with major depressive disorder or subthreshold forms of bipolar disorder who have a family history of bipolar I or bipolar II disorder).

As reviewed by Miklowitz and Chung (2016), there have been five randomized trials of FFT in adults with bipolar I or bipolar II disorder, two in adolescents with bipolar I or bipolar II disorder, and two in high-risk children or adolescents. In the various RCTs, FFT was combined with pharmacotherapy and compared with brief psychoeducation, individual supportive therapy, or other evidence-based psychosocial treatments, also combined with pharmacotherapy. In two trials, FFT was compared with comparably intensive individual therapies (see discussion of STEP-BD study later in this chapter). Across studies, FFT was associated with lower recurrence rates, greater reductions in depression and mania severity scores, and better psychosocial functioning over periods of 1–2 years compared with brief psychoeducational therapy.

There are several mechanisms by which family psychoeducation and skills training may lead to better outcomes of bipolar disorder. When families receive education about bipolar disorder, they are in a better position to recognize when the patient is developing prodromal symptoms of new episodes, and more likely to contact physicians and follow prevention plans focused on stress reduction. Trials that have examined family communication as a mechanism of action have concluded that FFT is associated with increases in positive/constructive communication in both caregivers and patients and decreases in family conflict (O'Brien et al. 2014; Simoneau et al. 1999; Sullivan et al. 2012).

Overall, RCTs have supported the use of FFT plus pharmacotherapy in the outpatient treatment of adults with bipolar disorder (Yatham et al. 2018). FFT may be particularly effective for the reduction and stabilization of depressive symptoms among patients, with some of the trials finding stronger effects of FFT in patients with high-

EE relatives than in patients with low-EE relatives (e.g., Miklowitz et al. 2009). One limitation to family therapy is the fact that engaging entire families can be a challenge, particularly when the patient has been struggling with the disorder for many years. Clinicians may find it challenging to get family members to understand the importance of their role in the success of treatment.

Case Example

Stefan was a 15-year-old boy diagnosed with bipolar I disorder, ADHD, and an expressive language disorder. He began FFT with his mother, Judy, following a bipolar, mixed episode that had led to his dismissal from a private school. At the beginning of family sessions, he was not attending school; he was taking one online course and met once weekly with a speech coach. Judy had quit her full-time job, and the two were home together most of every day. They both complained about excessive conflict in their relationship.

In initial psychoeducation sessions, Judy wondered aloud whether Stefan really had bipolar disorder. She expressed her doubts about whether his medications (aripiprazole and valproate), administered by a local psychiatrist, were helping or were even appropriate. Stefan, who had trouble attending to the content of sessions, was able to describe the initial phases of his manic escalation in the most basic of terms (e.g., "I got mad, I couldn't sleep"). His mother referred to his recent mixed symptoms as "behavior problems." Much of the content of psychoeducation revolved around whether they could agree on what aspects of Stefan's behavior were likely to be part of bipolar illness and what behaviors were within his control. The clinician helped clarify what a mixed episode was, how mood episodes differed from ordinary teen behavior, and what role medications and effective family communication might have in relapse prevention.

Judy began to consider the possibility that his anger and irritability were part of a manic syndrome. Stefan expressed some relief that his conflicts with his mother and his peers might have a biological as well as a psychological explanation. They discussed environmental triggers for his daily mood swings (e.g., being denied access to his phone), how these swings were different from his full manic or mixed episodes, and how Stefan and Judy might interrupt the sequence of events that precipitated or followed these mood changes and led to further family conflict.

The treatment "took off" at the introduction of communication skills training. The duo avidly participated in role-plays designed to increase their use of positive interpersonal feedback, active listening, and making positive requests for change in each other's behavior. Judy found the latter especially helpful; she noted that after a major conflict, Stefan would want her to hug him and tell him that everything would be all right, but she felt too alienated to do so. She was able to ask him to choose another means of self-soothing or to at least give her time to cool down before he asked her for comfort. In turn, Stefan expressed frustration that she would only listen to him for a few minutes and then would begin criticizing him, no matter what the topic. The clinician instructed him to express this frustration in a constructive way by tying it to ways she might be more patient with him. In turn, Judy learned to rephrase her criticisms as positive requests for change (e.g., "I'd appreciate your talking to me in a more respectful tone of voice"). With repeated practicing of these communication skills in the sessions and at home, they both reported reductions in their level of family conflict and a greater feeling of collaboration.

Toward the end of treatment, the focus shifted to Stefan's schooling. He expressed fear of telling others at school what had happened to him and avoided going as a result. The clinician normalized these fears, explaining that the experience of social stigma is common among people after a psychiatric illness episode. During problem solving, the pair discussed various options regarding whom Stefan should tell (e.g., friends, teachers, school health staff) about his bipolar disorder and what details he should give them. They role-played specific conversations he might have with friends. With the clinician's coaching, Stefan decided that he did not need to tell everyone that he had bipolar disorder or that he took antipsychotics, preferring to say he took "attention pills" and "mood medicines."

Upon discharge from FFT, Stefan's mood symptoms had largely stabilized, and he had enrolled in a new school. He reported some residual depression but was able to accomplish daily tasks with greater effort. His mother returned to her job at half-time. Stefan and Judy were regularly implementing the communication and problem-solving skills at home and reported that their original goal of reducing their level of conflict had been largely achieved. Both also felt they had benefited from understanding bipolar disorder as an illness that could affect one's relationships. Although Judy expressed a preference that Stefan continue with his medication regimen "for now," she continued to wonder whether he could get along without it. For follow-up care, Stefan was referred to his psychiatrist for further discussions of medication options and to a community mental health center for individual therapy. Judy was referred to a mindfulness-based cognitive therapy group for parents of teens with mood disorders.

Cognitive and Functional Remediation

Cognitive impairments have been found in 42%–64% of those with bipolar disorder, especially in the areas of executive functioning, memory, attention, and verbal learning (Reichenberg et al. 2009). Remediating cognitive deficits may be associated with improvements in social and occupational functioning and quality of life. Functional remediation (FR) consists of 21 weekly individual and group sessions providing psychoeducation and cognitive skills training (attention, memory, executive functioning) in daily life situations, plus communication, interpersonal effectiveness, and stress management training (Martínez-Arán et al. 2011). A 10-site RCT in Spain compared FR with psychoeducation (also 21 sessions) and TAU in 239 euthymic adults with bipolar I or bipolar II disorder. Patients with bipolar disorder who received FR showed greater improvements in social and occupational functioning than those in TAU, but no differences were detected between FR and psychoeducation alone (Torrent et al. 2013). At a 1-year follow-up, functional improvements persisted only for the FR group (Bonnin et al. 2016).

Computer-based cognitive remediation has also been evaluated. In a trial of 84 adults with bipolar disorder, patients were randomly allocated to a computer-based cognitive remediation treatment or a computer-based control condition, both consisting of three sessions per week for 24 weeks (Lewandowski et al. 2017). The computer-based cognitive remediation was associated with significantly greater improvements in cognitive domains (e.g., processing speed, visual learning, memory) over 12 months. Improvements in community functioning, however, occurred in both groups. Thus, both cognitive and functional remediation may reduce cognitive deficits for adults with bipolar disorder, but their unique role in improving psychosocial functioning is unclear.

The Systematic Treatment Enhancement Program

Few studies have addressed a key question in this literature: what treatment works best for whom? The Systematic Treatment Enhancement Program study, a 2-year multisite randomized clinical trial, compared three psychotherapies for bipolar disorder (FFT, IPSRT, or CBT), given in up to 30 sessions over 9 months, with three weekly sessions of individual psychoeducation guided by a self-care manual. Patients were 293 acutely depressed outpatients with bipolar I or bipolar II disorder who were treated by study psychiatrists with standardized pharmacotherapy algorithms. The study found that patients receiving intensive psychotherapy and medications had better outcomes than those in collaborative care across a range of measures (Miklowitz et al. 2007a, 2007b). Over 1 year, patients in the intensive therapy condition were more likely to recover from depression (64%) and recovered more rapidly (mean=169 days) than patients in collaborative care (52% and 279 days, respectively). One-year rates of recovery for the three intensive therapies, which did not statistically differ, were 77% for FFT, 65% for IPSRT, and 60% for CBT. Patients receiving the intensive therapies were also more likely to remain well in any given month of the 12-month study than patients in collaborative care, and had better overall psychosocial functioning, relationship functioning, and life satisfaction (Miklowitz et al. 2007a). Thus, the STEP-BD program validated earlier research indicating that intensive psychosocial treatments are more effective than brief psychoeducation for stabilization of depressive symptoms, although it did not clarify whether one of the treatments was more effective than the others.

Subsequent analyses of the STEP-BD data suggest the presence of moderating variables on these treatment outcomes. Notably, patients with comorbid anxiety disorders showed greater benefits from intensive therapy versus brief psychoeducation in rates of recovery from depression compared with patients without anxiety disorders, suggesting that comorbidity may be a selection factor determining who should receive intensive therapy in community care (Deckersbach et al. 2014).

Application of Psychosocial Treatments to Early-Onset and High-Risk Patients

Psychosocial interventions have been evaluated in patients who develop the full bipolar disorder syndrome before age 18 years. Childhood onset is a reliable predictor of a more pernicious course of bipolar disorder in adulthood (e.g., Perlis et al. 2009; Post et al. 2010). Two trials have compared FFT with brief psychoeducation in adolescents with bipolar I or bipolar II disorder; one of the trials showed an impact on the trajectory of depressive symptoms (Miklowitz et al. 2008), and the other showed an impact on manic symptoms (Miklowitz et al. 2014). The latter trial did not detect differences between FFT and brief psychoeducation on time to recovery or time to recurrence. However, patients in FFT reported higher quality-of-life scores over 2 years than patients in brief psychoeducation (O'Donnell et al. 2017).

For younger bipolar patients, psychoeducation given in an eight-session multifamily group format has been shown to improve the trajectory of mood symptoms among bipolar spectrum youth (ages 8–12) with bipolar I or II disorder or a bipolar disorder NOS diagnosis (Fristad et al. 2009). An 18-session protocol of individual CBT and FFT (known as the "Rainbow" program; West et al. 2014) consisted of alternating child-only, parent-only, and family sessions. Children in the Rainbow program showed greater improvement in parent-reported mania scores, lower parent-reported depression scores, and a steeper response curve for depressive symptoms at posttreatment and 6-month follow-up compared with an active, dose-matched individual psychotherapy control condition (West et al. 2014).

There has been increasing interest in the role of early psychosocial intervention for youth who are genetically at risk for bipolar disorder and show early signs of mood disturbance. The long-term goal of research studies is to determine whether early intervention can prevent or delay the onset of the full bipolar syndrome. In a 1-year RCT, 40 youth (ages 9–17) with major depressive disorder or unspecified bipolar disorder, all of whom had a first-degree relative with bipolar I or bipolar II disorder, were randomly allocated into one of two treatment groups: 12 sessions of FFT–high-risk (HR) version over 4 months, or 1–2 sessions of a brief psychoeducational control treatment. Compared with the control group, youth in FFT-HR experienced more rapid recovery from their initial mood symptoms, more weeks in remission, and greater improvement in hypomanic symptoms over 12 months (Miklowitz et al. 2013).

In a second, larger trial (N=127) of FFT-HR for high-risk youth—those with major depressive disorder or unspecified bipolar disorder and a familial history of bipolar disorder—family intervention was associated with a longer time to prospectively observed mood episodes (the majority of depressive polarity) than was seen with a 4-month psychoeducational comparison treatment. FFT-HR was not associated with a lower rate of conversion to bipolar I or II disorder, although the mean duration of follow-up (2 years) was not long enough to observe many conversions (Miklowitz et al. 2019).

In a 6-month pilot trial, Goldstein et al. (2018) randomly assigned 42 high-risk adolescents to receive eight sessions of IPSRT plus referrals to community care, or referrals alone. The adolescents had parents diagnosed with bipolar I or bipolar II disorder but, unlike the participants in the FFT high-risk trial, had not developed mood disorders themselves. None of the youth in either treatment group had had a mood episode (mania, hypomania, depression) by the 6-month follow-up, nor were there group differences in subthreshold depressive symptoms. Three adolescents developed subthreshold hypomanic or manic symptoms at follow-up, two in the referral-only arm and one in the IPSRT-plus-referral arm. Actigraphy data revealed that at baseline, the IPSRT group had more time awake after sleep onset compared with the referral-only group but had less time awake 6 months later. Thus, early intervention with IPSRT may have altered a key risk factor for mood episodes (sleep disturbance), but its effects on early symptoms were less clear.

Summary of Findings

The evidence reviewed in this chapter supports the use of bipolar-specific psychotherapies as adjuncts to pharmacotherapy in the stabilization and maintenance phases of bipolar disorder. Evidence is strongest for the long-term maintenance of bipolar disorder, including relapse prevention and restoring functioning for youth and adults. FFT and group psychoeducation have the strongest support and may be suitable for different phases of the illness: FFT for patients who are recovering from an episode of illness and group psychoeducation for patients in remission. No comparisons of group psychoeducation and family therapy have been undertaken, but this would be a potentially informative area for research.

The studies of CBT and IPSRT are less conclusive. However, there have been more trials of CBT across a broader array of settings than for other forms of psychotherapy. CBT,

FFT, and IPSRT were all more effective than brief psychoeducation in the STEP-BD study, although the trial was too underpowered to show differences between the treatments. A newer approach to adolescent bipolar disorder based on dialectical behavior therapy (DBT), which includes family and individual skills training components, has shown promise in a preliminary RCT (N=20). Adolescents who received DBT showed greater reductions in depression—and especially in suicidal ideation—over 1 year compared with a group that received supportive care (Goldstein et al. 2015).

Limitations Across Studies

Certain limitations of the extant literature must be emphasized. First, for ethical reasons, most RCTs examining psychotherapy also allow pharmacotherapy for patients in all treatment conditions, making it challenging to determine if improvements attributed to psychotherapy are due to different pharmacotherapy regimens (Yatham et al. 2018). Second, there is substantial heterogeneity in terms of the populations sampled (i.e., patients with bipolar I or bipolar II disorder vs. those with unspecified bipolar disorder, or patients in remission vs. those in episode), the number of therapy sessions (ranging from 6 to 30), length of follow-up periods (6 months to 5 years), and outcome measures (e.g., remission or relapse rates, symptom trajectories, hospitalizations, functional outcomes [Geddes and Miklowitz 2013; Yatham et al. 2018]). Thus, it is unclear whether certain approaches are more effective than others, whether certain subpopulations are less tractable, or whether the treatments are being compared on the same outcome domains. Third, in the majority of trials, notably several using FFT, the experimental treatment groups received a greater number of sessions than the control condition groups, raising the question of whether treatment gains can be attributed to amount rather than type of therapeutic contact.

Meta-analyses of the psychotherapy literature, especially those that take into account differences in treatment components, may be able to address some of these questions (Miklowitz et al. 2017). A recent meta-analysis of 39 randomized psychotherapy trials in bipolar disorder concluded that psychoeducation and skills training given in a family or a group format were more effective in preventing illness recurrences than psychoeducation and skills training given in an individual format (Miklowitz et al. 2021).

Future Directions

Identifying Active Ingredients

Few studies have examined the active ingredients of successful psychosocial treatment in bipolar disorder. Psychoeducation, which is common to all bipolar disorder psychotherapies, is consistently more effective than standard care without psychoeducation. Virtually all of the protocols involve some form of mood monitoring, relapse prevention planning, problem-solving regarding social and occupational reengagement, medication adherence monitoring, stress management, and intervening with substance use (Murray et al. 2017). The literature has not made clear how long psychoeducation needs to be in order to be effective, or whether effects differ as a function of delivery format (individuals, groups, or families).

There are other therapeutic ingredients that may explain the efficacy of some interventions over others. Involvement of the family in psychoeducation and skills training, stabilization of sleep/wake cycles, cognitive restructuring, and behavioral activation may have therapeutic benefits at different phases of the illness. For example, stabilizing sleep/wake cycles may play a greater role in mania stabilization, whereas behavioral activation may be more effective in alleviating depression. Clarification of the effective components of treatment at different stages or polarities of the illness may lead to the development of more effective forms of therapy.

Regarding treatment format, internet-based programs and phone apps are being increasingly used to remediate gaps in treatment access in many mental health populations. Patients with bipolar disorder are relatively adherent to web- or text-message-based tracking of mood states, whether given as a self-monitoring component of pharmacotherapy or as part of individual psychoeducation (Bilderbeck et al. 2016; Miklowitz et al. 2012). Preliminary evidence suggests that smartphone psychoeducation is well accepted among patients and can be delivered with good adherence to psychotherapeutic principles (e.g., Hidalgo-Mazzei et al. 2015; Leitan et al. 2015).

Mediation and Moderation

Treatment mediation—the ways in which psychotherapies work in bringing about clinical change—has received relatively little attention in the bipolar literature. Mediators are treatment targets that when modified help explain the statistical association between treatment and improved clinical outcomes. There are several candidates for mediators of psychosocial treatments for bipolar disorder: improvements in family interactions (for FFT), improved sleep/wake cycle regularity (IPSRT), and increased knowledge of coping strategies (psychoeducation). As an example of the latter, an Oxford University trial with 121 bipolar outpatients compared a five-session facilitator-guided psychoeducational therapy combined with electronic mood monitoring against an educational self-help guide with electronic mood monitoring (Bilderbeck et al. 2016). Although there were no between-group differences in self-rated depressive symptoms or relapse/readmission rates, the individual psychoeducation was associated with greater increases in knowledge about bipolar disorder from pre- to posttreatment (3 months) compared with the comparison condition. Further, increases in knowledge at 3 months were associated with more weeks in remission over the remainder of the study year. Identifying mediators of clinical improvement is an important direction for the next generation of psychosocial treatment studies, because there may be ways of modifying these mediators that will make treatment more effective and less costly.

We also know relatively little about whether various forms of psychotherapy are more versus less effective in illness subgroups (moderation). The current literature has yet to identify best-practice treatments for those with more severe forms of bipolar disorder—for example, patients with treatment-resistant depression who have active suicidal behaviors or self-harm, or patients with substance abuse, rapid cycling, or comorbidity with personality disorders or other major psychiatric disorders (e.g., ADHD). There has been some attention to the stage of illness as informing choice of treatments. It may be that therapies most applicable in the disorder's earliest stages (e.g., group psychoeducation, family skills training) may be less applicable later in the illness course, when patients may benefit more from functional remediation.

References

Bauer MS, McBride L, Williford WO, et al: Collaborative care for bipolar disorder, part II: impact on clinical outcome, function, and costs. Psychiatr Serv 57(7):937–945, 2006 16816277

Bilderbeck AC, Atkinson LZ, McMahon HC, et al: Psychoeducation and online mood tracking for patients with bipolar disorder: a randomised controlled trial. J Affect Disord 205:245–251, 2016 27454410

Bonnin CM, Torrent C, Arango C, et al: Functional remediation in bipolar disorder: 1-year follow-up of neurocognitive and functional outcome. Br J Psychiatry 208(1):87–93, 2016 26541692

Colom F, Vieta E, Martinez-Aran A, et al: A randomized trial on the efficacy of group psychoeducation in the prophylaxis of recurrences in bipolar patients whose disease is in remission. Arch Gen Psychiatry 60(4):402–407, 2003 12695318

Colom F, Vieta E, Sánchez-Moreno J, et al: Group psychoeducation for stabilised bipolar disorders: 5-year outcome of a randomised clinical trial. Br J Psychiatry 194(3):260–265, 2009 19252157

de Barros Pellegrinelli K, de O Costa LF, Silval KI, et al: Efficacy of psychoeducation on symptomatic and functional recovery in bipolar disorder. Acta Psychiatr Scand 127(2):153–158, 2013 22943487

Deckersbach T, Peters AT, Sylvia L, et al: Do comorbid anxiety disorders moderate the effects of psychotherapy for bipolar disorder? Results from STEP-BD. Am J Psychiatry 171(2):178–186, 2014 24077657

Deckersbach T, Peters AT, Shea C, et al: Memory performance predicts response to psychotherapy for depression in bipolar disorder: a pilot randomized controlled trial with exploratory functional magnetic resonance imaging. J Affect Disord 229:342–350, 2018 29331692

Ehlers CL, Frank E, Kupfer DJ: Social zeitgebers and biological rhythms. A unified approach to understanding the etiology of depression. Arch Gen Psychiatry 45(10):948–952, 1988 3048226

Frank E, Kupfer DJ, Thase ME, et al: Two-year outcomes for interpersonal and social rhythm therapy in individuals with bipolar I disorder. Arch Gen Psychiatry 62(9):996–1004, 2005 16143731

Fristad MA, Verducci JS, Walters K, et al: Impact of multifamily psychoeducational psychotherapy in treating children aged 8 to 12 years with mood disorders. Arch Gen Psychiatry 66(9):1013–1021, 2009 19736358

Geddes JR, Miklowitz DJ: Treatment of bipolar disorder. Lancet 381(9878):1672–1682, 2013 23663953

Gignac A, McGirr A, Lam RW, et al: Recovery and recurrence following a first episode of mania: a systematic review and meta-analysis of prospectively characterized cohorts. J Clin Psychiatry 76(9):1241–1248, 2015 25845021

Goldstein TR, Fersch-Podrat RK, Rivera M, et al: Dialectical behavior therapy for adolescents with bipolar disorder: results from a pilot randomized trial. J Child Adolesc Psychopharmacol 25(2):140–149, 2015 25010702

Goldstein TR, Merranko J, Krantz M, et al: Early intervention for adolescents at-risk for bipolar disorder: a pilot randomized trial of Interpersonal and Social Rhythm Therapy (IPSRT). J Affect Disord 235:348–356, 2018 29665518

Goodwin GM, Haddad PM, Ferrier IN, et al: Evidence-based guidelines for treating bipolar disorder: revised third edition recommendations from the British Association for Psychopharmacology. J Psychopharmacol 30(6):495–553, 2016 26979387

Hidalgo-Mazzei D, Mateu A, Reinares M, et al: Self-monitoring and psychoeducation in bipolar patients with a smart-phone application (SIMPLe) project: design, development and studies protocols. BMC Psychiatry 15:52, 2015 25884824

Hlastala SA, Kotler JS, McClellan JM, et al: Interpersonal and social rhythm therapy for adolescents with bipolar disorder: treatment development and results from an open trial. Depress Anxiety 27(5):457–464, 2010 20186968

Hooley JM, Miklowitz DJ: Families and mental disorders, in APA Handbook of Psychopathology, Vol 1: Psychopathology: Understanding, Assessing, and Treating Adult Mental Disorders. Edited by Butcher JN, Hooley JM, Kendall P. Washington, DC, American Psychological Association, 2018, pp 687–703

Inder ML, Crowe MT, Luty SE, et al: Randomized, controlled trial of Interpersonal and Social Rhythm Therapy for young people with bipolar disorder. Bipolar Disord 17(2):128–138, 2015 25346391

Inder ML, Crowe MT, Moor S, et al: Three-year follow-up after psychotherapy for young people with bipolar disorder. Bipolar Disord 20(5):441–447, 2017 29271072

Jones SH, Smith G, Mulligan LD, et al: Recovery-focused cognitive-behavioural therapy for recent-onset bipolar disorder: randomised controlled pilot trial. Br J Psychiatry 206(1):58–66, 2015 25213157

Kessing LV, Hansen HV, Christensen EM, et al: Do young adults with bipolar disorder benefit from early intervention? J Affect Disord 152–154:403–408, 2014 24268595

Lam DH, Watkins ER, Hayward P, et al: A randomized controlled study of cognitive therapy for relapse prevention for bipolar affective disorder: outcome of the first year. Arch Gen Psychiatry 60(2):145–152, 2003 12578431

Lam DH, Hayward P, Watkins ER, et al: Relapse prevention in patients with bipolar disorder: cognitive therapy outcome after 2 years. Am J Psychiatry 162(2):324–329, 2005 15677598

Leitan ND, Michalak EE, Berk L, et al: Optimizing delivery of recovery-oriented online self-management strategies for bipolar disorder: a review. Bipolar Disord 17(2):115–127, 2015 25238632

Lewandowski KE, Sperry SH, Cohen BM, et al: Treatment to enhance cognition in bipolar disorder (TREC-BD): efficacy of a randomized controlled trial of cognitive remediation versus active control. J Clin Psychiatry 78(9):e1242–e1249, 2017 29045770

Martínez-Arán A, Torrent C, Solé B, et al: Functional remediation for bipolar disorder. Clin Pract Epidemiol Ment Health 7(1):112–116, 2011 21687565

Meyer TD, Hautzinger M: Cognitive behaviour therapy and supportive therapy for bipolar disorders: relapse rates for treatment period and 2-year follow-up. Psychol Med 42(7):1429–1439, 2012 22099722

Miklowitz DJ: Bipolar Disorder: A Family Focused Treatment Approach, 2nd Edition. New York, Guilford, 2010

Miklowitz DJ, Chung B: Family-focused therapy for bipolar disorder: reflections on 30 years of research. Fam Process 55(3):483–499, 2016 27471058

Miklowitz DJ, Goldstein MJ, Nuechterlein KH, et al: Family factors and the course of bipolar affective disorder. Arch Gen Psychiatry 45(3):225–231, 1988 3341878

Miklowitz DJ, Otto MW, Frank E, et al: Intensive psychosocial intervention enhances functioning in patients with bipolar depression: results from a 9-month randomized controlled trial. Am J Psychiatry 164(9):1340–1347, 2007a 17728418

Miklowitz DJ, Otto MW, Frank E, et al: Psychosocial treatments for bipolar depression: a 1-year randomized trial from the Systematic Treatment Enhancement Program. Arch Gen Psychiatry 64(4):419–426, 2007b 17404119

Miklowitz DJ, Axelson DA, Birmaher B, et al: Family focused treatment for adolescents with bipolar disorder: results of a 2-year randomized trial. Arch Gen Psychiatry 65(9):1053–1061, 2008 18762591

Miklowitz DJ, Axelson DA, George EL, et al: Expressed emotion moderates the effects of family focused treatment for bipolar adolescents. J Am Acad Child Adolesc Psychiatry 48(6):643–651, 2009 19454920

Miklowitz DJ, Price J, Holmes EA, et al: Facilitated Integrated Mood Management for adults with bipolar disorder. Bipolar Disord 14(2):185–197, 2012 22420594
Miklowitz DJ, Schneck CD, Singh MK, et al: Early intervention for symptomatic youth at risk for bipolar disorder: a randomized trial of family focused therapy. J Am Acad Child Adolesc Psychiatry 52(2):121–131, 2013 23357439
Miklowitz DJ, Schneck CD, George EL, et al: Pharmacotherapy and family focused treatment for adolescents with bipolar I and II disorders: a 2-year randomized trial. Am J Psychiatry 171(6):658–667, 2014 24626789
Miklowitz DJ, Cipriani A, Goodwin GM: Network meta-analysis: drawing conclusions regarding trials of psychosocial interventions for bipolar disorder. Br J Psychiatry 211(6):334–336, 2017 29196390
Miklowitz DJ, Schneck CD, Walshaw PD et al: Early intervention for youth at high risk for bipolar disorder: a randomized clinical trial of family-focused therapy. Early Interv Psychiatry 13(2):208–216, 2019 28776930
Miklowitz DJ, Efthimiou O, Furukawa TA, et al: Adjunctive psychotherapy for bipolar disorder: a systematic review and component network meta-analysis. JAMA Psychiatry 78(2):141–150, 2021 33052390
Murray G, Leitan ND, Thomas N, et al: Towards recovery-oriented psychosocial interventions for bipolar disorder: quality of life outcomes, stage-sensitive treatments, and mindfulness mechanisms. Clin Psychol Rev 52:148–163, 2017 28129636
O'Brien MP, Miklowitz DJ, Candan KA, et al: A randomized trial of family focused therapy with populations at clinical high risk for psychosis: effects on interactional behavior. J Consult Clin Psychol 82(1):90–101, 2014 24188511
O'Donnell LA, Axelson DA, Kowatch RA, et al: Enhancing quality of life among adolescents with bipolar disorder: a randomized trial of two psychosocial interventions. J Affect Disord 219:201–208, 2017 28570966
Parikh SV, Zaretsky A, Beaulieu S, et al: A randomized controlled trial of psychoeducation or cognitive-behavioral therapy in bipolar disorder: a Canadian Network for Mood and Anxiety Treatments (CANMAT) study [CME]. J Clin Psychiatry 73(6):803–810, 2012 22795205
Perlis RH, Dennehy EB, Miklowitz DJ, et al: Retrospective age at onset of bipolar disorder and outcome during two-year follow-up: results from the STEP-BD study. Bipolar Disord 11(4):391–400, 2009 19500092
Post RM, Leverich GS, Kupka RW, et al: Early onset bipolar disorder and treatment delay are risk factors for poor outcome in adulthood. J Clin Psychiatry 71(7):864–872, 2010 20667291
Priebe S, Wildgrube C, Müller-Oerlinghausen B: Lithium prophylaxis and expressed emotion. Br J Psychiatry 154:396–399, 1989 2597843
Reichenberg A, Harvey PD, Bowie CR, et al: Neuropsychological function and dysfunction in schizophrenia and psychotic affective disorders. Schizophr Bull 35(5):1022–1029, 2009 18495643
Scott J, Paykel E, Morriss R, et al: Cognitive-behavioural therapy for severe and recurrent bipolar disorders: randomised controlled trial. Br J Psychiatry 188:313–320, 2006 16582056
Simon GE, Ludman EJ, Bauer MS, et al: Long-term effectiveness and cost of a systematic care program for bipolar disorder. Arch Gen Psychiatry 63(5):500–508, 2006 16651507
Simoneau TL, Miklowitz DJ, Richards JA, et al: Bipolar disorder and family communication: effects of a psychoeducational treatment program. J Abnorm Psychol 108(4):588–597, 1999 10609423
Sullivan AE, Judd CM, Axelson DA, et al: Family functioning and the course of adolescent bipolar disorder. Behav Ther 43(4):837–847, 2012 23046785
Swartz HA, Rucci P, Thase ME, et al: Psychotherapy alone and combined with medication as treatments for bipolar II depression: a randomized controlled trial. J Clin Psychiatry 79(2):7–15, 2018 28703949
Sylvia LG, Pegg SL, Dufour SC, et al: Pilot study of a lifestyle intervention for bipolar disorder: nutrition exercise wellness treatment (NEW Tx). J Affect Disord 250:278–283, 2019 30875669

Torrent C, del Mar Bonnin C, Martínez-Arán A, et al: Efficacy of functional remediation in bipolar disorder: a multicenter randomized controlled study. Am J Psychiatry 170(8):852–859, 2013 23511717

Wendel JS, Miklowitz DJ, Richards JA, et al: Expressed emotion and attributions in the relatives of bipolar patients: an analysis of problem-solving interactions. J Abnorm Psychol 109(4):792–796, 2000 11196006

West AE, Weinstein SM, Peters AT, et al: Child- and family-focused cognitive-behavioral therapy for pediatric bipolar disorder: a randomized clinical trial. J Am Acad Child Adolesc Psychiatry 53(11):1168–1178.e1, 2014 25440307

Yatham LN, Kennedy SH, Parikh SV, et al: Canadian Network for Mood and Anxiety Treatments (CANMAT) and International Society for Bipolar Disorders (ISBD) 2018 guidelines for the management of patients with bipolar disorder. Bipolar Disord 20(2):97–170, 2018 29536616

CHAPTER 27

Psychotherapy for Depression in Children and Adolescents

Jennifer L. Hughes, Ph.D., M.P.H.
Martha C. Tompson, Ph.D.
Adora Choquette, B.A.
Joan R. Asarnow, Ph.D.

Depressive disorders in youth are a major public health concern, causing significant morbidity and mortality, and rates of past-year major depressive episodes increased 52% between 2005 and 2017 (from 0.1% to 13.2%) among adolescents (Twenge et al. 2019). Within any given year, about 13% of youth have symptoms that meet diagnostic criteria for depression or another mood disorder, with some studies suggesting that 66%–75% of all lifetime depressive diagnoses begin during adolescence (Hankin 2015; National Institute of Mental Health 2017). Additionally, suicide is now the second leading cause of death in persons ages 10–24 in the United States. A recent Centers for Disease Control and Prevention (CDC) report focused on this age group highlighted the fact that after a stable trend in suicide rates from 2000 to 2007, the rate sharply increased from 2007 (6.8 per 100,000 persons) to 2017 (10.6 per 100,000 persons) (Curtin and Heron 2019).

Youth depression can be a life-altering illness, given that it is burdensome, often chronic, and disabling. Depressed youth, like depressed adults, have been shown to have thoughts and cognitive processing patterns that contribute to self-blame, self-deprecation, hopelessness, and negative attributions. Youth struggling with depression also frequently experience functional impairments, observed in school difficulties, social impairment, poorer family relationships, and substance misuse (Birmaher et al. 2007). Nearly all (approximately 80%–90%) of children and adolescents recover from an initial episode of major depressive disorder (MDD) within 1–2 years of onset (Emslie et al. 1997; Kovacs et al. 1984; McCauley et al. 1993; Strober et al. 1993). However, any time spent depressed during this important time of development can be impairing. While most youth recover, subsequent episodes of depression are common, with 50%–60% of youth experiencing a relapse of depression (Birmaher et al. 2007; Emslie et al. 2008; Kennard et al. 2009). Adolescence is a critical period for brain development, and depression can have adverse consequences for educational, social-emotional, and economic outcomes in adulthood (Trivedi et al. 2020). MDD in adolescence is also associated with elevated rates of suicide deaths and attempts (Weissman et al. 1999). The CDC estimates that mental illnesses among children result in an annual cost of $247 billion because of their impact not only on children but on families and communities (Perou et al. 2013).

In this chapter we provide an overview of psychotherapy approaches for addressing youth depression. Given the impact of depression on functioning, relationships, and key developmental tasks, as well as the frequently cited concerns about the use of antidepressants in children and adolescents, psychotherapy as a treatment approach is often preferred by youth and families. Interpersonal psychotherapy for adolescents (IPT-A) and cognitive-behavioral therapy (CBT) have the best evidence for efficacy in adolescent depression (American Psychological Association 2019; Viswanathan et al. 2020). The most current recommendations point to CBT, combination treatment with CBT and a selective serotonin reuptake inhibitor (SSRI), or medication management with fluoxetine as effective treatment options for adolescents with moderate to severe depression (Viswanathan et al. 2020). For children with depression, there is no psychotherapy with clear evidence of efficacy at present (Viswanathan et al. 2020). As described above, the course of depression in children and adolescents is marked by a trend toward recovery followed by risk of relapse and recurrence. Developing optimal treatment strategies, therefore, requires consideration of three treatment phases: acute treatment during a depressive episode to provide relief from depressive symptoms and promote episode remission; continuation treatment to consolidate response and prevent relapse; and maintenance treatment to prevent the recurrence of new depressive episodes. In this chapter, we review evidence-based therapies for child and adolescent depression and examine therapy outcomes across later stages of care (i.e., continuation and maintenance). We then review approaches for addressing the unmet need for evidence-based depression care by improving access to care in primary care and school-based settings. We close the chapter by exploring future directions.

Evidence-Based Psychotherapy Approaches

Acute treatment studies of psychotherapy alone for the treatment of pediatric depression demonstrate mixed results. There have been several systematic reviews and meta-analyses of these studies, with results generally concluding that there is support for efficacy and effectiveness of some psychotherapies. Perhaps the most comprehensive review is a comparative effectiveness review sponsored by the Agency for Healthcare Research and Quality (Viswanathan et al. 2020). This review concluded that evidence from studies evaluating treatment with children and adolescents experiencing depressive disorders supports improved depressive symptoms, response, and/or functional status with CBT or family therapy versus wait-list or active control conditions among adolescents or children (Clarke et al. 1999; Rosselló and Bernal 1999; Tompson et al. 2017b), and with family-based interpersonal psychotherapy versus active control conditions among children. However, the strength of evidence was rated as low (e.g., wide confidence intervals in estimates of treatment effects), raising questions regarding confidence that the evidence reflects a true effect and that estimated treatment effects will not be altered in future research. From a clinical perspective, this underscores the importance of additional research and adoption of measurement-based care with close monitoring of treatment response over time, and consideration of shifts in treatment strategies when a patient is not benefiting (e.g., adding medication if the patient is not responding to psychotherapy alone).

Several important points are worth noting in considering these results. First, although some studies comparing active treatment and a control condition (wait list, no treatment, pill placebo, usual care) indicate robust effects, the overall effect of psychotherapy for the acute management of depression in youth is modest. Second, findings from meta-analyses suggest no difference in efficacy between age groups, delivery modality, or type of therapy, although some differences have been identified in individual studies that were included in the meta-analyses (Eckshtain et al. 2020; Weisz et al. 2006). Findings from comprehensive reviews suggest that evidence for child treatments is notably weaker than that for adolescent interventions, with no child treatments achieving well-established status (Viswanathan et al. 2020; Weersing et al. 2017b). Weersing et al. (2017b) concluded that CBT for clinically depressed children appears to be possibly efficacious, with mixed findings across trials, and that both CBT and IPT-A are well-established interventions, with evidence of efficacy in several independent trials (Weersing et al. 2017b).

To date, for adolescents, CBT and combined fluoxetine and CBT may reduce symptoms in the short term, and CBT may improve symptoms and functioning (Viswanathan et al. 2020). The combination of pharmacotherapy and psychotherapy, specifically treatment with SSRIs and CBT, appears to be the most efficacious for moderate to severe depression in adolescents (March et al. 2004, 2006). As stated, there are no established treatments for children with depressive disorders (for reviews, see Forti-Buratti et al. 2016; Tompson et al. 2012). Several treatment options, with varying degrees of efficacy, are available for child and adolescent depression at this time and will be discussed here (for reviews, see Goodyer and Wilkinson 2019; Maalouf and Brent 2012; Sakolsky and Birmaher 2012; Tompson et al. 2012). The Association for Behavioral and Cognitive Therapies and the Society of Clinical Child and Adolescent Psychology have developed a useful website for patients, caregivers, and professionals about evidence-based mental health interventions (www.effectivechildtherapy.com).

Cognitive-Behavioral Therapy

CBT is the most commonly used specific therapy for child and adolescent depression, as well as the most widely studied (for reviews, see Curry 2001; Reinecke et al. 1998; Weersing and Brent 2006; Yang et al. 2017). CBT is generally time-limited and focuses on identifying thought and behavior patterns that contribute to the child's depressed mood. The goal of CBT is for the therapist and adolescent to collaboratively increase their understanding of how the adolescent's thoughts and behavior influence his or her emotions. Commonly used CBT manuals for depressed young people include the Primary and Secondary Control Enhancement Training (PASCET) manual (Weisz et al. 1997, 2005, 2009), the manual for the Coping with Depression course (Lewinsohn et al. 1990), and the Treatment for Adolescents with Depression Study (TADS) CBT Manual (Curry et al. 2000). Group CBT has been extensively studied and appears to be effective in both depressed and at-risk adolescents, as compared with a control group or activity comparator (for review, see Nardi et al. 2016). It has been suggested that CBT may not be as effective for children because of limitations imposed by their developing verbal and abstract thinking abilities. However, small studies of CBT in depressed children have found positive outcomes with this approach (for review, see Yang et al. 2017).

Important investigations of CBT for depressed adolescents include the single-site Adolescent Depression Antidepressants and Psychotherapy Trial (ADAPT; Goodyer et al. 2007, 2008), the multisite TADS (March et al. 2004), and Treatment of Resistant Depression in Adolescents trial (TORDIA; Brent et al. 2008). As mentioned above, CBT for adolescent depression has demonstrated mixed results across these large trials and in smaller studies. In the TADS (N=439) and TORDIA (N=334) studies, the combination treatment of CBT and medication management was superior to monotherapy medication management, suggesting an important adjunctive benefit (particularly related to suicidality in TADS). In the ADAPT trial (N=208), there was not a similar benefit for combined treatment (Goodyer et al. 2007, 2008). However, this trial excluded youth who had previously shown a positive response to a brief psychosocial intervention. In TADS, treatment with CBT alone was significantly less effective than treatment with medication management (fluoxetine) alone, and CBT alone was not superior to a medication placebo control (March et al. 2004). One benefit of CBT in combination with medication management may be an accelerated treatment response (March et al. 2007), though this was not found in all studies of combination treatment of CBT and medication (Dubicka et al. 2010).

However, not all CBT trials have yielded benefits relative to comparator conditions (Asarnow and Ougrin 2017; Goodyer et al. 2017), and there is some hint that trials that have used more flexible individually tailored and collaborative approaches result in greater benefits. The CBT used in randomized controlled trials (RCTs) has sometimes been criticized for being delivered in a too-rigid fashion and for not being individualized to the youth and family's problems and needs. A modular approach to CBT, with the flexible application of a manualized focused treatment of depression, anxiety, and behavior problems, has been shown to be more effective than treatment as usual (Weisz et al. 2012). This approach, Modular Approach to Therapy for Children with Anxiety, Depression, Trauma, or Conduct Problems (MATCH-ADTC; Chorpita and Weisz 2009), was developed by combining the results of meta-analysis of therapies with efforts to identify the most frequent common elements of evidence-based practices for youth used in clinical practice settings. Modules can be used in a flexible manner, based on an evidence-based algorithm, to address several diagnoses and comorbidities with one protocol. In the study comparing MATCH-ADTC with both usual care and a standard manualized treatment, youth in MATCH-ADTC showed significantly faster improvement on measures of internalizing symptoms, among other outcomes, than youth in the other conditions (Weisz et al. 2012). A recent systematic review and meta-regression analysis found that CBT containing a combination of behavioral activation and cognitive restructuring (specifically, challenging thoughts) or the involvement of caregivers in the intervention was associated with better long-term outcomes for depressed youth (Oud et al. 2019).

More recently, behavioral activation (BA) approaches to treating depression have received much attention. BA is defined as a "structured, brief psychotherapeutic approach that aims to (a) increase engagement in adaptive activities (which often are those associated with the experience of pleasure or mastery), (b) decrease engagement in activities that maintain depression or increase risk of depression, and (c) solve problems that limit access to reward or that maintain or increase aversive control" (Dimidjian et al. 2011, pp. 3–4). BA has demonstrated greater efficacy in treating depression in adults (Dimidjian et al. 2006; Jacobson et al. 2001; Martell et al. 2013), even when compared with full cognitive therapy (Gortner et al. 1998; Jacobson and Hollon 1996) and pharmacotherapy (Dimidjian et al. 2006; Dobson et al. 2008). This intervention has also shown promise for treating adolescent depression (McCauley et al. 2016; Ritschel et al. 2016). McCauley et al. (2016) adapted BA for use in a 14-session intervention for depressed adolescents, adding components for family engagement and more structured homework, to be delivered in an outpatient mental health setting. In an RCT of 60 depressed adolescents comparing the Adolescent Behavioral Activation Program (A-BAP) with uncontrolled evidence-based practice for depression, the A-BAP group reported statistically significant improvements in depression, global functioning, activation, and avoidance that were similar to those in the other condition. Ritschel et al. (2011, 2016) developed a similar BA treatment and pilot-tested this approach in an open trial with 28 adolescents; their intervention was up to 22 sessions over 18 weeks, and participants reported significant improvements in depression over the course of the intervention.

The mechanisms of depressive symptom change in CBT for youth with depression are not yet clear. In a review of potential mechanisms of change for cognitive-behavioral therapies for youth anxiety and depression, CBT for depression yielded small effects for cognitive processes but nonsignificant effects for behavioral and coping variables (Chu and Harrison 2007). A review of common process variables, such as therapeutic alliance, patient cognitive change, and therapist adherence to and competence in CBT, resulted in process-outcome correlations that were small and accounted for a small proportion of symptom change (Webb et al. 2012). With regard to brain changes associated with CBT for depressed youth, one small study (N=21) found CBT-related changes in adolescents with MDD, with observed regional cerebral blood flow increases in the right dorsolateral prefrontal cortex, an area related to self-regulation and cognitive control (Sosic-Vasic et al. 2017). In another small sample (N=13 in the post-CBT sample) of depressed youth, baseline increased activation in response to happy relative to neutral distractors was observed in the orbitofrontal cortex, and this activation was normalized after CBT (Chuang et al. 2016).

Interpersonal Therapy for Adolescents

Developed by Mufson et al. (1994, 1999), IPT-A has demonstrated efficacy for adolescents with depression, with recovery sustained through a 1-year follow-up (Mufson and Fairbanks 1996). The IPT model emphasizes that depression occurs in an interpersonal context and within the framework of one of four problem areas: grief, interpersonal role disputes, role transitions, and interpersonal deficits or, in IPT-A, issues with single-parent families (Klomek and Mufson 2006; Mufson and Sills 2006). Thus, the goal of IPT in treating depression is to understand the patient's current relationships and renegotiate interpersonal problems occurring at the onset of depressive symptoms. IPT-A encompasses three components: psychoeducation, affect identification and interpersonal skills techniques, and relapse prevention. The psychoeducation aspect incorporates parents.

IPT-A has demonstrated effectiveness in the treatment of depressive symptoms in adolescents. In a study of clinically referred depressed adolescents, IPT-A was found to be more effective than clinical monitoring for reducing depressive symptoms and improving social functioning (Mufson et al. 1999). Participants receiving IPT-A reported a greater decrease in depressive symptoms and greater improvements in social functioning when compared with the control group (Mufson et al. 1994). Similarly, in a 12-week open study of IPT-A for 25 moderately to severely depressed adolescents, 84% met criteria for remission by the end of the treatment (Santor and Kusumakar 2001). Rosselló and Bernal (1999) adapted IPT-A for Puerto Rican adolescents to add culturally sensitive elements, including an enhanced emphasis on family inclusion. They found this adaptation of IPT to be at least as efficacious as, and potentially more efficacious than, CBT in the management of adolescent depression. Clinical significance tests suggested that 82% of adolescents in IPT and 59% of those in CBT were functional after treatment (Rosselló and Bernal 1999).

More recently, an adapted treatment strategy utilizing IPT-A has been tested to provide empirical guidelines for sequential clinical decision making regarding IPT-A and medication use within a stepped-care model (Gunlicks-Stoessel et al. 2016). This pilot found that therapists implementing IPT-A should routinely monitor depression symptoms and consider augmenting treatment for insufficient responders as early as week 4 of IPT-A (Gunlicks-Stoessel et al. 2016).

IPT-A has recently been adapted as a family-based IPT (FB-IPT) for youth (ages 7–12) with depression (Dietz 2020; Dietz et al. 2008). In an RCT, 42 youths were randomly assigned to receive either FB-IPT or child-centered therapy; youth in the FB-IPT group showed higher rates of remission (66% vs. 31%) and greater decreases in depressive symptoms. The FB-IPT group also reported significant reductions in interpersonal impairment, a mechanism that is specifically targeted in FB-IPT (Dietz et al. 2015).

Potential mechanisms of change in IPT include change in dysfunctional thinking patterns and reductions in attachment anxiety and avoidance (Gunlicks-Stoessel et al. 2019b; Zhou et al. 2020). Additionally, hypothalamic–pituitary–adrenal axis functioning, as measured by cortisol response, has been found to be a predictor of IPT-A response, with higher cortisol levels after a conflict task associated with greater improvement in depressive symptoms after IPT-A treatment (Gunlicks-Stoessel et al. 2013).

Family-Focused Therapy

Family-focused treatments may be useful in addressing the interpersonal and family problems and symptoms; these approaches may be particularly helpful for depressed children. Family factors appear to play a role in relapse or depression maintenance in children and adolescents (Gillham et al. 2000). Often treatments for children and adolescents require intervention and guidance for parents or caregivers. Most successful intervention trials for depressed children and adolescents have included a family component, whether it be skills teaching for parents or a check-in associated with individual therapy sessions. There are few studies of family-focused treatments, and some studies in adolescents raise questions regarding the benefits of a family-focused approach (for review, see Asarnow et al. 2005a).

Family Focused Treatment for Childhood Depression (FFT-CD; Tompson et al. 2017a, 2017b) is a 15-session family treatment with both the youth and parents targeting two mechanisms involved in recovery: a) enhancing family support, specifically decreasing criticism and increasing supportive interactions; and b) strengthening specific cognitive-behavioral skills within a family context that have been central to CBT for depression, specifically BA, communication, and problem-solving. FFT-CD includes psychoeducation about depression and communication improvement techniques to enhance relationships and target stress factors for the child and family (Tompson et al. 2017a). FFT-CD was compared with individual supportive therapy for children ages 7–14 in an RCT. After 4 months of intervention, both groups demonstrated significant improvements in depressive symptoms, non-depressive symptoms, global response, and functioning; however, the FFT-CD group rated significantly higher on the outcome of adequate clinical depression response, defined as a 50% or more reduction on the Children's Depression Rating Scale—Revised (77.7% in FFT-CD vs. 59.9% in individual supportive therapy; Tompson et al. 2017b). More extended follow-up data indicated that while FFT-CD led to quicker depressive symptom improvement at 16 weeks in FFT-CD, there was a trend toward recovery over time, leading to similar outcomes for both FFT-CD and the comparator supportive psychotherapy by 1 year (Asarnow et al. 2020). However, depression recurrence after recovery and suicide attempts were less common in children receiving FFT-CD compared with supportive therapy.

Diamond and colleagues (Diamond and Siqueland 1995; Diamond et al. 2002) developed Attachment-Based Family Therapy (ABFT), grounded in attachment theory and aimed at using an interpersonal, process-oriented, trauma-focused approach to treating adolescent depression, as well as suicidality and trauma. ABFT aims to explicitly target improvement of attachment security through five therapeutic tasks: the relational reframe, adolescent alliance-building, parent alliance-building, the attachment task, and the autonomy-promoting task (Diamond et al. 2016). Initially, ABFT was developed with depressed adolescents, and in the first study 32 adolescents were randomly assigned to 12 weeks of ABFT or a 6-week, minimal-contact wait-list control group. At posttreatment, 81% of the patients treated with ABFT no longer had symptoms that met criteria for MDD (vs. 47% of patients in the wait-list group) (Diamond et al. 2002). Later iterations and examinations of ABFT focused on adolescent suicide attempters, and to date there have been four clinical trials, in addition to several pilot studies (Diamond et al. 2016). Two of these later studies reported outcomes related to depressive symptom improvement, demonstrating that ABFT leads to reductions in depression as compared with enhanced treatment as usual (Diamond et al. 2010) and treatment as usual (Israel and Diamond 2013).

Psychodynamic Psychotherapy

Psychodynamic psychotherapy focuses on interpersonal relationships, attachment, and life stresses and explicitly works on the therapeutic relationship between the client and therapist. Although widely utilized in clinical settings, psychodynamic psychotherapy lacks a strong evidence base. A large study in the United Kingdom compared CBT, short-term psychodynamic psychotherapy, and a manualized brief psychosocial intervention (BPI) delivered within the context of routine community care with some training and quality assurance procedures in an RCT of 465 adolescents with MDD (IMPACT study; Goodyer et al. 2017). There was no difference in the mean depressive symptom scores between treatments over the 86-week follow-up, with an average 49%–52% reduction in depressive symptoms by the end of the study. There was also no difference in cost or quality-of-life scores between groups (Goodyer et al. 2017). This suggests that both psychodynamic psychotherapy and BPI are as effective as CBT when delivered within community care. These findings were surprising, given that up to now CBT has appeared to be among the most widely supported and used treatments for adolescent depression. However, it is important to note that this was a pragmatic trial and intervention delivery was likely less rigorous than delivery in randomized controlled efficacy trials; in addition, there are differences across CBT versions for depression, and treatment benefits have varied across studies and sites (Asarnow and Ougrin 2017).

Acute Psychotherapy Long-Term Outcomes

There are numerous examples supporting the value of acute-phase psychosocial treatments in the short term, as well as that of combined psychotherapy and medication treatments for adolescents with severe and/or medication treatment–resistant depression. However, longer-term treatment benefits have been elusive, particularly given the natural tendency for youth to recover over time. Indeed, consistent with the frequent weakening of differences between treatment and comparator conditions over time as described in several studies above, naturalistic follow-up studies generally show similar outcomes for these specific therapies and control groups during follow-up periods of up to 2 years (Birmaher et al. 2000; Lewinsohn et al. 1990; Vostanis et al. 1998; Wood et al. 1996). However, there are hints of longer-term effects, such as the trend toward fewer recurrent episodes among children who recovered from depressive episodes with FFT-CD relative to supportive therapy (Asarnow et al. 2020), as well as the continuing low levels of depressive symptoms seen in a small 1-year naturalistic follow-up study of youth treated with IPT (Mufson and Fairbanks 1996).

After Acute Treatment: Continuation- and Maintenance-Phase Treatment

As noted earlier, the high risk of relapse and recurrence calls for attention to longer-term treatment strategies that address continuation- and maintenance-phase treatments. Whereas the emphasis in acute treatment is on achieving symptom reduction and remission, the goal of continuation treatment is to prevent relapses following recovery. Maintenance treatment emphasizes a longer-term view and prevention of recurrent depressive episodes. Attention to enhancing functioning in addition to monitoring for symptoms is also critical given the potential adverse impact of depressive symptoms on attainment of critical educational and social developmental milestones, risk of developing other, nondepressive disorders among children and adolescents who suffer from depression, and risk of suicide attempts and death by suicide as these youth mature (Weissman et al. 1999). While efforts to develop and evaluate later-phase treatments are lagging behind work on acute treatments, we review promising directions below.

Kennard et al. (2008b, 2016) developed a relapse-prevention CBT (RP-CBT) to address residual symptoms and prevent relapse in youth, utilizing a core set of CBT skills and wellness-focused strategies. RP-CBT included strategies to promote wellness along with adaptive coping strategies to enhance well-being in youth who were successfully treated for depression (Kennard et al. 2008a, 2014). The addition of RP-CBT treatment after response to antidepressant medication resulted in lower rates of relapse at both short- and long-term follow-ups (Emslie et al. 2015; Kennard et al. 2008a, 2014). Using a continuation CBT approach that included the wellness- and strengths-based strategies of RP-CBT, the researchers found that patients who were treated with the RP-CBT plus continued antidepressant medication had lower relapse rates over a 30-week treatment period compared with those treated with medication only (9% vs. 26.5%). The study also concluded that those who were treated with CBT spent a higher percentage of time well and required a lower antidepressant dosage (Kennard et al. 2014).

Another study examined continuation-phase CBT for 6 months following acute-phase treatment, demonstrating that the continuation-phase CBT significantly lowered relapse rates compared with historical controls (6% rate vs. 50% rate; Kroll et al. 1996). In the acute phase of treatment, 33 subjects (ages 9–17) received five to eight sessions of CBT. Twenty patients achieved remission, with an average time to remission of 10 weeks. Seventeen patients went on to participate in the continuation-phase CBT treatment. The CBT continuation-phase treatment sessions were biweekly to monthly for 6 months. Continuation-phase CBT sessions focused on preventing relapse by continuing to support the skills learned in the acute-phase CBT (i.e., cognitive, social problem-solving, and depression symptom management skills, such as sleep hygiene and activity scheduling), while emphasizing the risk factors associated with relapse such as poor peer and family relationships, continued elevated subsyndromal symptoms, and negative cognitions about the self (Kroll et al. 1996). By 6 months, only one of the subjects in the continuation phase had relapsed, compared with six of the control subjects. Of note, however, is that this study was not an RCT. In addition, the study was limited by a relatively small sample size and by the use of a historical control group for comparisons.

While the treatments described above that were developed specifically to address the need for continuation treatment have been promising, it should be noted that many trials have included booster sessions, with no indication of differential treatment benefits over the observed period. A study by Clarke et al. (1999) provided additional clarification of the needs of youth after acute treatment. Notably, the addition of booster sessions following 8 weeks of acute-phase treatment (group CBT, group CBT plus a parent group, or wait-list control), compared with assessments alone, indicated that although booster sessions did not reduce relapse, youth randomly assigned to receive the booster treatments who continued to suffer from depressive symptoms at the end of the acute phase showed accelerated remission. One limitation of this study is that the booster sessions were delivered only quarterly, a frequency that may be insufficient to prevent relapse.

Strategies for Improving Access to Evidence-Based Depression Care Through Primary Care and School-Based Health Clinics

Primary care is a major point of service; most children and adolescents have access to primary health care and attend at least one primary care visit annually. Hence, improving access to mental health care through primary care and school-based health clinics has potential for improving access to mental health care overall and for improving youth outcomes (Asarnow et al. 2017). Indeed, in 2016, the U.S. Preventive Services Task Force recommended screening for MDD for adolescents ages 12–18 years, with adequate systems "in place to ensure "accurate diagnosis, effective treatment, and appropriate follow-up" (Siu and U.S. Preventive Services Task Force 2016). This has resulted in an increased focus on depression screening within primary care and a need for attention to providing effective treatment options through primary care services. With accumulating data indicating that many children and adolescents referred to mental health services never link to specialty mental health care, alternative service models have been developed to strengthen access to care within primary care clinics such as pediatric patient-centered medical homes and services that support linkage to needed mental health services (Asarnow et al. 2017). Below, we review examples of approaches that have shown promise, because providing psychotherapy for youth in primary care settings can help improve accessibility.

In the Youth Partners in Care trial, Asarnow and colleagues developed and tested health information tools and strategies for improving access to evidence-based depression care (primarily CBT and antidepressant medications) through primary care. This randomized controlled effectiveness trial was conducted in primary care clinics within five diverse health care organizations and evaluated the collaborative quality improvement intervention, compared with usual care enhanced by primary care clinician education regarding depression evaluation and management (Asarnow et al. 2005a, 2009; Wells et al. 2001). Results indicated significantly greater improvement in depression, functioning, and patient satisfaction at a 6-month follow-up among youth in the intervention condition as compared with usual care (Asarnow et al. 2005a, 2009; Wells et al. 2001). While the primary effect of the intervention was to decrease the likelihood of severe depression at the 6-month outcome assessment, early intervention–related improvements conferred longer-term benefits through a favorable shift in the course of depression through 12 and 18 months. Interestingly, despite the fact that medication treatment is the most available treatment for depression in primary care, most youth indicated a preference for counseling (50%) over medication (22%) (Jaycox et al. 2006). This finding is consistent with treatment choices made within the trial, where medication treatment was less common than psychotherapy

(Asarnow et al. 2005a). Nevertheless, observational analyses indicating that receiving guideline-consistent psychotherapy and/or medication treatment was associated with a lower likelihood of severe depression further underscore the value of delivering evidence-based depression care (Wells et al. 2012). It is also important to note that this trial included a large proportion of minority youth, and results indicated strong benefits among minority youth (Ngo et al. 2009). This is important given the frequent disparities in access to evidence-based care among minority populations.

Clarke et al. (2016) demonstrated that a brief CBT delivered in primary care was effective in depressed adolescents who had declined medication treatment. Brief CBT was superior to the treatment-as-usual control condition on outcomes of depression recovery, depression diagnosis, and other secondary outcomes. However, the effect sizes were small, and the superiority of brief CBT did not hold over the 2-year-follow-up (Clarke et al. 2016). Yet, this study demonstrated that a brief CBT approach can be successfully delivered to depressed adolescents in a primary care setting with a positive impact on depression.

Integrated brief behavioral therapy (IBBT; Weersing et al. 2008) was specifically developed as an intervention to address depression and anxiety in pediatric primary care with providers seeing youth in the clinic setting. IBBT consists of 8–12 weekly sessions, and components include psychoeducation, relaxation and coping, problem solving, reducing avoidance and setting goals, increasing engagement/behavioral activation, and relapse prevention. The treatment components are designed for flexible use to address symptoms in youth with mild to moderate impairment. In a two-center RCT, 185 youths ages 8–17 years who met DSM-IV (American Psychiatric Association 1994) criteria for a full or probable diagnosis of anxiety (separation anxiety disorder, generalized anxiety disorder, or social phobia) or depression (MDD, dysthymic disorder, or minor depression) were randomly assigned to receive IBBT or assisted referral to care (Weersing et al. 2017a). Youth in the IBBT condition had significantly higher rates of clinical improvement (56.8% vs. 28.2%), greater reductions in symptoms, and better functioning at the 16-week follow-up. Additionally, Hispanic youth had stronger responses to IBBT (Weersing et al. 2017a). At the 32-week follow-up, IBBT remained superior to assisted referral to care on rate of clinical improvement (67.5% vs. 43.1%) and functioning; however, impact on depressive symptoms was not significantly different between the two groups at this time point (Brent et al. 2020).

Given the efficacy of IPT-A, Mufson et al. (2004) conducted a randomized effectiveness trial involving 63 adolescents referred for mental health treatment through school-based mental health clinics. Participants were randomly assigned to receive IPT-A or treatment as usual, and those treated with IPT-A experienced greater improvement in depressive symptoms, social functioning, and problem solving (Mufson et al. 2004). This study demonstrated that an evidence-based therapy for youth depression could be successfully delivered by school-based clinicians in school-based mental health clinics.

A brief version of IPT-A consisting of six weekly sessions was piloted in primary care with 10 low-income Latino adolescents and found to be feasible and acceptable, with significant improvements in depression, social and overall functioning, and overall severity of illness outcomes (Mufson et al. 2015). IPT-A has also been examined in primary care through a stepped collaborative care treatment model approach (stepped-care IPT-A) for adolescents with depression utilizing IPT-A and antidepressant medication. In a pilot study comparing this stepped-care IPT-A approach to enhanced treatment as usual in urban pediatric primary care clinics serving primarily Latino youth, Mufson et al. (2018) found that the stepped-care IPT-A model is feasible, acceptable, and potentially beneficial for urban Latino adolescents (Mufson et al. 2018).

In sum, we have accumulating evidence supporting the effectiveness of approaches that bring evidence-based depression care into primary care and school settings. Given the demonstrated benefits of treatment in minority youth (Mufson et al. 2018; Ngo et al. 2009; Weersing et al. 2017a), therapy provided in primary care and schools may provide an important means of addressing mental health needs of minority populations. This work underscores our readiness to bring our treatments into health and community settings, and service delivery approaches have been developed and tested.

Future Directions

It is also important to explore youth perspectives on managing depressed mood and helpful coping strategies. Recent work by Ng et al. (2016) found that the coping strategies adolescents reported using to help themselves feel better matched evidence-based therapy approaches 92.6% of the time, but that, conversely, 65% of the evidence-based therapy components included in the study did not match any of the coping strategies reported by adolescents.

A personalized approach to treatment for youth depression, with youth and families being matched to the best-fitting treatment, may be one way to improve on current treatments. In a recent latent class analysis of the TADS study, Gunlicks-Stoessel et al. (2019a) identified three subgroups of patients: 1) adolescents with high levels of problems in both family relationships and cognitions, 2) adolescents with moderate levels of problems in both domains, and 3) adolescents with low levels of problems in both domains. However, none of these subgroups predicted treatment outcome with the CBT or combination CBT and medication management condition (Gunlicks-Stoessel et al. 2019a). The analysis authors suggested considering other ways to personalize treatment, such as considering additional risk factors that might guide treatment decisions and weighting the malleability of a given risk factor against the magnitude of the risk factor before treatment. Comprehensive phenotyping of depression in youth will likely elucidate important biological and clinical risk factors to help optimize treatment assignment (Trivedi et al. 2020).

Conclusion

Effective psychotherapies for youth depression are available, particularly for treatment of acute episodes. These include CBT, IPT, family-focused therapy, and other approaches and offer encouragement that depression is a treatable condition and that our treatments can hasten relief and recovery. A family perspective with attention to the likelihood of depression in other family members is also important, given the high rates of depression and other problems observed in multiple family members, accumulating data indicating that depression in parents can adversely influence youth outcomes, and the importance of the family environment for supporting recovery and functioning in children and adolescents.

With recognition of the need to export treatments that work into community care settings and improve access to optimal evidence-based care approaches, there have been changes in health and behavioral health care systems to support care improvements. Approaches that emphasize implementation of evidence-based care within diverse service settings and measurement-based care that monitors patient outcomes and shifts treatment strategies when indicated by patient treatment response are increasingly emphasized in health and behavioral health systems (Asarnow et al. 2015, 2017). This work is supported by accumulating dissemination and effectiveness trials in youth depression, which provide strong examples of the use of evidence-based treatments in real-world practice settings, including primary care, schools, and other health, mental health, and community settings (Asarnow and Miranda 2014; Cheung et al. 2018; Kazdin 2008; Zuckerbrot et al. 2018). Future work to optimize these strategies and attend to longer-term care strategies to prevent chronic and recurrent depressions will be important for reducing suffering and premature death by suicide and other complications of depression and improving the lives of individuals who experience depression as children or adolescents. There is also a need to individualize the treatment based on severity, psychosocial stressors, and family circumstances and to develop algorithms for personalizing treatments so that individuals receive the "right treatment at the right time" to optimize outcomes. Given that care is not available to and/or accessed by many youths, and that personal and practical barriers can interfere with accessing care, future work is needed to improve treatment access and address barriers to care.

References

American Psychiatric Association: Diagnostic and Statistical Manual of Mental Disorders, 4th Edition. Washington, DC, American Psychiatric Association, 1994

American Psychological Association: Guideline Development Panel for the Treatment of Depressive Disorders: Clinical Practice Guideline for the Treatment Of Depression Across Three Age Cohorts. Washington, DC, American Psychological Association, 2019

Asarnow JR, Miranda J: Improving care for depression and suicide risk in adolescents: innovative strategies for bringing treatments to community settings. Annu Rev Clin Psychol 10:275–303, 2014 24437432

Asarnow J, Ougrin D: From efficacy to pragmatic trials: does the dodo bird verdict apply? Lancet Psychiatry 4(2):84–85, 2017 27914904

Asarnow JR, Jaycox LH, Duan N, et al: Effectiveness of a quality improvement intervention for adolescent depression in primary care clinics: a randomized controlled trial. JAMA 293(3):311–319, 2005a 15657324

Asarnow JR, Tompson MC, Berk MS: Adolescent depression: family focused treatment strategies, in Family Psychology: The Art of Science. Edited by Pinsof WM, Lebow JL. New York, Oxford University Press, 2005b, pp 425–450

Asarnow JR, Jaycox LH, Tang L, et al: Long-term benefits of short-term quality improvement interventions for depressed youths in primary care. Am J Psychiatry 166(9):1002–1010, 2009 19651711

Asarnow JR, Rozenman M, Wiblin J, et al: Integrated medical-behavioral care compared with usual primary care for child and adolescent behavioral health: a meta-analysis. JAMA Pediatr 169(10):929–937, 2015 26259143

Asarnow JR, Kolko DJ, Miranda J, Kazak AE: The Pediatric Patient-Centered Medical Home: innovative models for improving behavioral health. Am Psychol 72(1):13–27, 2017 28068135
Asarnow JR, Tompson MC, Klomhaus AM, et al: Randomized controlled trial of family focused treatment for child depression compared to individual psychotherapy: one-year outcomes. J Child Psychol Psychiatry 61(6):662–671, 2020 31840263
Birmaher B, Brent DA, Kolko D, et al: Clinical outcome after short-term psychotherapy for adolescents with major depressive disorder. Arch Gen Psychiatry 57(1):29–36, 2000 10632230
Birmaher B, Brent D, Bernet W, et al: Practice parameter for the assessment and treatment of children and adolescents with depressive disorders. J Am Acad Child Adolesc Psychiatry 46(11):1503–1526, 2007 18049300
Brent D, Emslie G, Clarke G, et al: Switching to another SSRI or to venlafaxine with or without cognitive behavioral therapy for adolescents with SSRI-resistant depression: the TORDIA randomized controlled trial. JAMA 299(8):901–913, 2008 18314433
Brent DA, Porta G, Rozenman MS, et al: Brief behavioral therapy for pediatric anxiety and depression in primary care: a follow-up. J Am Acad Child Adolesc Psychiatry 59(7):856–867, 2020 31278996
Cheung AH, Zuckerbrot RA, Jensen PS, et al: Guidelines for adolescent depression in primary care (GLAD-PC): part II. treatment and ongoing management. Pediatrics 141(3):e20174082, 2018 29483201
Chorpita BF, Weisz JR: Modular Approach to Therapy for Children With Anxiety, Depression, Trauma, or Conduct Problems (MATCH-ADTC). Satellite Beach, FL, PracticeWise, 2009
Chu BC, Harrison TL: Disorder-specific effects of CBT for anxious and depressed youth: a meta-analysis of candidate mediators of change. Clin Child Fam Psychol Rev 10(4):352–372, 2007 17985239
Chuang JY, J Whitaker K, Murray GK, et al: Aberrant brain responses to emotionally valent words is normalised after cognitive behavioural therapy in female depressed adolescents. J Affect Disord 189:54–61, 2016 26406969
Clarke GN, Rohde P, Lewinsohn PM, et al: Cognitive-behavioral treatment of adolescent depression: efficacy of acute group treatment and booster sessions. J Am Acad Child Adolesc Psychiatry 38(3):272–279, 1999 10087688
Clarke G, DeBar LL, Pearson JA, et al: Cognitive behavioral therapy in primary care for youth declining antidepressants: a randomized trial. Pediatrics 137(5):e20151851, 2016 27244782
Curry JF: Specific psychotherapies for childhood and adolescent depression. Biol Psychiatry 49(12):1091–1100, 2001 11430851
Curry JF, Wells KC, Brent DA, et al: Treatment for Adolescents With Depression Study (TADS): cognitive behavior therapy manual: introduction, rationale, and adolescent sessions. Duke University Medical Center, The TADS Team, March 15, 2000. Available at: aaronkrasner.com/wp-content/uploads/2017/10/TADS_CBT.pdf. Accessed November 25, 2020.
Curtin SC, Heron M: Death rates due to suicide and homicide among persons aged 10–24: United States, 2000–2017. NCHS Data Brief (352):1–8, 2019 31751202
Diamond G, Siqueland L: Family therapy for the treatment of depressed adolescents. Psychotherapy (Chic) 32:77–90, 1995
Diamond GS, Reis BF, Diamond GM, et al: Attachment-based family therapy for depressed adolescents: a treatment development study. J Am Acad Child Adolesc Psychiatry 41(10):1190–1196, 2002 12364840
Diamond GS, Wintersteen MB, Brown GK, et al: Attachment-based family therapy for adolescents with suicidal ideation: a randomized controlled trial. J Am Acad Child Adolesc Psychiatry 49(2):122–131, 2010 20215934
Diamond G, Russon J, Levy S: Attachment-based family therapy: a review of the empirical support. Fam Process 55(3):595–610, 2016 27541199
Dietz LJ: Family based interpersonal psychotherapy: an intervention for preadolescent depression. Am J Psychother 73(1):22–28, 2020 32050785
Dietz LJ, Mufson L, Irvine H, et al: Family based interpersonal psychotherapy for depressed preadolescents: an open-treatment trial. Early Interv Psychiatry 2(3):154–161, 2008 21352148

Dietz LJ, Weinberg RJ, Brent DA, et al: Family based interpersonal psychotherapy for depressed preadolescents: examining efficacy and potential treatment mechanisms. J Am Acad Child Adolesc Psychiatry 54(3):191–199, 2015 25721184

Dimidjian S, Hollon SD, Dobson KS, et al: Randomized trial of behavioral activation, cognitive therapy, and antidepressant medication in the acute treatment of adults with major depression. J Consult Clin Psychol 74(4):658–670, 2006 16881773

Dimidjian S, Barrera M Jr, Martell C, et al: The origins and current status of behavioral activation treatments for depression. Annu Rev Clin Psychol 7:1–38, 2011 21275642

Dobson KS, Hollon SD, Dimidjian S, et al: Randomized trial of behavioral activation, cognitive therapy, and antidepressant medication in the prevention of relapse and recurrence in major depression. J Consult Clin Psychol 76(3):468–477, 2008 18540740

Dubicka B, Elvins R, Roberts C, et al: Combined treatment with cognitive-behavioural therapy in adolescent depression: meta-analysis. Br J Psychiatry 197(6):433–440, 2010 21119148

Eckshtain D, Kuppens S, Ugueto A, et al: Meta-analysis: 13-year follow-up of psychotherapy effects on youth depression. J Am Acad Child Adolesc Psychiatry 59(1):45–63, 2020 31004739

Emslie GJ, Rush AJ, Weinberg WA, et al: Recurrence of major depressive disorder in hospitalized children and adolescents. J Am Acad Child Adolesc Psychiatry 36(6):785–792, 1997 9183133

Emslie GJ, Kennard BD, Mayes TL, et al: Fluoxetine versus placebo in preventing relapse of major depression in children and adolescents. Am J Psychiatry 165(4):459–467, 2008 18281410

Emslie GJ, Kennard BD, Mayes TL, et al: Continued effectiveness of relapse prevention cognitive-behavioral therapy following fluoxetine treatment in youth with major depressive disorder. J Am Acad Child Adolesc Psychiatry 54(12):991–998, 2015 26598474

Forti-Buratti MA, Saikia R, Wilkinson EL, et al: Psychological treatments for depression in preadolescent children (12 years and younger): systematic review and meta-analysis of randomised controlled trials. Eur Child Adolesc Psychiatry 25(10):1045–1054, 2016 26969618

Gillham JE, Shatte AJ, Freres DR: Preventing depression: a review of cognitive-behavioral and family interventions. Applied & Preventive Psychology 9(2):63–88, 2000

Goodyer IM, Wilkinson PO: Practitioner Review: Therapeutics of unipolar major depressions in adolescents. J Child Psychol Psychiatry 60(3):232–243, 2019 29939396

Goodyer I, Dubicka B, Wilkinson P, et al: Selective serotonin reuptake inhibitors (SSRIs) and routine specialist care with and without cognitive behaviour therapy in adolescents with major depression: randomised controlled trial. BMJ 335(7611):142, 2007 17556431

Goodyer IM, Dubicka B, Wilkinson P, et al: A randomised controlled trial of cognitive behaviour therapy in adolescents with major depression treated by selective serotonin reuptake inhibitors. The ADAPT trial. Health Technol Assess 12(14):iii–iv, iv–60, 2008 18462573

Goodyer IM, Reynolds S, Barrett B, et al: Cognitive behavioural therapy and short-term psychoanalytical psychotherapy versus a brief psychosocial intervention in adolescents with unipolar major depressive disorder (IMPACT): a multicentre, pragmatic, observer-blind, randomised controlled superiority trial. Lancet Psychiatry 4(2):109–119, 2017 27914903

Gortner ET, Gollan JK, Dobson KS, et al: Cognitive-behavioral treatment for depression: relapse prevention. J Consult Clin Psychol 66(2):377–384, 1998 9583341

Gunlicks-Stoessel M, Mufson L, Cullen KR, et al: A pilot study of depressed adolescents' cortisol patterns during parent-adolescent conflict and response to interpersonal psychotherapy (IPT-A). J Affect Disord 150(3):1125–1128, 2013 23774139

Gunlicks-Stoessel M, Mufson L, Westervelt A, et al: A pilot SMART for developing an adaptive treatment strategy for adolescent depression. J Clin Child Adolesc Psychol 45(4):480–494, 2016 25785788

Gunlicks-Stoessel M, Eckshtain D, Lee S, et al: Latent profiles of cognitive and interpersonal risk factors for adolescent depression and implications for personalized treatment. J Abnorm Child Psychol 47(12):1957–1967, 2019a 31102063

Gunlicks-Stoessel M, Westervelt A, Reigstad K, et al: The role of attachment style in interpersonal psychotherapy for depressed adolescents. Psychother Res 29(1):78–85, 2019b 28436756

Hankin BL: Depression from childhood through adolescence: risk mechanisms across multiple systems and levels of analysis. Curr Opin Psychol 4:13–20, 2015 25692174

Israel P, Diamond GS: Feasibility of Attachment Based Family Therapy for depressed clinic-referred Norwegian adolescents. Clin Child Psychol Psychiatry 18(3):334–350, 2013 22930777
Jacobson NS, Hollon SD: Prospects for future comparisons between drugs and psychotherapy: lessons from the CBT-versus-pharmacotherapy exchange. J Consult Clin Psychol 64(1):104–108, 1996 8907089
Jacobson NS, Martell CR, Dimidjian S: Behavioral activation treatment for depression: returning to contextual roots. Clin Psychol 8(3):255–270, 2001
Jaycox LH, Asarnow JR, Sherbourne CD, et al: Adolescent primary care patients' preferences for depression treatment. Adm Policy Ment Health 33(2):198–207, 2006 16502131
Kazdin AE: Evidence-based treatments and delivery of psychological services: shifting our emphases to increase impact. Psychol Serv 5(3):201–215, 2008
Kennard BD, Emslie GJ, Mayes TL, et al: Cognitive-behavioral therapy to prevent relapse in pediatric responders to pharmacotherapy for major depressive disorder. J Am Acad Child Adolesc Psychiatry 47(12):1395–1404, 2008a 18978634
Kennard BD, Stewart SM, Hughes JL, et al: Developing cognitive behavioral therapy to prevent depressive relapse in youth. Cognit Behav Pract 15(4):387–399, 2008b 20535241
Kennard BD, Silva SG, Mayes TL, et al: Assessment of safety and long-term outcomes of initial treatment with placebo in TADS. Am J Psychiatry 166(3):337–344, 2009 19147693
Kennard BD, Emslie GJ, Mayes TL, et al: Sequential treatment with fluoxetine and relapse-prevention CBT to improve outcomes in pediatric depression. Am J Psychiatry 171(10):1083–1090, 2014 24935082
Kennard BD, Hughes JL, Foxwell AA: CBT for Depression in Children and Adolescents: A Guide to Relapse Prevention. New York, Guilford, 2016
Klomek AB, Mufson L: Interpersonal psychotherapy for depressed adolescents. Child Adolesc Psychiatr Clin N Am 15(4):959–975, 2006 16952770
Kovacs M, Feinberg TL, Crouse-Novak MA, et al: Depressive disorders in childhood, I: a longitudinal prospective study of characteristics and recovery. Arch Gen Psychiatry 41(3):229–237, 1984 6367688
Kroll L, Harrington R, Jayson D, et al: Pilot study of continuation cognitive-behavioral therapy for major depression in adolescent psychiatric patients. J Am Acad Child Adolesc Psychiatry 35(9):1156–1161, 1996 8824059
Lewinsohn PM, Clarke GN, Hops H, et al: Cognitive-behavioral treatment for depressed adolescents. Behav Ther 21(4):385–401, 1990
Maalouf FT, Brent DA: Child and adolescent depression intervention overview: what works, for whom and how well? Child Adolesc Psychiatr Clin N Am 21(2):299–312, 2012 22537728
March J, Silva S, Petrycki S, et al: Fluoxetine, cognitive-behavioral therapy, and their combination for adolescents with depression: Treatment for Adolescents With Depression Study (TADS) randomized controlled trial. JAMA 292(7):807–820, 2004 15315995
March J, Silva S, Vitiello B: The Treatment for Adolescents with Depression Study (TADS): methods and message at 12 weeks. J Am Acad Child Adolesc Psychiatry 45(12):1393–1403, 2006 17135984
March JS, Silva S, Petrycki S, et al: The Treatment for Adolescents With Depression Study (TADS): long-term effectiveness and safety outcomes. Arch Gen Psychiatry 64(10):1132–1143, 2007 17909125
Martell CR, Dimidjian S, Herman-Dunn R: Behavioral Activation for Depression: A Clinician's Guide. New York, Guilford, 2013
McCauley E, Myers K, Mitchell J, et al: Depression in young people: initial presentation and clinical course. J Am Acad Child Adolesc Psychiatry 32(4):714–722, 1993 8340290
McCauley E, Gudmundsen G, Schloredt K, et al: The adolescent behavioral activation program: adapting behavioral activation as a treatment for depression in adolescence. J Clin Child Adolesc Psychol 45(3):291–304, 2016 25602170
Mufson L, Fairbanks J: Interpersonal psychotherapy for depressed adolescents: a one-year naturalistic follow-up study. J Am Acad Child Adolesc Psychiatry 35(9):1145–1155, 1996 8824058

Mufson L, Sills R: Interpersonal Psychotherapy for depressed adolescents (IPT-A): an overview. Nord J Psychiatry 60(6):431–437, 2006 17162450
Mufson L, Moreau D, Weissman MM, et al: Modification of interpersonal psychotherapy with depressed adolescents (IPT-A): phase I and II studies. J Am Acad Child Adolesc Psychiatry 33(5):695–705, 1994 8056733
Mufson L, Weissman MM, Moreau D, et al: Efficacy of interpersonal psychotherapy for depressed adolescents. Arch Gen Psychiatry 56(6):573–579, 1999 10359475
Mufson L, Dorta KP, Wickramaratne P, et al: A randomized effectiveness trial of interpersonal psychotherapy for depressed adolescents. Arch Gen Psychiatry 61(6):577–584, 2004 15184237
Mufson L, Yanes-Lukin P, Anderson G: A pilot study of Brief IPT-A delivered in primary care. Gen Hosp Psychiatry 37(5):481–484, 2015 25997880
Mufson L, Rynn M, Yanes-Lukin P, et al: Stepped care interpersonal psychotherapy treatment for depressed adolescents: a pilot study in pediatric clinics. Adm Policy Ment Health 45(3):417–431, 2018 29124527
Nardi B, Massei M, Arimatea E, Moltedo-Perfetti A: Effectiveness of group CBT in treating adolescents with depression symptoms: a critical review. Int J Adolesc Med Health 29(3):20150080, 2016 26812765
National Institute of Mental Health: Major depression. 2017. Available at: www.nimh.nih.gov/health/statistics/major-depression.shtml. Accessed November 25, 2020.
Ng MY, Eckshtain D, Weisz JR: Assessing fit between evidence-based psychotherapies for youth depression and real-life coping in early adolescence. J Clin Child Adolesc Psychol 45(6):732–748, 2016 26043230
Ngo VK, Asarnow JR, Lange J, et al: Outcomes for youths from racial-ethnic minority groups in a quality improvement intervention for depression treatment. Psychiatr Serv 60(10):1357–1364, 2009 19797376
Oud M, de Winter L, Vermeulen-Smit E, et al: Effectiveness of CBT for children and adolescents with depression: a systematic review and meta-regression analysis. Eur Psychiatry 57:33–45, 2019 30658278
Perou R, Bitsko RH, Blumberg SJ, et al: Mental health surveillance among children—United States, 2005–2011. MMWR Suppl 62(2):1–35, 2013 23677130
Reinecke MA, Ryan NE, DuBois DL: Cognitive-behavioral therapy of depression and depressive symptoms during adolescence: a review and meta-analysis. J Am Acad Child Adolesc Psychiatry 37(1):26–34, 1998 9444896
Ritschel LA, Ramirez CL, Jones M, et al: Behavioral activation for depressed teens: a pilot study. Cognit Behav Pract 18(2):281–299, 2011
Ritschel LA, Ramirez CL, Cooley JL, et al: Behavioral activation for major depression in adolescents: results from a pilot study. Clin Psychol 23(1):39–57, 2016
Rosselló J, Bernal G: The efficacy of cognitive-behavioral and interpersonal treatments for depression in Puerto Rican adolescents. J Consult Clin Psychol 67(5):734–745, 1999 10535240
Sakolsky D, Birmaher B: Developmentally informed pharmacotherapy for child and adolescent depressive disorders. Child Adolesc Psychiatr Clin N Am 21(2):313–325, 2012 22537729
Santor DA, Kusumakar V: Open trial of interpersonal therapy in adolescents with moderate to severe major depression: effectiveness of novice IPT therapists. J Am Acad Child Adolesc Psychiatry 40(2):236–240, 2001 11211373
Siu AL; U.S. Preventive Services Task Force: Screening for depression in children and adolescents: US Preventive Services Task Force recommendation statement. Pediatrics 137(3):e20154467, 2016 26908686
Sosic-Vasic Z, Abler B, Grön G, et al: Effects of a brief cognitive behavioural therapy group intervention on baseline brain perfusion in adolescents with major depressive disorder. Neuroreport 28(6):348–353, 2017 28328739
Strober M, Lampert C, Schmidt S, Morrell W: The course of major depressive disorder in adolescents: I. Recovery and risk of manic switching in a follow-up of psychotic and nonpsychotic subtypes. J Am Acad Child Adolesc Psychiatry 32(1):34–42, 1993 8428882

Tompson MC, Boger KD, Asarnow JR: Enhancing the developmental appropriateness of treatment for depression in youth: integrating the family in treatment. Child Adolesc Psychiatr Clin N Am 21(2):345–384, 2012 22537731

Tompson MC, Langer DA, Hughes JL, et al: Family-focused treatment for childhood depression: model and case illustrations. Cognit Behav Pract 24(3):269–287, 2017a 28966545

Tompson MC, Sugar CA, Langer DA, et al: A randomized clinical trial comparing family-focused treatment and individual supportive therapy for depression in childhood and early adolescence. J Am Acad Child Adolesc Psychiatry 56(6):515–523, 2017b 28545757

Trivedi MH, Chin Fatt CR, Jha MK, et al: Comprehensive phenotyping of depression disease trajectory and risk: rationale and design of Texas Resilience Against Depression study (T-RAD). J Psychiatr Res 122:22–32, 2020 31918350

Twenge JM, Cooper AB, Joiner TE, et al: Age, period, and cohort trends in mood disorder indicators and suicide-related outcomes in a nationally representative dataset, 2005–2017. J Abnorm Psychol 128(3):185–199, 2019 30869927

Viswanathan M, Kennedy SM, McKeeman J, et al: Treatment of Depression in Children and Adolescents: A Systematic Review. Comparative Effectiveness Review No 224 (AHRQ Publ No 20-EHC005-EF). Rockville, MD, Agency for Healthcare Research and Quality, 2020

Vostanis P, Feehan C, Grattan E: Two-year outcome of children treated for depression. Eur Child Adolesc Psychiatry 7(1):12–18, 1998 9563808

Webb CA, Auerbach RP, Derubeis RJ: Processes of change in CBT of adolescent depression: review and recommendations. J Clin Child Adolesc Psychol 41(5):654–665, 2012 22867130

Weersing VR, Brent DA: Cognitive behavioral therapy for depression in youth. Child Adolesc Psychiatr Clin N Am 15(4):939–957, 2006 16952769

Weersing VR, Gonzalez A, Campo JV, et al: Brief Behavioral Therapy for pediatric anxiety and depression: piloting an integrated treatment approach. Cognit Behav Pract 12(2):126–139, 2008

Weersing VR, Brent DA, Rozenman MS, et al: Brief Behavioral Therapy for pediatric anxiety and depression in primary care: a randomized clinical trial. JAMA Psychiatry 74(6):571–578, 2017a 28423145

Weersing VR, Jeffreys M, Do MT, et al: Evidence base update of psychosocial treatments for child and adolescent depression. J Clin Child Adolesc Psychol 46(1):11–43, 2017b 27870579

Weissman MM, Wolk S, Goldstein RB, et al: Depressed adolescents grown up. JAMA 281(18):1707–1713, 1999 10328070

Weisz JR, Thurber CA, Sweeney L, et al: Brief treatment of mild-to-moderate child depression using primary and secondary control enhancement training. J Consult Clin Psychol 65(4):703–707, 1997 9256573

Weisz JR, Moore PS, Southam-Gerow MA, et al: Therapist's Manual PASCET: Primary and Secondary Control Enhancement Training Program. Los Angeles, CA, University of California, 2005

Weisz JR, McCarty CA, Valeri SM: Effects of psychotherapy for depression in children and adolescents: a meta-analysis. Psychol Bull 132(1):132–149, 2006 16435960

Weisz JR, Southam-Gerow MA, Gordis EB, et al: Cognitive-behavioral therapy versus usual clinical care for youth depression: an initial test of transportability to community clinics and clinicians. J Consult Clin Psychol 77(3):383–396, 2009 19485581

Weisz JR, Chorpita BF, Palinkas LA, et al: Testing standard and modular designs for psychotherapy treating depression, anxiety, and conduct problems in youth: a randomized effectiveness trial. Arch Gen Psychiatry 69(3):274–282, 2012 22065252

Wells KB, Kataoka SH, Asarnow JR: Affective disorders in children and adolescents: addressing unmet need in primary care settings. Biol Psychiatry 49(12):1111–1120, 2001 11430853

Wells KB, Tang L, Carlson GA, et al: Treatment of youth depression in primary care under usual practice conditions: observational findings from Youth Partners in Care. J Child Adolesc Psychopharmacol 22(1):80–90, 2012 22251025

Wood A, Harrington R, Moore A: Controlled trial of a brief cognitive-behavioural intervention in adolescent patients with depressive disorders. J Child Psychol Psychiatry 37(6):737–746, 1996 8894955

Yang L, Zhou X, Zhou C, et al: Efficacy and acceptability of cognitive behavioral therapy for depression in children: a systematic review and meta-analysis. Acad Pediatr 17(1):9–16, 2017 27989281

Zhou Y, Arend J, Mufson L, et al: Change in dysfunctional attitudes and attachment in interpersonal psychotherapy for depressed adolescents. Psychother Res 30:1–9, 2020 32351173

Zuckerbrot RA, Cheung A, Jensen PS, et al: Guidelines for Adolescent Depression in Primary Care (GLAD-PC): Part I. Practice preparation, identification, assessment, and initial management. Pediatrics 141(3):e20174081, 2018 29483200

PART VI

Integrative Management of Mood Disorders

CHAPTER 28

Practice Guidelines for Major Depressive Disorder

Michael E. Thase, M.D.

Whereas the 1960s and 1970s were turbulent decades, rife with social unrest and political upheaval, they were also times of trailblazing advances in research on neurobiology and therapeutics of psychiatric disorders. With the publication of DSM-III (American Psychiatric Association 1980), a more reliable and operationally specified approach to diagnosis was introduced to psychiatric practice, and with respect to mood disorders, the several clinically meaningful nonbipolar depressive states were—for the first time—grouped together. By the early 1980s, there was growing therapeutic optimism that most people seeking treatment for moderate to severe episodes of major depressive disorder (MDD) could be treated effectively by a series of conscientiously delivered trials with the three proven forms of "somatic" therapy that were available at that time: tricyclic antidepressants (TCAs), monoamine oxidase inhibitors (MAOIs), and electroconvulsive therapy (ECT) (Klein et al. 1983). Parallel developments led to the first time-limited, manual-based models of psychotherapy specifically developed to treat MDD; these focused forms of psychotherapy appeared to have efficacy comparable to that of TCAs in the first generation of randomized controlled trials (RCTs) of depressed outpatients (Rush et al. 1977; Weissman et al. 1979). By the end of the 1980s, the initial members of a newer generation of antidepressant medications—fluoxetine and bupropion—were beginning to replace the TCAs as preferred options for depressed outpatients (American Psychiatric Association 2000; Depression Guideline Panel 1993a). These were times of exhilarating therapeutic optimism, as showcased by the National Institute of Mental Health (NIMH) Depression Awareness, Recognition, and Treatment (DART) Program, which aimed to reduce stigma, increase recognition, and improve access to treatment of MDD (Regier et al. 1988).

Not all in psychiatry was rosy, however, and there was growing recognition of a large gap between the evidence of what was possible in the treatment of MDD, as extrapolated from RCTs, and the care that was provided by clinicians working outside of research settings. This discrepancy was, in fact, broadly evident across areas of clinical medicine, leading a new federal organization, the Agency for Health Care Policy and Research (AHCPR), to ask the National Academy of Sciences Institute of Medicine to convene a work group on the development of practice guidelines (see Field and Lohr 1990). Their report (Institute of Medicine [US] Committee on Clinical Practice Guidelines 1992) acknowledged the importance of conventional methods used to derive expert consensus, but also embraced a process that incorporated strategies promulgated by the growing evidence-based medicine movement (i.e., systematic review, grading the strength of research evidence, and meta-analyses).

The report also provided a guideline for the development of practice guidelines (Institute of Medicine [US] Committee on Clinical Practice Guidelines 1992). The Institute of Medicine report suggested that the work groups charged with the development of practice guidelines (PGs) should be multidisciplinary, have the expertise in the field and a command of the relevant literature, and, to the extent possible, be gender and geographically balanced. The report suggested that the work group's leader should be an expert with strong skills in facilitating group processes and recommended adequate administrative support for note taking and writing. It also was suggested that the work groups include a methodologist or biostatistician with expertise in clinical research, a health care economist, and an expert in the process of guideline development. Involvement of patient/consumer representatives also was recommended, either as a member of the work group or as part of the prepublication review process. The report also advised editorial oversight to ensure that the recommendations were worded clearly and precisely, avoiding medical aphorisms such as "when clinically appropriate." Lastly, the report presciently warned about the need for the guideline process to be transparent both to professionals and to the public and readily available for dissemination to stakeholders.

The reports from the Institute of Medicine (Field and Lohr 1990; Institute of Medicine [US] Committee on Clinical Practice Guidelines 1992) set in motion a process that directly led to the development of what, to some, might have seemed like a veritable tidal wave of PGs, including some commissioned by the AHCPR (see McCormick and Fleming 1992) and others overseen by professional organizations. In the United States, the American Psychiatric Association (APA) established a Steering Committee on Practice Guidelines. Two of the inaugural group of PGs focused on the assessment and treatment of depressive disorders. One, which was funded by the AHCPR to specifically focus on primary care practitioners (PCPs), was developed by a multidisciplinary panel (Depression Guideline Panel 1993a, 1993b, 1993c). The other, primarily intended to guide the practice of psychiatrists in the United States, was prepared by a work group made up of psychiatrists who were members of the sponsoring organizations (American Psychiatric Association 2000).

In the nearly 30 years that have followed, a number of novel interventions for MDD have passed muster and have been introduced into practice; the methods, strategies, and tactics used in clinical practice have evolved; and the evidence base that underpins contemporary psychiatric practice has grown at a staggering pace. As predicted in the Institute of Medicine report (Institute of Medicine [US] Committee on Clinical Practice Guidelines 1992), guideline development has necessarily required an ongoing, iterative process, with periodic updates necessary to keep the PGs up to date, perhaps as often as every 5 years, given the rapid pace of discovery in clinical science.

It is also important to keep in mind that guideline development, like the practice of medicine itself, does not occur in a vacuum and is shaped by numerous societal and organizational forces. For example, in 1999, lawmakers judged that the initial mission of the AHCPR had been accomplished and, according to new federal legislation, the organization was renamed the Agency for Healthcare Research and Quality (AHRQ). Rather than having responsibility for directly supporting guideline development, the mission of the AHRQ was narrowed to supporting systematic reviews and meta-analyses and providing a clearinghouse for PGs prepared by professional organizations. The Institute of Medicine likewise counseled greater attention to recognition and management of potential conflicts of interest (Institute of Medicine 2009) and refinements in the methods used for guideline development (Institute of Medicine 2011a, 2011b); in 2015, this venerable organization underwent a name change, becoming the National Academy of Medicine.

This chapter reviews the progress in guideline development for the treatment of patients with MDD, with a particular focus on the PGs produced by the APA. Some of the limitations of these PGs are highlighted, as is the changing nature of the challenges faced by guideline development work groups. For context, the chapter begins with a brief review of the initial PG supported by the AHCPR (Depression Guideline Panel 1993a, 1993b, 1993c), followed by subsequent developments for PCPs. Next, the three editions of the APA PG for MDD are examined, paying greatest attention to the most recent edition (American Psychiatric Association 2010). As several confluent forces have led the APA's steering committee to put the development process "on hiatus," the third edition of the APA PG for MDD has become a bit "long in the tooth," and it is not certain when the fourth edition will be completed. As a result, more recently updated PGs, such as the ones produced by the Canadian Network for Mood and Anxiety Treatments (CANMAT; Lam et al. 2016), the U.S. Department of Veterans Affairs and U.S. Department of Defense (2016), and the American Psychological Association (2019), are called on as needed.

Primary Care Practice Guidelines

Chaired by A. John Rush, a psychiatrist with expertise in the treatment of depressive disorders, the initial PG was authored by a 12-member multidisciplinary panel that included representatives of most key stakeholders, including consultation-liaison psychiatry, primary care, nursing, social work, clinical psychology, and patient/consumer groups. The panel commissioned reports by expert consultants, who conducted narrative reviews of the literature (see, e.g., Jarrett and Rush 1994) or, when practicable, systematic reviews and meta-analyses of RCTs (see, e.g., Thase et al. 1995). The final document consisted of two main volumes, the first summarizing evidence pertaining to diagnosis and assessment (Depression Guideline Panel 1993b) and the second devoted to treatment (Depression Guideline Panel 1993c). A third, briefer volume also was produced to provide a concise guide to the PG's main recommendations (Depression Guideline Panel 1993a).

The recommendations of the Depression Guideline Panel (1993a, 1993c) for the treatment of MDD followed the three-phase temporal structure popularized by Kupfer (1991). From this perspective, the goals of each of the three treatment phases were tied to specific outcomes of particular interest: acute-phase therapy/response and remission; continuation-phase therapy/recovery and relapse prevention; and maintenance-phase therapy/sustained recovery and prevention of recurrent depressive episodes (Figure 28–1). The PG recommended use of standardized measures of depressive symptom severity to assess treatment outcomes, although it recognized that short, efficient, and freely available measures of patient-rated outcomes (PROs) were not yet available.

For most MDD patients encountered by PCPs, the Depression Guideline Panel (1993a, 1993c) recommended treatment with either antidepressant pharmacotherapy or—if available and preferred—a focused psychosocial intervention such as cognitive-behavioral therapy (CBT) or interpersonal psychotherapy (IPT). The guideline panel noted that a far greater weight of empirical support favored the used of antidepressant pharmacotherapy compared with focused psychotherapies and cautioned that issues with access to and reimbursement for services were barriers to use of all forms of psychotherapy. At the time the initial guidelines were developed, the panel recognized that the selective serotonin reuptake inhibitors (SSRIs) and bupropion—a norepinephrine-dopamine reuptake inhibitor (NDRI)—were likely better tolerated, safer in overdose, and easier for clinicians to prescribe than the TCAs. Yet, the panel also noted that the older antidepressants, which were widely available in generic formulations, were less costly than the newer medications. Although valid cost-effectiveness analyses comparing the older and newer antidepressants in primary care settings were not available to the panel, they recognized that for the patients for whom a TCA was both well tolerated and properly titrated to a therapeutic dosage, the use of TCAs likely resulted in lower treatment costs.

Eschewing the preferred practice of many psychiatrists, the panel noted that combining psychotherapy and pharmacotherapy was not commonly done in primary care and concluded, on the basis of a narrative review of RCTs conducted in psychiatric outpatients (Jarrett and Rush 1994), that combined treatment had only a modest added benefit for the average person seeking treatment for MDD. The PG thus recommended the combination of psychotherapy and pharmacotherapy for patients with more severe, chronic, or complicated forms of MDD.

With respect to the management of patients who were not responsive to standard pharmacotherapies—a clinical entity now widely referred to as *treatment-resistant depression* (TRD)—the PG recommended referral to specialty care but also provided recommendations for advanced or sequenced management strategies. Ironically, a PG developed for PCPs thus provided the impetus for the Thase-Rush classification system for TRD (Thase and Rush 1995, 1997). These efforts presaged the hierarchical or stepped-care paradigms for management of TRD that were implemented in the Texas Medication Algorithm Project (Trivedi et al. 2004) and tested prospectively by the massive Sequenced Treatment Alternatives to Relieve Depression (STAR*D) project funded by the National Institute of Mental Health (Fava et al. 2003; Rush et al. 2004, 2006).

Although influential and generally well received by stakeholders, the treatment recommendations of the Depression Guideline Panel (1993c) suffered from one unavoidable limitation—namely, the fact that the vast majority of the RCTs of antidepres-

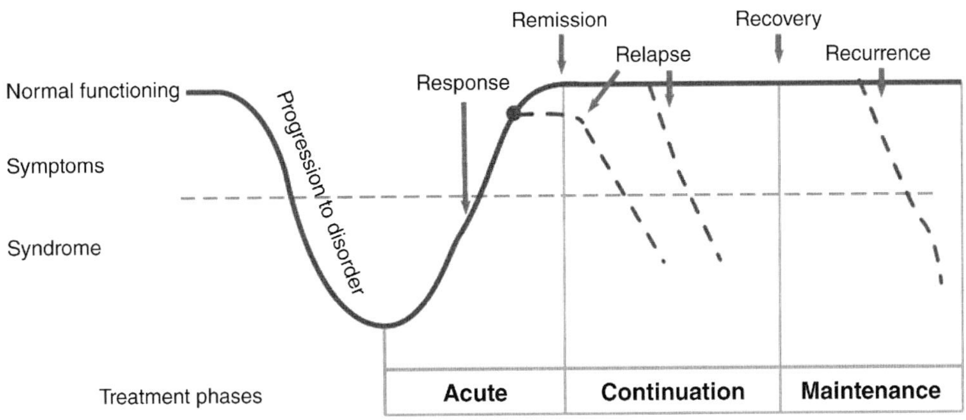

FIGURE 28–1. Temporal course of an episode of depression, pairing clinical milestones—or transitions in illness state—with phases of treatment.

The five treatment outcomes of interest include three sequential states reflecting progressively greater benefit (response, remission, and recovery) and two states reflecting hazards after response to treatment (relapse and recurrence). (Definitions for remission, recovery, relapse, and recurrence were first advanced by a working group in 1991 [Frank et al. 1991].) For pharmacotherapy, the phases of treatment are acute, continuation, and maintenance; whereas most patients who respond to antidepressants should receive 6–9 months of continuation-phase therapy, the maintenance phase—which can be indefinite in duration—is usually reserved for patients with a history of three or more lifetime episodes.

Source. Adapted from Kupfer DJ: "Long-Term Treatment of Depression." *The Journal of Clinical Psychiatry* 52 (Suppl):28–34, 1991.

sants and psychotherapies that populated its evidence tables had been conducted in specialty care settings (e.g., psychiatric or psychological research clinics). This shortcoming was slowly remedied over the next several decades, as reflected in the updated evidence tables prepared for the AHCPR (Mulrow et al. 1999; Schulberg et al. 1998). After the mission of the agency was somewhat revised and rebranded, the AHRQ supported a continuous process to update the evidence base for management of MDD in primary care (see, e.g., Gartlehner et al. 2008, 2011, 2016, 2017). These reviews helped to form the evidence base for a newer generation of PGs for the treatment of MDD in primary care settings, including those sponsored by the American College of Physicians (Qaseem et al. 2008, 2016) and one developed by the Institute for Clinical Systems Improvement (Trangle et al. 2016). Other brief, freely accessible and reasonably up-to-date PGs for PCPs can be found on the internet, including one developed for use by the University of Wisconsin Health Network (first released in April 2015) (UW Health 2015) and an adaptation found on the Dartmouth-Hitchcock Knowledge Map website (first released in 2017) (Dartmouth-Hitchcock 2017).

All of the newer PGs for PCPs explicitly incorporate the key features of collaborative care (American Psychiatric Association and Academy of Psychosomatic Medicine 2016), including routine use of care managers and PROs, such as the nine-item version of the Patient Health Questionnaire (PHQ-9; Kroenke et al. 2001). Guidelines thus provide templates to help ensure that adherence to treatment is maximized and outcomes are monitored on a timely basis and that when the initial choice of therapy is ineffective, there is a logical progression through evidence-based treatment algorithms (see American Psychiatric Association and Academy of Psychosomatic Medicine 2016). All contemporary PGs for PCPs also recognize that since the introduction of inexpensive, generic formulations of the SSRIs, bupropion, and several other newer-generation antidepressants, these medications have become the first line of pharmacotherapy for MDD. These PGs show increasing confidence that self-help strategies and exercise can have helpful effects, in combination both with "watchful waiting" and with conventional therapies. The use of focused forms of therapy, including CBT, IPT, and several newer adaptations of behavior therapy, as alternatives to pharmacotherapy is endorsed across PGs. In fact, the American College of Physicians PG concluded with a statement of equipoise with respect to selection of CBT or newer-generation antidepressants, with the caveat that patient preference needs to be taken into account after appropriate psychoeducation about the expected treatment effects, likely adverse effects, cost, and access to care options.

Practice Guidelines for Psychiatrists

APA Practice Guideline for Major Depressive Disorder

First Edition

The first edition of the APA PG for MDD (American Psychiatric Association 1993) was produced by a work group of six psychiatrists, led by T. Byram Karasu, M.D. The work group members volunteered their time across nearly 2 years. Although not an interventions researcher, Professor Karasu was well versed in contemporary treatment research, having edited a massive two-volume text on psychiatric therapeutics published by the APA (Karasu 1984a, 1984b). He also was the editor-in-chief of the *American Journal of Psychotherapy* and was widely known for his advocacy of biopsychosocial models of treatment. APA staff performed literature searches, which were reviewed by assigned group members, who in turn wrote narrative reviews. The work group members did not conduct their own systematic reviews and did not have access to the systematic reviews and meta-analyses conducted as part of the development of the AHCPR's PG. The group's expert consensus was used to rate confidence in each specific recommendation made by the PG using three levels or grades: I (substantial clinical confidence), II (moderate clinical confidence), and III (may be recommended in some clinical circumstances). An abridged version of their final product, a slim 26-page summary of the PG's recommendations and the state of the evidence in the areas reviewed, was published as a supplement in the April 1993 issue of the *American Journal of Psychiatry* (American Psychiatric Association 1993). It is no longer possible to retrieve this document from the journal's web-based archives. By design, separate PGs for management of bipolar disorder and suicidal behavior contemporaneously developed by the steering committee (see psychiatryonline.org/guidelines).

The first edition of the APA PG for MDD provided a concise and well-reasoned summary of many aspects of psychiatric care for depressed patients at the beginning of the final decade of the twentieth century. At the time, TCAs were the best-proven antidepressants, though clinical experience was growing with fluoxetine (introduced in 1987 as the first member of the SSRI class of antidepressants in the United States) and bupropion (a drug with an aminoketone structure thought to work as an NDRI).

For patients who did not respond to these first lines of pharmacotherapy, MAOIs and ECT were recommended with highest confidence. There was growing certainty in the value of longer-term or maintenance-phase pharmacotherapy for the prevention of recurrent depressive episodes when the benefits were judged to outweigh the risks.

Some dissenters suggested that the APA PG for MDD, with its reliance on the consensus of a small group of psychiatrists, suffered in comparison to the PG produced by the multidisciplinary Depression Guideline Panel (1993a). This suggested difference was particularly evident in recommendations pertaining to use of the newer, time-limited psychotherapies (see, e.g., Persons et al. 1996). It was asserted that by relying too heavily on clinical experience and expert consensus, the PG overestimated confidence in more traditional, longer-term dynamic and supportive approaches to psychotherapy, which had not been subjected to more rigorous controlled studies (Persons et al. 1996). In contrast to the AHCPR PG, the initial APA PG recommended combined psychotherapy and pharmacotherapy regimens "with highest confidence." The strength of this recommendation, without definitive meta-analytic support, was noteworthy because psychiatrists are the one group of mental health care providers who are trained to routinely provide combined treatment.

Second Edition

An updated revision of the APA PG for MDD was published as a supplement to the *American Journal of Psychiatry* in 2000 (American Psychiatric Association 2000). Professor Karasu again led a small work group of APA members who volunteered their efforts, strengthened by the addition of a consulting methodologist who was an early-career psychiatrist, Philip Wang. The wisdom of the choice of Dr. Wang, who had just completed advanced training in psychiatric epidemiology, is illustrated by his subsequent career trajectory, which has included stints as deputy director of NIMH and director of research for the APA.

Although the development process did not include conducting or commissioning new systematic reviews or meta-analyses, work group members were provided comprehensive literature searches in key content areas, which included—to the extent available—the most recently published meta-analyses. Evidence tables thus were prepared to summarize a progressively growing treatment literature. In particular, the work group relied heavily on systematic review and meta-analysis of the efficacy of newer-generation antidepressants supported by the AHCPR (Mulrow et al. 1999). On the basis of the evidence review, clinical experience, and the expert consensus of the work group, the level of confidence in various PG recommendations was again graded using the three-category ranking.

At 45 pages, the published summary of the PG was nearly twice the length of its progenitor (American Psychiatric Association 2000). Although the abridged version is no longer retrievable from the *American Journal of Psychiatry*'s web-based archives, the full version of the PG can be found in a published compendium of the APA's PGs (American Psychiatric Association 2006). The greater length and more extensive literature review of the second edition of the PG reflected the growing evidence base and larger number of options for the treatment of MDD at the beginning of the twenty-first century. The second edition also incorporated the transition in the nomenclature to DSM-IV (American Psychiatric Association 1994). The PG implicitly reflected the field's growing emphasis on outpatient care, even for many patients with more severe or treatment-resistant episodes of illness. The decreasing role of inpatient treatment was one by-product of converging societal forces to reduce the cost of health care.

Like its predecessor, the second edition of the APA PG for MDD was divided into three main parts. Part A summarized the main treatment recommendations, formulation and implementation of a treatment plan, and special clinical considerations that were known to influence the treatment process. Part B provided more detailed summaries of the evidence that underpinned the PG's recommendations. A short third section, Part C, outlined areas of unmet need and made recommendations for future research.

With respect to treatment recommendations, the second edition of the PG provided a more balanced review of the evidence supporting the use of newer, time-limited psychotherapies, noting a growing number of RCTs of increasing methodological sophistication (see, e.g., Thase 2001). Time-limited psychotherapy was now recommended with greater confidence as an alternative to pharmacotherapy for outpatients across a broader range of severity of MDD. The revised PG also provided a more tempered view of the additive benefits of psychotherapy and pharmacotherapy combinations. Although the PG continued to have the highest confidence for combined treatment, this treatment approach was recommended as "most useful" for individuals with moderate to severe MDD episodes and social/interpersonal problems or personality disorders.

Looking back at the document 20 years later, it is sobering to be reminded that all but two of today's most widely prescribed antidepressants—the SSRI escitalopram and the serotonin-norepinephrine reuptake inhibitor (SNRI) duloxetine—were already in common use in 2000. That said, none of the newer generation antidepressants were yet available in generic formulations. As a result, questions pertaining to cost-effectiveness and cost-benefit were quite topical for clinicians consulting the PG. It is therefore unfortunate that the APA PG development process did not include an expert in health care economics in the work group. On the basis of the literature reviewed, clinical experience, and expert opinion, the PG recommended as first-line therapies the entire group of SSRIs, venlafaxine (the first SNRI to reach the U.S. market), and bupropion (which was available in immediate- and sustained-release formulations), as well as two older drugs available in generic formulations, the secondary-amine TCAs desipramine and nortriptyline. Several other less widely prescribed newer antidepressants—mirtazapine and nefazodone—and the remaining TCAs were recommended as second-line interventions, with the MAOIs generally reserved for third- our fourth-line use.

Although not buttressed by pharmacoeconomic calculations, the PG's recommendations were consistent with the state of the art and reflected the field's growing confidence that the newer-generation antidepressants conveyed advantages over the TCAs in terms of tolerability and safety, without offering a significant loss of efficacy for depressed outpatients (see Mulrow et al. 1999). In fact, it is now known that by 2000, when the second edition of the PG was published, the newer-generation antidepressants already accounted for a large majority of new prescriptions for antidepressants in the United States (Luo et al. 2020).

The second edition of the APA PG for MDD also provided a brief summary of the state of the art for patients with TRD. The PG recommendations showed higher confidence for older strategies, such as switching from an SSRIs to a TCA or—with appropriate washout—from a TCA to an MAOIs, use of lithium or thyroid hormone to "augment" an ineffective antidepressant, or ECT. It is interesting to note that the practice of combining antidepressants—now commonplace—is barely discussed. It is noteworthy that when the second edition of the PG was published, there were no data yet in the published literature to support the use of second-generation antipsychotics as adjuncts to antidepressants. With respect to neuromodulation strategies, the therapeutic applications of transcranial magnetic stimulation (TMS) were just beginning to be explored, and vagus nerve stimulation (VNS) was only being studied as an alternative for treatment-resistant epilepsy. The therapeutic potential of ketamine for patients with more advanced levels of treatment resistance also was largely unknown; the first report on the rapid antidepressant effects of an intravenous infusion of ketamine (0.5 mg/kg) in an eight-patient study using a crossover design had just gone to press (Berman et al. 2000).

Third Edition

Work on the third edition of the APA PG for MDD (American Psychiatric Association 2010) began in 2005. The work group had a new chair, Alan Gelenberg, a "veteran" of the first two editions, the editor-in-chief of the *Journal of Clinical Psychiatry*, and an expert psychopharmacologist. The work group was still limited to only psychiatrists and, as such, did not include a biostatistician or health care economist. The composition of the work group was expanded to include new members with expertise in a broader range of areas of intervention research, including focused psychotherapies, complementary medicine, and women's mental health.

The years between publication of the second and third editions of the APA PG for MDD were a time of important developments in psychiatric therapeutics, including both the introduction of new medications and the publication of the results of several of the large-scale intervention studies supported by NIMH, most notably STAR*D (see Rush et al. 2006). In 2004 the FDA had affixed a "black box warning" to all antidepressant medications that advised of the risk of onset or exacerbation of suicidal ideation and behavior, based on RCTs, in children, adolescents, and young adults (Hammad et al. 2006). Although the pace of introduction of new antidepressants had slowed, the last two members of the newer generation of antidepressants that would become commercial "blockbusters," escitalopram and duloxetine, were approved by the FDA and assimilated into practitioners' personal algorithms and various formularies. Two other "new" antidepressants that would not reach this exalted commercial milestone also were introduced to clinical practice: a transdermal or skin patch formulation of the MAOI selegiline, first synthesized in the 1970s, and the SNRI desvenlafaxine, the principal active metabolite of venlafaxine. Other events in antidepressant development included approval of a once-daily (XL) formulation of bupropion and controlled release (CR) formulations of the SSRIs paroxetine and fluvoxamine. Conversely, evidence of hepatic toxicity had largely ended the use of nefazodone.

The appellation "newer-generation antidepressants" had become increasingly hackneyed in the years leading up to the third edition of the PG; November 2007 marked the twentieth anniversary of the introduction of Prozac. From the overlapping perspectives of patients, prescribers, and organizational payers of pharmaceuticals, a more important development was that, beginning with citalopram and fluoxetine, generic formulations began to become available for the most widely prescribed antidepressants. As the number of generic options increased and the cost of antidepressants predictably tumbled, brand loyalty was rapidly supplanted by market force economics, and by 2010, most of the antidepressant therapy in the United States was conducted with generic medications (Cheng et al. 2017).

Another sea change in the therapeutics of depressive disorders involved the expanding roles of medications originally developed to treat schizophrenia and mania. Although the recommended use of first-generation antipsychotic medications was largely limited to adjunctive treatment of patients with psychotic features in the second edition of the APA PG for MDD (American Psychiatric Association 2000), several members of the class of second-generation antipsychotics (SGAs) were increasingly used to treat patients with difficult-to-treat depressive disorders (Thase 2002). By the end of the decade, a large body of research demonstrated the value of SGAs for adjunctive therapy of nonpsychotic depressive episodes that did not benefit from standard antidepressants (Nelson and Papakostas 2009), and two of these medications—aripiprazole in 2007 and quetiapine in 2009—had received FDA approval for this indication. Parallel developments in the therapeutics of bipolar depression led to FDA approval of a combination of olanzapine and fluoxetine for bipolar I depressive episodes (in 2003) and quetiapine monotherapy for treatment of bipolar I and bipolar II depressive episodes (in 2007).

Data from a number of smaller studies began to emerge to support the use of TMS as a nonpharmacological alternative for patients who did not respond adequately to antidepressants (Holtzheimer et al. 2001; Loo and Mitchell 2005). Although the pivotal study of one device for administration of TMS failed to show a meaningful benefit (as compared with a double-blind sham intervention) for MDD patients with more advanced levels of TRD (O'Reardon et al. 2007), the FDA judged that the benefits outweighed the relatively low risks of this intervention and approved the device in 2007. For patients with nonresponse to only one adequate trial of antidepressant pharmacotherapy, the efficacy of 4–6 weeks of week TMS was generally comparable to that of other second-line therapies (Demitrack and Thase 2009).

VNS was approved by the FDA in 2005 for the treatment of more advanced states of TRD (O'Reardon et al. 2006). Although results of the double-blind portion of a larger-scale RCT of VNS were not positive on the primary dependent measure (Rush et al. 2005), the outcomes of the 1-year controlled follow-up study did suggest a slowly emerging benefit for a significant minority of patients compared with those in a matched historical comparison group (George et al. 2005). Despite FDA approval, use of this more invasive and expensive intervention in clinical practice was greatly inhibited by the fact that few, if any, insurance companies would pay for treatment.

The primary responsibilities of the work group members, including reviewing the evidence tables prepared for their assigned content areas and updating or drafting the corresponding sections of the PG, were essentially completed by midyear 2009. However, as the work of the group was winding down, several confluent developments cast doubts on the integrity of the process of guideline development and shook confidence in the value of the particular PG that was under development. First, there was increasing mistrust of the research conducted by the pharmaceutical industry (Angell 2008) and of the ways that the industry interacted with physicians to promote their products (see, e.g., Angell 2009). In fact, dating back to the phenomenal commercial success of Prozac, antidepressants had been one of the most profitable classes of medications, yet several highly publicized reports (see, e.g., Fournier et al. 2010; Kirsch et al. 2008) suggested that the specific value of these medications (over and above nonspecific factors) had been grossly exaggerated. Such assertions were not without merit, as the actual mean drug versus placebo difference in meta-analyses, as derived from complete datasets from Phase III studies submitted by the pharmaceutical industry for review by the FDA, was relatively modest, perhaps even below the margin of clinical significance (Kirsch et al. 2008). A meta-analysis of individual patient data from six studies funded by NIMH or foundations, which was in press at the time, yielded strikingly similar results (Fournier et al. 2010).

Second, another in-press paper using FDA submission data showed that overestimation of the specific benefits of antidepressants occurred, at least in part, because the sponsors of the research—the pharmaceutical industry—had selectively published their studies with positive results (and, by implication, systematically suppressed publication of studies with negative results or failed studies) (Turner et al. 2008). A subsequent report from the FDA (Khin et al. 2011) confirmed that almost one-half of the Phase III trials of newer-generation antidepressants had failed to detect significant drug versus placebo differences (Khin et al. 2011). Because the data tables used by the PG work group were based on computer searches of the published literature, the conclusions about the strength of the evidence were likely to be inflated by publication bias.

Third, there were growing concerns about the propriety of academicians—perhaps most particularly those who were members of PG work groups—having any income-earning relationships with the pharmaceutical industry (Institute of Medicine 2009). Similar concerns were voiced about the propriety of industry funding received by professional organizations (see, e.g., Rothman et al. 2009). As NIMH, universities, and professional organizations such as the APA endeavored throughout the decade to develop and implement methods to manage the potential for bias resulting from industry relations, Cosgrove et al. (2009) reported that nearly 90% of the authors of the second editions of the APA PGs on schizophrenia, bipolar disorder, and MDD had had "undisclosed financial ties" to the pharmaceutical industry. In the zeitgeist of that moment, it mattered only a little that the ties were "undisclosed" because the APA did not report potential conflicts of interests when these second edition PGs were written. Nor was it noted that—commencing in the early 2000s—most academicians had been routinely reporting the nature and extent of their earnings to their universities and NIMH.

Tarring the volunteer efforts of the participants with the broad charge of "undisclosed industry ties" also ignored legitimate ongoing debate about distinctions among the various types of collaborations with the pharmaceutical industry, including several that had widely acknowledged benefits for society, such as unrestricted research grants to investigate the mechanism of action of novel compounds or the opportunity to consult on the best methodology for detecting drug effects in RCTs (see, e.g., Healy and Thase 2003). Nevertheless, the findings of Cosgrove et al. (2009) resonated with the recommendations of a contemporaneous report from the Institute of Medicine (2009), leading some to call for a particularly draconian remedy to manage apparent conflicts of interest: forbidding experts with any "financial ties" to industry from participating in PG development.

Concerns about the impact of conflicts of interest on the integrity of guideline development were germane to the ongoing work of the APA Steering Committee for Development of Clinical Practice Guidelines: Professor Gelenberg and all but one member of the work group for the third edition of the PG for MDD had "financial ties" to the pharmaceutical industry. In fact, throughout the 4-plus years of the guideline development process, the work group members had dutifully disclosed their financial relationships with pharmaceutical companies; these relationships were summarized in the report (American Psychiatric Association 2010). After some review and debate, the steering committee chose to ignore the Institute of Medicine's draconian recommendation, which would have necessitated scuttling the almost complete third edition of the APA PG for MDD. Instead, the steering committee recruited an independent review panel of experts without significant industry ties to review drafts of the PG and to provide feedback if and when questions arose. This iterative process had to bring about satisfactory resolution of all questions before the next draft of the PG could move forward.

In addition to this process to try to eliminate industry bias, successive drafts of the PG were next reviewed by members of the steering committee, other relevant APA committees and work groups, and the APA's governing bodies. Next, reviews and suggestions were solicited from representatives of numerous other professional organizations and patient advocacy groups. Lastly, an "open call" for comments was made in trade newspapers and e-mail blasts; 15 organizations and 71 individuals ultimately provided written comments. The work group members and the APA's professional editorial staff carefully reviewed and, as necessary, revised the drafts in response to these rounds of comments. The PG received final prepublication approval by the APA in May 2010 (about 6 months later than originally planned), and a summary of the PG was published as a supplement to the October issue of the *American Journal of Psychiatry*. A copy of the PG can be downloaded from the APA's website (psychiatryonline.org/guidelines).

In response to changing perceptions of the use and misuse of PGs, the third edition of the APA PG for MDD began with an expanded statement of intent. Caveats included a disclaimer that the PG was not intended to represent the standard of medical care and a cautionary note that the recommendations of the PG were not intended to be followed in a lockstep or rigid manor. The authors of the PG reminded readers that, ultimately, patient care and treatment recommendations were the responsibility of the treating psychiatrist, who should take into account all available information about that particular person and all other relevant sources of knowledge that might specifically affect his or her care. Lastly, it was acknowledged that guideline adherence was not proven to improve patient outcomes and that newer treatment options may become available to change treatment practices.

The third edition of the APA PG for MDD (American Psychiatric Association 2010) was again structured in three segments: Part A summarized treatment recommendations, Part B provided more detailed reviews of the evidence underpinning the recommendations, and Part C offered recommendations for future research to address areas of unmet need or knowledge gaps in the literature. Confidence in the specific recommendations summarized in Part A was again rated using the three ordinally ranked grades (levels I, II, and III), as determined by the work group's consensus ratings. At 152 pages in length, the PG was more than three times the length of its immediate predecessor. The recommendations of the PG were supported by nearly 1,200 references, including hundreds of citations from research conducted in the preceding decade. Although some sections are now outdated, the third edition of the PG for MDD provided a fairly broad yet detailed summary of an approach to psychiatric management that is still reflective of the state of the art as we enter the third decade of the twenty-first century. The following subsections provide a synopsis of the major recommendations.

Overview of psychiatric management. More so than in earlier editions, the third edition of the MDD PG went to some length to outline the recommended components of the clinical management provided by psychiatrists. For most recommendations about clinical management, the PG work group had level I certainty. The PG emphasized that clinical management was the foundation of the care provided by psychiatrists and that establishing and maintaining a therapeutic alliance was a key component of care. The specific direction of the care provided should be guided by a comprehensive and individualized treatment plan, which in turn should be based on a thorough assessment. The assessment should include the tasks necessary to make a psychiatric diagnosis and gain understanding about the patient's developmental, medical, and social histories as well as current vocational and social functioning (Table 28–1). The psychiatric evaluation should be accompanied by a physical examination and laboratory tests if clinically indicated to rule out the role of a general medical illness. A comprehensive treatment plan also should include attention to the behaviors and routines that promote a healthy lifestyle, such as regular aerobic exercise, attention to sleep hygiene and nutrition, and curbing use of tobacco, alcohol, marijuana, and other intoxicating substances.

Recognizing that many depressed people experience a sense of hopelessness and/or least some thoughts of the futility of life or actual suicidal ideation and that most people who commit suicide are suffering from depression, the PG emphasized that evaluation of safety was one of the most critical aspects of the initial assessment. The safety assessment should include directly asking the patient about his or her current suicidal thoughts and any past history of suicidal behavior. When suicidal thoughts are evident, the assessment should include determining the strength of intent, whether or not plans have been made, and/or whether there are means available. Identification of means, commonly including access to large supplies of medication or firearms, conveys the obligation to incorporate means restriction into a safety plan. Assessment of moderating or potentially exacerbating factors, such as level of current social support, living alone, or recent interpersonal or vocational losses, is also recommended. As part of the safety assessment, the psychiatrist should ascertain if there are particular clinical features present that are known to heighten the risk of suicidal behavior or completed suicide, including psychosis, severe anxiety, or substance abuse. The PG noted that on occasion, a safety assessment may need to include the risk of homicidal or other physically dangerous behavior and, in more severe depressive states, to ensure that dehydration or self-starvation are not jeopardizing the individual's life.

As directly informed by the safety assessment, the psychiatrist next should establish the most clinically appropriate setting to begin treatment. Choice of treatment setting—outpatient, inpatient, or some setting in between (e.g., intensive outpatient or partial hospital programs)—is guided by the risk of suicide or other dangerous be-

TABLE 28–1. Key elements of psychiatric clinical management

The initial visit

1. Establish rapport and address the patient's concerns and questions as the basis for fostering a therapeutic alliance.
2. Conduct as complete a psychiatric assessment as practicable.
   - Establish a likely diagnosis or construct a hierarchical differential diagnosis.
   - Collect baseline measures of symptom intensity.
   - Identify contributing comorbidities.
   - Assess functional status and areas of critical role impairment.
   - Perform a safety assessment for suicidality and threats to others.
   - Determine the most appropriate level of care based on the above considerations.
3. When indicated, either conduct a physical exam and appropriate laboratory studies or ensure prompt referral for a more expert assessment.
4. Present impressions and recommendations, taking patient preference into account.
5. Provide psychoeducation about the condition and recommended treatment (to the patient and, if relevant and the patient consents, to significant others):
   - Likelihood and time course of benefit
   - Possible side effects
   - Plans for emergency or answering questions
6. Coordinate care with other health care providers (i.e., counselor, therapist, or primary care practitioner).
7. Plan for follow-up.

Follow-up visits

1. Assess progress, including collecting follow-up measures of symptom intensity.
2. Recheck safety and level of care assessments.
3. Query for side effects and ascertain severity and impact.
4. Gauge patient's level of satisfaction with treatment plan.
5. Revise treatment plan in relation to items 1–3.
6. Provide ongoing psychoeducation.
7. Plan for ongoing follow-up.

havior, the level of care that is judged to be most likely to promote recovery, and the ethical principle of recommending the least restrictive care setting appropriate for the patient's condition. By 2010, inpatient care for patients with MDD was largely reserved for those who posed a serious and imminent threat to themselves or others or, less commonly, patients who were so severely ill that they were unable to care for themselves. The fortunately uncommon need for involuntary treatment was outlined, particularly for a depressed patient judged to be at great risk for self-harm but refusing to accept treatment voluntarily, and it was noted that the criteria for commitment and the parameters of involuntary hospitalization varied by state and by other jurisdictions. Although not explicitly discussed in the PG, the average length of emergency involuntary hospitalization for suicidal patients has decreased substantially in the United States, and is typically in the range of 7 days or less.

The evolving role of psychiatric management was evident in sections on coordinating care with other clinicians and monitoring patients' status on an ongoing basis. By 2010, only a minority of psychiatrists practiced in private offices, where they routinely provided both psychotherapy and pharmacotherapy; most collaborated with psychologists, social workers, or other mental health specialists whose services often included psychotherapy. The principles of measurement-based care—embedded within the STAR*D trial (Trivedi et al. 2006)—were now incorporated into psychiatric management, including the use of brief PROs at each follow-up visit to ascertain progress vis à vis symptom reduction and as an explicit means to prompt decision making. Although the PG did not recommend use of a particular PRO, the aforementioned PHQ-9 was being increasingly used for this purpose in primary care settings, and a number of investigators affiliated with STAR*D had developed a 16-item self-report version of the Quick Inventory for Depressive Symptomatology (QIDS-SR; Rush et al. 2003). Because the QIDS-SR was freely available in the public domain and provided broader symptom coverage than the PHQ-9, it was arguably better suited for psychiatric practices than the PHQ-9. The value of routinely assessing side effects also was recognized in the PG as a way to minimize treatment burden and improve treatment adherence. The PG also recognized the increasing evidence that the treating psychiatrist could improve treatment outcomes by taking a more active role in the adherence process through asking about medication-taking and addressing potential barriers to pharmacotherapy.

More so than earlier editions, the 2010 PG endorsed the value of patient education about the illness and its treatment, including—with the patient's explicit permission—involving family members, significant others, and caregivers. It was recommended that such efforts include discussing expectations about treatment options, the expected duration of treatment, and the likely benefits and side effects of the various treatment options. As acceptance of a psychiatric diagnosis and the decision to take a psychiatric medication were recognized to sometimes involve emotion-laden or "overdetermined" psychological complexities, the term *psychoeducation* was used to underscore the sophistication of this component of psychiatric management. The PG encouraged the treating psychiatrist to explore and, when evident, address common beliefs and misperceptions about treatment (e.g., "Are antidepressant medications habit-forming?" or "Will I become addicted to this drug?").

Acute-phase treatment: choosing the initial intervention. The initial phase of treatment—still referred to as *acute-phase therapy*—was described as extending from the first prescription medication or first session of psychotherapy until the desired treatment outcome is achieved. So defined, the acute phase of treatment might last as little as a few weeks or, for patients with more difficult-to-treat depressive episodes, extend for months or even years. Reflecting both greater clinical sophistication and recognition of the outcome qualities that patients value most, remission was recommended as the ideal goal of acute-phase therapy, and the definition was broadened to include normalization of psychosocial and vocational functioning in addition to a virtually complete relief of symptoms.

Based on a comprehensive assessment that included the patient's past treatment history and current preferences, the PG recommended that—in most cases—acute-phase therapy would begin with antidepressant pharmacotherapy, depression-focused psychotherapy, or a combination of the two. As in previous editions of the APA PG for MDD, antidepressant medication was implicitly recommended as the cornerstone of the treatment provided by psychiatrists for nonpsychotic episodes of MDD and was recommended with level I confidence across the full range of symptom severity. The PG included detailed tables summarizing dosing, side effects, and potential drug-drug interactions for all of the antidepressants in use in 2010.

For most patients with no prior treatment history, the PG recommended with level I certainty a relatively large group of newer antidepressants as first-line options, including the SSRIs and the SNRIs venlafaxine and duloxetine, as well as mirtazapine and bupropion. The PG noted that some people might prefer to try a "complementary" medication or a nutraceutical, such as *S*-adenosyl methionine (SAMe), St. John's wort, or omega-3 fatty acids, before agreeing to treatment with a conventional antidepressant. However, the PG had little confidence in this option, affixing a level III rating (i.e., may be useful in selected cases). Bright white light (aka phototherapy) also was rated as a level III alternative to pharmacotherapy for patients with a seasonal (fall-winter) pattern of recurrent MDD despite several positive sham-controlled studies. The PG did note that bright white light could be a useful adjunct to antidepressant medication.

By 2010, nortriptyline and desipramine had joined the other TCAs in the bin of second- or third-line therapies, with the important caveat that patients who had previously experienced a good response and minimal tolerability issues with TCA therapy were candidates for first-line use. The nonselective MAOIs—phenelzine, tranylcypromine, and isocarboxazid—similarly slid further down the PG's hierarchical ordering of treatments and were now largely recommended for patients with more advanced levels of TRD. The PG considered the recently introduced transdermally delivered form of selegiline as a potentially better-tolerated option for patients being considered for MAOI therapy.

The PG did not recommend a specific frequency of follow-up pharmacotherapy visits, but it did state that patients should be "carefully and systematically monitored" during acute-phase therapy. The practitioner thus should use factors such as urgency and safety or tolerability concerns to determine which patients should be seen weekly, every other week, or monthly. Some of the strategies woven into collaborative care protocols originally developed for primary care practices, including check-ins with office staff by telephone or e-mail, were recommended to streamline care, improve follow-up, and foster treatment adherence. The PG also recommended that the practice of pharmacotherapy could be enhanced by efforts to promote and encourage depressed patients to adopt healthier lifestyles.

As part of a recommendation to incorporate the tools of measurement-based care, the strategies used to facilitate more follow-up would also facilitate more frequent assessment of symptomatic response, recognizing and addressing side effects, providing clinical support, and supporting adherence and engagement in healthy lifestyle changes. In this regard, there was already emerging evidence that a lack of even modest symptom relief during the first few weeks of treatment had ominous prognostic implications (Szegedi et al. 2009). However, the PG did not actually provide temporal cues or threshold scores on standard PROs to define important clinical outcomes, such as early nonresponse, response, and remission. In the most global terms, people who obtain very little symptomatic relief during the first 2 weeks of treatment will likely require some change in treatment, and those who are judged by their treating clinicians to be "much" or "very much" improved are almost certain to have obtained at least a 50% drop in symptom severity. Ideally, people whose depressive episode has remitted would be essentially indistinguishable from someone who has never suffered from depression, although the many comorbidities that can complicate the life histories of our patients often get in the way of that level of improvement.

Recognizing important differences among antidepressants with respect to pharmacokinetics (e.g., fluoxetine vs. the rest of the SSRIs) and pharmacodynamics (e.g., TCAs or mirtazapine vs. SSRIs), the PG contains relatively general recommendations about upward titration of antidepressants during acute-phase therapy. Such imprecision was largely justified by the fact that ascending dose-response relationships had not been convincingly established for most of the antidepressants recommended for first-line use. That said, and reflecting both clinical experience and expert consensus circa 2010, the PG did recommend upward titration if a minimal effective dosage of an antidepressant was well tolerated but only minimally effective after 4–6 weeks of treatment. In the case of antidepressants with three or more FDA-approved dosages with established efficacy, such as fluoxetine (20–60 mg/day), sertraline (50–200 mg/day), paroxetine (20–50 mg/day), and venlafaxine (75–375 mg/day), upward titration might extend the acute-phase trial to 10 or 12 weeks.

Confidence in the use of depression-focused psychotherapies alone as an initial treatment choice for outpatients with mild to moderate MDD continued to grow, with CBT and IPT recommended with level I ratings. Support for use of time-limited psychodynamic therapy as an alternative to CBT or IPT similarly grew, garnering a level II rating in the third edition. Several other forms of psychotherapy, including problem-solving therapy, couples therapy, and family therapy, also were recommended with moderate (level II) confidence.

Across three editions of APA PGs for MDD, focused psychotherapy—as a monotherapy—was not recommended for treatment of the most severe episodes of MDD (e.g., inpatients, those with psychotic features, those grossly incapacitated by the depressive illness). However, beyond these most extreme cases, it is noteworthy that by 2010, most of the older and historically influential notions of differential therapeutics, such as using symptoms of a more classical or "endogenous" depressive episode to determine the need for pharmacotherapy or, conversely, using symptoms or other clinical characteristics of more reactive, neurotic, or atypical depressions to gauge the need for psychotherapy, were no longer endorsed with high confidence. The third edition of the PG concluded that head-to-head trials had generally demonstrated comparable efficacy for pharmacotherapy and focused psychotherapy across 8–12 weeks and noted that there were few—if any—well-replicated indicators of response to one form of treatment versus the other. Instead, the PG considered patient preference to be the major determinant of selecting psychotherapy alone instead of pharmacotherapy or the combination as a treatment of first choice. The PG noted that many women who were pregnant or breastfeeding expressed particularly strong preferences to minimize exposure to medication, as did some patients with a history of intolerance and/or nonresponse to several courses of antidepressant medication.

With respect to which form of psychotherapy to recommend, the PG concluded that there were no reliable empirical criteria for picking CBT over IPT or vice versa. In such a situation, simply the availability of a capable therapist with expertise in the delivery of a focused psychotherapy could be the deciding factor in making a referral. Consistent with the RCTs that established the efficacy of these forms of psychotherapy, the PG recommended the use of the same general time course to judge the effectiveness of the selected therapy (e.g., weekly sessions across 2–3 months), and likewise recommended the use of similar milestones and symptom measures to evaluate outcome. The occasional use of more frequent sessions of psychotherapy for patients with more severe/complex depressions and, when practicable, the use of group formats for delivery of psychotherapy were recommended with level II confidence.

As in previous editions of the PG, the combination of psychotherapy and pharmacotherapy continued to be recommended with highest confidence for patients with more severe, recurrent, and complicated depressive episodes. Although no longer recommended as the treatment of first choice for outpatients with milder, uncomplicated depressive episodes, the PG did recommend the addition of psychotherapy to pharmacotherapy when patients had more pressing interpersonal or psychosocial difficulties. For the first time, the PG recommended indications for sequential uses of combined treatment, such as adding psychotherapy to ongoing pharmacotherapy to target residual symptoms of incompletely remitted depressive episodes as a means to ensure a more durable recovery or reduce the risk of subsequent relapse and recurrence.

Antidepressant pharmacotherapy and psychotherapy were not the alpha and omega of therapeutics in the third edition of the APA PG for MDD. In fact, the PG recommended ECT (with high confidence) as a first-line option in specific circumstances. For example, ECT was recommended with level I confidence for patients with a past history of TRD and subsequent relapse/recurrence after a good response to ECT. Such a first-line use not only would have the highest probability of a successful outcome but also would reduce the patient's time spent ill by bypassing further—and likely futile—attempts to find an effective pharmacotherapy regimen. Other level I recommendations for the first-line use of ECT included its use for inpatient treatment of patients who manifested florid psychotic symptoms (i.e., delusions, hallucinations, or catatonic features) and for those who were too severely depressed to able to care for themselves or who were refusing to eat or drink, as well as for depressed patients experiencing compellingly strong suicidal intent. Despite FDA approval of two other neuromodulation strategies for patients with difficult-to-treat depressions, neither TMS nor VNS were recommended for first-line use in the 2010 PG.

Other options for nonresponders to first-line therapies. For patients who did not benefit from an adequate trial of a first-line antidepressant, the PG recommended switching to a different antidepressant or adding a focused psychotherapy with level I confidence. When severity or urgency justified it, ECT also was recommended with high confidence for antidepressant nonresponders. By contrast, none of the adjunctive strategies that were more commonly used in 2010 were recommended with level I confidence; lithium and thyroid hormone, which had been used off-label for years, and aripiprazole, quetiapine, and olanzapine (the last mentioned combined with fluoxetine), which either had been recently approved by the FDA or were being considered for approval, were recommended with level II confidence. The other adjunctive strategies typically found within a psychopharmacologist's toolbox, including anticonvulsant mood stabilizers, omega-3 fatty acids, folate, psychostimulants, buspirone, and benzodiazepines, were only recommended for selected patients (with level III confidence).

Continuation-phase therapy. By 2010, continuation-phase therapy had become a standard of care for essentially all antidepressant responders. Routinely extending for 6–9 months after the patient reached the desired outcome of acute-phase antidepressant pharmacotherapy, the two key aims of continuation-phase therapy were to prevent relapse and to support consolidation of response or remission so that the patient could truly recover from the index episode of depression. The recommended course of continuation-phase pharmacotherapy included seeing patients at a regular, albeit lower, frequency (e.g., transitioning from every other week to monthly) and continuing therapy with the medication that was judged to be effective in the acute phase at the full dosage that was used (level I confidence). Continuation-phase pharmacotherapy sessions were recommended to employ the same clinical management strategies outlined for acute-phase therapy for ongoing assessments of symptoms and side effects, adherence, and functional status. As noted above, there was growing confidence in the use of sequential courses of psychotherapy to improve the quality of remission or reduce the risk of relapse, and it was noted that CBT might be used in this manner to reduce the risk of relapse after discontinuation of an antidepressant (level II confidence). For responders to time-limited psychotherapy, parallel models of continuation-phase psychotherapy were gaining some empirical support for relapse prevention (level II confidence). For ECT responders, the combination of lithium and nortriptyline was recommended with level I confidence, and for those patients who relapsed despite ongoing pharmacotherapy, continuation-phase therapy with ECT was recommended with moderate (level II) confidence.

Maintenance-phase therapy. The third edition of the PG for MDD also reflected growing certainty that some patients with more highly recurrent and/or chronic forms of MDD benefited from indefinite, perhaps even lifelong, preventive pharmacotherapy. Echoing broad expert consensus in the literature, maintenance-phase pharmacotherapy was recommended with level I confidence for patients who had had three or more lifetime episodes of MDD or for those who had relapsed during continuation-phase pharmacotherapy during use of or after withdrawal from the antidepressant. Other factors recommended for consideration with moderate confidence included the presence of residual symptoms, ongoing psychosocial stressors, early age at onset, and family history of mood disorders.

Full-dosage therapy with antidepressant medication was recommended for maintenance-phase pharmacotherapy (level I evidence). The PG recognized that during a longer-term course of pharmacotherapy, it was sometimes necessary to reduce the medication dosage to mitigate side effects. Although the state of the evidence indicated that dosage reduction did increase the risk of relapse/recurrence, this practice was judged to be indicated in selected cases (level III evidence).

There was growing confidence in the value of longer-term adaptations of depression-focused psychotherapy for relapse or recurrence prevention (level II evidence). Such adaptations, which generally "thinned" the frequency of visits to every other week, and then to once a month, might also be sequenced to facilitate subsequent discontinuation of pharmacotherapy.

Planned discontinuation of longer-term pharmacotherapy. The PG recognized that even for patients with less highly recurrent depressive disorders, the risk of relapse/recurrence was particularly high during the first 6 months after stopping an antidepressant. Beyond the possibility of hastening a depressive relapse, the PG also recognized that abrupt cessation of antidepressant medication could cause a characteristic set of discontinuation symptoms (e.g., nausea, autonomic symptoms, headaches, paresthesias, insomnia, irritability). Although such reactions following abrupt cessation of therapy with TCAs or MAOIs had been described for decades (see, e.g., Dilsaver and Greden 1984), they were commonplace following treatment with newer-generation antidepressants, most particularly paroxetine and venlafaxine (Haddad and Anderson 2007). The PG therefore recommended patient education—namely, that all patients prescribed antidepressants should know not to stop them abruptly, and that, outside of clinical emergencies, when it was time to stop antidepressant therapy, the medication should be tapered over at least several weeks; these recommendations were made with highest confidence. When education and a simple tapering schedule did not suffice, the PG recommended either prolonging the taper or switching to a medication with a longer elimination half-life (i.e., fluoxetine) (level II evidence).

Aftermath and epilogue. In the month following acceptance for publication of the third edition of the APA PG for MDD, an influential article in the *Annals of Internal Medicine* called for new methods to minimize the impact of potential conflicts pertaining to both financial and intellectual interests (Guyatt et al. 2010). A few months after the PG was released, the same work group published a paper summarizing a new system of grading the strength of evidence underpinning guideline recommendations (Guyatt et al. 2011). Shortly thereafter, an updated set of recommendations for guideline development was released by the Institute of Medicine (2011a). The new Institute of Medicine recommendations were even more strident about the importance of increasing transparency in the process and minimizing potential conflicts of interest as means of increasing public trust in the process. The Institute of Medicine reaffirmed and strengthened their earlier recommendations that PGs be written by multidisciplinary panels that included the input of health economists and representatives of patient/consumer groups. To further strengthen the empirical basis of the process, a companion monograph was released summarizing the recommended methods for conducting systematic reviews, meta-analyses, and related approaches to data synthesis (Institute of Medicine 2011b). It was even suggested that a document that did not use this approach to validated recommendations should not be called a practice guideline, but rather should be referred to as an "expert consensus."

Despite the best intentions of all involved with the development of the third edition of the APA PG for MDD, it did not meet a number of the Institute of Medicine's updated criteria. The concerted efforts of the work group to disclose and responsibly manage their relationships with industry, the steering committee's oversight, the independent review group's efforts to ensure that the report was not biased, and the multi-tiered review process to elicit and incorporate the input from all interested stakeholders similarly did not preclude concerns about the integrity of the process of APA guideline development. Cosgrove and Shaughnessy (2011), for example, opined that the PG gave a "privileged" ranking to pharmacotherapy by recommending antidepressant medication for even "mild depression" and ignoring "growing concerns" about the risks of antidepressants. Subsequently, Cosgrove et al. (2013) made a not-so-veiled accusation of bias by reporting that the APA PG for MDD work group authors had an average of 20.5 industry relationships. They also declared that they had detected that one of the members of the independent review group had an "undisclosed financial tie" to the pharmaceutical industry and that because several other members had previously had various relationships with the industry, they could not be confident in the process. They further suggested that their "independent" review of the PG's scholarship reflected bias in the following ways: 1) more than half of the studies cited to support guideline recommendations did not meet criteria for "high quality," 2) nearly 20% of the studies cited actually had results that were "not congruent" with the recommendations, and 3) about 17% of the supporting citations did not report "clinically meaningful" results. Finally, Cosgrove and colleagues concluded that the APA PG for MDD also showed intellectual bias because the work group consisted only of psychiatrists who were members of the sponsoring organization, "all" had conducted research involving antidepressant medications, and group members had authored or coauthored 9.1% of the literature cited in support of the PG's recommendations.

In such a climate, the APA's steering committee recommended suspension of work on other PGs, including those on bipolar disorder and schizophrenia. After a long hiatus, the steering committee recommended resuming guideline development, largely following the Academy of Medicine's revised guidelines, as amended for PGs produced by specialty societies. As this chapter was being written, a completely reworked and reformatted edition of the APA PG for schizophrenia was nearing publication and is now published (American Psychiatric Association 2021).

Developments Since the Third Edition: Does Missing a Decade Make a Difference?

In the 11+ years since the publication of the third edition of the APA PG for MDD, there have been a number of important developments, beginning with the publication of the fifth edition of the APA's Diagnostic and Statistical Manual (American Psychiatric Association 2013) (Table 28–2). Efforts to improve the interpersonal aspects of medication management have continued (see, e.g., Rush and Thase 2018), and many health care systems have now systematized aspects of measurement-based care. Although a number of new antidepressant medications have been introduced, the change with the greatest impact on the day-to-day practice of U.S. psychiatrists was the almost universal acceptance of a small group of generic antidepressants as the standard of care for first-line pharmacotherapy. In such an inhospitable climate for branded medications, only four novel antidepressants were approved by the FDA as treatments for MDD, and of these, only three were introduced in the marketplace. The first, vilazodone, which pairs serotonin reuptake inhibition with potent partial agonism of serotonin (5-hydroxytryptamine [5-HT]) type 1A (5-HT_{1A}) receptors, was approved in 2011. The second, vortioxetine (approved in 2013), is a serotonin reuptake inhibitor with up to five clinically relevant effects on serotonin receptors. The third, levomilnacipran, a stereoisomer of a drug introduced a decade earlier, also was approved in 2013 as the fourth member of the SNRI class. Although each of these medications may have benefits for selected patients as an alternative to generic anti-

TABLE 28–2. Developments since the 2010 publication of the American Psychiatric Association Practice Guideline for the Treatment of Patients With Major Depressive Disorder, 3rd Edition

1. New DSM episode specifiers with treatment indications (introduced in DSM-5; American Psychiatric Association 2013)
   - "With anxious features"
   - "With mixed features"
2. Novel reuptake-inhibiting antidepressants
   - Vilazodone (FDA approved in 2011)
   - Vortioxetine (FDA approved in 2013)
   - Levomilnacipran (FDA approved in 2013)
3. Novel second-generation antipsychotics
   - Lurasidone (bipolar I depression) (indication approved by FDA in 2014)
   - Brexpiprazole (adjunctive therapy for MDD) (FDA approved in 2015)
   - Cariprazine (bipolar I depression) (indication approved by FDA in 2019)
4. Refinements to transcranial magnetic stimulation (TMS)
   - "Deep" TMS device (FDA approved in 2013)
5. Novel infusion therapy for postpartum depression
   - Brexanolone, a neurosteroid (FDA approved for postpartum depression in 2019)
6. Clinical use of ketamine and esketamine
   - APA Task Force Report on intravenous ketamine (2015)
   - FDA approves an intranasal formulation of esketamine for TRD (2019)

depressants, truly unique "heads above" advantages have not—at least yet—been demonstrated to the satisfaction of regulatory agencies or those who manage the pharmacy benefits for third-party payers (see, e.g., Wagner et al. 2018). As a result, the almost universal use of prior authorization procedures by third-party payers to reduce expenditures has functionally precluded first- or even second-line use of these medications (Hodgkin et al. 2015).

For more specific treatment indications, a broader array of newer medications have been introduced in the past decade. In 2015 the FDA approved brexpiprazole—a direct descendant of the SGA aripiprazole—for adjunctive treatment of MDD patients who have not obtained adequate benefit from antidepressants alone. Although technically off-label for MDD, two other SGAs were approved by the FDA for treatment of major depressive episodes in people with bipolar disorder: lurasidone (approved in 2014) and cariprazine (approved in 2019). Given the inclusion of a "with mixed features" episode specifier in DSM-5 (American Psychiatric Association 2013) and the absence of proven treatments for this relatively common presentation (Stahl et al. 2017), it is noteworthy that lurasidone monotherapy showed a strong efficacy signal in a placebo-controlled RCT delimited to MDD patients with mixed features (Suppes et al. 2016).

In 2019, brexanolone—an intravenous formulation of the neurosteroid allopregnanolone—became the first drug specifically approved by the FDA for treatment of postpartum episodes of MDD. Although the results of RCTs suggest that this drug's antidepressant effects were evident within 4–5 days (Meltzer-Brody et al. 2018), the cost of this truly novel treatment, estimated at about $38,500 per course of therapy, precludes widespread use (Eldar-Lissai et al. 2020). For this reason, brexanolone's cost-effectiveness would be questionable even if its use were limited to inpatient settings or to treatment of women with severe peripartum depression who had not benefited from conventional antidepressants.

As evidence accumulated that off-label use of subanesthetic doses of intravenous ketamine produced rapid antidepressant effects and concerns about tolerance of antidepressant effects or late-emerging toxicities slowly lessened (see, e.g., Newport et al. 2015), the field was primed for a more conventional, commercially available treatment option. Into this void came esketamine, an intranasal formulation of the *S*-enantiomer of racemic ketamine, which was approved by the FDA in 2019 for adjunctive therapy of patients with TRD. Not unlike brexanolone, esketamine therapy is substantially more expensive than other options for adjunctive treatment of TRD. For example, at about $600–$800 per intranasal treatment, the drug cost for a recommended 4-week course of twice-weekly therapy could be as high as $6,400. The cost of treatment with esketamine would also include at least $200 per treatment to cover the 2 hours of clinical care required to comply with the Risk Evaluation and Mitigation Strategy that accompanies esketamine therapy. The total cost for a successful course of esketamine would be much higher for the subgroup of patients who received ongoing weekly sessions for relapse prevention (Daly et al. 2019). Negotiations pertaining to reimbursement have been further complicated by a report funded by the Institute for Clinical and Economic Review, which concluded that intranasal esketamine was not a cost-effective option for TRD (Agboola et al. 2020). Although some of the assumptions of this particular analysis may have been biased in favor of the standard comparators (Karkare et al. 2020), the absence of strong comparative efficacy data for patients presenting with more advanced levels of TRD also continues to inhibit broader insurance coverage for esketamine therapy.

There also have been further developments in neuromodulation therapies for MDD. Results of a large-scale multicenter study on continuation-phase ECT for older patients with difficult-to-treat depression further established the value of this time-honored strategy for selected patients (Kellner et al. 2016). The evidence base supporting the utility of TMS for MDD continued to expand (Gaynes et al. 2011, 2014), insurance coverage steadily grew, and a number of new devices were approved by the FDA (McClintock et al. 2018). Although TMS does not yet consistently rank as a preferred option for TRD throughout the world (Bayes and Parker 2018), there is growing consensus in the United States that, when feasible, TMS is a useful second- or third-line strategy for patients who did not tolerate or who did not respond to antidepressants (McClintock et al. 2018). There is also a slowly growing database supporting the value of VNS for treatment of chronically depressed patients with the most advanced levels of TRD, although this treatment is still not widely covered by third-party payers (Bottomley et al. 2019).

Other Practice Guidelines for Psychiatrists

Because it is uncertain when the next iteration of the APA PG for MDD will be published, stakeholders may consult several other, more up-to-date guidelines, as briefly summarized below.

CANMAT Guidelines

There are many similarities between the practice of psychiatry in the United States and Canada, and to no surprise, the most recent update of the CANMAT PG provides a very close approximation to what an updated version of the APA PG for MDD would look like. Written by a multidisciplinary group of experts, the third edition of the CANMAT PG comprises six concise executive summary reports published together in a special issue of the *Canadian Journal of Psychiatry*. The updated PG includes reports summarizing the state of the art for principles of care/clinical management (Lam et al. 2016), psychotherapy (Parikh et al. 2016), pharmacotherapy (Kennedy et al. 2016), neuromodulation therapies (Milev et al. 2016), complementary and alternative treatments (Ravindran et al. 2016) and treatment of special clinical populations (i.e., youth, women, and the elderly) (MacQueen et al. 2016). Although the evidence-based review in the CANMAT PG is quickly becoming dated, most of the recommendations short of ketamine and esketamine continue to reflect the state of the art in the United States. Of note, a "pocket book" adaptation of CANMAT tailored specifically to the United States is nearing completion (S. Parikh, personal communication, November 2, 2021).

Veterans Affairs and Department of Defense Guideline

This Veterans Affairs (VA) and Department of Defense (DoD) Clinical Practice Guideline for the Management of Major Depressive Disorder (VA-DoD CPG for MDD) was developed jointly under the auspices of the VA and the DoD. Chaired by noted VA researcher David Oslin and most recently updated in 2016 (U.S. Department of Veterans Affairs and U.S. Department of Defense 2016), this PG was written by a multidisciplinary panel, and scrupulous attention was paid to minimizing potential conflicts of industry. As was the case with earlier iterations, the VA-DoD CPG for MDD was developed to assist clinicians from a broad range of disciplines (physicians, advanced practice nurses, psychologists, social workers, and other health care providers) in their work with depressed patients—both veterans and those on active duty in the military (U.S. Department of Veterans Affairs and U.S. Department of Defense 2016). In perfect step with the cost-containing exigencies of the parent organizations, the VA-DoD CPG for MDD utilizes a somewhat more restricted formulary but is noteworthy for embracing strategies to improve the delivery of care, almost seamlessly blending in the methods of measurement-based care, collaborative care, and stepped-care strategies. For example, an appendix summarizes use of the PHQ-9 (Kroenke et al. 2001) to monitor outcomes and to help ensure timely progression through treatment hierarchies. Among the evidence-based psychotherapies, CBT receives particular emphasis, no doubt reflecting the VA's considerable efforts over the past decade focused on training of psychotherapists (see www.mentalhealth.va.gov/depression/cbt-d.asp). Although the VA-DoD CPG for MDD is now 5 years old, recent developments in psychiatric therapeutics that address unmet needs are incorporated into VA practice on an ongoing basis, as illustrated by rapid incorporation of adjunctive aripiprazole in VA formularies following the results of the large-scale VA Augmentation and Switching Treatments for Improving Depression Outcomes (VAST-D) trial (Mohamed et al. 2017) and new initiatives to improve access to TMS and intranasal esketamine.

American Psychological Association Guideline

The recently updated guideline from the American Psychological Association (2019) provides much useful information about the role of various forms of psychotherapy for the treatment of outpatients with MDD. Chaired by the accomplished VA depression researcher John McQuaid (Elizabeth Lin, a PCP with an established research track record in primary care settings, was the vice chair), the multidisciplinary panel primarily focused on the role of psychotherapy across three age groups: youth, adults, and older adults. The guideline generally followed the Institute of Medicine's (2011b) road map and used the Grading of Recommendations Assessment, Development and Evaluation (GRADE) approach to calibrate the weight of evidence supporting each treatment recommendation (Guyatt et al. 2011).

With respect to treatment of uncomplicated MDD in adults, the PG noted that survey data from outpatients suggested a strong preference for treatment with psychotherapy alone (McHugh et al. 2013). For patients preferring this option, the PG considered six forms of therapy to be reasonable choices: behavioral therapy, CBT, IPT, mindfulness-based cognitive therapy, psychodynamic therapy, and supportive therapy. Because of a dearth of evidence for most of the options, the PG recommended only CBT and IPT for use in combination with antidepressants. The potential value of focused psychotherapy after inadequate response to pharmacotherapy, either alone or sequentially added to pharmacotherapy, was also noted, with an intermediate grade of empirical support. Of perhaps greatest importance to the field, the PG concluded with a call for support for more rigorous research on comparative effectiveness (both between psychotherapies and across modalities, singly and in combination with pharmacotherapy) and careful research to further refine identification of variables to better match depressed people with the specific treatments most likely to be helpful.

Conclusion

Since the early 1990s, there has been growing recognition of the need to align more closely the treatments that are provided in everyday care with the best practices recommended by expert consensus and the best available evidence derived from RCTs. This unmet need has been addressed in part by a movement that has spanned literally all areas of clinical medicine, namely, the development of clinical practice guidelines. As evidenced by the several generations of reports promulgated by the Institute of Medicine, the guidelines or best practices for PG development have steadily evolved and, along the way, have gained sophistication in the empirical methods used to rank or grade treatments. There has also been greater appreciation of the potential hazards that a lack of scientific transparency and concerns about undue influence of outside interests can have on the process. In parallel, there has been growing appreciation of the benefits of incorporating multidisciplinary perspectives and input from patients/consumers and other stakeholders. Despite obvious imperfections, the third edition of the APA PG for MDD—as complemented by several more recent PGs prepared by multidisciplinary groups—provides a useful overview of the best practices for the assessment and treatment of depressed patients. The debate over whether or not to exclude the input of experts who have relationships with commercial entities is ongoing, though the vitriol expressed by a relatively small number of critics with obvious anti-industry bias has had a disproportionately large effect on the process of guideline development. Of arguably far greater importance is the need to continue to implement, refine, and evaluate new ways to ensure that the clinical care provided to depressed patients more closely and more consistently follow the recommendations provided by these documents.

References

Agboola F, Atlas SJ, Touchette DR, et al: The effectiveness and value of esketamine for the management of treatment-resistant depression. J Manag Care Spec Pharm 26(1):16–20, 2020 31880219

American Psychiatric Association: Diagnostic and Statistical Manual for Mental Disorders, 3rd Edition. Washington, DC, American Psychiatric Association, 1980

American Psychiatric Association: Practice guideline for the treatment of patients with major depressive disorder. Am J Psychiatry 150 (4 suppl):1–26, 1993

American Psychiatric Association: Diagnostic and Statistical Manual for Mental Disorders, 4th Edition. Washington, DC, American Psychiatric Association, 1994

American Psychiatric Association: Practice guideline for the treatment of patients with major depressive disorder (revision). Am J Psychiatry 157 (4 suppl):1–45, 2000 10767867

American Psychiatric Association: Practice Guidelines for the Treatment of Psychiatric Disorders Compendium 2006. Washington, DC, American Psychiatric Association, 2006

American Psychiatric Association: Practice Guideline for the Treatment of Patients With Major Depressive Disorder, 3rd Edition. Washington, DC, American Psychiatric Association, 2010

American Psychiatric Association: Diagnostic and Statistical Manual for Mental Disorders, 5th Edition. Arlington, VA, American Psychiatric Association, 2013

American Psychiatric Association: Practice Guideline for the Treatment of Patients With Schizophrenia, 3rd Edition. Washington, DC, American Psychiatric Association, 2021. Available at: https://psychiatryonline.org/doi/book/10.1176/appi.books.9780890424841. Accessed April 23, 2021.

American Psychiatric Association, Academy of Psychosomatic Medicine: Dissemination of integrated care within adult primary care setting: the collaborative care model. 2016. Available at: www.psychiatry.org/File%20Library/Psychiatrists/Practice/Professional-Topics/Integrated-Care/APA-APM-Dissemination-Integrated-Care-Report.pdf. Accessed November 27, 2020.

American Psychological Association: Clinical Practice Guideline for the Treatment of Depression Across Three Age Cohorts. Guideline Development Panel for the Treatment of Depressive Disorders, 2019. Available at: www.apa.org/depression-guideline/guideline.pdf. Accessed November 27, 2020.

Angell M: Industry-sponsored clinical research: a broken system. JAMA 300(9):1069–1071, 2008 18768418

Angell M: Drug companies and doctors: a story of corruption. The New York Review, January 15, 2009. Available at: https://www.nybooks.com/articles/2009/01/15/drug-companies-doctorsa-story-of-corruption/. Accessed November 27, 2020.

Bayes AJ, Parker GB: Comparison of guidelines for the treatment of unipolar depression: a focus on pharmacotherapy and neurostimulation. Acta Psychiatr Scand 137(6):459–471, 2018 29577229

Berman RM, Cappiello A, Anand A, et al: Antidepressant effects of ketamine in depressed patients. Biol Psychiatry 47(4):351–354, 2000 10686270

Bottomley JM, LeReun C, Diamantopoulos A, et al: Vagus nerve stimulation (VNS) therapy in patients with treatment resistant depression: a systematic review and meta-analysis. Compr Psychiatry 98:152156, 2019 31978785
Cheng N, Banerjee T, Qian J, et al: Association of authorized generic marketing with prescription drug spending on antidepressants from 2000 to 2011. J Am Pharm Assoc 57(3):341–348, 2017 28400255
Cosgrove L, Shaughnessy AF: Conflicts of interest in clinical practice guidelines. Int J Pers Cent Med 1:668–674, 2011
Cosgrove L, Bursztajn HJ, Krimsky S, et al: Conflicts of interest and disclosure in the American Psychiatric Association's clinical practice guidelines. Psychother Psychosom 78(4):228–232, 2009 19401623
Cosgrove L, Bursztajn HJ, Erlich DR, et al: Conflicts of interest and the quality of recommendations in clinical guidelines. J Eval Clin Pract 19(4):674–681, 2013 23731207
Daly EJ, Trivedi MH, Janik A, et al: Efficacy of esketamine nasal spray plus oral antidepressant treatment for relapse prevention in patients with treatment-resistant depression: a randomized clinical trial. JAMA Psychiatry 76(9):893–903, 2019 31166571
Dartmouth-Hitchcock: Knowledge Map: Depression Management Adult, Ambulatory Clinical Practice Guideline. 2017. Available at: https://www.dartmouth-hitchcock.org/sites/default/files/2021-02/depression-clinical-practice-guideline.pdf. Accessed November 27, 2020.
Demitrack MA, Thase ME: Clinical significance of transcranial magnetic stimulation (TMS) in the treatment of pharmacoresistant depression: synthesis of recent data. Psychopharmacol Bull 42(2):5–38, 2009 19629020
Depression Guideline Panel: Depression in Primary Care: Detection, Diagnosis, and Treatment. Washington, DC, Agency for Health Care Policy and Research, 1993a
Depression Guideline Panel: Depression in Primary Care, Vol 1: Detection and Diagnosis. AHCPR Clinical Practice Guideline No 5.1. Rockville, MD, US Department of Health and Human Services, Public Health Service, Agency for Health Care Policy and Research, 1993b. Available at: www.ncbi.nlm.nih.gov/books/NBK52213. Accessed November 27, 2020.
Depression Guideline Panel: Depression in Primary Care, Vol 2: Treatment of Major Depression. AHCPR Clinical Practice Guideline No 5.2. Rockville, MD, US Department of Health and Human Services, Public Health Service, Agency for Health Care Policy and Research, 1993c. Available at: www.ncbi.nlm.nih.gov/books/NBK52234. Accessed November 27, 2020.
Dilsaver SC, Greden JF: Antidepressant withdrawal phenomena. Biol Psychiatry 19(2):237–256, 1984 6324897
Eldar-Lissai A, Cohen JT, Meltzer-Brody S, et al: Cost-effectiveness of brexanolone versus selective serotonin reuptake inhibitors for the treatment of postpartum depression in the United States. J Manag Care Spec Pharm 26(5):627–638, 2020 32191592
Fava M, Rush AJ, Trivedi MH, et al: Background and rationale for the sequenced treatment alternatives to relieve depression (STAR*D) study. Psychiatr Clin North Am 26(2):457–494, 2003 12778843
Field MJ, Lohr KN (eds): Clinical Practice Guidelines: Directions for a New Program. Washington, DC, National Academies Press, 1990
Fournier JC, DeRubeis RJ, Hollon SD, et al: Antidepressant drug effects and depression severity: a patient-level meta-analysis. JAMA 303(1):47–53, 2010 20051569
Frank E, Prien RF, Jarrett RB, et al: Conceptualization and rationale for consensus definitions of terms in major depressive disorder. Remission, recovery, relapse, and recurrence. Arch Gen Psychiatry 48(9):851–855, 1991 1929776
Gartlehner G, Gaynes BN, Hansen RA, et al: Comparative benefits and harms of second-generation antidepressants: background paper for the American College of Physicians. Ann Intern Med 149(10):734–750, 2008 19017592

Gartlehner G, Hansen RA, Morgan LC, et al: Second-generation antidepressants in the pharmacologic treatment of adult depression: an update of the 2007 comparative effectiveness review. AHRQ Comparative Effectiveness Review No 46. Agency for Healthcare Research and Quality, 2011. Available at: https://effectivehealthcare.ahrq.gov/sites/default/files/pdf/antidepressants-update_research.pdf. Accessed November 27, 2020.

Gartlehner G, Gaynes BN, Amick HR, et al: Comparative benefits and harms of antidepressant, psychological, complementary, and exercise treatments for major depression: an evidence report for a clinical practice guideline from the American College of Physicians. Ann Intern Med 164(5):331–341, 2016 26857743

Gartlehner G, Wagner G, Matyas N, et al: Pharmacological and non-pharmacological treatments for major depressive disorder: review of systematic reviews. BMJ Open 7(6):e014912, 2017 28615268

Gaynes BN, Lux LJ, Lloyd SW, et al: Nonpharmacologic Interventions for Treatment-Resistant Depression in Adults. Rockville, MD, Agency for Healthcare Research and Quality, 2011

Gaynes BN, Lloyd SW, Lux L, et al: Repetitive transcranial magnetic stimulation for treatment-resistant depression: a systematic review and meta-analysis. J Clin Psychiatry 75(5):477–489, quiz 489, 2014 24922485

George MS, Rush AJ, Marangell LB, et al: A one-year comparison of vagus nerve stimulation with treatment as usual for treatment-resistant depression. Biol Psychiatry 58(5):364–373, 2005 16139582

Guyatt G, Akl EA, Hirsh J, et al: The vexing problem of guidelines and conflict of interest: a potential solution. Ann Intern Med 152(11):738–741, 2010 20479011

Guyatt G, Oxman AD, Akl EA, et al: GRADE guidelines: 1. Introduction—GRADE evidence profiles and summary of findings tables. J Clin Epidemiol 64(4):383–394, 2011 21195583

Haddad P, Anderson I: Recognising and managing antidepressant discontinuation symptoms. Adv Psychiatr Treat 13:447–457, 2007

Hammad TA, Laughren T, Racoosin J: Suicidality in pediatric patients treated with antidepressant drugs. Arch Gen Psychiatry 63(3):332–339, 2006 16520440

Healy D, Thase ME: Is academic psychiatry for sale? Br J Psychiatry 182:388–390, 2003 12724241

Hodgkin D, Horgan CM, Creedon TB, et al: Management of newer antidepressant medications in U.S. commercial health plans. J Ment Health Policy Econ 18(4):165–173, 2015 26729008

Holtzheimer PE 3rd, Russo J, Avery DH: A meta-analysis of repetitive transcranial magnetic stimulation in the treatment of depression. Psychopharmacol Bull 35(4):149–169, 2001 12397863

Institute of Medicine: Conflict of Interest in Medical Research, Education, and Practice. Washington, DC, National Academies Press, 2009

Institute of Medicine: Clinical Practice Guidelines We Can Trust. Washington, DC, National Academies Press, 2011a

Institute of Medicine: Finding What Works in Health Care: Standard for Systematic Reviews. Washington, DC, National Academies Press, 2011b

Institute of Medicine (US) Committee on Clinical Practice Guidelines: Guidelines for clinical practice: from development to use. Field MJ, Lohr KN, editors. Washington, DC, National Academies Press, 1992. Available at: www.ncbi.nlm.nih.gov/books/NBK234503/. Accessed November 27, 2020.

Jarrett RB, Rush AJ: Short-term psychotherapy of depressive disorders: current status and future directions. Psychiatry 57(2):115–132, 1994 7938331

Karasu TB: The Psychiatric Therapies, Part I: The Somatic Therapies. Washington, DC, American Psychiatric Association, 1984a

Karasu TB: The Psychiatric Therapies, Part II: The Psychosocial Therapies. Washington, DC, American Psychiatric Association, 1984b

Karkare S, Le HH, Sheehan JJ, et al: Pitfalls of cost-effectiveness analysis in practice: a TRD case example in the United States with esketamine versus oral antidepressants. J Manag Care Spec Pharm 26(4):568–569, 2020 32223604

Kellner CH, Husain MM, Knapp RG, et al: A novel strategy for continuation ECT in geriatric depression: phase 2 of the PRIDE study. Am J Psychiatry 173(11):1110–1118, 2016 27418381

Kennedy SH, Lam RW, McIntyre RS, et al: Canadian Network for Mood and Anxiety Treatments (CANMAT) 2016 clinical guidelines for the management of adults with major depressive disorder: Section 3. Pharmacological treatments. Can J Psychiatry 61(9):540–560, 2016 27486148

Khin NA, Chen YF, Yang Y, et al: Exploratory analyses of efficacy data from major depressive disorder trials submitted to the US Food and Drug Administration in support of new drug applications. J Clin Psychiatry 72(4):464–472, 2011 21527123

Kirsch I, Deacon BJ, Huedo-Medina TB, et al: Initial severity and antidepressant benefits: a meta-analysis of data submitted to the Food and Drug Administration. PLoS Med 5(2):e45, 2008 18303940

Klein DF, Gittelman R, Quitkin F, et al: Diagnosis and Drug Treatment of Psychiatric Disorders: Adults and Children. Baltimore, MD, Williams & Wilkins, 1983

Kroenke K, Spitzer RL, Williams JB: The PHQ-9: validity of a brief depression severity measure. J Gen Intern Med 16(9):606–613, 2001 11556941

Kupfer DJ: Long-term treatment of depression. J Clin Psychiatry 52 (suppl):28–34, 1991 1903134

Lam RW, McIntosh D, Wang J, et al: Canadian Network for Mood and Anxiety Treatments (CANMAT) 2016 clinical guidelines for the management of adults with major depressive disorder: Section 1. Disease burden and principles of care. Can J Psychiatry 61(9):510–523, 2016 27486151

Loo CK, Mitchell PB: A review of the efficacy of transcranial magnetic stimulation (TMS) treatment for depression, and current and future strategies to optimize efficacy. J Affect Disord 88(3):255–267, 2005 16139895

Luo Y, Kataoka Y, Ostinelli EG, et al: National prescription patterns of antidepressants in the treatment of adults with major depression in the US between 1996 and 2015: a population representative survey based analysis. Front Psychiatry 11:35, 2020 32116850

MacQueen GM, Frey BN, Ismail Z, et al: Canadian Network for Mood and Anxiety Treatments (CANMAT) 2016 clinical guidelines for the management of adults with major depressive disorder: Section 6. Special populations: youth, women, and the elderly. Can J Psychiatry 61(9):588–603, 2016 27486149

McClintock SM, Reti IM, Carpenter LL, et al: Consensus recommendations for the clinical application of repetitive transcranial magnetic stimulation (rTMS) in the treatment of depression. J Clin Psychiatry 79(1):16cs10905, 2018 28541649

McCormick KA, Fleming B: Clinical practice guidelines. The Agency for Health Care Policy and Research fosters the development of evidence-based guidelines. Health Prog 73(10):30–34, 1992 10122521

McHugh RK, Whitton SW, Peckham AD, et al: Patient preference for psychological vs pharmacologic treatment of psychiatric disorders: a meta-analytic review. J Clin Psychiatry 74(6):595–602, 2013 23842011

Meltzer-Brody S, Colquhoun H, Riesenberg R, et al: Brexanolone injection in post-partum depression: two multicentre, double-blind, randomised, placebo-controlled, phase 3 trials. Lancet 392(10152):1058–1070, 2018 30177236

Milev RV, Giacobbe P, Kennedy SH, et al: Canadian Network for Mood and Anxiety Treatments (CANMAT) 2016 clinical guidelines for the management of adults with major depressive disorder: Section 4. Neurostimulation treatments. Can J Psychiatry 61(9):561–575, 2016 27486154

Mohamed S, Johnson GR, Chen P, et al: Effect of antidepressant switching vs augmentation on remission among patients with major depressive disorder unresponsive to antidepressant treatment: the VAST-D randomized clinical trial. JAMA 318(2):132–145, 2017 28697253

Mulrow CD, Williams JW Jr, Trivedi M, et al: Treatment of depression—newer pharmacotherapies: summary. AHRQ Evidence Report Summaries, No 7. Agency for Healthcare Research and Quality, 1999. Available at: www.ncbi.nlm.nih.gov/books/NBK11912/. Accessed November 27, 2020.

Nelson JC, Papakostas GI: Atypical antipsychotic augmentation in major depressive disorder: a meta-analysis of placebo-controlled randomized trials. Am J Psychiatry 166(9):980–991, 2009 19687129

Newport DJ, Carpenter LL, McDonald WM, et al: Ketamine and other NMDA antagonists: early clinical trials and possible mechanisms in depression. Am J Psychiatry 172(10):950–966, 2015 26423481

O'Reardon JP, Cristancho P, Peshek AD: Vagus nerve stimulation (VNS) and treatment of depression: to the brainstem and beyond. Psychiatry (Edgmont) 3(5):54–63, 2006 21103178

O'Reardon JP, Solvason HB, Janicak PG, et al: Efficacy and safety of transcranial magnetic stimulation in the acute treatment of major depression: a multisite randomized controlled trial. Biol Psychiatry 62(11):1208–1216, 2007 17573044

Parikh SV, Quilty LC, Ravitz P, et al; CANMAT Depression Work Group: Canadian Network for Mood and Anxiety Treatments (CANMAT) 2016 clinical guidelines for the management of adults with major depressive disorder: Section 2. Psychological treatments. Can J Psychiatry 61(9):524–539, 2016 27486150

Persons JB, Thase ME, Crits-Christoph P: The role of psychotherapy in the treatment of depression: review of two practice guidelines. Arch Gen Psychiatry 53(4):283–290, 1996 8634003

Qaseem A, Snow V, Denberg TD, et al: Using second-generation antidepressants to treat depressive disorders: a clinical practice guideline from the American College of Physicians. Ann Intern Med 149(10):725–733, 2008 8634003

Qaseem A, Barry MJ, Kansagara D: Nonpharmacologic versus pharmacologic treatment of adult patients with major depressive disorder: a clinical practice guideline from the American College of Physicians. Ann Intern Med 164(5):350–359, 2016 26857948

Ravindran AV, Balneaves LG, Faulkner G, et al: Canadian Network for Mood and Anxiety Treatments (CANMAT) 2016 clinical guidelines for the management of adults with major depressive disorder: Section 5. Complementary and alternative medicine treatments. Can J Psychiatry 61(9):576–587, 2016 27486153

Regier DA, Hirschfeld RM, Goodwin FK, et al: The NIMH depression awareness, recognition, and treatment program: structure, aims, and scientific basis. Am J Psychiatry 145(11):1351–1357, 1988 2847566

Rothman DJ, McDonald WJ, Berkowitz CD, et al: Professional medical associations and their relationships with industry: a proposal for controlling conflict of interest. JAMA 301(13):1367–1372, 2009 19336712

Rush AJ, Thase ME: Improving depression outcome by patient-centered medical management. Am J Psychiatry 175(12):1187–1198, 2018 30220219

Rush AJ, Beck AT, Kovacs M, et al: Comparative efficacy of cognitive therapy and pharmacotherapy in the treatment of depressed outpatients. Cognit Ther Res 1:17–37, 1977

Rush AJ, Trivedi MH, Ibrahim HM, et al: The 16-Item Quick Inventory of Depressive Symptomatology (QIDS), clinician rating (QIDS-C), and self-report (QIDS-SR): a psychometric evaluation in patients with chronic major depression. Biol Psychiatry 54(5):573–583, 2003 12946886

Rush AJ, Fava M, Wisniewski SR, et al: Sequenced treatment alternatives to relieve depression (STAR*D): rationale and design. Control Clin Trials 25(1):119–142, 2004 15061154

Rush AJ, Marangell LB, Sackeim HA, et al: Vagus nerve stimulation for treatment-resistant depression: a randomized, controlled acute phase trial. Biol Psychiatry 58(5):347–354, 2005 16139580

Rush AJ, Trivedi MH, Wisniewski SR, et al: Acute and longer-term outcomes in depressed outpatients requiring one or several treatment steps: a STAR*D report. Am J Psychiatry 163(11):1905–1917, 2006 17074942

Schulberg HC, Katon W, Simon GE, et al: Treating major depression in primary care practice: an update of the Agency for Health Care Policy and Research Practice Guidelines. Arch Gen Psychiatry 55(12):1121–1127, 1998 9862556

Stahl SM, Morrissette DA, Faedda G, et al: Guidelines for the recognition and management of mixed depression. CNS Spectr 22(2):203–219, 2017 28421980

Suppes T, Silva R, Cucchiaro J, et al: Lurasidone for the treatment of major depressive disorder with mixed features: a randomized, double-blind, placebo-controlled study. Am J Psychiatry 173(4):400–407, 2016 26552942

Szegedi A, Jansen WT, van Willigenburg APP, et al: Early improvement in the first 2 weeks as a predictor of treatment outcome in patients with major depressive disorder: a meta-analysis including 6562 patients. J Clin Psychiatry 70(3):344–353, 2009 19254516
Thase ME: Depression-focused psychotherapies, in Treatment of Psychiatric Disorders, 3rd Edition, Vol 2. Edited by Gabbard GO. Washington, DC, American Psychiatric Press, 2001, pp 1181–1227
Thase ME: What role do atypical antipsychotic drugs have in treatment-resistant depression? J Clin Psychiatry 63(2):95–103, 2002 11874227
Thase ME, Rush AJ: Treatment resistant depression, in Psychopharmacology: The Fourth Generation of Progress. Edited by Bloom FE, Kupfer DJ. New York, Raven, 1995, pp 1081–1097
Thase ME, Rush AJ: When at first you don't succeed: sequential strategies for antidepressant nonresponders. J Clin Psychiatry 58 (suppl 13):23–29, 1997 9402916
Thase ME, Trivedi MH, Rush AJ: MAOIs in the contemporary treatment of depression. Neuropsychopharmacology 12(3):185–219, 1995 7612154
Trangle M, Gursky J, Haight R, et al: Adult Depression in Primary Care, 17th Edition. Institute for Clinical Systems Improvement, 2016. Available at: www.icsi.org/wp-content/uploads/2019/01/Depr.pdf. Accessed November 27, 2020.
Trivedi MH, Rush AJ, Crismon ML, et al: Clinical results for patients with major depressive disorder in the Texas Medication Algorithm Project. Arch Gen Psychiatry 61(7):669–680, 2004 15237079
Trivedi MH, Rush AJ, Wisniewski SR, et al: Evaluation of outcomes with citalopram for depression using measurement-based care in STAR*D: implications for clinical practice. Am J Psychiatry 163(1):28–40, 2006 16390886
Turner EH, Matthews AM, Linardatos E, et al: Selective publication of antidepressant trials and its influence on apparent efficacy. N Engl J Med 358(3):252–260, 2008 18199864
U.S. Department of Veterans Affairs; U.S. Department of Defense: VA/DoD Clinical Practice Guideline for the Management of Major Depressive Disorder. Management of Major Depressive Disorder Working Group, 2016. Available at: www.healthquality.va.gov/guidelines/MH/mdd/VADoDMDDCPGFINAL82916.pdf. Accessed November 27, 2020.
UW Health: Diagnosing and Treating Depression—Pediatric/Adult—Ambulatory Clinical Practice Guideline. 2015. Available at: https://ghcscw.com/SiteCollectionDocuments/Clinical_Practice_Guidelines/15_CPG_Diagnosis_Depression.pdf. Accessed November 27, 2020.
Wagner G, Schultes MT, Titscher V, et al: Efficacy and safety of levomilnacipran, vilazodone and vortioxetine compared with other second-generation antidepressants for major depressive disorder in adults: a systematic review and network meta-analysis. J Affect Disord 228:1–12, 2018 29197738
Weissman MM, Prusoff BA, Dimascio A, et al: The efficacy of drugs and psychotherapy in the treatment of acute depressive episodes. Am J Psychiatry 136(4B):555–558, 1979 371421

CHAPTER 29

Treatment Guidelines for Bipolar Disorder

Jorge Renner Cardoso de Almeida, M.D., Ph.D.
Lakshmi N. Yatham, M.B.B.S., FRCPC
Benjamin Goldstein, M.D., Ph.D.

Bipolar spectrum disorders, which affect up to 2.4% of the population, are associated with a high disease burden and cost. Despite having a distinguishing phenotype (i.e., mania and hypomania), bipolar disorder is associated with high rates of misdiagnosis—particularly misdiagnosis with major depressive disorder (Almeida and Phillips 2013). For about 30% of individuals, it takes about 10 years from the first appearance of symptoms to receive a correct diagnosis (Hirschfeld et al. 2003b). Accurate diagnosis is of central importance for optimal treatment. Bipolar disorder is associated with the highest rate of suicide—up to 15% among individuals with the illness—of any psychiatric disorder (Goodwin and Jamison 2007a; Schaffer et al. 2015; Strakowski 2014). Individuals with bipolar disorder frequently experience a relapsing and remitting course of illness that requires purposeful medication management, with special attention to avoiding polypharmacy as the illness course changes. Furthermore, the illness course is typically associated with progressive cognitive decline as the patient continues to experience mood episodes (Burdick et al. 2014, 2019; López-Jaramillo et al. 2010; Molina et al. 2016), with neurocognitive deficits often worse when the patient is symptomatic yet still present during the remission phase of the illness (Burdick et al. 2019). However, a recent meta-analysis did not find evidence that progressive cognitive decline occurs in most patients with bipolar disorder (Szmulewicz et al. 2020). Cognitive impairment is often an indicator of relapse, a decreased level of functioning, and risk for future hospitalization (Bonnín et al. 2010; Martino et al. 2009). Functional recovery is often slow, and long-term disability is often present. Taken together, these challenges can be hard to treat if not considered systematically. Centers of excellence that specialize in treating bipolar disorder have grown in number in recent years, especially in academic settings, allowing individuals with bipolar disorder to receive evidence-based, optimal care early in the course of their illness. In this chapter, we delineate the different components necessary to provide optimal treatment for bipolar disorder.

Considerations in Bipolar Disorder Diagnosis

The diagnosis of bipolar disorder remains a clinical endeavor because no biologically relevant diagnostic markers of bipolar disorder are currently available (Almeida and Phillips 2013). The clinical diagnosis is associated with high rates of misdiagnosis, especially with major depressive disorder, and in about 30% of individuals it takes approximately 10 years and assessment by three or more psychiatrists to receive an accurate diagnosis (Goodwin and Jamison 2007b). Only 20% of individuals with bipolar disorder seeking care during a depressive episode receive the correct diagnosis of bipolar disorder within the first year of seeking treatment, and close to 60% of individuals with bipolar disorder are initially diagnosed as having unipolar depression (Hirschfeld et al. 2003b). Unfortunately, misdiagnosis of bipolar depression as unipolar depression has many potentially deleterious consequences, including inappropriate medication, which in turn might lead to a poorer prognosis, increased suicidal ideation/suicide attempts, and increased risk of switching to mania, as well as greater health care costs (Hirschfeld et al. 2003b; Perlis et al. 2010; Valentí et al. 2012). Two main reasons for the difficulty in distinguishing between bipolar and unipolar depression are the higher prevalence of depressive relative to hypomanic or manic symptoms over the course of bipolar disorder (with hypomanic/manic symptoms experienced only about 1% of the time in bipolar II disorder and 9% of the time in bipolar I disorder [Judd et al. 2002, 2003]) and the presence of subthreshold manic symptoms in up to 30%–55% of individuals during a depressive episode (Akiskal and Mallya 1987; Angst et al. 2010; Judd et al. 2012). Furthermore, patients tend to seek care during the depressive phase, rather than during the hypomanic or manic phase, and patients often do not mention having previously experienced manic symptoms (for instance, patients may perceive times marked by such symptoms as their "good days" or have a negative bias that is commonly seen during a depressive episode) (Goodwin and Jamison 2007b). Although there is some controversy in the literature, clinicians may want to consider using the Mood Disorder Questionnaire as a screening tool to further prompt reporting of symptomatology, especially if they do not typically ask about such symptoms during routine clinical care (Hirschfeld et al. 2003a). More recently, as in DSM-5 (American Psychiatric Association 2013), experts have argued for the bipolar disorder diagnosis to be considered on a continuum, while the search for empirically based clinical criteria and objective markers continues (Almeida and Phillips 2013). However, there are several features of depression that may increase suspicion of bipolarity and prompt more careful investigation, including earlier age at illness onset; high recurrence of depressive episodes; a family history of bipolar disorder; depression with psychotic features; psychomotor agitation; atypical depressive symptoms such as hypersomnia, hyperphagia, and leaden paralysis; postpartum depression or psychosis; past suicide attempts; and antidepressant-induced manic symptoms or rapid cycling (Yatham et al. 2018). Ultimately, a comprehensive clinical assessment is of fundamental importance in identifying depression with features suggestive of bipolar disorder; the clinician commits to looking for signs and symptoms of previous mania and other comorbidities for an accurate diagnosis. Although not always feasible, this assessment is optimally achieved with the use of a structured or semistructured diagnostic interview designed to be administered by a trained clinician, such as the Structured Clinical Interview for DSM-5 (SCID-5; First et al. 2016), the Schedule for Affective Disorders and Schizophrenia for School-Age Children (K-SADS; Kaufman et al. 1997), or the Diagnostic Interview for Genetics Studies (DIGS; Nurnberger et al. 1994). Zimmerman (2016) described use of the SCID-5 in intake visits at a large general academic psychiatric practice, with good results.

Evidence-Based Medicine

In this chapter, we classify the different treatment options according to current medical evidence across illness course (i.e., acute mania, acute depression, relapse prevention). Typically, the highest evidence designation (i.e., first-line) is given to approaches that have received FDA approval or for which there is evidence of efficacy from replicated positive double-blind, randomized controlled trials (RCTs); in assigning this level, we also consider the safety and tolerability profile of the treatment modality, including risk of a treatment-emergent switch. Options designated as second-line are those that have received FDA approval but have a problematic side-effect profile and/or poor evidence of efficacy in another illness phase. We also designate as second-line those options that have not received FDA approval but have accrued enough evidence to be considered for off-label use. Medications with lower-level or controversial evidence of efficacy and/or an unfavorable side-effect profile are designated as third-line options. In making this determination, we also considered other illness phases. The approaches used here are similar to those described by Strakowski et al. (2020), and by Yatham et al. (2018) in the Canadian Network for Mood and Anxiety Treatments (CANMAT) guideline for bipolar disorder (adapted to U.S. readership to take into account FDA recommendations).

The general approach when initiating new treatment or evaluating current treatment for bipolar disorder is to select and start one of the first-line medication options for treating the current illness phase (while also considering whether the chosen medication is effective for relapse prevention), gradually increasing the dosage to at least the middle of the recommended dosage range, per individual tolerance. Even though the clinician should give preference to medications that the person (or even a family member with bipolar disorder) responded to previously, selection of the best medication regimen is ultimately based on a few important factors. For instance, the clinician should consider the efficacy and adverse-event profile of the medication, the patient's previous history of treatment response or nonresponse, and clinical features of the episode that may predict response (e.g., classic euphoric mania responds better to lithium, whereas mania with psychotic symptoms responds better to antipsychotics). The process should be carried out systematically until the patient's symptoms resolve, because persistence of symptoms, even if subsyndromal, predicts a poor outcome. Once remission is achieved for 2 months (sometimes a longer period is used for individuals with more chronic symptoms), the clinician should consider tapering acute-phase medications with less evidence of efficacy in maintenance treatment and, when necessary, replacing them with medications with more evidence for efficacy in maintenance. However, as a general rule, the treatment that works for the acute phase is typically also effective in preventing relapse of that phase of illness. The clinician should consider reducing the medication dosage if there are tolerability concerns, while bearing in mind the risk of relapse or recurrence. Because management of bipolar disorder is a lifelong process, the clinician should consider whether polypharmacy is truly indicated, given that no clinical trial has tested three or more concurrent medications and there are concerns regarding the generalizability of clinical trials in bipolar disorder to community samples (Hoertel et al. 2013). Furthermore, the side effects may trigger other medical problems (e.g., olanzapine leading to metabolic syndrome). Importantly, there is no cure for bipolar disorder, and the relapse rate is high (within 6–12 months) if maintenance treatment is discontinued, even after several years of mood stability (Kessing et al. 2004; Murru et al. 2019).

In acute mania, it is reasonable to expect a 50% response rate with any of the first-line options (or in combination with a first-line option for maintenance treatment in individuals with more chronic illness) within 3–6 weeks at the recommended dosage. If there is no evidence of response after 2–3 weeks, the clinician should consider a further dosage increase or a switch to a different compound. Given that fewer studies are available to provide guidance on treatment of hypomania, it is reasonable to use the same approach used to treat acute mania.

Similarly, in acute depression, it is reasonable to expect a 50% response rate with any of the first-line options (or in combination with a first-line option for maintenance in individuals with more chronic illness) within 6–12 weeks at the recommended dosage. If there is no evidence of response after 4–6 weeks, the clinician should consider switching to a different compound or increasing the dosage, while keeping in mind that depression typically responds to lower- to mid-range medication dosages (unlike acute mania, which usually requires higher medication dosage ranges). Again, because fewer studies are available on the treatment of depression in the context of bipolar II disorder, it is reasonable to use the approach delineated for depression in bipolar I disorder, with the exception that an antidepressant might be considered as a higher-evidence-level option or even as monotherapy (Yatham et al. 2018). However, until more evidence is available and this controversy is resolved, the general clinician should continue to use antidepressants as an adjunctive option only.

Acute Mania

As shown in Table 29–1 (modified from Yatham et al. 2018), first-line therapies for acute mania in adults with bipolar disorder are lithium, quetiapine, cariprazine, asenapine, risperidone, aripiprazole, and divalproex (in men). Second-line therapies for acute mania in adults with bipolar disorder are olanzapine, ziprasidone, carbamazepine, paliperidone, divalproex (in women), and electroconvulsive therapy (ECT). Third-line therapies for acute mania in adults with bipolar disorder are clozapine, chlorpromazine, and haloperidol.

All first-line therapies for acute mania that are FDA approved show good evidence during this illness phase, as well as for treating bipolar disorder in general. Lithium remains a first-line treatment for acute mania but is unfortunately disfavored in acute inpatient settings because of its relatively slower action compared with other first-line options for acute mania. However, we recommend keeping lithium as a go-to choice because of its overall better action in bipolar disorder. Quetiapine is also a first-line option, given its efficacy in acute mania and also in treating acute bipolar depression, as well as its role in preventing both manic and depressive relapses. Cariprazine is a first-line option for acute mania and depression, but it is a relatively new medication with no evidence in relapse prevention yet. In addition to their efficacy in acute mania, both risperidone and asenapine also have good evidence for maintenance, but neither has been studied for efficacy in acute depression in large RCTs. Aripiprazole is also FDA approved for acute mania and maintenance treatment, but trials for bipolar depression, which is the most common presentation of the illness, have been negative. Finally, divalproex is a good option for men, with some evidence of efficacy for acute depression and maintenance, but it should be considered a second-line option in women because of its unfavorable side-effect profile.

Olanzapine has been downgraded to second line because of its problematic side-effect profile (Yatham et al. 2018), despite being FDA approved for acute mania, maintenance treatment, and acute depression (in combination with fluoxetine). Ziprasidone is considered a second-line option because the evidence is positive only when ziprasidone is combined with lithium or divalproex for maintenance. Ziprasidone's potential cardiac effects (QTc prolongation) are another factor in the decision to designate it as a second-line option. Despite its FDA-approved indication for treating acute mania, carbamazepine also is not classified as a first-line option because of its unfavorable adverse-effect profile. Paliperidone is not FDA approved for treatment of acute mania despite several positive studies, and in fact, a meta-analysis has questioned its efficacy (Chang et al. 2017). Finally, ECT is relatively effective in the treatment of acute mania (Yatham et al. 2018), but because of its cognitive effects, the stigma related to its use, and the requirement of medical support for administration, it is classified as a second-line option. However, ECT might be the best option for pregnant patients or those with psychosis, or for medically complicated patients.

Third-line options with evidence of effectiveness in acute mania include clozapine (although there are only limited data on clozapine's efficacy in acute depression and maintenance treatment, and it has an unfavorable side-effect profile), chlorpromazine (despite having FDA approval for acute mania), and haloperidol (which may worsen depression long term, and has an unfavorable side-effect profile) (Yatham et al. 2018).

Acute Depression

As described in Table 29–1, first-line therapies for acute depression in adults with bipolar disorder are quetiapine, lurasidone, cariprazine, and lithium. Second-line acute depression therapies for adults with bipolar disorder are cognitive-behavioral therapy, family-focused therapy, interpersonal and social rhythm therapy, lamotrigine, olanzapine/fluoxetine combination, divalproex (in men), and adjunctive antidepressants (i.e., selective serotonin reuptake inhibitors, bupropion). Third-line therapies for acute depression in adults with bipolar disorder are olanzapine (monotherapy), divalproex (in women), carbamazepine, asenapine, risperidone, stimulants (adjunctive), and ECT.

TABLE 29–1. Therapies typically used in bipolar disorder, with corresponding dosage ranges, evidence-based indications (i.e., first- vs. second- vs. third-line) during each illness phase, and safety/tolerability profile

Medication	Range (daily dosage, mg)	Acute mania	Acute depression	Relapse and recurrence prevention	Safety concerns[a]		Tolerability concerns[a]		Risk of treatment-emergent switch[a]	
					A	RRP	A	RRP	Mania	Depression
Antidepressants										
SSRIs	Variable		Second (adj)		–	–	+	+	+	–
Bupropion	300–450		Second (adj)		+	–	+	–	+	–
Aripiprazole	5–20	First[b]		First (mono[b] and adj with Li/DVP)	–	–	+	+	–	–
Asenapine	5–20	First[b]	Third	First	–	–	+	+	–	–
Carbamazepine[c]	200–1,600	Second[b]	Third	Third	++	++[d]	+	++	–	–
Cariprazine	3–6	First[b]	First[b]		–	–	+	–	–	–
Chlorpromazine	300–900	Third[b]			NA	NA	NA	NA	NA	NA
Clozapine	300–900	Third		Third	++	+++	++	+++	–	–
Divalproex[e]	500–2,500	First[b,d]	Second[d]	Second[d]	–	++[d]	+	+	–	–
ECT		Second	Third		+	++	+	++	–	–
Haloperidol	5–15	Third			+	+++	++	++	–	++
Lamotrigine	100–300		Second	First[b]	++	–	–	–	–	–
Lithium[f]	600–2,400	First[b]	First	First[b]	+	++	+	++	–	–
Lurasidone	20–160		First[b]	Third	–	–	+	+	–	–
Modafinil	200–400		Third (adj)		–	–	–	–	++	Not known
Olanzapine	5–30	Second[b]	Third	Second[b]	+	+++	++	++	–	–

TABLE 29–1. Therapies typically used in bipolar disorder, with corresponding dosage ranges, evidence-based indications (i.e., first- vs. second- vs. third-line) during each illness phase, and safety/tolerability profile *(continued)*

Medication	Range (daily dosage, mg)	Acute mania	Acute depression	Relapse and recurrence prevention	Safety concerns[a]		Tolerability concerns[a]		Risk of treatment-emergent switch[a]	
					A	RRP	A	RRP	Mania	Depression
Olanzapine/fluoxetine	6–12/25–50		Second[b]		+	+++	++	++	–	–
Paliperidone	3–12	Second		Third	–	+	+	++	–	–
Quetiapine	200–800[g]	First[b]	First[b]	First (mono and adj[b] with Li/DVP)	+	++	++	++	–	–
Risperidone	2–6	First[b]	Third		–	+	+	++	–	–
Risperidone LAI	12.5–50			First (mono and adj[b] with Li/DVP)	–	+	+	++	–	–
Ziprasidone	40–160	Second		Second (adj[b] with Li/DVP)	++	++	++	+	–	–

Note. A=acute; adj=adjunctive therapy; DVP=divalproex; ECT=electroconvulsive therapy; mono=monotherapy; LAI=long-acting injectable; Li=lithium; NA=not available; RPR=relapse and recurrence prevention; SSRI=selective serotonin reuptake inhibitor.

[a]Concerns/risks: –=limited impact on treatment selection; +=minor impact on treatment selection; ++=moderate impact on treatment selection; +++=significant impact on treatment selection.

[b]FDA approved.

[c]Carbamazepine therapeutic range: 4–12 µg/mL.

[d]In women of childbearing age, carbamazepine and divalproex should be downgraded one level and used with caution.

[e]Divalproex therapeutic range: 50–150 µg/mL.

[f]Lithium therapeutic range: 0.6–1.2 mEq/L.

[g]If used for mania, quetiapine daily dosage should exceed 500 mg.

Source. Adapted from Yatham et al. 2018.

All of the first-line therapies that are FDA approved for acute depression show good evidence for efficacy during this illness phase. Quetiapine is also a first-line option for maintenance treatment when combined with lithium or divalproex (and as monotherapy), and it is an efficacious antimanic agent as well. Positive open-label extension trial data support the use of lurasidone in maintenance treatment; however, in the only double-blind RCT examining lurasidone for this indication, the medication failed on the primary efficacy measure. Nevertheless, post hoc analysis revealed that in patients with an index depressive episode, lurasidone adjunctive therapy was more effective than placebo adjunctive therapy in preventing relapse of mood episodes. Therefore, it is reasonable to consider maintenance therapy with lurasidone as an adjunct to mood stabilizers in patients with bipolar depression who respond to lurasidone augmentation for acute depression. Cariprazine recently received FDA approval for acute depression (Pinto et al. 2020; Saraf et al. 2019; Stahl et al. 2020), and it is also approved for acute mania; however, it is a relatively new medication and has not yet been studied as a relapse prevention agent. Lithium remains in this category because of its historical evidence, despite the lack of FDA approval and despite reported negative trials (Yatham et al. 2018).

The olanzapine/fluoxetine combination is not included as a first-line therapy because of its significant adverse-effect profile, despite being FDA approved for acute depression. Lamotrigine is not FDA approved for treatment of acute depression because data from trials were mixed (Yatham et al. 2018); moreover, it requires a slow titration, and there is poor-quality evidence for its effectiveness in treating acute mania. However, lamotrigine is approved as a maintenance option and thus should be considered a second-line therapy for acute depression. Divalproex also is not FDA approved despite positive evidence. It is, however, a first-line option for acute mania, although it carries risk for women of reproductive age, so we included it as second-line therapy for men but a third-line therapy for women. When combined with an antimanic agent, antidepressants could be considered a second-line treatment for bipolar depression. Despite the ongoing controversy about their use in bipolar disorder (McGirr et al. 2016), antidepressants are still widely used in clinical practice, possibly because of their role in treating anxiety, which is highly comorbid with bipolar disorder.

Third-line options for treating acute depression include olanzapine monotherapy or olanzapine in combination with fluoxetine (because of olanzapine's significant adverse-effect profile, it is classified as a third-line option despite having FDA approval) (Yatham et al. 2018); carbamazepine (also designated third line because of its adverse-effect profile despite reasonably good evidence for its effectiveness in acute depression); asenapine; and risperidone (for which data are lacking but there is some evidence of effectiveness in treating acute mania; risperidone is also a good maintenance option). The evidence supporting use of stimulants in the treatment of acute depression is still controversial, but this class of medications should be considered for patients who have not responded to other options or patients who have comorbid ADHD; however, stimulants should not be considered for patients with a history of psychosis. ECT is an effective antidepressant for both unipolar and bipolar depression, but because of its cognitive effects and associated stigma, it is considered a third-line option. However, ECT may be considered first line in certain situations, including for individuals with suicidal intent or behavior or severely psychotic or medically compromised individuals. ECT may also have a unique role in pregnancy (Yatham et al. 2018).

Relapse and Recurrence Prevention

As previously noted, bipolar disorder often manifests a relapsing and remitting illness trajectory that requires purposeful medication management with special attention to avoiding polypharmacy as symptoms change. As a clinician considers the different treatment options, it is important to aim toward relapse and recurrence prevention (i.e., maintenance treatment) when selecting treatment for the acute phase of the illness. Moreover, functional recovery typically follows symptom improvement by weeks or months after a major affective episode, so preventing recurrences is critical for good long-term outcomes.

As described in Table 29–1, first-line maintenance monotherapies for adults with bipolar disorder are lithium, lamotrigine, quetiapine, aripiprazole, and asenapine; adjunctive therapies with lithium or divalproex are quetiapine and aripiprazole. Adjunctive psychoeducation is also considered a first-line maintenance treatment. Risperidone (both long-acting injectable monotherapy and adjunctive therapy) can also be considered here. Second-line maintenance therapies for adults with bipolar disorder include psychological strategies used as adjuncts to pharmacotherapy (e.g., cognitive-behavioral therapy, family-focused therapy, interpersonal social rhythm therapy), olanzapine, divalproex (third line in women), and ziprasidone (used as an adjunct to lithium or divalproex). Third-line maintenance therapies for adults with bipolar disorder include adjunctive peer support specialist (PSS) involvement, lurasidone, paliperidone, carbamazepine, and clozapine.

Lithium continues to be the medication with the most evidence for relapse prevention in bipolar disorder. It reduces the frequency of, and extends the time until, recurrence of both mania and depression, and there is some evidence suggesting that it decreases suicidality. Other FDA-approved first-line choices are lamotrigine (best used to prevent depression [Strakowski et al. 2020; Yatham et al. 2018]); aripiprazole (best used to prevent mania); long-acting risperidone (as monotherapy or adjunctive therapy; best used to prevent mania); and quetiapine (as monotherapy or an adjunct to therapy with lithium or divalproex; probably a good option to prevent depression and mania [Strakowski et al. 2020; Yatham et al. 2018] and shows evidence of effectiveness as monotherapy [Strakowski et al. 2020; Yatham et al. 2018]). Finally, asenapine is also a first-line choice, given that it prevents both mania and depression (McIntyre et al. 2010; Szegedi et al. 2018).

Olanzapine is FDA approved for relapse prevention in bipolar disorder, but because of its side-effect profile, it should be considered a second-line option (Strakowski et al. 2020; Yatham et al. 2018). When added to lithium or divalproex, ziprasidone is FDA approved as maintenance treatment, but the data are weak regarding its efficacy in preventing depression, so we have listed it as a second-line treatment. Divalproex is likewise listed as a second-line option, and despite its frequent use in clinical practice for relapse prevention, it has not received FDA approval for this indication because of the lack of large positive RCTs. In addition, divalproex can lead to polycystic ovary syndrome in reproductive-age women, so it should be considered a third-line option in this population group (Strakowski et al. 2020; Yatham et al. 2018).

Third-line options for relapse prevention include lurasidone (best for acute depression), paliperidone (not properly studied in bipolar disorder), carbamazepine (inadequate evidence for efficacy and a problematic side-effect profile), and clozapine. The use of antidepressants or stimulants for maintenance treatment in clinical practice remains controversial, and use of these agents is not an evidence-based approach to relapse prevention and may lead to mood switching.

Ongoing Safety Evaluation, Mood Monitoring, and Comorbidity Assessment

As noted earlier, bipolar disorder is associated with the highest rate of suicide of any psychiatric illness, occurring in up to 15% of individuals with the disorder, and this rate is even higher if the person is receiving no treatment at all (Fiedorowicz et al. 2009, 2019; Leon et al. 2014; Persons et al. 2018). Therefore, keeping individuals with bipolar disorder alive is a major treatment goal. The watchful clinician should evaluate the patient for safety at every visit and consider a higher level of care if actual risk is identified, always being conservative (i.e., choosing hospitalization rather than outpatient care) when in doubt. Safety should be evaluated not only for suicidal behavior but also for psychosis (including catatonia) and aggressive/impulsive behavior, which are often under-evaluated.

Because of the relapsing-remitting nature of bipolar disorder, it is important to use mood charts or other tracking tools throughout the illness course. Monitoring for triggers and vulnerabilities, identifying early signs and symptoms, and implementing prevention and intervention strategies as early as possible constitute the "relapse-prevention triangle" of essential tactics to avoid a new full-blown mood episode. Optimally, these efforts should be documented in a written plan that is shared with members of the individual's safety net.

Important triggers to monitor include the disorders that are frequently comorbid with bipolar disorder, such as substance use disorders, anxiety disorders, and other medical conditions. If possible, a primary care provider should be included as part of the treatment team for individuals with bipolar disorder, because physical complaints are often not properly evaluated in individuals with a documented psychiatric history. A savvy provider should advocate for the patient to receive high-quality care and also be prepared to identify and manage comorbid medical problems (beyond substance use and anxiety disorders), because these can trigger a relapse or a new episode.

Attention to comorbid medical conditions is especially important because these conditions are frequently untreated despite their high prevalence and negative impact on a patient's longevity (Chesney et al. 2014; Crump et al. 2013; Forty et al. 2014; Gomes et al. 2013; Kemp et al. 2014; Schoepf and Heun 2015; Smith et al. 2013; Wu et al. 2013). In particular, metabolic syndrome is common in patients with bipolar disorder (occurring in 20%–65% of these individuals), leading to premature mortality due to increased risk for cardiovascular disease and diabetes mellitus (Gans 2006). This risk highlights the necessity for vigilance when treating all patients with bipolar disorder, including regular assessments of their metabolic parameters (for comprehensive guidelines, see Ng et al. 2009). Treatment strategies that target metabolic disorders should include nonpharmacological and pharmacological interventions in collaboration with a primary care provider and/or specialist.

A New Care Model for Treating Bipolar Disorder: Preliminary Results

At the Dell Medical School at the University of Texas at Austin, within the Mulva Clinics for Neurosciences, Almeida and colleagues used the principles described in the book *Redefining Health Care* by Porter and Teisberg (2006) to design an integrated practice unit (IPU). (Porter and Teisberg provided a road map [designed from the perspective of the person receiving care] for improving care while also striving to achieve the highest possible quality at the lowest cost.) The bipolar disorder–specific IPU implemented by Almeida and colleagues provided a predetermined care pathway organized around the individual with bipolar disorder (J. Almeida, K. Casey, R. Day, et al.: "A New Care Model to Treat Bipolar Disorder Using a 6-Week Cycle Organized in an Integrated Practice Unit: Preliminary Results of 100 Individuals Into the First Cycle," manuscript in preparation). Specialization of care may produce improved syndromic, symptomatic, and functional recovery outcomes, and it is typically achieved in so-called centers of excellence (Kessing et al. 2013; Kuiper et al. 2014; Macritchie et al. 2019; Vieta 2013). Such centers help to increase the depth and sophistication of treatment by supplying high concentrations of expertise and resources focused on a particular medical area (e.g., bipolar disorder) and delivered in a comprehensive, interdisciplinary fashion.

The multidisciplinary team includes psychiatrist, therapist, pharmacist, nurse, and peer support specialist. The care pathway is modeled on a 6-week cycle (Figure 29–1), with systematic integration of evidence-based pharmacological and psychosocial treatments. The term *cycle* is deliberately used within the team and between the team and the person receiving care to create a limited time frame that is measurable and repeatable (i.e., one may enter into subsequent cycles if no improvement is achieved). Each week, the individual receiving care meets with a psychiatrist for up 30 minutes and with a therapist for up to 60 minutes. These two visits are provided in the same room, one after the other ("in tandem"), to reinforce the person-centered nature of the care delivery. Prior to entering a cycle, each person participates in a comprehensive diagnostic evaluation that includes a structured clinical interview. In the first visit of the cycle, the team develops a personalized psychosocial treatment plan based on the six most problematic areas identified by the individual out of a menu of 24 problems typically seen in bipolar disorder. Each problem is managed using predetermined treatments that are evidence-based. Moreover, any medication change is based on the latest guidelines. Finally, as part of the standard of care at every visit, each individual also completes a patient-reported outcome (PRO) that provides a current picture of the patient's health status and care experience from his or her own perspective and helps to guide treatment decisions. Consistent with IPU principles, these PROs are dynamic and subject to change based on perceived value to the patient and clinician (i.e., if measured outcomes are not sensitive or informative, they will be dropped in a subsequent IPU generation). The first generation of this program, which yielded very good results, is illustrated in Figure 29–2 for the first 67 participants (J. Almeida, K. Casey, R. Day, et al: "A New Care Model to Treat Bipolar Disorder Using a 6-Week Cycle Organized in an Integrated Practice Unit: Preliminary Results of 100 Individuals Into the First Cycle," manuscript in preparation). This type of integrative model may be the future of psychiatric care.

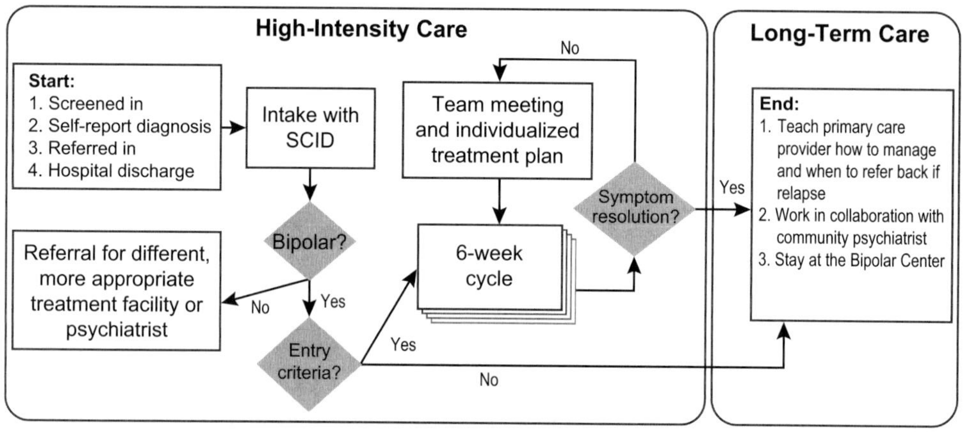

FIGURE 29–1. Six-week care pathway plus intake with comprehensive diagnostic assessment.

SCID=Structured Clinical Interview for DSM.

Source. J. Almeida, K. Casey, R. Day, et al.: "A New Care Model to Treat Bipolar Disorder Using a 6-Week Cycle Organized in an Integrated Practice Unit: Preliminary Results of 100 Individuals Into the First Cycle," manuscript in preparation.

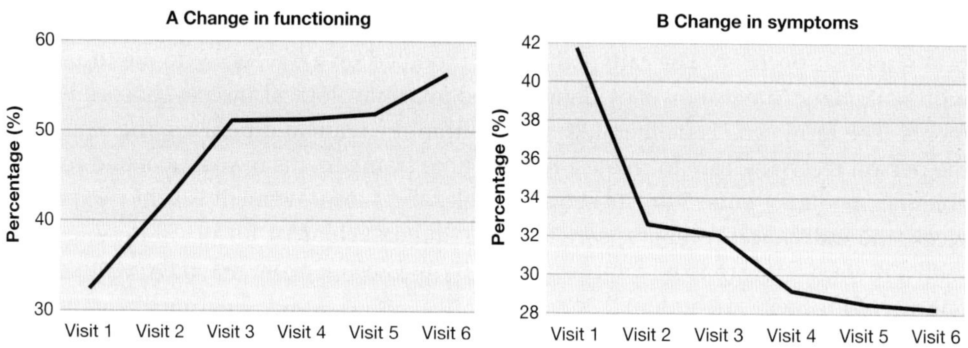

FIGURE 29–2. First-cycle outcomes for patients in a novel bipolar disorder integrated practice unit (IPU).

Outcome results for the first 67 patients with bipolar disorder who entered the novel bipolar disorder IPU demonstrated marked improvement as a percentage of baseline assessments in **(A)** functioning, as measured by the Sheehan Disability Scale (Sheehan et al. 1996), and in **(B)** symptoms, as measured by the Affective Self Rating Scale (Adler et al. 2008).

Source. J. Almeida, K. Casey, R. Day, et al.: "A New Care Model to Treat Bipolar Disorder Using a 6-Week Cycle Organized in an Integrated Practice Unit: Preliminary Results of 100 Individuals Into the First Cycle," manuscript in preparation.

References

Adler M, Liberg B, Andersson S, et al: Development and validation of the Affective Self Rating Scale for manic, depressive, and mixed affective states. Nord J Psychiatry 62(2):130–135, 2008 18569776

Akiskal HS, Mallya G: Criteria for the "soft" bipolar spectrum: treatment implications. Psychopharmacol Bull 23(1):68–73, 1987 3602332

Almeida JRC, Phillips ML: Distinguishing between unipolar depression and bipolar depression: current and future clinical and neuroimaging perspectives. Biol Psychiatry 73(2):111–118, 2013 22784485

American Psychiatric Association: Diagnostic and Statistical Manual of Mental Disorders, 5th Edition. Arlington, VA, American Psychiatric Association, 2013

Angst J, Cui L, Swendsen J, et al: Major depressive disorder with subthreshold bipolarity in the National Comorbidity Survey Replication. Am J Psychiatry 167(10):1194–1201, 2010 20713498

Bonnín CM, Martínez-Arán A, Torrent C, et al: Clinical and neurocognitive predictors of functional outcome in bipolar euthymic patients: a long-term, follow-up study. J Affect Disord 121(1–2):156–160, 2010 19505727

Burdick KE, Russo M, Frangou S, et al: Empirical evidence for discrete neurocognitive subgroups in bipolar disorder: clinical implications. Psychol Med 44(14):3083–3096, 2014 25065409

Burdick KE, Millett CE, Bonnín CDM, et al: The International Consortium Investigating Neurocognition in Bipolar Disorder (ICONIC-BD). Bipolar Disord 21(1):6–10, 2019 30720913

Chang HY, Tseng PT, Stubbs B, et al: The efficacy and tolerability of paliperidone in mania of bipolar disorder: a preliminary meta-analysis. Exp Clin Psychopharmacol 25(5):422–433, 2017 29048190

Chesney E, Goodwin GM, Fazel S: Risks of all-cause and suicide mortality in mental disorders: a meta-review. World Psychiatry 13(2):153–160, 2014 24890068

Crump C, Sundquist K, Winkleby MA, et al: Comorbidities and mortality in bipolar disorder: a Swedish national cohort study. JAMA Psychiatry 70(9):931–939, 2013 23863861

Fiedorowicz JG, Leon AC, Keller MB, et al: Do risk factors for suicidal behavior differ by affective disorder polarity? Psychol Med 39(5):763–771, 2009 18667100

Fiedorowicz JG, Persons JE, Assari S, et al: Depressive symptoms carry an increased risk for suicidal ideation and behavior in bipolar disorder without any additional contribution of mixed symptoms. J Affect Disord 246:775–782, 2019 30623823

First MB, Williams JBW, Karg RS, Spitzer RL: Structured Clinical Interview for DSM-5 Disorders, Clinician Version (SCID-5-CV). Arlington, VA, American Psychiatric Association, 2016

Forty L, Ulanova A, Jones L, et al: Comorbid medical illness in bipolar disorder. Br J Psychiatry 205(6):465–472, 2014 25359927

Gans RO: The metabolic syndrome, depression, and cardiovascular disease: interrelated conditions that share pathophysiologic mechanisms. Med Clin North Am 90(4):573–591, 2006 16843763

Gomes FA, Almeida KM, Magalhães PV, et al: Cardiovascular risk factors in outpatients with bipolar disorder: a report from the Brazilian Research Network in Bipolar Disorder. Br J Psychiatry 35(2):126–130, 2013 23904016

Goodwin FK, Jamison KR: Clinical management of suicide risk, in Manic-Depressive Illness: Bipolar Disorders and Recurrent Depression, 2nd Edition. New York, Oxford University Press, 2007a, pp 953–976

Goodwin FK, Jamison KR: Introduction, in Manic-Depressive Illness: Bipolar Disorders and Recurrent Depression, 2nd Edition. New York, Oxford University Press, 2007b, p xxvi

Hirschfeld RM, Holzer C, Calabrese JR, et al: Validity of the Mood Disorder Questionnaire: a general population study. Am J Psychiatry 160(1):178–180, 2003a 12505821

Hirschfeld RM, Lewis L, Vornik LA: Perceptions and impact of bipolar disorder: how far have we really come? Results of the national depressive and manic-depressive association 2000 survey of individuals with bipolar disorder. J Clin Psychiatry 64(2):161–174, 2003b 12633125

Hoertel N, Le Strat Y, Lavaud P, et al: Generalizability of clinical trial results for bipolar disorder to community samples: findings from the National Epidemiologic Survey on Alcohol and Related Conditions. J Clin Psychiatry 74(3):265–270, 2013 23561233

Judd LL, Akiskal HS, Schettler PJ, et al: The long-term natural history of the weekly symptomatic status of bipolar I disorder. Arch Gen Psychiatry 59(6):530–537, 2002 12044195

Judd LL, Akiskal HS, Schettler PJ, et al: A prospective investigation of the natural history of the long-term weekly symptomatic status of bipolar II disorder. Arch Gen Psychiatry 60(3):261–269, 2003 12622659

Judd LL, Schettler PJ, Akiskal H, et al: Prevalence and clinical significance of subsyndromal manic symptoms, including irritability and psychomotor agitation, during bipolar major depressive episodes. J Affect Disord 138(3):440–448, 2012 22314261

Kaufman J, Birmaher B, Brent D, et al: Schedule for Affective Disorders and Schizophrenia for School-Age Children-Present and Lifetime Version (K-SADS-PL): initial reliability and validity data. J Am Acad Child Adolesc Psychiatry 36(7):980–988, 1997 9204677

Kemp DE, Sylvia LG, Calabrese JR, et al: General medical burden in bipolar disorder: findings from the LiTMUS comparative effectiveness trial. Acta Psychiatr Scand 129(1):24–34, 2014 23465084

Kessing LV, Hansen MG, Andersen PK: Course of illness in depressive and bipolar disorders. Naturalistic study, 1994–1999. Br J Psychiatry 185:372–377, 2004 15516544

Kessing LV, Hansen HV, Hvenegaard A, et al: Treatment in a specialised out-patient mood disorder clinic v. standard out-patient treatment in the early course of bipolar disorder: randomised clinical trial. Br J Psychiatry 202(3):212–219, 2013 23349295

Kuiper S, Fritz K, Tanious M, et al: Psychiatric tertiary referral and clinical decision making. Aust N Z J Psychiatry 48(3):219–223, 2014 24425795

Leon AC, Fiedorowicz JG, Solomon DA, et al: Risk of suicidal behavior with antidepressants in bipolar and unipolar disorders. J Clin Psychiatry 75(7):720–727, 2014 25093469

López-Jaramillo C, Lopera-Vásquez J, Gallo A, et al: Effects of recurrence on the cognitive performance of patients with bipolar I disorder: implications for relapse prevention and treatment adherence. Bipolar Disord 12(5):557–567, 2010 20712758

Macritchie K, Mantingh T, Hidalgo-Mazzei D, et al: A new inner-city specialist programme reduces readmission rates in frequently admitted patients with bipolar disorder. BJPsych Bull 43(2):58–60, 2019 30481491

Martino DJ, Marengo E, Igoa A, et al: Neurocognitive and symptomatic predictors of functional outcome in bipolar disorders: a prospective 1 year follow-up study. J Affect Disord 116(1–2):37–42, 2009 19033081

McGirr A, Vöhringer PA, Ghaemi SN, et al: Safety and efficacy of adjunctive second-generation antidepressant therapy with a mood stabiliser or an atypical antipsychotic in acute bipolar depression: a systematic review and meta-analysis of randomised placebo-controlled trials. Lancet Psychiatry 3(12):1138–1146, 2016 28100425

McIntyre RS, Cohen M, Zhao J, et al: Asenapine for long-term treatment of bipolar disorder: a double-blind 40-week extension study. J Affect Disord 126(3):358–365, 2010 20537396

Molina M, Palacio JD, Vargas C, et al: Neurocognitive performance in euthymic bipolar I patients with and without history of psychosis from a multimodal intervention program: PRISMA [in Spanish]. Rev Colomb Psiquiatr 45(4):230–237, 2016 27842735

Murru A, Verdolini N, Anmella G, et al: A 12-month prospective study on the time to hospitalization and clinical management of a cohort of bipolar type I and schizoaffective bipolar patients. Eur Psychiatry 61:1–8, 2019 31255957

Ng F, Mammen OK, Wilting I, et al: The International Society for Bipolar Disorders (ISBD) consensus guidelines for the safety monitoring of bipolar disorder treatments. Bipolar Disord 11(6):559–595, 2009 19689501

Nurnberger JI Jr, Blehar MC, Kaufmann CA, et al: Diagnostic interview for genetic studies. Rationale, unique features, and training. NIMH Genetics Initiative. Arch Gen Psychiatry 51(11):849–859; discussion 863–864, 1994 7944874

Perlis RH, Ostacher MJ, Goldberg JF, et al: Transition to mania during treatment of bipolar depression. Neuropsychopharmacology 35(13):2545–2552, 2010 20827274

Persons JE, Coryell WH, Solomon DA, et al: Mixed state and suicide: is the effect of mixed state on suicidal behavior more than the sum of its parts? Bipolar Disord 20(1):35–41, 2018 20827274

Pinto JV, Saraf G, Vigo D, et al: Cariprazine in the treatment of bipolar disorder: a systematic review and meta-analysis. Bipolar Disord 22(4):360–371, 2020 31618503

Porter ME, Teisberg EO: Redefining Health Care: Creating Value-Based Competition on Results. Boston, MA, Harvard Business School Press, 2006

Saraf G, Pinto JV, Yatham LN: Efficacy and safety of cariprazine in the treatment of bipolar disorder. Expert Opin Pharmacother 20(17):2063–2072, 2019 31644326

Schaffer A, Isometsä ET, Tondo L, et al: Epidemiology, neurobiology and pharmacological interventions related to suicide deaths and suicide attempts in bipolar disorder: part I of a report of the International Society for Bipolar Disorders Task Force on Suicide in Bipolar Disorder. Aust N Z J Psychiatry 49(9):785–802, 2015 26185269

Schoepf D, Heun R: Comorbid medical illness in bipolar disorder. Br J Psychiatry 206(6):522–523, 2015 26034186

Sheehan DV, Harnett-Sheehan K, Raj BA: The measurement of disability. Int Clin Psychopharmacol 11 (suppl 3):89–95, 1996 8923116

Smith DJ, Martin D, McLean G, et al: Multimorbidity in bipolar disorder and undertreatment of cardiovascular disease: a cross sectional study. BMC Med 11:263, 2013 24359325

Stahl SM, Laredo S, Morrissette DA: Cariprazine as a treatment across the bipolar I spectrum from depression to mania: mechanism of action and review of clinical data. Ther Adv Psychopharmacol 10:2045125320905752, 2020 32110377

Strakowski S: Epidemiology of bipolar disorder, in Bipolar Disorder (Oxford American Psychiatry Library). New York, Oxford University Press, 2014, pp 17–22

Strakowski SM, Almeida JRC, DelBello MP: Psychopharmacologic treatments for bipolar disorder, in Primer On: Bipolar Disorder. Edited by Strakowski SM, DelBello MP, Adler CM, et al. New York, Oxford University Press, 2020, pp 189–228

Szegedi A, Durgam S, Mackle M, et al: Randomized, double-blind, placebo-controlled trial of asenapine maintenance therapy in adults with an acute manic or mixed episode associated with bipolar I disorder. Am J Psychiatry 175(1):71–79, 2018 28946761

Szmulewicz A, Valerio MP, Martino DJ: Longitudinal analysis of cognitive performances in recent-onset and late-life bipolar disorder: a systematic review and meta-analysis. Bipolar Disord 22(1):28–37, 2020 31541587

Valentí M, Pacchiarotti I, Bonnín CM, et al: Risk factors for antidepressant-related switch to mania. J Clin Psychiatry 73(2):e271–e276, 2012 22401488

Vieta E: Pros and cons of specialised care in bipolar disorder: an international perspective. Br J Psychiatry 202(3):170–171, 2013 23457179

Wu HC, Chou FH, Tsai KY, et al: The incidence and relative risk of stroke among patients with bipolar disorder: a seven-year follow-up study. PLoS One 8(8):e73037, 2013 24023667

Yatham LN, Kennedy SH, Parikh SV, et al: Canadian Network for Mood and Anxiety Treatments (CANMAT) and International Society for Bipolar Disorders (ISBD) 2018 guidelines for the management of patients with bipolar disorder. Bipolar Disord 20(2):97–170, 2018 29536616

Zimmerman M: A review of 20 years of research on overdiagnosis and underdiagnosis in the Rhode Island Methods to Improve Diagnostic Assessment and Services (MIDAS) project. Can J Psychiatry 61(2):71–79, 2016 27253697

CHAPTER 30

Understanding and Preventing Suicide

J. John Mann, M.D.
Mina M. Rizk, M.B.B.Ch., M.Sc.

Suicide is the tenth leading cause of death in the United States. The age-adjusted suicide rate rose 36.7% between 2000 and 2018 (based on WISQARS data from the Centers for Disease Control and Prevention [2020]). Up to 4.6% of Americans attempt suicide at some time in their life (Kessler et al. 1999; Nock and Kessler 2006). For each suicide death, there are about 30 adults who report making a suicide attempt (Centers for Disease Control and Prevention 2015), although the ratio of nonfatal to fatal suicide attempts decreases with age from about 30:1 in young adults to 6:1 in later life. Suicidal ideation is more frequent than suicide attempts and deaths; about 9.5 million U.S. adults experience serious thoughts of suicide, and 2.7 million make plans to die by suicide every year (Park-Lee et al. 2018).

Worldwide, despite a decrease in suicide deaths of 16% in men and 20% in women between 2000 and 2016, suicide still claims the lives of over 800,000 people every year (World Health Organization 2019). The incidence of suicide attempts is highest in individuals 15–24 years of age. Although suicide attempts are about two to four times more frequent among females (Wolff and Puts 2009), suicide mortality rates are 1.75 times higher in men than in women because men use more lethal methods.

Findings from reviews of psychological autopsy studies of suicide deaths indicate that decedents for whom no psychiatric disorders are detected account for a relatively high percentage of suicides in Asian countries (e.g., up to 50% in China) but lower proportions of total suicides in Western countries (~13%) (Arsenault-Lapierre et al. 2004; Phillips et al. 2002). In a systematic review of studies using the psychological autopsy method, Cavanagh et al. (2003) found that approximately 60% of individuals with a diagnosable psychiatric illness who died by suicide had a mood disorder. Notwithstanding these findings, it is worth noting that among individuals with psychiatric disorders, only approximately 14% of those with major depressive disorder and 34% of those with bipolar disorder attempt suicide, and that more generally, most people with major psychiatric disorders never manifest suicidal behavior (Dong et al. 2019; Hasin et al. 2018). The presence of a psychiatric disorder alone is thus insufficient as an explanation for suicidal behavior, and there appear to be other risk factors that, if identified and targeted appropriately, would help curb the increasing suicide rates.

Stress-Diathesis Model of Suicidal Behavior

The stress-diathesis model of suicidal behavior—first proposed by Mann and Arango (1992) and further developed and refined over the years (Mann and Rizk 2020; Mann et al. 1999; van Heeringen 2012; van Heeringen and Mann 2014)—offers an explanation of the pathway to suicidal behavior. This model views suicidal behavior not solely as a symptom of mood and other psychiatric disorders but rather as an interaction between acute stressors (i.e., *proximal* risk factors) and a pre-existing vulnerability, or *diathesis* (i.e., *distal* risk factors). Stressors could be external in the form of relationship or financial problems, or internal such as a major depressive episode. In this model, *diathesis* refers to a set of suicide-related traits that may include mood dysregulation or sensitivity, impulsive aggression related to impaired decision making, social distortions, and learning difficulties. Genetic effects and epigenetic mechanisms may underlie these traits. Familial pathways to suicidal behavior include genetic effects (Brent and Mann 2006; Mann and Haghighi 2010), and childhood adversity (e.g., emotional, physical, or sexual abuse) may lead to epigenetic changes (Althoff et al. 2012), thereby increasing risk of suicidal behavior. The stronger the diathesis, the higher the likelihood that an individual will engage in suicidal behavior when faced with internal or environmental stressors.

Is Suicidal Behavior/Ideation a Distinct Mental Disorder?

The extant body of evidence for a suicide-related diathesis and associated neurobiological markers (e.g., the serotonergic system, white matter integrity, resting-state functional connectivity, other molecular and neuroimaging findings) (Mann and Rizk 2020; van Heeringen and Mann 2014) supports the idea that suicidal behavior and ideation are not exclusively a symptom of a small subset of psychiatric disorders. Suicidal behavior is found in many psychiatric disorders, and its presence or absence is determined by psychopathological and cognitive domains associated with a diathesis for suicidal behavior that are different from domains associated with the psychopathology of associated psychiatric illnesses. Researchers have thus begun to question whether suicidal ideation and suicidal behavior should be included as a distinct mental disorder in diagnostic manuals of psychiatric disorders (Sisti et al. 2020). Making it a distinct diagnosis would reinforce research aimed at identifying suicide-related diatheses in order to develop interventions for individuals at risk for suicide. Furthermore, identification of biological correlates of suicide-related traits/diatheses could provide biomarkers for suicide risk that are distinguishable from biomarkers of co-occurring psychiatric disorders and that might help to predict risk in individuals exposed to stressors.

Suicide Risk Assessment

Defining Suicidal Ideation and Behavior

Several suicide-related terms need to be understood for a proper risk assessment to take place. *Suicidal ideation* refers to thoughts of harming or killing oneself and is the first step on a path toward dying by suicide (Nock et al. 2008). Suicidal ideation can vary considerably in terms of frequency, intensity, and duration, as well as underlying biology (Lan et al. 2019; Linehan 1986, 2019a) and can range from transient thoughts that life is not worth living to persistent ruminations about death (Oquendo et al. 2003). Although more persistent and severe suicidal ideation carries a higher risk for suicidal behavior, individuals with brief, fleeting suicidal ideation can still attempt suicide at any time (Pfeffer et al. 1993; Witte et al. 2005).

Suicide attempts are self-injurious acts carried out by an individual with the intent to die. Suicide attempts vary in lethality (i.e., the degree of medical consequences). They also vary in the degree of suicidal intent (i.e., the balance between the desire to die and the desire to live) (Beck et al. 1975). A higher level of suicide intent is associated with a more lethal, or more medically damaging, suicide attempt. Higher lethality of suicide attempts is also associated with a greater degree of planning (Chaudhury et al. 2016) (including taking measures to avoid detection) and the use of more lethal methods, such as firearms (Mann and Michel 2016). Individuals who make high-lethality suicide attempts share demographical, clinical, and neurobiological similarities with suicide decedents, and differ from those who make lower-lethality suicide attempts (Linehan 1986; Rizk et al. 2019b; Stengel 1964). Lower-lethality suicide attempts likely occur in the context of an interpersonal crisis, usually contain a strong element of appeal for help, and are conducted in a manner that favors discovery and rescue (Linehan 1986; Stengel 1964). Although lower-lethality suicide attempts are usually impulsive, they are not necessarily carried out by impulsive individuals. Attempter impulsivity is not always a reliable predictor of attempt impulsivity (Baca-Garcia et al. 2005). Attempters who spend greater amounts of time planning for their suicide attempts, which can result in a higher-lethality attempt, can also have greater trait impulsivity; in other words, impulsive individuals who plan and prepare for a suicide attempt over weeks or longer may carry out a more lethal suicide attempt within minutes of having decided to act on their plans and feelings (Chaudhury et al. 2016).

Assessment Tools

The Beck Scale for Suicide Ideation (SSI; Beck et al. 1979) and the Columbia-Suicide Severity Rating Scale (C-SSRS; Oquendo et al. 2003) are the two most widely used tools for assessment and follow-up of individuals at risk for suicide. Both are validated, have a quantitative component, can be repeated, are not diagnosis-specific, and are available in a variety of formats and in different languages (Oquendo and Bernanke 2017).

The SSI is a 19-item scale administered by clinicians and includes questions about the individual's wish to die, wish to live, and the characteristics of suicidal thoughts. Each item is rated on a 3-point scale from 0 to 2, with a total score ranging from 0 to 38. The SSI can be administered at initial evaluation and subsequently repeated to assess improvement.

The C-SSRS goes beyond the SSI because it characterizes suicidal thoughts and past suicidal behaviors. It comes in a clinician-administered version and as a self-report form (both can be administered as an "initial evaluation" or as a "since last visit" follow-up). Studies have shown the C-SSRS to be sensitive, specific, and reflective of changes in patients' conditions (Posner et al. 2011).

Another useful and brief measure for suicide risk assessment is the P4 Screener (Dube et al. 2010). The P4 Screener is usually used in primary care settings, where patients are asked an initial question about thoughts of self-harm. Any individual who responds "yes" to this question is asked four additional questions—the 4 Ps: *past* suicide attempts, *plan* for a past or future attempt, *probability* of completing suicide in the next month, and *preventive* factors. Individuals are then classified into minimal, lower, and higher risk categories based on their responses.

One limitation to these risk assessment tools is that they are retrospective and are therefore affected by recall bias. Some individuals at risk for suicide experience only transient but intense suicidal thoughts. These thoughts may not be captured at the time of assessment, although they still carry risk for a suicide attempt. Recent technological advances allow for the use of ecological momentary assessment (EMA) to measure individuals' thoughts, feelings, and behaviors in real time, outside of the clinical setting (Husky et al. 2014). Individuals receive questionnaires at multiple time points during the day on their own electronic devices (e.g., cell phone, iPad, other tablets). The use of EMA in clinical settings may boost the efforts of suicide prevention by identifying suicidal individuals who are at their peak risk for attempting suicide.

Another challenge for clinicians while conducting suicide risk assessment is that some individuals at risk for suicide may not reveal their suicidal thoughts in order to avoid hospitalization and clinical care. Others may be unconsciously using the defense mechanism of denial, which renders them unaware of their suicidal impulses. The Death/Suicide Implicit Association Test (IAT) has been proposed in such situations. The Death/Suicide IAT provides an objective measure of individuals' cognitive processes that may provide insight into their suicide risk. By asking individuals to categorize words associated with life and suicide as fast as they can, the Death/Suicide IAT predicted suicidal behavior in some prospective studies (Millner et al. 2019; Nock et al. 2010), but not others (Glenn et al. 2017).

Suicide Prevention

Suicidal behavior is heterogeneous, with a variety of underlying biological and risk factors. Research shows that no single suicide prevention strategy clearly stands above the others in terms of efficacy (Zalsman et al. 2016). Combinations of evidence-based suicide prevention strategies at population, institutional, and individual levels are needed to curb the increasing suicide rates.

Population-Level Strategies

Public Awareness and Education

Raising the public awareness about suicide causes and risk factors has been proposed as an approach to suicide prevention. Lack of appropriate information about mental illness and suicidal behavior may increase stigmatization, result in shame or fear of help-seeking, and discourage an individual from reporting psychological symptoms or suicidal tendencies. Furthermore, at-risk individuals who lack knowledge about suicide are more likely to accept it as inevitable or as the only solution to a serious life problem such as a financial crisis or a terminal illness. Public education can help reduce the stigma associated with psychiatric disorders and encourage individuals to seek help for their suicidal thoughts and behavior. For example, a significant—and sustained—reduction in suicidal acts of approximately 25% was observed during a 2-year public education program in Nuremberg (480,000 inhabitants) compared with both the baseline year and a control region (Wuerzburg, 270,000 inhabitants) (Hegerl et al. 2006, 2010). Similar effects have been observed in other regions in Germany and Hungary (Hübner-Liebermann et al. 2010; Székely et al. 2013). A more recent study in several European countries found that large-scale approaches involving public education about mental illnesses reduced suicidal acts in some—but not all—countries (Hegerl et al. 2019).

Media Reporting of Suicide

The term *suicide contagion* has been defined as imitative suicidal behavior by vulnerable individuals in response to exposure to sensationalized reports of suicide (Cheng et al. 2014), such as high-visibility media coverage that employs dramatic language, glamorizes the individual, and/or provides detailed information on the method used or the site of the death (Gould 2011). Responsible coverage of news about suicide can change social perceptions of suicide as a stigma and inform the public on its complexity. Use of appropriate language (e.g., "died by suicide" or "completed suicide" or "killed him/herself") and avoidance of stigmatizing terms (e.g., "committed suicide" or "successful or failed attempt") may be beneficial in this regard. Media reporting should include stories on hope and recovery and should provide links to mental health care information and services, which may reduce the risk of contagion effects. Responsible reporting should also include information on warning signs of suicide risk as well as emergency hotline and treatment resources.

Restriction of Lethal Means of Suicide

Means restriction is another important approach to reducing suicide rates (Mann et al. 2005). The more determined the individual is to kill himself or herself, the more lethal are the methods used. In addition, suicide attempters are more likely to use a method that is at hand, as 70% of attempters take less than 1 hour between deciding to kill themselves and the actual suicidal act (Chaudhury et al. 2016; Simon et al. 2001). Restricting access to highly lethal means could allow the suicidal crisis to pass or result in an attempt with a less lethal method. Survivors of a suicide attempt have a more than 80% chance of not dying from a suicide attempt in the future (Owens et al. 2002). Through means restriction, in which the most lethal methods are made less available, there will be a decrease in suicide deaths. Examples of successful programs of means restriction include barbiturate restriction in Australia (Oliver and Hetzel 1972), pesticide regulations in Sri Lanka (Gunnell et al. 2007), and detoxification of domestic gas and packaging changes for analgesics in the United Kingdom (Hawton et al. 2013; Kreitman 1976; Lester 1991). Erection of barriers at sites popular for jumping resulted in an 86% reduction in rates of suicide by jumping between 2005 and 2014 (Zalsman et al. 2016). In the United States, firearms account for up to half of suicides every year (Centers for Disease Control and Prevention 2020), with greater availability of firearms associated with higher firearm suicide rates. Most suicides involve guns purchased years earlier. Targeted initiatives like gun violence restraining orders, smart gun technology, and gun safety education campaigns can potentially reduce access to already purchased firearms by individuals at risk of suicide (Mann and Michel 2016).

Institutional Strategies

Gatekeeper Education and Interventions

Instead of seeking professional help, a person in suicidal crisis may turn to family, friends, or work and school colleagues for advice. These community and social network members may serve as "gatekeepers" for at-risk persons and may be able to refer them to mental health professionals for assessment and help. Gatekeepers include staff in institutional settings such as the military, police, personnel in prisons, staff in schools, staff in personnel departments of businesses, geriatric caregivers, and clergy. Training such personnel on providing direct, specific, and supportive assistance to an at-risk individual is a promising approach for suicide prevention. A number of factors may influence an individual's decision to intervene with an at-risk person and can be affected by effective gatekeeper training: 1) knowledge about suicide and depression and resources available for at-risk individuals, 2) beliefs and attitudes about suicide being preventable, 3) ability to overcome reluctance to intervene (i.e., due to perceived stigma or individuals' perceptions that it is not their responsibility or that it is inappropriate to intervene), and 4) self-confidence in intervening (i.e., being comfortable and competent to identify, empathize with, and facilitate referral for a person at risk of suicide). Several gatekeeper training programs have been developed and include Mental Health First Aid, Applied Suicide Intervention Skills Training (ASIST), Signs of Suicide (SOS), and Question, Persuade, and Refer (QPR) (Aseltine et al. 2007; Gould et al. 2013; Wyman et al. 2008). For example, QPR consists of a brief standardized role-play exercise and a 1-hour didactic training with a short video that teaches three gatekeeper skills (i.e., questioning, persuading, and referring). The QPR program has been shown to improve suicide-related knowledge and self-efficacy among veterans (Matthieu et al. 2008) and secondary school staff (Wyman et al. 2008). Additionally, school-based awareness programs that include selective interventions designed to reduce bullying and social isolation may prevent suicide attempts (Zalsman et al. 2016). Some of these school-based programs are tailored toward particular subgroups, such as LGBTQ+ young people, and report positive effects in reducing suicidal ideation and deaths (Saewyc et al. 2014).

Primary Care Physician Education and Awareness

Primary care physicians (or general practitioners) are usually the contact point in the health care system for individuals at risk for suicide. About 45% of individuals who die by suicide have visited their primary care physician within a month of their death (Luoma et al. 2002). However, a study of physician-patient interactions indicated that primary care physicians discussed depression with only 52% of patients who had depressive symptoms, and discussed suicide with 11% of depressed patients, although the majority had experienced suicidal ideation (Vannoy and Robins 2011). Educating primary care clinicians can help protect against suicide, primarily by improving the recognition of depression, which leads to the increased prescribing of antidepressants (Szanto et al. 2007). Collaborative care models of depression treatment are used in an effort to improve depression recognition and treatment (Gilbody et al. 2006).

Individual-Level Strategies

Prompt diagnosis and effective treatment of suicidal ideation and behavior—and underlying psychiatric illnesses—are considered crucial for suicide prevention (Zalsman et al. 2016). Most depressed patients with a history of suicide attempts, who are at higher risk for future suicide and suicide attempts, receive inadequate treatment (Oquendo et al. 1999). Individuals at risk for suicide often present to the emergency department seeking aid for suicidal thoughts or treatment after low-lethality suicide attempts. A combination of effective psychological and pharmacological treatment of depressive illnesses and suicidal thoughts and behavior, as well as appropriate interventions and follow-up care, could prevent more-lethal suicide attempts in the future.

Pharmacotherapy

Antidepressants. There has been a long-standing belief that the early activating effects of some antidepressants might increase suicidal thoughts and give depressed patients the energy to act on suicidal impulses. However, a systematic review of suicide prevention studies published between 2005 and 2014 reported that effective treatment of depression is crucial for suicide prevention (Zalsman et al. 2016). Additionally, population-level studies show that selective serotonin reuptake inhibitors and other, newer antidepressants are associated with an overall decrease in suicide rates in the United States (Gibbons et al. 2005; Grunebaum et al. 2004). The findings in non-U.S. studies were generally similar (Hall and Lucke 2006).

Lithium. Several observational studies have reported the effectiveness of lithium in reducing the incidence of a variety of suicide-related events (Coppen et al. 1991; Felber et al. 2018). A longitudinal cohort study examined the electronic health records of more than 14,000 individuals with bipolar disorder and found that self-harm rates were lower in patients prescribed lithium compared with those prescribed other mood stabilizers (olanzapine, valproate, or quetiapine) (Hayes et al. 2016). In addition, an 8-year prospective follow-up study in Sweden involving more than 50,000 individuals with bipolar disorder found that lithium treatment, but not valproate treatment, was associated with a significant reduction in suicide-related events (e.g., suicide attempts, death by suicide, hospitalization for suicide attempts) (Song et al. 2017). However, randomized controlled clinical trials that compared lithium with either placebo or other mood stabilizers failed to demonstrate this effect (Girlanda et al. 2014; Lauterbach et al. 2008; Oquendo et al. 2011), probably because of inadequate statistical power due to small sample size. It is important to note that the use of lithium is somewhat limited by its toxicity in overdose and its relatively narrow therapeutic window. Alternatively, increased monitoring of patients who receive lithium, including monitoring of lithium blood levels, may improve treatment efficiency and compliance and decrease suicide risk.

Clozapine. Clozapine is the first medication to get FDA approval for use in prevention of suicidal behavior. It is an antipsychotic medication used for treatment-resistant schizophrenia, in which around half of patients attempt suicide. Clozapine reduces the risk for suicide attempts compared with other antipsychotics (Meltzer et al. 2003; Vermeulen et al. 2019). Nevertheless, given the risk of neutropenia and agranulocytosis associated with clozapine use, clozapine remains relatively underutilized for the prevention of suicidal behavior.

Ketamine. Ketamine is a rapidly acting treatment for depressive symptoms and suicidal ideation (Reinstatler and Youssef 2015). Randomized clinical trials of adjunctive ketamine in mood disorders and for suicidal ideation found that a single subanesthetic ketamine infusion, adjunctive to ongoing pharmacotherapy, produced a greater reduction in suicidal thoughts in one day compared with midazolam in both bipolar depression (Grunebaum et al. 2017) and major depressive disorder (Grunebaum et al. 2018). Ketamine reduces suicidal ideation independent of improvement in other mood symptoms (Grunebaum et al. 2017, 2018; Murrough et al. 2015), and its effect on suicidal ideation is sustained for 5–6 weeks in patients who continue to take other oral psychotropic medications (Grunebaum et al. 2017). Intranasal ketamine (or esketamine) shows promise as an antisuicidal treatment in various populations (Canuso et al. 2018). It uses a less invasive route of administration but, like intravenous ketamine, is administered in medical settings. Questions remain about the duration of ketamine effects and the safety and efficacy of repeated administration.

Buprenorphine. Buprenorphine is a mu opioid receptor partial agonist (Dum et al. 1981; Greenwald et al. 2007; Lee et al. 1999) and a kappa receptor antagonist (Butler 2013) used for relapse prevention in opioid use disorder (Lee et al. 2018). There has been an opioid epidemic in the United States since the 1990s that has contributed significantly to the climbing suicide rates. Treating suicidal ideation and behavior in individuals with opioid use disorder may help reduce risk in this vulnerable population. Buprenorphine has antidepressant effects when used for both opioid use disorder and treatment-resistant depression (Bodkin et al. 1995; Ehrich et al. 2015; Fava et al. 2016; Latif et al. 2019; Nyhuis et al. 2008; Serafini et al. 2018) and may reduce suicidal ideation (Ahmadi and Abtahi 2017; Ahmadi et al. 2018; Serafini et al. 2018; Striebel and Kalapatapu 2014; Yovell et al. 2016). In a trial in which severely suicidal patients without opioid use disorder were randomly assigned to 4 weeks of treatment with either low-dosage buprenorphine (0.1–0.8 mg/day) or placebo as an adjunct to their ongoing medication regimen, Yovell et al. (2016) found that patients receiving buprenorphine showed greater reductions in suicidal ideation than patients receiving placebo, both after 2 weeks and after 4 weeks. In another study in individuals with opioid use disorder, Ahmadi et al. (2018) reported a greater than 80% reduction in suicidal ideation in response to a 3-day course of high-dose buprenorphine (32 mg, 64 mg, or 96 mg) administered as a single sublingual daily dose.

Psychotherapy

A meta-analysis of over 30 randomized controlled trials reported that psychotherapies, irrespective of type, administered to individuals at risk for suicide with varying clinical presentations were associated with fewer suicide attempts during follow-up compared with treatment as usual (Calati and Courtet 2016). Moreover, a population-based study found that those who received a psychosocial intervention after self-harm were less likely to have died by suicide at long-term follow-up (Erlangsen et al. 2015).

Cognitive-behavioral therapy (CBT) and dialectical behavior therapy (DBT) are the most intensively studied psychotherapies in terms of suicidal behavior. CBT targeting suicidal thoughts and behaviors in adults at high risk for suicide reduces the incidence of self-harm at 6 months and 1 year (Hawton et al. 2016). Brief CBT (12.5 hours per patient) also reduced the odds of suicide attempts at 2 years compared with treatment as usual (Rudd et al. 2015). Similarly, a recent meta-analysis demonstrated the effectiveness of DBT in reducing suicidal behavior (DeCou et al. 2019). Other psychotherapies with evidence of beneficial effects for preventing suicide attempts or self-directed violence in adults include problem-solving therapy (Hatcher et al. 2011), mentalization-based treatment (Bateman and Fonagy 1999), and psychodynamic interpersonal therapy (Guthrie et al. 2001).

Follow-Up Care for Persons Who Attempt Suicide

The first 6–12 months after discharge from a psychiatric hospital or an emergency department visit is the period of greatest risk for suicidal behavior (Angst et al. 2002). In addition to provision of follow-up treatment for underlying psychiatric disorders, there are brief psychological and educational interventions that have shown effectiveness in suicide prevention among persons who have attempted suicide soon after discharge from a hospital (Turecki et al. 2019). These brief interventions are inexpensive and easy to implement, and do not require extensive resources. These interventions are administered either in one session or via several brief in-person contacts by phone, e-mail, or mail. The interventions focus on helping suicidal individuals to 1) be informed about suicidal ideation and behavior; 2) become aware of problems and events linked to the behavior; 3) be motivated to engage in safety planning, help-seeking, and problem solving; and 4) develop practical strategies to manage future suicidal crises. In general, these brief interventions have a greater effect on behavioral outcomes than on symptom outcomes; that is, patients may still be experiencing suicidal ideation but make fewer suicide attempts and are less likely to die by suicide. For example, Safety Planning Intervention (SPI) (Stanley and Brown 2012) helps engage individuals at risk for suicide in a suicide-related narrative aimed at identifying warning signs. Furthermore, it provides individuals with a prioritized and specific set of coping strategies and sources of support that they can use if suicidal thoughts reemerge, which may lower their imminent risk for suicidal behavior. SPI has six steps: 1) recognize warning signs, 2) employ internal coping strategies, 3) make use of people or social settings that could serve as a distraction, 4) reach out to friends and family members who can provide support, 5) contact professionals and agencies, and 6) limit access to lethal means. SPI, combined with follow-up calls (known as SPI+),

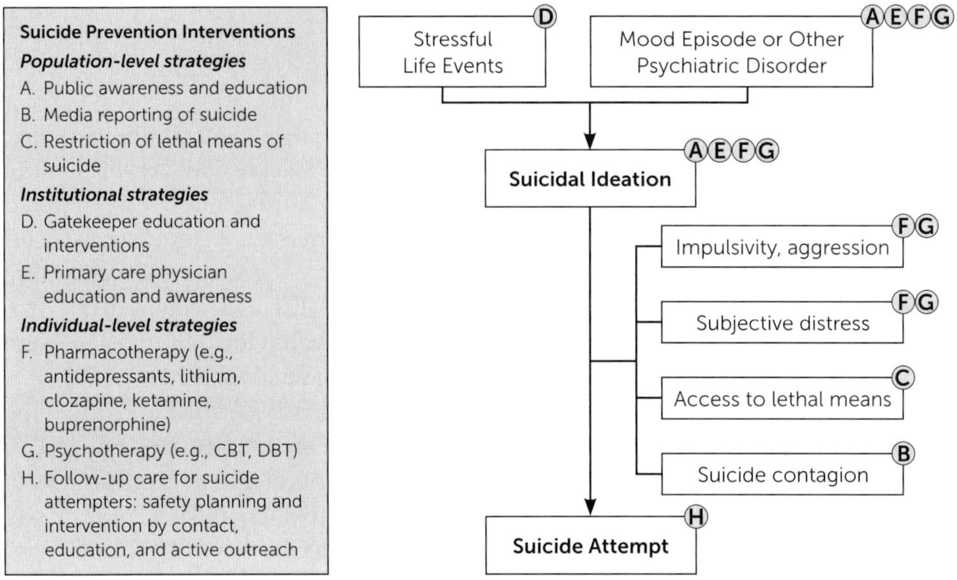

FIGURE 30–1. Targets of suicide prevention interventions.

CBT=cognitive-behavioral therapy; DBT=dialectical behavior therapy.

is effective in reducing the incidence of suicidal behavior and increasing treatment engagement in the 6 months after discharge from the emergency department (Stanley et al. 2018). Crisis response planning (Bryan et al. 2017) is an abbreviated form of SPI that has been shown to be effective in preventing suicide attempts, resolving suicidal ideation, and reducing inpatient hospitalization among high-risk active-duty military personnel (Bryan et al. 2017). Other brief interventions that have shown efficacy in reducing suicide attempt rates following discharge from a hospital or an emergency department include Emergency Department Safety Assessment and Follow-up Evaluation (ED-SAFE) (Miller et al. 2017), Attempted Suicide Short Intervention Program (ASSIP) (Gysin-Maillart et al. 2016), brief intervention and contact (BIC) (Bertolote et al. 2010; Fleischmann et al. 2008), and volitional help sheet (VHS) (O'Connor et al. 2017).

Conclusion

Identifying at-risk individuals and implementing treatment and intervention strategies are crucial for suicide prevention (Figure 30–1). This involves addressing both the long-term traits that predispose individuals to suicidal behavior and the more transient states that might acutely precipitate that behavior. Effective pharmacological and psychological treatments of underlying psychiatric disorders, including depression, are important in prevention. The antisuicidal effects of clozapine and lithium are well established, but both medications need close monitoring. Ketamine and buprenorphine are new antisuicidal agents that show promise for reducing suicidal ideation, but they have not been tested in preventing suicide attempts. Hospitalization and removal of the means of suicide may reduce risk in individuals with intense current suicidal ideation and active planning, and follow-up care with education and active outreach my prevent future suicide attempts. Other approaches such as increasing awareness and education of primary care physicians and gatekeepers can help with early detection of suicidal individuals. Given the heterogeneity of suicidal behavior and related underlying cognitive and biological processes, more research is needed on tailoring psychological or pharmacological treatments for subsets of individuals at risk for suicide that share the same risk pattern. Additionally, studies should validate implementation strategies of suicide risk assessment tools more broadly in clinical practice.

References

Ahmadi J, Abtahi S: Eight-milligram single dose of buprenorphine as an expeditious treatment for severe suicidal ideation: a case report. Iran Red Crescent Med J 19(9):e59999, 2017

Ahmadi J, Jahromi MS, Ehsaei Z: The effectiveness of different singly administered high doses of buprenorphine in reducing suicidal ideation in acutely depressed people with co-morbid opiate dependence: a randomized, double-blind, clinical trial. Trials 19(1):462, 2018 30157924

Althoff RR, Hudziak JJ, Willemsen G, et al: Genetic and environmental contributions to self-reported thoughts of self-harm and suicide. Am J Med Genet B Neuropsychiatr Genet 159B(1):120–127, 2012 22162437

Angst F, Stassen HH, Clayton PJ, et al: Mortality of patients with mood disorders: follow-up over 34–38 years. J Affect Disord 68(2–3):167–181, 2002 12063145

Arsenault-Lapierre G, Kim C, Turecki G: Psychiatric diagnoses in 3275 suicides: a meta-analysis. BMC Psychiatry 4(1):37, 2004 15527502

Aseltine RH Jr, James A, Schilling EA, et al: Evaluating the SOS suicide prevention program: a replication and extension. BMC Public Health 7:161, 2007 17640366

Baca-Garcia E, Diaz-Sastre C, García Resa E, et al: Suicide attempts and impulsivity. Eur Arch Psychiatry Clin Neurosci 255(2):152–156, 2005 15549343

Bateman A, Fonagy P: Effectiveness of partial hospitalization in the treatment of borderline personality disorder: a randomized controlled trial. Am J Psychiatry 156(10):1563–1569, 1999 10518167

Beck AT, Beck R, Kovacs M: Classification of suicidal behaviors: I. Quantifying intent and medical lethality. Am J Psychiatry 132(3):285–287, 1975 1115273

Beck AT, Kovacs M, Weissman A: Assessment of suicidal intention: the Scale for Suicide Ideation. J Consult Clin Psychol 47(2):343–352, 1979 469082

Bertolote JM, Fleischmann A, De Leo D, et al: Repetition of suicide attempts: data from emergency care settings in five culturally different low- and middle-income countries participating in the WHO SUPRE-MISS Study. Crisis 31(4):194–201, 2010 20801749

Bodkin JA, Zornberg GL, Lukas SE, et al: Buprenorphine treatment of refractory depression. J Clin Psychopharmacol 15(1):49–57, 1995 7714228

Brent DA, Mann JJ: Familial pathways to suicidal behavior—understanding and preventing suicide among adolescents. N Engl J Med 355(26):2719–2721, 2006 17192535

Bryan CJ, Mintz J, Clemans TA, et al: Effect of crisis response planning vs. contracts for safety on suicide risk in U.S. Army soldiers: a randomized clinical trial. J Affect Disord 212:64–72, 2017 28142085

Butler S. Buprenorphine: clinically useful but often misunderstood. Scand J Pain 4(3):148–152, 2013 29913911

Calati R, Courtet P: Is psychotherapy effective for reducing suicide attempt and non-suicidal self-injury rates? Meta-analysis and meta-regression of literature data. J Psychiatr Res 79:8–20, 2016 27128172

Canuso CM, Singh JB, Fedgchin M, et al: Efficacy and safety of intranasal esketamine for the rapid reduction of symptoms of depression and suicidality in patients at imminent risk for suicide: results of a double-blind, randomized, placebo-controlled study. Am J Psychiatry 175(7):620–630, 2018 29656663

Cavanagh JT, Carson AJ, Sharpe M, et al: Psychological autopsy studies of suicide: a systematic review. Psychol Med 33(3):395–405, 2003 12701661

Centers for Disease Control and Prevention: National Center for Injury Prevention and Control. Web-Based Injury Statistics Query and Reporting System (WISQARS). 2015. Available at: https://www.cdc.gov/injury/wisqars/index.html. Accessed November 30, 2020.

Centers for Disease Control and Prevention: Web-Based Injury Statistics Query and Reporting System (WISQARS): Fatal Injury Reports, National and Regional, 1999–2018. Atlanta, CA, Centers for Disease Control and Prevention, 2014. Available at: https://webappa.cdc.gov/sasweb/ncipc/mortrate.html. Accessed January 19, 2022.

Chaudhury SR, Singh T, Burke A, et al: Clinical correlates of planned and unplanned suicide attempts. J Nerv Ment Dis 204(11):806–811, 2016 27105457

Cheng Q, Li H, Silenzio V, Caine ED: Suicide contagion: a systematic review of definitions and research utility. PLoS One 9(9):e108724, 2014 25259604

Coppen A, Standish-Barry H, Bailey J, et al: Does lithium reduce the mortality of recurrent mood disorders? J Affect Disord 23(1):1–7, 1991 1774419

DeCou CR, Comtois KA, Landes SJ: Dialectical behavior therapy is effective for the treatment of suicidal behavior: a meta-analysis. Behav Ther 50(1):60–72, 2019 30661567

Dong M, Lu L, Zhang L, et al: Prevalence of suicide attempts in bipolar disorder: a systematic review and meta-analysis of observational studies. Epidemiol Psychiatr Sci 29:e63, 2019 31648654

Dube P, Kurt K, Bair MJ, et al: The p4 screener: evaluation of a brief measure for assessing potential suicide risk in 2 randomized effectiveness trials of primary care and oncology patients. Prim Care Companion J Clin Psychiatry 12(6):PCC.10m00978, 2010 21494337

Dum J, Bläsig J, Herz A: Buprenorphine: demonstration of physical dependence liability. Eur J Pharmacol 70(3):293–300, 1981 6262095

Ehrich E, Turncliff R, Du Y, et al: Evaluation of opioid modulation in major depressive disorder. Neuropsychopharmacology 40(6):1448–1455, 2015 25518754

Erlangsen A, Lind BD, Stuart EA, et al: Short-term and long-term effects of psychosocial therapy for people after deliberate self-harm: a register-based, nationwide multicentre study using propensity score matching. Lancet Psychiatry 2(1):49–58, 2015 26359612

Fava M, Memisoglu A, Thase ME, et al: Opioid modulation with buprenorphine/samidorphan as adjunctive treatment for inadequate response to antidepressants: a randomized double-blind placebo-controlled trial. Am J Psychiatry 173(5):499–508, 2016 26869247

Felber W, Bauer M, Lewitzka U, et al: Lithium clinics in Berlin and Dresden: a 50-year experience. Pharmacopsychiatry 51(5):166–171, 2018 29902821

Fleischmann A, Bertolote JM, Wasserman D, et al: Effectiveness of brief intervention and contact for suicide attempters: a randomized controlled trial in five countries. Bull World Health Organ 86(9):703–709, 2008 18797646

Gibbons RD, Hur K, Bhaumik DK, et al: The relationship between antidepressant medication use and rate of suicide. Arch Gen Psychiatry 62(2):165–172, 2005 15699293

Gilbody S, Bower P, Fletcher J, et al: Collaborative care for depression: a cumulative meta-analysis and review of longer-term outcomes. Arch Intern Med 166(21):2314–2321, 2006 17130383

Girlanda F, Cipriani A, Agrimi E, et al: Effectiveness of lithium in subjects with treatment-resistant depression and suicide risk: results and lessons of an underpowered randomised clinical trial. BMC Res Notes 7(1):731, 2014 25326163

Glenn CR, Kleiman EM, Coppersmith DDL, et al: Implicit identification with death predicts change in suicide ideation during psychiatric treatment in adolescents. J Child Psychol Psychiatry 58(12):1319–1329, 2017 28675456

Gould MS: Suicide and the media. Ann N Y Acad Sci 932:200–221, discussion 221–224, 2001 11411187

Gould MS, Cross W, Pisani AR, et al: Impact of applied suicide intervention skills training on the National Suicide Prevention Lifeline. Suicide Life Threat Behav 43(6):676–691, 2013 23889494

Greenwald M, Johanson CE, Bueller J, et al: Buprenorphine duration of action: mu-opioid receptor availability and pharmacokinetic and behavioral indices. Biol Psychiatry 61(1):101–110, 2007 16950210

Grunebaum MF, Ellis SP, Li S, et al: Antidepressants and suicide risk in the United States, 1985–1999. J Clin Psychiatry 65(11):1456–1462, 2004 15554756

Grunebaum MF, Ellis SP, Keilp JG, et al: Ketamine versus midazolam in bipolar depression with suicidal thoughts: a pilot midazolam-controlled randomized clinical trial. Bipolar Disord 19(3):176–183, 2017 28452409

Grunebaum MF, Galfalvy HC, Choo TH, et al: Ketamine for rapid reduction of suicidal thoughts in major depression: a midazolam-controlled randomized clinical trial. Am J Psychiatry 175(4):327–335, 2018 29202655

Gunnell D, Fernando R, Hewagama M, et al: The impact of pesticide regulations on suicide in Sri Lanka. Int J Epidemiol 36(6):1235–1242, 2007 17726039

Guthrie E, Kapur N, Mackway-Jones K, et al: Randomised controlled trial of brief psychological intervention after deliberate self poisoning. BMJ 323(7305):135–138, 2001 11463679

Gysin-Maillart A, Schwab S, Soravia L, et al: A novel brief therapy for patients who attempt suicide: a 24-months follow-up randomized controlled study of the Attempted Suicide Short Intervention Program (ASSIP). PLoS Med 13(3):e1001968, 2016 26930055

Hall WD, Lucke J: How have the selective serotonin reuptake inhibitor antidepressants affected suicide mortality? Aust N Z J Psychiatry 40(11–12):941–950, 2006 17054562

Hasin DS, Sarvet AL, Meyers JL, et al: Epidemiology of adult DSM-5 major depressive disorder and its specifiers in the United States. JAMA Psychiatry 75(4):336–346, 2018 29450462

Hatcher S, Sharon C, Parag V, et al: Problem-solving therapy for people who present to hospital with self-harm: Zelen randomised controlled trial. Br J Psychiatry 199(4):310–316, 2011 21816868

Hawton K, Bergen H, Simkin S, et al: Long term effect of reduced pack sizes of paracetamol on poisoning deaths and liver transplant activity in England and Wales: interrupted time series analyses. BMJ 346:f403, 2013 23393081

Hawton K, Witt KG, Salisbury TLT, et al: Psychosocial interventions following self-harm in adults: a systematic review and meta-analysis. Lancet Psychiatry 3(8):740–750, 2016 27422028

Hayes JF, Pitman A, Marston L, et al: Self-harm, unintentional injury, and suicide in bipolar disorder during maintenance mood stabilizer treatment: a UK population-based electronic health records study. JAMA Psychiatry 73(6):630–637, 2016 27167638

Hegerl U, Althaus D, Schmidtke A, et al: The Alliance Against Depression: 2-year evaluation of a community-based intervention to reduce suicidality. Psychol Med 36(9):1225–1233, 2006 16707028

Hegerl U, Mergl R, Havers I, et al: Sustainable effects on suicidality were found for the Nuremberg Alliance Against Depression. Eur Arch Psychiatry Clin Neurosci 260(5):401–406, 2010 19921299

Hegerl U, Maxwell M, Harris F, et al: Prevention of suicidal behaviour: results of a controlled community-based intervention study in four European countries. PLoS One 14(11): e0224602, 2019 31710620

Hübner-Liebermann B, Neuner T, Hegerl U, et al: Reducing suicides through an alliance against depression? Gen Hosp Psychiatry 32(5):514–518, 2010 20851273

Husky M, Olié E, Guillaume S, et al: Feasibility and validity of ecological momentary assessment in the investigation of suicide risk. Psychiatry Res 220(1–2):564–570, 2014 25155939

Kessler RC, Borges G, Walters EE: Prevalence of and risk factors for lifetime suicide attempts in the National Comorbidity Survey. Arch Gen Psychiatry 56(7):617–626, 1999 10401507

Kreitman N: The coal gas story. United Kingdom suicide rates, 1960–71. Br J Prev Soc Med 30(2):86–93, 1976 953381

Lan MJ, Rizk MM, Pantazatos SP, et al: Resting-state amplitude of low-frequency fluctuation is associated with suicidal ideation. Depress Anxiety 36(5):433–441, 2019 30900329

Latif ZE, Šaltyte Benth J, Solli KK, et al: Anxiety, depression, and insomnia among adults with opioid dependence treated with extended-release naltrexone vs buprenorphine-naloxone: a randomized clinical trial and follow-up study. JAMA Psychiatry 76(2):127–134, 2019 30566177

Lauterbach E, Felber W, Müller-Oerlinghausen B, et al: Adjunctive lithium treatment in the prevention of suicidal behaviour in depressive disorders: a randomised, placebo-controlled, 1-year trial. Acta Psychiatr Scand 118(6):469–479, 2008 18808400

Lee JD, Nunes EV Jr, Novo P, et al: Comparative effectiveness of extended-release naltrexone versus buprenorphine-naloxone for opioid relapse prevention (X:BOT): a multicentre, open-label, randomised controlled trial. Lancet 391(10118):309–318, 2018 29150198

Lee KO, Akil H, Woods JH, et al: Differential binding properties of oripavines at cloned mu- and delta-opioid receptors. Eur J Pharmacol 378(3):323–330, 1999 10493109

Lester D: Effects of detoxification of domestic gas on suicide in The Netherlands. Psychol Rep 68(1):202, 1991 2034761

Linehan MM: Suicidal people. One population or two? Ann N Y Acad Sci 487:16–33, 1986 3471160

Luoma JB, Martin CE, Pearson JL: Contact with mental health and primary care providers before suicide: a review of the evidence. Am J Psychiatry 159(6):909–916, 2002 12042175

Mann JJ, Arango V: Integration of neurobiology and psychopathology in a unified model of suicidal behavior. J Clin Psychopharmacol 12(2) (suppl):2S–7S, 1992 1374433

Mann JJ, Haghighi F: Genes and environment: multiple pathways to psychopathology. Biol Psychiatry 68(5):403–404, 2010 20705146

Mann JJ, Michel CA: Prevention of firearm suicide in the United States: what works and what is possible. Am J Psychiatry 173(10):969–979, 2016 27444796

Mann JJ, Rizk MM: A brain-centric model of suicidal behavior. Am J Psychiatry 177(10):902–916, 2020 32998550

Mann JJ, Waternaux C, Haas GL, et al: Toward a clinical model of suicidal behavior in psychiatric patients. Am J Psychiatry 156(2):181–189, 1999 9989552

Mann JJ, Apter A, Bertolote J, et al: Suicide prevention strategies: a systematic review. JAMA 294(16):2064–2074, 2005 16249421

Matthieu MM, Cross W, Batres AR, et al: Evaluation of gatekeeper training for suicide prevention in veterans. Arch Suicide Res 12(2):148–154, 2008 18340597

Meltzer HY, Alphs L, Green AI, et al: Clozapine treatment for suicidality in schizophrenia: International Suicide Prevention Trial (InterSePT). Arch Gen Psychiatry 60(1):82–91, 2003 12511175

Miller IW, Camargo CA Jr, Arias SA, et al: Suicide prevention in an emergency department population: the ED-SAFE Study. JAMA Psychiatry 74(6):563–570, 2017 28456130

Millner AJ, Augenstein TM, Visser KH, et al: Implicit cognitions as a behavioral marker of suicide attempts in adolescents. Arch Suicide Res 23(1):47–63, 2019 29482489

Murrough JW, Soleimani L, DeWilde KE, et al: Ketamine for rapid reduction of suicidal ideation: a randomized controlled trial. Psychol Med 45(16):3571–3580, 2015 26266877

Nock MK, Kessler RC: Prevalence of and risk factors for suicide attempts versus suicide gestures: analysis of the National Comorbidity Survey. J Abnorm Psychol 115(3):616–623, 2006 16866602

Nock MK, Borges G, Bromet EJ, et al: Cross-national prevalence and risk factors for suicidal ideation, plans and attempts. Br J Psychiatry 192(2):98–105, 2008 18245022

Nock MK, Park JM, Finn CT, et al: Measuring the suicidal mind: implicit cognition predicts suicidal behavior. Psychol Sci 21(4):511–517, 2010 20424092

Nyhuis PW, Gastpar M, Scherbaum N: Opiate treatment in depression refractory to antidepressants and electroconvulsive therapy. J Clin Psychopharmacol 28(5):593–595, 2008 18794671

O'Connor RC, Ferguson E, Scott F, et al: A brief psychological intervention to reduce repetition of self-harm in patients admitted to hospital following a suicide attempt: a randomised controlled trial. Lancet Psychiatry 4(6):451–460, 2017 28434871

Oliver RG, Hetzel BS: Rise and fall of suicide rates in Australia: relation to sedative availability. Med J Aust 2(17):919–923, 1972 4639963

Oquendo MA, Bernanke JA: Suicide risk assessment: tools and challenges. World Psychiatry 16(1):28–29, 2017 28127916

Oquendo MA, Malone KM, Ellis SP, et al: Inadequacy of antidepressant treatment for patients with major depression who are at risk for suicidal behavior. Am J Psychiatry 156(2):190–194, 1999 9989553

Oquendo MA, Halberstam B, Mann JJ: Risk factors for suicidal behavior: utility and limitations of research instruments, in Standardized Evaluation in Clinical Practice. Edited by First MB. Washington, DC, American Psychiatric Publishing, 2003, pp 103–130

Oquendo MA, Galfalvy HC, Currier D, et al: Treatment of suicide attempters with bipolar disorder: a randomized clinical trial comparing lithium and valproate in the prevention of suicidal behavior. Am J Psychiatry 168(10):1050–1056, 2011 21768611

Owens D, Horrocks J, House A: Fatal and non-fatal repetition of self-harm. Systematic review. Br J Psychiatry 181(3):193–199, 2002 12204922

Park-Lee E, Hedden SL, Lipari RN: Suicidal Thoughts and Behavior in 33 Metropolitan Statistical Areas Update: 2013 to 2015. The CBHSQ Report: March 14, 2018. Rockville, MD, Center for Behavioral Health Statistics and Quality, Substance Abuse and Mental Health Services Administration, 2018

Pfeffer CR, Klerman GL, Hurt SW, et al: Suicidal children grow up: rates and psychosocial risk factors for suicide attempts during follow-up. J Am Acad Child Adolesc Psychiatry 32(1):106–113, 1993 8428862

Phillips MR, Li X, Zhang Y: Suicide rates in China, 1995–99. Lancet 359(9309):835–840, 2002 11897283

Posner K, Brown GK, Stanley B, et al: The Columbia-Suicide Severity Rating Scale: initial validity and internal consistency findings from three multisite studies with adolescents and adults. Am J Psychiatry 168(12):1266–1277, 2011 22193671

Reinstatler L, Youssef NA: Ketamine as a potential treatment for suicidal ideation: a systematic review of the literature. Drugs R D 15(1):37–43, 2015 25773961

Rizk MM, Galfalvy H, Singh T, et al: Toward subtyping of suicidality: brief suicidal ideation is associated with greater stress response. J Affect Disord 230:87–92, 2018 29407544

Rizk MM, Choo TH, Galfalvy H, et al: Variability in suicidal ideation is associated with affective instability in suicide attempters with borderline personality disorder. Psychiatry 82(2):173–178, 2019a 31013205

Rizk MM, Rubin-Falcone H, Lin X, et al: Gray matter volumetric study of major depression and suicidal behavior. Psychiatry Res Neuroimaging 283:16–23, 2019b 30469094

Rudd MD, Bryan CJ, Wertenberger EG, et al: Brief cognitive-behavioral therapy effects on post-treatment suicide attempts in a military sample: results of a randomized clinical trial with 2-year follow-up. Am J Psychiatry 172(5):441–449, 2015 25677353

Saewyc EM, Konishi C, Rose HA, et al: School-based strategies to reduce suicidal ideation, suicide attempts, and discrimination among sexual minority and heterosexual adolescents in Western Canada. Int J Child Youth Family Stud 5(1):89–112, 2014 26793284

Serafini G, Adavastro G, Canepa G, et al: The efficacy of buprenorphine in major depression, treatment-resistant depression and suicidal behavior: a systematic review. Int J Mol Sci 19(8):2410, 2018 30111745

Simon OR, Swann AC, Powell KE, et al: Characteristics of impulsive suicide attempts and attempters. Suicide Life Threat Behav 32(1) (suppl):49–59, 2001 11924695

Sisti D, Mann JJ, Oquendo MA: Toward a distinct mental disorder—suicidal behavior. JAMA Psychiatry 77(7):661–662, 2020 32186693

Song J, Sjölander A, Joas E, et al: Suicidal behavior during lithium and valproate treatment: a within-individual 8-year prospective study of 50,000 patients with bipolar disorder. Am J Psychiatry 174(8):795–802, 2017 28595491

Stanley B, Brown GK: Safety planning intervention: a brief intervention to mitigate suicide risk. Cognit Behav Pract 19(2):256–264, 2012

Stanley B, Brown GK, Brenner LA, et al: Comparison of the safety planning intervention with follow-up vs usual care of suicidal patients treated in the emergency department. JAMA Psychiatry 75(9):894–900, 2018 29998307

Stengel E: Suicide and Attempted Suicide. Oxford, England, Penguin Books, 1964

Striebel JM, Kalapatapu RK: The anti-suicidal potential of buprenorphine: a case report. Int J Psychiatry Med 47(2):169–174, 2014 25084802

Szanto K, Kalmar S, Hendin H, et al: A suicide prevention program in a region with a very high suicide rate. Arch Gen Psychiatry 64(8):914–920, 2007 17679636

Székely A, Konkolÿ Thege B, Mergl R, et al: How to decrease suicide rates in both genders? An effectiveness study of a community-based intervention (EAAD). PLoS One 8(9):e75081, 2013 24086443

Turecki G, Brent DA, Gunnell D, et al: Suicide and suicide risk. Nat Rev Dis Primers 5(1):74, 2019 31649257

van Heeringen K: Stress-diathesis model of suicidal behavior, in The Neurobiological Basis of Suicide. Edited by Dwivedi Y. Boca Raton, FL, CRC Press, 2012, pp 113–125

van Heeringen K, Mann JJ: The neurobiology of suicide. Lancet Psychiatry 1(1):63–72, 2014 26360403

Vannoy SD, Robins LS: Suicide-related discussions with depressed primary care patients in the USA: gender and quality gaps. A mixed methods analysis. BMJ Open 1(2):e000198, 2011 22021884

Vermeulen JM, van Rooijen G, van de Kerkhof MPJ, et al: Clozapine and long-term mortality risk in patients with schizophrenia: a systematic review and meta-analysis of studies lasting 1.1–12.5 years. Schizophr Bull 45(2):315–329, 2019 29697804

Witte TK, Fitzpatrick KK, Joiner TE Jr, et al: Variability in suicidal ideation: a better predictor of suicide attempts than intensity or duration of ideation? J Affect Disord 88(2):131–136, 2005 16054227

Wolff S, Puts DA: Sex differences: summarizing more than a century of scientific research. Arch Sex Behav 38(6):1070–1072, 2009

World Health Organization: World Health Statistics 2019: Monitoring Health for the SDGs. Geneva, World Health Organization, 2019

Wyman PA, Brown CH, Inman J, et al: Randomized trial of a gatekeeper program for suicide prevention: 1-year impact on secondary school staff. J Consult Clin Psychol 76(1):104–115, 2008 18229988

Yovell Y, Bar G, Mashiah M, et al: Ultra-low-dose buprenorphine as a time-limited treatment for severe suicidal ideation: a randomized controlled trial. Am J Psychiatry 173(5):491–498, 2016 26684923

Zalsman G, Hawton K, Wasserman D, et al: Suicide prevention strategies revisited: 10-year systematic review. Lancet Psychiatry 3(7):646–659, 2016 27289303

CHAPTER 31

Suicide in Children and Adolescents

Christine Yu Moutier, M.D.
Joan Asarnow, Ph.D.

Suicide among youth is a major public health concern around the globe. Although suicide rates among youth are generally lower than those among middle-age and older adult populations in most countries (with American Indian youth in the United States being one exception), any early loss of life to a preventable cause of death such as suicide is tragic and warrants a major national public health response plan. Suicide is the second leading cause of death among youth ages 15–24 years in the United States, and rates of suicide have been rising in recent years. Only unintentional injuries, including car accidents and drug overdoses, take more lives among young people every year (National Institute of Mental Health 2020). Suicide takes more young lives in the United States than all of the other leading health-related causes of death combined (Figure 31–1). The recognition that young people are more likely to die by suicide than by any other single medical illness underscores the need for increased emphasis on medical education regarding suicide and the potential life-saving impact of identifying and providing effective care for young people who are at elevated risk for suicide. Because suicidal ideation and behavior tend to make their first appearance during adolescence, this developmental period may offer an important window of opportunity for interventions aimed at preventing the development of suicidal tendencies that may lead to elevated risk of premature death, mental health and functioning problems, and psychological pain and distress. Recent data further underscore the point that youths who struggle with suicidal ideation, suicidal behavior, and other forms of deliberate self-harm (e.g., nonsuicidal self-injury [NSSI] such as cutting or burning oneself without suicidal intent) are at increased risk for both death by suicide and death by other non-natural causes (e.g., alcohol or drug overdose, accidents) (King et al. 2019; Morgan et al. 2017). Indeed, it may be that suicidality and/or

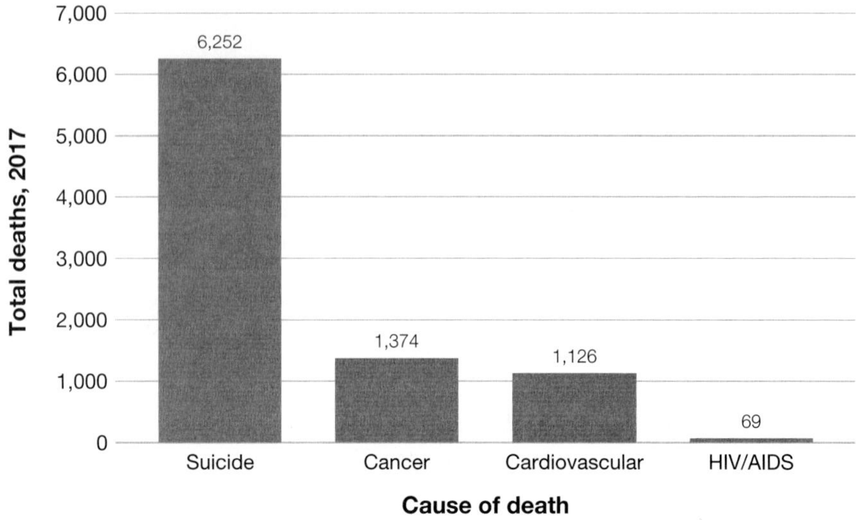

FIGURE 31–1. Number of deaths from selected causes, youth ages 15–24 years: United States, 2017.

Source. Data from Table 6 ("Number of deaths from selected causes, by age: United States, 2017"; pp. 34–35) in Kochanek KD, Murphy SL, Xu JQ, Arias E: Deaths: Final data for 2017. National Vital Statistics Reports, Vol. 68, No. 9. Hyattsville, MD, National Center for Health Statistics, 2019. Available at: https://www.cdc.gov/nchs/data/nvsr/nvsr68/nvsr68_09-508.pdf. Accessed July 6, 2021.

deliberate self-harm in youths signals the presence of active mechanisms such as risk-taking and health risk behaviors that contribute to premature death.

Among the 38 countries that have National Suicide Prevention Strategies (World Health Organization 2018), many use a public health approach in targeting youth suicide that includes universal education about mental health, suicide risk factors and warning signs, and how to change culture and stigma, particularly surrounding help seeking. Additionally, efforts are under way to augment peer support training, engage high-risk populations, and better prepare health professionals and systems to appropriately identify and care for youth at risk of suicide.

We begin this chapter with an overview of the epidemiology and scope of the problem. We then review the knowledge base regarding risk and protective factors, warning signs, screening and assessment strategies, treatment approaches, and communitywide suicide prevention interventions.

Epidemiology

Suicide is a leading cause of death among youth and a major public health crisis, as illustrated by the following epidemiological survey findings:

- Suicide is a leading cause of death among youth worldwide (Figure 31–2).
- Suicide is the second leading cause of death for people ages 10–34 years in the United States.

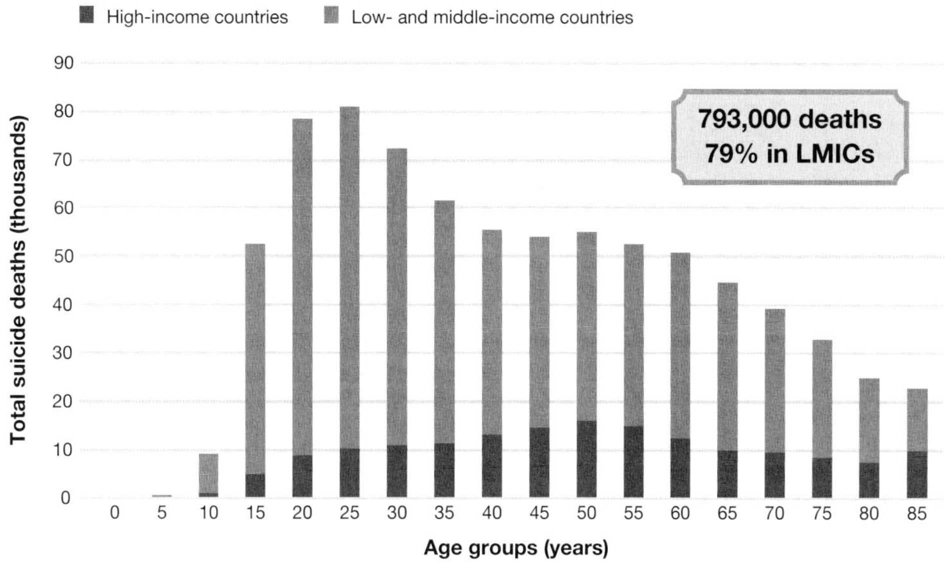

FIGURE 31–2. Global suicides by age and country income level,[a] 2016.

Globally, the majority of deaths by suicide in 2016 (79%) occurred in low- and middle-income countries (LMICs), where most (i.e., 84%) of the world's population lives. Regarding age, more than half (52.1%) of global suicides occurred in individuals younger than 45 years. Most adolescents who died by suicide (90%) were from LMICs, where nearly 90% of the world's adolescents live.

[a]World Bank income groups, 2017.

Source. Reprinted from Figure 5 (p. 11) in World Health Organization: Suicide in the World: Global Health Estimates (WHO/MSD/MER/19.3). Geneva, World Health Organization, 2019. License: CC BY-NC-SA 3.0 IGO. Available at: https://apps.who.int/iris/rest/bitstreams/1244794/retrieve. Accessed July 6, 2021.

- In epidemiological surveys conducted in the United States, approximately 1 in 6 teenagers reports having seriously considered suicide over the past 12 months (Centers for Disease Control and Prevention 2019).
- Youth suicide attempts are a major U.S. public health concern; it is estimated that 100–200 youth attempt suicide for every death by suicide. The suffering and trauma that suicidal behavior causes for the young person and their parents, siblings, and peers, and for schools and communities, is enormous. In the United States, the kindergarten through grade 12 education system has become increasingly involved in suicide prevention among youth through school suicide prevention policies, mandatory suicide prevention training of teachers and staff, and procedures for handling suicidal students and re-entry to school after inpatient or intensive mental health care treatment for individuals who have attempted suicide.
- Girls are more likely than boys to attempt suicide, but as with the adult population, boys are more likely to die by suicide than are girls. A 2019 study (Ruch et al. 2019) of the 40-year youth suicide trends in the United States found that youth suicide rates increased from 1975 to 1992, decreased from 1992 to 2007, and increased from 2007 to 2016.
- The gender gap is narrowing, especially for youth ages 10–14 years. Over the past decade, use of high-lethality methods (e.g., suffocation/hanging) has been increasing, particularly among girls (Ruch et al. 2019).

- Girls between the ages of 10 and 19 years attempt suicide at twice the rate of boys, but suicide rates among boys are higher than those among girls. However, a U.S. trend shows that the gender gap is shrinking, as suicide rates in girls have risen at a disproportionate pace compared with rates in boys, leading to a narrowing of the gender ratio from 3:1 to 2:1 (male: female suicide rate) from 1975 to 2016 (Ruch et al. 2019).

According to death certificate data from 1999 through 2016 collected by the National Center for Health Statistics (Curtin et al. 2018), the most commonly used methods for suicide in teenagers are suffocation (mostly hanging), accounting for 43% of all youth suicides, closely followed by firearm suicide, accounting for 42%. Less common are the methods of poisoning (6%) and falling (3%).

Risk and Protective Factors for Youth Suicide

Risk Factors

Suicide is a complex health outcome with multiple risk factors dynamically converging to culminate in a period of acute risk for suicidal behavior. There is rarely a single factor that leads to suicide, and there are diverse pathways that lead to this tragic outcome. Factors such as depression, anxiety, trauma, early childhood adversity, perfectionism, and genetic loading combine with external life circumstances to push the young person toward a sense of hopelessness and feelings of being overwhelmed, trapped, or a burden to others. The same factors—notably, previous suicide attempts or deliberate self-harm, suicidal ideation, depression, and other signs of mental health deterioration, including substance abuse—are as powerful in increasing suicide risk for adolescents and teenagers as they are for adults. However, young people who die by suicide are more likely than adult suicide decedents to have been experiencing undetected mental health deterioration. Lack of recognition of mental health problems in youth is a significant but addressable barrier in preventing suicide. There are also particular risk factors that are more critical for suicide risk in youth than for risk in adults; these include early-life adversity or maltreatment, child-parent conflict and negative family dynamics, parental substance use or mental illness, LGBTQ (lesbian, gay, bisexual, transgender, queer [or questioning]) status leading to rejection by family and others, bullying and cyberbullying, heavy use of online screen time, and impulsivity, all of which contribute to suicide risk in teens in a more significant way than in adults (Brent 2019; Kaess 2018).

As is the case for adults, access to lethal means plays a major part in increasing risk for youth. An important risk factor is the presence of guns and other lethal means in the home. Studies show that access to guns in the home increases suicide risk; the risk of death by suicide is two to five times higher for youth in gun-owning homes compared with youth in non-gun-owning homes (Baxley and Miller 2006; Grossman et al. 2005). A 2018 study of state-level gun ownership and suicide rates found that for each 10-percentage-point increase in statewide household gun ownership, the youth suicide rate increased by 26.9% (Knopov et al. 2018).

Psychosocial stressors that increase suicide risk include the following:

- Family violence
- Physical abuse
- Sexual abuse
- Rejection related to sexual orientation or gender identity
- Experiences with loss or humiliation
- Bullying

Protective Factors

Protective factors play an important role in preventing suicide. Suicide risk is multifaceted and dynamic, and protective factors do not exist in a vacuum. Thus, even when protective factors have been developed, suicide risk can still increase when other risk factors emerge, such as risk factors related to brain physiology, psychological status, and environmental pressures. Creative and robust coping strategies and flexible responses to one's own flaws and failings are key ways of reducing risk and should be taught and reinforced in youth. However, it is also true that during a period of escalating crisis or depression, these protective factors can be temporarily diminished or dismantled. Factors that have been shown to reduce suicide risk in youth overall (Brent et al. 2013) include the following:

- Parental support
- Parental positive mental health and affect
- Healthy family dynamics
- Help-seeking behaviors and attitudes
- Mental health care treatment for psychiatric illness or stress
- Good sleep patterns
- Sobriety

Warning Signs of Suicide Risk in Youth

A variety of warning signs have been identified that may indicate increased risk of suicide, especially when these signs occur in the context of stress or loss. Clinicians should avoid the trap of viewing significant behavior changes in teens, such as the following warning signs, as normal teenage behavior:

- Talking about suicide or about being dead—*Expressing thoughts of killing oneself should never be discounted.*
- Experiencing overwhelming emotional pain—*While teens generally have a heightened sense of emotional intensity and greater difficulty seeing the long view compared with adults, serious emotional pain should be followed up on.*
- Feeling trapped or as if one is a burden to others
- Feeling hopeless or worthless or having a sense of futility
- Showing significant changes in behavior or "personality"—*Behavior or mood changes to pay attention to include sadness or flat affect, withdrawal, tiredness, apathy,*

anger, agitation, irritability, and anxiety. Behavior changes can also include inability to focus on school, work, or routine tasks. It is important to note that any change in mood can be a sign for concern, as dysphoric mood may lift once a teen decides to take his or her life, and the youth may appear happier and more peaceful.
- Showing changes in daily routine, eating, and sleep habits

Clinical Care Strategies in Youth Suicide Prevention: Screening and Assessment

Major advances have been made in knowledge regarding effective treatment and care. While risk for suicide involves a complex interplay of risk and protective factors, and any single risk factor accounts for a relatively small level of the variance in suicide death outcomes, a history of prior suicide attempts or deliberate self-harm is still the most robust predictor of future fatal and nonfatal attempts (Ribeiro et al. 2016). Moreover, health care professionals often encounter youths struggling with suicidal thoughts and behaviors and nonsuicidal self-harm in clinical settings, and contacts with the health system provide important opportunities to identify youths with risk and provide lifesaving care.

There are a number of validated screening tools that can be used in clinical practice, including the Columbia–Suicide Severity Rating Scale (C-SSRS), which can be administered to adolescents and adults, and the Ask About Suicide Questionnaire (ASQ), which has been used with patients ages 8–21 years (Ballard et al. 2017; Horowitz et al. 2012, 2020). Such instruments can be incorporated as a component of a care process model that includes screening using an evidence-based questionnaire or rating scale, more extensive evaluation for youths with positive screens, and recommendations regarding risk stratification and care (U.S. Department of Health and Human Services 2019). This screening approach is increasingly used in health care systems as part of "Zero Suicide (ZS)" quality improvement programs that aim to advance the aspirational goal of making suicide a "never event" within health care systems. Findings from open evaluation trials (Layman et al. 2021) have supported the ZS approach, which includes efforts to 1) change culture and obtain an organizational leadership commitment to reducing suicide, 2) train the workforce in suicide prevention, 3) identify high-risk individuals through screening/assessment, 4) engage high-risk individuals in suicide prevention care management plans, 5) offer evidence-based treatment, 6) attend to transition points between services as high-risk points, and 7) use data-driven continuous quality improvement strategies (https://zerosuicide.edc.org/).

A major challenge for youth presenting with suicidal episodes is that these youths tend to have difficulty transitioning to care after emergency treatment and often receive inadequate doses of care. A variety of interventions have been developed to improve continuity of care of all patients treated for suicide risk (i.e., Objective 8.4 of the U.S. National Strategy for Suicide Prevention [U.S. Department of Health and Human Services Office of the Surgeon General and National Action Alliance for Suicide Prevention 2012]). For example, the Family Intervention for Suicide Prevention (Asarnow et al. 2009, 2011) offers a brief "therapeutic" behavioral assessment that serves the dual functions of enhancing linkage to further follow-up treatment and offering further assessment of risk by examining whether the therapist can elicit behaviors from the youth and family that are inconsistent with attempting suicide (e.g., hope, reasons for living, use of safety plan by youth with family support, commitments to living, protective support and monitoring, parent/caregiver restriction of youth access to lethal suicide methods, youth and parent engagement in treatment). This developmentally informed approach to safety planning and activation of protective processes has been found to be associated with improved linkage to follow-up treatment and continuity of care, and when combined with evidence-informed treatment, led to improved clinical outcomes, including fewer suicide attempts (Asarnow et al. 2011). Other therapeutic assessment and motivational enhancement interventions have also been shown to address the important problem of increasing the likelihood that youths will receive care following a suicidal or self-harm episode (Grupp-Phelan et al. 2012; Ougrin et al. 2011, 2015; Spirito et al. 2002).

Figure 31–3 depicts a care process model based on what we have learned about approaches for reducing suicide risk and improving continuity of care after an emergency department or other visit where suicidal thoughts or behaviors require emergency intervention (Asarnow et al. 2017a; U.S. Department of Health and Human Services, Health Resources and Services Administration, Maternal and Child Health Bureau 2019). This approach begins with identification of risk (screening or other information), notes the need for safety precautions (do not leave youth alone), provides medical treatment for any injury, and conducts a mental health evaluation to determine disposition. Based on current knowledge, there are benefits for youth stabilization and further assessment of whether the youth requires inpatient care or can be discharged home under the care and supervision of parents/caregivers, using a brief intervention such as the Family Intervention for Suicide Prevention (FISP) model (Asarnow et al. 2009, 2011, 2017a) (see Figure 31–3). The FISP model aims to strengthen or activate reasons for living and hope, initiate safety planning and obtain from the youth a commitment to use the safety plan in place of suicidal behavior if a suicidal urge emerges, increase protective support and monitoring of the youth, provide counseling to parents regarding the importance of restricting access to potentially dangerous/lethal self-harm methods (it is strongly recommended that parents be counseled separately in further detail to ensure that the youth does not learn more about available self-harm methods), and educate the parents and youth regarding the potential dangers of disinhibition associated with substance use.

If the response of the youth and parents to this secondary evaluation (in combination with the standard mental health evaluation) supports a decision to send the youth home under the supervision of a responsible adult, it is important to further educate the youth about the value and importance of follow-up treatment; provide a follow-up appointment if possible, or refer to mental health; obtain a commitment from the youth and parents/caregivers to attend follow-up treatment; and follow up with the youth and parents with caring contacts until they have been linked to follow-up treatment. Caring contacts are brief, nondemanding messages of support (e.g., "I want you to know that I am thinking of you and hope that you are having a good day") that aim to strengthen connectedness between the youth/parents and a "caring health system," thereby increasing the likelihood that the youth and parents will turn to the health care system should the need arise (Miller et al. 2017). Following their health care setting policy and Health Insurance Portability and Accountability Act

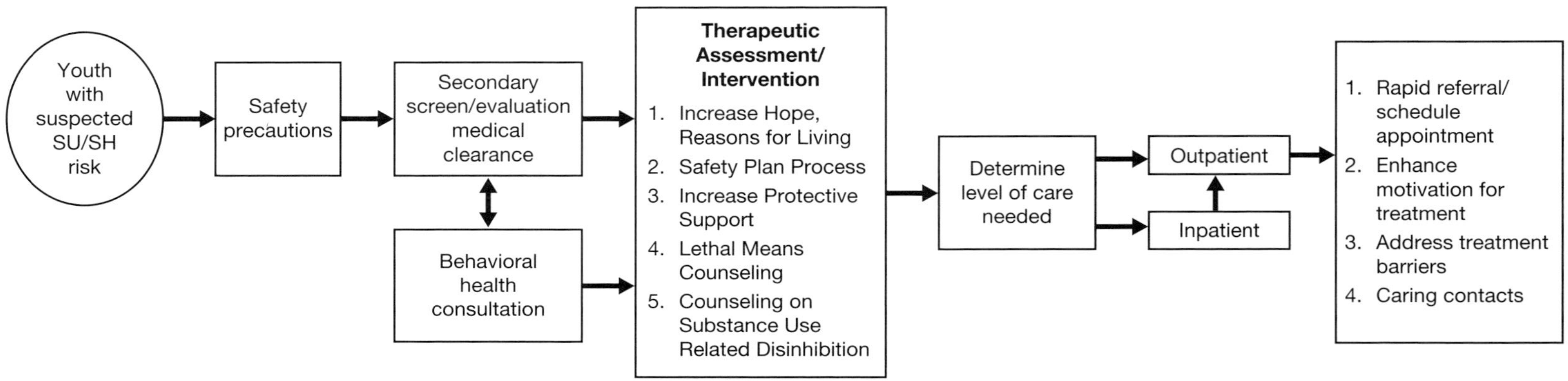

FIGURE 31–3. Care process: Family Intervention for Suicide Prevention (FISP) model.

SH=self-harm; SU=suicide.

Source. Copyright © 2019, Joan Asarnow.

regulations, health providers or health systems can provide these messages by phone, mail, text, or email. If difficulties with connecting to outpatient care are identified, these contacts can also include communication to enhance motivation for treatment and can problem-solve practical and individual barriers to follow-up care.

Role of Psychosocial Treatment and Medications in Youth Suicide Prevention

Psychosocial Interventions

There are currently a number of treatment approaches that in randomized controlled trials and open trials have shown promise for reducing self-injurious thoughts and behaviors (Glenn et al. 2019). It is important to note that in the United Kingdom and Europe, there is a tendency to combine suicidal and nonsuicidal self-harm into a single overall self-harm variable. This trend of combining both types of self-harm is based on the challenges of determining intent, the mixed intent behind many self-harm behaviors, and data indicating that self-harm predicts subsequent repeat self-harm and death by self-harm (Hawton et al. 2012). In the United States, by contrast, we tend to distinguish between self-harm with suicidal intent (defined as suicide attempts) and other forms of nonsuicidal and unclear self-harm. These cross-national differences complicate review of the treatment research, although accumulating evidence that nonsuicidal self-harm/NSSI is a strong predictor of suicide attempts and that self-harm behaviors predict repeat fatal and nonfatal self-harm provides some confidence that we can interpret studies showing positive outcomes for both suicidal and nonsuicidal self-harm interventions as all contributing to strategies that can prevent suicide (Hawton et al. 2012; King et al. 2019; Morgan et al. 2017).

Two independent trials examining dialectical behavior therapy (DBT), a treatment that has shown efficacy in reducing future suicide attempts in adults (Linehan et al. 2006), found that DBT led to lower rates of subsequent self-harm in youths relative to active comparator conditions. The Norwegian trial (Mehlum et al. 2014, 2016, 2019), which used active clinic treatment as usual as the comparator condition, found that DBT had a sustained effect, with youths receiving DBT showing lower levels of self-harm behaviors 3 years following the start of the trial, although the two treatment groups showed similar improvements on other clinical outcomes, such as depression, at the 3-year endpoint (Mehlum et al. 2019). There was also evidence of greater cost-effectiveness for DBT (Haga et al. 2018).

The larger U.S. trial (McCauley et al. 2018), which used individual and group supportive psychotherapy matched to DBT for dose intensity as the comparator condition, found a significant advantage for DBT in reducing suicide attempts as well as NSSI and overall rates of self-harm, both soon after the 6-month DBT treatment and at follow-up 12 months after the start of treatment. Moreover, the U.S. study results indicated that in comparison with youths receiving supportive psychotherapy, significantly more youths receiving DBT were free of self-harm at follow-up (McCauley et al. 2018).

In considering the results of the DBT trials, it is important to note that DBT is an intensive treatment that requires strong time commitments from youths, parents, and therapists. The treatment involves 1 hour of individual DBT psychotherapy with youths weekly, 2 hours of multifamily group skills training weekly, phone coaching available 24 hours a day to youths and parents, and weekly team meetings for therapist support. The Norwegian and U.S. trials, however, used somewhat different DBT approaches. Whereas the Norwegian trial (Mehlum et al. 2019) had a moderately less severely ill patient sample and used a briefer, 19-week adaptation of DBT for adolescents (Miller et al. 2017), the U.S. trial (McCauley et al. 2018), which was led by Linehan, had a more severely ill patient sample and multifamily skills groups and used the Linehan skills training manual (Linehan 2015).

Although replication is critical, particularly when evaluating rare outcomes such as suicide attempts, and several subsequent studies of DBT failed to replicate the robust findings described above, three additional treatments have produced evidence supporting efficacy: 1) Safe Alternatives for Teens and Youths (SAFETY), a DBT-informed cognitive-behavioral treatment with a strong family focus, was associated with reduced risk of suicide attempts both at posttreatment (3 months) and through 6–12 months of follow-up (Asarnow et al. 2017b); 2) integrated cognitive-behavioral therapy (CBT) for suicidality and substance abuse was found to be associated with fewer suicide attempts and improvement in substance abuse (Esposito-Smythers et al. 2011); and 3) mentalization-based treatment was associated with reduced levels of self-harm (Rossouw and Fonagy 2012). Other treatments that have also shown promise include parent training, which was associated with reductions in an overall scale of suicidality in a randomized controlled trial (Pineda and Dadds 2013), and CBT for Suicide Prevention (a therapy modeled on the Beck and Brown treatment for adults [Brown et al. 2005), which was associated with decreases in suicidal ideation, suicidal behaviors, and hopelessness in a nonrandomized trial (Stanley et al. 2009). Meta-analyses and systematic reviews also have been conducted, and the results of a large meta-analysis (Glenn et al. 2019; Ougrin et al. 2015) indicated small but statistically significant advantages for a diverse range of treatments in reducing rates of self-harm, with a need to treat approximately 14 youths to prevent 1 episode of self-harm (number needed to treat [NNT]=14, 95% confidence interval [CI]=7.7–100). The strongest effects in the Ougrin et al. (2015) meta-analysis, which included studies through May 2014, were for DBT, CBT, and mentalization-based therapy. When only the smaller number of studies evaluating suicide attempt outcomes were examined, no statistically significant advantage for any of the diverse study treatments was observed. This analysis was conducted prior to the availability of data from the U.S. DBT trial, which showed a DBT advantage, relative to a strong comparator condition (see earlier description), in reducing suicide attempts at the posttreatment assessment (McCauley et al. 2018).

These data can guide clinicians in identifying and delivering effective psychosocial treatments, although there remains a strong need for additional treatment research to inform care, particularly given failures to replicate and evidence that continued care is needed after 6 months of treatment for many youths, particularly those in severely ill populations. For example, in the U.S. DBT trial, which involved severely suicidal adolescents with high levels of suicidal ideation, prior suicide attempts, and multiple self-harm episodes, the researchers found that only slightly more than half of the youths receiving DBT were self-harm-free at 12 months (McCauley et al. 2018). Measurement-based care approaches, in which treatment response is closely monitored to support shifts in treatment strategy when youths are not benefiting from a treatment, offer an important mechanism for improving outcomes. Such approaches can also inform efforts to combine psychosocial and medication treatments as needed.

Before we turn to the topic of medication treatments, it is also important to note that DBT is an intensive treatment that is burdensome for clinics, youths, and families. Offering DBT is not feasible in care settings in which the clinical workforce is too limited to provide DBT and in U.S. locales where access to DBT is not available, and DBT may be more intensive than is appropriate for some youths, particularly because time in therapy means time away from other activities important for youth development. These significant limitations in access to DBT and other evidence-based, intensive treatments have led to interest in stepped-care models wherein the intensity of services is matched to the level of the assessed patient need or risk. Other treatments, such as SAFETY and integrated CBT, use two therapists, one for the youth and one for the parent. This two-therapist approach is not typical in clinical settings and may present feasibility problems in community settings. However, potential justification for this stepped-care approach will become clearer with more research evidence. Current evidence does suggest that a strong family focus is needed to effectively treat youths after a suicide attempt, given that such a focus is an integral part of the three treatments with evidence supporting their efficacy for this population. Elsewhere, we have suggested that this family work allows parents to function as protective "seat belts" when youths experience unbearable pain and suicidal urges and to safeguard their children from acting on potentially life-threatening urges (Asarnow et al. 2017a).

No discussion of psychosocial treatment targeting suicide risk reduction would be complete without emphasizing the importance of restricting access to potentially lethal means of self-harm, such as firearms, when a youth is struggling with suicidality and self-harm urges. As discussed earlier, if a gun is available, the likelihood of death is greatly increased. Therefore, it is the standard of care to counsel parents about the importance of restricting access to potentially lethal methods and to assist them in finding ways to eliminate or safely store weapons or potentially dangerous implements. Although access to firearms and medicines can be restricted, it is not possible to eliminate access to all means of hanging or suffocation, or even access to all medicines, poisons, or firearms. Therefore, parents must be counseled on the importance of support, strengthening communication, protective monitoring, and enlisting other responsible adults or even youths in efforts to sustain and protect the vulnerable youth.

Medication Treatment

Medication treatment is an important tool for treating youths with mental health conditions. One in four Americans will have a mental disorder in their lifetime; 50% of these conditions have their onset by age 14, and 75% by age 24 years (Kessler et al. 2007; World Health Organization 2020). Therefore, the need to identify and treat mental health deterioration and mental illness in children and adolescents is compelling, and yet fewer than half of young people with depression or other psychiatric disorders receive treatment. For individuals with mood disorders and other psychiatric conditions, the average length of time between onset of symptoms and diagnosis is more than 10 years (Baldessarini et al. 2020).

Many suicidal and self-harming youths meet criteria for major depressive disorder (McCauley et al. 2018), and many are treated with antidepressant medications. A special consideration that was introduced in the early 2000s was the FDA decision to place a black box warning on all antidepressants for patients younger than 24 years for "increased risk of suicidal thinking, feeling, and behavior" in young people. During the years following the black box warning in 2004, there was a documented decrease in diagnosing and treating depression in primary care. A large cohort study that included 1.1 million adolescents, 1.4 million young adults, and 5 million older adults collected mental health–related data over the 10-year period from 2000 to 2010 (Lu et al. 2014). The study revealed significant reductions in antidepressant use within 2 years of the FDA advisory release—relative reductions of 31.0%, 24.3%, and 14.5% among adolescents, young adults, and middle-age/older adults, respectively. Notably, the study found that the rate of suicide attempts *significantly increased*—by 22% in adolescents and by 34% in young adults (Lu et al. 2014). Even though the black box warning was for youth and young adults younger than 24 years, the effect of the warning seemed to spill over into the identification and treatment of depression across all ages. Moreover, the use of nonpharmacological treatments such as CBT for depression and anxiety did not increase to replace the decreases in treatment with medications. These reductions in diagnosing and treating depression were thought to be associated with fear and new confusion regarding the use of antidepressants among pediatricians and other health care providers, as well as among parents and the general population, leading to reluctance among health care practitioners to appropriately treat depression with antidepressant medication.

The FDA's decision to place the black box warning on antidepressant labeling for use in young people younger than 24 years was based on findings from a series of meta-analyses of 372 randomized clinical trials of antidepressants, involving nearly 100,000 participants, which showed that the rate of suicidal thinking or suicidal behavior was 4% among patients assigned to receive an antidepressant, as compared with 2% among those assigned to receive placebo, although none of the suicide attempts documented in the trials were fatal (Hammad 2004). However, the methodology in the FDA series of meta-analyses did not allow for examination of potential positive effects on suicide risk or for incorporation of premedication levels of suicidal ideation or behaviors (Baldessarini et al. 2006). Notably, there were no suicide deaths and extremely few attempts in the dataset on which the FDA based its decision (Friedman 2014).

According to the American Academy of Pediatrics, the benefits of antidepressants outweigh the potential risks for most young patients (Cheung et al. 2018; March et al. 2004). Many studies support this opinion. For example, one research team conducted a reanalysis of all the trials related to two medications, fluoxetine and venlafaxine (Gibbons et al. 2012). The researchers did not find any evidence of increased suicidal ideation or behavior among patients who received the medications. They did find a significant impact on depression for all age groups, but especially for youth, with 46.6% of young patients treated with fluoxetine experiencing a decrease in their depression, compared with 16.5% of young patients treated with placebo (Bridge et al. 2005).

Additionally, a review by Walkup (2017) concluded that much of the controversy surrounding the efficacy of antidepressants for the treatment of depression in children and adolescents was related to methodological and implementation problems with industry-sponsored depression trials in children. Walkup made a strong case for the appropriate use and efficacy of antidepressants related to the National Institute of Mental Health (NIMH)–sponsored trials—which, in contrast to industry trials, have many methodological strengths, lower placebo response rates (30%–35%), and meaningful between-group differences that support antidepressant efficacy. These compelling arguments for the superiority of the NIMH trials over industry drug trials, combined with the clear efficacy of selective serotonin reuptake inhibitors for childhood-onset obsessive-compulsive disorder and anxiety disorders, suggest that appropriate use of antidepressants plays an important role in the treatment of child and adolescent mental health conditions (Walkup 2017).

Role of Social Media

Emerging research on the impact of social media and screen time in general on youth mental health is complex and shows mixed findings. On the one hand, social media and online sites can provide a source of connection and encouragement related to mental health topics for many people, and use of these resources is often needed for completion of school assignments. However, findings are emerging that suggest that heavy and/or pathological use of the internet and social media can have a negative impact on mental health (Durkee et al. 2016; Kaess et al. 2014). Examples of problematic use include heavy internet or online gaming (defined as multiple hours of screen time per day, leading to addictive behavioral changes and impairments in fulfilling school or family obligations [Brand et al. 2019]); screen use at bedtime (which may contribute to disruptions in sleep, depressed mood, and anxiety); and heavy social media use with potential for exposure to cyberbullying or risky contacts (e.g., sexting), which can contribute to distress and suicidal thoughts or urges. According to many child experts, including Dr. Benjamin Shain, who led the American Academy of Pediatrics Committee on Adolescence in developing guidelines for addressing suicide risk (Shain and Committee on Adolescence 2016), suicide risk in vulnerable teens may be impacted by social media use.

Heavy internet use can also contribute to the risk of suicide contagion following the suicide death or attempt of a peer or a celebrity (Shain and Committee on Adolescence 2016). Additionally, there are publicly accessible pro-suicide websites (not only on the dark web) that encourage suicide and provide specific methods for suicide. Advocacy efforts to have these sites closed down have proven challenging to date, despite the fact that one element contributing to the increased rate of suicide deaths, particularly in younger individuals, may be easy access to information regarding deadly methods.

Research data on the relationship between social media use and mental health point to several mediators between social media use and mental health outcomes: nighttime use of screens is known to disrupt sleep, and youth with mental health vulnerabilities may be particularly susceptible to the adverse mood and anxiety effects of social comparison, fear of missing out, and negative online interactions. Some youths may also interpret online peer interactions in more negative ways. Finally, heavy internet use can contribute to screen or online gaming addiction. Clinicians may consider providing parents with guidance such as the following:

- Parents should consider limiting their children's screen time (on recreational sites such as social media and YouTube-type platforms). For youth with mental health conditions or other vulnerabilities, parents should consider monitoring and even further limiting the child's online and social media use.
- Parents should be advised to think carefully about the age at which their children should initially be provided with a smartphone and to consider methods for monitoring the child's online and cellphone contacts, as they would other interactions.
- Clinicians should inquire about child and teen patients' social media use because such use is often as "real" a part of their lives as what we adults think of as "real life." Clinicians are encouraged to incorporate social media use into history taking and similarly utilize it as part of psychoeducation and treatment planning.

Many "mental health–savvy" young people are practicing social media pauses—taking breaks from social media, limiting their use in a number of ways (e.g., reducing amount of time spent per day, being more selective in types of platforms used, avoiding toxic interactions), and seeking out rewarding interactions with positive, encouraging individuals and platforms.

It is also important to note that electronic health (eHealth) and mobile health (mHealth) technologies show strong promise for improving mental health generally and for delivering suicide prevention interventions. Online treatments and technology-enhanced treatment strategies are receiving increasing attention, have shown benefits, and may be particularly valuable for teens and young adults, who tend to be very comfortable with these technologies. One promising approach that uses ecological momentary assessments in tandem with interventions[1] is the As Safe As Possible intervention, which combines brief in-person treatment with a smartphone app featuring cued daily ratings of current emotional distress followed by personalized safety planning strategy messages with suggestions regarding emotion regulation (Kennard et al. 2018). The promising results of these eHealth and mHealth strategies underscores the fact that there is potential for benefit as well as harm from smartphone and internet access.

Suicide Contagion

Suicide contagion is a real phenomenon for vulnerable individuals, given that humans are social creatures that are hardwired for imitation (vis-à-vis mirror neurons), and youth are more highly susceptible than adults because of their stage of psycho-

---

[1] Ecological momentary assessment (EMA) is a form of real-world psychological assessment that involves repeated sampling of subjects' current behaviors and experiences in real time, in subjects' natural environments. It aims to minimize recall bias and provide nuanced data that can be assessed for ecological or environmental influences and associations. Ecological momentary interventions (EMI) are brief interventions individuals employ based on real-time self-monitoring and customized feedback, with the goal of improving health in a personalized manner.

CHAPTER 32

Combination Pharmacological Strategies for Antidepressant Treatment

Adel Farah, M.D., M.Sc.
Pierre Blier, M.D., Ph.D.

Approximately two-thirds of depressed patients will experience various degrees of improvement in response to a medication trial (Belmaker and Agam 2008; Cipriani et al. 2018). The response criterion, generally accepted to be a 50% improvement, has, however, not been the clinical standard used to assess the effectiveness of antidepressant treatments (Nierenberg and DeCecco 2001). This is largely based on the observation that patients who have responded to their therapeutic regimen but still show significant residual symptoms have a higher relapse rate than do patients treated to remission (Judd et al. 2000; Paykel et al. 1995). Consequently, more than half of depressed patients will require additional measures after a first drug treatment or a monotherapy. Nevertheless, whether remission is the target or full functional recovery is the end goal, it is unlikely that a single pharmacological agent will achieve this outcome(s) in patients with treatment-resistant depression.

Classically, the available options for additional measures consist of medication substitution, combination, and augmentation. A *medication substitution* consists of switching a medication indicated for depression for another of the same or a different class, with or without a washout period. The *combination* strategy entails keeping the first drug and adding a second agent that is endowed with antidepressant activity when used on its own. The *augmentation*, or *potentiation*, approach consists of adding a second agent that is not an established monotherapy for depression. In this chapter, no distinction is made between combination and augmentation or potentiation, because all of these strategies involve the use of different mechanism(s) of action to improve symptomatic benefits. For instance, even some *substitutions* can be considered as *combinations*, as is the case with switching from a selective serotonin reuptake inhibitor (SSRI) to a serotonin-norepinephrine reuptake inhibitor (SNRI). Consequently, when a clinician is managing patients with an insufficient response to a first pharmacotherapeutic trial, it is most important to consider the neuronal target(s) of the additional or alternative medication and not merely the initial clinical indication for which it was introduced on the market. In this perspective, the different strategies described in this chapter follow the neuroscience-based nomenclature (Zohar et al. 2015) that was endorsed by the American Psychiatric Association in July 2019.

This chapter is not an exhaustive review of all the pharmacological strategies ever reported. Rather, we concentrate on the more commonly used approaches and emphasize their biological targets. Even for such strategies, the focus is on the main findings and how to implement them safely and effectively rather than describing and analyzing every single report. These approaches are those that have been supported by controlled designs.

Targets for Antidepressant Strategies

The antidepressant response achieved with currently marketed drugs relies almost entirely on the enhancement of serotonin (5-hydroxytryptamine [5-HT]), norepinephrine, or to some extent the dopamine system. This is best exemplified by the depletion studies of serotonin and catecholamines in patients with treatment-responsive depression. Basically, a significant proportion of the patients who respond to an SSRI will experience, typically within a few hours, a return of some depressive symptoms with a dietary depletion of tryptophan, the amino acid precursor for serotonin (Booij et al. 2002; Delgado et al. 1990, 1999). Of note, even patients who respond to monoamine oxidase inhibitors (MAOIs), which enhance brain levels of serotonin, norepinephrine, and dopamine, will also experience a partial relapse with this challenge (Delgado et al. 1990). In contrast, patients with a favorable response to a norepinephrine reuptake inhibitor can experience a return of symptoms with the inhibition of dopamine and norepinephrine but not serotonin synthesis (Miller et al. 1996).

Transmission in these systems can be modulated in multiple ways. These approaches may lead to differential effects in various brain structures and different side effects. For instance, when serotonin availability is increased with an SSRI, typically 20%–30% of patients will experience nausea to various degrees. When MAOIs are used, whether reversible (moclobemide) or irreversible (phenelzine or tranylcypromine), serotonin levels are elevated, yet they rarely produce nausea. Furthermore, nausea triggered by SSRIs generally fades away within 1–2 weeks, whereas the sexual dysfunction they cause in at least half of patients persists over time (Montejo-González et al. 1997).

Another example of the differential synaptic effects of agents that act on these specific neurotransmission systems is illustrated by the prolactin-enhancing effect of serotonin agents. Tryptophan increases prolactin release, which is blocked by serotonin type 1A (5-HT_{1A}) receptor antagonists, whereas the effect of the serotonin releaser/reuptake blocker fenfluramine on prolactin is blocked by a serotonin type 2 (5-HT_2)

receptor antagonist (Goodall et al. 1993; Park and Cowen 1995). Consequently, the use of two agents may alter serotonin transmission through different mechanisms even within the same brain structure. It is therefore conceivable that targeting two different neuronal elements on the same types of neurons may lead to a much greater effect on that specific neurotransmission than does either agent used alone, yielding greater clinical benefits. For instance, it is well known that norepinephrine reuptake inhibitors enhance the synaptic availability of norepinephrine (by about twofold), whereas α_2-adrenergic antagonists have a more modest effect. Their combined use leads, however, to a more than fivefold increase in the levels of norepinephrine (Dennis et al. 1987). A concrete example of such a synergy possibly contributing to a superior antidepressant response is the combination of the SNRI venlafaxine with the α_2-adrenoceptor antagonist mirtazapine (Blier et al. 2010).

Treatment strategies in patients with an inadequate response should, therefore, be attempted with this framework in mind because targeting any neuronal elements of a specific neurotransmitter will not necessarily produce the same synaptic alterations. There can be at the very least a summation, or even a synergy of effects, as described earlier, whereby the net action of two drugs when used together is greater than the sum of the actions of the drugs used alone.

Choosing a Combination Antidepressant Strategy

The first step in choosing a combination approach is to identify possible medical contraindications of the agents that are contemplated. An absolute contraindication would be the concomitant use of a potent serotonin reuptake inhibitor (i.e., clomipramine or any of the SSRIs) and an irreversible MAOI. In the early 1990s, the underestimation of the long elimination of fluoxetine and its active metabolite norfluoxetine, which has a much longer half-life than the parent drug, led to fatalities when irreversible MAOIs were prematurely introduced (Boyer and Shannon 2005; Sternbach 1991). This combination of drugs neutralizes the only two inactivation pathways for serotonin and leads to an excessive accumulation of this neurotransmitter, thereby producing a serotonin syndrome.

Most other drug combinations can still target the serotonin system to produce safe pharmacodynamic actions. In the process, serotonergic adverse effects (nausea, increased anxiety, and agitation) may be triggered, as can be the case even with SSRIs used alone. These can be easily managed by dosage reduction or the cessation of one of the two drugs, and they are not life-threatening because monoamine oxidase can inactivate excessive serotonin. Potentially lethal drug interactions should not occur when a norepinephrine reuptake inhibitor is used with an MAOI. In fact, the combination of such drugs was reported to be effective in cases of treatment-resistant depression (Schmauss et al. 1988). The relative safety of the latter approach is the result of catechol-*O*-methyltransferase providing an alternative metabolic inactivation pathway for norepinephrine and dopamine. Such a drug combination even protects patients from hypertensive crises produced by the ingestion of tyramine in the presence of an MAOI. Indeed, norepinephrine reuptake inhibitors prevent the entry of tyramine into norepinephrine terminals, which normally would produce a calcium-independent release of norepinephrine, leading to blood pressure spiking (Blier et al.

Bupropion

The addition of bupropion has been one of the most popular strategies in North America because of its ease of use and because of studies rather consistently showing efficacy when combined with other drugs (Blier et al. 2010; Lam et al. 2004; Mischoulon et al. 2000; Trivedi et al. 2006; Zuilhof et al. 2018). It is well tolerated at an initial dosage of 150 mg/day, which has been shown to be effective by itself in monotherapy in a placebo-controlled trial (Reimherr et al. 1998). A maximum dosage of 450 mg/day can be used in patients without contraindications and will avoid reaching plasma levels that could be in the range of those producing epileptic activity (Connarn et al. 2017; Davidson 1989).

Bupropion can be considered as acting primarily on the norepinephrine and dopamine system but also on the serotonin system (Dong and Blier 2001; Ghanbari et al. 2011; Li et al. 2002). The drug does not act, however, as a dopamine reuptake blocker, as evidenced by its very low affinity for the human dopamine transporter (Tatsumi et al. 1997). Furthermore, four positron emission tomography studies have shown that in usual clinical regimens, bupropion occupies only about 20% of dopamine transporters in the brain (see Argyelán et al. 2005). Furthermore, it does not alter the firing rate of rat dopamine neurons, which would be expected from a dopamine reuptake blocker (Dong and Blier 2001). Bupropion is a norepinephrine releaser, which initially decreases norepinephrine neuronal firing through an excess activation of the norepinephrine cell body autoreceptors. Because it also increases norepinephrine release on serotonin neurons, it drives up the firing rate of serotonin neurons in a sustained fashion. With treatment prolongation, the firing rate of norepinephrine neurons gradually recovers (El Mansari et al. 2010). Consequently, bupropion can be considered an agent that increases monoaminergic transmission but not via reuptake inhibition. Therefore, the clinical benefits of adding bupropion to SSRIs described earlier is theoretically supported by preclinical data. Furthermore, the combination of bupropion with escitalopram promptly doubles the normal firing rate of rat serotonin neurons, rather than decreasing it by half as with the SSRI alone (Ghanbari et al. 2010).

Given the norepinephrine-releasing action of bupropion, this strategy would appear more conservative than using agents like methylphenidate, dexedrine, lisdexamfetamine, or mixed amphetamine salts. Indeed, these medications have abuse potential in some individuals, may worsen insomnia and anxiety, and do not have intrinsic antidepressant activity as does bupropion. Nevertheless, these individual agents, despite not showing consistent antidepressant activity in add-on controlled designs, can be useful for the management of residual symptoms of anergia and cognitive symptoms (Giacobbe et al. 2018; McIntyre et al. 2017).

Modafinil

In contrast with bupropion, modafinil is a dopamine reuptake inhibitor, as shown in a brain imaging study (Volkow et al. 2009). Initially, data suggested that addition of this drug, at dosages of 100–400 mg/day, to the therapeutic regimen of depressed patients with incomplete responses had beneficial actions on fatigue and sleepiness (Fava et al. 2005). Subsequently, a meta-analysis of controlled studies showed a significant improvement in overall depression scores (Goss et al. 2013). In addition, modafinil was efficacious in improving episodic and working memory functioning in patients with remitted depression in a controlled study (Kaser et al. 2017).

Alpha-2 Adrenergic Antagonists

Positive results have been reported in double-blind studies with α_2-adrenergic antagonists when mianserin, mirtazapine, and yohimbine were used in combination with SSRIs (Henssler et al. 2016). These α_2-adrenergic receptors are located on both norepinephrine and serotonin terminals, and therefore have the potential to influence the release of both neurotransmitters (Blier and El Mansari 2013; El Mansari et al. 2010).

Blockade of α_2-adrenergic autoreceptors on the cell body of norepinephrine neurons increases their firing activity in the locus coeruleus (see Figure 32–2). This enhanced activity of norepinephrine neurons is likely partially offset by their reuptake transporters in projection areas. Indeed, the excitatory effect of norepinephrine on serotonin neurons in the rat dorsal raphe nucleus produced by mirtazapine is only transient. It becomes sustained, however, after 3 weeks of administration. Again, this enhanced activity of serotonin neurons may be partially offset by their reuptake transporters, which are not affected by mirtazapine (Blier and El Mansari 2013). It would thus appear that the antidepressant action of mirtazapine would depend on some degree of combined enhancement of both serotonin and norepinephrine transmission, and furthermore its therapeutic effect can be reversed by either serotonin or norepinephrine synthesis inhibition in improved depressed patients (Delgado et al. 2002). The beneficial action of mianserin and mirtazapine addition in patients with SSRI-resistant depression thus may stem from their ability to counteract the dampening action of the SSRIs on the firing rate of norepinephrine neurons described earlier.

It is important to note that these drugs also may exert their beneficial action in SSRI-resistant depression through their potent 5-HT_2 receptor antagonism. Indeed, it was reported that the combination of serotonin reuptake inhibition and 5-HT_{2A} receptor antagonism acutely increases norepinephrine release in the rat frontal cortex and in the locus coeruleus (Hatanaka et al. 2000). Consistent with the latter alteration, the firing rate of norepinephrine neurons is initially dampened by administration of an SSRI/5-HT_{2A} receptor antagonist, but it recovers gradually to normal after 3 weeks of sustained administration (Szabo and Blier 2002). This combined mechanism may, in part, underlie the mechanism of action of the addition of D_2/5-HT_{2A} receptor antagonists in patients with SSRI-resistant depression.

Dopamine and Serotonin Antagonists: Addition to Selective Serotonin Reuptake Inhibitors

Ample evidence now indicates that the addition of psychotropic medications that inhibit dopamine D_2 and 5-HT_2 receptor signaling to the regimen of depressed patients not responding to an SSRI may produce a rapid and robust antidepressant response. Double-blind studies support the marked beneficial effect of olanzapine, risperidone, and quetiapine addition (Nelson and Papakostas 2009). Such a positive response to the addition of a dopamine antagonist does not rely on the presence of psychotic symptoms to manifest itself. Because it is widely accepted that pure D_2 receptor antagonists are not useful adjuncts in the management of treatment-resistant unipolar depression without psychotic features, these medications must not exert their therapeutic action via the antagonism of D_2 receptors that is common to all of these drugs.

Microdialysis studies examining the levels of extracellular serotonin, norepinephrine, and dopamine following the coadministration of fluoxetine and olanzapine have shown that these medications markedly enhance the synaptic availability of the three neurotransmitters (Koch et al. 2004). By comparing the neurochemical profile of olanzapine, risperidone, and quetiapine at various receptor sites, it would seem that the antagonism of 5-HT_{2A} and/or 5-HT_{2C} receptors in the presence of serotonin reuptake inhibition is a likely candidate (Blier 2014) (Table 32–3). As described earlier, the combination of these two actions leads to increased norepinephrine release. Given that SSRIs can decrease the norepinephrine tone in the central nervous system (Coplan et al. 1997; Sheline et al. 1997), the norepinephrine system could thus contribute to a significant extent to the therapeutic action of this strategy (see Table 32–3).

Other properties of some medications that antagonize D_2 and 5-HT_2 receptors may also contribute their beneficial action when used in combination. These would include α_2-adrenoceptor antagonism and 5-HT_{1A} receptor agonism, which are the mechanisms exerted by mirtazapine and buspirone, respectively.

Dopamine Type 2 Receptor Agonists

Full Dopamine Agonists

Combination studies with dopamine agonists, such as bromocriptine, pergolide, and pramipexole, that demonstrate their antidepressant action provide additional evidence that D_2 receptor antagonism cannot serve as a basis for the therapeutic effects of adjuvant drugs such olanzapine (Cusin et al. 2013; Inoue et al. 1996; Izumi et al. 2000). The $D_{2/3}$ receptor full agonist pramipexole increases signaling at D_2 and D_3 receptors, which decreases the firing of dopamine neurons in the ventral tegmental area. With repeated administration over 14 days in rats, however, these neurons regain their normal firing activity because of D_2 autoreceptor desensitization, at which time dopamine transmission is increased in the medial prefrontal cortex (Chernoloz et al. 2009, 2012). Given the reciprocal interactions between the dopamine and serotonin systems, pramipexole can alter the firing activity of serotonin neurons in the dorsal raphe through their excitatory D_2 receptors on their cell bodies (Aman et al. 2007). Indeed, the same 14-day pramipexole regimen mentioned above increases the firing rate of serotonin neurons, at which time 5-HT_{1A} transmission is increased in the hippocampus (Chernoloz et al. 2009, 2012). The antidepressant activity of pramipexole used alone in a placebo-controlled trial gives credence to this approach (Corrigan et al. 2000). Although taking pramipexole may be somewhat cumbersome because it has to be administered more than once a day, it does not impair sexual function and may even help reverse an SSRI-induced dysfunction (Sporn et al. 2000). In addition, it may help simplify the therapeutic regimen of patients with Parkinson's disease. In treatment-resistant depression, it can be prescribed at 0.125 mg three times a day and doubled every week, according to side effects and response, up to 3–4 mg/day, its effective dosage as monotherapy in depression (Corrigan et al. 2000). It is nevertheless important to warn patients that it may trigger compulsive behaviors, such as pathological gambling and hypersexuality, especially in older individuals (Grall-Bronnec et al. 2016).

TABLE 32–3. **Properties of antipsychotic drugs used in the treatment of unipolar and bipolar mood disorders**

Drugs	$5\text{-}HT_{2A/2C}$ antagonism	α_2-Adrenoceptor antagonism	$5\text{-}HT_{1A}$ agonism	D_2 partial agonism	NE uptake inhibition
Aripiprazole	+	0	+	+	0
Asenapine	+	+	+	0	0
Brexpiprazole	+	+	+	+	0
Cariprazine	+/0	0	+	+	0
Lurasidone	+/0	+	+	0	0
Olanzapine	+	0	0	0	0
Quetiapine	+	+	+	0	+
Risperidone	+	+	0	0	0
Ziprasidone	+	0	+	0	0

Note. NE=norepinephrine; 0=no activity; +=significant activity at clinical regimens. Pharmacological properties of medications demonstrated to be effective in depressive episodes in major depressive disorder and bipolar disorder, used either alone or in combination with other drugs. Effective dosages in depressive episodes are generally lower than those necessary to treat psychosis or mania, presumably to avoid decreasing overall dopamine transmission.

Partial Dopamine Agonists

Two partial dopamine agonists are now approved in the United States and Canada as adjunctive treatment for inadequate response in MDD (Citrome 2018). Aripiprazole was first introduced for the treatment of schizophrenia in dosages of 10–30 mg/day, with a mean daily dosage of 25 mg/day, and was thought to compete with and displace excessive synaptic dopamine (full agonist). The net effect on dopamine transmission is thus a decrease, without lowering it too much, thereby limiting extrapyramidal motor symptoms. Several years later, aripiprazole was shown to be efficacious in unipolar depression in dosages of 2–20 mg/day, with a mean daily dosage of 10 mg/day. Following clinical experience and more studies, the most useful dosage range is 2–5 mg/day, with a mean dosage of about 4 mg/day (Cheon et al. 2017; Han et al. 2015; Kennedy et al. 2019). These results indicate that in MDD, dosages in the antipsychotic range should be avoided so as not to decrease dopamine transmission, presumably keeping its effects in an agonistic range. Another feature of this medication, in contrast with its D_2 antagonist predecessors, is its long half-life (3 days). Therefore, in MDD, the usual initial dosage of 2 mg/day should not be increased before 2 weeks, the time required to achieve a steady-state level in plasma, certainly longer in the brain. As was the case for lithium, patients need not have had a partial response to their previous medication for aripiprazole to be effective. Nelson et al. (2014) showed in post hoc analyses that even patients who experienced a worsening of their depressive symptoms in a prospective verification of inadequate response to a different medication still had significant improvement with aripiprazole addition. Furthermore, in a study carried out in Japan, patients taking 3 mg/day presented a significant improvement on 5 of 10 items of the Montgomery-Åsberg Depression Rating

Scale after only 1 week, thereby indicating prompt improvement at low dosages before achievement of a plasma steady state (Ozaki et al. 2015).

The putative mechanism of action of this partial agonist is consistent with decreased dopamine transmission, in at least some patients with MDD (Belujon and Grace 2017; Dunlop and Nemeroff 2007). Aripiprazole is not solely a D_2 receptor partial agonist; it also exerts potent 5-$HT_{2A/2C}$ functional antagonism and 5-HT_{1A} agonism, which could contribute to its therapeutic benefits (see Table 32–3).

Brexpiprazole is the other partial dopamine agonist with an indication for MDD as adjunctive treatment. It has subnanomolar affinity for D_2, 5-HT_{1A}, and 5-HT_{2A} receptors, but unlike aripiprazole, it also has a similar affinity for α_{2C}-adrenoceptors, an effect exerted by mirtazapine (Maeda et al. 2014; Oosterhof et al. 2014). Brexpiprazole should be started at a dosage of 0.5 mg/day or 1 mg/day and gradually increased to 2 mg/day over an interval of about 3 weeks, given its 4-day half-life. Post hoc analyses reported more side effects with a dosage of 3 mg/day without more therapeutic benefits (Kishi et al. 2019).

Cariprazine has yet to be approved for MDD but is approved in the United States for schizophrenia, acute mania, and bipolar I depression as monotherapy. The main benefit of this partial dopamine agonist over its two predecessors is its preferential affinity for D_3 over D_2 receptors. In addition, it has an active metabolite with a half-life of 7 days, indicating that precipitous dosage adjustments should be avoided when treating a depressive episode. Taking into account the clinical experience gained with aripiprazole and brexpiprazole, cariprazine appears to have its greatest therapeutic benefits in depressive episodes with dosages somewhat lower than its effective range in schizophrenia, that is, 1.5–3 mg/day versus 3–6 mg/day, respectively (Citrome 2018; Durgam et al. 2016; Earley et al. 2019).

Rare cases of pathological gambling have been reported with aripiprazole, but they cannot solely be attributable to its dopaminergic pharmacodynamic effects. Indeed, aripiprazole is used in patients with diagnoses associated with a higher prevalence of this problem than in the general population, and therefore vulnerability factors such as a history of gambling, impulsivity, and substance misuse must be taken into consideration (Bergamini et al. 2018; Grall-Bronnec et al. 2016). It is important to mention that after years of treatment with brexpiprazole and cariprazine, no cases of treatment-emergent pathological gambling have been reported with these two partial dopamine agonists.

Ketamine and Esketamine

Ketamine is a dissociative anesthetic agent approved by the FDA in 1970. It was first used in a low subanesthetic dose to treat resistant depression two decades ago by Berman et al. (2000), and its efficacy for this indication has been widely replicated since then, always in combination with other medications for MDD (Krystal et al. 2019; Zarate et al. 2006). The most commonly used antidepressant dose of ketamine is 0.5 mg/kg given intravenously over 40 minutes, and the efficacy of different doses of intravenous ketamine for the treatment of depression also has been examined. Low-dose infusions of 0.1 and 0.2 mg/kg are not efficacious, whereas 0.5, 0.75, and 1.0 mg/kg are effective, but with no clear evidence of the higher of these doses providing additional benefits over 0.5 mg/kg (Fava et al. 2020; Su et al. 2017). Subsequent characterization of the antidepressant effects of ketamine has shown that a single dose according to this regimen will produce rapid-acting improvement in depressive symptoms, reaching a maximum effect up to 24 hours after infusion (Newport et al. 2015). Importantly, it also has a robust effect in decreasing suicidal ideation that does not always coincide with its overall antidepressant action (Phillips et al. 2020; Wilkinson et al. 2018). Although the antidepressant action of ketamine has a quick onset and is robust, it generally lasts only about 1 week. With repeated infusions, however, its effects can be sustained and even enhanced over time (Murrough 2012; Phillips et al. 2019). The American Psychiatric Association Council of Research Task Force on Novel Biomarkers and Treatments has released a consensus statement on the use of ketamine in the treatment of mood disorders (Sanacora et al. 2017).

Ketamine is an *N*-methyl-D-aspartate (NMDA) receptor antagonist. Its main effect is believed to be primarily mediated by the prevention of the depolarization of GABA neurons, which normally exert an inhibitory effect on pyramidal neurons of the frontal cortex. This results in a surge of glutamate release that preferentially increases α-amino-3-hydroxy-5-methyl-4-isoxazolepropionic acid (AMPA) receptor signaling, promptly triggering neurotrophic phenomena in the frontal cortex (Krystal et al. 2019). Ketamine also may act through interactions between the glutamate and monoamine systems, for instance, by enhancing dopamine neuronal activity, and also through an AMPA-dependent mechanism (Belujon and Grace 2017; El Iskandrani et al. 2015).

Intranasal esketamine has emerged as an alternative form of achieving the antidepressant effects of ketamine while being less cumbersome than the intravenous infusions (Daly et al. 2018). The *S*-enantiomer of racemic ketamine has a greater affinity than the *R*-enantiomer for the NMDA binding site. It was approved by the FDA and the European Medicines Agency in 2019 and by Health Canada in 2020. Such approvals were based on double-blind acute studies and a maintenance study. In brief, patients had failed to respond to two to five medications and were randomly assigned to either fixed or flexible doses of 56-mg or 84-mg intranasal spray or placebo twice weekly for 4 weeks, while initiating yet another oral SSRI or SNRI (Fedgchin et al. 2019; Popova et al. 2019). In the maintenance study, patients were first stabilized in response or remission for 16 weeks on an optimized oral medication and intranasal esketamine, after which they were randomly assigned to continue esketamine or to switch to a placebo inhaler while continuing the oral medication. The risk of relapse was decreased by 51% in remitted patients and by 70% in patients who had achieved a stable response. The median time to relapse after discontinuation of the intranasal spray in patients who had achieved a stable remission was 88 days and in those with a stable response was 273 days (Daly et al. 2019).

Combining Medications From Treatment Initiation

Although depressed patients have likely been ill for weeks, if not months or years, when they first seek help, there may be a state of urgency. Therefore, a drug combination from treatment initiation may be considered in the hope of achieving earlier relief. There is no consensus on what a rapid onset of action is, but some studies suggest that within a standard antidepressant drug trial, a superior outcome may be achieved with a drug combination. Although initiating treatment with two drugs is somewhat unconventional for depression, combination treatment is the norm for some medical illnesses. For example, asthma is treated at the outset with inhaled β_2-adrenergic agonists and steroids. In the treatment of depression, a benzodiazepine receptor ligand in combination with an SSRI is commonly prescribed to improve sleep and decrease anxiety. Therefore, the prescription of two medications at treatment initiation may not seem that unusual from that perspective.

Positive results when two medications are used from treatment onset have been reported in double-blind studies: fluoxetine and mianserin (Maes et al. 1999), fluoxetine and desipramine (Nelson et al. 2004), fluoxetine and olanzapine (Tohen et al. 2010), and mirtazapine and paroxetine (Blier et al. 2009, 2010). The combination of an SSRI and bupropion initially produced significant results in open-label studies, but variable outcomes have been reported in single-blind and double-blind studies, depending on dosages and patient characteristics (Rush et al. 2011; Stewart et al. 2014; Zuilhof et al. 2018). Although a pindolol combination is not recommended in patients with treatment-resistant depression (Kennedy et al. 2016), 8 of 11 double-blind studies have reported an acceleration of the antidepressant response when pindolol is used from treatment onset (Portella et al. 2011). This action of pindolol is believed to result from prevention of an initial suppression of firing of serotonin neurons on SSRI initiation via 5-HT_{1A} autoreceptor antagonism (Blier and El Mansari 2013).

Even if a drug combination is not used from treatment initiation, it can still be considered early on. This is supported by the observation in 41 double-blind trials using various types of medication for MDD that if an onset of action has not taken place in the first 2 weeks (i.e., a 20% improvement), there is only about a 5% chance of achieving response by the end of a standard trial duration (Szegedi et al. 2009). Furthermore, even if optimization of dosages of a single drug occurs within a week, the odds of failure of the current monotherapy remain the same (Benkert et al. 2006).

How Long Should Effective Combined Pharmacotherapies Be Used?

Once the patient achieves remission, the next concern becomes the duration of the treatment. Clear guidelines are available for treatment with a single agent. No such recommendations exist for combined treatments because this issue has not been thoroughly studied. Only a few studies have examined this problem. For instance, lithium cessation immediately after achieving remission or after a short-term treatment has produced about a 50% relapse rate in two studies (Bauer et al. 2003; de Montigny et al. 1983). In a combination mirtazapine study that used two drugs from treatment initiation, double-blind discontinuation of one medication resulted in about a 50% relapse rate over the following 6 months, with most patients relapsing within 1 month (Blier et al. 2010). Thus, it would be prudent to continue the combined therapies for about 6 months before considering tapering off one of the two drugs. It is wise to err on the side of safety, because no data are available on the rate of resistance following reintroduction of the previous drug regimen. Such observations have been reported for single agents, such as tricyclics and lithium, in mood disorders and should constitute sufficient evidence for clinicians to avoid early discontinuation of drug combinations after achieving the desired goal (Sim et al. 2015).

Conclusion

Numerous strategies are now available to treat depression that does not respond or remit to a first medication trial. Although the number of possibilities may be limited by consideration of undesired side effects, several options remain to bring patients to recovery. When managing the care of patients with treatment-resistant depression, it is imperative to reassure them that a treatment that will not fail them can be found. Indeed, after the clinician makes a proper diagnosis, he or she should tell the patient that medications, when taken adequately, may fail them, but not the reverse. The uncertainty about which strategy will bring about the targeted improvement, however, needs to be emphasized. Such clear and supportive explanations generally enhance compliance with the treatment plan. When compliant patients do not achieve remission with sequential and rational drug combinations, clinicians should consider whether there are complicating issues preventing a favorable outcome. These may include alcohol abuse, illicit drug use, unresolved psychosocial issues, and undiagnosed medical illnesses (McAllister-Williams et al. 2020).

Although new treatment strategies are still eagerly awaited, the vast majority of depressed patients can be brought to remission with the present pharmacopoeia. Novel pharmacological strategies, even if not superior in terms of effectiveness to the current medications, will help increase the potential of treatment approaches to improve outcome and comfort. Given the heterogeneity of depression, it is unlikely that a single drug will ever be able to treat all patients with this syndrome. Therefore, the basic principles of drug management covered in this chapter must always be retained, albeit modified and improved with new developments in this field. For instance, research into predictors of response may help shorten the time necessary to achieve remission. All in all, the burden of depression can be markedly attenuated with rational site-directed pharmacotherapy.

References

Aman TK, Shen RY, Haj-Dahmane S: D2-like dopamine receptors depolarize dorsal raphe serotonin neurons through the activation of nonselective cationic conductance. J Pharmacol Exp Ther 320(1):376–385, 2007 17005915

Argyelán M, Szabó Z, Kanyó B, et al: Dopamine transporter availability in medication free and in bupropion treated depression: a 99mTc-TRODAT-1 SPECT study. J Affect Disord 89(1–3):115–123, 2005 16213028

Aronson R, Offman HJ, Joffe RT, et al: Triiodothyronine augmentation in the treatment of refractory depression: a meta-analysis. Arch Gen Psychiatry 53(9):842–848, 1996 8792761

Auclair AL, Martel JC, Assié MB, et al: Levomilnacipran (F2695), a norepinephrine-preferring SNRI: profile in vitro and in models of depression and anxiety. Neuropharmacology 70:338–347, 2013 23499664

Bauer M, Forsthoff A, Baethge C, et al: Lithium augmentation therapy in refractory depression-update 2002. Eur Arch Psychiatry Clin Neurosci 253(3):132–139, 2003 12904977

Belmaker RH, Agam G: Major depressive disorder. N Engl J Med 358(1):55–68, 2008 18172175

Belpaire FM, Wijnant P, Temmerman A, et al: The oxidative metabolism of metoprolol in human liver microsomes: inhibition by the selective serotonin reuptake inhibitors. Eur J Clin Pharmacol 54(3):261–264, 1998 9681670

Belujon P, Grace AA: Dopamine system dysregulation in major depressive disorders. Int J Neuropsychopharmacol 20(12):1036–1046, 2017 29106542

Benkert O, Szegedi A, Philipp M, et al: Mirtazapine orally disintegrating tablets versus venlafaxine extended release: a double-blind, randomized multicenter trial comparing the onset of antidepressant response in patients with major depressive disorder. J Clin Psychopharmacol 26(1):75–78, 2006 16415711

Bergamini A, Turrina C, Bettini F, et al: At-risk gambling in patients with severe mental illness: prevalence and associated features. J Behav Addict 7(2):348–354, 2018 29865864

Berman RM, Cappiello A, Anand A, et al: Antidepressant effects of ketamine in depressed patients. Biol Psychiatry 47(4):351–354, 2000 10686270

Blier P: Rational site-directed pharmacotherapy for major depressive disorder. Int J Neuropsychopharmacol 17(7):997–1008, 2014 23745670

Blier P, Abbott FV: Putative mechanisms of action of antidepressant drugs in affective and anxiety disorders and pain. J Psychiatry Neurosci 26(1):37–43, 2001 11212592

Blier P, de Montigny C: Electrophysiological investigations on the effect of repeated zimelidine administration on serotonergic neurotransmission in the rat. J Neurosci 3(6):1270–1278, 1983 6304261

Blier P, de Montigny C: Short-term lithium administration enhances serotonergic neurotransmission: electrophysiological evidence in the rat CNS. Eur J Pharmacol 113(1):69–77, 1985 2995061

Blier P, El Mansari M: Serotonin and beyond: therapeutics for major depression. Philos Trans R Soc Lond B Biol Sci 368(1615):20120536, 2013 23440470

Blier P, Saint-André E, Hébert C, et al: Effects of different doses of venlafaxine on serotonin and norepinephrine reuptake in healthy volunteers. Int J Neuropsychopharmacol 10(1):41–50, 2007 16690005

Blier P, Gobbi G, Turcotte JE, et al: Mirtazapine and paroxetine in major depression: a comparison of monotherapy versus their combination from treatment initiation. Eur Neuropsychopharmacol 19(7):457–465, 2009 19345072

Blier P, Ward HE, Tremblay P, et al: Combination of antidepressant medications from treatment initiation for major depressive disorder: a double-blind randomized study. Am J Psychiatry 167(3):281–288, 2010 20008946

Booij L, Van der Does W, Benkelfat C, et al: Predictors of mood response to acute tryptophan depletion: a reanalysis. Neuropsychopharmacology 27(5):852–861, 2002 12431859

Bouwer C, Stein DJ: Buspirone is an effective augmenting agent of serotonin selective re-uptake inhibitors in severe treatment-refractory depression. S Afr Med J 87 (4 suppl):534–537, 540, 1997 9180827

Boyer EW, Shannon M: The serotonin syndrome. N Engl J Med 352(11):1112–1120, 2005 15784664

Brøsen K, Hansen JG, Nielsen KK, et al: Inhibition by paroxetine of desipramine metabolism in extensive but not in poor metabolizers of sparteine. Eur J Clin Pharmacol 44(4):349–355, 1993 8513845

Cheon EJ, Lee KH, Park YW, et al: Comparison of the efficacy and safety of aripiprazole versus bupropion augmentation in patients with major depressive disorder unresponsive to selective serotonin reuptake inhibitors: a randomized, prospective, open-label study. J Clin Psychopharmacol 37(2):193–199, 2017 28129308

Chernoloz O, El Mansari M, Blier P: Sustained administration of pramipexole modifies the spontaneous firing of dopamine, norepinephrine, and serotonin neurons in the rat brain. Neuropsychopharmacology 34(3):651–661, 2009 18688211

Chernoloz O, El Mansari M, Blier P: Long-term administration of the dopamine D3/2 receptor agonist pramipexole increases dopamine and serotonin neurotransmission in the male rat forebrain. J Psychiatry Neurosci 37(2):113–121, 2012 22023785

Cipriani A, Furukawa TA, Salanti G, et al: Comparative efficacy and acceptability of 21 antidepressant drugs for the acute treatment of adults with major depressive disorder: a systematic review and network meta-analysis. Lancet 391(10128):1357–1366, 2018 29477251

Citrome L: Aripiprazole, brexpiprazole, and cariprazine: not all the same. Curr Psychiatry Rev 17:24–33, 2018
Connarn JN, Flowers S, Kelly M, et al: Pharmacokinetics and pharmacogenomics of bupropion in three different formulations with different release kinetics in healthy human volunteers. AAPS J 19(5):1513–1522, 2017 28685396
Cooper-Kazaz R, Apter JT, Cohen R, et al: Combined treatment with sertraline and liothyronine in major depression: a randomized, double-blind, placebo-controlled trial. Arch Gen Psychiatry 64(6):679–688, 2007 17548749
Coplan JD, Papp LA, Pine D, et al: Clinical improvement with fluoxetine therapy and noradrenergic function in patients with panic disorder. Arch Gen Psychiatry 54(7):643–648, 1997 9236548
Corrigan MH, Denahan AQ, Wright CE, et al: Comparison of pramipexole, fluoxetine, and placebo in patients with major depression. Depress Anxiety 11(2):58–65, 2000 10812530
Cusin C, Iovieno N, Iosifescu DV, et al: A randomized, double-blind, placebo-controlled trial of pramipexole augmentation in treatment-resistant major depressive disorder. J Clin Psychiatry 74(7):e636–e641, 2013 23945458
Daly EJ, Singh JB, Fedgchin M, et al: Efficacy and safety of intranasal esketamine adjunctive to oral antidepressant therapy in treatment-resistant depression: a randomized clinical trial. JAMA Psychiatry 75(2):139–148, 2018 29282469
Daly EJ, Trivedi MH, Janik A, et al: Efficacy of esketamine nasal spray plus oral antidepressant treatment for relapse prevention in patients with treatment-resistant depression: a randomized clinical trial. JAMA Psychiatry 76:893–903, 2019 31166571
Davidson J: Seizures and bupropion: a review. J Clin Psychiatry 50(7):256–261, 1989 2500425
Debonnel G, Saint-André E, Hébert C, et al: Differential physiological effects of a low dose and high doses of venlafaxine in major depression. Int J Neuropsychopharmacol 10(1):51–61, 2007 16690006
Delgado PL, Charney DS, Price LH, et al: Serotonin function and the mechanism of antidepressant action: reversal of antidepressant-induced remission by rapid depletion of plasma tryptophan. Arch Gen Psychiatry 47(5):411–418, 1990 2184795
Delgado PL, Miller HL, Salomon RM, et al: Tryptophan-depletion challenge in depressed patients treated with desipramine or fluoxetine: implications for the role of serotonin in the mechanism of antidepressant action. Biol Psychiatry 46(2):212–220, 1999 10418696
Delgado PL, Moreno FA, Onate L, et al: Sequential catecholamine and serotonin depletion in mirtazapine-treated depressed patients. Int J Neuropsychopharmacol 5(1):63–66, 2002 12057033
de Montigny C, Cournoyer G, Morissette R, et al: Lithium carbonate addition in tricyclic antidepressant-resistant unipolar depression: correlations with the neurobiologic actions of tricyclic antidepressant drugs and lithium ion on the serotonin system. Arch Gen Psychiatry 40(12):1327–1334, 1983 6418109
Dennis T, L'Heureux R, Carter C, et al: Presynaptic alpha-2 adrenoceptors play a major role in the effects of idazoxan on cortical noradrenaline release (as measured by in vivo dialysis) in the rat. J Pharmacol Exp Ther 241(2):642–649, 1987 3033221
Dinan TG, Barry S: A comparison of electroconvulsive therapy with a combined lithium and tricyclic combination among depressed tricyclic nonresponders. Acta Psychiatr Scand 80(1):97–100, 1989 2504034
Dong J, Blier P: Modification of norepinephrine and serotonin, but not dopamine, neuron firing by sustained bupropion treatment. Psychopharmacology (Berl) 155(1):52–57, 2001 11374336
Dostert P, Castelli MG, Cicioni P, et al: Reboxetine prevents the tranylcypromine-induced increase in tyramine levels in rat heart. J Neural Transm Suppl 41:149–153, 1994 7931221
Dremencov E, El Mansari M, Blier P: Effects of sustained serotonin reuptake inhibition on the firing of dopamine neurons in the rat ventral tegmental area. J Psychiatry Neurosci 34(3):223–229, 2009 19448853
Dunlop BW, Nemeroff CB: The role of dopamine in the pathophysiology of depression. Arch Gen Psychiatry 64(3):327–337, 2007 17339521

Durgam S, Earley W, Guo H, et al: Efficacy and safety of adjunctive cariprazine in inadequate responders to antidepressants: a randomized, double-blind, placebo-controlled study in adult patients with major depressive disorder. J Clin Psychiatry 77(3):371–378, 2016 27046309

Earley W, Burgess MV, Rekeda L, et al: Cariprazine treatment of bipolar depression: a randomized double-blind placebo-controlled phase 3 study. Am J Psychiatry 176(6):439–448, 2019 30845817

El Iskandrani KS, Oosterhof CA, El Mansari M, et al: Impact of subanesthetic doses of ketamine on AMPA-mediated responses in rats: an in vivo electrophysiological study on monoaminergic and glutamatergic neurons. J Psychopharmacol 29(7):792–801, 2015 25759403

El Mansari M, Guiard BP, Chernoloz O, et al: Relevance of norepinephrine-dopamine interactions in the treatment of major depressive disorder. CNS Neurosci Ther 16(3):e1–e17, 2010 20406250

Fava M, Thase ME, DeBattista C: A multicenter, placebo-controlled study of modafinil augmentation in partial responders to selective serotonin reuptake inhibitors with persistent fatigue and sleepiness. J Clin Psychiatry 66(1):85–93, 2005 15669893

Fava M, Freeman MP, Flynn M, et al: Double-blind, placebo-controlled, dose-ranging trial of intravenous ketamine as adjunctive therapy in treatment-resistant depression (TRD). Mol Psychiatry 25(7):1592–1603, 2020 30283029

Fedgchin M, Trivedi M, Daly EJ, et al: Efficacy and safety of fixed-dose esketamine nasal spray combined with a new oral antidepressant in treatment-resistant depression: results of a randomized, double-blind, active-controlled study (TRANSFORM-1). Int J Neuropsychopharmacol 22(10):616–630, 2019 31290965

Ghanbari R, El Mansari M, Blier P: Electrophysiological effects of the co-administration of escitalopram and bupropion on rat serotonin and norepinephrine neurons. J Psychopharmacol 24(1):39–50, 2010 18719044

Ghanbari R, El Mansari M, Blier P: Enhancement of serotonergic and noradrenergic neurotransmission in the rat hippocampus by sustained administration of bupropion. Psychopharmacology (Berl) 217(1):61–73, 2011 21445565

Giacobbe P, Rakita U, Lam R, et al: Efficacy and tolerability of lisdexamfetamine as an antidepressant augmentation strategy: a meta-analysis of randomized controlled trials. J Affect Disord 226:294–300, 2018 29028590

Goodall EM, Cowen PJ, Franklin M, et al: Ritanserin attenuates anorectic, endocrine and thermic responses to d-fenfluramine in human volunteers. Psychopharmacology (Berl) 112(4):461–466, 1993 7871058

Goss AJ, Kaser M, Costafreda SG, et al: Modafinil augmentation therapy in unipolar and bipolar depression: a systematic review and meta-analysis of randomized controlled trials. J Clin Psychiatry 74(11):1101–1107, 2013 24330897

Grall-Bronnec M, Sauvaget A, Perrouin F, et al: Pathological gambling associated with aripiprazole or dopamine replacement therapy: do patients share the same features? A review. J Clin Psychopharmacol 36(1):63–70, 2016 26658263

Gur E, Lerer B, Newman ME: Chronic clomipramine and triiodothyronine increase serotonin levels in rat frontal cortex in vivo: relationship to serotonin autoreceptor activity. J Pharmacol Exp Ther 288(1):81–87, 1999 9862756

Haddjeri N, Szabo ST, de Montigny C, et al: Increased tonic activation of rat forebrain 5-HT(1A) receptors by lithium addition to antidepressant treatments. Neuropsychopharmacology 22(4):346–356, 2000 10700654

Han C, Wang SM, Kwak KP, et al: Aripiprazole augmentation versus antidepressant switching for patients with major depressive disorder: a 6-week, randomized, rater-blinded, prospective study. J Psychiatr Res 66–67:84–94, 2015 26013203

Happe S, Trenkwalder C: Role of dopamine receptor agonists in the treatment of restless legs syndrome. CNS Drugs 18(1):27–36, 2004 14731057

Harvey AT, Preskorn SH: Cytochrome P450 enzymes: interpretation of their interactions with selective serotonin reuptake inhibitors, part II. J Clin Psychopharmacol 16(5):345–355, 1996 8889906

Hatanaka K, Yatsugi S, Yamaguchi T: Effect of acute treatment with YM992 on extracellular serotonin levels in the rat frontal cortex. Eur J Pharmacol 395(1):23–29, 2000 10781669

Henssler J, Bschor T, Baethge C: Combining antidepressants in acute treatment of depression: a meta-analysis of 38 studies including 4511 patients. Can J Psychiatry 61(1):29–43, 2016 27582451

Hyttel J: Citalopram—pharmacological profile of a specific serotonin uptake inhibitor with antidepressant activity. Prog Neuropsychopharmacol Biol Psychiatry 6(3):277–295, 1982 6128769

Inoue T, Tsuchiya K, Miura J, et al: Bromocriptine treatment of tricyclic and heterocyclic antidepressant-resistant depression. Biol Psychiatry 40(2):151–153, 1996 8793048

Izumi T, Inoue T, Kitagawa N, et al: Open pergolide treatment of tricyclic and heterocyclic antidepressant-resistant depression. J Affect Disord 61(1–2):127–132, 2000 11099751

Judd LL, Paulus MJ, Schettler PJ, et al: Does incomplete recovery from first lifetime major depressive episode herald a chronic course of illness? Am J Psychiatry 157(9):1501–1504, 2000 10964869

Kaser M, Deakin JB, Michael A, et al: Modafinil improves episodic memory and working memory cognition in patients with remitted depression: a double-blind, randomized, placebo-controlled study. Biol Psychiatry Cogn Neurosci Neuroimaging 2(2):115–122, 2017 28299368

Katzman MA, Bleau P, Blier P, et al: Canadian clinical practice guidelines for the management of anxiety, posttraumatic stress and obsessive-compulsive disorders. BMC Psychiatry 14 (suppl 1):S1, 2014 25081580

Keller MB, Lavori PW, Mueller TI, et al: Time to recovery, chronicity, and levels of psychopathology in major depression: a 5-year prospective follow-up of 431 subjects. Arch Gen Psychiatry 49(10):809–816, 1992 1417434

Kennedy SH, Lam RW, McIntyre RS, et al: Canadian Network for Mood and Anxiety Treatments (CANMAT) 2016 clinical guidelines for the management of adults with major depressive disorder, section 3: pharmacological treatments. Can J Psychiatry 61(9):540–560, 2016 27486148

Kennedy SH, Lam RW, Rotzinger S, et al: Symptomatic and functional outcomes and early prediction of response to escitalopram monotherapy and sequential adjunctive aripiprazole therapy in patients with major depressive disorder: a CAN-BIND-1 report. J Clin Psychiatry 80(2):18m12202, 2019 30840787

Kishi T, Sakuma K, Nomura I, et al: Brexpiprazole as adjunctive treatment for major depressive disorder following treatment failure with at least one antidepressant in the current episode: a systematic review and meta-analysis. Int J Neuropsychopharmacol 22(11):698–709, 2019 31350882

Koch S, Perry KW, Bymaster FP: Brain region and dose effects of an olanzapine/fluoxetine combination on extracellular monoamine concentrations in the rat. Neuropharmacology 46(2):232–242, 2004 14680761

Krystal JH, Abdallah CG, Sanacora G, et al: Ketamine: a paradigm shift for depression research and treatment. Neuron 101(5):774–778, 2019 30844397

Kurtz DL, Bergstrom RF, Goldberg MJ, et al: The effect of sertraline on the pharmacokinetics of desipramine and imipramine. Clin Pharmacol Ther 62(2):145–156, 1997 9284850

Lam RW, Hossie H, Solomons K, et al: Citalopram and bupropion-SR: combining versus switching in patients with treatment-resistant depression. J Clin Psychiatry 65(3):337–340, 2004 15096072

Li SXM, Perry KW, Wong DT: Influence of fluoxetine on the ability of bupropion to modulate extracellular dopamine and norepinephrine concentrations in three mesocorticolimbic areas of rats. Neuropharmacology 42(2):181–190, 2002 11804614

Maeda K, Sugino H, Akazawa H, et al: Brexpiprazole I: in vitro and in vivo characterization of a novel serotonin-dopamine activity modulator. J Pharmacol Exp Ther 350(3):589–604, 2014 24947465

Maes M, Libbrecht I, van Hunsel F, et al: Pindolol and mianserin augment the antidepressant activity of fluoxetine in hospitalized major depressed patients, including those with treatment resistance. J Clin Psychopharmacol 19(2):177–182, 1999 10211920

McAllister-Williams RH, Arango C, Blier P, et al: The identification, assessment and management of difficult-to-treat depression: an international consensus statement. J Affect Disord 267:264–282, 2020 32217227

McCabe C, Mishor Z, Cowen PJ, et al: Diminished neural processing of aversive and rewarding stimuli during selective serotonin reuptake inhibitor treatment. Biol Psychiatry 67(5):439–445, 2010 20034615

McIntyre RS, Lee Y, Zhou AJ, et al: The efficacy of psychostimulants in major depressive episodes: a systematic review and meta-analysis. J Clin Psychopharmacol 37(4):412–418, 2017 28590365

Meyer JH, Wilson AA, Sagrati S, et al: Serotonin transporter occupancy of five selective serotonin reuptake inhibitors at different doses: an [11C]DASB positron emission tomography study. Am J Psychiatry 161(5):826–835, 2004 15121647

Miller HL, Delgado PL, Salomon RM, et al: Clinical and biochemical effects of catecholamine depletion on antidepressant-induced remission of depression. Arch Gen Psychiatry 53(2):117–128, 1996 8629887

Mischoulon D, Nierenberg AA, Kizilbash L, et al: Strategies for managing depression refractory to selective serotonin reuptake inhibitor treatment: a survey of clinicians. Can J Psychiatry 45(5):476–481, 2000 10900529

Montejo-González AL, Llorca G, Izquierdo JA, et al: SSRI-induced sexual dysfunction: fluoxetine, paroxetine, sertraline, and fluvoxamine in a prospective, multicenter, and descriptive clinical study of 344 patients. J Sex Marital Ther 23(3):176–194, 1997 9292833

Murrough JW: Ketamine as a novel antidepressant: from synapse to behavior. Clin Pharmacol Ther 91(2):303–309, 2012 22205190

Nelson JC, Papakostas GI: Atypical antipsychotic augmentation in major depressive disorder: a meta-analysis of placebo-controlled randomized trials. Am J Psychiatry 166(9):980–991, 2009 19687129

Nelson JC, Mazure CM, Jatlow PI, et al: Combining norepinephrine and serotonin reuptake inhibition mechanisms for treatment of depression: a double-blind, randomized study. Biol Psychiatry 55(3):296–300, 2004 14744472

Nelson JC, Rahman Z, Laubmeier KK, et al: Efficacy of adjunctive aripiprazole in patients with major depressive disorder whose symptoms worsened with antidepressant monotherapy. CNS Spectr 19(6):528–534, 2014 24642260

Newport DJ, Carpenter LL, McDonald WM, et al: Ketamine and other NMDA antagonists: early clinical trials and possible mechanisms in depression. Am J Psychiatry 172(10):950–966, 2015 26423481

Nierenberg AA, DeCecco LM: Definitions of antidepressant treatment response, remission, nonresponse, partial response, and other relevant outcomes: a focus on treatment-resistant depression. J Clin Psychiatry 62 (suppl 16):5–9, 2001 11480882

Nutt DJ: Tolerability and safety aspects of mirtazapine. Hum Psychopharmacol 17 (suppl 1):S37–S41, 2002 12404669

Oluboka OJ, Katzman MA, Habert J, et al: Functional recovery in major depressive disorder: providing early optimal treatment for the individual patient. Int J Neuropsychopharmacol 21(2):128–144, 2018 29024974

Oosterhof CA, El Mansari M, Blier P: Acute effects of brexpiprazole on serotonin, dopamine, and norepinephrine systems: an in vivo electrophysiologic characterization. J Pharmacol Exp Ther 351(3):585–595, 2014 25225185

Ozaki N, Otsubo T, Kato M, et al: Efficacy of aripiprazole augmentation in Japanese patients with major depressive disorder: a subgroup analysis and Montgomery-Åsberg Depression Rating Scale and Hamilton Rating Scale for Depression item analyses of the Aripiprazole Depression Multicenter Efficacy study. Psychiatry Clin Neurosci 69(1):34–42, 2015 24965202

Park SBG, Cowen PJ: Effect of pindolol on the prolactin response to d-fenfluramine. Psychopharmacology (Berl) 118(4):471–474, 1995 7568634

Paykel ES, Ramana R, Cooper Z, et al: Residual symptoms after partial remission: an important outcome in depression. Psychol Med 25(6):1171–1180, 1995 8637947

Phillips JL, Norris S, Talbot J, et al: Single, repeated, and maintenance ketamine infusions for treatment-resistant depression: a randomized controlled trial. Am J Psychiatry 176(5):401–409, 2019 30922101

Phillips JL, Norris S, Talbot J, et al: Single and repeated ketamine infusions for reduction of suicidal ideation in treatment-resistant depression. Neuropsychopharmacology 45(4):606–612, 2020 31759333

Poirier M-F, Boyer P: Venlafaxine and paroxetine in treatment-resistant depression: double-blind, randomised comparison. Br J Psychiatry 175:12–16, 1999 10621762

Popova V, Daly EJ, Trivedi M, et al: Efficacy and safety of flexibly dosed esketamine nasal spray combined with a newly initiated oral antidepressant in treatment-resistant depression: a randomized double-blind active-controlled study. Am J Psychiatry 176(6):428–438, 2019 31109201

Portella MJ, de Diego-Adeliño J, Ballesteros J, et al: Can we really accelerate and enhance the selective serotonin reuptake inhibitor antidepressant effect? A randomized clinical trial and a meta-analysis of pindolol in nonresistant depression. J Clin Psychiatry 72(7):962–969, 2011 21034693

Reimherr FW, Cunningham LA, Batey SR, et al: A multicenter evaluation of the efficacy and safety of 150 and 300 mg/d sustained-release bupropion tablets versus placebo in depressed outpatients. Clin Ther 20(3):505–516, 1998 9663366

Rush AJ, Trivedi MH, Carmody TJ, et al: Response in relation to baseline anxiety levels in major depressive disorder treated with bupropion sustained release or sertraline. Neuropsychopharmacology 25(1):131–138, 2001 11377926

Rush AJ, Trivedi MH, Wisniewski SR, et al: Bupropion-SR, sertraline, or venlafaxine-XR after failure of SSRIs for depression. N Engl J Med 354(12):1231–1242, 2006 16554525

Rush AJ, Trivedi MH, Stewart JW, et al: Combining medications to enhance depression outcomes (CO-MED): acute and long-term outcomes of a single-blind randomized study. Am J Psychiatry 168(7):689–701, 2011 21536692

Sagman D, McIntosh D, Lee MS, et al: Attributes of response in depressed patients switched to treatment with duloxetine. Int J Clin Pract 65(1):73–81, 2011 21078010

Sanacora G, Frye MA, McDonald W, et al: A consensus statement on the use of ketamine in the treatment of mood disorders. JAMA Psychiatry 74(4):399–405, 2017 28249076

Schmauss M, Kapfhammer HP, Meyr P, Hoff P: Combined MAO-inhibitor and tri- (tetra) cyclic antidepressant treatment in therapy resistant depression. Prog Neuropsychopharmacol Biol Psychiatry 12(4):523–532, 1988 3406429

Sheline Y, Bardgett ME, Csernansky JG: Correlated reductions in cerebrospinal fluid 5-HIAA and MHPG concentrations after treatment with selective serotonin reuptake inhibitors J Clin Psychopharmacol 17(1):11–14, 1997 9004051

Sim K, Lau WK, Sim J, et al: Prevention of relapse and recurrence in adults with major depressive disorder: systematic review and meta-analyses of controlled trials. Int J Neuropsychopharmacol 19(2):pyv076, 2015 26152228

Sporn J, Ghaemi SN, Sambur MR, et al: Pramipexole augmentation in the treatment of unipolar and bipolar depression: a retrospective chart review. Ann Clin Psychiatry 12(3):137–140, 2000 10984002

Sternbach H: The serotonin syndrome. Am J Psychiatry 148(6):705–713, 1991 2035713

Stewart JW, McGrath PJ, Blondeau C, et al: Combination antidepressant therapy for major depressive disorder: speed and probability of remission. J Psychiatr Res 52:7–14, 2014 24485847

Su T-P, Chen M-H, Li C-T, et al: Dose-related effects of adjunctive ketamine in Taiwanese patients with treatment-resistant depression. Neuropsychopharmacology 42(13):2482–2492, 2017 28492279

Szabadi E: Functional neuroanatomy of the central noradrenergic system. J Psychopharmacol 27(8):659–693, 2013 23761387

Szabo ST, Blier P: Effects of serotonin (5-hydroxytryptamine, 5-HT) reuptake inhibition plus 5-HT(2A) receptor antagonism on the firing activity of norepinephrine neurons. J Pharmacol Exp Ther 302(3):983–991, 2002 12183655

Szabo ST, de Montigny C, Blier P: Progressive attenuation of the firing activity of locus coeruleus noradrenergic neurons by sustained administration of selective serotonin reuptake inhibitors. Int J Neuropsychopharmacol 3(1):1–11, 2000 11343573

Szegedi A, Jansen WT, van Willigenburg APP, et al: Early improvement in the first 2 weeks as a predictor of treatment outcome in patients with major depressive disorder: a meta-analysis including 6562 patients. J Clin Psychiatry 70(3):344–353, 2009 19254516

Tatsumi M, Groshan K, Blakely RD, et al: Pharmacological profile of antidepressants and related compounds at human monoamine transporters. Eur J Pharmacol 340(2–3):249–258, 1997 9537821

Tohen M, Case M, Trivedi MH, et al: Olanzapine/fluoxetine combination in patients with treatment-resistant depression: rapid onset of therapeutic response and its predictive value for subsequent overall response in a pooled analysis of 5 studies. J Clin Psychiatry 71(4):451–462, 2010 20361905

Trivedi MH, Fava M, Wisniewski SR, et al: Medication augmentation after the failure of SSRIs for depression. N Engl J Med 354(12):1243–1252, 2006 16554526

Turcotte JE, Debonnel G, de Montigny C, et al: Assessment of the serotonin and norepinephrine reuptake blocking properties of duloxetine in healthy subjects. Neuropsychopharmacology 24(5):511–521, 2001 11282251

Vincent S, Bieck PR, Garland EM, et al: Clinical assessment of norepinephrine transporter blockade through biochemical and pharmacological profiles. Circulation 109(25):3202–3207, 2004 15184278

Volkow ND, Fowler JS, Logan J, et al: Effects of modafinil on dopamine and dopamine transporters in the male human brain: clinical implications. JAMA 301(11):1148–1154, 2009 19293415

Wagner G, Schultes MT, Titscher V, et al: Efficacy and safety of levomilnacipran, vilazodone and vortioxetine compared with other second-generation antidepressants for major depressive disorder in adults: a systematic review and network meta-analysis. J Affect Disord 228:1–12, 2018 29197738

Wilkinson ST, Ballard ED, Bloch MH, et al: The effect of a single dose of intravenous ketamine on suicidal ideation: a systematic review and individual participant data meta-analysis. Am J Psychiatry 175(2):150–158, 2018 28969441

Zarate CA Jr, Singh JB, Carlson PJ, et al: A randomized trial of an N-methyl-D-aspartate antagonist in treatment-resistant major depression. Arch Gen Psychiatry 63(8):856–864, 2006 16894061

Zerbe RL, Rowe H, Enas GG, et al: Clinical pharmacology of tomoxetine, a potential antidepressant. J Pharmacol Exp Ther 232(1):139–143, 1985 3965689

Zohar J, Stahl S, Moller HJ, et al: A review of the current nomenclature for psychotropic agents and an introduction to the neuroscience-based nomenclature. Eur Neuropsychopharmacol 25(12):2318–2325, 2015 26527055

Zuilhof Z, Norris S, Blondeau C, et al: Optimized regimens of combined medications for the treatment of major depressive disorder: a double-blind, randomized-controlled trial. Neuropsychiatr Dis Treat 14:3209–3218, 2018 30538479

CHAPTER 33

Management of Treatment-Resistant Depression

Samuel J. Collier, M.D.
Charles B. Nemeroff, M.D., Ph.D.

The operational definition of treatment-resistant depression (TRD) remains debatable among mood disorder researchers and clinicians. Proposed definitions range from one to several failed antidepressant trials (with a failed trial defined as minimal or no response to an adequate trial of evidence-based treatment), and because consensus on a definition is lacking, comparative treatment research is limited (Conway et al. 2017). A widely accepted view is that two failed antidepressant trials of adequate dosage and duration represents treatment resistance. This definition largely stems from results of the National Institute of Mental Health (NIMH)–funded Sequenced Treatment Alternatives to Relieve Depression (STAR*D) trial (Gaynes et al. 2009), which showed a marked decline in remission rates (i.e., from 31% to 14%) after two failed trials of antidepressant treatment, both within and outside the selective serotonin reuptake inhibitor (SSRI) medication class, including cognitive-behavioral therapy (CBT). This "inflection point" predicts steadily declining remission rates, higher relapse risks, and greater medication intolerance with subsequent trials (Conway et al. 2017; Rush et al. 2006a). Various staging systems have been proposed to further stratify TRD (akin to cancer-staging paradigms), but no official system for grading TRD has yet been adopted. For the purposes of this chapter, we will adhere to the "two failed antidepressant trials" definition of TRD because it is grounded in clinical trial outcome data.

Epidemiology and Burden

Major depressive disorder (MDD) is a common illness with an annual prevalence of 7.1% in the United States, as reported by NIMH in 2017 (Center for Behavioral Health Statistics and Quality 2018). The World Health Organization (2021) has recognized MDD as a major public health issue, commenting that "depression is the leading cause of disability worldwide, and is a major contributor to the overall global burden of disease." The estimated economic burden of MDD in the United States exceeds $200 billion annually, and the incremental annual health care costs for an individual with MDD are approximately $6,400 more than costs for an individual without MDD (Greenberg et al. 2015). The percentage of depressed patients who are likely to experience treatment resistance ranges from 29% to 46%; therefore, TRD imposes a major burden on society (Fava and Davidson 1996).

Diagnostic Accuracy, Pseudoresistance, and Comorbidity

The primary task in evaluating TRD is differentiating true treatment resistance from pseudoresistance. *Pseudoresistance* is defined as perceived treatment resistance in the setting of inaccurate diagnosis, subtherapeutic antidepressant or psychotherapy trials, or unrecognized comorbidity—medical or psychiatric, including substance use disorder—that interferes with treatment. Clinical assessment should prioritize diagnostic accuracy, physician factors, patient factors, and relevant comorbidities that can complicate treatment and reduce its effectiveness (Kornstein and Schneider 2001).

The lack of validated biomarkers for MDD perpetuates a significant diagnostic limitation, because clinicians exclusively rely on the narrative interview and mental status examination for diagnosis. Indeed, two patients meeting DSM-5 (American Psychiatric Association 2013) criteria for a major depressive episode (MDE) may exhibit starkly different symptom profiles and illness courses, which raises concern that MDD represents a phenotypic endpoint of a genetically heterogeneous illness group with differential treatment response. This hypothesis is grounded in genome-wide association studies of MDD that have identified more than 40 relevant genetic loci and more than 100 independent genetic variants, each of which confers a very small contribution to risk (Gerring et al. 2019; Howard et al. 2019). The ramifications of large heterogeneous genetic risk are incompletely understood with respect to successful biological interventions, but a positive correlation between the magnitude of symptom severity and the chance of response to biological interventions exists, likely because a sicker patient group represents a more homogeneous sample of biologically responsive MDD. One of the most severe depressive subtypes is psychotic depression, which responds to electroconvulsive therapy (ECT) impressively well (i.e., >90% [Petrides et al. 2001]). Mild to moderate depressions probably represent a more heterogeneous group (i.e., MDD plus mood disturbances) that is less likely to respond to biological interventions; therefore, psychotherapy alone is typically indicated in this context, as the treatment effect is more generalized. TRD evaluation should be considered in this context so that lower-grade illness states are not managed purely through the lens of biological intervention; rather, expectations are set around the utility of biologics (i.e., antidepressants, ECT) while psychosocial therapies are aggressively employed.

Because physician practice patterns vary widely, two major causes of pseudoresistance are prescribing inadequate antidepressant dosages and treating for too short a duration. Learning from STAR*D and other clinical trials, we know that approximately half of the patients who ultimately experienced symptom remission in level 1 did so after week 6 of therapy, and 40% of those who experienced remission required 8 or more weeks to do so. This timing suggests the need for antidepressant trials lasting 8 weeks or longer, with even longer exposure periods in the setting of multiple antidepressant failures (Gaynes et al. 2009). A careful evaluation of the adequacy of past treatments by antidepressant dosage and duration is therefore essential in the assessment of TRD. Systematic utilization of research questionnaires such as the Antidepressant Treatment History Form (ATHF) and the Antidepressant Treatment Response Questionnaire (ATRQ) can operationalize the assessment of trial adequacy via comprehensive screening of all past antidepressant exposures by agent/class, dosage, and duration. However, there is no formal consensus on the lowest acceptable antidepressant dosage to qualify as adequate, and minimum adequate dosages vary between instruments.

Patient factors may also influence the risk for TRD. Pharmacokinetic variance (i.e., cytochrome P450 [CYP] enzyme mutation, differential absorption, pregnancy) may lead to lower serum antidepressant levels with consequent poor efficacy. Ultrarapid CYP metabolizers account for fewer than 1% of the population. Slow or poor CYP metabolizers (fewer than 5% of the population) may be more prone to treatment-emergent side effects in comparison with normal metabolizers. As a general rule, given the low risk of metabolic variance, nonmetabolic factors are more commonly implicated in TRD. Titration to the highest tolerable FDA-approved antidepressant dosage, or even to higher dosages, remains advisable for TRD, and this strategy was modeled in the STAR*D trial. Indeed, it is often advisable to exceed the maximum FDA-approved dosage, mainly in the setting of stepwise symptom improvement (but not remission) at escalating dosages with adequate tolerance. Nonetheless, achievement of adequate exposure time at a standard dosage should precede more heroic dosing targets; treatment tolerability and patient safety should be prioritized. Of concern, medication-induced side effects can limit dosage optimization or lead to nonadherence, and the prescriber will not be aware of this situation. Clinician inquiry into treatment tolerability and collateral verification of treatment adherence via companion interview—or, rarely, measurement of serum levels—are useful considerations. Despite industry claims, pharmacogenomic testing has not been found to be helpful in predicting antidepressant efficacy, yet many practitioners continue to routinely prescribe such testing explicitly for that purpose, in spite of recent FDA warnings that companies are illegally marketing genetic tests that claim to predict patient response to specific medications (Greden et al. 2019; U.S. Food and Drug Administration 2019b; Zeier et al. 2018).

Recognition of MDD subtypes is also diagnostically important because different subtypes may require different treatment strategies. For example, it may be difficult to differentiate psychotic depression from nonpsychotic depression but it is important to do so, given that psychotic depression is very unlikely to respond to antidepressant therapy alone. A preferable strategy with better efficacy in this subset of patients would be a trial of an antidepressant combined with an antipsychotic or a course of ECT (Charney and Nelson 1981).

Bipolar depression is also important to recognize, given that guidelines for first-line interventions do not include traditional antidepressants at all. In one chart review (N=281), "occult" bipolar disorder was reportedly present in 47.1% of patients with TRD, compared with 3.8% of depressed patients without TRD (Correa et al. 2010). A family history of bipolar disorder, early age at onset of depressive symptoms, a high number of recurrent mood episodes, and atypical features all increase the likelihood of bipolarity (van der Linden et al. 2019). Treatment with a mood stabilizer, preferably a data-supported agent for bipolar depression, is advisable. The introduction of novel agents for bipolar depression with increasingly favorable metabolic profiles (e.g., lurasidone, cariprazine) has improved pharmacological options. The Canadian Network for Mood and Anxiety Treatments (CANMAT) and the International Society for Bipolar Disorders (ISBD) jointly released updated treatment guidelines for bipolar disorder in 2018 (Yatham et al. 2018), and the summary document serves as a useful reference for clinicians seeking evidence-based strategies for managing bipolar disorder.

Atypical depression, characterized by hyperphagia, hypersomnia, leaden limb paralysis, extreme mood reactivity, and rejection sensitivity, is thought to respond more favorably to monoamine oxidase inhibitors (MAOIs) than to tricyclic antidepressants (TCAs); however, because the clinical trials evaluating the pharmacological response of atypical depression to MAOIs and TCAs preceded the introduction of SSRIs and serotonin-norepinephrine reuptake inhibitors (SNRIs), their findings may be somewhat less relevant today, with the current widespread first-line use of these newer agents (Liebowitz et al. 1988).

MDD with seasonal pattern, previously known as seasonal affective disorder, may benefit from standard antidepressant therapy and/or bright light therapy (BLT) during the fall and winter months. BLT can be initiated with a 30-minute exposure to a 10,000-lux-intensity light box. Early-morning administration improves the chance of remission. Lower light intensities also show efficacy, at the cost of a prolonged exposure duration (Maruani and Geoffroy 2019).

Finally, premenstrual dysphoric disorder (PMDD) in women with luteal-phase depressive symptoms responds preferentially to serotonergic antidepressants, often at a low dosage. Findings from a Cochrane systematic review of PMDD treatment supported the use of traditional SSRIs, either taken continuously or taken in the luteal phase only (Marjoribanks et al. 2013).

Multiple additional factors—in particular, comorbid psychiatric or medical conditions—are associated with treatment resistance. Anxiety disorders, PTSD, personality disorders, obsessive-compulsive disorder, eating disorders, and body dysmorphic disorder are important psychiatric comorbidities that have been associated with markedly lower MDD remission rates. Hypothyroidism (grades I–IV), glucocorticoid exposure, isotretinoin therapy, and other common medical exposures and conditions, including uncontrolled diabetes, coronary artery disease, Parkinson's disease, HIV, cancer, chronic pain syndromes, fibromyalgia, chronic fatigue syndrome, and irritable bowel syndrome, may also contribute to TRD if not properly diagnosed and managed.

Chronicity of depression increases the likelihood of treatment resistance (Kornstein and Schneider 2001). The DSM-IV Chronic specifier was used when full criteria for an MDE had been continuously met for at least 2 years (Blanco et al. 2010). Double depression—defined as the coexistence of MDD with persistent depressive disorder (dysthymia)—and MDD with incomplete interepisode recovery are two other forms of chronic depression. Several clinical studies have reported that chronic depression is associated with comorbid psychiatric disorders (including personality disorders), a family history of mood disorders, a history of psychiatric hospitalization, and a lifetime history of substance use disorders (Kornstein and Schneider 2001). Chronic depression also is associated with more severe functional impairment, more frequent suicide attempts, earlier illness onset, and a worse prognosis. Significant efforts should be made to prevent chronic depression, given that the chance of response plummets with extended illness time.

Pharmacological Management

In the third edition of the American Psychiatric Association's (APA's) *Practice Guideline for the Treatment of Patients With Major Depressive Disorder*, the recommended first-line pharmacological treatment for mild to moderate MDEs was monotherapy with an SSRI, an SNRI, mirtazapine, or bupropion (American Psychiatric Association 2010). Section 3 ("Pharmacological Treatments") of the CANMAT 2016 *Clinical Guidelines for the Management of Adults With Major Depressive Disorder* echoed these recommendations, with the addition of vortioxetine and agomelatine for MDEs with moderate or greater severity (Kennedy et al. 2016). In the case of nonresponse to an initial agent, it is incumbent on the clinician to first rule out factors that can cause pseudoresistance. After confirming the absence of pseudoresistance, the clinician can address the central questions of therapeutic strategies and their optimal sequence (Dold and Kasper 2017). We know from STAR*D that an initial SSRI trial (i.e., citalopram at an approximate dosage of 40 mg/day) resulted in a Hamilton Depression Rating Scale (HAM-D)–based remission rate of 27% (Gaynes et al. 2009); however, that trial was not designed for direct comparison of switching (either within or outside the antidepressant class) versus augmentation. Because patients were allowed to choose between switching strategies (sertraline, bupropion sustained release [SR], or venlafaxine extended release [XR]) and augmentation strategies (bupropion-SR or buspirone), a selection bias was introduced into the level 2 treatment groups such that patients who chose the augmentation option represented a less-ill subgroup compared with those who opted to switch to a different medication class. Therefore, clinical outcome data examining switching, combination, and augmentation strategies must be derived from studies other than STAR*D. Notably, the patient symptom profile (e.g., anxious, atypical, melancholic features) did not appear to influence outcomes in level 2 therapy (Rush et al. 2008).

Switching Strategies

The switching strategy entails transitioning from an ineffective antidepressant to a new antidepressant either within the same or in a new class. This strategy is generally favored in the setting of nonresponse or intolerance (as opposed to partial response) to the current agent. Following a failed SSRI trial, the clinician might choose a within-class switch to an alternative SSRI or a between-class switch to an SNRI, bupropion, or mirtazapine. However, it remains unclear which option is superior.

A 2008 meta-analysis of four clinical trials analyzed pooled data from 1,496 subjects and found a very modest statistical advantage in remission rates after switching patients to a non-SSRI (bupropion, mirtazapine, venlafaxine) instead of to a second SSRI (28% vs. 23.5%) (Papakostas et al. 2008). In this study, the number needed to treat (NNT) was calculated at 22, meaning that 22 SSRI nonresponders would have to be switched to a non-SSRI to obtain 1 additional symptom remission outcome—a slight advantage at best.

The STAR*D study showed that 25% of subjects who did not experience symptom remission with citalopram did respond to either a within-class switch (i.e., citalopram to sertraline) or a between-class switch (i.e., citalopram to venlafaxine or bupropion), and there were no significant efficacy differences between the strategies (Rush et al. 2006b). However, this subset of citalopram nonremitters likely represented a more treatment-resistant group, given that most STAR*D subjects who experienced some symptomatic relief (but not remission) with citalopram elected to receive augmentation rather than switch agents. Another large open-label study of nonresponders to first-line antidepressants in a primary care setting (N=3,097) compared the strategies of switching to an alternative first-line antidepressant and switching to venlafaxine-XR for 24 weeks, finding remission rates of 51.5% and 59.3%, respectively (Baldomero et al. 2005). Although the study did not utilize a randomized controlled design, the large sample size and substantial 24-week follow-up period support the likelihood of a small efficacy advantage for the SNRI venlafaxine over first-line antidepressants. Table 33–1 lists factors that should be weighed when choosing between switching and augmentation strategies.

As a final point, a 2017 review of evidence-based pharmacotherapy for TRD recommended that a switching strategy be implemented only if there is "absolutely no response" to the current antidepressant and/or "severe side effects are present" (Dold and Kasper 2017). In the scenario of partial response to the first antidepressant, other treatment strategies are likely more appropriate (Dold and Kasper 2017).

Consideration of TCAs as a switch option remains a viable therapeutic strategy; however, there are limited data examining the efficacy of such a maneuver. Meta-analytic data confirm that TCAs appear largely equivalent to SSRIs in terms of efficacy. The APA practice guideline for MDD (American Psychiatric Association 2010) commented on the potential for the superior efficacy of TCAs in hospitalized patients with more severe depression, but this finding has not been seen in less impaired outpatients. The STAR*D trial compared response and remission rates between nortriptyline and mirtazapine after two consecutive antidepressant failures, with no statistical difference reported, although nortriptyline was nonstatistically superior, with 20% remission based on the HAM-D compared with 12% for mirtazapine (Fava et al. 2006). Notably, the mean nortriptyline dosage was reportedly 96.8 mg/day, but no measured therapeutic blood levels were obtained. One practical advantage of TCAs is the ease of measuring a serum TCA trough level to confirm adherence and therapeutic levels as well as to rule out aberrant hepatic metabolism. Because STAR*D did not report TCA serum drug levels, it is impossible to know whether personalizing the nortriptyline dosage via a target plasma level might have improved outcomes.

The use of MAOIs has become increasingly rare in clinical practice due to the risk of potentially serious dietary and drug-drug interactions, namely serotonin syndrome and hypertensive crisis (Thase 2012). For this reason, MAOIs are not recom-

TABLE 33–1. Factors to consider in choosing between switching to monotherapy with another antidepressant and adding an adjunctive medication (level 3 evidence)

Consider switching to another antidepressant when

- It is the first antidepressant trial.
- There are poorly tolerated side effects with the initial antidepressant.
- There is no response (i.e., <25% improvement) to the initial antidepressant.[a]
- There is more time to wait for a response (less severe symptoms, less functional impairment).
- The patient prefers to switch to another antidepressant.

Consider an adjunctive medication when

- There have been two or more antidepressant trials.
- The initial antidepressant is well tolerated.
- There is partial response (i.e., >25% improvement) to the initial antidepressant.
- There are specific residual symptoms or side effects with the initial antidepressant that can be targeted.
- There is less time to wait for a response (more severe symptoms, more functional impairment).
- The patient prefers to add on another medication.

[a]For the initial antidepressant trial. In subsequent trials, lack of response (<25% improvement) may not be a factor in choosing between switching and adjunctive strategies.

Source. Adapted from Kennedy SH, Lam RW, McIntyre RS, et al: "Canadian Network for Mood and Anxiety Treatments (CANMAT) 2016 Clinical Guidelines for the Management of Adults With Major Depressive Disorder: Section 3. Pharmacological Treatments." *Canadian Journal of Psychiatry* 61(9):540–560, 2016, Table 12. Copyright © 2016 The Authors. Used with permission.

mended as a first-line class for the treatment of depression; rather, they are typically employed as third- through fifth-line treatment steps, depending on the specific treatment guideline referenced. A Canadian population based observational cohort study examining the prevalence and incidence of irreversible MAOI use from 1997 to 2007 found a decreasing yearly incidence of new MAOI prescriptions, from 3.1 per 100,000 to 1.4 per 100,000, while the overall prevalence of MAOI use decreased from 400 per 100,000 to 216 per 100,000 (Shulman et al. 2009). These data suggest that most contemporary psychiatrists have very limited experience with MAOI therapy. The efficacy of oral MAOIs has been studied in comparison with placebo and TCAs, with MAOIs showing inferior efficacy to TCAs in inpatients with MDD (Thase et al. 1995). Oral MAOIs were found to have superior efficacy relative to TCAs in MDD outpatients with atypical depressive features (Rapaport 2007; Thase et al. 1995). The CANMAT 2016 clinical guidelines for MDD recommended MAOI therapy as a third-line choice because of its higher risks for side effects and serious dietary/drug interactions (Kennedy et al. 2016). There are no clear head-to-head data comparing the efficacy of MAOIs against that of first- or second-line antidepressants. The STAR*D trial compared tranylcypromine against combination mirtazapine plus venlafaxine at level 4 treatment after three prior antidepressant failures. The HAM-D-based remission rate for the combination of mirtazapine plus venlafaxine was 14%, compared with a remission rate of 7% for tranylcypromine, a non-statistically-significant result, although the MAOI had poorer tolerability (Gaynes et al. 2009). Notably, the low mean dosage of tranylcypromine (36.9 mg/day) was criticized as being potentially subtherapeutic. In practice, MAOI therapy should be considered for patients who have failed to respond to two or more previous adequate antidepressant trials, have prominent atypical symptoms, have historically responded to MAOIs, communicate a clear preference for MAOIs, and are able to follow the necessary dietary and medication restrictions to maintain safety.

Adjunctive Strategies

The CANMAT 2016 clinical guidelines for MDD defined *adjunctive therapy* as "the addition of a second medication to an initial medication" (Kennedy et al. 2016, p. 552). Furthermore, the CANMAT working group prefers the term *adjunctive* over *combination* (i.e., adding a second antidepressant to the first) or *augmentation* (i.e., adding a non-antidepressant to an antidepressant), because some mood-stabilizing agents (i.e., lithium, quetiapine) have independent antidepressant effects. Nevertheless, clinicians should be aware of the nomenclature (i.e., combination, augmentation) that is commonly used.

Combination therapy involves the addition of a second antidepressant, typically from a novel class with a different mechanism of action, to the initial antidepressant. The clinical rationale for this strategy has long held that combining medications that enhance monoamine availability (e.g., serotonin, norepinephrine, dopamine) via differential mechanisms may provide an efficacy advantage over single-monoamine modulators such as SSRIs. However, efficacy data are lacking in this regard. In a trial investigating the utility of combination antidepressant therapy as an initial treatment for MDD, Stewart et al. (2014) randomly assigned 245 outpatients to escitalopram monotherapy, bupropion monotherapy, or combination escitalopram plus bupropion. There was no reported advantage for any treatment group at 12 weeks. A similar study by Rush et al. (2011) compared escitalopram monotherapy against combination therapy with either escitalopram plus bupropion or venlafaxine plus mirtazapine in 665 patients with moderate to severe MDD. Response and remission rates did not differ at either the 12-week or the 7-month endpoint; however, tolerability was worse in the two combination therapy groups. A final study by Kessler et al. (2018) examined the utility of combining mirtazapine with SSRIs or SNRIs for treating TRD. Four hundred eighty primary care MDD patients in the United Kingdom were randomly assigned to either treatment as usual with first-line antidepressant therapy or treatment with an SSRI or SNRI plus mirtazapine. Seventy-two percent of the subjects had been taking standard antidepressants for more than 1 year, with 25% meeting criteria for severe MDD. Unfortunately, the study "did not find convincing evidence of a clinically important benefit for mirtazapine given in addition to an SSRI or SNRI antidepressant over placebo in primary care patients with TRD" (Kessler et al. 2018, p. 73). This finding conflicts with the conclusions of Dold and Kasper (2017), whose interpretation of the data led them to recommend initial antidepressant therapy with an SSRI or SNRI, followed by combination treatment with "inhibitors of presynaptic autoreceptors or serotonin antagonist and reuptake inhibitors" (i.e., mirtazapine or trazodone) (Dold and Kasper 2017). Overall, the evidence for antidepressant combination therapy remains relatively weak, and such therapy clearly cannot be recommended at treatment initiation (Kennedy et al. 2016). A practical role for combination antidepressant therapy may exist in clinical scenarios in which a second antidepressant with a novel mechanism of action is added to improve isolated target symptoms in addition to mood (e.g., bupropion augmentation for fatigue, mirtazapine for insomnia).

Adjunctive therapy with atypical antipsychotics has become an increasingly popular treatment choice in the United States, with prescribing rates (assessed by percentage of physician visits in which an adjunctive atypical antipsychotic was prescribed for an outpatient with nonpsychotic depression) increasing from 4.6% in 1999/2000 to 12.5% in 2009/2010 (Gerhard et al. 2014). An abundance of randomized controlled trial (RCT) data with atypical antipsychotics has enabled systematic reviews of augmentation outcomes with various antipsychotic medications. Spielmans et al. (2013) examined 14 short-term trials of aripiprazole, olanzapine-fluoxetine combination (OFC), quetiapine, and risperidone. All four agents had a statistically significant effect on remission, with an NNT of 9 for aripiprazole, quetiapine, and risperidone. OFC had an NNT of 19, a finding of more questionable clinical relevance. Adverse effects were present and included akathisia (aripiprazole), sedation (quetiapine, OFC, and aripiprazole), metabolic derangement (quetiapine and OFC), and weight gain (all four agents, particularly OFC). Overall, the benefits of atypical antipsychotic augmentation were "small to moderate," with no clear benefit in regard to quality of life or functional impairment.

Zhou et al. (2015b) analyzed data from 48 augmentation trials (involving 6,654 subjects) including atypical antipsychotics along with lithium, thyroid hormone, lamotrigine, pindolol, bupropion, buspirone, and methylphenidate. They concluded that quetiapine and aripiprazole were the "most robust evidence-based options for augmentation therapy in patients with treatment-resistant depression" but warned of treatment-related side effects. Another meta-analysis by Zhou et al. (2015a) that examined atypical antipsychotic augmentation for depression found that "standard dosage" augmentation with aripiprazole, risperidone, OFC, or quetiapine was superior to "low dosage" augmentation with these agents. In this analysis, both aripiprazole and risperidone demonstrated benefit with respect to quality of life and functioning.

Comorbid anxiety symptoms often accompany MDD and deserve attention from clinicians when considering augmentation options. One post hoc analysis of STAR*D data that compared remission outcomes among individuals with anxious (defined as an anxiety/somatization factor score on the 17-item HAM-D of 7 or higher at baseline) versus nonanxious depression revealed that patients with anxious MDD were significantly less likely to achieve remission (22.2% vs. 32.4% in level 1) and on average took a longer time to achieve response or remission (Fava et al. 2008). This finding highlights the need for better anxiety symptom management in the setting of TRD. In this context, short-term use of an intermediate- or long-acting benzodiazepine (i.e., clonazepam or alprazolam-ER) can be considered as a "bridge" for patients who are waiting for medications to take effect in a new antidepressant trial (Coplan et al. 2015). Notably, benzodiazepine therapy should generally be avoided in patients with known substance use problems, with quetiapine serving as an alternative.

The most recent addition to the atypical antipsychotic armamentarium is brexpiprazole, a compound related to aripiprazole. In a systematic review and meta-analysis, Kishi et al. (2019) concluded that brexpiprazole was a useful adjunct to antidepressant treatment for patients with MDD who had failed to respond to at least one previous trial of an antidepressant. However, with NNTs of 17 for response and 25 for remission, brexpiprazole appears to be relatively less effective than the approved alternatives.

Clinically and medicolegally, it is important to be aware of which atypical antipsychotics are FDA-approved for MDD augmentation. Currently, aripiprazole, quetiapine, brexpiprazole, and OFC are FDA approved for this indication.

The CANMAT 2016 clinical guidelines for MDD commented on the outcomes of two additional meta-analyses examining atypical antipsychotic augmentation of antidepressants in addition to those previously discussed (Kennedy et al. 2016). Aripiprazole, olanzapine, quetiapine, and risperidone all demonstrated small to moderate effect sizes and no evidence of differential efficacy. Brexpiprazole and ziprasidone also demonstrated efficacy in RCTs as adjunctive agents, but ziprasidone has not been included in meta-analytic evaluations. Tolerability of adjunctive atypical antipsychotics was shown to be worse than that of placebo.

The addition of lithium to an antidepressant is a long-standing strategy originating from findings of studies evaluating lithium augmentation of TCAs (Bauer et al. 2014). A comprehensive review by Bauer et al. (2014) reported a clear benefit from lithium augmentation versus placebo, with an odds ratio (OR) of 3.11, an NNT of 5, and a mean response rate of 41.2% (vs. 12.4% in the placebo group). However, these researchers acknowledged the limitation that the majority of these outcome data were derived from studies examining lithium augmentation of TCAs, noting that TCAs are no longer in widespread use (Bauer et al. 2014). Another systematic review and meta-analysis by Nelson et al. (2014) examined the efficacy of lithium augmentation as an adjunct to second-generation antidepressants as well as to TCAs. Lithium augmentation was found to be superior to TCAs or second-generation antidepressants, with a pooled OR of 2.89 and a remission rate of 46.1% (compared with 25.4% in the placebo group) (Nelson et al. 2014). In a 2015 review, Tundo et al. (2015) noted that the STAR*D outcome data on level 3 lithium augmentation revealed a 16% remission rate after a failed citalopram trial plus a failed switch or augmentation in 142 patients. Tundo and colleagues warned that "methodological limits including low lithium dosage" may have negatively influenced the outcome (Tundo et al. 2015). The World Federation of Societies of Biological Psychiatry guidelines for treatment of MDD (Bauer et al. 2013) noted that "lithium augmentation should be administered for 2–4 weeks in order to allow assessment of the patient's response. The recommended lithium serum target levels are 0.6 to 0.8 mmol/L. In the case of response, lithium augmentation should be continued for at least 12 months" (Bauer et al. 2013, p. 356). Finally, lithium is well known to reduce the odds of suicide completion, a finding that originated from outcome studies in patients with bipolar disorder (Grof and Müller-Oerlinghausen 2009). A separate meta-analysis evaluating the antisuicidal properties of lithium using pooled data from 329 patients with MDD and found that the overall risk of suicide completions and attempts was 88.5% lower among patients exposed to lithium compared with those without lithium exposure (Guzzetta et al. 2007).

Thyroid hormone augmentation with triiodothyronine (T_3) is yet another augmentation strategy for TRD. The STAR*D trial included T_3 augmentation versus lithium at level 3 and reported a 24.7% remission rate (with a nonsignificant trend toward superiority) and better relative tolerability (Gaynes et al. 2009). A review by Connolly and Thase (2011) concluded that T_3 augmentation has efficacy for TCA nonresponders, with an NNT "essentially equivalent to that of lithium." However, the authors noted that there remains a paucity of positive RCTs that support the routine use of T_3 augmentation in euthyroid patients. Notably, for patients with high-normal thyroid-stimulating hormone (TSH) levels or subclinical hypothyroidism along with depressive symptoms (especially TRD), there may be a treatment advantage for adding either T_3 or thyroxine (T_4), with a target TSH below 2.5 mIU/mL, and perhaps below 2 mIU/mL (Cohen et al. 2018).

Finally, the dopamine (primarily D_3) receptor agonist pramipexole is sometimes used as an augmentation agent with traditional antidepressants in patients with TRD. However, the evidence for pramipexole augmentation of an antidepressant in MDD is scant, as pramipexole has been evaluated more often as monotherapy for MDD, sometimes against an active antidepressant comparator, or as augmentation of a mood stabilizer in bipolar depression (Tundo et al. 2019). Kleeblatt et al. (2017) highlighted conflicting results from two small trials examining pramipexole augmentation—one trial (N=13 patients) that failed to show an accelerated response or enhanced efficacy for pramipexole added to escitalopram, and another trial (N=60 patients) that showed a superior response rate of 40% for subjects who received pramipexole (vs. 27% for those who received an unaugmented antidepressant) (Kleeblatt et al. 2017). Overall, the evidence for pramipexole augmentation in TRD remains limited.

Psychotherapy

The combination of psychotherapeutic treatments, namely CBT, and psychotropic medication has historically shown efficacy in short-term RCTs of MDD (Thase et al. 1997). The utility and effectiveness of psychotherapy, as well as the most efficacious modality, remain unclear. One U.K. trial (CoBalT [**Co**gnitive **B**ehaviour**al** **T**herapy as an adjunct to pharmacotherapy for primary care patients with TRD) randomly assigned 469 primary care patients with TRD to usual care or usual care plus CBT, with a primary outcome of response at 6 months (Wiles et al. 2014). The response rate for the intervention group was 46.1% (vs. 21.6% for the comparison group), and the benefit of adjunctive CBT persisted at 12 months. The intervention was also deemed to be cost-effective in accordance with the National Institute for Health and Care Excellence (NICE) definition (Wiles et al. 2014). Another systematic review by Trivedi et al. (2011) examined psychotherapy as an adjunctive or substitution strategy for 592 patients with TRD. The authors concluded that although psychotherapy showed some efficacy in TRD, the evidence was sparse, and results were mixed (Trivedi et al. 2011).

Neuromodulation

Neuromodulation therapies for MDD remain a key area of interest, especially in the setting of treatment resistance. The oldest and most efficacious form of neuromodulation is ECT, a procedure wherein an electrical stimulus is applied to the brain, with subsequent induction of a brief generalized seizure. ECT is generally used when antidepressant therapy fails to adequately ameliorate severe depressive symptoms. However, ECT can be used as a first-line therapy in situations of high clinical urgency, such as imminent suicidality, malignant catatonia, malnutrition, severe postpartum depression, or agitated psychosis (American Psychiatric Association 2001; Kellner et al. 2012). A patient's past response to ECT should also be considered, because certain patients may prefer a known, previously effective therapy. Rates of response to ECT range from 70% to 80% and are significantly higher than rates of response to pharmacological interventions (Milev et al. 2016). Despite significant improvements in the delivery of ECT (i.e., anesthesia, neuromuscular blockade, unilateral electrode placement), concerns about tolerability—namely, short-term amnesia or other cognitive impairment—serve as barriers to its consideration. For this reason, many practitioners delay referring patients for ECT consultation until an illness episode has lasted many months or years, and this reluctance and delay has been questioned in light of ECT's unequivocally superior efficacy for MDD compared with other therapies (Beale and Kellner 2000). Additionally, because data suggest that the more chronic a depressive episode becomes, the more likely it is to become treatment resistant, this delay in considering use of ECT can contribute to long-term morbidity (Perugi et al. 2012). The CANMAT 2016 clinical guidelines for MDD summarized the evidence for ECT as follows: "ECT remains a second-line treatment for patients with treatment-resistant depression, although in some situations, it may be considered first line" (Milev et al. 2016, p. 561).

Brain stimulation with repetitive transcranial magnetic stimulation (rTMS) is an alternative FDA-approved nonpharmacological option for MDD, albeit one that is inferior to ECT (Ren et al. 2014). Traditional rTMS involves the application of strong (1–2.5 Tesla), focused magnetic field pulses via a "figure-of-eight" magnetic coil to the left or right dorsolateral prefrontal cortex (DLPFC), resulting in depolarization of underlying cortical neural tissue at a depth of approximately 2 cm. Whereas high-frequency rTMS is considered "excitatory" and is delivered to the left DLPFC, low-frequency rTMS is "inhibitory" and delivered to the right DLPFC. Both stimulation paradigms have demonstrated efficacy in treating MDD (Berlim et al. 2014). A standard course of rTMS involves administration of a minimum of 3,000 pulses per session, delivered 5 days per week on an outpatient basis without anesthesia, for a total of 20–30 sessions (McClintock et al. 2018). Because anesthesia is not required, patients may drive themselves home after treatment, a significant advantage over ECT. Recent advances in rTMS have led to novel protocols such as intermittent theta-burst stimulation (iTBS), which reduces the total treatment time per session from 15–45 minutes to 1–3 minutes (Milev et al. 2016). Additionally, new rTMS coil configurations (e.g., H1, "deep" TMS coil) with documented efficacy and FDA approval have been developed that reach deeper cortical areas (Filipčić et al. 2019). The CANMAT 2016 clinical guidelines for MDD concluded that rTMS is now a first-line recommendation for patients with MDD who have failed to respond to at least one antidepressant (Milev et al. 2016).

Transcranial direct current stimulation (tDCS) is another noninvasive, non-FDA-approved neuromodulation option for MDD that delivers low-amplitude electrical current to a defined cortical target using scalp electrodes (Milev et al. 2016). Whereas anodal stimulation increases cortical excitability, cathodal stimulation decreases excitability via hyperpolarization of neuronal membrane potentials (Stagg and Nitsche 2011). The optimal tDCS stimulation parameters remain unclear, although data suggest that 2 mA stimulation for 30 minutes daily for at least 2 weeks is necessary for an antidepressant effect (Shiozawa et al. 2014). Various outcome studies and meta-analyses have examined tDCS efficacy, including a recent systematic review and meta-analysis by Wang (2019) that confirmed a significant, albeit modest, effect of tDCS on HAM-D and Montgomery-Åsberg Depression Rating Scale (MADRS) score reduction. This study followed a failed single-center double-blind RCT of 245 patients randomly assigned to receive tDCS plus placebo versus sham tDCS plus escitalopram versus sham tDCS plus placebo (Brunoni et al. 2017). In that trial, the investigators were unable to demonstrate noninferiority of tDCS to the SSRI comparator. All said, the CANMAT 2016 clinical guidelines for MDD (Milev et al. 2016) consider tDCS to be a third-line intervention, and its use remains off-label.

Vagus nerve stimulation (VNS) is an FDA-approved therapy for TRD recommended by the APA practice guideline for MDD (American Psychiatric Association 2010) as a treatment option after four failed trials of antidepressant therapy, including ECT. VNS involves surgically implanting a small lead wire in the neck attached to the afferent fibers of the left vagus nerve and stimulating it with an implanted pulse generator (i.e., a battery) placed subcutaneously in the chest or axilla. A prospective, open-label, nonrandomized observational study in a registry of patients with TRD that compared VNS against treatment as usual (TAU) found a significantly higher 5-year cumulative MADRS response rate (67.6%) among patients who received implanted VNS devices compared with those who received TAU (40.9%) (Aaronson et al. 2017). Patients in the study sample had failed to respond to an average of 8.2 trials of antidepressant treatment and therefore represented a highly treatment-resistant group. A new long-term clinical trial of VNS funded by the Centers for Medicare and Medicaid Services is under way (ClinicalTrials.gov Identifier NCT03887715).

Novel Therapies

Ketamine

The newest pharmacological intervention for TRD to date is ketamine, delivered either by intravenous (IV) infusion (racemic ketamine) or intranasally (isomeric esketamine). The IV racemic formulation is not FDA approved. IV delivery of a single subanesthetic ketamine dose (e.g., 0.5 mg/kg) is known to antagonize the *N*-methyl-D-aspartate (NMDA) receptor in the brain, resulting in a rapid but nonsustained antidepressant effect (Berman et al. 2000). A systematic review and meta-analysis of NMDA antagonists conducted by Newport et al. (2015) concluded that the antidepressant effects of ketamine infusion are "both rapid and robust, albeit transient," with the OR of transient symptomatic remission peaking at postinfusion day 1 (OR=14.5) but no longer remaining statistically significant by day 7. Ketamine use is known to cause psychotomimetic and dissociative symptoms, which can complicate the effects of ketamine therapy. The optimal method of prolonging ketamine response and remission is still under investigation (Xu et al. 2016). Phillips et al. (2019) conducted a trial comparing single, repeated, and maintenance ketamine infusions for TRD. In comparison with subjects who received midazolam as an active comparator, those who received a single ketamine infusion showed significantly greater depressive symptom reduction that peaked at 24 hours and had abated by day 7. Resumption of the 3-times-per-week ketamine infusion regimen restored antidepressant efficacy over the next 2 weeks, with more than half of the group responding and almost one-quarter achieving symptom remission. Benefits were maintained in responders over the next month with weekly maintenance infusions (Phillips et al. 2019).

Apart from its NMDA antagonism, ketamine has also been shown to modulate the endogenous opioid system, and a small trial demonstrated that ketamine's acute antidepressant effects in humans are effectively blocked with oral naltrexone (Williams et al. 2018). The authors of this trial concluded that "ketamine produces its acute antidepressant response primarily through direct and/or indirect actions at the mu opioid receptors" (p. 1210). The opiate modulation from ketamine, together with its known historic abuse as a "club drug," raises concerns about abusability, especially with long-term use (Schatzberg 2019). Concerns surrounding ketamine's potential for abuse, poor screening practices for patients with substance abuse, and widespread off-label use prompted the Task Force on Novel Biomarkers and Treatments of the American Psychiatric Association Research Council to develop a consensus statement on the use of ketamine in the treatment of mood disorders (Sanacora et al. 2017). This document serves as a platform for the development of responsible intravenous ketamine treatment programming.

Intranasal esketamine received FDA approval for use in the treatment of TRD in 2019, with efficacy demonstrated in a single Phase III trial comparing esketamine plus a novel antidepressant against placebo plus a novel antidepressant (Popova et al. 2019). Esketamine's FDA approval was unusual in that two positive Phase III trials are generally required to gain an FDA indication. Although two previous Phase III trials (Fedgchin et al. 2019; Ochs-Ross et al. 2020) had demonstrated MADRS change scores similar to those in the pivotal trial, these did not achieve statistical separation from placebo, and the effect size of the positive study was notably in the mild range (Schatzberg 2019). Multiple concerns have been raised about the quality and/or the design of the original industry-supported trials. In a published commentary, Turner (2019) pointed out several specific criticisms, including an "arguably lax regulatory definition" of TRD that included subjects with two within-class antidepressant failures (i.e., SSRIs only), a modest MADRS reduction of 4 points, enrichment of the randomized withdrawal trial (Study 3003) with esketamine responders, an outlier trial site in Poland with a 100% rate of placebo-arm relapses, and a standardized mean difference of change in MADRS score that was inferior to that for aripiprazole or quetiapine augmentation (Turner 2019). Adding to those concerns, three patients in the initial esketamine trials arm died by suicide, as opposed to none in the placebo arm (U.S. Food and Drug Administration 2019a). According to the FDA report, "the patients who committed suicide 12 and 4 days after their last dose both appeared to be improving based on their MADRS scores (from baseline of 27 to 9, and 41 to 25, respectively)" (p. 42). This finding is difficult to interpret, especially with one subject nearly meeting remission criteria on the MADRS. Oddly, the two patients, whose last ketamine doses prior to suicide completion were at 12 and 20 days, respectively, screened negative on the primary suicide rating instrument (Columbia–Suicide Severity Rating Scale) at baseline and at last assessment. Additionally, there were three other deaths, one involving a motorcycle accident occurring 26 hours after the last ketamine exposure, another involving sudden death in a 60-year-old male with hypertension and obesity who exhibited normal vital signs at a study visit 5 days prior to death, and the third involving a 74-year-old woman with hypertension and hyperlipidemia who died of a myocardial infarction 6 days after her last esketamine dose. Although none of the six total trial deaths was ultimately considered to be directly related to esketamine, the mortality in the clinical studies does raise significant concerns.

The risk-benefit ratio of maintenance esketamine therapy for relapse prevention remains largely unclear due to mixed outcomes. In a study by Daly et al. (2019), 297 patients with TRD who had achieved either a stable response or remission after 16 weeks of esketamine plus antidepressant treatment were randomly assigned (1:1) to continue esketamine augmentation (once weekly for 4 weeks, then every 1–2 weeks based on severity of depressive symptoms) or to switch to intranasal placebo for a minimum of 32 weeks. Among patients entering the study with a stable remission on esketamine augmentation, 26.7% of those assigned to resume esketamine augmentation treatment experienced a relapse, compared with 45.3% of those assigned to receive placebo augmentation. Similarly, among patients entering the study with a stable response to esketamine augmentation, 25.8% of those assigned to resume esketamine experienced a relapse, compared with 57.6% of those assigned to receive placebo plus antidepressant. Notably, relapse in the placebo plus antidepressant group occurred abruptly, within the first 4 weeks, raising questions about a ketamine withdrawal effect (Daly et al. 2019).

Overall, the clinical utility of esketamine remains in question because of uncertainties about its side effects associated with long-term exposure, rapid relapse, addictive potential, and maintenance efficacy; therefore, clinicians are advised to exercise caution when considering esketamine as a therapeutic option (Schatzberg 2019). As a further complication, the average cost of esketamine exceeds $4,700 for the first month (excluding FDA-required monitoring costs), a clear barrier to widespread patient access (Institute for Clinical and Economic Review 2019).

Brexanolone

Brexanolone, a novel neuroactive steroid, was approved by the FDA in March 2019 for the treatment of postpartum depression as a 60-hour intravenous infusion. This new agent combines an aqueous formulation of allopregnanolone (a positive allosteric modulator of synaptic and extrasynaptic $GABA_A$ receptors) with a delivery vehicle (sulfobutylether-β-cyclodextrin) designed to improve intravenous bioavailability (Kanes et al. 2017a). Allopregnanolone is the major metabolite of progesterone and increases throughout pregnancy, reaching peak concentrations in the third trimester and undergoing a precipitous drop after delivery (Kanes et al. 2017b). With parturition, the abrupt decline in allopregnanolone levels is postulated to negatively influence the adaptive function of $GABA_A$ receptors, triggering postpartum depression (Kanes et al. 2017a). The FDA approval of brexanolone was propelled by two positive RCTs (reviewed in Meltzer-Brody et al. 2018) involving 246 adult women up to 6 months postpartum who experienced a major depressive episode between the third pregnancy trimester and 4 weeks postdelivery. One of the RCTs (ClinicalTrials.gov Identifier NCT02942004) included patients with severe postpartum depression (HAM-D score ≥26), and the second RCT (ClinicalTrials.gov Identifier NCT02942017) included women with moderate depression (HAM-D score=20–25); in both trials, the primary outcome was change in HAM-D score at the terminus of the 60-hour infusion. In both RCTs, the active-treatment group separated modestly from placebo at the primary endpoint, with only the severely depressed group retaining benefit after 30 days (Meltzer-

Brody et al. 2018). Excessive sedation and sudden loss of consciousness (occurring in fewer than 5% of patients) are the primary side-effect concerns with brexanolone; therefore, continuous inpatient observation and concurrent continuous pulse oximetry monitoring are required. A minimum of five vials of the drug, at a cost of $34,000, is required to complete the 60-hour infusion. An oral derivative of brexanolone, zuranolone, is currently under development, with positive findings in one Phase III trial (Deligiannidis et al. 2021).

Experimental Therapies

Deep Brain Stimulation

Deep brain stimulation (DBS) involves the surgical implantation of paired electrodes into specific bilateral brain structures (i.e., subcallosal cingulate, ventral capsule/ventral striatum, medial forebrain bundle) in an effort to modulate the neural network implicated in MDD (Drobisz and Damborská 2019). The electrodes are programmed to deliver small electrical pulses to the target areas via an implanted pulse generator (battery) in an effort to positively influence mood network dysfunction noted in prior neuroimaging studies. Helen Mayberg and colleagues evaluated stimulation of the bilateral subcallosal cingulate (SCC/Cg25) in the first large-scale DBS RCT, published in 2017 (Holtzheimer et al. 2017). Participants with TRD were randomly assigned to active or sham stimulation, with a primary outcome of "frequency of response," defined as a score reduction of at least 40% on the 17-item HAM-17 averaged over 4–6 months. A planned futility analysis was performed after approximately half of the sample (90 patients) had received implantation and completed the double-blind phase. Unfortunately, the active stimulation group failed to separate from the sham stimulation group at that juncture, and the industry sponsor halted the study. This result contributed to a negative perception of the efficacy of DBS for TRD, in both the scientific and the public spheres, a criticism challenged by Widge et al. (2018). In their commentary, Widge and colleagues argued that early trials of DBS for TRD were "limited by the heterogeneity of depressive illness, poorly understood mechanism(s) of action, and limitations of a common 'front end' trial design" (p. 2). Their review outlined other DBS targets for depression, including the ventral capsule/ventral striatum (VC/VS) target studied in the RECLAIM (Reclaim DBS System) trial, which also was stopped early because of futility after 30 subjects "showed no separation between active and sham stimulation at that 4-month timepoint, either on the continuous MADRS outcome or [on the] response rate" (Widge et al. 2018, p. 3). However, after the 24-month follow-up, data revealed a 23% response rate in patients who received active DBS, with 6 of 7 responders going on to achieve remission (Widge et al. 2018). This finding raised questions about the required period of stimulation for depressive symptom response, suggesting that longer-term stimulation may be required for efficacy.

A DBS target used more recently in TRD is the superolateral branch of the medial forebrain bundle (slMFB). Coenen et al. (2019) reported on the outcomes of 16 patients with TRD who were randomly assigned to active or sham DBS of the slMFB for the first 2 months postimplantation, with all patients receiving active stimulation thereafter. Although the sample size was small, significant reductions were seen in MADRS scores, from 29.6 at baseline to 12.9 after 12 months of DBS, with all patients achieving response. Ten patients responded within 1 week of receiving stimulation. A novel aspect of Coenen et al.'s approach involved the application of diffusion tensor imaging to individualize the targeting of slMFB fiber tracts rather than using standard anatomical targeting.

In summary, DBS outcomes for TRD have been mixed because of variable stimulation targets, problems with study design and surgical planning, and incomplete understanding of brain networks implicated in TRD on a general and an individual level (Filkowski and Sheth 2019). However, improved imaging techniques, individualized targeting, and a shift to a "systems/circuits perspective" in psychiatric neuroscience research hold great promise for this intervention (Widge et al. 2018).

Magnetic Seizure Therapy

Magnetic seizure therapy (MST) is another investigational treatment for TRD that combines aspects of rTMS and ECT. A strong magnetic field is used to induce a generalized seizure in a patient under anesthesia and muscle relaxation. The electric field induced by MST is more focal and less impeded than the field induced by ECT; therefore, the hope is that MST can approximate the efficacy of ECT while producing fewer cognitive side effects (Lisanby 2002). A systematic review of MST confirmed the antidepressant efficacy of MST, reporting response rates ranging from 40% to 60% and remission rates ranging from 15% to 30%; however, outcomes from MST remained inferior to those from ECT (Cretaz et al. 2015). Nevertheless, MST does have considerable advantages over ECT in terms of cognitive side-effect risk. It is hoped that additional studies evaluating MST dosing parameters will further optimize the efficacy and tolerability of this technique, thereby moving it from the experimental realm to real-world clinical practice.

Conclusion

TRD remains a formidable foe for clinicians, research scientists, and society. Despite a host of different treatment options, a significant proportion of patients continue to suffer, often struggling to function in the most basic of ways. However, a systematic approach to MDD treatment does have a meaningful effect on outcomes, and a comprehensive understanding of therapeutic options is critical to achieving clinical success. Careful attention to diagnosis; comorbidity; antidepressant trial adequacy; and switching, combination, and augmentation strategies can improve outcomes. Furthermore, consideration of neuromodulation strategies earlier in the course of illness can reduce the chance of illness chronicity. New advances in psychiatric neuroscience promise further growth in the understanding of this complex brain illness through advanced neuroimaging techniques and individualized brain stimulation targeting, and this prospect inspires hope, an essential element for our patients who suffer from stigmatized illness.

References

Aaronson ST, Sears P, Ruvuna F, et al: A 5-year observational study of patients with treatment-resistant depression treated with vagus nerve stimulation or treatment as usual: comparison of response, remission, and suicidality. Am J Psychiatry 174(7):640–648, 2017 28359201

American Psychiatric Association: The Practice of Electroconvulsive Therapy: Recommendations for Treatment, Training, and Privileging: A Task Force Report of the American Psychiatric Association, 2nd Edition. Washington, DC, American Psychiatry Association, 2001

American Psychiatric Association: Practice Guideline for the Treatment of Patients With Major Depressive Disorder, 3rd Edition. Washington, DC, American Psychiatric Association, 2010

American Psychiatric Association: Diagnostic and Statistical Manual of Mental Disorders, 5th Edition. Arlington, VA, American Psychiatric Publishing, 2013

Baldomero EB, Ubago JG, Cercós CL, et al: Venlafaxine extended release versus conventional antidepressants in the remission of depressive disorders after previous antidepressant failure: ARGOS study. Depress Anxiety 22(2):68–76, 2005 16094658

Bauer M, Pfennig A, Severus E, et al: World Federation of Societies of Biological Psychiatry (WFSBP) guidelines for biological treatment of unipolar depressive disorders, part 1: update 2013 on the acute and continuation treatment of unipolar depressive disorders. World J Biol Psychiatry 14(5):334–385, 2013 23879318

Bauer M, Adli M, Ricken R, et al: Role of lithium augmentation in the management of major depressive disorder. CNS Drugs 28(4):331–342, 2014 24590663

Beale MD, Kellner CH: ECT in treatment algorithms: no need to save the best for last. J ECT 16(1):1–2, 2000 10735326

Berlim MT, van den Eynde F, Tovar-Perdomo S, et al: Response, remission and drop-out rates following high-frequency repetitive transcranial magnetic stimulation (rTMS) for treating major depression: a systematic review and meta-analysis of randomized, double-blind and sham-controlled trials. Psychol Med 44(2):225–239, 2014 23507264

Berman RM, Cappiello A, Anand A, et al: Antidepressant effects of ketamine in depressed patients. Biol Psychiatry 47(4):351–354, 2000 10686270

Blanco C, Okuda M, Markowitz JC, et al: The epidemiology of chronic major depressive disorder and dysthymic disorder: results from the National Epidemiologic Survey on Alcohol and Related Conditions. J Clin Psychiatry 71(12):1645–1656, 2010 21190638

Brunoni AR, Moffa AH, Sampaio-Junior B, et al: Trial of electrical direct-current therapy versus escitalopram for depression. N Engl J Med 376(26):2523–2533, 2017 28657871

Charney DS, Nelson JC: Delusional and nondelusional unipolar depression: further evidence for distinct subtypes. Am J Psychiatry 138(3):328–333, 1981 6110345

Center for Behavioral Health Statistics and Quality: Results from the 2017 National Survey on Drug Use and Health: Detailed Tables. Rockville, MD, Substance Abuse and Mental Health Services Administration, Center for Behavioral Health Statistics and Quality, September 7, 2018. Available at: https://www.samhsa.gov/data/sites/default/files/cbhsq-reports/NSDUHDetailedTabs2017/NSDUHDetailedTabs2017.pdf. Accessed October 26, 2021.

Coenen VA, Bewernick BH, Kayser S, et al: Superolateral medial forebrain bundle deep brain stimulation in major depression: a gateway trial. Neuropsychopharmacology 44(7):1224–1232, 2019 30867553

Cohen BM, Sommer BR, Vuckovic A: Antidepressant-resistant depression in patients with comorbid subclinical hypothyroidism or high-normal TSH levels. Am J Psychiatry 175(7):598–604, 2018 29961367

Connolly KR, Thase ME: If at first you don't succeed: a review of the evidence for antidepressant augmentation, combination and switching strategies. Drugs 71(1):43–64, 2011 21175239

Conway CR, George MS, Sackeim HA: Toward an evidence-based, operational definition of treatment-resistant depression: when enough is enough. JAMA Psychiatry 74(1):9–10, 2017 27784055

Coplan JD, Aaronson CJ, Panthangi V, et al: Treating comorbid anxiety and depression: Psychosocial and pharmacological approaches. World J Psychiatry 5(4):366–378, 2015 26740928

Correa R, Akiskal H, Gilmer W, et al: Is unrecognized bipolar disorder a frequent contributor to apparent treatment resistant depression? J Affect Disord 127(1–3):10–18, 2010 20655113
Cretaz E, Brunoni AR, Lafer B: Magnetic seizure therapy for unipolar and bipolar depression: a systematic review. Neural Plast 2015:521398, 2015 26075100
Daly EJ, Trivedi MH, Janik A, et al: Efficacy of esketamine nasal spray plus oral antidepressant treatment for relapse prevention in patients with treatment-resistant depression: a randomized clinical trial. JAMA Psychiatry 76(9):893–903, 2019 31166571
Deligiannidis KM, Meltzer-Brody S, Gunduz-Bruce H, et al: Effect of zuranolone vs placebo in postpartum depression: a randomized clinical trial. JAMA Psychiatry 78(9):951–959, 2021 34190962
Dold M, Kasper S: Evidence-based pharmacotherapy of treatment-resistant unipolar depression. Int J Psychiatry Clin Pract 21(1):13–23, 2017 27848269
Drobisz D, Damborská A: Deep brain stimulation targets for treating depression. Behav Brain Res 359:266–273, 2019 30414974
Fava M, Davidson KG: Definition and epidemiology of treatment-resistant depression. Psychiatr Clin North Am 19(2):179–200, 1996 8827185
Fava M, Rush AJ, Wisniewski SR, et al: A comparison of mirtazapine and nortriptyline following two consecutive failed medication treatments for depressed outpatients: a STAR*D report. Am J Psychiatry 163(7):1161–1172, 2006 16816220
Fava M, Rush AJ, Alpert JE, et al: Difference in treatment outcome in outpatients with anxious versus nonanxious depression: a STAR*D report. Am J Psychiatry 165(3):342–351, 2008 18172020
Fedgchin M, Trivedi M, Daly EJ, et al: Efficacy and safety of fixed-dose esketamine nasal spray combined with a new oral antidepressant in treatment-resistant depression: results of a randomized, double-blind, active-controlled study (TRANSFORM-1). Int J Neuropsychopharmacol 22(10):616–630, 2019 31290965
Filipčić I, Šimunović Filipčić I, Milovac Ž, et al: Efficacy of repetitive transcranial magnetic stimulation using a figure-8-coil or an H1-coil in treatment of major depressive disorder: a randomized clinical trial. J Psychiatr Res 114:113–119, 2019 31059991
Filkowski MM, Sheth SA: Deep brain stimulation for depression: an emerging indication. Neurosurg Clin N Am 30(2):243–256, 2019 30898275
Gaynes BN, Warden D, Trivedi MH, et al: What did STAR*D teach us? Results from a large-scale, practical, clinical trial for patients with depression. Psychiatr Serv 60(11):1439–1445, 2009 19880458
Gerhard T, Akincigil A, Correll CU, et al: National trends in second-generation antipsychotic augmentation for nonpsychotic depression. J Clin Psychiatry 75(5):490–497, 2014 24500284
Gerring ZF, Gamazon ER, Derks EM: A gene co-expression network-based analysis of multiple brain tissues reveals novel genes and molecular pathways underlying major depression. PLoS Genet 15(7):e1008245, 2019 31306407
Greden JF, Parikh SV, Rothschild AJ, et al: Impact of pharmacogenomics on clinical outcomes in major depressive disorder in the GUIDED trial: a large, patient- and rater-blinded, randomized, controlled study. J Psychiatr Res 111:59–67, 2019 30677646
Greenberg PE, Fournier AA, Sisitsky T, et al: The economic burden of adults with major depressive disorder in the United States (2005 and 2010). J Clin Psychiatry 76(2):155–162, 2015 25742202
Grof P, Müller-Oerlinghausen B: A critical appraisal of lithium's efficacy and effectiveness: the last 60 years. Bipolar Disord 11 (suppl 2):10–19, 2009 19538682
Guzzetta F, Tondo L, Centorrino F, et al: Lithium treatment reduces suicide risk in recurrent major depressive disorder. J Clin Psychiatry 68(3):380–383, 2007 17388706
Holtzheimer PE, Husain MM, Lisanby SH, et al: Subcallosal cingulate deep brain stimulation for treatment-resistant depression: a multisite, randomised, sham-controlled trial. Lancet Psychiatry 4(11):839–849, 2017 28988904
Howard DM, Adams MJ, Clarke TK, et al: Genome-wide meta-analysis of depression identifies 102 independent variants and highlights the importance of the prefrontal brain regions. Nat Neurosci 22(3):343–352, 2019 30718901

Institute for Clinical and Economic Review: Esketamine for the treatment of treatment-resistant depression: effectiveness and value: evidence report. May 9, 2019. Available at: icer.org/wp-content/uploads/2020/10/ICER_TRD_Evidence_Report_050919.pdf. Accessed December 16, 2020.

JAMA: Brexanolone (Zulresso) for postpartum depression. JAMA 322(1):73–74, 2019 31265098

Kanes SJ, Colquhoun H, Doherty J, et al: Open-label, proof-of-concept study of brexanolone in the treatment of severe postpartum depression. Hum Psychopharmacol 32(2):e2576, 2017a 28370307

Kanes S, Colquhoun H, Gunduz-Bruce H, et al: Brexanolone (SAGE-547 injection) in post-partum depression: a randomised controlled trial. Lancet 390(10093):480–489, 2017b 28619476

Kellner CH, Greenberg RM, Murrough JW, et al: ECT in treatment-resistant depression. Am J Psychiatry 169(12):1238–1244, 2012 23212054

Kennedy SH, Lam RW, McIntyre RS, et al: Canadian Network for Mood and Anxiety Treatments (CANMAT) 2016 clinical guidelines for the management of adults with major depressive disorder: Section 3. Pharmacological treatments. Can J Psychiatry 61(9):540–560, 2016 27486148

Kessler D, Burns A, Tallon D, et al: Combining mirtazapine with SSRIs or SNRIs for treatment-resistant depression: the MIR RCT. Health Technol Assess 22(63):1–136, 2018 30468145

Kishi T, Sakuma K, Nomura I, et al: Brexpiprazole as adjunctive treatment for major depressive disorder following treatment failure with at least one antidepressant in the current episode: a systematic review and meta-analysis. Int J Neuropsychopharmacol 22(11):698–709, 2019 31350882

Kleeblatt J, Betzler F, Kilarski LL, et al: Efficacy of off-label augmentation in unipolar depression: a systematic review of the evidence. Eur Neuropsychopharmacol 27(5):423–441, 2017 28318897

Kornstein SG, Schneider RK: Clinical features of treatment-resistant depression. J Clin Psychiatry 62 (suppl 16):18–25, 2001 11480880

Liebowitz MR, Quitkin FM, Stewart JW, et al: Antidepressant specificity in atypical depression. Arch Gen Psychiatry 45(2):129–137, 1988 3276282

Lisanby SH: Update on magnetic seizure therapy: a novel form of convulsive therapy. J ECT 18(4):182–188, 2002 12468992

Marjoribanks J, Brown J, O'Brien PM, et al: Selective serotonin reuptake inhibitors for premenstrual syndrome. Cochrane Database Syst Rev (6):CD001396, 2013 23744611

Maruani J, Geoffroy PA: Bright light as a personalized precision treatment of mood disorders. Front Psychiatry 10:85, 2019 30881318

McClintock SM, Reti IM, Carpenter LL, et al: Consensus recommendations for the clinical application of repetitive transcranial magnetic stimulation (rTMS) in the treatment of depression. J Clin Psychiatry 79(1):16cs10905, 2018 28541649

Meltzer-Brody S, Colquhoun H, Riesenberg R, et al: Brexanolone injection in post-partum depression: two multicentre, double-blind, randomised, placebo-controlled, phase 3 trials. Lancet 392(10152):1058–1070, 2018 30177236

Milev RV, Giacobbe P, Kennedy SH, et al: Canadian Network for Mood and Anxiety Treatments (CANMAT) 2016 clinical guidelines for the management of adults with major depressive disorder: Section 4. Neurostimulation treatments. Can J Psychiatry 61(9):561–575, 2016 27486154

Nelson JC, Baumann P, Delucchi K, et al: A systematic review and meta-analysis of lithium augmentation of tricyclic and second generation antidepressants in major depression. J Affect Disord 168:269–275, 2014 25069082

Newport DJ, Carpenter LL, McDonald WM, et al: Ketamine and other NMDA antagonists: early clinical trials and possible mechanisms in depression. Am J Psychiatry 172(10):950–966, 2015 26423481

Ochs-Ross R, Daly EJ, Zhang Y, et al: Efficacy and safety of esketamine nasal spray plus an oral antidepressant in elderly patients with treatment-resistant depression—TRANSFORM-3. Am J Geriatr Psychiatry 28(2):121–141, 2020 31734084

Papakostas GI, Fava M, Thase ME: Treatment of SSRI-resistant depression: a meta-analysis comparing within- versus across-class switches. Biol Psychiatry 63(7):699–704, 2008 17919460

Perugi G, Medda P, Zanello S, et al: Episode length and mixed features as predictors of ECT nonresponse in patients with medication-resistant major depression. Brain Stimul 5(1):18–24, 2012 22037132

Petrides G, Fink M, Husain MM, et al: ECT remission rates in psychotic versus nonpsychotic depressed patients: a report from CORE. J ECT 17(4):244–253, 2001 11731725

Phillips JL, Norris S, Talbot J, et al: Single, repeated, and maintenance ketamine infusions for treatment-resistant depression: a randomized controlled trial. Am J Psychiatry 176(5):401–409, 2019 30922101

Popova V, Daly EJ, Trivedi M, et al: Efficacy and safety of flexibly dosed esketamine nasal spray combined with a newly initiated oral antidepressant in treatment-resistant depression: a randomized double-blind active-controlled study. Am J Psychiatry 176(6):428–438, 2019 31109201

Rapaport MH: Translating the evidence on atypical depression into clinical practice. J Clin Psychiatry 68(4):e11, 2007 17474801

Ren J, Li H, Palaniyappan L, et al: Repetitive transcranial magnetic stimulation versus electroconvulsive therapy for major depression: a systematic review and meta-analysis. Prog Neuropsychopharmacol Biol Psychiatry 51:181–189, 2014 24556538

Rush AJ, Trivedi MH, Wisniewski SR, et al: Acute and longer-term outcomes in depressed outpatients requiring one or several treatment steps: a STAR*D report. Am J Psychiatry 163(11):1905–1917, 2006a 17074942

Rush AJ, Trivedi MH, Wisniewski SR, et al: Bupropion-SR, sertraline, or venlafaxine-XR after failure of SSRIs for depression. N Engl J Med 354(12):1231–1242, 2006b 16554525

Rush AJ, Wisniewski SR, Warden D, et al: Selecting among second-step antidepressant medication monotherapies: predictive value of clinical, demographic, or first-step treatment features. Arch Gen Psychiatry 65(8):870–880, 2008 18678792

Rush AJ, Trivedi MH, Stewart JW, et al: Combining medications to enhance depression outcomes (CO-MED): acute and long-term outcomes of a single-blind randomized study. Am J Psychiatry 168(7):689–701, 2011 21536692

Sanacora G, Frye MA, McDonald W, et al; American Psychiatric Association (APA) Council of Research Task Force on Novel Biomarkers and Treatments: A consensus statement on the use of ketamine in the treatment of mood disorders. JAMA Psychiatry 74(4):399–405, 2017 28249076

Schatzberg AF: A word to the wise about intranasal esketamine. Am J Psychiatry 176(6):422–424, 2019 31109197

Shiozawa P, Fregni F, Benseñor IM, et al: Transcranial direct current stimulation for major depression: an updated systematic review and meta-analysis. Int J Neuropsychopharmacol 17(9):1443–1452, 2014 24713139

Shulman KI, Fischer HD, Herrmann N, et al: Current prescription patterns and safety profile of irreversible monoamine oxidase inhibitors: a population-based cohort study of older adults. J Clin Psychiatry 70(12):1681–1686, 2009 19852903

Spielmans GI, Berman MI, Linardatos E, et al: Adjunctive atypical antipsychotic treatment for major depressive disorder: a meta-analysis of depression, quality of life, and safety outcomes. PLoS Med 10(3):e1001403, 2013 23554581

Stagg CJ, Nitsche MA: Physiological basis of transcranial direct current stimulation. Neuroscientist 17(1):37–53, 2011 21343407

Stewart JW, McGrath PJ, Blondeau C, et al: Combination antidepressant therapy for major depressive disorder: speed and probability of remission. J Psychiatr Res 52:7–14, 2014 24485847

Thase ME: The role of monoamine oxidase inhibitors in depression treatment guidelines. J Clin Psychiatry 73 (suppl 1):10–16, 2012 22951237

Thase ME, Trivedi MH, Rush AJ: MAOIs in the contemporary treatment of depression. Neuropsychopharmacology 12(3):185–219, 1995 7612154

Thase ME, Greenhouse JB, Frank E, et al: Treatment of major depression with psychotherapy or psychotherapy-pharmacotherapy combinations. Arch Gen Psychiatry 54(11):1009–1015, 1997 9366657

Trivedi RB, Nieuwsma JA, Williams JW Jr: Examination of the utility of psychotherapy for patients with treatment resistant depression: a systematic review. J Gen Intern Med 26(6):643–650, 2011 21184287

Tundo A, Filippis R, Proietti L: Pharmacological approaches to treatment resistant depression: evidences and personal experience. World J Psychiatry 5(3):330–341, 2015 26425446

Tundo A, de Filippis R, De Crescenzo F: Pramipexole in the treatment of unipolar and bipolar depression. A systematic review and meta-analysis. Acta Psychiatr Scand 140(2):116–125, 2019 31111467

Turner EH: Esketamine for treatment-resistant depression: seven concerns about efficacy and FDA approval. Lancet Psychiatry 6(12):977–979, 2019 31680014

U.S. Food and Drug Administration: Psychopharmacologic Drugs Advisory Committee (PDAC) and Drug Safety and Risk Management (DSaRM) Advisory Committee Meeting. Agenda topic: the committees will discuss the efficacy, safety, and risk-benefit profile of New Drug Application (NDA) 211243, esketamine 28 mg single-use nasal spray device, submitted by Janssen Pharmaceuticals, Inc., for the treatment of treatment-resistant depression. FDA Briefing Document, February 12, 2019a. Available at: https://www.fda.gov/media/121376/download. Accessed December 16, 2020.

U.S. Food and Drug Administration: FDA issues warning letter to genomics lab for illegally marketing genetic test that claims to predict patients' responses to specific medications. FDA News Release, April 04, 2019b. Available at: https://www.fda.gov/news-events/press-announcements/fda-issues-warning-letter-genomics-lab-illegally-marketing-genetic-test-claims-predict-patients. Accessed January 23, 2022.

van der Linden GGH, Lochmann van Bennekom MWH, Spijker J: Prevalence and recognition of bipolarity in patients with a treatment-resistant depressive disorder: a systematic review [in Dutch]. Tijdschr Psychiatr 61(2):104–111, 2019 30793271

Wang Y: Transcranial direct current stimulation for the treatment of major depressive disorder: a meta-analysis of randomized controlled trials. Psychiatry Res 276:186–190, 2019 31100509

Widge AS, Malone DA Jr, Dougherty DD: Closing the loop on deep brain stimulation for treatment-resistant depression. Front Neurosci 12:175, 2018 29618967

Wiles N, Thomas L, Abel A, et al: Clinical effectiveness and cost-effectiveness of cognitive behavioural therapy as an adjunct to pharmacotherapy for treatment-resistant depression in primary care: the CoBalT randomised controlled trial. Health Technol Assess 18(31):1–167, vii–viii, 2014 24824481

Williams NR, Heifets BD, Blasey C, et al: Attenuation of antidepressant effects of ketamine by opioid receptor antagonism. Am J Psychiatry 175(12):1205–1215, 2018 30153752

World Health Organization: Depression (fact sheet). 13 September 2021. Available at: https://www.who.int/news-room/fact-sheets/detail/depression. Accessed December 12, 2021.

Xu Y, Hackett M, Carter G, et al: Effects of low-dose and very low-dose ketamine among patients with major depression: a systematic review and meta-analysis. Int J Neuropsychopharmacol 19(4):pyv124, 2016 26578082

Yatham LN, Kennedy SH, Parikh SV, et al: Canadian Network for Mood and Anxiety Treatments (CANMAT) and International Society for Bipolar Disorders (ISBD) 2018 guidelines for the management of patients with bipolar disorder. Bipolar Disord 20(2):97–170, 2018 29536616

Zeier Z, Carpenter LL, Kalin NH, et al: Clinical implementation of pharmacogenetic decision support tools for antidepressant drug prescribing. Am J Psychiatry 175(9):873–886, 2018 29690793

Zhou X, Keitner GI, Qin B, et al: Atypical antipsychotic augmentation for treatment-resistant depression: a systematic review and network meta-analysis. Int J Neuropsychopharmacol 18(11):pyv060, 2015a 26012350

Zhou X, Ravindran AV, Qin B, et al: Comparative efficacy, acceptability, and tolerability of augmentation agents in treatment-resistant depression: systematic review and network meta-analysis. J Clin Psychiatry 76(4):e487–e498, 2015b 25919841

PART VII

Subtypes of Mood Disorders

CHAPTER 34

Seasonal Affective Disorder and Light Therapy

Norman E. Rosenthal, M.D.
Dan A. Oren, M.D.

Seasonal affective disorder (SAD) was first described in the mid-1980s (Rosenthal et al. 1984). Patients with SAD report a close relationship between their mood changes and the changing seasons. Typically, depressive episodes occur regularly in autumn and winter and respond when patients with SAD are exposed to bright environmental light. Later, a summer version of SAD was described by two groups (Boyce and Parker 1988; Wehr et al. 1991). In this chapter, the term *SAD* is used to describe winter SAD, and the summer version is referred to as *summer SAD*. We also discuss a milder version of SAD, often termed *subsyndromal SAD* (Kasper et al. 1989a). This condition is also known as "winter blues." We deal with the clinical and epidemiological features of SAD in adults, children, and adolescents and its treatments.

Bright light therapy (BLT), which is a first-line treatment for SAD (Lam and Levitt 1999), has also been found to be useful for nonseasonal depression (Golden et al. 2005), including major depressive disorder (MDD) and bipolar depression (Lam et al. 2016). We discuss the use of BLT for these conditions.

Diagnosis of Seasonal Affective Disorder

Shortly after SAD was defined, the diagnosis entered the next edition of DSM, DSM-III-R (American Psychiatric Association 1987), as MDD "with seasonal pattern," an adjectival modifier designed to enable seasonality to be incorporated alongside any

TABLE 34–1. Side-by-side comparison of original seasonal affective disorder (SAD) criteria and DSM-5 specifier "with seasonal pattern" criteria

SAD criteria of Rosenthal et al. 1984	DSM-5 criteria for major depressive disorder "with seasonal pattern"
A pattern of winter depressions, at least two of which developed during consecutive winters.	A regular temporal relationship between the onset of major depressive episodes and a particular time of the year (e.g., fall or winter).
At least one of these depressions was severe enough to meet the criteria for major depression.	In the past 2 years, two major depressive episodes have occurred that demonstrate the temporal seasonal relationships defined above, and no nonseasonal major depressive episodes have occurred during the same period.
Nondepressed periods in spring and summer.	Full remissions (or a change from major depressive disorder to mania or hypomania) also occur at a characteristic time of the year (e.g., depression disappears in the spring).
No other major psychiatric disorder present.	Seasonal major depressive episodes (as described above) substantially outnumber the nonseasonal major depressive episodes that may have occurred over the individual's lifetime.
No clear-cut recurring social or psychological reasons to account for the recurrent winter depression.	No obvious effect of season-related psychosocial stressors (e.g., regularly being unemployed every winter).
Source. Rosenthal et al. 1984.	*Source.* American Psychiatric Association 2013.

recurrent mood disorder. "Seasonal pattern" has not been enthusiastically embraced by the field, which has generally preferred the diagnosis of SAD, as have those diagnosed with the condition. Nevertheless, the adjectival modifier has proven extremely durable among classifying committees, which have passed it down from one generation to the next despite vigorous arguments to the contrary (Rosenthal 2009). The original criteria for SAD are shown in Table 34–1 alongside the DSM-5 (American Psychiatric Association 2013) version of the MDD specifier "with seasonal pattern."

Criteria for summer SAD have been loosely based on those for winter SAD, but the paucity of systematic studies on this condition make these criteria more theoretical than data-based. Criteria for subsyndromal winter SAD, colloquially known as "the winter blues" were defined as regularly occurring winter difficulties that fall short of prompting those with the condition to seek medical help (Kasper et al. 1989a).

Clinical and Demographic Profiles

The clinical and demographic features of SAD for 662 patients that we studied at the National Institute of Mental Health (NIMH) between 1981 and 2001 are shown in Tables 34–2 and 34–3.

As shown in the tables, over the 20 years during which the NIMH seasonality program operated, averages indicated that people with SAD presented more often in

TABLE 34–2. Demographic and clinical features of seasonal affective disorder, National Institute of Mental Health, 1981–2001 (*N*=662)

Age (years)	38.8±9.8
Age of onset (years)	23.3±10.5 (*N*=495)
Sex ratio (female:male)	3.1:1 (502:160)
Length of depressive episodes (months)	4.9±1.4
Psychiatric diagnosis (% of patients)	
Bipolar II	34%
Bipolar I	5%
Major depressive disorder	61%
Family history (more than one affected first-degree relative)	
Major depressive disorder	46%
Seasonal affective disorder	19%
Substance abuse	38%

TABLE 34–3. Winter symptoms of seasonal affective disorder, National Institute of Mental Health Seasonal Studies Program, 1981–2001 (*N*=662)

Symptom	Percentage
Decreased activity	96
Affect	
Sadness	96
Anxiety	86
Appetite	
Increased	65
Decreased	15
Carbohydrate craving	70
Weight	
Increase	74
Decrease	7
Decreased libido	68
Sleep: increased duration	76
Menstrual difficulties	66
Work difficulties	84
Symptoms better nearer equator	94

their late 30s, with a reported onset of the illness in their early 20s. They had experienced seasonal mood changes for more than 15 years before presenting for treatment. One can only hope that with the spread of knowledge about the condition in recent decades, current and future patients will not have to wait so long to be diagnosed with SAD and treated accordingly. As Table 34–2 shows, women with SAD outnumber men by about three to one, a preponderance that has been found elsewhere in the literature (Modell et al. 2005). The reported average duration of depression was about 5 months. Most patients with SAD have recurrent MDD, although some suffer from bipolar disorder, with bipolar II disorder being more common than bipolar I disorder.

People with SAD typically report onset of their fall-winter symptoms as the days get shorter and darker. Although days become longer after the winter solstice in December, symptoms often worsen in January and February, which tend to be cloudy months in the northern hemisphere. *Paradoxically, the severity of SAD symptoms may correlate more closely with the lack of environmental light than with the length of day.* This is important for patients and clinicians to remember in order to recognize and properly treat SAD symptoms that arise unexpectedly at atypical times of year. A case in point would be midsummer, when people may be staying indoors with their blinds drawn to escape the heat only to fall prey to the depressing effects of poorly lit interiors. Likewise, erratic weather in the spring may result in unexpected mood swings at a time when days are rapidly getting longer. Despite these exceptions, mood and energy generally improve in the summer.

As seen in Table 34–3, people with SAD generally develop atypical vegetative symptoms of depression—increased appetite, carbohydrate craving, weight gain, and increased sleep duration—along with depression and anxiety. Often, vegetative symptoms occur early in the course of the illness, followed by depression, anxiety, and difficulties at work and interpersonally. SAD has also been reported in children and adolescents (Rosenthal et al. 1986) and appears to persist over time (Giedd et al. 1998) and continue to respond to light therapy.

Epidemiology

Most epidemiological studies of SAD have used the Seasonal Pattern Assessment Questionnaire (SPAQ) (Hardin et al. 1991; Rosenthal 2013). Using the SPAQ, Kasper et al. (1989b) found the prevalence of SAD in Montgomery County, Maryland, to be 4.3%. Using Kasper's criteria, the NIMH group (Rosen et al. 1990) estimated the prevalence of SAD and subsyndromal SAD in locations at four different latitudes: Sarasota, Florida (27°N), Montgomery County, Maryland (39°N), New York City (40°N), and Nashua, New Hampshire (42°N). The researchers found the estimated prevalence of SAD to be 1.4%, 6.3%, 4.7%, and 9.7%, respectively; for subsyndromal SAD, the prevalences were 2.6%, 10.4%, 12.5%, and 11.0%, respectively. Thus, they found a correlation between latitude and prevalence of winter depressive symptoms. This correlation increased when SAD and subsyndromal SAD were combined, underscoring the fact that these are two arbitrary categories of severity on a continuum of seasonal variation seen in the general population.

The SPAQ has also been used in Europe, Japan, and China. Results in European countries have yielded prevalence estimates comparable with those in the United States (Magnússon 1996, 2000; Magnússon et al. 1997). An outlier was Iceland, where prevalence rates were considerably lower despite the high latitude (Magnússon and Stefánsson 1993). Magnússon found that Canadian immigrants of Icelandic origin also had lower-than-expected rates of SAD and subsyndromal SAD. They suggested that this may reflect a genetic protection against SAD in the small and homogeneous population of Icelanders (Magnússon and Axelsson 1993). Rates of winter SAD in studies conducted Japan (Ozaki et al. 1995) and China (Han et al. 2000) were lower than those at comparable latitudes in the United States, but the reverse was true in both those countries for summer SAD.

The SPAQ was later modified for use in middle- and high-school children (Rosenthal 2013; Swedo et al. 1995) to assess the prevalence of SAD in these age groups in Maryland middle and high schools (Swedo et al. 1995). Overall, the estimated rate of SAD was 3%, which is comparable with the estimated rate of attention-deficit disorder in a similar population. The rate of SAD increased with age, so that by the senior year of high school it was 5%, roughly equivalent to the prevalence in the adult population at the same latitude. The researchers estimated the effects of puberty on rates of SAD and found an approximately threefold increase in the rate of SAD in girls after puberty compared with before, but no analogous sudden increase in boys. This suggests that some aspect of mature female physiology is associated with the increased prevalence of SAD among women.

Light Therapy

BLT is regarded by researchers in the field as the first-line treatment for SAD (Wirz-Justice 2016). Many studies of light therapy have been modeled on the initial published paradigm (Rosenthal et al. 1984) and have focused on establishing the efficacy of the treatment, as well as the formal properties that modify efficacy. A PubMed search using the terms "light therapy" and "seasonal affective disorder" yielded 790 publications. We cite just a small percentage of these, which either were of landmark significance or expanded our understanding of mechanisms underlying efficacy.

Efficacy

After the initial positive study of light therapy for SAD, several replication studies followed from the NIMH group (Rosenthal et al. 1985) and others in Portland, Oregon (Lewy et al. 1988), New York City (Terman et al. 1989b), and elsewhere. The question of a possible placebo effect, most eloquently articulated by Eastman et al. (1992), remained an outstanding question until Eastman herself came up with a placebo condition that satisfied most other workers in the field: an inactivated negative ion generator. In a curious aside, when functioning ion generators were later used as a control treatment for light therapy, Terman and Terman (1995) found negative ions to have antidepressant effects. Using an *inactivated* negative ion generator as a control, Eastman et al. (1998) replicated the efficacy of BLT; this research, along with two other publications in *Archives of General Psychiatry* (now *JAMA Psychiatry*) (Lewy et al. 1998; Terman et al. 1998), paved the way for the general acceptance of BLT as an effective treatment for SAD, a conclusion also reached in a later meta-analysis (Golden et al. 2005).

A series of light therapy studies followed, whose goal was to investigate what formal elements of light therapy were necessary or optimal for achieving a therapeutic effect. These properties involved 1) intensity, 2) time of administration, 3) anatomical pathways involved, and 4) wavelength. We discuss each in turn.

Intensity

The earliest studies of BLT for SAD involved the use of 2,500 lux, which was the intensity that Lewy et al. (1980) found sufficient to suppress melatonin secretion in humans. Terman et al. (1990) went on to study light of higher intensity (10,000 lux), which is roughly equivalent to the intensity of light from the sun cresting the horizon on a summer day. These researchers found that light at the higher intensity was more effective and therefore allowed for shorter durations of administration than the durations used in the earlier studies at the lower intensity. Following the success of these higher-intensity studies, the brighter (10,000 lux) treatments became the clinical standard.

Time of Day

Lewy et al. (1998) first emphasized the superiority of light therapy administered in the morning versus the evening (Sack et al. 1990), a finding replicated by Terman et al. (1998). This led to the general recommendation that patients with SAD begin treatment with morning BLT. Nevertheless, BLT can also be effective in the evening (James et al. 1985; Terman et al. 1998) and may even be effective when administered at midday (Jacobsen et al. 1987). In practice, BLT is often used at various times of the day if morning BLT is insufficient.

Anatomical Pathways Involved

Although researchers suspected that the benefits of light therapy for SAD were mediated via the eyes, not the skin, Wehr et al. (1987) put the question to the test by comparing these two modes of administration in a crossover study. As expected from extensive prior chronobiological studies in animals, the eyes had it, from which researchers concluded that BLT for SAD is mediated via the eyes. This does not exclude the possibility that sunlight might also have effects on mood mediated via the skin, perhaps by the activation of melanocytes, which are known to secrete beta-endorphin under the influence of ultraviolet (UV) light (Jussila et al. 2016).

Wavelength

The earliest studies of BLT involved "full-spectrum" fluorescent light (roughly equivalent to the spectrum of sunlight), raising the question of whether this particular spectrum was necessary for efficacy. Later studies used fluorescent bulbs that had the spectrum of ordinary office lighting (less blue than full spectrum) and seemed to produce results of comparable efficacy. Although no formal studies compared these two similar wavelengths, a consensus emerged in the field that full-spectrum light was not necessary. Likewise, screens that filtered out most UV light produced good results and became standard, yielding a consensus in the field that UV light was also unnecessary for the efficacy of BLT. Further studies of efficacy of different wavelengths revealed that green light was superior to red (Oren et al. 1991), as was blue light (Glickman et al. 2006).

Dawn Simulation

Based on studies of human circadian system responses to cycles of light and dark, Terman et al. (1989a) hypothesized that exposing people with SAD to a slowly increasing light environment at dawn before they wake up would have antidepressant effects. Avery et al. (1993, 1994) followed up on this hypothesis and found in controlled studies that exposing patients with SAD to a light stimulus that slowly increased to 250 lux had antidepressant effects and helped them feel more alert during the day. This led to the production of commercially available dawn simulators that increase ambient light gradually in the morning before wakeup time and are a useful supplementary treatment for people with SAD.

Constructing a Light Therapy Program for Patients With SAD

Although each patient is different, the following are some general guidelines for constructing a light therapy program. *All measures outlined here may also be helpful for people with subsyndromal SAD (the winter blues).*

1. *Discuss improving your patient's general light environment.* Not all therapeutic light should come from a box. Encourage walking outdoors, especially in the morning, which has been shown by Wirz-Justice et al. (1996) to have antidepressant effects. Even on a winter day, much light can be enjoyed from a cloudy sky, not to mention reflection off the snow-covered ground. The combination of exercise plus light seems to have synergistic effects.
2. When choosing a light box, encourage the patient to use the type of fixture that has been tested and found to be effective in most research studies. Authors of a recent study evaluating light produced by various commercially available devices warned that many models on the market may not meet research-supported specifications (Oldham et al. 2019). In practice, this means obtaining a fixture from an established manufacturer in which white fluorescent lights emit approximately 10,000 lux at a specified distance through a plastic diffusing screen that includes a UV light filter. Light therapy boxes used in most research studies conducted to date have an illuminated surface area of at least 1 square foot. Although the question of surface area has not specifically been tested, clinical impressions suggest that light fixtures with larger illuminated surface areas are generally better than those with smaller ones. If the surface area is small, it can be expected to irradiate a smaller area of the retina and can also be less forgiving of head movements that result in variable illuminance.

   Smaller fixtures, including those that have white light–emitting diodes (LEDs) embedded in plastic that diffuses light across the irradiating surface, have become popular because of their lower cost, greater portability, and ease of use since they fit more easily into small spaces. Many patients report benefits from these boxes, although those with more severe SAD and veteran light box users often prefer the larger boxes. In time, we expect that larger light fixtures using LED sources will be developed and be useful.

   Be sure to remind patients that most manufacturers allow light fixtures to be returned for some time after purchase. It is therefore important to keep the box and packaging. These tips are often helpful in allaying anxiety about the cost of light fixtures because, in practice, they allow people a free trial.

Light Therapy for Other Types of Depression

Perhaps the most common misconception about the antidepressant effects of light is that they are confined to people with SAD or seasonal exacerbations of their mood disorder. In fact, light therapy has been found to be effective for many types of depression other than SAD. This misconception is unfortunate because light therapy can easily be added to any other antidepressant treatment with salutary effects.

A meta-analysis by Golden et al. (2005) published in the *American Journal of Psychiatry* concluded that exposure to bright light is effective for nonseasonal depression. In the three studies of nonseasonal depression that they included in their meta-analysis, they found a modest effect size of 0.5, as compared with an effect size of 0.8 for seasonal depression. A more recent meta-analysis of nine trials by Al-Karawi and Jubair (2016) confirmed these earlier conclusions, finding an overall effect size of 0.62, which was higher when BLT was administered for 2–5 weeks (0.78) and when it was administered as monotherapy (0.71). A meta-analysis by Perera et al. (2016) also found significant evidence of light therapy's efficacy in nonseasonal depression. Other meta-analyses have examined this question and have reached negative conclusions. Such discrepancies are not uncommon in relation to meta-analyses, the outcomes of which depend heavily on the inclusion criteria. Yet the two meta-analyses cited here were well done, and their conclusions are in line with both clinical experience and the individual studies cited in the following discussion.

In a randomized controlled trial, Lam et al. (2016) studied the efficacy of BLT, fluoxetine, and the combination in patients with nonseasonal MDD. A total of 122 patients were randomly assigned to the following conditions: BLT alone, fluoxetine alone, fluoxetine plus BLT, and placebo. The mean changes in Montgomery-Åsberg Depression Rating Scale scores for the light, fluoxetine, combination, and placebo groups were 13.4, 8.8, 16.9, and 6.5, respectively. Effect sizes were 0.8, 0.24, 1.1, and 0.2, respectively. BLT and the combination were statistically superior to placebo, but fluoxetine was not. This well-designed study is particularly important because it involved people with nonseasonal MDD and was conducted at major academic centers by clinical researchers skilled in the use of both light therapy and antidepressant medications.

For readers who might like to replicate the exact parameters of light therapy used in this study, they are as follows: daily exposure to a fluorescent light box for 30 minutes as soon as possible after awakening, preferably between 7:00 A.M. and 8:00 A.M. (Carex Day-Light Classic, emitting 4,000 Kelvin white light rated at 10,000 lux, 36 cm from screen to cornea, with a UV filter). Patients used the light box at home and were given standardized verbal and written instructions.

One important difference between the response to BLT in people with SAD and those with nonseasonal depression is the time course of response. Whereas people with SAD typically respond to BLT within 2–4 days, those with nonseasonal depression have a time course response resembling that seen when they are treated with antidepressants, *namely 2–4 weeks*. It is therefore important when using BLT to treat nonseasonal depression to allow for this longer interval before expecting improvement and to manage the patient's expectations accordingly.

Light therapy might be of particular use for people in whom antidepressant medications are regarded as less desirable, such as the elderly, adolescents, and pregnant women. Regarding nonseasonal depression in the elderly, the best available meta-analysis of light therapy to date was conducted by Chang et al. (2018) in Taiwan. Out of eight trials that met inclusion criteria involving 395 participants, light therapy was significantly more effective than comparative treatments, including placebo or dim light (effect size 0.4). The results of this meta-analysis were essentially replicated by another meta-analysis conducted by Zhao et al. (2018) in mainland China. In a crossover study of 28 adolescents, Niederhofer and von Klitzing (2012) found that 1 hour of BLT (2,500 lux) for a week was superior to a dim light (50 lux) control. No significant adverse events were observed.

Regarding perinatal depression, Wirz-Justice et al. (2011) studied 27 pregnant women with nonseasonal MDD who were randomly assigned to BLT (7,000 lux white light) or placebo (70 lux dim red light) for 1 hour in the morning over 5 weeks. BLT improved depression scores significantly compared with placebo. Although this is the only controlled study published to date, given the presumed safety of light therapy for the fetus and the ease of administration and favorable side-effect profile for the mother, light therapy should certainly be considered for treating pregnant women with depression, seasonal or nonseasonal.

Recently, there have been favorable reports of the use of BLT for the treatment of bipolar depression. Sit et al. (2018) from the University of Pittsburgh found that bright white light therapy administered *at midday* adjunctively with an antimanic medication was significantly superior to a dim red light control in 46 people with bipolar depression. In their pilot work, these researchers found that light therapy in the morning, which has been the standard time of presentation for MDD (as opposed to bipolar disorder), seemed less helpful in bipolar disorder, paradoxically because of the risk of light therapy being "too effective" in the early morning and risking the induction of mania in this vulnerable population. These favorable results are consistent with a meta-analysis of light therapy for bipolar depression by Tseng et al. (2016) and a more recent one by Lam et al. (2020). These findings are especially significant because depression is a major problem for people with bipolar disorder, even those receiving excellent medical care.

Bright Light Augmentation of Antidepressant Treatment

Although meta-analyses have not substantiated the value of BLT as an augmentation strategy, clinical experience suggests that it is likely to be beneficial. This synergistic effect is supported by the findings of Lam et al. (2020) in nonseasonal depression and suggested by a controlled study of bright green light versus an inactive control in conjunction with antidepressants in MDD and bipolar disorder in a European study (Benedetti et al. 2003). Likewise, a Danish controlled trial yielded similar potentiating effects for bright white light versus dim red light (Martiny 2004). Given the favorable side-effect profile of BLT and the absence of drug interactions associated with this means of potentiation, light therapy should be high on a clinician's list for potentiating antidepressant responses in nonseasonal depression. It goes without saying that the same applies for MDD and bipolar disorder with winter exacerbations. Using mood stabilizers in conjunction with BLT is sensible when treating depressed patients with a history of mania.

Wake Therapy, Phase Advance, and Triple Chronotherapy

Sleep deprivation, also known these days as "wake therapy," has long been known to induce rapid antidepressant responses (Wirz-Justice and Van den Hoofdakker 1999). Unfortunately, remissions are generally short lived, and repeated sleep deprivation is unsustainable. Further research into this area has found that sleep deprivation in the *second* half of the night is most instrumental in the antidepressant effect. This line of research led Wehr et al. (1979) to test whether phase-advancing sleep (moving it earlier), even in the absence of sleep deprivation, might also induce antidepressant effects. They found this strategy, now known as *phase-advance treatment of depression,* to be effective in reversing depression. Partial sleep deprivation in the second half of the night has been combined in various ways with phase advancing of sleep and BLT administered in the morning, a composite treatment generally known as *triple chronotherapy.* Although it can be surprisingly effective in some people, in practice this treatment is difficult to implement and sustain. Humpston et al. (2020) conducted a meta-analysis of circadian manipulations, also known as *chronotherapy,* for depression, and those interested in learning more about this line of treatment can find further information in Wirz-Justice et al.'s (2013) *Chronotherapeutics for Affective Disorders: A Clinician's Manual for Light and Wake Therapy,* Second Revised Edition.

We have not addressed putative biological mechanisms by which BLT may regulate brain systems and circadian rhythms. These mechanisms are thought to be mediated via the retina, hypothalamic nuclei, and their connections to relevant mood-regulating centers.

Conclusion

In summary, SAD is a common condition that responds well to bright light therapy (BLT), environmental modification, CBT, stress reduction, and exercise. It is important to ask all patients with mood or energy problems about a history of seasonal variation in symptoms, or the diagnosis can easily be missed. A less severe variant of the condition, known as subsyndromal SAD or the winter blues, also responds to similar interventions.

BLT can also help people with nonseasonal depression (MDD or bipolar disorder) in many groups, including the young, the elderly, and pregnant women, both as a solo treatment and in conjunction with antidepressant medications. We have discussed those aspects of BLT that appear to be important for its therapeutic effects and provided practical advice about BLT administration. Because BLT has a favorable side-effect profile and does not interact adversely with other treatments, it deserves prominent consideration in a broad range of clinical situations.

References

Al-Karawi D, Jubair L: Bright light therapy for nonseasonal depression: meta-analysis of clinical trials. J Affect Disord 198:64–71, 2016 27011361

American Psychiatric Association: Diagnostic and Statistical Manual of Mental Disorders, 3rd Edition, Revised. Washington, DC, American Psychiatric Association, 1987

American Psychiatric Association: Diagnostic and Statistical Manual of Mental Disorders, 5th Edition. Arlington, VA, American Psychiatric Association, 2013

Avery DH, Bolte MA, Dager SR, et al: Dawn simulation treatment of winter depression: a controlled study. Am J Psychiatry 150(1):113–117, 1993 8417552

Avery DH, Bolte MA, Wolfson JK, et al: Dawn simulation compared with a dim red signal in the treatment of winter depression. Biol Psychiatry 36(3):180–188, 1994 7948455

Benedetti F, Colombo C, Pontiggia A, et al: Morning light treatment hastens the antidepressant effect of citalopram: a placebo-controlled trial. J Clin Psychiatry 64(6):648–653, 2003 12823078

Boyce P, Parker G: Seasonal affective disorder in the southern hemisphere. Am J Psychiatry 145(1):96–99, 1988 3422138

Center for Environmental Therapeutics: Automated Morningness-Eveningness Questionnaire (AutoMEQ). 2021. Available at: https://www.cet-surveys.com/index.php?sid=61524and-newtest=Y. Accessed August 25, 2021.

Chang CH, Liu CY, Chen SJ, et al: Efficacy of light therapy on nonseasonal depression among elderly adults: a systematic review and meta-analysis. Neuropsychiatr Dis Treat 14:3091–3102, 2018 30532540

Eastman CI, Lahmeyer HW, Watell LG, et al: A placebo-controlled trial of light treatment for winter depression. J Affect Disord 26(4):211–221, 1992 1479133

Eastman CI, Young MA, Fogg LF, et al: Bright light treatment of winter depression: a placebo-controlled trial. Arch Gen Psychiatry 55(10):883–889, 1998 9783558

Frandsen TB, Pareek M, Hansen JP, et al: Vitamin D supplementation for treatment of seasonal affective symptoms in healthcare professionals: a double-blind randomised placebo-controlled trial. BMC Res Notes 7:528, 2014 25125215

Giedd JN, Swedo SE, Lowe CH, et al: Case series: pediatric seasonal affective disorder. A follow-up report. J Am Acad Child Adolesc Psychiatry 37(2):218–220, 1998 9473919

Glickman G, Byrne B, Pineda C, et al: Light therapy for seasonal affective disorder with blue narrow-band light-emitting diodes (LEDs). Biol Psychiatry 59(6):502–507, 2006 16165105

Golden RN, Gaynes BN, Ekstrom RD, et al: The efficacy of light therapy in the treatment of mood disorders: a review and meta-analysis of the evidence. Am J Psychiatry 162(4):656–662, 2005 15800134

Han L, Wang K, Du Z, et al: Seasonal variations in mood and behavior among Chinese medical students. Am J Psychiatry 157(1):133–135, 2000 10618029

Hardin TA, Wehr TA, Brewerton T, et al: Evaluation of seasonality in six clinical populations and two normal populations. J Psychiatr Res 25(3):75–87, 1991 1941711

Humpston C, Benedetti F, Serfaty M, et al: Chronotherapy for the rapid treatment of depression: a meta-analysis. J Affect Disord 261:91–102, 2020 31606606

Jacobsen FM: Waking in a lighted room. Biol Psychiatry 27(3):372–374, 1990 2302443

Jacobsen FM, Wehr TA, Skwerer RA, et al: Morning versus midday phototherapy of seasonal affective disorder. Am J Psychiatry 144(10):1301–1305, 1987 3310669

James SP, Wehr TA, Sack DA, et al: Treatment of seasonal affective disorder with light in the evening. Br J Psychiatry 147:424–428, 1985 4075032

Jussila A, Huotari-Orava R, Ylianttila L, et al: Narrow-band ultraviolet B radiation induces the expression of beta-endorphin in human skin in vivo. J Photochem Photobiol B 155:104–108, 2016 26774381

Kasper S, Rogers SLB, Yancey A, et al: Phototherapy in individuals with and without subsyndromal seasonal affective disorder. Arch Gen Psychiatry 46(9):837–844, 1989a 2774849

Kasper S, Wehr TA, Bartko JJ, et al: Epidemiological findings of seasonal changes in mood and behavior. A telephone survey of Montgomery County, Maryland. Arch Gen Psychiatry 46(9):823–833, 1989b 2789026

Lam RW, Levitt AJ (eds): Canadian Consensus Guidelines for the Treatment of Seasonal Affective Disorder. Vancouver, BC, Clinical & Academic Publishing, 1999

Lam RW, Levitt AJ, Levitan RD, et al: Efficacy of bright light treatment, fluoxetine, and the combination in patients with nonseasonal major depressive disorder: a randomized clinical trial. JAMA Psychiatry 73(1):56–63, 2016 26580307

Lam RW, Teng MY, Jung YE, et al: Light therapy for patients with bipolar depression: systematic review and meta-analysis of randomized controlled trials. Can J Psychiatry 65(5):290–300, 2020 31826657

Lewy AJ, Wehr TA, Goodwin FK, et al: Light suppresses melatonin secretion in humans. Science 210(4475):1267–1269, 1980 7434030

Lewy AJ, Sack RL, Singer CM, et al: Winter depression and the phase-shift hypothesis for bright light's therapeutic effects: history, theory, and experimental evidence. J Biol Rhythms 3(2):121–134, 1988 2979635

Lewy AJ, Bauer VK, Cutler NL, et al: Morning vs evening light treatment of patients with winter depression. Arch Gen Psychiatry 55(10):890–896, 1998 9783559

Magnusson A: Validation of the Seasonal Pattern Assessment Questionnaire (SPAQ). J Affect Disord 40(3):121–129, 1996 8897111

Magnusson A: An overview of epidemiological studies on seasonal affective disorder. Acta Psychiatr Scand 101(3):176–184, 2000 10721866

Magnússon A, Axelsson J: The prevalence of seasonal affective disorder is low among descendants of Icelandic emigrants in Canada. Arch Gen Psychiatry 50(12):947–951, 1993 8250680

Magnússon A, Stefánsson JG: Prevalence of seasonal affective disorder in Iceland. Arch Gen Psychiatry 50(12):941–946, 1993 8250679

Magnusson A, Friis S, Opjordsmoen S: Internal consistency of the Seasonal Pattern Assessment Questionnaire (SPAQ). J Affect Disord 42(2–3):113–116, 1997 9105952

Martiny K: Adjunctive bright light in non-seasonal major depression. Acta Psychiatr Scand Suppl (425):7–28, 2004 15527426

Modell JG, Rosenthal NE, Harriett AE, et al: Seasonal affective disorder and its prevention by anticipatory treatment with bupropion XL. Biol Psychiatry 58(8):658–667, 2005 16271314

Niederhofer H, von Klitzing K: Bright light treatment as mono-therapy of non-seasonal depression for 28 adolescents. Int J Psychiatry Clin Pract 16(3):233–237, 2012 22809107

Oldham MA, Oldham MB, Desan PH: Commercially available phototherapy devices for treatment of depression: physical characteristics of emitted light. Psychiatric Research & Clinical Practice 1(2):49–57, 2019. Available at: https://onlinelibrary.wiley.com/doi/abs/10.1176/appi.prcp.2019.20180011. Accessed October 26, 2021.

Oren DA, Brainard GC, Johnston SH, et al: Treatment of seasonal affective disorder with green light and red light. Am J Psychiatry 148(4):509–511, 1991 2006698

Ozaki N, Ono Y, Ito A, et al: Prevalence of seasonal difficulties in mood and behavior among Japanese civil servants. Am J Psychiatry 152(8):1225–1227, 1995 7625479

Perera S, Eisen R, Bhatt M, et al: Light therapy for non-seasonal depression: systematic review and meta-analysis. BJPsych Open 2(2):116–126, 2016 27703764

Rohan KJ, Mahon JN, Evans M, et al: Randomized trial of cognitive-behavioral therapy versus light therapy for seasonal affective disorder: acute outcomes. Am J Psychiatry 172(9):862–869, 2015 25859764

Rosen LN, Targum SD, Terman M, et al: Prevalence of seasonal affective disorder at four latitudes. Psychiatry Res 31(2):131–144, 1990 2326393

Rosenthal NE: Issues for DSM-V: seasonal affective disorder and seasonality. Am J Psychiatry 166(8):852–853, 2009 19651748

Rosenthal NE: Winter Blues: Everything You Need to Know to Beat Seasonal Affective Disorder, 4th Edition. New York, Guilford, 2013, pp 52–58

Rosenthal NE, Sack DA, Gillin JC, et al: Seasonal affective disorder. A description of the syndrome and preliminary findings with light therapy. Arch Gen Psychiatry 41(1):72–80, 1984 6581756

Rosenthal NE, Sack DA, Carpenter CJ, et al: Antidepressant effects of light in seasonal affective disorder. Am J Psychiatry 142(2):163–170, 1985 3882000

Rosenthal NE, Carpenter CJ, James SP, et al: Seasonal affective disorder in children and adolescents. Am J Psychiatry 143(3):356–358, 1986 3953872

Sack RL, Lewy AJ, White DM, et al: Morning vs evening light treatment for winter depression. Evidence that the therapeutic effects of light are mediated by circadian phase shifts. Arch Gen Psychiatry 47(4):343–351, 1990 2322085

Sit DK, McGowan J, Wiltrout C, et al: Adjunctive bright light therapy for bipolar depression: a randomized double-blind placebo-controlled trial. Am J Psychiatry 175(2):131–139, 2018 28969438

Swedo SE, Pleeter JD, Richter DM, et al: Rates of seasonal affective disorder in children and adolescents. Am J Psychiatry 152(7):1016–1019, 1995 7793436

Swedo SE, Allen AJ, Glod CA, et al: A controlled trial of light therapy for the treatment of pediatric seasonal affective disorder. J Am Acad Child Adolesc Psychiatry 36(6):816–821, 1997 9183137

Terman JS, Terman M, Schlager D, et al: Efficacy of brief, intense light exposure for treatment of winter depression. Psychopharmacol Bull 26(1):3–11, 1990 2371371

Terman M, Terman JS: Treatment of seasonal affective disorder with a high-output negative ionizer. J Altern Complement Med 1(1):87–92, 1995 9395604

Terman M, Schlager D, Fairhurst S, et al: Dawn and dusk simulation as a therapeutic intervention. Biol Psychiatry 25(7):966–970, 1989a 2720008

Terman M, Terman JS, Quitkin FM, et al: Light therapy for seasonal affective disorder. A review of efficacy. Neuropsychopharmacology 2(1):1–22, 1989b 2679625

Terman M, Terman JS, Ross DC: A controlled trial of timed bright light and negative air ionization for treatment of winter depression. Arch Gen Psychiatry 55(10):875–882, 1998 9783557

Tseng PT, Chen YW, Tu KY, et al: Light therapy in the treatment of patients with bipolar depression: a meta-analytic study. Eur Neuropsychopharmacol 26(6):1037–1047, 2016 26993616

Vicente-Tejedor J, Marchena M, Ramírez L, et al: Removal of the blue component of light significantly decreases retinal damage after high intensity exposure. PLoS One 13(3):e0194218, 2018 29543853

Wehr TA, Wirz-Justice A, Goodwin FK, et al: Phase advance of the circadian sleep-wake cycle as an antidepressant. Science 206(4419):710–713, 1979 227056

Wehr TA, Skwerer RG, Jacobsen FM, et al: Eye versus skin phototherapy of seasonal affective disorder. Am J Psychiatry 144(6):753–757, 1987 3591996

Wehr TA, Giesen HA, Schulz PM, et al: Contrasts between symptoms of summer depression and winter depression. J Affect Disord 23(4):173–183, 1991 1791262

Wirz-Justice A: A history of light therapy (A65), in Abstracts of the Society for Light Treatment and Biological Rhythms 29th Annual Meeting, Berlin, June 23–25, 2017. Neuropsychobiology 74(4):255–256, 2016. Available at: https://www.karger.com/Article/Pdf/477426. Accessed July 6, 2021.

Wirz-Justice A, Van den Hoofdakker RH: Sleep deprivation in depression: what do we know, where do we go? Biol Psychiatry 46(4):445–453, 1999 10459393

Wirz-Justice A, Graw P, Kräuchi K, et al: "Natural" light treatment of seasonal affective disorder. J Affect Disord 37(2–3):109–120, 1996 8731073

Wirz-Justice A, Bader A, Frisch U, et al: A randomized, double-blind, placebo-controlled study of light therapy for antepartum depression. J Clin Psychiatry 72(7):986–993, 2011 21535997

Wirz-Justice A, Benedetti F, Terman M: Chronotherapeutics for Affective Disorders: Clinician's Manual for Light and Wake Therapy, 2nd Revised Edition. New York, Karger, 2013

Zhao X, Ma J, Wu S, et al: Light therapy for older patients with non-seasonal depression: a systematic review and meta-analysis. J Affect Disord 232:291–299, 2018 29500957

CHAPTER 35

Atypical Depression, Dysthymia, and Cyclothymia

John T.P. Liggins, M.D., M.S.
William Coryell, M.D.

In this chapter we discuss three mood disorders: depression with atypical features, persistent depressive disorder (dysthymia), and cyclothymia. Atypical depression and dysthymia are conceptualized as subtypes of major depressive disorder and are in part defined on the basis of how they differ from a "typical" major depressive episode; cyclothymia is considered a subtype of bipolar disorder and is defined on the basis of its differences from the usual presentations of bipolar hypomanic and major depressive episodes. In addition to considering the history and evolution of each of these disorder categories, we describe their clinical features, biological correlates, and treatment options and discuss their future directions.

Atypical Depression

West and Dally (1959) were the first to use the term *atypical* to describe a group of depressed patients who manifested a constellation of symptoms that differed from symptoms in patients with endogenous depression (defined as nonreactive depression with prominent *vegetative symptoms* [e.g., early-morning awakening, marked psychomotor disturbance, reduced appetite or weight loss]) and who appeared to have a better response to the monoamine oxidase inhibitor (MAOI) iproniazid than to tricyclic antidepressants (TCAs). On the basis of findings in subsequent investigations that depressed patients with atypical features have a distinct treatment response, biology, clinical features, and course of illness, DSM-IV (American Psychiatric Association

1994) was the first DSM edition to include "with atypical features" as a specifier for a major depressive episode or for dysthymia. DSM-5 (American Psychiatric Association 2013) continued this practice. To qualify for this specifier, a patient must demonstrate mood reactivity, defined as mood brightening in response to actual or potential positive events, along with two or more of four Criterion B symptoms—significant weight gain or increase in appetite (i.e., hyperphagia), hypersomnia, leaden paralysis (a heavy or leaden feeling in arms or legs), and interpersonal rejection sensitivity that is chronic and that also occurs outside of the depressive episode. The patient cannot meet criteria for melancholic features or catatonia.

Clinical Features

Several clinical and epidemiological variables have been associated with depression with atypical features. Lifetime prevalence rates have ranged from 0.7% (as estimated in the Epidemiologic Catchment Area study [Horwath et al. 1992]) to up to 10.23% (in the 2012 National Epidemiologic Survey on Alcohol and Related Conditions [Blanco et al. 2012]). Among patients with a major depressive episode diagnosis, the prevalence of depression with atypical features has been estimated to be as high as 39% (Henkel et al. 2004; Horwath et al. 1992; Levitan et al. 1998; Matza et al. 2003; Parker et al. 2005; Posternak and Zimmerman 2002). These data suggest that the presence of atypical symptoms in a major depressive episode is more common than the name *atypical* implies.

In comparison with depression without atypical symptoms, depression with atypical features is associated with female gender, family history of depression, earlier age at onset of depression, longer duration of depressive episodes, and a greater number of depressive episodes (Blanco et al. 2012; Horwath et al. 1992). In the National Comorbidity Survey, a nationally representative community survey based on DSM-III (American Psychiatric Association 1980) criteria, depression with atypical features was associated with an increase in both suicidal thoughts and suicide attempts in comparison with non-atypical depression (Matza et al. 2003). A large community study conducted in Ontario, Canada, found an association between a history of childhood physical or sexual abuse and the presence of reverse vegetative symptoms (hypersomnia and hyperphagia) (Levitan et al. 1998). Studies examining depressive symptoms in twins and nontwin siblings have shown a low concordance rate for atypical symptoms, suggesting a low heritability for these symptoms (Korszun et al. 2004).

In their original study, West and Dally (1959) observed that patients with atypical depression symptoms also had higher amounts of comorbid anxiety. Other studies have similarly found higher rates of comorbid social anxiety disorder and panic disorder in depressed patients with atypical features compared with depressed patients without atypical features (Horwath et al. 1992; Matza et al. 2003). Depression with atypical features has also been associated with higher rates of comorbid drug use disorders and personality disorders, including avoidant and dependent personality disorders (Blanco et al. 2012; Matza et al. 2003; Parker et al. 2005). Some studies have found higher rates of bipolar II disorder among patients with atypical depression (Perugi et al. 1998).

At the level of individual symptoms of depression with atypical features, there continues to be disagreement about the optimal grouping of symptoms to differentiate depression with atypical features from other putative depressive subtypes. Factor analyses of samples of depressed patients have revealed a cluster of symptoms (including reverse vegetative symptoms) that are distinct from other clusters of depression symptoms (Kendler et al. 1996; Korszun et al. 2004). One of the main areas of disagreement pertains to mood reactivity as an obligate criterion, given that there is evidence that patients with and without mood reactivity do not differ in regard to the presence of other atypical symptoms, comorbidities, or course-of-illness variables (Parker et al. 2005; Posternak and Zimmerman 2002). In contrast, the presence of either of the reverse vegetative symptoms of hypersomnia and hyperphagia during a major depressive episode appears to reliably delineate a separate subgroup of depressed patients with a distinct profile of these same variables (Matza et al. 2003; Thase et al. 1991); therefore, only one of these symptoms may be sufficient to identify atypical depression (Blanco et al. 2012).

The presence of atypical symptoms is at least moderately stable across episodes, with a particularly high concordance of the direction of self-reported weight change across depressive episodes (Stunkard et al. 1990). Nierenberg et al. (1996) found that up to 90% of patients with reverse vegetative symptoms during the index depressive episode experienced the same symptoms upon relapse. Taken together, this evidence suggests that depression with atypical features is distinct from depression with the more typical vegetative symptoms.

Biology

In comparison with patients with non-atypical depression, patients with atypical depression may be more likely to have abnormalities in hypothalamic-pituitary-adrenal (HPA) axis functioning. Anisman et al. (1999) showed that patients with atypical depression had elevated plasma adrenocorticotropic hormone (ACTH) levels and lower cortisol levels compared with nondepressed control subjects. In a challenge study that used desipramine to stimulate cortisol release, patients with depression with atypical features had higher cortisol responses in comparison with both depressed patients with mood reactivity only and depressed patients with neither mood reactivity nor atypical features (McGinn et al. 1996). Cerebrospinal fluid measurements of HPA axis components in a small sample of depressed patients, the majority of whom had atypical symptoms, showed lower levels of both ACTH and corticotropin-releasing hormone (CRH) but no difference in cortisol levels compared with healthy control subjects (Geracioti et al. 1997). Intriguingly, Stewart et al. (2005) found that both younger age at onset of depressive symptoms and chronicity were associated with abnormalities in HPA axis function. Specifically, patients with depression with atypical features and an early-onset/chronic course had lower baseline and post–dexamethasone suppression test cortisol levels compared with patients with depression with atypical features and a late-onset/nonchronic course. Collectively, these findings suggest the presence of hypoactive HPA axis functioning in depressed patients with atypical symptoms that contrasts with the hyperactive HPA axis functioning often seen in depressed patients with melancholic features.

There is some electrophysiological evidence that hemispheric differences in information processing distinguish depressed patients with atypical features from those with melancholic features. On a dichotic listening task involving nonsense syllables and complex tones, patients with melancholic depression showed abnormal perceptual asymmetry, whereas depressed patients with atypical features and healthy control subjects did not (Bruder et al. 1989). Patients with atypical depression instead had larger right-hemisphere biases in processing emotionally chimeric faces in comparison with both depressed patients with non-atypical or melancholic features and healthy control subjects (Bruder et al. 2002). A right-hemisphere bias was also found on a dichotic listening task but was more prominent in patients with atypical depression who had an early onset and chronic dysphoria (Stewart et al. 2003). Assessment of pattern-reversed visual evoked potentials, used as a proxy for speed of information processing in the CNS, showed that patients with atypical depression had shorter N80 and P100 latencies compared with patients with melancholic depression (Fotiou et al. 2003).

Treatment

In their seminal investigation, West and Dally (1959) observed that a group of depressed patients with atypical features responded more quickly and fully to the MAOI iproniazid than did patients with the more characteristic endogenous depressive symptoms. West and Dally's description of atypical features identified a profile opposite to that of endogenous depression (e.g., early-morning awakening, weight loss). West and Dally also noted that patients with atypical depression had higher levels of comorbid anxiety.

Subsequent studies used a narrower definition of atypical symptoms, and many were based on the criteria for atypical depression of McGinn et al. (1996) and colleagues at Columbia University. These criteria required the presence of mood reactivity along with two of four associated symptoms (hyperphagia, hypersomnolence, rejection sensitivity, and leaden paralysis). Several studies found a difference in treatment response to MAOIs versus TCAs among patients who met criteria for depression with atypical features compared with patients with melancholic features or patients who lacked atypical symptoms (Himmelhoch et al. 1991; Liebowitz et al. 1988; McGrath et al. 1992; Quitkin et al. 1988, 1991, 1993). For example, Quitkin et al. (1993), in a summary of the results of multiple trials conducted by associates at Columbia, noted that 269 patients with atypical features had a superior response to phenelzine compared with imipramine. In contrast, depressed patients without atypical symptoms had responses to phenelzine and to imipramine that were equivalent. The same superiority of MAOIs over TCAs was also found in patients with bipolar depression (Himmelhoch et al. 1991). Furthermore, Stewart et al. (2002) reported that among patients with atypical depression, those with an earlier onset and a more chronic course demonstrated a poorer response to TCAs in comparison with those without an early onset or chronic course.

Studies of selective serotonin reuptake inhibitors (SSRIs) in the treatment of depression with atypical features found evidence of equal efficacy between the SSRIs and MAOIs. For example, in a small head-to-head comparison trial following a single-blind placebo lead-in phase, Pande et al. (1996) found no difference in treatment response between patients with atypical depression who received fluoxetine and those who received phenelzine. A meta-analysis by Henkel et al. (2006) based on a small number of good-quality trials in patients with atypical depression found no differences in treatment response to SSRIs compared with MAOIs, but did find evidence of an advantage for MAOIs over TCAs, with an effect size of 0.27. In a comparison of fluoxetine and nortriptyline in an outpatient group of depressed patients, the presence of depression with atypical features predicted a poorer response to nortriptyline (Joyce et al. 2002). Collectively, these results suggest that patients who have depression with atypical features tend to respond more poorly to TCAs than to MAOIs or SSRIs and that MAOIs and SSRIs are equivalent in efficacy in this patient population. The poorer response to TCAs could be related to the side effects of this class of medications, particularly sedation, which might be less tolerable for patients with atypical depression, who are already experiencing hypersomnolence.

Future Directions

The DSM-5 specifier "with atypical features" is based on multiple lines of epidemiological, biological, and treatment-response evidence suggesting the existence of a distinct subgroup of depressed patients who experience reverse vegetative symptoms (listed in Criterion B for the specifier) that are superimposed on a stable trait of interpersonal rejection sensitivity (Criterion A). There is some evidence that mood reactivity might not be as central to the diagnosis of atypical depression as was previously thought. For example, mood reactivity does not appear to have a strong correlation with the other atypical symptoms (Parker et al. 2005), and treatment response does not differ between patients with mood reactivity and patients without such reactivity (Quitkin et al. 1989). Future editions of DSM will need to evaluate whether the presence of mood reactivity (Criterion A) remains essential to the diagnosis of atypical depression or, alternatively, whether it would be sufficient to require any two of the four atypical symptoms listed in Criterion B. Emerging evidence regarding the importance of the timing of onset of mood symptoms (early versus late) and of the course of illness (chronic versus nonchronic) in depression with atypical features should also be considered in conceptualizations of this subtype.

Persistent Depressive Disorder (Dysthymia)

Early work by Akiskal et al. (1981) sought to characterize subgroups of chronic depressive states and influenced the inclusion of *intermittent depressive disorder* in the Research Diagnostic Criteria (RDC; Spitzer et al. 1975). The criteria for intermittent depressive disorder, in turn, shaped the definition of *dysthymic disorder* in DSM-III. The RDC specified that a minimum of 2 symptoms (from a list of 16) be present, in addition to dysphoria or anhedonia, and DSM-III similarly required 3 symptoms from a list of 13. DSM-III-R (American Psychiatric Association 1987) and DSM-IV definitions narrowed the list to two out of six symptoms. The RDC and the first three DSM editions, however, required that the number of symptoms present over the first 2 years of the episode not rise to a number that would satisfy criteria for a major depressive episode.

Many individuals seeking treatment for depressive symptoms, however, cannot recall experiencing clear remissions from their symptoms, and symptom onset may have been decades in the past. The inherent unreliability of requiring patients to recollect whether the number of their depressive symptoms has risen from fewer than five to five or more for any 2-week period during the first 2 years of illness led DSM-5 to combine dysthymia with chronic major depressive disorder (MDD), both as defined in DSM-IV, creating the single category of persistent depressive disorder (dysthymia). This combination of dysthymia and chronic MDD was also based on the recognition that few differences exist between these conditions in patterns of comorbidity (Blanco et al. 2010; Klein et al. 2004, 2008; McCullough et al. 2000, 2003; Vandeleur et al. 2017), in morbid risks for mood or anxiety disorders among family members (Blanco et al. 2010; Klein et al. 2004; McCullough et al. 2000, 2003), or in likelihood of response to various types of treatment (McCullough et al. 2000, 2003).

Clinical Features

Community surveys conducted in the United States (Blanco et al. 2010; Kessler et al. 1994, 2005; Weissman et al. 1988), Canada (Satyanarayana et al. 2009), and Australia (Murphy and Byrne 2012) have estimated lifetime prevalence rates for persistent depressive disorder (PDD) of 2%–4.6%. Kessler et al. (2005) used the early-onset (i.e., before age 21 years) versus late-onset (i.e., 21 years or later) distributions for DSM-III-R dysthymia to project a lifetime estimated prevalence of 3.5%. A survey of 75 individuals seen in an outpatient psychiatric clinic found that one-third met criteria for dysthymia (Markowitz et al. 1992).

A community survey from Switzerland found a much higher lifetime prevalence rate for PDD of 18% (Vandeleur et al. 2017). The difference between this rate and the rates reported in earlier surveys may reflect the use of a diagnostic interview that was semistructured rather than highly structured and that had screening questions for the depressive disorder section with lower thresholds that allowed raters to more readily follow up on subtle evidence of depressive illness.

Studies have found that in comparison with patients with more acute and episodic MDD, patients with either dysthymia or chronic MDD have earlier onsets of illness (Akiskal et al. 1981; Gilmer et al. 2005; Hölzel et al. 2011; Markowitz et al. 1992), higher rates of mood disorders among family members (Akiskal et al. 1981; Hölzel et al. 2011; Klein et al. 1988; Scott et al. 1988), higher numbers of comorbid personality disorders (Garyfallos et al. 1999; Klein and Kotov 2016; Klein et al. 1988; Markowitz et al. 1992), greater severity of childhood adversity (Angst et al. 2011; Barnhofer et al. 2014; Brown et al. 1994; Klein and Kotov 2016), higher levels of neuroticism and impairment of social functioning (Rhebergen et al. 2010), and more suicide attempts (Garvey et al. 1986; Gilmer et al. 2005; Satyanarayana et al. 2009).

DSM-III, DSM-III-R, and DSM-IV each specified a distinction between early-onset (i.e., before 21 years of age) and later-onset dysthymia. DSM-5 continued this practice for PDD. In comparison with those with later symptom onset, individuals with early-onset dysthymia or chronic MDD are more likely to be female (Barzega et al. 2001; Klein et al. 1999b), to have a longer-duration index episode (Barzega et al. 2001; Klein et al. 1999a, 1999b), to have higher morbid risks for mood disorders among relatives (Klein et al. 1988, 1999a), and to have higher rates of comorbid personality disorders (Klein et al. 1999a, 1999b).

Treatment

A meta-analysis of 22 studies examining antidepressant treatments for dysthymia or chronic MDD showed that TCAs and SSRIs produced outcomes that were equally superior to those of placebo but that SSRI treatment had significantly better acceptability, as reflected in dropout rates that were approximately one-half those with TCA treatment (von Wolff et al. 2013). Even though patients with dysthymia can be expected to exhibit less severe symptoms than patients with MDD when they present for treatment (because of the lower requisite number of symptoms for the diagnosis), the efficacy of antidepressant treatment relative to placebo appears to be greater for patients with dysthymia than for patients with MDD. In a meta-analysis that compared outcomes from placebo-controlled trials in MDD with outcomes from trials in dysthymia, placebo response rates were 21% higher among MDD patients than they were among patients with dysthymia (Levkovitz et al. 2011). Response rates for patients treated with antidepressants were nearly identical in the two groups—52.4% for those with dysthymia and 54.3% for those with MDD.

Fewer comparisons of treatment response to pharmacotherapy versus psychotherapy have been undertaken for dysthymia than for nonchronic MDD; however, two of the largest comparison studies in patients with dysthymia found that antidepressant treatment was more efficacious than psychotherapy. In both studies, the therapy modality used was interpersonal psychotherapy (IPT) (Browne et al. 2002; Markowitz et al. 2005). In neither study was the combination of IPT with SSRI treatment more efficacious than SSRI treatment alone. A meta-analysis involving 39 studies of MDD and 5 of dysthymia found that pharmacotherapy was significantly superior to psychotherapy for dysthymia but observed no difference between these modalities for nonchronic MDD (Cuijpers et al. 2013).

In contrast to IPT, the Cognitive Behavioral Analysis System of Psychotherapy (CBASP) is a psychotherapeutic approach designed specifically for individuals with early-onset chronic depression. In one of the earliest trials of CBASP in chronically depressed patients, those treated with a combination of CBASP and antidepressant therapy had better outcomes at 12 weeks than did those treated with only CBASP or only antidepressant therapy (Keller et al. 2000). A study evaluating the efficacy of CBASP monotherapy versus nonspecific supportive monotherapy in outpatients with early-onset chronic depression who were not taking antidepressant medication found that CBASP was moderately more effective than supportive therapy in this patient population (Schramm et al. 2017). However, another trial comparing 1) CBASP augmentation, 2) brief supportive therapy augmentation, or 3) no augmentation of patients' ongoing medication regimens over a 12-week period failed to find added benefit for CBASP (Kocsis et al. 2009). The importance of therapy duration was demonstrated by Wiersma et al. (2014) in a comparison of CBASP versus care as usual (CAU)—consisting of various evidence-based psychotherapies and pharmacotherapies—in patients with chronic depression. The superiority of CBASP emerged at 53 weeks but was not evident at 8, 16, or 32 weeks. Because the CAU condition included cognitive-behavioral therapy (CBT) or IPT, these results are important in that they show that CBASP performs well when comparatively tested against a "high standard" active treatment control condition (Wiersma et al. 2014). Moreover, this study, in contrast to the others described here, included patients with DSM-IV dysthymia as well as patients with chronic MDD. This diagnostic mix thus closely approximated the DSM-5 diagnosis of PDD. Taken together, these study findings present evidence that treatment provided to patients with chronic depression should be tailored to that disorder and that full benefits may require a year or longer to manifest.

Future Directions

Chronic MDD and dysthymia were combined in DSM-5 largely because a number of diagnostic validators failed to show differences between these groups. Nevertheless, because PDD is a new diagnostic category, additional studies are needed that compare long-term outcomes, family histories, comorbidity patterns, and treatment response characteristics between patients with PDD and patients with nonchronic MDD.

Efforts to identify candidate genes associated with MDD have been thwarted by the well-recognized heterogeneity of the disorder. While recurrence and early age at onset have been widely used to isolate samples with higher heritability, evidence exists that the study of chronically depressed cohorts may serve this purpose as well (Luo et al. 2016).

Treatment studies that target PDD are also likely to be rewarding. Higher rates of placebo response have plagued randomized controlled trials for antidepressants, but placebo response rates are substantially lower among individuals with dysthymia (Levkovitz et al. 2011) or with chronic MDD (Papakostas et al. 2015) compared with those with nonchronic MDD. Patients with PDD are thus likely to show true drug effects in placebo trials with lower numbers of participants. The number of controlled antidepressant trials targeting chronic depressive conditions is surprisingly low. In light of this deficiency and of the high prevalence of these conditions, it seems clear that antidepressants should be tested much more frequently in this patient population.

Cyclothymic Disorder

The term *cyclothymia* has been applied to forms of mood disorder that contain a cyclical variation in mood over time. Ewald Hecker, a student of the German psychiatrist Karl Ludwig Kahlbaum, first used the term *cyclothymia* in 1877 to describe patients with manic-depressive illness (Brieger and Marneros 1997), and Emil Kraepelin subsequently applied the term *cyclothymia* to a milder form of manic-depressive illness. Kraepelin also brought forward the idea of affective temperaments that predisposed individuals to the development of manic-depressive illness (Brieger and Marneros 1997). There continues to be disagreement about whether cyclothymia represents a distinct mood disorder, a personality or temperament style, or a prodromal syndrome of bipolar disorder (Akiskal et al. 2000; Parker et al. 2012; Perugi et al. 2015).

DSM-5 considers cyclothymia to be a distinct mood disorder that is part of the bipolar spectrum. to qualify for the diagnosis, an individual must experience chronic and fluctuating mood symptoms that do not meet criteria for either a hypomanic or a major depressive episode. The mood fluctuations must have been present for at least 2 years, although this period is reduced to 1 year for children and adolescents. The individual must experience mood symptoms for at least half of the time and cannot be symptom-free for longer than 2 months. If the person subsequently develops a full-blown mood episode, the diagnosis changes to MDD, bipolar I or II disorder, or other specified/unspecified bipolar and related disorder, and the cyclothymic disorder diagnosis is discontinued.

Clinical Features

Patients with cyclothymic disorder experience chronic mood instability characterized by frequent shifts among irritable, elevated, and depressed moods (Akiskal et al. 1977). These mood shifts can occur over the span of a single day or over the course of multiple days. Patients can experience a mixture of both depressive and hypomanic symptoms as well (Akiskal et al. 1977). There is considerable overlap between the constellation of symptoms present in cyclothymic disorder and those present in personality disorders such as borderline personality disorder, although there is some evidence that borderline personality disorder can be distinguished from subthreshold bipolar symptoms on the basis of the frequency, intensity, and quality of affective shifts (Reich et al. 2012). Cyclothymic disorder appears to have an early age at onset, with the first mood symptoms commonly developing in childhood or adolescence (Kurumaji et al. 2014; Van Meter et al. 2011).

The few studies that have directly examined prevalence of cyclothymic disorder have reported rates ranging from 0.4% to 2.5% (Angst et al. 2005; Faravelli et al. 1990). It is unclear whether prevalence rates of cyclothymic disorder differ by sex. Cyclothymic disorder is commonly found in the first-degree relatives of patients with bipolar disorder, a circumstance that has been used to support the idea that this disorder is part of the bipolar spectrum (Akiskal et al. 1985; Edvardsen et al. 2008; Klein et al. 1985).

Suicide rates have not been directly examined in cohorts of patients with cyclothymic disorder, although suicidal ideation has been found to be similarly high in youth with cyclothymic disorder and youth with other bipolar spectrum disorders (Van Meter et al. 2017). In comparison with healthy control subjects (Tomba et al. 2012) or patients with other psychiatric diagnoses (Van Meter et al. 2011, 2017), patients with cyclothymic disorder have higher rates of several comorbid psychiatric conditions, including anxiety disorders, ADHD, and substance use disorders. In a few studies, patients with a diagnosis of cyclothymic disorder were found to experience subsequent episodes of depression, mania, and hypomania at high rates (Akiskal et al. 1979, 1985; Lewinsohn et al. 2000).

Biology

Scant research is available on the potential biological underpinnings of cyclothymic disorder. In an older study, individuals who were diagnosed with the General Behavior Inventory were found to have elevated cortisol levels compared with healthy control subjects (Depue et al. 1985). No studies have assessed biological correlates of cyclothymic disorder as defined by DSM criteria.

Treatment

Few studies have examined treatment response in patients with cyclothymic disorder. In a retrospective study, Peselow et al. (1982) found that lithium was less effective for depression prophylaxis in cyclothymic patients compared with patients with either unipolar depression or bipolar II disorder, as assessed by the probability of remaining free from depressive episodes for up to 3 years of follow-up. The percentage of patients remaining free from depressive episodes was not significantly different when the patients with cyclothymic disorder were stratified by family history of mood disorder (Peselow et al. 1982). Two double-blind, placebo-controlled drug studies have been conducted in youth who were deemed to be at high risk of developing bipolar disorder (because of a positive family history [i.e., a first-degree relative with bipolar disorder]) and who also met criteria for either DSM-IV cyclothymic disorder or DSM-IV bipolar disorder not otherwise specified (BP-NOS). In the first study (Findling et al. 2007), divalproex monotherapy was not found to be superior to placebo in reducing either depression or mania ratings. In the second study (Findling et al. 2017), aripiprazole significantly reduced mania ratings on the Young Mania Rating Scale (YMRS) compared with placebo, but it did not reduce depression ratings. Taken together, these studies provide only weak evidence for the efficacy of mood stabilizers in patients with cyclothymic disorder.

Future Directions

Some evidence indicates that patients with cyclothymic disorder have distinct clinical features and a high familial loading for mood disorders. However, no high-quality studies have examined the potential biological correlates of cyclothymic disorder, and only a few studies have examined treatment response. Research in this area is complicated by the use of varying definitions for cyclothymia, depending on whether it is considered to represent a temperament or a distinct disorder or is categorized as a DSM-5 other specified/unspecified bipolar and related disorder to tap into "subsyndromal" features of bipolar disorder. Future studies should consider using the DSM-5 criteria to facilitate better comparisons among studies and to further investigate the illness course, potential biological underpinnings, and response to treatment of cyclothymic disorder.

Conclusion

Of the three disorders discussed in this chapter, atypical depression may be the most prevalent. Reverse vegetative symptoms appear to be the most important distinguishing feature, and patients with this disorder may have hypoactive HPA axis functioning, in contrast to the hyperactive functioning present in many individuals with melancholic depression. Much of the initial interest in atypical depression centered on the finding that MAOIs were more effective in treating atypical depression than were TCAs (which at that time were the standard treatment for depression). MAOIs do not appear to be more effective than SSRIs, however, and interest in differential antidepressant response in atypical depression has subsided accordingly.

PDD, a merging of dysthymia with chronic MDD, was a new category introduced in DSM-5. Given the lack of differences between the two parent conditions in comorbidity, family history patterns, and treatment response, most of the previous research pertaining to dysthymia or chronic MDD can probably be applied to PDD. In comparison with patients with nonchronic MDD, patients with dysthymia or chronic MDD have earlier onsets, more childhood adversity, more severe underlying neuroticism, and a higher likelihood of suicide attempts. CBASP, a psychotherapeutic approach developed specifically for the treatment of early-onset chronic depression, has been shown to be more effective than other forms of psychotherapy for this condition. Because patients with chronic MDD or PDD have lower placebo response rates than do patients with nonchronic depression, placebo-controlled trials in these patients are more likely to show true drug effects. Antidepressant trials in patients with PDD are sorely needed and are likely to be fruitful.

The literature describing cyclothymia is relatively limited. Cyclothymia has been linked to bipolar disorder in family studies and in many cases may represent a prodromal state for a full manic or hypomanic episode. Patients with cyclothymia appear to be less responsive to mood stabilizers than are patients with bipolar I or bipolar II disorder.

References

Akiskal HS, Djenderedjian AM, Rosenthal RH, et al: Cyclothymic disorder: validating criteria for inclusion in the bipolar affective group. Am J Psychiatry 134(11):1227–1233, 1977 910973

Akiskal H, Khani M, Scott-Strauss A: Cyclothymic temperamental disorders. Psychiatr Clin North Am 2:527–554, 1979

Akiskal HS, King D, Rosenthal TL, et al: Chronic depressions, part 1: clinical and familial characteristics in 137 probands. J Affect Disord 3(3):297–315, 1981 6456296

Akiskal HS, Downs J, Jordan P, et al: Affective disorders in referred children and younger siblings of manic-depressives. Mode of onset and prospective course. Arch Gen Psychiatry 42(10):996–1003, 1985 4037989

Akiskal HS, Bourgeois ML, Angst J, et al: Re-evaluating the prevalence of and diagnostic composition within the broad clinical spectrum of bipolar disorders. J Affect Disord 59 (suppl 1):S5–S30, 2000 11121824

American Psychiatric Association: Diagnostic and Statistical Manual of Mental Disorders, 3rd Edition. Washington, DC, American Psychiatric Association, 1980

American Psychiatric Association: Diagnostic and Statistical Manual of Mental Disorders, 3rd Edition, Revised. Washington, DC, American Psychiatric Association, 1987

American Psychiatric Association: Diagnostic and Statistical Manual of Mental Disorders, 4th Edition. Washington, DC, American Psychiatric Association, 1994

American Psychiatric Association: Diagnostic and Statistical Manual of Mental Disorders, 5th Edition. Arlington, VA, American Psychiatric Association, 2013

Angst J, Gamma A, Neuenschwander M, et al: Prevalence of mental disorders in the Zurich Cohort Study: a twenty year prospective study. Epidemiol Psichiatr Soc 14(2):68–76, 2005 16001703

Angst J, Gamma A, Rössler W, et al: Childhood adversity and chronicity of mood disorders. Eur Arch Psychiatry Clin Neurosci 261(1):21–27, 2011 20589507

Anisman H, Ravindran AV, Griffiths J, et al: Endocrine and cytokine correlates of major depression and dysthymia with typical or atypical features. Mol Psychiatry 4(2):182–188, 1999 10208451

Barnhofer T, Brennan K, Crane C, et al: A comparison of vulnerability factors in patients with persistent and remitting lifetime symptom course of depression. J Affect Disord 152–154:155–161, 2014 24183488

Barzega G, Maina G, Venturello S, et al: Dysthymic disorder: clinical characteristics in relation to age at onset. J Affect Disord 66(1):39–46, 2001 11532531

Blanco C, Okuda M, Markowitz JC, et al: The epidemiology of chronic major depressive disorder and dysthymic disorder: results from the National Epidemiologic Survey on Alcohol and Related Conditions. J Clin Psychiatry 71(12):1645–1656, 2010 21190638

Blanco C, Vesga-López O, Stewart JW, et al: Epidemiology of major depression with atypical features: results from the National Epidemiologic Survey on Alcohol and Related Conditions (NESARC). J Clin Psychiatry 73(2):224–232, 2012 21939615

Brieger P, Marneros A: Dysthymia and cyclothymia: historical origins and contemporary development. J Affect Disord 45(3):117–126, 1997 9298424
Brown GW, Harris TO, Hepworth C, et al: Clinical and psychosocial origins of chronic depressive episodes, II: a patient enquiry. Br J Psychiatry 165(4):457–465, 1994 7804659
Browne G, Steiner M, Roberts J, et al: Sertraline and/or interpersonal psychotherapy for patients with dysthymic disorder in primary care: 6-month comparison with longitudinal 2-year follow-up of effectiveness and costs. J Affect Disord 68(2–3):317–330, 2002 12063159
Bruder GE, Quitkin FM, Stewart JW, et al: Cerebral laterality and depression: differences in perceptual asymmetry among diagnostic subtypes. J Abnorm Psychol 98(2):177–186, 1989 2708661
Bruder GE, Stewart JW, McGrath PJ, et al: Atypical depression: enhanced right hemispheric dominance for perceiving emotional chimeric faces. J Abnorm Psychol 111(3):446–454, 2002 12150420
Cuijpers P, Sijbrandij M, Koole SL, et al: The efficacy of psychotherapy and pharmacotherapy in treating depressive and anxiety disorders: a meta-analysis of direct comparisons. World Psychiatry 12(2):137–148, 2013 23737423
Depue RA, Kleiman RM, Davis P, et al: The behavioral high-risk paradigm and bipolar affective disorder, VIII: serum free cortisol in nonpatient cyclothymic subjects selected by the General Behavior Inventory. Am J Psychiatry 142(2):175–181, 1985 3970242
Edvardsen J, Torgersen S, Røysamb E, et al: Heritability of bipolar spectrum disorders. Unity or heterogeneity? J Affect Disord 106(3):229–240, 2008 17692389
Faravelli C, Guerrini Degl'Innocenti B, Aiazzi L, et al: Epidemiology of mood disorders: a community survey in Florence. J Affect Disord 20(2):135–141, 1990 2148328
Findling RL, Frazier TW, Youngstrom EA, et al: Double-blind, placebo-controlled trial of divalproex monotherapy in the treatment of symptomatic youth at high risk for developing bipolar disorder. J Clin Psychiatry 68(5):781–788, 2007 17503990
Findling RL, Youngstrom EA, Rowles BM, et al: A double-blind and placebo-controlled trial of aripiprazole in symptomatic youths at genetic high risk for bipolar disorder. J Child Adolesc Psychopharmacol 27(10):864–874, 2017 28759262
Fotiou F, Fountoulakis KN, Iacovides A, Kaprinis G: Pattern-reversed visual evoked potentials in subtypes of major depression. Psychiatry Res 118(3):259–271, 2003 12834820
Garvey MJ, Tollefson GD, Tuason VB: Is chronic primary major depression a distinct depression subtype? Compr Psychiatry 27(5):446–448, 1986 3757492
Garyfallos G, Adamopoulou A, Karastergiou A, et al: Personality disorders in dysthymia and major depression. Acta Psychiatr Scand 99(5):332–340, 1999 10353448
Geracioti TD Jr, Loosen PT, Orth DN: Low cerebrospinal fluid corticotropin-releasing hormone concentrations in eucortisolemic depression. Biol Psychiatry 42(3):165–174, 1997 9232208
Gilmer WS, Trivedi MH, Rush AJ, et al: Factors associated with chronic depressive episodes: a preliminary report from the STAR-D project. Acta Psychiatr Scand 112(6):425–433, 2005 16279871
Henkel V, Mergl R, Coyne JC, et al: Depression with atypical features in a sample of primary care outpatients: prevalence, specific characteristics and consequences. J Affect Disord 83(2–3):237–242, 2004 15555720
Henkel V, Mergl R, Allgaier AK, et al: Treatment of depression with atypical features: a meta-analytic approach. Psychiatry Res 141(1):89–101, 2006 16321446
Himmelhoch JM, Thase ME, Mallinger AG, et al: Tranylcypromine versus imipramine in anergic bipolar depression. Am J Psychiatry 148(7):910–916, 1991 2053632
Hölzel L, Härter M, Reese C, et al: Risk factors for chronic depression—a systematic review. J Affect Disord 129(1–3):1–13, 2011 20488546
Horwath E, Johnson J, Weissman MM, et al: The validity of major depression with atypical features based on a community study. J Affect Disord 26(2):117–125, 1992 1447429
Joyce PR, Mulder RT, Luty SE, et al: Patterns and predictors of remission, response and recovery in major depression treated with fluoxetine or nortriptyline. Aust N Z J Psychiatry 36(3):384–391, 2002 12060188

Keller MB, McCullough JP, Klein DN, et al: A comparison of nefazodone, the cognitive behavioral-analysis system of psychotherapy, and their combination for the treatment of chronic depression. N Engl J Med 342(20):1462–1470, 2000 10816183
Kendler KS, Eaves LJ, Walters EE, et al: The identification and validation of distinct depressive syndromes in a population-based sample of female twins. Arch Gen Psychiatry 53(5):391–399, 1996 8624182
Kessler RC, McGonagle KA, Zhao S, et al: Lifetime and 12-month prevalence of DSM-III-R psychiatric disorders in the United States. Results from the National Comorbidity Survey. Arch Gen Psychiatry 51(1):8–19, 1994 8279933
Kessler RC, Berglund P, Demler O, et al: Lifetime prevalence and age-of-onset distributions of DSM-IV disorders in the National Comorbidity Survey Replication. Arch Gen Psychiatry 62(6):593–602, 2005 15939837
Klein DN, Kotov R: Course of depression in a 10-year prospective study: evidence for qualitatively distinct subgroups. J Abnorm Psychol 125(3):337–348, 2016 26845258
Klein DN, Depue RA, Slater JF: Cyclothymia in the adolescent offspring of parents with bipolar affective disorder. J Abnorm Psychol 94(2):115–127, 1985 3998280
Klein DN, Taylor EB, Dickstein S, Harding K: The early–late onset distinction in DSM-III-R dysthymia. J Affect Disord 14(1):25–33, 1988 2963049
Klein DN, Schatzberg AF, McCullough JP, et al: Early- versus late-onset dysthymic disorder: comparison in out-patients with superimposed major depressive episodes. J Affect Disord 52(1–3):187–196, 1999a 10357032
Klein DN, Schatzberg AF, McCullough JP, et al: Age of onset in chronic major depression: relation to demographic and clinical variables, family history, and treatment response. J Affect Disord 55(2–3):149–157, 1999b 10628884
Klein DN, Shankman SA, Lewinsohn PM, et al: Family study of chronic depression in a community sample of young adults. Am J Psychiatry 161(4):646–653, 2004 15056510
Klein DN, Shankman SA, Rose S: Dysthymic disorder and double depression: prediction of 10-year course trajectories and outcomes. J Psychiatr Res 42(5):408–415, 2008 17466334
Kocsis JH, Gelenberg AJ, Rothbaum BO, et al; REVAMP Investigators: Cognitive behavioral analysis system of psychotherapy and brief supportive psychotherapy for augmentation of antidepressant nonresponse in chronic depression: the REVAMP Trial. Arch Gen Psychiatry 66(11):1178–1188, 2009 19884606
Korszun A, Moskvina V, Brewster S, et al: Familiality of symptom dimensions in depression. Arch Gen Psychiatry 61(5):468–474, 2004 15123491
Kurumaji A, Narushima K, Ooshima K, et al: Clinical course of the bipolar II disorder in a Japanese sample. J Affect Disord 168:363–366, 2014 25103632
Levitan RD, Parikh SV, Lesage AD, et al: Major depression in individuals with a history of childhood physical or sexual abuse: relationship to neurovegetative features, mania, and gender. Am J Psychiatry 155(12):1746–1752, 1998 9842786
Levkovitz Y, Tedeschini E, Papakostas GI: Efficacy of antidepressants for dysthymia: a meta-analysis of placebo-controlled randomized trials. J Clin Psychiatry 72(4):509–514, 2011 21527126
Lewinsohn PM, Klein DN, Seeley JR: Bipolar disorder during adolescence and young adulthood in a community sample. Bipolar Disord 2(3 Pt 2):281–293, 2000 11249806
Liebowitz MR, Quitkin FM, Stewart JW, et al: Antidepressant specificity in atypical depression. Arch Gen Psychiatry 45(2):129–137, 1988 3276282
Luo X, Stavrakakis N, Penninx BW, et al: Does refining the phenotype improve replication rates? A review and replication of candidate gene studies on major depressive disorder and chronic major depressive disorder. Am J Med Genet B Neuropsychiatr Genet 171B(2):215–236, 2016 26566975
Markowitz JC, Moran ME, Kocsis JH, et al: Prevalence and comorbidity of dysthymic disorder among psychiatric outpatients. J Affect Disord 24(2):63–71, 1992 1541768
Markowitz JC, Kocsis JH, Bleiberg KL, et al: A comparative trial of psychotherapy and pharmacotherapy for "pure" dysthymic patients. J Affect Disord 89(1–3):167–175, 2005 16263177

Matza LS, Revicki DA, Davidson JR, et al: Depression with atypical features in the National Comorbidity Survey: classification, description, and consequences. Arch Gen Psychiatry 60(8):817–826, 2003 12912765
McCullough JP Jr, Klein DN, Keller MB, et al: Comparison of DSM-III-R chronic major depression and major depression superimposed on dysthymia (double depression): validity of the distinction. J Abnorm Psychol 109(3):419–427, 2000 11016111
McCullough JP Jr, Klein DN, Borian FE, et al: Group comparisons of DSM-IV subtypes of chronic depression: validity of the distinctions, part 2. J Abnorm Psychol 112(4):614–622, 2003 14674873
McGinn LK, Asnis GM, Rubinson E: Biological and clinical validation of atypical depression. Psychiatry Res 60(2–3):191–198, 1996 8723310
McGrath PJ, Stewart JW, Harrison WM, et al: Predictive value of symptoms of atypical depression for differential drug treatment outcome. J Clin Psychopharmacol 12(3):197–202, 1992 1629387
Murphy JA, Byrne GJ: Prevalence and correlates of the proposed DSM-5 diagnosis of chronic depressive disorder. J Affect Disord 139(2):172–180, 2012 22381955
Nierenberg AA, Pava JA, Clancy K, et al: Are neurovegetative symptoms stable in relapsing or recurrent atypical depressive episodes? Biol Psychiatry 40(8):691–696, 1996 8894060
Pande AC, Birkett M, Fechner-Bates S, et al: Fluoxetine versus phenelzine in atypical depression. Biol Psychiatry 40(10):1017–1020, 1996 8915561
Papakostas GI, Østergaard SD, Iovieno N; The nature of placebo response in clinical studies of major depressive disorder. J Clin Psychiatry 76(4):456–466, 2015 25700292
Parker G, Parker K, Mitchell P, et al: Atypical depression: Australian and US studies in accord. Curr Opin Psychiatry 18(1):1–5, 2005 16639176
Parker G, McCraw S, Fletcher K: Cyclothymia. Depress Anxiety 29(6):487–494, 2012 22553122
Perugi G, Akiskal HS, Lattanzi L, et al: The high prevalence of "soft" bipolar (II) features in atypical depression. Compr Psychiatry 39(2):63–71, 1998 9515190
Perugi G, Hantouche E, Vannucchi G, Pinto O: Cyclothymia reloaded: a reappraisal of the most misconceived affective disorder. J Affect Disord 183:119–133, 2015 26005206
Peselow ED, Dunner DL, Fieve RR, et al: Lithium prophylaxis of depression in unipolar, bipolar II, and cyclothymic patients. Am J Psychiatry 139(6):747–752, 1982 6805339
Posternak MA, Zimmerman M: Partial validation of the atypical features subtype of major depressive disorder. Arch Gen Psychiatry 59(1):70–76, 2002 11779285
Quitkin FM, Stewart JW, McGrath PJ, et al: Phenelzine versus imipramine in the treatment of probable atypical depression: defining syndrome boundaries of selective MAOI responders. Am J Psychiatry 145(3):306–311, 1988 3278631
Quitkin FM, McGrath PJ, Stewart JW, et al: Phenelzine and imipramine in mood reactive depressives. Further delineation of the syndrome of atypical depression. Arch Gen Psychiatry 46(9):787–793, 1989 2673130
Quitkin FM, Harrison W, Stewart JW, et al: Response to phenelzine and imipramine in placebo nonresponders with atypical depression. A new application of the crossover design. Arch Gen Psychiatry 48(4):319–323, 1991 2009033
Quitkin FM, Stewart JW, McGrath PJ, et al: Columbia atypical depression. A subgroup of depressives with better response to MAOI than to tricyclic antidepressants or placebo. Br J Psychiatry 163 (suppl 21):30–34, 1993 8217065
Reich DB, Zanarini MC, Fitzmaurice G: Affective lability in bipolar disorder and borderline personality disorder. Compr Psychiatry 53(3):230–237, 2012 21632042
Rhebergen D, Beekman AT, de Graaf R, et al: Trajectories of recovery of social and physical functioning in major depression, dysthymic disorder and double depression: a 3-year follow-up. J Affect Disord 124(1–2):148–156, 2010 19945171
Satyanarayana S, Enns MW, Cox BJ, Sareen J: Prevalence and correlates of chronic depression in the Canadian community health survey: mental health and well-being. Can J Psychiatry 54(6):389–398, 2009 19527559

Schramm E, Kriston L, Zobel I, et al: Effect of disorder-specific vs nonspecific psychotherapy for chronic depression: a randomized clinical trial. JAMA Psychiatry 74(3):233–242, 2017 28146251

Scott J, Barker WA, Eccleston D: The Newcastle Chronic Depression Study. Patient characteristics and factors associated with chronicity. Br J Psychiatry 152:28–33, 1988 3167350

Spitzer RL, Endicott J, Robins E: Clinical criteria for psychiatric diagnosis and DSM-III. Am J Psychiatry 132(11):1187–1192, 1975 1172654

Stewart JW, McGrath PJ, Quitkin FM: Do age of onset and course of illness predict different treatment outcome among DSM IV depressive disorders with atypical features? Neuropsychopharmacology 26(2):237–245, 2002 11790519

Stewart JW, Bruder GE, McGrath PJ, et al: Do age of onset and course of illness define biologically distinct groups within atypical depression? J Abnorm Psychol 112(2):253–262, 2003 12784835

Stewart JW, Quitkin FM, McGrath PJ, Klein DF: Defining the boundaries of atypical depression: evidence from the HPA axis supports course of illness distinctions. J Affect Disord 86(2–3):161–167, 2005 15935235

Stunkard AJ, Fernstrom MH, Price A, et al: Direction of weight change in recurrent depression. Consistency across episodes. Arch Gen Psychiatry 47(9):857–860, 1990 2393344

Thase ME, Carpenter L, Kupfer DJ, et al: Clinical significance of reversed vegetative subtypes of recurrent major depression. Psychopharmacol Bull 27(1):17–22, 1991 1862201

Tomba E, Rafanelli C, Grandi S, et al: Clinical configuration of cyclothymic disturbances. J Affect Disord 139(3):244–249, 2012 22551912

Vandeleur CL, Fassassi S, Castelao E, et al: Prevalence and correlates of DSM-5 major depressive and related disorders in the community. Psychiatry Res 250:50–58, 2017 28142066

Van Meter A, Youngstrom EA, Youngstrom JK, et al: Examining the validity of cyclothymic disorder in a youth sample. J Affect Disord 132(1–2):55–63, 2011 21396717

Van Meter AR, Youngstrom EA, Birmaher B, et al: Longitudinal course and characteristics of cyclothymic disorder in youth. J Affect Disord 215:314–322, 2017 28365522

von Wolff A, Hölzel LP, Westphal A, et al: Selective serotonin reuptake inhibitors and tricyclic antidepressants in the acute treatment of chronic depression and dysthymia: a systematic review and meta-analysis. J Affect Disord 144(1–2):7–15, 2013 22963896

Weissman MM, Leaf PJ, Tischler GL, et al: Affective disorders in five United States communities. Psychol Med 18(1):141–153, 1988 3363034

West ED, Dally PJ: Effects of iproniazid in depressive syndromes. BMJ 1(5136):1491–1494, 1959 13651775

Wiersma JE, Van Schaik DJ, Hoogendorn AW, et al: The effectiveness of the cognitive behavioral analysis system of psychotherapy for chronic depression: a randomized controlled trial. Psychother Psychosom 83(5):263–269, 2014 25116461

CHAPTER 36

Major Depressive Disorder With Psychotic Features

Alan F. Schatzberg, M.D.

In DSM-5 (American Psychiatric Association 2013), psychotic depression is classified as major depressive disorder (MDD) with psychotic features. In DSM-IV-TR (American Psychiatric Association 2000), the disorder was characterized as severe MDD with psychotic features (in the context of a severity dimension that spanned mild, moderate, severe without psychotic features, and severe with psychotic features). Both DSM editions required the usual criteria for a major depressive episode, with the additional symptoms of hallucinations or delusions, which could be either mood congruent or mood incongruent. The change in the severity dimension criterion reflected data indicating that severity in terms of other depressive symptoms does not always overlap with the presence of psychosis (discussed later in chapter). Data continue to emerge that support psychotic depression as a distinct clinical entity when compared with nonpsychotic depression. This distinction is based on statistically significant differences in presenting features, biology, familial transmission, course, and response to treatment between unipolar MDD with psychotic features and nonpsychotic MDD.

Epidemiology

In a sample of nearly 19,000 subjects across five European countries, approximately 19% of those who fulfilled criteria for MDD reported psychotic features (Ohayon and Schatzberg 2002). In this latter study, unipolar MDD with psychotic features was found to affect 4 in 1,000 individuals in the community (Ohayon and Schatzberg 2002). In a large-scale Finnish study, a prevalence rate of 0.35% was reported for MDD with psychotic features (Perälä et al. 2007), confirming findings in the European study (Schatzberg 2015). Cross-sectional and 1-year prospective data from the Epidemiologic Catchment Area study indicated that 14% of the patients with MDD were classified as having psychotic features (Johnson et al. 1991). A recent study of nonhospitalized first-episode, drug-naive patients with MDD in China reported a 10% rate of psychotic features (Zhou et al. 2020). In a recent European multicenter study of refractory depression, psychotic features were found in 11% of patients with MDD (Dold et al. 2019). Higher rates of psychotic features have been reported in cohorts of hospitalized patients with MDD, with Coryell et al. (1984) reporting approximately 25% as psychotically depressed.

Genetics and Family History

Psychotic MDD is associated with a 10% concordance rate (Cardno et al. 1999), and specific patterns of familial transmission have been noted. A family history of schizophrenia has been reported to be more typically associated with psychotic depression than with nonpsychotic depression (Coryell et al. 1984). First-degree relatives of those with psychotic MDD also have been shown to have a greater likelihood of having both MDD and psychotic MDD compared with first-degree relatives of subjects with nonpsychotic MDD (Leckman et al. 1984; Simpson et al. 1999). A higher rate of bipolar disorder also has been reported among first-degree relatives of subjects with psychotic MDD as compared with first-degree relatives of subjects with nonpsychotic MDD (Schatzberg and Rothschild 1992; Weissman et al. 1988).

Interestingly, subjects with severe MDD with mood-incongruent psychotic features appear to have family histories more similar to histories reported for patients with schizophrenia than to histories reported for patients with nonpsychotic MDD (Coryell et al. 1982, 1985). Furthermore, data have suggested a trend toward a much lower risk for family history of affective illness among subjects in this group compared with those with mood-congruent psychotic features (Maj et al. 1991). In contrast, subjects with severe MDD with mood-congruent psychotic features have been found to have family histories more consistent with those found among patients with nonpsychotic MDD and significantly different from those found in patients with schizophrenia (Coryell et al. 1982).

Efforts to determine specific genetic risks for MDD with psychotic features have been limited because large-scale genetic studies have generally not concentrated on this subtype. As described later in the "Psychoneuroendocrinology" section, our group has hypothesized that excessive glucocorticoid activity underlies the development of psychosis in depression. In that context, we have explored the contribution of genetic variation in the hypothalamic-pituitary-adrenal (HPA) axis to psychotic symptoms and have reported that variations in the genes for glucocorticoid and corticotropin-releasing hormone 1 receptors contribute significantly to psychosis in MDD (Schatzberg et al. 2014). Variation in the glucocorticoid receptor contributed to cortisol activity.

Symptomatology

Differences Between Psychotic and Nonpsychotic Major Depressive Disorder in Symptomatology and Comorbidity

Subjects with psychotic MDD have been reported to experience more severe depressive symptoms than those with nonpsychotic MDD (Coryell et al. 1985). Psychotic MDD has also been associated with younger age at onset (Black et al. 1992).

Psychotic MDD in patients older than 50 years is associated with both a longer duration of illness and lower comorbidity compared with that in patients younger than 50 years (Benazzi 1999b). Among patients with a major depressive episode who are older than 50 years, psychotic MDD is associated with significantly greater severity, lower comorbidity, greater likelihood of a diagnosis of bipolar I disorder, and lower likelihood of unipolar depressive disorder as compared with nonpsychotic MDD (Benazzi 1999b).

Bipolar and unipolar depression with psychotic features have been reported to show no significant differences in age, gender, duration of illness, severity, recurrences, chronicity, comorbidity, hallucinations, or delusions (Benazzi 1999a).

Our group (Keller et al. 2006b) has reported that patients with MDD who are delusional and those who are nondelusional can be separated with a high degree of sensitivity and specificity by applying the psychotic subscale of the Brief Psychiatric Rating Scale (BPRS). Among the four subscale items, unusual thought content provided the most robust test characteristics.

Symptoms Correlated With Psychotic Major Depressive Disorder; Measurement of Symptom Severity

A retrospective study of patients with MDD found that subjects with the psychotic form were more ruminative, had more feelings of guilt, and showed more psychomotor agitation (Charney and Nelson 1981). Overall, feelings of worthlessness, guilt, and suicidal ideation have been found to be highly associated with symptoms of psychosis in psychotic depression (Ohayon and Schatzberg 2002). In a study of patients with MDD, those with psychosis were more likely to report psychomotor disturbance, feeling sinful and guilty, feeling deserving of punishment, constipation, terminal insomnia, appetite and weight loss, and loss of pleasure and interest (Parker et al. 1995). In fact, both of these latter studies suggested that the presence of these highly associated nonpsychotic features may be indicative of the diagnosis of psychotic MDD in the absence of psychosis being elicited or acknowledged (Ohayon and Schatzberg 2002; Parker et al. 1995).

Measurement of severity of MDD with psychotic features has been demonstrated using a combined scale (named the HAMD-BPRS11) consisting of the six-item melancholia subscale of the Hamilton Depression Rating Scale (HAM-D6) plus five items from the BPRS (Østergaard et al. 2014).

Mood Congruence in Psychotic Features

Psychotic depression appears to show a high rate of stability of diagnosis on follow-up (Schwartz et al. 2000), with the form and content of delusional thinking being consistent across recurrent episodes (Charney and Nelson 1981). As. stated earlier, DSM-IV-TR classified the psychotic features in psychotic MDD as either mood congruent or mood incongruent. Interestingly, a study of patients hospitalized for a diagnosis of psychotic MDD found that 50%–60% of the subjects experienced both mood-congruent and mood-incongruent psychotic features (Burch et al. 1994). In addition, this study reported that approximately half of the subjects with mood-incongruent features experienced at least one mood-congruent symptom (Burch et al. 1994). Also, approximately two-thirds of the individuals with primarily mood-congruent features experienced at least one mood-incongruent symptom (Burch et al. 1994). Thus, it has been suggested that the subclassification of severe MDD with psychotic features into mood-congruent and mood-incongruent types may be artificial, given that features of both types are commonly encountered together (Burch et al. 1994).

Among patients with MDD, those with psychotic features have greater levels of both morbidity and impairment in insight than do those without psychotic features. For example, relative to patients with nonpsychotic depression, patients with psychotic depression are more likely to have been ill for a longer time and to have experienced more episodes of depression (Leyton et al. 1995). An analysis of data from the Netherlands Mental Health Survey and Incidence Study (NEMESIS) found that patients with psychotic MDD had the highest levels of impairment in physical, psychological, and social functioning among all patients with depression, including those with severe nonpsychotic depression (Kruijshaar et al. 2003). Furthermore, when the Scale to Assess Unawareness of Mental Disorders was used to compare insight into illness among individuals with various psychotic disorders, subjects with psychotic depression showed a lack of insight into the presence of symptoms such as hallucinations, delusions, and thought disorder comparable to that shown by patients with schizophrenia, schizoaffective disorder, or bipolar disorder (Pini et al. 2001).

Neuropsychological Dysfunction in Psychotic Depression

Patients with psychotic MDD have been shown to have a pattern of neuropsychological dysfunction that is distinct from that of nonpsychotic MDD (Belanoff et al. 2001b; Fleming et al. 2004; Hill et al. 2004; Jeste et al. 1996; Schatzberg et al. 2000). They have been shown to perform significantly more poorly on measures of visual memory and visual-spatial perception (Hill et al. 2004). Significantly greater impairment on measures of psychomotor speed, motor skills, attention, and learning has been reported in elderly subjects with psychotic MDD compared with those with nonpsychotic MDD (Jeste et al. 1996). Subjects with psychotic MDD have also been shown to have significantly greater impairment on tests of attention, response inhibition, and verbal declarative memory (Schatzberg et al. 2000). In addition, they have been found to show significantly greater impairment in verbal recognition memory than subjects with nonpsychotic MDD (Belanoff et al. 2001b). Overall, the most consistently reported deficits in cognitive performance that have been associated with psychotic MDD as compared with the nonpsychotic form occur on measures of verbal memory, executive functioning, and psychomotor speed (Fleming et al. 2004). A recent meta-analysis indicated these deficits were clearly seen in elderly adults (55+ years) but, as noted here, are also seen in patients of all ages with psychotic MDD (Vermeulen et al. 2019).

Interestingly, the pattern of neuropsychological dysfunction among subjects with psychotic MDD appears to be similar to that seen in schizophrenia (Hill et al. 2004; Jeste et al. 1996). In a study of first-episode, antipsychotic-naive patients, both those with psychotic depression and those with schizophrenia showed a similar pattern of neuropsychological impairment on measures of verbal memory, visual memory, motor skills, and visual-spatial abilities (Hill et al. 2004). This latter study, however, found a degree of impairment in subjects with psychotic MDD that was less severe than that in subjects with schizophrenia (Hill et al. 2004). In contrast, another study comparing neuropsychological performance in elderly subjects with schizophrenia and those with psychotic MDD reported comparable degrees of neuropsychological impairment for both groups (Jeste et al. 1996). Our group recently confirmed this lack of difference in neuropsychological deficits between nonelderly cohorts of patients with psychotic MDD and those with schizophrenia (Cherian et al. 2019). Numerous studies have demonstrated that cortisol levels are major contributors to neuropsychological impairment in depression and schizophrenia (Gomez et al. 2006; Keller et al. 2017).

Pathogenesis

Psychotic depression is more frequently and consistently associated with biological abnormalities than is nonpsychotic depression. For instance, negative life events are less likely to be associated with psychotic depression than with nonpsychotic depression (Kohn et al. 2001).

Neurophysiology

Psychotic MDD is associated with significantly increased wakefulness, decreased rapid eye movement (REM) sleep percentage, decreased REM activity, and decreased sleep-onset REM latencies as compared with nonpsychotic MDD (Thase et al. 1986).

Abnormalities of the P300 component of event-related potentials have been suggested as clinical correlates of psychotic depression. For instance, although prolonged P300 latency has been associated with clinical depression, decreased P300 amplitude has been correlated with paranoid ideation in psychotic MDD (Karaaslan et al. 2003). In addition, it also has been shown that P300 abnormalities, both prolonged latency and decreased amplitude, resolve with successful drug treatment of psychotic MDD (Karaaslan et al. 2003).

Psychoneuroendocrinology

Cortisol Physiology

Psychotic MDD is consistently and commonly associated with more severe abnormalities of the HPA axis compared with nonpsychotic MDD (Arana et al. 1985; Coryell et al. 1984; Nelson and Davis 1997; Stetler and Miller 2011). Patients with psychotic MDD also have been shown to have significantly higher rates of nonsuppression on the dexamethasone suppression test (Arana et al. 1985; Nelson and Davis 1997; Rihmer et al. 1984) and significantly higher cortisol levels after administration of dexamethasone compared with individuals with nonpsychotic MDD and control subjects (Evans et al. 1983; Maes et al. 1989; Rothschild et al. 1982; Schatzberg et al. 1983). A positive dexamethasone suppression test result has been reported to be a statistically significant correlate of psychotic depression (Vythilingam et al. 2003). Predexamethasone studies of cortisol (e.g., urinary free cortisol) have reported it to be significantly elevated in patients with psychotic MDD (Anton 1987; Nelson et al. 1984).

In a study assessing 24-hour cortisol and corticotropin secretion over 3 days, patients with nonpsychotic MDD showed reduced levels of cortisol secretion relative to control subjects (Posener et al. 2000). In contrast, the same study found that patients with psychotic MDD had significantly increased corticotropin secretion compared with control subjects (Posener et al. 2000). In a study assessing patterns of afternoon cortisol secretion among patients with depression and healthy subjects, patients with psychotic MDD were found to have a significantly higher mean and a nonlinear pattern of cortisol levels throughout the afternoon (Belanoff et al. 2001b). Furthermore, evening cortisol levels were significantly elevated in those with psychotic MDD compared with nondelusional individuals with depression and healthy control subjects (Keller et al. 2006a). More recently, we observed in a 15-hour study from 6 P.M. to 9 A.M. that cortisol levels in subjects with psychotic depression were particularly elevated between 6 P.M. and 1 A.M. in comparison with levels in the nonpsychotic depression and healthy control groups (Keller et al. 2017; Schatzberg et al. 2014).

Some time ago, we hypothesized that increased cortisol activity could enhance mesolimbic dopamine and could explain the development of psychosis in psychotic MDD (Schatzberg et al. 1985). Significantly higher plasma dopamine levels have been reported among subjects with psychotic MDD compared with those with a nonpsychotic form (Rothschild et al. 1987). Significantly higher plasma dopamine levels in response to a 1-mg dose of dexamethasone have also been reported among subjects with psychotic MDD compared with those with nonpsychotic MDD (Rothschild et al. 1987). Lupien et al. (1995) have reported that metyrapone, a glucocorticoid synthesis blocker, results in increases in plasma homovanillic acid, a dopamine metabolite, in healthy control subjects, suggesting that cortisol may result in decreased dopamine activity. Thus, the earlier reported effects of dexamethasone on plasma dopamine may have reflected a rebound effect of rising corticotropin-releasing hormone levels on dopamine. In rats, we reported that corticosterone decreases prefrontal dopamine metabolism, an effect that could account for the prefrontal cognitive deficits seen in psychotic MDD (Lindley et al. 1999, 2002). In squirrel monkeys, cortisol administration can produce prefrontal cognitive defects similar to those seen with dopamine depletion (Lyons et al. 2000).

In addition, the mean plasma activity of dopamine β-hydroxylase, the enzyme that converts dopamine to norepinephrine, has been reported to be significantly lower among patients with psychotic MDD than those with nonpsychotic MDD (Cubells et al. 2002). However, no association between specific dopamine β-hydroxylase alleles and psychotic MDD was observed (Cubells et al. 2002). Thus, further investigation is required to ferret out possible cortisol-dopamine interactions in psychotic depression.

Neuroimaging

Structural

Psychotic MDD has been explored using both structural and functional imaging. An early computed tomography study of subjects with depression found significantly larger ventricle-to-brain ratios and inferior parietal brain atrophy that were associated with nonsuppression on the dexamethasone suppression test and greater impairment on cognitive testing (Rothschild et al. 1989). MRI studies of late-life depression have reported significant atrophy in specific brain regions; in one study, Simpson et al. (1999) found the strongest correlates of psychotic features to be with diencephalic atrophy, reticular activating system lesions, brain stem atrophy, and left-sided frontotemporal atrophy. Similarly, Kim et al. (1999) reported prefrontal atrophy in elderly patients with psychotic depression. Of interest, in a review of studies examining cognitive deficits in psychotic depression, we noted that the areas of impairment most commonly reported corresponded to cognitive domains thought to be mediated by frontal and medial temporal brain regions (Fleming et al. 2004).

Hippocampal volume has been reported to be decreased in patients with MDD. Early studies may have included assessment of the amygdala in combination with the hippocampus. In a study by our group, we did not observe smaller hippocampal volumes in psychotic depression but did see significant reductions in amygdalar volumes (Keller et al. 2008).

Functional

A single-photon emission computed tomography study of subjects with MDD compared with healthy control subjects found that those with psychotic MDD had significantly decreased regional cerebral blood flow in both the left subgenual anterior cingulate cortex and the right inferior frontal cortex as compared with those with nonpsychotic MDD (Skaf et al. 2002). In a study that included subjects with delusional or nondelusional depression, we reported that default mode functional connectivity in severe depression was increased in a circuit that included the anterior cingulate, thalamus, and subgenual region (Greicius et al. 2007). Resting-state functional connectivity was not increased in subjects with psychotic depression who were in remission (Neufeld et al. 2018).

In a study that used task-mediated imaging to examine working memory, Garrett et al. (2011) found that participants with psychotic MDD showed increased activation of the parahippocampal region at lower demand on the N-back task in comparison with participants with nonpsychotic MDD and healthy control subjects. Patients with psychosis also showed abnormalities in temporoparietal regions with extraneous stimuli, pointing to sensory gating deficits in the disorder (Garrett et al. 2011). Another report on verbal memory from the same study found that deficits in verbal retrieval of memories may reflect difficulties in encoding because decreased activation in the hippocampus, insula, and prefrontal cortex during encoding was seen in those with psychotic depression (Kelley et al. 2013). Higher prefrontal and parietal activation observed in those with psychotic depression was thought to reflect a means of compensating for difficulty in encoding.

Treatment

Various data have been put forth supporting the efficacy of electroconvulsive therapy (ECT) and combination antidepressant and antipsychotic therapies in the treatment of psychotic MDD. Most studies clearly indicate that ECT and combination antidepressant and antipsychotic interventions are superior to antidepressant therapy alone. Psychotic MDD has, in general, also been associated with a lower placebo response rate when compared with nonpsychotic MDD. Furthermore, ECT appears more likely to be effective in the psychotic than the nonpsychotic form, but relapse rates are high.

Placebo Response

Originally, data examining placebo response in psychotic MDD had been derived from single-blind run-in studies. Spiker and Kupfer (1988) reviewed placebo response rates in psychotic versus nonpsychotic MDD and found response rates of 0% and 13.3%, respectively. Over time, with accumulation of data from double-blind randomized controlled trials (RCTs), much higher placebo response rates have been observed. This was first evident in a controlled comparison of olanzapine, fluoxetine, and placebo that reported higher placebo response rates (approximately 28%) in a parallel nonplacebo washout design (Rothschild et al. 2004). Furthermore, a placebo response rate of approximately 30% was reported in a combined analysis of data from five double-blind studies of mifepristone in psychotic MDD (Block et al. 2018).

Antidepressant Monotherapy

Glassman et al. (1977), in their classic study on imipramine blood levels and response in hospitalized patients with depression, noted that those with psychotic MDD had poor responses to imipramine monotherapy. Two early retrospective studies of patients with MDD (Brown et al. 1982; Charney and Nelson 1981) reported that, in contrast to patients with nonpsychotic depression, those with psychotic depression had a poor response to antidepressant monotherapy but a good response either to a combination of antidepressant and antipsychotic or to ECT. These observations were followed by a prospective comparison study of 35 patients with psychotic depression who received amitriptyline, perphenazine, or a combination of the two (Spiker et al. 1986). In this latter study, combination therapy was found to be significantly more effective than either component alone. A 6-week study of imipramine, dosed to a target blood level of 200–300 μg/L, in the treatment of MDD found response rates of 69% and 44%, respectively, for subjects with psychotic depression and those with nonpsychotic depression (Bruijn et al. 2001).

More recent antidepressant studies have concentrated on the selective serotonin reuptake inhibitors (SSRIs). An 8-week open-label study of patients with MDD treated with sertraline monotherapy found a significantly lower likelihood of achieving a 50% reduction in or a complete remission of symptoms among patients with psychotic compared with nonpsychotic MDD (Simpson et al. 2003). In this study, psychosis was found to be a predictor of poor response to SSRI treatment independent of degree of depression and general psychopathology.

In contrast, a 6-week study of patients with psychotic depression found a response rate of 84% for open-label fluvoxamine monotherapy (Gatti et al. 1996). Similarly, a 6-week prospective, randomized, double-blind study of subjects with psychotic MDD treated with either venlafaxine or fluvoxamine monotherapy found response rates of 58% and 79%, respectively (Zanardi et al. 2000). A 6-week double-blind study of subjects with psychotic MDD found response rates of 75% and 46% for sertraline and paroxetine monotherapy, respectively (Zanardi et al. 1996). Overall, however, these data do not agree with the general United States experience, and questions have been raised as to the consistency in diagnoses between Europe and the United States. It is interesting that there are relatively few RCT data on antidepressant monotherapy in the U.S. trials of psychotic MDD.

Antipsychotic Monotherapy and Combination Antidepressant and Antipsychotic Therapy

The early study by Spiker et al. (1985b) reported response rates of approximately 78%, 41%, and 19%, respectively, for amitriptyline plus perphenazine, amitriptyline alone, and perphenazine alone. Similarly, a response rate of 73% was reported for patients with psychotic depression who were treated for 5 weeks with fluoxetine plus perphenazine (Rothschild et al. 1993a). It is notable that this latter study found an overall lower likelihood of side effects with this combination as compared with a combination of a tricyclic antidepressant and an antipsychotic (Rothschild et al. 1993a).

A 6-week study comparing the efficacy of combination treatment with haloperidol plus amitriptyline with that of risperidone monotherapy found the former to be significantly superior in the treatment of psychotic depression on measures of depression and the BPRS (Müller-Siecheneder et al. 1998).

Olanzapine was at one time thought to be both an effective adjunctive therapy and monotherapy intervention in the treatment of psychotic MDD because of its antipsychotic and potential antidepressant properties (Nelson et al. 2001; Rothschild et al. 1999). An open-label study of patients with psychotic MDD treated with olanzapine combined with fluoxetine found an overall response rate of 55.6% and a remission rate of 40.7% at 6 weeks (Matthews et al. 2002). However, a report on combined data from two parallel 8-week double-blind studies of patients with MDD with psychotic features reported response rates of 63.6% for those treated with a combination of olanzapine and fluoxetine, 34.9% for olanzapine monotherapy, and 28.0% for placebo treatment (Rothschild et al. 2004). Interestingly, when this single analysis was divided into two studies, one of the two trials failed to show statistically significant superiority for the combination of olanzapine and fluoxetine (Rothschild et al. 2004). These trials were devised to demonstrate that olanzapine monotherapy was effective in the disorder, but that was not observed. Furthermore, in a double-blind comparison of olanzapine plus sertraline vs. olanzapine plus placebo, the combination with sertraline produced a significantly greater remission rate (42%) compared with that of olanzapine alone (24%) (Meyers et al. 2009). Greater weight gain and glucose increases were observed in younger patients. These data thus demonstrate that olanzapine monotherapy is not particularly effective in psychotic MDD, but it does appear to be effective in combination with either fluoxetine or sertraline. Monitoring for weight gain and metabolic effects is needed.

Electroconvulsive Therapy

In a study of 55 consecutively admitted inpatients with MDD, ECT was associated with a significantly greater likelihood of achieving a 50% reduction (92% vs. 55%) and complete remission (57% vs. 24%) of symptoms among patients with psychotic depression than among those with nonpsychotic depression (Birkenhäger et al. 2003). Similarly, a study of 37 patients with psychotic depression found a response rate of 86% for ECT (Spiker et al. 1985a). More recently, Prudic et al. (2004) reported that psychosis was a positive predictor of response; however, it also augured more rapid relapse on follow-up. In contrast, a recent epidemiological study pointed to lower mortality on follow-up among patients with severe MDD who received ECT (Jorgensen et al. 2020), as discussed later in the section "Course and Follow-Up."

Treatment-Refractory Psychotic Depression

Among patients with psychotic depression refractory to combined antidepressant and antipsychotic therapy, lithium has been reported as an effective augmentation strategy (Nelson and Mazure 1986; Price et al. 1983). In an open-label study of six patients with psychotic depression refractory to combination therapy, lithium augmentation resulted in significant improvement in symptoms in three subjects and a more gradual improvement in two (Price et al. 1983). In contrast, another study reported lithium augmentation to be effective in 8 of 9 patients with bipolar but only 3 of 12 with unipolar refractory psychotic depression (Nelson and Mazure 1986).

Adequacy and Duration of Treatment

Data have suggested that psychotic MDD is often inadequately treated. In a study of 187 patients with depression referred for ECT, only 4% of the subjects with psychotic depression had received at least one adequate antidepressant and antipsychotic medication trial, and 47% had received either no antipsychotic medication or antipsychotic treatment for less than 3 weeks (Mulsant et al. 1997). In contrast, the same study reported that more than 50% of the subjects with nonpsychotic MDD had received at least one adequate medication trial (Mulsant et al. 1997). On the basis of these data, it has been suggested that several of the patients classified as having treatment-refractory depression, especially among those referred for ECT, actually had unidentified psychosis and had been prescribed inadequate pharmacotherapy (Fink 2003a, 2003b). These latter concerns underscore the importance of both distinguishing psychotic from nonpsychotic depression and improving the diagnostic criteria by which psychotic depression is defined.

An early study that followed up with patients with psychotic depression for 11 months after discontinuation of both antidepressant and antipsychotic therapy suggested that antipsychotic therapy should be continued for at least 4 months after remission of psychosis symptoms (Rothschild and Duval 2003). A recent study compared continuation therapy for up to 9 months with sertraline plus olanzapine or sertraline plus placebo in patients who showed a response to 12 weeks of combination treatment (Flint et al. 2019). A 55% relapse rate was observed with sertraline plus placebo, compared with 20% with sertraline plus olanzapine. Continuation combined therapy was associated with a significantly greater risk of weight gain and increased cholesterol levels, but not with other metabolic effects (e.g., glucose and triglyceride levels). This may reflect the relatively high percentage of older subjects included in the trial. These data do suggest that antipsychotic therapy needs to be continued for several months past the point of response.

Novel Strategies

Amoxapine has been suggested as a potential monotherapy in the treatment of psychotic depression because of its combined antidepressant and antipsychotic properties. A double-blind study comparing amoxapine monotherapy with amitriptyline plus perphenazine in the treatment of psychotic depression found overall comparable improvements in depression and psychosis but significantly fewer extrapyramidal side effects among those receiving amoxapine (Anton and Burch 1990).

Following our findings that subjects with psychotic MDD had extremely high post-dexamethasone cortisol levels on the dexamethasone suppression test, we pursued whether administering an agent that blocked the glucocorticoid receptor could rapidly reverse the psychotic symptoms in MDD. In a 9-day double-blind, placebo-controlled crossover study (4 days in each condition), five subjects with psychotic depression treated with the glucocorticoid receptor antagonist mifepristone, at 600 mg/day, had greater improvement in BPRS, 21-item HAM-D (HAM-D-21), and Clinical Global Impression Scale scores while receiving the active drug (Belanoff et al. 2001a). Interestingly, this study found that at the conclusion of the 9-day study, four of the five patients were no longer psychotic, and all subjectively noted improved cognitive abilities (Belanoff et al. 2001a).

In a randomized but open-label study that compared the efficacy of 50 mg, 600 mg, and 1,200 mg of mifepristone for 7 days in subjects with psychotic MDD, 13 of 19 individuals (68.4%) in the 600-mg and 1,200-mg groups showed at least a 30% decline in BPRS score, 12 of 19 (63.2%) showed a 50% decrease in BPRS positive symptoms subscale score, and 8 of 19 (42.1%) had a 50% decline in HAM-D-21 score (Belanoff et al. 2002). In contrast, among those in the 50-mg group, 4 of 11 (36.4%) showed at least a 30% decline in BPRS score, 3 of 11 (27.3%) had a 50% decrease in BPRS positive symptoms subscale score, and 2 of 11 (18.2%) had a 50% decline in HAM-D-21 score (Belanoff et al. 2002). These data have led to several double-blind RCTs by our research group and by an industry sponsor. In the study by our group (Flores et al. 2006), 30 patients were randomly assigned to receive 600 mg/day of mifepristone or placebo for 7 days; by day 8, significantly more mifepristone-treated patients showed a 50% reduction in BPRS positive symptoms than those given placebo. In the industry-sponsored trials (Block et al. 2018), mifepristone was compared with placebo for 7 days, and response was assessed at day 7 and at scheduled intervals thereafter up to day 56. Dosages ranged from 300 mg/day to 1,200 mg/day. None of the trials met the primary endpoint, but in individual studies and in a combined analysis, attainment of a therapeutic blood level greater than 1,637 ng/mL was associated with clinical response and statistical separation from placebo. Specifically, 43% of the subjects who attained that concentration met the criterion of response (psychosis improvement) at 1 week, with response continuing to 8 weeks, in contrast to 29% of those who received placebo and 31% of those who attained lower plasma levels on mifepristone (Block et al. 2018). Of particular importance was that patients who attained the so-called therapeutic level also demonstrated significantly greater increases in adrenocorticotropic hormone and cortisol than did patients in the other two groups. These data indicate that increases in these hormones are associated with attaining therapeutic drug levels and are in keeping with the notion that blocking the HPA axis is associated with improvement in psychosis in response to treatment with mifepristone.

Course and Follow-Up

In a study examining diagnostic predictors among 45 inpatients with MDD, psychotic features were found to predict an unfavorable course (Maier et al. 1989). According to 1-year prospective data from the Epidemiological Catchment Area study, psychotic MDD was associated with an overall more severe course, increased risk of relapse, persistence of symptoms over 1 year, more suicide attempts, more hospitalization, more comorbid psychiatric diagnoses, and greater impairment in psychosocial functioning compared with nonpsychotic MDD (Johnson et al. 1991). Similarly, a study of patients with either psychotic or nonpsychotic MDD assessed 1 year after discharge from inpatient treatment found that those with the psychotic form had an overall poorer clinical course, a greater likelihood of depression lasting longer than 9 months, and a greater likelihood of being in a depressive episode at follow-up (Robinson and Spiker 1985). We reported that at the 1-year follow-up, patients with psychotic MDD had significantly poorer psychosocial functioning than did those with nonpsychotic MDD (Rothschild et al. 1993b). In this study, the two groups did not differ on measures of depression or psychosis at follow-up.

In a study examining the risk of symptom relapse in subjects with psychotic depression treated with fluoxetine and perphenazine, it was reported that patients who had signs of relapse after discontinuation of antipsychotic therapy at 4 months were more likely to have had a longer duration of the current episode, to have had a history of more frequent episodes, and to be younger (Rothschild and Duval 2003). Despite an initial response rate of 80%–90% to acute treatment with ECT, patients with psychotic depression were found to have a high relapse rate (50%) at the 1-year follow-up (Spiker et al. 1985a), a finding replicated in Prudic et al. (2004).

A 2-year follow-up study of patients with MDD found significantly greater levels of psychosocial impairment among subjects with psychotic MDD compared with those with nonpsychotic MDD both in the 5 years preceding study entry and at the 6-month follow-up (Coryell et al. 1987). Interestingly, this study also reported that at the 2-year follow-up, the significant differences in psychosocial impairment between psychotic and nonpsychotic MDD had resolved (Coryell et al. 1987).

A 40-year follow-up study of patients with psychotic depression found that mood-incongruent psychotic features were associated with a long-term outcome intermediate between that of nonpsychotic depression and that of schizophrenia (Coryell and Tsuang 1985). In contrast, subjects with MDD with mood-congruent psychotic features in this study had a long-term outcome that was similar to that of subjects with nonpsychotic depression (Coryell and Tsuang 1985). However, an 8-year follow-up of patients with psychotic depression found the prognosis of those with mood-incongruent psychotic features to be comparable to the prognosis of those with mood-congruent psychotic features (Tsuang and Coryell 1993).

In a study of patients with MDD who were followed for up to 15 years after a hospital admission, patients with psychotic features had a twofold greater mortality rate compared with those without psychotic features (41% vs. 20%) (Vythilingam et al. 2003). This greater mortality was thought to reflect co-occurring or resultant cardiac disease, but it might have reflected poor response to treatment. A recent study indicated that despite demonstrating marked impairment in health-related quality of life on the 36-Item Short Form Survey (SF-36) before acute treatment, patients with psychotic depression showed normalized SF-36 scores after successful therapy (Bingham et al. 2019). Another study in Europe reported that treatment with ECT was associated with lower mortality on follow-up in patients with severe MDD with psychotic features (Jorgensen et al. 2020).

In a study of patients admitted for a first episode of psychotic depression, nearly one in eight developed symptoms of mania or hypomania within 2 years after discharge (DelBello et al. 2003). Interestingly, this study also found that antidepressant treatment was associated with a significantly reduced risk of developing a manic or hypomanic episode (DelBello et al. 2003).

Suicide

Elevated suicide risk in patients with psychotic depression was first reported in a retrospective study at the New York State Psychiatric Institute (Roose et al. 1983). This increased risk has also been reported by others. For example, psychotic depression was associated with a greater lifetime risk of suicide attempts compared with schizophrenia—rates were 42.4% and 27.3%, respectively (Radomsky et al. 1999). Furthermore, a violent means of suicide appears to be more commonly associated with psychotic MDD than with nonpsychotic MDD (Isometsä et al. 1994). A retrospective study of 45 inpatients with a diagnosis of psychotic depression found delusions of persecution and guilt to be significantly associated with a greater likelihood of making a medically serious suicide attempt (Miller and Chabrier 1987, 1988). In contrast, psychotic depression with delusions of bodily disease, damage, and malfunction has been found to be associated with a significantly lower likelihood of a medically serious suicide attempt (Miller and Chabrier 1987). Although these data pointed to an increased risk of suicide in psychotic depression, the Collaborative Depression Study failed to find an increased rate at 5-year follow-up (Fawcett et al. 1987). More recently, a systematic review of 24 studies in the literature indicated that hospitalized patients with psychotic depression had higher rates of suicide during their acute episodes than did nonpsychotic subjects. Longer-term follow-up did not demonstrate a consistently elevated suicide risk, perhaps reflecting treatment effects (Zalpuri and Rothschild 2016). A large-scale Danish study of some 35,000 patients with severe depression treated in the hospital indicated that psychosis was not a significant predictor of suicide risk above severity (Leadholm et al. 2014).

Conclusion

Psychotic depression is a relatively common psychiatric condition that affects up to 20% of patients with MDD. It is more commonly associated with feelings of guilt, worthlessness, and suicidal ideation in addition to, and highly correlated with, symptoms of psychosis. Psychotic depression also has been found to be characterized by a specific pattern of neuropsychological impairment that appears to overlap with that observed in schizophrenia. Psychotic depression distinguishes itself from nonpsychotic depression, particularly in neuroendocrine and neuroimaging findings.

Psychotic depression has generally been associated with a low placebo response rate and poor response to antidepressant monotherapy, although recent data have raised questions, particularly about the validity of this low placebo response. Data thus far best support efficacy for the combination of an antidepressant and an antipsychotic or for ECT in the treatment of psychotic depression. Data are limited on the utility of lithium augmentation in treatment-refractory psychotic depression. Recent findings suggest the possible utility of glucocorticoid receptor antagonists in the treatment of psychotic depression.

In addition, studies have shown that psychotic depression is associated with a greater risk of relapse, suicide, mortality, and poor long-term psychosocial functioning as compared with nonpsychotic depression. Unfortunately, data also have been put forth suggesting that psychotic depression may be frequently underdiagnosed and undertreated. Such findings greatly underscore the importance of both distinguishing psychotic depression from nonpsychotic depression and improving the diagnostic criteria for and treatment of this condition. In summary, data support psychotic depression as a distinct clinical entity from nonpsychotic depression. This distinction is based on statistically significant differences in presenting features, biology, familial transmission, course, and response to treatment between psychotic and nonpsychotic depression.

References

American Psychiatric Association: Diagnostic and Statistical Manual of Mental Disorders, 4th Edition, Text Revision. Washington, DC, American Psychiatric Association, 2000

American Psychiatric Association: Diagnostic and Statistical Manual of Mental Disorders, 5th Edition. Arlington, VA, American Psychiatric Association, 2013

Anton RF: Urinary free cortisol in psychotic depression. Biol Psychiatry 22(1):24–34, 1987 3790638

Anton RF Jr, Burch EA Jr: Amoxapine versus amitriptyline combined with perphenazine in the treatment of psychotic depression. Am J Psychiatry 147(9):1203–1208, 1990 2201223

Arana GW, Baldessarini RJ, Ornsteen M: The dexamethasone suppression test for diagnosis and prognosis in psychiatry. Commentary and review. Arch Gen Psychiatry 42(12):1193–1204, 1985 3000317

Belanoff JK, Flores BH, Kalezhan M, et al: Rapid reversal of psychotic depression using mifepristone. J Clin Psychopharmacol 21(5):516–521, 2001a 11593077

Belanoff JK, Kalehzan M, Sund B, et al: Cortisol activity and cognitive changes in psychotic major depression. Am J Psychiatry 158(10):1612–1616, 2001b 11578992

Belanoff JK, Rothschild AJ, Cassidy F, et al: An open label trial of C-1073 (mifepristone) for psychotic major depression. Biol Psychiatry 52(5):386–392, 2002 12242054

Benazzi F: Bipolar versus unipolar psychotic outpatient depression. J Affect Disord 55(1):63–66, 1999a 10512608

Benazzi F: Psychotic late-life depression: a 376-case study. Int Psychogeriatr 11(3):325–332, 1999b 10547132

Bingham KS, Whyte EM, Mulsant BH, et al: Health-related quality of life in remitted psychotic depression. J Affect Disord 256:373–379, 2019 31207561

Birkenhäger TK, Pluijms EM, Lucius SAP: ECT response in delusional versus non-delusional depressed inpatients. J Affect Disord 74(2):191–195, 2003 12706521
Black DW, Winokur G, Nasrallah A, et al: Psychotic symptoms and age of onset in affective disorders. Psychopathology 25(1):19–22, 1992 1603906
Block TS, Kushner H, Kalin N, et al: Combined analysis of mifepristone for psychotic depression: plasma levels associated with clinical response. Biol Psychiatry 84(1):46–54, 2018 29523415
Brown RP, Frances A, Kocsis JH, et al: Psychotic vs. nonpsychotic depression: comparison of treatment response. J Nerv Ment Dis 170(10):635–637, 1982 6125562
Bruijn JA, Moleman P, Mulder PGH, et al: Treatment of mood-congruent psychotic depression with imipramine. J Affect Disord 66(2–3):165–174, 2001 11578669
Burch EA Jr, Anton RF, Carson WH: Mood congruent and incongruent psychotic depressions: are they the same? J Affect Disord 31(4):275–280, 1994 7989642
Cardno AG, Marshall EJ, Coid B, et al: Heritability estimates for psychotic disorders: the Maudsley twin psychosis series. Arch Gen Psychiatry 56(2):162–168, 1999 10025441
Charney DS, Nelson JC: Delusional and nondelusional unipolar depression: further evidence for distinct subtypes. Am J Psychiatry 138(3):328–333, 1981 6110345
Cherian K, Schatzberg AF, Keller J: HPA axis in psychotic major depression and schizophrenia spectrum disorders: cortisol, clinical symptomatology, and cognition. Schizophr Res 213:72–79, 2019 31307859
Coryell W, Tsuang MT: Major depression with mood-congruent or mood-incongruent psychotic features: outcome after 40 years. Am J Psychiatry 142(4):479–482, 1985 3976922
Coryell W, Tsuang MT, McDaniel J: Psychotic features in major depression. Is mood congruence important? J Affect Disord 4(3):227–236, 1982 6215441
Coryell W, Pfohl B, Zimmerman M: The clinical and neuroendocrine features of psychotic depression. J Nerv Ment Dis 172(9):521–528, 1984 6470694
Coryell W, Endicott J, Keller M, Andreasen NC: Phenomenology and family history in DSM-III psychotic depression. J Affect Disord 9(1):13–18, 1985 3160743
Coryell W, Endicott J, Keller M: The importance of psychotic features to major depression: course and outcome during a 2-year follow-up. Acta Psychiatr Scand 75(1):78–85, 1987 3577843
Cubells JF, Price LH, Meyers BS, et al: Genotype-controlled analysis of plasma dopamine beta-hydroxylase activity in psychotic unipolar major depression. Biol Psychiatry 51(5):358–364, 2002 11904129
DelBello MP, Carlson GA, Tohen M, et al: Rates and predictors of developing a manic or hypomanic episode 1 to 2 years following a first hospitalization for major depression with psychotic features. J Child Adolesc Psychopharmacol 13(2):173–185, 2003 12880511
Dold M, Bartova L, Kautzky A, et al: Psychotic features in patients with major depressive disorder: a report from the European group for the study of resistant depression. J Clin Psychiatry 80(1):17m12090, 2019 30677267
Evans DL, Burnett GB, Nemeroff CB: The dexamethasone suppression test in the clinical setting. Am J Psychiatry 140(5):586–589, 1983 6342422
Fawcett J, Scheftner W, Clark D, et al: Clinical predictors of suicide in patients with major affective disorders: a controlled prospective study. Am J Psychiatry 144(1):35–40, 1987 3799837
Fink M: Electroconvulsive therapy update: recognizing and treating psychotic depression. J Clin Psychiatry 64(3):232–234, 2003a 12716262
Fink M: Separating psychotic depression from nonpsychotic depression is essential to effective treatment. J Affect Disord 76(1–3):1–3, 2003b 12943927
Fleming SK, Blasey C, Schatzberg AF: Neuropsychological correlates of psychotic features in major depressive disorders: a review and meta-analysis. J Psychiatr Res 38(1):27–35, 2004 14690768
Flint AJ, Meyers BS, Rothschild AJ, et al: Effect of continuing olanzapine vs placebo on relapse among patients with psychotic depression in remission: the STOP-PD II randomized clinical trial. JAMA 322(7):622–631, 2019 31429896
Flores BH, Kenna H, Keller J, et al: Clinical and biological effects of mifepristone treatment for psychotic depression. Neuropsychopharmacology 31(3):628–636, 2006 16160710

Garrett A, Kelly R, Gomez R, et al: Aberrant brain activation during a working memory task in psychotic major depression. Am J Psychiatry 168(2):173–182, 2011 21078708
Gatti F, Bellini L, Gasperini M, et al: Fluvoxamine alone in the treatment of delusional depression. Am J Psychiatry 153(3):414–416, 1996 8610832
Glassman AH, Perel JM, Shostak M, et al: Clinical implications of imipramine plasma levels for depressive illness. Arch Gen Psychiatry 34(2):197–204, 1977 843179
Gomez RG, Fleming SH, Keller J, et al: The neuropsychological profile of psychotic major depression and its relation to cortisol. Biol Psychiatry 60(5):472–478, 2006 16483550
Greicius MD, Flores BH, Menon V, et al: Resting-state functional connectivity in major depression: abnormally increased contributions from subgenual cingulate cortex and thalamus. Biol Psychiatry 62(5):429–437, 2007 17210143
Hill SK, Keshavan MS, Thase ME, et al: Neuropsychological dysfunction in antipsychotic-naive first-episode unipolar psychotic depression. Am J Psychiatry 161(6):996–1003, 2004 15169687
Isometsä E, Henriksson M, Aro H, et al: Suicide in psychotic major depression. J Affect Disord 31(3):187–191, 1994 7963071
Jeste DV, Heaton SC, Paulsen JS, et al: Clinical and neuropsychological comparison of psychotic depression with nonpsychotic depression and schizophrenia. Am J Psychiatry 153(4):490–496, 1996 8599396
Johnson J, Horwath E, Weissman MM: The validity of major depression with psychotic features based on a community study. Arch Gen Psychiatry 48(12):1075–1081, 1991 1845225
Jorgensen MB, Rozing MP, Kellner CH, et al: Electroconvulsive therapy, depression severity and mortality: data from the Danish National Patient Registry. J Psychopharmacol 34(3):273–279, 2020 31909674
Karaaslan F, Gonul AS, Oguz A, et al: P300 changes in major depressive disorders with and without psychotic features. J Affect Disord 73(3):283–287, 2003 12547298
Keller J, Flores B, Gomez RG, et al: Cortisol circadian rhythm alterations in psychotic major depression. Biol Psychiatry 60(3):275–281, 2006a 16458262
Keller J, Gomez RG, Kenna HA, et al: Detecting psychotic major depression using psychiatric rating scales. J Psychiatr Res 40(1):22–29, 2006b 16165160
Keller J, Shen L, Gomez RG, et al: Hippocampal and amygdalar volumes in psychotic and non-psychotic unipolar depression. Am J Psychiatry 165(7):872–880, 2008 18450931
Keller J, Gomez R, Williams G, et al: HPA axis in major depression: cortisol, clinical symptomatology and genetic variation predict cognition. Mol Psychiatry 22(4):527–536, 2017 27528460
Kelley R, Garrett A, Cohen J, et al: Altered brain function underlying verbal memory encoding and retrieval in psychotic major depression. Psychiatry Res 211(2):119–126, 2013 23149036
Kim DK, Kim BL, Sohn SE, et al: Candidate neuroanatomic substrates of psychosis in old-aged depression. Prog Neuropsychopharmacol Biol Psychiatry 23(5):793–807, 1999 10509375
Kohn Y, Zislin J, Agid O, et al: Increased prevalence of negative life events in subtypes of major depressive disorder. Compr Psychiatry 42(1):57–63, 2001 11154717
Kruijshaar ME, Hoeymans N, Bijl RV, et al: Levels of disability in major depression: findings from the Netherlands Mental Health Survey and Incidence Study (NEMESIS). J Affect Disord 77(1):53–64, 2003 14550935
Leadholm AK, Rothschild AJ, Nielsen J, et al: Risk factors for suicide among 34,671 patients with psychotic and non-psychotic severe depression. J Affect Disord 156:119–125, 2014 24388683
Leckman JF, Weissman MM, Prusoff BA, et al: Subtypes of depression. Family study perspective. Arch Gen Psychiatry 41(9):833–838, 1984 6466042
Leyton M, Corin E, Martial J, Meaney M: Psychotic symptoms and vulnerability to recurrent major depression. J Affect Disord 33(2):107–115, 1995 7759658
Lindley SE, Bengoechea TG, Schatzberg AF, et al: Glucocorticoid effects on mesotelencephalic dopamine neurotransmission. Neuropsychopharmacology 21(3):399–407, 1999 10457537
Lindley SE, Bengoechea TG, Wong DL, et al: Mesotelencephalic dopamine neurochemical responses to glucocorticoid administration and adrenalectomy in Fischer 344 and Lewis rats. Brain Res 958(2):414–422, 2002 12470878

Lupien S, Richter R, Risch SC, et al: Time course of the corticosteroid-dopaminergic interaction during metyrapone and dexamethasone administration. Psychiatry Res 58(1):23–35, 1995 8539309

Lyons DM, Lopez JM, Yang C, et al: Stress-level cortisol treatment impairs inhibitory control of behavior in monkeys. J Neurosci 20(20):7816–7821, 2000 11027246

Maes M, Minner B, Suy E: The influences of dexamethasone levels on the predictive value of the DST for unipolar major depression and the relationships between post-dexamethasone cortisol and ACTH levels. J Affect Disord 17(1):39–46, 1989 2544636

Maier W, Philipp M, Schlegel S, et al: Diagnostic determinants of response to treatment with tricyclic antidepressants: a polydiagnostic approach. Psychiatry Res 30(1):83–93, 1989 2594875

Maj M, Starace F, Pirozzi R: A family study of DSM-III-R schizoaffective disorder, depressive type, compared with schizophrenia and psychotic and nonpsychotic major depression. Am J Psychiatry 148(5):612–616, 1991 2018162

Matthews JD, Bottonari KA, Polania LM, et al: An open study of olanzapine and fluoxetine for psychotic major depressive disorder: interim analyses. J Clin Psychiatry 63(12):1164–1170, 2002 12523877

Meyers BS, Flint AJ, Rothschild AJ, et al: A double-blind randomized controlled trial of olanzapine plus sertraline vs olanzapine plus placebo for psychotic depression: the study of pharmacotherapy of psychotic depression (STOP-PD). Arch Gen Psychiatry 66(8):838–847, 2009 19652123

Miller F, Chabrier LA: The relation of delusional content in psychotic depression to life-threatening behavior. Suicide Life Threat Behav 17(1):13–17, 1987 3590269

Miller FT, Chabrier LA: Suicide attempts correlate with delusional content in major depression. Psychopathology 21(1):34–37, 1988 3222430

Müller-Siecheneder F, Müller MJ, Hillert A, et al: Risperidone versus haloperidol and amitriptyline in the treatment of patients with a combined psychotic and depressive syndrome. J Clin Psychopharmacol 18(2):111–120, 1998 9555596

Mulsant BH, Haskett RF, Prudic J, et al: Low use of neuroleptic drugs in the treatment of psychotic major depression. Am J Psychiatry 154(4):559–561, 1997 9090348

Nelson EB, Rielage E, Welge JA, Keck PE Jr: An open trial of olanzapine in the treatment of patients with psychotic depression. Ann Clin Psychiatry 13(3):147–151, 2001 11791952

Nelson JC, Davis JM: DST studies in psychotic depression: a meta-analysis. Am J Psychiatry 154(11):1497–1503, 1997 9356556

Nelson JC, Mazure CM: Lithium augmentation in psychotic depression refractory to combined drug treatment. Am J Psychiatry 143(3):363–366, 1986 2869701

Nelson WH, Khan A, Orr WW Jr: Delusional depression. Phenomenology, neuroendocrine function, and tricyclic antidepressant response. J Affect Disord 6(3–4):297–306, 1984 6235261

Neufeld NH, Mulsant BH, Dickie EW, et al: Resting state functional connectivity in patients with remitted psychotic depression: a multi-centre STOP-PD study. EBioMedicine 36:446–453, 2018 30287158

Ohayon MM, Schatzberg AF: Prevalence of depressive episodes with psychotic features in the general population. Am J Psychiatry 159(11):1855–1861, 2002 12411219

Østergaard SD, Meyers BS, Flint AJ, et al; STOP-PD Study Group: Measuring psychotic depression. Acta Psychiatr Scand 129(3):211–220, 2014 23799875

Parker G, Hadzi-Pavlovic D, Brodaty H, et al: Sub-typing depression, II: clinical distinction of psychotic depression and non-psychotic melancholia. Psychol Med 25(4):825–832, 1995 7480460

Perälä J, Suvisaari J, Saarni SI, et al: Lifetime prevalence of psychotic and bipolar I disorders in a general population. Arch Gen Psychiatry 64(1):19–28, 2007 17199051

Pini S, Cassano GB, Dell'Osso L, et al: Insight into illness in schizophrenia, schizoaffective disorder, and mood disorders with psychotic features. Am J Psychiatry 158(1):122–125, 2001 11136644

Posener JA, DeBattista C, Williams GH, et al: 24-Hour monitoring of cortisol and corticotropin secretion in psychotic and nonpsychotic major depression. Arch Gen Psychiatry 57(8):755–760, 2000 10920463

Price LH, Conwell Y, Nelson JC: Lithium augmentation of combined neuroleptic-tricyclic treatment in delusional depression. Am J Psychiatry 140(3):318–322, 1983 6131612

Prudic J, Olfson M, Marcus SC, et al: Effectiveness of electroconvulsive therapy in community settings. Biol Psychiatry 55(3):301–312, 2004 14744473

Radomsky ED, Haas GL, Mann JJ, et al: Suicidal behavior in patients with schizophrenia and other psychotic disorders. Am J Psychiatry 156(10):1590–1595, 1999 10518171

Rihmer Z, Arató M, Szádoczky E, et al: The dexamethasone suppression test in psychotic versus non-psychotic endogenous depression. Br J Psychiatry 145:508–511, 1984 6498417

Robinson DG, Spiker DG: Delusional depression. A one year follow-up. J Affect Disord 9(1):79–83, 1985 3160751

Roose SP, Glassman AH, Walsh BT, et al: Depression, delusions, and suicide. Am J Psychiatry 140(9):1159–1162, 1983 6614220

Rothschild AJ, Duval SE: How long should patients with psychotic depression stay on the antipsychotic medication? J Clin Psychiatry 64(4):390–396, 2003 12716238

Rothschild AJ, Schatzberg AF, Rosenbaum AH, et al: The dexamethasone suppression test as a discriminator among subtypes of psychotic patients. Br J Psychiatry 141:471–474, 1982 7150883

Rothschild AJ, Schatzberg AF, Langlais PJ, et al: Psychotic and nonpsychotic depressions, I: comparison of plasma catecholamines and cortisol measures. Psychiatry Res 20(2):143–153, 1987 2883694

Rothschild AJ, Benes F, Hebben N, et al: Relationships between brain CT scan findings and cortisol in psychotic and nonpsychotic depressed patients. Biol Psychiatry 26(6):565–575, 1989 2790096

Rothschild AJ, Samson JA, Bessette MP, et al: Efficacy of the combination of fluoxetine and perphenazine in the treatment of psychotic depression. J Clin Psychiatry 54(9):338–342, 1993a 8104930

Rothschild AJ, Samson JA, Bond TC, et al: Hypothalamic-pituitary-adrenal axis activity and 1-year outcome in depression. Biol Psychiatry 34(6):392–400, 1993b 8218607

Rothschild AJ, Bates KS, Boehringer KL, et al: Olanzapine response in psychotic depression. J Clin Psychiatry 60(2):116–118, 1999 10084638

Rothschild AJ, Williamson DJ, Tohen MF, et al: A double-blind, randomized study of olanzapine and olanzapine/fluoxetine combination for major depression with psychotic features. J Clin Psychopharmacol 24(4):365–373, 2004 15232326

Schatzberg AF: Anna-Monika Award Lecture, DGPPN Kongress, 2013: The role of the hypothalamic-pituitary-adrenal (HPA) axis in the pathogenesis of psychotic major depression. World J Biol Psychiatry 16(1):2–11, 2015 24933348

Schatzberg AF, Rothschild AJ: Psychotic (delusional) major depression: should it be included as a distinct syndrome in DSM-IV? Am J Psychiatry 149(6):733–745, 1992 1590491

Schatzberg AF, Rothschild AJ, Stahl JB, et al: The dexamethasone suppression test: identification of subtypes of depression. Am J Psychiatry 140(1):88–91, 1983 6847992

Schatzberg AF, Rothschild AJ, Langlais PJ, et al: A corticosteroid/dopamine hypothesis for psychotic depression and related states. J Psychiatr Res 19(1):57–64, 1985 2859366

Schatzberg AF, Posener JA, DeBattista C, et al: Neuropsychological deficits in psychotic versus nonpsychotic major depression and no mental illness. Am J Psychiatry 157(7):1095–1100, 2000 10873917

Schatzberg AF, Keller J, Tennakoon L, et al: HPA axis genetic variation, cortisol and psychosis in major depression. Mol Psychiatry 19(2):220–227, 2014 24166410

Schwartz JE, Fennig S, Tanenberg-Karant M, et al: Congruence of diagnoses 2 years after a first-admission diagnosis of psychosis. Arch Gen Psychiatry 57(6):593–600, 2000 10839338

Simpson GM, El Sheshai A, Rady A, et al: Sertraline as monotherapy in the treatment of psychotic and nonpsychotic depression. J Clin Psychiatry 64(8):959–965, 2003 12927014

Simpson S, Baldwin RC, Jackson A, et al: The differentiation of DSM-III-R psychotic depression in later life from nonpsychotic depression: comparisons of brain changes measured by multispectral analysis of magnetic resonance brain images, neuropsychological findings, and clinical features. Biol Psychiatry 45(2):193–204, 1999 9951567

Skaf CR, Yamada A, Garrido GE, et al: Psychotic symptoms in major depressive disorder are associated with reduced regional cerebral blood flow in the subgenual anterior cingulate cortex: a voxel-based single photon emission computed tomography (SPECT) study. J Affect Disord 68(2–3):295–305, 2002 12063157

Spiker DG, Kupfer DJ: Placebo response rates in psychotic and nonpsychotic depression. J Affect Disord 14(1):21–23, 1988 2963048

Spiker DG, Stein J, Rich CL: Delusional depression and electroconvulsive therapy: one year later. Convuls Ther 1(3):167–172, 1985a 11940820

Spiker DG, Weiss JC, Dealy RS, et al: The pharmacological treatment of delusional depression. Am J Psychiatry 142(4):430–436, 1985b 3883815

Spiker DG, Perel JM, Hanin I, et al: The pharmacological treatment of delusional depression, part II. J Clin Psychopharmacol 6(6):339–342, 1986 3805326

Stetler C, Miller GE: Depression and hypothalamic-pituitary-adrenal activation: a quantitative summary of four decades of research. Psychosom Med 73(2):114–126, 2011 21257974

Thase ME, Kupfer DJ, Ulrich RF: Electroencephalographic sleep in psychotic depression. A valid subtype? Arch Gen Psychiatry 43(9):886–893, 1986 3753166

Tsuang D, Coryell W: An 8-year follow-up of patients with DSM-III-R psychotic depression, schizoaffective disorder, and schizophrenia. Am J Psychiatry 150(8):1182–1188, 1993 8328561

Vermeulen T, Lauwers T, Van Diermen L, et al: Cognitive deficits in older adults with psychotic depression: a meta-analysis. Am J Geriatr Psychiatry 27(12):1334–1344, 2019 31378679

Vythilingam M, Chen J, Bremner JD, et al: Psychotic depression and mortality. Am J Psychiatry 160(3):574–576, 2003 12611843

Weissman MM, Warner V, John K, et al: Delusional depression and bipolar spectrum: evidence for a possible association from a family study of children. Neuropsychopharmacology 1(4):257–264, 1988 3251505

Zalpuri I, Rothschild AJ: Does psychosis increase the risk of suicide in patients with major depression? A systematic review. J Affect Disord 198:23–31, 2016 26998793

Zanardi R, Franchini L, Gasperini M, et al: Double-blind controlled trial of sertraline versus paroxetine in the treatment of delusional depression. Am J Psychiatry 153(12):1631–1633, 1996 8942464

Zanardi R, Franchini L, Serretti A, et al: Venlafaxine versus fluvoxamine in the treatment of delusional depression: a pilot double-blind controlled study. J Clin Psychiatry 61(1):26–29, 2000 10695642

Zhou Y, Li Z, Wang Y, et al: Prevalence and clinical correlates of psychotic depression in first-episode and drug-naïve outpatients with major depressive disorder in a Chinese Han population. J Affect Disord 263:500–506, 2020 31759662

CHAPTER 37

Pediatric Mood Disorders

Manpreet K. Singh, M.D., M.S.

Mood disorders among youth are on the rise (Avenevoli et al. 2015), and there is increased recognition that mood disorders commonly have their onset in childhood or adolescence. An early onset of mood disorders frequently portends a chronic, treatment-refractory, and complicated course and outcome (Johnson et al. 2018). In comparison with adults with mood disorders, youth with mood disorders are four times more likely to attempt suicide (Ballesteros et al. 2018; Kann et al. 2018), are more likely to have co-occurring psychiatric disorders that impact treatment course (Weintraub et al. 2019), and more frequently experience family maladjustment and early-life stress. Mood disorders can lead to academic impairment, lower life satisfaction, and reductions in overall functioning in youth. Despite advances in the accurate diagnosis of childhood-onset mood disorders as well as an increasing number of available interventions, objective diagnostic and therapeutic biomarkers anchored in the biological underpinnings of these disorders are only beginning to emerge.

Juxtaposed with these concerns, new evidence provides an alternative, optimistic outlook for childhood-onset mood disorders. For pediatric-onset bipolar disorders, prevalence rates are not higher in the United States than in other Western countries, as was previously assumed, and do not appear to be increasing over time, although prevalence rates of pediatric bipolar disorders continue to vary due to inconsistent operationalization of standard diagnostic criteria (Van Meter et al. 2019). Furthermore, individuals with pediatric-onset bipolar disorders spend most of their time in euthymic mood states (Weintraub et al. 2020) and may have better outcomes than individuals with adult-onset bipolar disorders (Frahm Laursen et al. 2019). Although female sex, high polygenic risk scores for depressive symptoms, and maternal postnatal depression have been associated with persistent forms of unipolar depressive disorders (i.e., major depressive disorder [MDD]), exposure to parental domestic violence and bullying appears to be associated with discrete, nonrecurrent, and time-limited forms of depression (Kwong et al. 2019). These findings suggest opportunities for providing early preventive interventions for most youth, and for providing concentrated, specialized therapeutic interventions during critically sensitive windows in development for those children and adolescents who are at greatest risk of negative outcomes (de Lijster et al. 2019).

In this chapter I briefly summarize known brain-based models of mood disorders in youth, discuss developmentally sensitive approaches to diagnosing mood disorders, and review current FDA-approved and off-label treatments. Although youth, in comparison with adults, may be less diagnostically differentiated into unipolar versus bipolar subtypes, points of divergence among these subtypes are attracting increasing interest as part of the search for improved personalized strategies for treatment. Here, I describe representative studies in youth with or at risk for MDD and bipolar disorder that attempt to characterize both broad and specific features of each of these populations. The focus in this chapter is on diagnostic definitions, as operationalized in the Diagnostic and Statistical Manual of Mental Disorders (DSM), because clinical research and practice frequently espouse the use of consistent and reliable diagnostic criteria for sample selection and characterization. I conclude with recommendations on future directions for the field of pediatric mood disorders.

Neural Network Models of Mood Disorders in Youth

Unipolar Depressive Disorders

Key regional and network-based structural and functional brain characteristics have been described in pediatric-onset depressive disorders, leading to the proposal that early-onset depression is a syndrome of corticolimbic and striatal network dysfunction, with points of developmental divergence and convergence with features of adult-onset depression (Hulvershorn et al. 2011). Some brain characteristics are evident before the onset of clinical symptoms in youth at risk for depression. For example, Shapero et al. (2019) found that resting-state functional connectivity abnormalities in the default mode and cognitive control networks that differentiated high-risk from low-risk youth predicted the onset of MDD during adolescence. Indeed, perinatal exposure to maternal depression was shown to influence the functional organization of the cortico-striato-amygdala circuitry, which is critical for the development of emotional perception and regulation (Soe et al. 2018). Furthermore, distinct risk- and disorder-specific patterns of limbic resting state functional connectivity have been found to differentiate youth with depressive disorders, youth at risk for depression, and healthy comparison youth (Singh et al. 2018). Recent evidence that antidepressant treatment may normalize aberrant functional connectivity in neural networks, producing improvement of mood symptoms (Bansal et al. 2018), also supports the crucial role of these networks in the pathophysiology of pediatric depression. Youth share some regional brain regional and network-based formulations of depression with adults; however, there are some key differences that may help explain phenotypic differences in symptom expression, timing of onset of symptoms, and trajectories (Ellis et al. 2017). These differences suggest a dynamic model of depression in which the developmental timing and duration of depression symptoms during adolescence may affect brain structural outcomes, with potential implications for future illness severity and chronicity.

Bipolar Disorders

A neurodevelopmental model of pediatric bipolar disorders suggests an imbalance between prefrontal and limbic neural system function over the course of development, leading to progressive symptom expression and consequent impairments in daily function (Roybal et al. 2012). Although the model is likely more complex than an imbalance of function, it provides clinicians with an accessible place to start the conversation with youth, who frequently deny symptoms or have poor insight into the necessity for mood stabilization. Individual differences and multiple-cognitive-domain dysfunction in pediatric bipolar disorders provide context for the complexity of symptom presentations. However, findings from studies of youth with and at risk for bipolar disorders consistently suggest that risk endophenotypes can be identified and targeted with prevention measures (Wiggins et al. 2017). Moreover, discussions of neural network dysfunction are understandable to many youth, who may be perturbed by the cognitive (most commonly attentional) dysfunction frequently experienced during mania. This perturbation in their usual cognitive function can motivate them to seek timely multimodal (medication, psychotherapy, educational) treatment approach for mania, which may be a state of relatively poor illness insight.

As in the case of depression, youth and adults with bipolar disorder engage different neural mechanisms (Wegbreit et al. 2014). Among the most replicated findings in pediatric bipolar disorders is reduction in amygdala volume (Pfeifer et al. 2008), which has not been documented in adults with bipolar disorder, and which suggests that pediatric-onset bipolar disorders have a developmentally distinct neurobiology. However, other lines of evidence suggest that pediatric-onset bipolar disorder is continuous with adult-onset bipolar disorder (Chang 2007). More recently, there has been increasing recognition that clinical and biological features of bipolar disorders vary with stage of illness development (Berk et al. 2017). Youth at familial risk for bipolar disorders show neural risk markers of vulnerability (Singh et al. 2014a) and resilience (Singh et al. 2014b). These markers have been observed in early presymptomatic stages and may change over time, leading to multiple potential developmental outcomes (Kapczinski et al. 2017). It is clear that the amygdala-prefrontal networks in youth with bipolar disorders differ from those in typically developing youth, and also from the amygdala-prefrontal networks in children with other psychiatric disorders (Hafeman et al. 2017). Furthermore, psychiatric conditions that commonly co-occur, such as anxiety disorders and ADHD, may, for some youth, reflect subclinical or clinical prodromes of threshold bipolar development (Faedda et al. 2014).

Diagnosis of Pediatric Mood Disorders

The diagnosis of childhood-onset mood disorders is complicated by a number of factors. Variation in symptom presentations over the course of development can lead to misdiagnosis. Discerning the subtle differences between normal and abnormal moods in youth requires experience and a contextual understanding that many clinicians do not sufficiently acquire in training. Mood disorders by definition require characterization of the patterns of mood symptom onset and offset, which can be tricky for youth and parents to recall, making the establishment of an episode challenging. Moreover, comorbidity seems to be a rule rather than an exception in pediatric psychopathology, frequently leading to diagnostic confusion. Finally, discrepancies between youth and caregiver reports of symptoms can also complicate the establishment of diagnostic criteria. Although these factors add "noise" to a well-intended diagnostic assessment, a clinician who focuses on DSM criteria and who uses available diagnostic tools to facilitate a systematic assessment can improve her chances of capturing a diagnostic formulation that is reliable and consistent both with observable clinical signs and with the patient's experience of symptoms.

Even with the burgeoning field of neuroscience and the availability of multiple valid screening and assessment tools, the gold standard approach to the diagnosis of mood disorders in youth is still the clinical interview, ideally involving multiple informants (Singh 2019b). Clinicians in a variety of settings can ask simple but key questions to assess for mood symptoms in youth, determine their severity, and evaluate how these symptoms relate to a child's functioning. Once a core low or elevated mood is endorsed, its persistence, associated factors, and functional impact can help a clinician efficiently decide whether the mood falls within the scope of psychiatric practice. Underlying neurophysiological contributors (e.g., anemia, altered thyroid function) and vitamin D and lead levels can all be assessed with a single blood draw while referrals for more in-depth evaluations are being considered. Furthermore, asking youth about recreational drug use individually and directly is generally preferred over ordering urine toxicology screening in an outpatient setting. Because no validated diagnostic biomarkers or confirmatory tests currently exist for mood disorders, health care providers must rely on their interviewing skills and clinical acumen to diagnose youth early and accurately.

Because symptoms of mood disorders may resemble and co-occur with symptoms of other conditions or psychiatric problems, a comprehensive assessment of pertinent positive and negative symptoms endorsed will likely yield the most accurate primary and secondary diagnoses and may merit a more in-depth interview or referral to a mental health care professional. Life problems such as a relationship breakup, academic stress, or bullying can trigger and perpetuate mood symptoms. One goal of a careful diagnostic assessment is to help a patient develop insight about factors that contribute to triggering, perpetuating, or alleviating mood symptoms. Helping the patient describe symptoms in his or her own words facilitates this goal and establishes an early alliance between the patient and the clinician to understand mood symptoms and their impact, and to collaboratively monitor these symptoms as they evolve with treatment.

Children and adolescents may experience a spectrum of mood symptoms that in the early stages of development may be ill-defined diagnostically and may change over time or be influenced by specific contextual factors. For example, treatment of a depressive episode with an antidepressant may trigger mania or mania-like symptoms. To ensure that the full spectrum of mood disorders is considered at any and all clinical evaluations of a child presenting with mood symptoms, all presenting mood symptoms (hereafter referred to as *index* mood symptoms)—ranging from sad mood, anhedonia, and irritability for MDD to euphoria and explosive irritability for bipolar disorder—should be considered and explored. Index mood symptoms are solicited (in the patient's own words) first, followed by secondary or "Criterion B" symptoms of depression and mania as defined in DSM-5 (American Psychiatric Association 2013).

For MDD, "SIGECAPS" remains a popular mnemonic, where **S** generally stands for sleep abnormalities (insomnia or hypersomnia; initial/middle/terminal), **I** for diminished interest or pleasure in the things the youth normally experiences as fun, **G** for guilt or self-blame, **E** for low energy, **C** for concentration difficulties or poor decision making, **A** for appetite changes (increases or decreases, sometimes corresponding with weight changes), **P** for psychomotor agitation or retardation, and **S** for suicidal ideation or suicide-related behavior. A major depressive episode (MDE) requires at least 2 weeks of an index low or irritable mood and four additional Criterion B symptoms. A manic episode requires index euphoria daily for more than 50% of the day, lasting at least 1 week and accompanied by at least three additional Criterion B symptoms (four if the index mood is explosive irritability). For bipolar disorder, the mnemonic "DIGFAST" may be used to remember secondary symptoms, where **D** may stand for distractibility or motor hyperactivity, **I** for increased goal-directed activity, **G** for grandiosity, **F** for flight of ideas and racing thoughts, **A** for accelerated speech, **S** for decreased need for sleep, and **T** for "trouble," or engagement in impulsive, risk-taking behaviors, including hypersexuality, that have the potential for dangerous consequences for the patient or others. In youth, examples of high-risk behaviors might include staying out all night, spending a lot of money, or taking unplanned trips. Adolescents might report that during a manic episode, they got involved in relationships quickly, had a lot of one-night stands, or drove recklessly. Preadolescents might report jumping from elevated places, going on long trips without planning or supervision, playing serious pranks in school, or engaging in inappropriate sexual behavior during mania. Because these symptoms manifest differently depending on the child's age, they should be contextualized with typical development in mind.

Establishing the timeline of onset and offset of mood symptoms early in the interview allows a clinician to quickly and easily rule in or rule out a major mood disorder such as bipolar I disorder or MDD. The clinician can then proceed systematically down a list of potential diagnoses of exclusion, as well as evaluate for the presence of co-occurring conditions. Unfortunately, clinicians in often-busy clinical settings tend to underuse DSM criteria, frequently neglecting to collect sufficient information to establish a correct diagnosis for most psychiatric disorders (Nakash et al. 2015). Moreover, studies have found that agreement between research diagnostic assessments and clinical evaluations is low to moderate for most disorders (Rettew et al. 2009). Incomplete diagnostic information may result in poor diagnostic reliability and biased clinical decision making (Jensen-Doss et al. 2014), delaying initiation of treatment or resulting in the implementation of inappropriate, excessively costly, or potentially harmful treatments. Thus, an accurate and timely diagnosis can prevent adverse clinical and financial outcomes at multiple levels.

Efforts to systematically evaluate clinicians' assessment processes in naturalistic settings may help to identify the best diagnostic probes to use in clinical practice to improve diagnostic accuracy and efficiency. For the busy clinician, a toolkit of feasible assessments that are integrated into practice and supported by billing structures may facilitate use of systematic diagnostic approaches. Several measurement-based care models are being developed by for-profit and not-for-profit organizations; these are aimed at improving real-time clinical decision making, facilitating reimbursement, and optimizing resource utilization in behavioral health care. Because measurement-based care is still relatively new, data demonstrating its efficacy in improving diagnostic accuracy and treatment outcomes are still emerging. Indeed, validation of measurement-based care approaches is well justified in pediatric settings, given the diagnostic challenges described above. Resources such as the recently published *Clinical Handbook on the Diagnosis and Treatment of Pediatric Mood Disorders* detail commonly used screening tools, self-assessments, diagnostic assessments, and structured and semistructured interviews (Singh 2019a).

Treatment of Pediatric Mood Disorders

Pediatric Depressive Disorders

Providing psychoeducation about depressive symptoms; helping patients to implement sleep, dietary, exercise, and other lifestyle habits that promote optimal mood function; and initiating psychotherapy are the first-line interventions for youth presenting with depression (Weersing et al. 2017). Youth with severe and persistent forms of depression may require pharmacotherapy in addition to these interventions to achieve symptom response or remission. Multiple factors must be considered in the process of selecting the most appropriate treatment, including the patient's age, family and social environment, cultural context, cognitive development, severity and subtype of depression, degree of chronicity, comorbid conditions, and family psychiatric history. Additional considerations include the patient's preferences for and expectations of treatment and the availability of expert pharmacotherapy and/or psychotherapy practitioners. Consequently, a multimodal approach that includes family and school psychoeducation and involvement throughout all stages of treatment is critical. Indeed, the Treatment for Adolescents With Depression Study (TADS [March et al. 2004]) and the Treatment of Resistant Depression in Adolescents (TORDIA [Brent et al. 2008]) study have shown that combining pharmacotherapy with psychotherapy is more efficacious, results in higher remission rates, and shows greater rates of symptom reduction than monotherapy.

Available evidence for optimal pharmacological management of depression in pediatric populations generally lags behind that in adults. The greatest weight of the available evidence for the treatment of pediatric depression supports the use of selective serotonin reuptake inhibitors (SSRIs), which have demonstrated relatively similar effect sizes for efficacy and safety. SSRIs that are currently marketed for use in pediatric populations include fluoxetine, sertraline, paroxetine, fluvoxamine, citalopram, and escitalopram, as well as the serotonin partial agonist and reuptake inhibitor vilazodone. As of 2019, fluoxetine and escitalopram were the only two FDA-approved antidepressants for the treatment of MDD in youths younger than 18 years. A systematic review and meta-analysis of 13 pediatric MDD trials involving a total of 3,004 patients revealed that the greatest improvement with SSRIs versus placebo was observed early in the course of treatment (e.g., within 2 weeks) (Varigonda et al. 2015). There were no significant differences based on maximum SSRI dosages or between particular SSRI agents. SSRIs were demonstrated to have a smaller benefit in pediatric compared with adult MDD. Selection of an antidepressant should include consideration of previous antidepressant response, family treatment history, patient/family preference, avoidance of specific side effects, comorbid psychiatric illness, drug-drug interactions, and cost. In general, the dosages of SSRIs prescribed for youths are similar to those prescribed for adult patients. However, SSRIs are generally started at lower dosages in youth, and dosages for preadolescent youth are based on patient weight to ensure tolerability. Clinical response should be assessed at 4- to 6-week intervals, and dosages should be gradually increased as tolerated and should be maximized if a complete response has not been obtained. Table 37–1 presents medications commonly used to treat depression in children and adolescents, organized according to their main mechanisms of action (Alvano and Zieher 2020), and lists the adverse effects reported for these drugs in pediatric clinical trials. Table 37–2 summarizes the dosage ranges and efficacy evidence for antidepressants used in pediatric patients.

In comparison with adults, youth are more susceptible to placebo effects, have lower rates of medication adherence, and are more vulnerable to the adverse side effects of medications. Among the most worrisome of the adverse side effects associated with antidepressants is the potential for treatment-emergent suicidal ideation and/or behavior. In 2004, the FDA issued a public warning about an increased risk of suicidal thoughts or behavior (i.e., suicidality) in children and adolescents treated with antidepressants. This warning was based on a meta-analysis of 24 randomized, placebo-controlled antidepressant clinical trials in which suicidal thoughts or behavior were experienced by 4% of the children and adolescents assigned to active drug compared with 2% of those assigned to placebo (Hammad et al. 2006). Although the FDA reported few suicide attempts and no suicide completions, findings of follow-up studies examining the relative risk of suicide attempts and suicide deaths in children and adults with severe depression who were treated with antidepressants versus those not so treated suggested that antidepressants were significantly related to suicide attempts or suicide deaths in children but not in adults. As a result of these findings, the FDA mandated a black box warning recommending that depressed children and adolescents treated with antidepressants receive careful clinical monitoring for suicidal ideation/suicide attempts. However, the risk of suicidal thoughts and/or behavior needs to be balanced against the risks associated with untreated depression.

About a third of youth with MDD do not experience adequate clinical response to initial treatment. When a clinician is confronted with a pediatric patient with treatment-resistant depression, a reevaluation of the clinical diagnosis can be helpful, along with evaluation and treatment of co-occurring conditions and contributing factors, including family dynamics and sociocultural issues. In the acute setting, the presence of severe and chronic depression, suicidal ideation or nonsuicidal self-injury, and hopelessness may predict poor outcomes. The presence of co-occurring disorders such as ADHD, persistent depressive disorder (dysthymia), anxiety disorders, and substance use disorders has been correlated with poor treatment response. Medical comorbidity, such as anemia, vitamin B_{12} deficiency, hypothyroidism, diabetes mellitus, fibromyalgia, and other chronic medical conditions, is also related to functional impairment and may lead to exacerbation of depressive symptoms in children and adolescents. Environmental factors such as a history of abuse, family discord, parental mood disorders, bullying, same-sex attraction, peer victimization, or family rejection are known risk factors for depression and are predictors of poorer treatment response for depression in adolescents.

Thus, for first-line pharmacotherapy, the antidepressant class with the highest level of evidence is the SSRIs—in particular, fluoxetine and escitalopram, which are FDA approved for use in pediatric patients. Once response is achieved, there is a limited evidence base to guide continuation and maintenance phases of treatment. In the

TABLE 37–1. Main mechanisms of action and reported adverse effects of monoamine[a]–modulating drugs commonly used to treat pediatric depression

Main mode of action	Main monoaminergic target(s)[b]	Drug class	Adverse effects reported in pediatric clinical trials[c]
Neuronal reuptake inhibitor	Serotonergic	SSRIs Fluoxetine Sertraline Paroxetine Citalopram Escitalopram Fluvoxamine	**Common:** headache and gastrointestinal adverse effects such as nausea, diarrhea, anorexia, vomiting, flatulence, dyspepsia **Other:** somnolence, anxiety, agitation, tremor, sweating, dry mouth, dizziness, sexual dysfunction
Neuronal reuptake inhibitor	Serotonergic and noradrenergic	SNRIs Venlafaxine Desvenlafaxine Duloxetine Levomilnacipran	*Venlafaxine—* **Common (in RCTs):** anorexia, abdominal pain **Serious (in RCTs):** hostility, suicide-related events **Other:** tachycardia, hypertension, sweating, weight loss, loss of appetite, nausea, constipation, dizziness, headache, insomnia, somnolence, blurred vision **Serious (rare):** hyponatremia, hepatitis, seizure, neuroleptic malignant syndrome *Desvenlafaxine—* **Children (100 mg/day):** headache, upper abdominal pain, vomiting, cough, oropharyngeal pain **Adolescents (200 mg/day):** nausea, somnolence, upper abdominal pain, vomiting, dysmenorrhea

TABLE 37–1. Main mechanisms of action and reported adverse effects of monoamine[a]–modulating drugs commonly used to treat pediatric depression *(continued)*

Main mode of action	Main monoaminergic target(s)[b]	Drug class	Adverse effects reported in pediatric clinical trials[c]
Neuronal reuptake inhibitor	Noradrenergic and dopaminergic	NDRI Bupropion	**Common:** insomnia, weight loss **Other:** hypertension, tachycardia, headache, tremors, dizziness **Serious (rare):** seizures, cardiac dysrhythmia, anaphylaxis
Alpha-2 (α_2) receptor antagonist	Noradrenergic and serotonergic (receptor antagonist)	NaSSA Mirtazapine	**Common:** Sedation, weight gain, hypercholesterolemia, constipation, liver dysfunction, dizziness **Serious (rare):** agranulocytosis, neutropenia, seizures
Multimodal	Serotonergics	Vortioxetine	**Common:** headache, nausea, sedation
		Vilazodone	**Rare:** several case reports of seizures with toxic ingestion
Multimodal	Noradrenergic and serotonergic (with significant muscarinic antagonism)	TCAs	**Common:** Weight change, bloating, constipation, appetite loss, nausea, dry mouth, dizziness, headache, somnolence, blurred vision, fatigue **Serious (rare):** cardiac dysrhythmia, agranulocytosis, myocardial infarction
Monoamine oxidase inhibitor	Serotonergic, noradrenergic, and dopaminergic	MAOIs, irreversible selective (MAO-B) Selegiline (transdermal patch)	Application site reactions, headache, nausea

Note. 5-HT = 5-hydroxytryptamine (serotonin); NaSSA = noradrenergic and specific serotonergic antidepressant; NDRI = norepinephrine and dopamine reuptake inhibitor; RCT = randomized controlled trial; SNRIs = serotonin-norepinephrine reuptake inhibitor; SSRIs = selective serotonin reuptake inhibitor; TCAs = tricyclic antidepressants.

(continued on following page)

TABLE 37–1. Main mechanisms of action and reported adverse effects of monoamine[a]–modulating drugs commonly used to treat pediatric depression *(continued)*

[a]Monoamines: serotonin, norepinephrine, and dopamine.

[b]In comparison with adverse drug reaction (ADR) patterns in adults, patterns in pediatric populations are far less clearly established to be linked to known mechanisms of action, possibly because ADR reporting can be complex in youth, given the low level of the available evidence (i.e., mostly case reports) and the paucity of quantification studies (Coates et al. 2018; Egberts et al. 2011; Strawn et al. 2021).Although methods for aligning ADRs with drug mechanisms of action are still evolving, knowledge of an antidepressant's main monoaminergic target(s)—serotonergic, noradrenergic, or both—can offer the clinician some insight into its important ADRs and pharmacodynamic interactions, as shown below:

- Sexual dysfunction appears to mainly involve the 5-HT_2 receptor, and among drugs with serotonergic action, those with mechanisms that block or bypass that receptor are less likely to cause this ADR.
- Most drugs with noradrenergic action are capable of causing antimuscarinic effects, such as dry mouth, blurred vision, or dry skin.
- Among drugs with noradrenergic action, those that antagonize the α_1-adrenergic receptor carry a very low risk of causing serious hypertension, and in some cases can even cause orthostatic hypotension.
- Among drugs with noradrenergic action, urinary retention has been reported. Other drugs with noradrenergic action by different mechanisms can partially counteract this effect or can increase it through antimuscarinic action.
- Combining drugs with serotonergic action can cause a potentially fatal pharmacodynamic interaction.

Future Directions: To enable the field to move beyond trial-and-error prescribing, novel therapeutic drug monitoring strategies are being developed (Strawn et al. 2021) that provide improved guidance for pediatric dosing and dose pacing to help mitigate ADRs.

[c]The listed adverse effects were *observed* rather than *expected* (i.e., by virtue of being listed in the manufacturer's prescribing information).
Antidepressant precautions and warnings that are highlighted in the full prescribing information (as mandated by regulatory agencies) are as follows:

- All antidepressants can increase the risk of suicide in children, adolescents, and young adults under 24 years of age.
- All antidepressants can increase the risk of switching to hypomania or mania.
- Most antidepressants decrease the convulsive threshold. This ADR has been less reported with the NaSSA mirtazapine and the SSRI citalopram.
- Extension of the QTc interval has been reported with the SSRIs fluoxetine, citalopram, and escitalopram and the NaSSA mirtazapine.
- Elevation of hepatic enzymes and sporadic cases of toxic hepatitis have been reported with the SNRI duloxetine.

Sources. Nomenclature used in columns 1 and 2 is derived from the updated classification of antidepressants proposed by Alvano and Zieher (2020); Adverse effects reported in pediatric clinical trials are from Singh (2019a).

TABLE 37–2. Characteristics of antidepressants commonly used in pediatric patients

Drug class/ Medication	Dosage range	Pediatric efficacy data	Types of evidence
Selective serotonin reuptake inhibitors			
Fluoxetine (Prozac)	10–80 mg/day	Four positive studies in 6- to 17-year-olds	RCTs; FDA approved
Escitalopram (Lexapro)	10–40 mg/day	One positive study in 12- to 17-year-olds; one negative study in 6- to 17-year-olds	RCTs; FDA approved
Sertraline (Zoloft)	25–300 mg/day	One positive pooled analysis in 6- to 17-year-olds	A priori pooled analysis, individual trials negative
Citalopram (Celexa)	10–40 mg/day	One negative study in 13- to 18-year-olds	RCT
Paroxetine (Paxil)	10–60 mg/day	Four negative studies in 7- to 17-year-olds	RCTs
Fluvoxamine (Luvox)	25–300 mg/day	Positive studies in 6- to 17-year-olds for anxiety	Open-label MDD trials
Serotonin-norepinephrine reuptake inhibitors			
Venlafaxine (Effexor)	37.5–375 mg/day	Two negative studies in 7- to 17-year-olds	RCTs
Desvenlafaxine (Pristiq)	10–50 mg/day	Two negative studies in 7- to 17-year-olds	RCTs
Duloxetine (Cymbalta)	30–120 mg/day	Two negative studies in youth with MDD	RCT; FDA approved for pediatric GAD
Levomilnacipran (Fetzima)	10–40 mg/day	Unavailable; FDA approved in adults in 2013	Multisite Phase III study anticipated
Norepinephrine and dopamine reuptake inhibitor			
Bupropion (Wellbutrin)	150–400 mg/day	Three positive studies; not effective for anxiety	Open-label trials
Noradrenergic and specific serotonergic antidepressant			
Mirtazapine (Remeron)	15–45 mg/day	Two negative studies in 7- to 17-year-olds	RCT
Multimodal serotonergics			
Vortioxetine (Trintellix)	5–20 mg/day	Negative in 12- to 17-year-olds	12-week fluoxetine-referenced, fixed-dose RCT (Findling et al. 2022)
Vilazodone (Viibryd)	15–30 mg/day	One negative study in 12- to 17-year-olds; FDA approved in adults in 2011	10-week double-blind, placebo-controlled trial in adolescents with depression (Phase III)
Multimodal noradrenergic and serotonergics			
Tricyclic antidepressants	Variable	Multiple negative studies	RCTs for pediatric depressive disorders

TABLE 37–2. Characteristics of antidepressants commonly used in pediatric patients *(continued)*

Drug class/ Medication	Dosage range	Pediatric efficacy data	Types of evidence
Selective norepinephrine reuptake inhibitor			
Atomoxetine (Strattera)	10–80 mg/day	Seven negative studies in 5- to 18-year-olds	RCTs; equally effective in reducing symptoms of ADHD in patients with and without comorbid depression
Monoamine oxidase inhibitor			
Selegiline (Emsam)	Transdermal patch	No separation from placebo	RCT
Glutamatergic modulator (investigational)			
Ketamine/ esketamine	0.5 mg/kg infusion	Possibly positive	Case reports; multisite clinical trial for intranasal esketamine under way for acute suicidal ideation

Note. GAD=generalized anxiety disorder; MDD=major depressive disorder; RCT=randomized controlled trial.

Recommended Sources. Dwyer et al. 2020 (research review on pediatric treatment-resistant depression); Meister et al. 2020 (meta-analysis of RCTs of antidepressants for MDD in children and adolescents); Weersing et al. 2017 (evidence-based update on pediatric psychosocial treatment for depression); Zhou et al. 2020 (meta-analysis of comparative studies of antidepressants, psychotherapies, and their combination for pediatric depression).

treatment of pediatric depression, the goals are to achieve response and remission and to prevent future depressive episodes. Because subsyndromal depression is particularly vulnerable to recurrence, treatment should aim to eliminate or minimize residual symptoms. Most studies in pediatric depression have evaluated acute-phase treatments, with fewer studies evaluating continuation-phase treatment. In the continuation phase (usually defined as any time between 6 and 20 weeks after the index episode), the goal is to consolidate remission to prevent relapse. Antidepressants are generally maintained at the same dosage, provided that there are no significant side effects. Once the patient has been asymptomatic for approximately 6–12 months, the clinician must decide whether maintenance therapy is indicated and, if so, select the type and duration of therapy. Discontinuation of medications should be done gradually (generally over a period of 6 weeks) to avoid withdrawal effects. Maintenance treatment is recommended for patients with a history of at least two previous MDEs as well as patients with double depression (i.e., those with both major depressive episodes and persistent depressive disorder), severe suicidality, or severe impairment during the episodes. One severe episode or multiple chronic episodes of depression may require maintenance treatment for longer than 1 year. In the maintenance phase, the goal is to prevent recurrence, particularly for patients with a history of more severe, recurrent, or chronic disorder. Limited information is available to guide clinicians on the next steps after a youth with depression has achieved remission. The Guidelines for Adolescent Depression in Primary Care (GLAD-PC; Cheung et al. 2018) recommend that treatment be continued for 6–12 months to consolidate the patient's response and avoid relapse. In addition, pending publication of prospective data on treatment outcomes, expert opinion (Singh 2019a) recommends combining antidepressants with psychotherapy, especially in cases that have not responded to an adequate SSRI trial alone. More research is needed to guide treatment decisions for youth who have not responded to multiple interventions, and to guide management of depression once a response is achieved.

Pediatric Bipolar Disorders

Treating bipolar disorder in children and adolescents is challenging because youth often require immediate intervention not only to reduce symptom severity but also to reduce academic impairment and psychosocial morbidity associated with acute illness. For this reason, early detection and treatment are critical, because earlier onset and longer duration of illness tend to be associated with lower rates of recovery. Currently, there are several pharmacological interventions available for the treatment of pediatric bipolar disorder. Although treatment of acute mania is the primary treatment target in most clinical trials, there is a need for further clarification regarding optimal approaches to pharmacotherapy for acute depression in pediatric bipolar disorder as well as pharmacotherapy for maintenance treatment of mania and depression.

FDA-approved treatments for pediatric bipolar disorder are summarized in Table 37–3. Several review articles (most recently, one by Stepanova and Findling [2017]) have summarized the available pharmacological interventions for pediatric bipolar disorders. Here, I briefly review the research data regarding the efficacy and safety of pharmacological interventions for pediatric bipolar disorders, with particular emphasis on identifying the mood state being treated—depression, mania, or both—and the treatment phase—acute, continuation, or maintenance. I also provide recommendations for treatment based on the level of evidence available.

Second-generation antipsychotics (SGAs) are considered the first-line treatment for children and adolescents with acute mania. SGAs are more effective than lithium and other mood stabilizers used in the treatment of acute pediatric mania, showing the largest effect sizes and consistency in findings across studies, and supported by higher-quality evidence. Most SGAs are associated with weight gain and metabolic adverse effects, requiring active surveillance and monitoring. Much remains unknown regarding the long-term consequences of these side effects in terms of morbidity and mortality. There are a number of studies currently investigating treatment options for managing metabolic side effects, including lifestyle modifications and adjunctive pharmacological options such as metformin. In youth in whom use of SGAs is contraindicated or there is a failure to achieve response or remission, lithium is considered to be the second-line treatment choice, either monotherapeutically or in combination with an SGA. Lithium monotherapy has a moderate effect size, and although no double-blind, placebo-controlled studies have examined the use of lithium in combination with SGAs, large effect sizes and consistent findings in open-label studies support lithium's recommendation as a second-line treatment. Lithium response may run in families (Grof et al. 2002) and can reduce the risk of suicidal behavior in youth. Divalproex and lamotrigine are third-line agents for treatment of acute mania in youth due to negative results from a double-blind, placebo-controlled trial and demonstrated inferiority to SGAs (risperidone and quetiapine). Thus, use of divalproex for acute mania should be limited to those individuals who have already failed to respond

TABLE 37–3. FDA-approved medications for pediatric bipolar disorder, with years of initial approvals

Acute mania	Acute bipolar depression	Bipolar maintenance
1970, Lithium[a(e)]	2014, Olanzapine + fluoxetine[b]	1974, Lithium[a(e)]
2007, Risperidone[b]	2018, Lurasidone[b]	2008, Aripiprazole[b(e)]
2008, Aripiprazole[b,*(e)]		
2009, Quetiapine[b]	Unmet Clinical Need	
2009, Olanzapine[c]		
2015, Asenapine[b]		

*Adjunctive therapy (as well as monotherapy).
[a]Ages 12 to 17; [b]Ages 10 to 17; [c]Ages 13 to 17.
[(e)]Indication extrapolated from adult data.
Source. Adapted and updated from Ketter TA: Advances in the Treatment of Bipolar Disorder. Washington, DC, American Psychiatric Publishing, 2015. Copyright © 2015 American Psychiatric Association. Used with permission.

to SGAs and lithium (either as monotherapy or in combination with an SGA). Divalproex combined with quetiapine has shown large response and remission rates and may be considered. Lamotrigine has practical limitations in the treatment of acute mania due to the protracted dosage titration required to prevent Stevens-Johnson syndrome, and because of the limited evidence supporting its use in acute mania.

Large placebo responses are common in pediatric bipolar depression, highlighting the importance of psychosocial interventions (Vallarino et al. 2015) as an initial treatment approach in mild to moderate bipolar depression. Lurasidone received FDA approval in 2018 for use in pediatric bipolar depression, with moderate treatment effect sizes. After up to 2 years of follow-up from the acute phase, treatment with lurasidone was associated with continued improvement in depressive symptoms, resulting in progressively higher rates of response, remission, and recovery (Singh et al. 2021). Because of its favorable risk-benefit profile, lurasidone is considered a first-line treatment choice for pediatric bipolar depression. Olanzapine-fluoxetine combination (OFC) has shown similarly moderate effect sizes for response and remission, but because of its metabolic and weight-gain side effects, it is considered a second-line choice for pediatric bipolar depression, reserved for those with a lack of response to psychosocial intervention and lurasidone treatment. Lithium has established efficacy in adults with bipolar depression or treatment-resistant unipolar depression, and it may be effective in preventing suicidal behavior in adults; however, there is limited evidence to support its use in youth. Adjunctive lamotrigine has yielded positive results in open-label pediatric studies, but its long titration period and potentially serious side effects limit its use in youth. Finally, although antidepressants are well tolerated in unipolar pediatric depression, the efficacy of these agents in pediatric bipolar depression has not been well established. Thus, antidepressants as monotherapy or adjunctive therapy should be used only in settings where the potential benefits outweigh the known risks (e.g., activation or worsening of mania symptoms or increased suicide risk).

To maintain youth in euthymic mood states, aripiprazole monotherapy and lamotrigine used adjunctively are recommended as first-line options. Aripiprazole performed better than placebo in extending time to emergence of a mood event and showed in an extension study that it can maintain its effect over time (Findling et al. 2013). Similarly, lamotrigine has evidence to support its use as a maintenance agent both as monotherapy and as an adjunctive agent, with the latter use having a stronger level of evidence, particularly in preventing depressive relapses. Extension studies for aripiprazole, asenapine, quetiapine, and ziprasidone in youth have shown that continuing these agents leads to maintenance of the response, which merits replication. Similarly, in studies evaluating lithium for long-term symptom reduction and relapse prevention for pediatric patients with bipolar disorders, lithium showed moderate success as a maintenance therapy for youth who achieved response and remission during the acute phase of treatment. These studies demonstrate that maintenance therapy in pediatric bipolar disorders has a limited evidence base. Additional studies are sorely needed to establish the optimal first-line strategy for long-term treatment of pediatric bipolar disorders. Indeed, current pharmacotherapies are associated with high relapse rates and frequent residual symptoms, and the long-term safety and tolerability in youth is unknown. Ultimately, clinicians must select treatments based on the available empirical evidence, individual clinical characteristics, and safety concerns in the immediate and long term.

Future Directions

Mood disorders are increasingly being recognized and treated in youth. Although the field has received increased research attention in recent years, there remain key uncertainties that merit investigation through carefully designed prospective follow-up research. Indeed, the preponderance of data on the efficacy of pharmacological interventions come from adult studies, and from studies targeting acute rather than prolonged mood states. The FDA has approved fluoxetine (ages 7+) and escitalopram (ages 12+) for the treatment of acute unipolar depression; lithium (ages 12+), aripiprazole (ages 10+), asenapine (ages 10+), olanzapine (ages 13+), quetiapine (ages 10+), and risperidone (ages 10+) for the treatment of acute mania; and OFC (ages 10+) and lurasidone (age 10+) for the treatment of acute bipolar depression. However, we know that youth with mood disorders experience full episodes or subsyndromal symptoms of depression variably and frequently for extended periods of time, and with a high likelihood of relapse, and there is a dearth of controlled data to support the long-term management of mood disorders in youth to guide relapse prevention.

We need evidence for additional pharmacological and nonpharmacological treatment options for pediatric mood disorders, because rarely does one size fit all youth. Studies aimed at investigating individual differences in symptom presentation and predictors of treatment response are central for the development of personalized treatment approaches. A combination of clinical and biological predictive factors—encompassing demographic characteristics, symptom clusters, family history, pharmacogenomic markers, cognitive impairments, and neuroimaging-derived trait and state phenotypes—may contribute to risk stratification (Birmaher et al. 2018). Efforts to pool data derived from multiple studies in the search for those predictors should be supported (Vieta et al. 2018), facilitated by standardized data collection, design, and analytic procedures. Indeed, if future research endeavors to investigate personalized treatment strategies by including a systematic evaluation of markers of treatment response and tolerability, perhaps more definitive guidance for specific and sequential interventions can be provided to patients who do not respond to the first treatment offered. It is hoped that preliminary studies on brain-responsive biomarkers of treatment will yield interventions that will help to normalize brain structure and function, principally in prefrontal, limbic, and striatal regions and networks critical for adaptive functioning and regulation of emotion and reward. Future studies informed by these neuroimaging biomarkers may lead to improved early identification and treatment.

The scientific mechanisms underlying risk for developing a lifelong mood disorder and risk for acute versus chronic symptoms are largely unknown, as are the mechanisms underlying response to treatment. However, in recent years, with the development and application of novel neuroscience tools to better understand brain and behavior, the field has seen dramatic and accelerated advances. Numerous researchers are now conducting and reporting on prospective longitudinal observations of youth with or at risk for mood disorders throughout the course of their neurodevelopment, alongside treatment, and as youth transition into adulthood. These longitudinal studies will increase the field's capacity to predict which youth are most vulnerable to suffering from mood disorders throughout their lives and which youth are most likely to respond to treatment. With a strong movement in medicine toward evidence-based practice, clinicians and patients alike are seeking guidance from contemporary observational and intervention studies to establish clinical best practices and to usher in the development of novel treatments for pediatric mood disorders that will outperform the current standard of care and lead to optimal long-term outcomes.

References

Alvano SA, Zieher LM: An updated classification of antidepressants: a proposal to simplify treatment. Personalized Medicine in Psychiatry (19–20):100042, 2020. Available at: https://www.personalizedmedpsych.com/article/S2468-1717(18)30028-0/fulltext.

American Psychiatric Association: Diagnostic and Statistical Manual of Mental Disorders, 5th Edition. Arlington, VA, American Psychiatric Association, 2013

Avenevoli S, Swendsen J, He J-P, et al: Major depression in the National Comorbidity Survey—adolescent supplement: prevalence, correlates, and treatment. J Am Acad Child Adolesc Psychiatry 54(1):37.e2–44.e2, 2015 25524788

Ballesteros MF, Williams DD, Mack KA, et al: The epidemiology of unintentional and violence-related injury morbidity and mortality among children and adolescents in the United States. Int J Environ Res Public Health 15(4):E616, 2018 29597289

Bansal R, Hellerstein DJ, Peterson BS: Evidence for neuroplastic compensation in the cerebral cortex of persons with depressive illness. Mol Psychiatry 23(2):375–383, 2018 28265119

Berk M, Post R, Ratheesh A, et al: Staging in bipolar disorder: from theoretical framework to clinical utility. World Psychiatry 16(3):236–244, 2017 28941093

Birmaher B, Merranko JA, Goldstein TR, et al: A risk calculator to predict the individual risk of conversion from subthreshold bipolar symptoms to bipolar disorder I or II in youth. J Am Acad Child Adolesc Psychiatry 57(10):755.e4–763.e4, 2018 30274650

Brent D, Emslie G, Clarke G, et al: Switching to another SSRI or to venlafaxine with or without cognitive behavioral therapy for adolescents with SSRI-resistant depression: the TORDIA randomized controlled trial. JAMA 299(8):901–913, 2008 18314433

Chang K: Adult bipolar disorder is continuous with pediatric bipolar disorder. Can J Psychiatry 52(7):418–425, 2007 17688005

Cheung AH, Zuckerbrot RA, Jensen PS, et al: Guidelines for Adolescent Depression in Primary Care (GLAD-PC), part II. Pediatrics 141(3):e20174082, 2018 29483201

Coates M, Spanos M, Parmar P, et al: A review of methods for monitoring adverse events in pediatric psychopharmacology clinical trials. Drug Saf 41(5):465–471, 2018 29318515

de Lijster JM, van den Dries MA, van der Ende J, et al: Developmental trajectories of anxiety and depression symptoms from early to middle childhood: a population-based cohort study in the Netherlands. J Abnorm Child Psychol 52(7):418–425, 2019 31069583

Dwyer JB, Stringaris A, Brent DA, Bloch MH: Annual research review: defining and treating pediatric treatment-resistant depression. J Child Psychol Psychiatry 61(3):312–332, 2020 32020643

Egberts KM, Mehler-Wex C, Gerlach M: Therapeutic drug monitoring in child and adolescent psychiatry. Pharmacopsychiatry 44(6):249–253, 2011 21959786

Ellis R, Seal ML, Adamson C, et al: Brain connectivity networks and longitudinal trajectories of depression symptoms in adolescence. Psychiatry Res Neuroimaging 260:62–69, 2017 28038362

Faedda GL, Serra G, Marangoni C, et al: Clinical risk factors for bipolar disorders: a systematic review of prospective studies. J Affect Disord 168:314–321, 2014 25086290

Findling RL, Correll CU, Nyilas M, et al: Aripiprazole for the treatment of pediatric bipolar I disorder: a 30-week, randomized controlled study. Bipolar Disord 15(2):138–149, 2013 23437959

Findling RL, DelBello MP, Zuddas A, et al: Vortioxetine for major depressive disorder in adolescents: 12-week randomized, placebo-controlled, fluoxetine-referenced, fixed-dose study. J Am Acad Child Adolesc Psychiatry January 11, 2022 [Online ahead of print] 35033635

Frahm Laursen M, Valentin JB, Licht RW, et al: Longitudinal outcomes in pediatric- and adult-onset bipolar patients compared to healthy and schizophrenia controls. Bipolar Disord 21(6):514–524, 2019 31069923

Grof P, Duffy A, Cavazzoni P, et al: Is response to prophylactic lithium a familial trait? J Clin Psychiatry 63(10):942–947, 2002 12416605

Hafeman D, Bebko G, Bertocci MA, et al: Amygdala-prefrontal cortical functional connectivity during implicit emotion processing differentiates youth with bipolar spectrum from youth with externalizing disorders. J Affect Disord 208:94–100, 2017 27756046

Hammad TA, Laughren T, Racoosin J: Suicidality in pediatric patients treated with antidepressant drugs. Arch Gen Psychiatry 63(3):332–339, 2006 16520440

Hulvershorn LA, Cullen K, Anand A: Toward dysfunctional connectivity: a review of neuroimaging findings in pediatric MDD. Brain Imaging Behav 5(4):307–328, 2011 21901425

Jensen-Doss A, Youngstrom EA, Youngstrom JK, et al: Predictors and moderators of agreement between clinical and research diagnoses for children and adolescents. J Consult Clin Psychol 82(6):1151–1162, 2014 24773574

Johnson D, Dupuis G, Piche J, et al: Adult mental health outcomes of adolescent depression: a systematic review. Depress Anxiety 35(8):700–716, 2018 29878410

Kann L, McManus T, Harris WA, et al: Youth risk behavior surveillance—United States, 2017. MMWR Surveill Summ 67(8):1–114, 2018 29878410

Kapczinski NS, Mwangi B, Cassidy RM, et al: Neuroprogression and illness trajectories in bipolar disorder. Expert Rev Neurother 17(3):277–285, 2017 27659841

Ketter TA: Advances in the Treatment of Bipolar Disorder. Washington, DC, American Psychiatric Publishing, 2015

Kwong ASF, López-López JA, Hammerton G, et al: Genetic and environmental risk factors associated with trajectories of depression symptoms from adolescence to young adulthood. JAMA Netw Open 2(6):e196587, 2019 31251383

March J, Silva S, Petrycki S, et al; TADS Team: Fluoxetine, cognitive-behavioral therapy, and their combination for adolescents with depression: Treatment for Adolescents With Depression Study (TADS) randomized controlled trial. JAMA 292(7):807–820, 2004 15315995

Meister R, Abbas M, Antel J, et al: Placebo response rates and potential modifiers in double-blind randomized controlled trials of second and newer generation antidepressants for major depressive disorder in children and adolescents: a systematic review and meta-regression analysis. Eur Child Adolesc Psychiatry 29(3):253–273, 2020 30535589

Nakash O, Nagar M, Kanat-Maymon Y: Clinical use of the DSM categorical diagnostic system during the mental health intake session. J Clin Psychiatry 76(7):e862–e869, 2015 26231013

Pfeifer JC, Welge J, Strakowski SM, et al: Meta-analysis of amygdala volumes in youth with bipolar disorder. J Am Acad Child Adolesc Psychiatry 47(11):1289–1298, 2008 18827720
Rettew DC, Lynch AD, Achenbach TM, et al: Meta-analyses of agreement between diagnoses made from clinical evaluations and standardized diagnostic interviews. Int J Methods Psychiatr Res 18(3):169–184, 2009 19701924
Roybal DJ, Singh MK, Cosgrove VE, et al: Biological evidence for a neurodevelopmental model of pediatric bipolar disorder. Isr J Psychiatry Relat Sci 49(1):28–43, 2012 22652927
Shapero BG, Chai XJ, Vangel M, et al: Neural markers of depression risk predict the onset of depression. Psychiatry Res Neuroimaging 285:31–39, 2019 30716688
Singh MK (ed): Clinical Handbook for the Diagnosis and Treatment of Pediatric Mood Disorders. Washington, DC, American Psychiatric Association Publishing, 2019a
Singh MK: Using screening tools and diagnosing bipolar disorder in pediatric patients. J Clin Psychiatry 80(1):SU18023BR1C, 2019b 30865786
Singh MK, Chang KD, Kelley RG, et al: Early signs of anomalous neural functional connectivity in healthy offspring of parents with bipolar disorder. Bipolar Disord 16(7):678–689, 2014a 24938878
Singh MK, Kelley RG, Howe ME, et al: Reward processing in healthy offspring of parents with bipolar disorder. JAMA Psychiatry 71(10):1148–1156, 2014b 25142103
Singh MK, Leslie SM, Packer MM, et al: Limbic intrinsic connectivity in depressed and high-risk youth. J Am Acad Child Adolesc Psychiatry 57(10):775.e3–785.e3, 2018 30274652
Singh M, Tocco M, Schweizer E, Pikalov A: Long-term effectiveness of lurasidone in pediatric bipolar depression: response, remission and recovery. CNS Spectr 26(2):148, 2021 34127107
Soe NN, Wen DJ, Poh JS, et al: Perinatal maternal depressive symptoms alter amygdala functional connectivity in girls. Hum Brain Mapp 39(2):680–690, 2018 29094774
Stepanova E, Findling RL: Psychopharmacology of bipolar disorders in children and adolescents. Pediatr Clin North Am 64(6):1209–1222, 2017 29173781
Strawn JR, Poweleit EA, Uppugunduri CRS, Ramsey LB: Pediatric therapeutic drug monitoring for selective serotonin reuptake inhibitors. Front Pharmacol 12:749692, 2021 34658889
Vallarino M, Henry C, Etain B, et al: An evidence map of psychosocial interventions for the earliest stages of bipolar disorder. Lancet Psychiatry 2(6):548–563, 2015 26360451
Van Meter A, Moreira ALR, Youngstrom E: Updated meta-analysis of epidemiologic studies of pediatric bipolar disorder. J Clin Psychiatry 80(3):18r12180, 2019 30946542
Varigonda AL, Jakubovski E, Taylor MJ, et al: Systematic review and meta-analysis: early treatment responses of selective serotonin reuptake inhibitors in pediatric major depressive disorder. J Am Acad Child Adolesc Psychiatry 54(7):557–564, 2015 26088660
Vieta E, Arango C, Rush AJ: The need for paediatric registries to assess long-term brain effects of psychotropic medications: the case of bipolar disorder. Eur Neuropsychopharmacol 28(11):1181–1184, 2018 30193832
Weersing VR, Jeffreys M, Do M-CT, et al: Evidence base update of psychosocial treatments for child and adolescent depression. J Clin Child Adolesc Psychol 46(1):11–43, 2017 27870579
Wegbreit E, Cushman GK, Puzia ME, et al: Developmental meta-analyses of the functional neural correlates of bipolar disorder. JAMA Psychiatry 71(8):926–935, 2014 25100166
Weintraub MJ, Axelson DA, Kowatch RA, et al: Comorbid disorders as moderators of response to family interventions among adolescents with bipolar disorder. J Affect Disord 246:754–762, 2019 30623821
Weintraub MJ, Schneck CD, Axelson DA, et al: Classifying mood symptom trajectories in adolescents with bipolar disorder. J Am Acad Child Adolesc Psychiatry 59(3):381–390, 2020 31150753
Wiggins JL, Brotman MA, Adleman NE, et al: Neural markers in pediatric bipolar disorder and familial risk for bipolar disorder. J Am Acad Child Adolesc Psychiatry 56(1):67–78, 2017 27993231
Zhou X, Teng T, Zhang Y, et al: Comparative efficacy and acceptability of antidepressants, psychotherapies, and their combination for acute treatment of children and adolescents with depressive disorder: a systematic review and network meta-analysis. Lancet Psychiatry 7(7):581–601, 2020 32563306

CHAPTER 38

Geriatric Mood Disorders

Kristina F. Zdanys, M.D.
David C. Steffens, M.D., M.H.S.

Mood disorders are common among older adults and are associated with a variety of negative outcomes, including suicide, functional impairment, cognitive decline and dementia, and increased mortality risk. In this chapter we highlight several mood disorders, including major depressive disorder, persistent depressive disorder (dysthymia), adjustment disorder with depressed mood, bereavement-related depression, and bipolar disorder, that are important to recognize and treat in older adults. A variety of biological, psychological, and social factors have been identified that increase the risk of depression and limit treatment response in this population. Examples of such factors include cerebrovascular disease, personality traits (e.g., neuroticism), and low social support. Evidence-based treatments—including psychotherapy, pharmacotherapy, and neurostimulation—are available for mood disorders in older adults, and in the final portion of this chapter we review these treatments and offer guidelines for their use.

Differential Diagnosis of Late-Life Mood Disorders

The differential diagnosis of mood disorders in late life is summarized in Table 38–1.

Major Depressive Disorder

An episode of major depressive disorder (MDD) is defined as the presence, over a 2-week period, of five or more of the following symptoms: depressed mood, diminished interests, insomnia or hypersomnia, psychomotor agitation or retardation, loss of energy, feelings of worthlessness or guilt, and recurrent thoughts of death with or without suicidal ideation or a specific plan (American Psychiatric Association 2013). At least one of the five symptoms present must be depressed mood or loss of interest

TABLE 38–1. Differential diagnosis of mood disorders in late life

Primary psychiatric illness
Major depressive disorder
Persistent depressive disorder (dysthymia)
Adjustment disorder with depressed mood
Bereavement-related depression
Bipolar disorder
Mixed psychiatric/medical illness
Vascular depression
Primary neurocognitive disorder
Alzheimer's disease
Vascular dementia
Other dementia
Depression in the setting of medical illness
Examples: stroke, Parkinson's disease, coronary artery disease

or pleasure. These symptoms cause clinically significant distress and impair functioning (American Psychiatric Association 2013). These criteria, as defined in the *Diagnostic and Statistical Manual of Mental Disorders*, 5th Edition (DSM-5), are applied across age groups. In the older adult population, it is especially important to consider underlying medical and physiological conditions that may contribute to the patient's presentation, to ensure that symptoms are not strictly a consequence of one of these factors (Aziz and Steffens 2013; Casey 2017). In the Cache County study in 2000, the point prevalence of MDD in community-dwelling elderly (ages 65–100 years) was estimated to be 4.4% in women and 2.7% in men (Steffens et al. 2000); the Institute of Medicine reported in 2010 a 12-month prevalence rate of 3.0%–4.3% for major depressive episodes in older adults (Committee on the Mental Health Workforce for Geriatric Populations et al. 2012). Rates of MDD are higher in non-community-dwelling older adult populations, with MDD reported in approximately 14.4% of older adults in nursing homes (Teresi et al. 2001) and 11.5% of those hospitalized (Koenig et al. 1988).

A complex relationship exists between cognitive impairment and late-life depression. MDD in the elderly is associated with prominent executive dysfunction, which can impair judgment and limit functional ability (Alexopoulos et al. 2002). When present with depression, executive dysfunction may be helped by specific treatment aimed at improving problem-solving abilities (Alexopoulos 2019; Alexopoulos et al. 2008). Historically, the term *pseudodementia* referred to cognitive impairment present in the context of a depressive episode, which would resolve with remission of the mood symptoms. However, studies have found that even when cognitive symptoms initially improve following resolution of a depressive episode, the affected patient has a greater than 40% chance of developing an irreversible dementia within 3 years (Alexopoulos et al. 1993). In addition, evidence suggests that patients with depression-associated cognitive dysfunction are over four times more likely to develop dementia than are older adults who experienced depression without cognitive changes (Alexopoulos et al. 1993). Longitudinal studies in older adults show higher rates of

Alzheimer's disease, vascular dementia, mild cognitive impairment, and all-cause dementia among patients who have depression (Diniz et al. 2013; Gao et al. 2013). Therefore, the term *pseudodementia* has fallen out of favor with many geriatric psychiatrists. Conceptually, depression may be considered as not just a prodrome of, but also a risk factor for, development of dementia (Jorm 2001; Ownby et al. 2006; Spira et al. 2012).

Among older adults, MDD is associated with increased disability and mortality (Hybels et al. 2016; Schulz et al. 2000). In a longitudinal study of patients referred for a geriatric psychiatry consultation (Royall et al. 2007), older adults with Geriatric Depression Scale (GDS) (Yesavage et al. 1982–1983) scores greater than 6 died an average of almost 3 years sooner than those with GDS scores of 6 or less. Late-life depression is also associated with suicide risk, especially among older white men (Jack et al. 2018).

MDD may also manifest with mood-congruent or mood-incongruent psychotic features. There is evidence that delusions are more commonly observed among depressed adults older than 60 years than among younger depressed adults (Meyers et al. 1984). Prognostically, the presence of delusions in MDD is associated with high rates of MDD relapse and chronicity of depression in older adults (Meyers et al. 2001). Psychotic depression in later life is associated with poor social support and symptomatically has been associated with feelings of guilt and worthlessness, suicidal ideation and intent, and a prior history of delusions (Thakur et al. 1999).

Persistent Depressive Disorder (Dysthymia)

Persistent depressive disorder (PDD), or dysthymia, is characterized by the presence of depressed mood for more days than not, for at least 2 years, in addition to two or more of the following symptoms: change in appetite, insomnia or hypersomnia, low energy, low self-esteem, poor concentration, and feelings of hopelessness (American Psychiatric Association 2013). The diagnostic criteria additionally specify that the symptoms must not have been absent for more than 2 consecutive months at a time and must not be attributable to a substance or a medical condition, and also that the patient must not have a history of mania. The symptoms must affect the patient's functioning and cause clinically significant distress (American Psychiatric Association 2013). Although the severity of symptoms is lower than that in a full major depressive episode, patients with dysthymia may also experience intermittent episodes of MDD superimposed on their chronic illness (American Psychiatric Association 2013).

The prevalence of PDD among older adults is estimated at approximately 2%, but true rates may be as high as 8% (Blazer and Steffens 2015; Blazer et al. 1987). PDD is less commonly associated with psychiatric comorbidity in older adults than in younger adults and is less frequently associated with a family history of depression (Devanand et al. 1994). Among patients for whom the onset of PDD occurs in later life, there is a roughly equal gender distribution (Devanand et al. 2004). Later age at onset is associated with the presence of significant psychosocial stressors (Devanand 2014).

Older patients with PDD often first present to primary care, a setting in which their illness may not be recognized or treated (Fann et al. 2009; Piek et al. 2012). In the elderly, PDD is associated with increased disability and poor medical outcomes (Devanand 2014); thus, identification and treatment of this disorder is important for the patient's overall health.

Adjustment Disorder With Depressed Mood

In DSM-5, adjustment disorder with depressed mood is classified in the category of trauma- and stressor-related disorders rather than among the depressive disorders (American Psychiatric Association 2013). Adjustment disorders involve "the development of emotional or behavioral symptoms in response to an identifiable stressor(s) occurring within 3 months of the onset of the stressor(s)" (American Psychiatric Association 2013, p. 286). These symptoms must be associated with marked distress and/or impairment in functioning and must not last for more than 6 months after the stressor and its consequences have ended (American Psychiatric Association 2013). Little is known about the epidemiology of adjustment disorder in older adults.

Stressors for older adults may be medical (e.g., a new diagnosis of illness), social (e.g., interpersonal difficulty with family, a move to a new living situation), or functional (e.g., loss of the ability to drive or to manage finances); stressors may also entail an unexpected new responsibility (e.g., caregiving for an ill relative). In adjustment disorder with depressed mood, the degree of depressive symptomatology exceeds what would be expected as a response to these stressors (Blazer and Steffens 2015).

Bereavement-Related Depression

Bereavement refers to a person's response to the death of someone close to him or her, which may be characterized as a grief reaction that includes feelings of longing, loss of interests, and frequent thoughts of the deceased (Shear et al. 2013). Virtually all older adults have experienced the death of a spouse or a member of their immediate family, or of a friend or colleague; in a study using longitudinal data from 839 community-dwelling older adults, more than 70% reported having experienced bereavement over the 2.5-year period (Williams et al. 2007). Historically, MDD was not diagnosed if symptoms occurred in the context of bereavement; however, DSM-5 removed this so-called bereavement exclusion, thereby indicating that individuals experiencing bereavement may also meet criteria for MDD (American Psychiatric Association 2013). Symptoms of grief in older adults typically resolve within a few months, and the individual regains baseline functioning (Chentsova Dutton and Zisook 2005). If severe grief and mourning reactions persist, the individual may be experiencing "complicated grief" (Shear et al. 2013) or *persistent complex bereavement disorder* (American Psychiatric Association 2013), a disorder listed in the DSM-5 Trauma- and Stressor-Related Disorders chapter as an example of a presentation qualifying for a diagnosis of "other specified trauma- and stressor-related disorder" and also listed under "Conditions for Further Study" in DSM-5 Section III.

Bipolar Disorder

A new diagnosis of bipolar I disorder in a older adult requires a history of an episode of mania. The manic episode may have occurred in early adulthood or may have had a later-life onset. A late-life manic episode may resemble delirium, catatonia, or dementia with behavioral disturbances or may manifest as a prominent dysphoria; because of these variable presentations, mania in an older adult may be challenging to diagnose (Blazer and Steffens 2015).

Although the prevalence of bipolar disorder decreases as age increases, bipolar disorder has an estimated prevalence of between 0.08% and 0.5% among community-dwelling older adults and of between 4.7% and 18.5% among older adults in inpatient settings (Beyer 2015; Depp and Jeste 2004; Dols et al. 2014). After adjustment for overall gender ratio, bipolar disorder among older adults appeared to be equally distributed between genders (Depp and Jeste 2004). Late-onset bipolar disorder is often associated with underlying neurological illness (Beyer 2015; Depp and Jeste 2004; Shulman et al. 1992), and older adults with bipolar disorder may be at higher risk of cognitive decline than their peers (Dhingra and Rabins 1991; Kocsis et al. 1993). Bipolar disorder in older adults is associated with the presence of hyperintensities on magnetic resonance imaging (MRI) (Altshuler et al. 1995; Botteron et al. 1995; Dupont et al. 1987, 1995; Figiel et al. 1991; Krabbendam et al. 2000). Medical comorbidity and mortality are higher among older adults with bipolar disorder relative to their peers (Beyer 2015).

Factors That Influence Late-Life Mood Disorders

Biological Factors

Age-related cerebrovascular disease has long been observed to be related to depressive syndromes in older adults. More than a century ago, Binswanger noted that subcortical microvascular disease was a critical factor in the development of neurocognitive symptoms (Mathers et al. 1987), but the presence of depression symptoms in this condition did not become a major focus of study until much later in the twentieth century (Venna et al. 1988). In the late 1990s, investigators studying mood disorders in elderly adults proposed the concept of *vascular depression* (which posits that cerebrovascular disease may predispose to, precipitate, or perpetuate geriatric mood disorders) as a research subtype of late-life unipolar depression (Andreescu and Reynolds 2011). Two pivotal papers that spurred further studies of vascular depression focused on a clinical definition (Alexopoulos et al. 1997a) and a definition derived from MRI findings (Krishnan et al. 1997) to operationalize its features. Subsequent research testing the vascular depression hypothesis (Alexopoulos et al. 1997b) has capitalized on advances in neuroimaging techniques to further refine this clinical construct. The capacity of MRI-based diffusion tensor imaging to examine white matter integrity has allowed exploration of the relationship between damage to white matter and the development and maintenance of depressive symptoms (Reppermund et al. 2014). Despite a large volume of research supporting the contribution of subcortical microvascular disease to the development of depression, vascular depression was not represented in the DSM-5 classification, and some have strongly urged that it be included in the next revision of the diagnostic nomenclature (Steffens 2019). Cerebrovascular changes have also been reported in late-onset bipolar disorder (Tamashiro et al. 2008).

In addition to chronic cerebrovascular changes, acute cerebrovascular events are also associated with the development of late-life depression. Depression may be seen in 29%–52% of patients in the 5 years following a stroke (Ayerbe et al. 2014; Hackett and Pickles 2014). Increased depression has been observed among patients with a severe stroke and mild, moderate, or severe poststroke disability, relative to patients with a mild stroke and no poststroke disability (Kutlubaev and Hackett 2014). The role of lesion location in the development of depression has been studied, with inconsistent results (Folstein et al. 1977; Kutlubaev and Hackett 2014; Robinson et al. 1984; Starkstein et al. 1987). Other neurological illnesses are associated with development of depression. For example, depressive symptoms are observed in 40%–50% of patients with Parkinson's disease (Reijnders et al. 2008); while poorly understood, these symptoms may be related to neurobiological changes secondary to the underlying Parkinson's disease that affect mood and reward systems in the brain (Aarsland et al. 2011) in addition to reflecting the influence of other factors (e.g., disability, life events, level of social support) (Rod et al. 2013).

Non-neurological medical illnesses found to be associated with late-life depression include coronary artery disease (Sullivan et al. 1997), hypotension (Briggs et al. 2016), and diabetes (Black et al. 1998; Blazer et al. 2002b). Changes in endocrine function, such as subclinical hypothyroidism (Schindler 2003) or low testosterone (Harman et al. 2001), may be associated with depression in older adults. Overall medical burden and associated disability may play a larger role in development of late-life depression than specific medical diagnoses (Koenig et al. 1991). The association between medical illness and late-life depression may be bidirectional, such that depression may contribute to or exacerbate the presentation of medical symptoms, and medical symptoms also may lead to depressive symptoms (Gleason et al. 2013).

Depression often co-occurs with other psychiatric disorders, but the association of depression with comorbid psychiatric illness is more commonly observed among younger adults than older adults (Blazer and Steffens 2015). Anxiety and alcohol use disorder are commonly associated with late-life depression (Devanand 2002; Hybels and Blazer 2003).

Genetics appear to play less of a role in late-life depression than in depression of earlier onset. Certain genetically inherited conditions, such as cerebral autosomal dominant arteriopathy with subcortical infarcts and leukoencephalopathy (CADASIL), often manifest with symptoms suggestive of vascular depression (Park et al. 2017). Another possible relationship involving genes, cerebrovascular disease, and depression was proposed in the homocysteine depression hypothesis, which speculated that genetic variations in enzymes affecting homocysteine metabolism may contribute to cerebrovascular disease and, consequently, to vascular depression (Folstein et al. 2007). There is some evidence that serotonin transporter polymorphisms may influence the efficacy and tolerability of antidepressants in older adults (Pollock 2000). The apolipoprotein E epsilon 4 allele (*APOE*E4*), one of the most frequently studied genes in older adults because of its relationship with Alzheimer's disease, does not appear to have an association with the development of late-life depression (Blazer et al. 2002a).

Psychological Factors

Personality attributes are associated with late-life depression. Neuroticism (a personality trait associated with a tendency to experience negative affects, such as anger, anxiety, depression, and emotional instability) is considered to be a personality construct rather than a personality disorder. Facets of this trait include anxiety, anger, depression, self-consciousness, and vulnerability to stress (Costa and McCrae 1992). Neuroticism is associated with a predisposition toward negative mood states and an increased risk of depression in older adults (Costa and McCrae 1980; Henderson et al. 1993; Kendler et al. 2006; Lyness et al. 2002). The trait of neuroticism is additionally associated with poorer response to treatment for depression, and vulnerability to stress, a facet of neuroticism, is associated with cognitive impairment (Manning et al. 2017). Late-life depression is also associated with personality disorder clusters A (odd/eccentric personality disorders) and C (anxious/fearful personality disorders) (Morse and Lynch 2004).

A history of negative life events such as abuse or neglect or socioeconomic stress may predispose patients to depression in late life (Kraaij and de Wilde 2001). Maladaptive coping strategies such as rumination and catastrophizing may play a role in how life events influence the development of depression (Kraaij et al. 2002). *Self-efficacy* is a term referring to an individual's sense of control over events and situations (Bandura 1994). Older adults who have a high level of self-efficacy have fewer depressive symptoms, and are less disabled by depressive symptoms, than are those who have a lower sense of individual control (Jang et al. 2002). There appears to be a relationship between perceived self-efficacy and social support, which may mediate the relationship between self-efficacy and depression (Holahan and Holahan 1987).

Social Factors

Acute and chronic life stressors are associated with depressive symptoms in late life. Examples of stressors include death of a spouse or child, life-threatening illness in oneself or a close relation, financial or material loss, personal assault, emotional abuse, and a change of residence outside one's control (Kraaij and de Wilde 2001; Murphy 1982). As previously discussed, bereavement often correlates with the onset of significant depressive symptoms in late life (Chentsova Dutton and Zisook 2005). There is evidence that the association of bereavement with depressive symptoms may be mediated by the level of social support available to the patient, such that patients with less social support are at higher risk of developing depression while experiencing bereavement grief (Prigerson et al. 1994). In general, older adults facing life stressors who lack meaningful social contact are at higher risk of developing depressive symptoms (Bruce and Hall 1994; Murphy 1982; Prince et al. 1998), although not all studies have demonstrated this association (Schoevers et al. 2000). There is evidence that patients who are socioeconomically disadvantaged are at higher risk of developing depressive symptomatology than are those with greater financial means (Mojtabai and Olfson 2004). In one study, socioeconomic stressors even in early life were significantly associated with late-life depression (Kraaij et al. 1997).

Caregiving takes many forms but represents a particularly challenging stressor in late life that is often associated with caregiver burden, burnout, and depression. Elderly caregivers may be providing care for spouses, family members, or others with medical, cognitive, and psychiatric illnesses. Additionally, older adults often are responsible for the care of younger generations, such as grandchildren. Finally, dementia care is one of the most taxing forms of caregiving. Often, the role of primary dementia caregiver is taken on not by choice but rather due to circumstance and necessity (Pertl et al. 2019). Factors that appear to increase the risk of caregiver burden and depression include disruptive neuropsychiatric symptoms in the care recipient (e.g., agitation, aggression, irritability), higher numbers of caregiving hours per day, and (less significantly) the care recipient's level of functional dependence (Cheng 2017).

Diagnostic Workup for Late-Life Mood Disorders

The diagnostic workup of mood symptoms in older adults begins with a thorough history, physical examination, and laboratory testing (Blazer 2003). The goal of the evaluation is to narrow the differential diagnosis while considering medical, cognitive, and substance-related factors that may contribute to the clinical presentation. Key focal points of the interview include current symptoms (including details on nature, severity, and duration); history of prior episodes (including response to previous treatment strategies); medical history and current medications; substance use history; and family history (particularly in regard to treatment response of family members and history of suicide) (Blazer and Steffens 2015). Involvement of family members or other caregivers in the interview often yields additional information (e.g., on symptom onset and course of illness) to clarify the clinical picture; however, the patient should first be interviewed alone whenever possible (Glover and Srinivasan 2013). A thorough suicide risk assessment is important at the initial and subsequent visits to determine the severity and urgency of the risk and the level of care that may be most appropriate for the patient (Raue et al. 2014).

Screening tools helpful in the assessment of depression in older adults may focus on mood symptoms as well as cognitive functioning. The GDS (Yesavage et al. 1982–1983) has both a long form and a short form and uses a yes/no format to assess symptoms of depression commonly observed among older adults. Assessments typically used in younger adults, such as the 9-item Patient Health Questionnaire (PHQ-9; Kroenke et al. 2001) may also be helpful. Screening instruments for cognitive functioning that can be integrated into an office visit include the Mini-Mental State Examination (MMSE; Folstein et al. 1975), the Montreal Cognitive Assessment (MoCA; Nasreddine et al. 2005), and the Saint Louis University Mental Status exam (SLUMS; Tariq et al. 2006). Scores lower than would be expected for a patient's age and education level may warrant further assessment by a neuropsychologist to determine whether cognitive performance problems are more likely related to an underlying neurocognitive disorder than to a primary mood disorder or another etiology. Additionally, a functional assessment focusing on instrumental activities of daily living (IADLs) and activities of daily living (ADLs) (Katz 1983) is important to determine the degree to which a patient is independent or is relying on the assistance of others for day-to-day tasks. Reliance on others may reflect the impact of the mood disorder, cognitive impairment, or physical limitations.

Key components of a physical examination include a neurological examination (to assess possible cerebrovascular involvement), vital signs, and weight (as older adults often experience significant weight loss during depressive episodes) (Blazer and Steffens 2015). Laboratory workup typically includes complete blood count; blood chemistries; thyroid function; and B_{12}, vitamin D, and folate levels (Blazer and Steffens 2015; Glover and Srinivasan 2013). The laboratory workup is useful for identifying factors that may be contributing to the clinical presentation (e.g., patients with anemia, hypothyroidism, or low B_{12} levels may "appear" depressed), as well as for establishing a baseline against which to monitor the patient for possible changes due to medication side effects (e.g., hyponatremia secondary to certain antidepressant medications) (Glover and Srinivasan 2013). Additional studies that may be relevant in the assessment of mood symptoms in older adults include MRI (to establish a diagnosis of vascular depression) and polysomnography (to assess persistent sleep abnormalities) (Blazer and Steffens 2015). An electrocardiogram may also be indicated if medications with the potential to prolong the QTc interval are being considered (Blazer and Steffens 2015). Components of the workup for late-life depression are presented in Table 38–2.

Treatment of Late-Life Mood Disorders

Psychotherapy

Psychotherapy is a well-accepted treatment approach among older adults with depression (Gum et al. 2006; Raue et al. 2009, 2011). It is an effective alternative to antidepressants for older adults who are reluctant to take medications or are unable to tolerate them because of side effects (Jayasekara et al. 2015). Psychotherapy is also useful as an adjunctive treatment for patients taking medications. The psychotherapeutic modality with the strongest evidence in older adults is cognitive-behavioral therapy (CBT) (Areán et al. 1993; Floyd et al. 2004; Gould et al. 2012; Huang et al. 2015; Jayasekara et al. 2015; Scogin et al. 1989; Steuer et al. 1984). CBT is a skills-based intervention that focuses on modifying dysfunctional thinking and behavior (Beck 1964). There is specific evidence supporting the use of CBT for patients with comorbid medical illnesses, such as type 2 diabetes (Lustman et al. 1998), stroke (Broomfield et al. 2011; Kneebone and Dunmore 2000), Parkinson's disease (Calleo et al. 2015; Egan et al. 2015), chronic obstructive pulmonary disease (Cully et al. 2010; Kunik et al. 2008), and heart disease (Freedland et al. 2015; Jeyanantham et al. 2017). Additionally, CBT techniques may benefit patients with mood symptoms and comorbid neurocognitive disorders (Teri and Gallagher-Thompson 1991). An advantage of CBT in older adults is that the therapy is structured and time-limited, generally consisting of between 16 and 20 sessions (Laidlaw et al. 2003). Although there is evidence supporting the use of CBT as a standalone treatment approach in older adults, it is also beneficial for patients who have had a less-than-complete response to medication treatment (Scott et al. 2000).

Besides CBT, several other psychotherapeutic modalities have been studied in older adults with mood disorders. Problem-solving therapy (PST) has some of the most robust evidence in older adults with depression (Alexopoulos et al. 2003, 2011; Areán et al. 1993; Choi et al. 2016; Gustavson et al. 2016; Kasckow et al. 2014). In this approach, patients are taught specific skills to address their individual problems, rather than general skills (D'Zurilla and Goldfried 1971). PST has demonstrated some benefit among patients with executive dysfunction (Alexopoulos et al. 2003, 2011; Gustavson et al. 2016), patients who have had a stroke (Robinson et al. 2008), and patients on hemodialysis (Erdley et al. 2014). There is also evidence that patients who receive PST sessions delivered by telephone, videophone, or the internet experience

TABLE 38–2. Workup for late-life depression

Screening tools for mood:
Geriatric Depression Scale (GDS; Yesavage et al. 1982–1983)
9-item Patient Health Questionnaire (PHQ-9; Kroenke et al. 2001)
Screening tools for cognition:
Mini-Mental State Examination (MMSE; Folstein et al. 1975)
Montreal Cognitive Assessment (MoCA; Nasreddine et al. 2005)
Saint Louis University Mental Status exam (SLUMS; Tariq et al. 2006)
Functional assessment:
Instrumental activities of daily living (IADLs) (Katz 1983)
Activities of daily living (ADLs) (Katz 1983)
Physical examination (key components):
Vital signs
Weight
Neurological examination
Laboratory workup:
Complete blood count
Blood chemistries
Thyroid-stimulating hormone
B_{12} level
Folate level
Vitamin D level
Other studies (as indicated):
Brain MRI
Electrocardiogram
Polysomnography

reductions in depressive symptoms similar to those experienced by patients who receive in-person PST sessions (Kiosses and Alexopoulos 2014).

Interpersonal psychotherapy (IPT) is a psychotherapeutic approach that explores the relationship between mood and interpersonal relationships in a patient's current social context (Weissman et al. 2000). Although IPT has been less studied than CBT or PST in older adults, there is some evidence that IPT is effective for the treatment of depressive symptoms in this population (Miller et al. 2001; van Schaik et al. 2006) and that it may be adapted to older adults to reduce risk of suicide (Heisel et al. 2015). Additional evidence suggests that for maintenance treatment of MDD, combination antidepressant treatment and IPT is superior to either approach used alone (Reynolds et al. 1999a). However, research findings have been mixed, as some studies of acute depression treatment and maintenance treatment with IPT do not support its use, while active and maintenance pharmacotherapy in the same studies demonstrate benefit (Dombrovski et al. 2007; Reynolds et al. 1999b). It is possible that patient characteristics, such as severity of depression at baseline and robustness of treatment response, may play a role in these differing findings (Taylor et al. 1999).

There are practical and systematic challenges for the older adult seeking psychotherapy for treatment of a late-life mood disorder. Often, older adults are treated for late-life depression in the primary care setting (Klap et al. 2003), where psychotherapy is usually not offered. Older adults may be housebound and unable to attend psychotherapy on a regular basis; to address this need, there has been a recent movement to expand access to psychotherapy via telephone- and computer-based technologies (Choi et al. 2014a, 2014b; Egede et al. 2015). Additionally, lack of economic resources may affect an individual's ability to establish care with a psychotherapist, a problem that warrants particular concern, given that low-income older adults are at higher risk for developing MDD (Areán and Alvidrez 2001).

Pharmacotherapy

Several systematic reviews and meta-analyses that have compared different classes of antidepressant medications in the treatment of late-life depression have generally found antidepressant treatment to be more effective than placebo but have not found substantial differences in rates of response to any one medication class compared with another (Kok et al. 2012; Mittmann et al. 1997; Mottram et al. 2006; Taylor and Doraiswamy 2004; Tham et al. 2016; Thorlund et al. 2015). Therefore, the choice of antidepressant depends on other factors, such as the patient's predominant symptoms, medical comorbidities, and history of response to previous medication trials, as well as medication factors such as side-effect profile and potential drug or food interactions.

Selective serotonin reuptake inhibitors (SSRIs) are considered the first-line choice for treating mild to moderate depression in older adults (Alamo et al. 2014; Blazer and Steffens 2015; Taylor 2014). SSRIs as a class carry a lower risk of cardiac, anticholinergic, and orthostatic side effects and are less sedating than certain other classes of antidepressants (e.g., tricyclic antidepressants [TCAs]) (Kok and Reynolds 2017; Montgomery et al. 1994; Song et al. 1993), making them the preferred class for use in the elderly. However, SSRIs are not without risk, given that gastrointestinal symptoms, weight loss, hyponatremia, sexual dysfunction, and tremor are all potential side effects (Alamo et al. 2014; Blazer and Steffens 2015). Although there is limited evidence to suggest that any one SSRI would be more efficacious than any other SSRI among older adults, paroxetine is generally avoided because of its anticholinergic effects, and fluoxetine is generally avoided because of its long half-life (Alamo et al. 2014). Additionally, concern has been raised regarding the risk of QTc prolongation associated with higher dosages of citalopram (McClelland and Mathys 2016), although this adverse effect has been infrequently reported (Tampi et al. 2015) and appears to be less of a risk with citalopram than with TCAs (Beach et al. 2014).

Serotonin-norepinephrine reuptake inhibitors (SNRIs)—including duloxetine (Raskin et al. 2008), venlafaxine (Staab and Evans 2000), and desvenlafaxine (Kornstein et al. 2010)—similarly have shown benefit for treatment of depression in older adults. Duloxetine is FDA approved for use in the treatment of musculoskeletal and neuropathic pain, an effect that offers an additional benefit for many older adults. Side effects of the SNRIs include nausea, dizziness, hyperhidrosis, hypertension (for venlafaxine), and decreased libido (Kornstein et al. 2010). A recent systematic review also identified an association between duloxetine and an increased incidence of falls (Sobieraj et al. 2019).

Another frequently prescribed antidepressant medication for older adults is mirtazapine, whose side-effect profile of weight gain and sedation may benefit patients who present with anorexia, weight loss, or insomnia (Roose et al. 2003). However, there are limited data on how mirtazapine compares with other antidepressant classes. There is also limited evidence supporting the use of bupropion in older adults, although this agent is generally considered to have a favorable side-effect profile and has demonstrated efficacy in the treatment of depression in adults older than 60 years (Weihs et al. 2000).

TCAs are less commonly prescribed for the treatment of older adults because of their adverse side effects (particularly anticholinergic effects, orthostasis, risk of falls, risk of overdose, and cardiovascular effects such as QTc prolongation) (Blazer and Steffens 2015; Kok and Reynolds 2017; Taylor 2014). However, TCAs remain efficacious and are used for patients with more severe depression who may have failed to respond to other medication trials and who are able to tolerate the adverse effects (Taylor 2014). Monoamine oxidase inhibitors (MAOIs) are generally avoided in older adults because of their side-effect profile and risk of interaction with other medications (Alamo et al. 2014; Blazer and Steffens 2015).

Approximately one-third of older adults who are treated with an antidepressant experience remission of their symptoms (Kok et al. 2012). For the other two-thirds, another antidepressant class may be considered. For treatment-refractory depression, additional strategies for use in older adults include augmentation of antidepressant treatment with lithium (Cooper et al. 2011) or with an atypical antipsychotic such as aripiprazole (Lenze et al. 2015; Rutherford et al. 2007; Sheffrin et al. 2009).

When prescribing antidepressants for older adults, clinicians should be guided by several important principles. Antidepressants should be started at lower dosages than are used in younger adult populations, and dosages should be gradually increased to optimal effect while remaining mindful of side-effect risk, although higher dosages may be required for clinical benefit (Taylor 2014). Polypharmacy, defined as regular use of five or more prescription medications, is associated with an increased risk of many adverse outcomes in older adults, including falls, delirium, cognitive impairment, frailty, weight loss, and dangerous interactions with other medications (Saraf et al. 2016). For this reason, if a patient's first medication trial is ineffective, it may be preferable to switch medications rather than to augment the first medication with one or more additional medications. Given that no one medication or class of antidepressant is consistently more effective than any other in the treatment of late-life mood disorders, the choice of medication should be based on the patient's presenting symptoms and treatment history, as well as the side-effect profiles of the agents being considered and their risk of interacting with other medications the patient is taking.

Neurostimulation

Electroconvulsive therapy (ECT) is a mainstay of depression treatment in older adults. It is particularly effective for patients who have MDD with psychotic symptoms or catatonia, patients who have severe symptoms such as suicidality or refusal to eat, and patients who have not responded to or cannot tolerate antidepressant medications (Blazer and Steffens 2015; Geduldig and Kellner 2016; Meyer et al. 2018). ECT requires a thorough medical workup prior to treatment; however, it is safe for use even in frail older adults with multiple medical comorbidities (Dong et al. 2018; Geduldig and Kellner 2016; Kellner et al. 2012). Medical side effects of ECT of concern in older adults include transient hypertension, arrhythmias, transient posttreatment confusion, and, in rare cases, compression fractures (Blazer and Steffens 2015; Burke et al. 1985; Geduldig and Kellner 2016). Although cognitive impairment is a side effect that warrants concern in patients of all ages, research suggests that in many older adults, cognitive functioning often stays the same or improves following ECT, and cognitive impairment following treatment is usually transient (Bosboom and Deijen 2006; Frith et al. 1983; Meyer et al. 2018; Verwijk et al. 2014). Patients with neurocognitive disorders have shown high rates of response to ECT (Price and McAllister 1989). Although one might be concerned about worsening cognition in this group, there is evidence that ECT-related cognitive effects are limited, and that overall improvement is seen in both depression and cognitive scores following ECT treatment (Price and McAllister 1989; Rao and Lyketsos 2000). Overall, older adults show higher rates of response and remission of depression with ECT in comparison with younger patients, making it a safe and efficacious treatment option for this age group (Kellner et al. 2012; Meyer et al. 2018).

In comparison with the large amount of research evidence on ECT in older patients, less is known about the utility of repetitive transcranial magnetic stimulation (rTMS) in the elderly. From the few studies that are available, rTMS appears to be a safe and well-tolerated treatment option (Iriarte and George 2018). Potential advantages of rTMS in comparison with ECT for older adults are that rTMS does not require general sedation and has no evidence of cognitive side effects (Nardone et al. 2014). Some studies have demonstrated cognitive benefits for patients undergoing rTMS (Guse et al. 2010; Nardone et al. 2014). Side effects are uncommon but can include muscle twitching, headaches, pain at the site of stimulation, and, in rare cases, seizures (Gálvez et al. 2015). Although few studies have examined the role of rTMS in the treatment of late-life depression, one study of rTMS in geriatric patients with vascular depression demonstrated benefit in the active stimulation group in comparison with the sham group (Jorge et al. 2008). Several studies have demonstrated roughly equivalent treatment responses to rTMS among older and younger adults (Conelea et al. 2017; Herwig et al. 2007; Lisanby et al. 2009).

Conclusion

In sum, mood disorders are prevalent among older adults and are related to several negative health outcomes. Because the origins of geriatric mood disorders for individual patients are often heterogeneous, clinicians caring for older adults must incorporate treatment approaches that consider biological, psychological, and social factors. Careful assessment involves not just a history of the present illness but also a past history (including prior response to stress, quality of interpersonal relationships, and losses), a review of medical conditions, a physical examination, and appropriate laboratory testing. Treatment should be tailored to the patient and may include psychotherapy, pharmacotherapy, and/or neurostimulation. Monitoring of functional status, overall health maintenance, and cognition is a key element in the management of late-life mood disorders in order to optimize long-term outcomes.

References

Aarsland D, Påhlhagen S, Ballard CG, et al: Depression in Parkinson disease—epidemiology, mechanisms and management. Nat Rev Neurol 8(1):35–47, 2011 22198405

Alamo C, López-Muñoz F, García-García P, et al: Risk-benefit analysis of antidepressant drug treatment in the elderly. Psychogeriatrics 14(4):261–268, 2014 25495088

Alexopoulos GS: Mechanisms and treatment of late-life depression. Transl Psychiatry 9(1):188, 2019 31383842

Alexopoulos GS, Meyers BS, Young RC, et al: The course of geriatric depression with "reversible dementia": a controlled study. Am J Psychiatry 150(11):1693–1699, 1993 8105707

Alexopoulos GS, Meyers BS, Young RC, et al: Clinically defined vascular depression. Am J Psychiatry 154(4):562–565, 1997a 9090349

Alexopoulos GS, Meyers BS, Young RC, et al: "Vascular depression" hypothesis. Arch Gen Psychiatry 54(10):915–922, 1997b 9337771

Alexopoulos GS, Kiosses DN, Klimstra S, et al: Clinical presentation of the "depression-executive dysfunction syndrome" of late life. Am J Geriatr Psychiatry 10(1):98–106, 2002 11790640

Alexopoulos GS, Raue P, Areán P: Problem-solving therapy versus supportive therapy in geriatric major depression with executive dysfunction. Am J Geriatr Psychiatry 11(1):46–52, 2003 12527539

Alexopoulos GS, Raue PJ, Kanellopoulos D, et al: Problem solving therapy for the depression-executive dysfunction syndrome of late life. Int J Geriatr Psychiatry 23(8):782–788, 2008 18213605

Alexopoulos GS, Raue PJ, Kiosses DN, et al: Problem-solving therapy and supportive therapy in older adults with major depression and executive dysfunction: effect on disability. Arch Gen Psychiatry 68(1):33–41, 2011 21199963

Altshuler LL, Curran JG, Hauser P, et al: T2 hyperintensities in bipolar disorder: magnetic resonance imaging comparison and literature meta-analysis. Am J Psychiatry 152(8):1139–1144, 1995 7625460

American Psychiatric Association: Diagnostic and Statistical Manual of Mental Disorders, 5th Edition. Arlington, VA, American Psychiatric Association, 2013

Andreescu C, Reynolds CF 3rd: Late-life depression: evidence-based treatment and promising new directions for research and clinical practice. Psychiatr Clin North Am 34(2):335–355, 2011 21536162

Areán PA, Alvidrez J: The prevalence of psychiatric disorders and subsyndromal mental illness in low-income, medically ill elderly. Int J Psychiatry Med 31(1):9–24, 2001 11529394

Areán PA, Perri MG, Nezu AM, et al: Comparative effectiveness of social problem-solving therapy and reminiscence therapy as treatments for depression in older adults. J Consult Clin Psychol 61(6):1003–1010, 1993 8113478

Ayerbe L, Ayis SA, Crichton S, et al: Natural history, predictors and associated outcomes of anxiety up to 10 years after stroke: the South London Stroke Register. Age Ageing 43(4):542–547, 2014 24375225

Aziz R, Steffens DC: What are the causes of late-life depression? Psychiatr Clin North Am 36(4):497–516, 2013 24229653

Bandura A: Self-efficacy, in Encyclopedia of Human Behaviour. Edited by Ramachaudran VS. New York, Academic Press, 1994, pp 71–81

Beach SR, Kostis WJ, Celano CM, et al: Meta-analysis of selective serotonin reuptake inhibitor-associated QTc prolongation. J Clin Psychiatry 75(5):e441–e449, 2014 24922496

Beck AT: Thinking and depression, II: theory and therapy. Arch Gen Psychiatry 10:561–571, 1964 14159256

Beyer JL: Bipolar and related disorders, in The American Psychiatric Publishing Textbook of Geriatric Psychiatry. Edited by Steffens DC, Blazer D, Thakur ME. Washington, DC, American Psychiatric Association, 2015, pp 283–308

Black SA, Markides KS, Miller TQ: Correlates of depressive symptomatology among older community-dwelling Mexican Americans: the Hispanic EPESE. J Gerontol B Psychol Sci Soc Sci 53(4):S198–S208, 1998 9679521

Blazer DG: Depression in late life: review and commentary. J Gerontol A Biol Sci Med Sci 58(3):249–265, 2003 12634292

Blazer DG, Steffens DC: Depressive disorders, in The American Psychiatric Publishing Textbook of Geriatric Psychiatry. Edited by Steffens DC, Blazer D, Thakur ME. Washington, DC, American Psychiatric Publishing, 2015, pp 243–282.

Blazer D, Hughes DC, George LK: The epidemiology of depression in an elderly community population. Gerontologist 27(3):281–287, 1987 3609795

Blazer DG, Burchett BB, Fillenbaum GG: APOE epsilon4 and low cholesterol as risks for depression in a biracial elderly community sample. Am J Geriatr Psychiatry 10(5):515–520, 2002a 12213685

Blazer DG, Moody-Ayers S, Craft-Morgan J, et al: Depression in diabetes and obesity: racial/ethnic/gender issues in older adults. J Psychosom Res 53(4):913–916, 2002b 12377303

Bosboom PR, Deijen JB: Age-related cognitive effects of ECT and ECT-induced mood improvement in depressive patients. Depress Anxiety 23(2):93–101, 2006 16400627

Botteron KN, Vannier MW, Geller B, et al: Preliminary study of magnetic resonance imaging characteristics in 8- to 16-year-olds with mania. J Am Acad Child Adolesc Psychiatry 34(6):742–749, 1995 7608047

Briggs R, Kenny RA, Kennelly SP: Systematic review: the association between late life depression and hypotension. J Am Med Dir Assoc 17(12):1076–1088, 2016 27523406

Broomfield NM, Laidlaw K, Hickabottom E, et al: Post-stroke depression: the case for augmented, individually tailored cognitive behavioural therapy. Clin Psychol Psychother 18(3):202–217, 2011 20632301

Bruce ML, Hoff RA: Social and physical health risk factors for first-onset major depressive disorder in a community sample. Soc Psychiatry Psychiatr Epidemiol 29(4):165–171, 1994 7939965

Burke WJ, Rutherford JL, Zorumski CF, Reich T: Electroconvulsive therapy and the elderly. Compr Psychiatry 26(5):480–486, 1985 4028698

Calleo JS, Amspoker AB, Sarwar AI, et al: A pilot study of a cognitive-behavioral treatment for anxiety and depression in patients with Parkinson disease. J Geriatr Psychiatry Neurol 28(3):210–217, 2015 26047635

Casey DA: Depression in older adults: a treatable medical condition. Prim Care 44(3):499–510, 2017 28797375

Cheng ST: Dementia caregiver burden: a research update and critical analysis. Curr Psychiatry Rep 19(9):64, 2017 28795386

Chentsova Dutton Y, Zisook S: Adaptation to bereavement. Death Stud 29(10):877–903, 2005 16265796

Choi NG, Hegel MT, Marti N, et al: Telehealth problem-solving therapy for depressed low-income homebound older adults. Am J Geriatr Psychiatry 22(3):263–271, 2014a 23567376

Choi NG, Marti CN, Bruce ML, et al: Six-month postintervention depression and disability outcomes of in-home telehealth problem-solving therapy for depressed, low-income homebound older adults. Depress Anxiety 31(8):653–661, 2014b 24501015

Choi NG, Marti CN, Conwell Y: Effect of problem-solving therapy on depressed low-income homebound older adults' death/suicidal ideation and hopelessness. Suicide Life Threat Behav 46(3):323–336, 2016 26456016

Committee on the Mental Health Workforce for Geriatric Populations, Board on Health Care Services, Institute of Medicine, et al: Assessing the service needs of older adults with mental health and substance use conditions, in The Mental Health and Substance Use Workforce for Older Adults: In Whose Hands? Washington, DC, National Academies Press, 2012, pp 39–158

Conelea CA, Philip NS, Yip AG, et al: Transcranial magnetic stimulation for treatment-resistant depression: Naturalistic treatment outcomes for younger versus older patients. J Affect Disord 217:42–47, 2017 28388464

Cooper C, Katona C, Lyketsos K, et al: A systematic review of treatments for refractory depression in older people. Am J Psychiatry 168(7):681–688, 2011 21454919

Costa PT Jr, McCrae RR: Influence of extraversion and neuroticism on subjective well-being: happy and unhappy people. J Pers Soc Psychol 38(4):668–678, 1980 7381680

Costa PT, McCrae RR: NEO PI-R Professional Manual. Odessa, FL, Psychological Assessment Resources: 1992

Cully JA, Stanley MA, Deswal A, et al: Cognitive-behavioral therapy for chronic cardiopulmonary conditions: preliminary outcomes from an open trial. Prim Care Companion J Clin Psychiatry 12(4):PCC.09m00896, 2010 21085552

Depp CA, Jeste DV: Bipolar disorder in older adults: a critical review. Bipolar Disord 6(5):343–367, 2004 15383127

Devanand DP: Comorbid psychiatric disorders in late life depression. Biol Psychiatry 52(3):236–242, 2002 12182929

Devanand DP: Dysthymic disorder in the elderly population. Int Psychogeriatr 26(1):39–48, 2014 24152873

Devanand DP, Nobler MS, Singer T, et al: Is dysthymia a different disorder in the elderly? Am J Psychiatry 151(11):1592–1599, 1994 7943446

Devanand DP, Adorno E, Cheng J, et al: Late onset dysthymic disorder and major depression differ from early onset dysthymic disorder and major depression in elderly outpatients. J Affect Disord 78(3):259–267, 2004 15013252

Dhingra U, Rabins PV: Mania in the elderly: a 5-7 year follow-up. J Am Geriatr Soc 39(6):581–583, 1991 2037748

Diniz BS, Butters MA, Albert SM, et al: Late-life depression and risk of vascular dementia and Alzheimer's disease: systematic review and meta-analysis of community-based cohort studies. Br J Psychiatry 202(5):329–335, 2013 23637108

Dols A, Rhebergen D, Beekman A, et al: Psychiatric and medical comorbidities: results from a bipolar elderly cohort study. Am J Geriatr Psychiatry 22(11):1066–1074, 2014 24495405

Dombrovski AY, Lenze EJ, Dew MA, et al: Maintenance treatment for old-age depression preserves health-related quality of life: a randomized, controlled trial of paroxetine and interpersonal psychotherapy. J Am Geriatr Soc 55(9):1325–1332, 2007 17767673

Dong M, Zhu XM, Zheng W, et al: Electroconvulsive therapy for older adult patients with major depressive disorder: a systematic review of randomized controlled trials. Psychogeriatrics 18(6):468–475, 2018 30073725

Dupont RM, Jernigan TL, Gillin JC, et al: Subcortical signal hyperintensities in bipolar patients detected by MRI. Psychiatry Res 21(4):357–358, 1987 3628618

Dupont RM, Butters N, Schafer K, et al: Diagnostic specificity of focal white matter abnormalities in bipolar and unipolar mood disorder. Biol Psychiatry 38(7):482–486, 1995 8672610

D'Zurilla TJ, Goldfried MR: Problem solving and behavior modification. J Abnorm Psychol 78(1):107–126, 1971 4938262

Egan SJ, Laidlaw K, Starkstein S: Cognitive Behaviour Therapy for Depression and Anxiety in Parkinson's Disease. J Parkinsons Dis 5(3):443–451, 2015 26406124

Egede LE, Acierno R, Knapp RG, et al: Psychotherapy for depression in older veterans via telemedicine: a randomised, open-label, non-inferiority trial. Lancet Psychiatry 2(8):693–701, 2015 26249300

Erdley SD, Gellis ZD, Bogner HA, et al: Problem-solving therapy to improve depression scores among older hemodialysis patients: a pilot randomized trial. Clin Nephrol 82(1):26–33, 2014 24755106

Fann JR, Fan MY, Unützer J: Improving primary care for older adults with cancer and depression. J Gen Intern Med 24 (suppl 2):S417–S424, 2009 19838842

Figiel GS, Krishnan KR, Doraiswamy PM, et al: Subcortical hyperintensities on brain magnetic resonance imaging: a comparison between late age onset and early onset elderly depressed subjects. Neurobiol Aging 12(3):245–247, 1991 1876230

Floyd M, Scogin F, McKendree-Smith NL, et al: Cognitive therapy for depression: a comparison of individual psychotherapy and bibliotherapy for depressed older adults. Behav Modif 28(2):297–318, 2004 14997954

Folstein MF, Folstein SE, McHugh PR: "Mini-mental state": a practical method for grading the cognitive state of patients for the clinician. J Psychiatr Res 12(3):189–198, 1975 1202204
Folstein MF, Maiberger R, McHugh PR: Mood disorder as a specific complication of stroke. J Neurol Neurosurg Psychiatry 40(10):1018–1020, 1977 591971
Folstein M, Liu T, Peter I, et al: The homocysteine hypothesis of depression. Am J Psychiatry 164(6):861–867, 2007 17541043
Freedland KE, Carney RM, Rich MW, et al: Cognitive behavior therapy for depression and self-care in heart failure patients: a randomized clinical trial. JAMA Intern Med 175(11):1773–1782, 2015 26414759
Frith CD, Stevens M, Johnstone EC, et al: Effects of ECT and depression on various aspects of memory. Br J Psychiatry 142:610–617, 1983 6882984
Gálvez V, Ho KA, Alonzo A, et al: Neuromodulation therapies for geriatric depression. Curr Psychiatry Rep 17(7):59, 2015 25995098
Gao Y, Huang C, Zhao K, et al: Depression as a risk factor for dementia and mild cognitive impairment: a meta-analysis of longitudinal studies. Int J Geriatr Psychiatry 28(5):441–449, 2013 22815126
Geduldig ET, Kellner CH: Electroconvulsive therapy in the elderly: new findings in geriatric depression. Curr Psychiatry Rep 18(4):40, 2016 26909702
Gleason OC, Pierce AM, Walker AE, Warnock JK: The two-way relationship between medical illness and late-life depression. Psychiatr Clin North Am 36(4):533–544, 2013 24229655
Glover J, Srinivasan S: Assessment of the person with late-life depression. Psychiatr Clin North Am 36(4):545–560, 2013 24229656
Gould RL, Coulson MC, Howard RJ: Cognitive behavioral therapy for depression in older people: a meta-analysis and meta-regression of randomized controlled trials. J Am Geriatr Soc 60(10):1817–1830, 2012 23003115
Gum AM, Areán PA, Hunkeler E, et al: Depression treatment preferences in older primary care patients. Gerontologist 46(1):14–22, 2006 16452280
Guse B, Falkai P, Wobrock T: Cognitive effects of high-frequency repetitive transcranial magnetic stimulation: a systematic review. J Neural Transm (Vienna) 117(1):105–122, 2010 19859782
Gustavson KA, Alexopoulos GS, Niu GC, et al: Problem-solving therapy reduces suicidal ideation in depressed older adults with executive dysfunction. Am J Geriatr Psychiatry 24(1):11–17, 2016 26743100
Hackett ML, Pickles K: Part I: frequency of depression after stroke: an updated systematic review and meta-analysis of observational studies. Int J Stroke 9(8):1017–1025, 2014 25117911
Harman SM, Metter EJ, Tobin JD, et al: Longitudinal effects of aging on serum total and free testosterone levels in healthy men. J Clin Endocrinol Metab 86(2):724–731, 2001 11158037
Heisel MJ, Talbot NL, King DA, et al: Adapting interpersonal psychotherapy for older adults at risk for suicide. Am J Geriatr Psychiatry 23(1):87–98, 2015 24840611
Henderson AS, Jorm AF, MacKinnon A, et al: The prevalence of depressive disorders and the distribution of depressive symptoms in later life: a survey using Draft ICD-10 and DSM-III-R. Psychol Med 23(3):719–729, 1993 8234578
Herwig U, Fallgatter AJ, Höppner J, et al: Antidepressant effects of augmentative transcranial magnetic stimulation: randomised multicentre trial. Br J Psychiatry 191:441–448, 2007 17978325
Holahan CK, Holahan CJ: Self-efficacy, social support, and depression in aging: a longitudinal analysis. J Gerontol 42(1):65–68, 1987 3794199
Huang AX, Delucchi K, Dunn LB, Nelson JC: A systematic review and meta-analysis of psychotherapy for late-life depression. Am J Geriatr Psychiatry 23(3):261–273, 2015 24856580
Hybels CF, Blazer DG: Epidemiology of late-life mental disorders. Clin Geriatr Med 19(4):663–696, v, 2003 15024807
Hybels CF, Pieper CF, Payne ME, et al: Late-life depression modifies the association between cerebral white matter hyperintensities and functional decline among older adults. Am J Geriatr Psychiatry 24(1):42–49, 2016 25863558

Iriarte IG, George MS: Transcranial magnetic stimulation (TMS) in the elderly. Curr Psychiatry Rep 20(1):6, 2018 29427050
Jack SPD, Petrosky E, Lyons BH, et al: Surveillance for violent deaths—national violent death reporting system, 27 states, 2015. MMWR Surveill Summ 67(11):1–32, 2018 30260938
Jang Y, Haley WE, Small BJ, Mortimer JA: The role of mastery and social resources in the associations between disability and depression in later life. Gerontologist 42(6):807–813, 2002 12451162
Jayasekara R, Procter N, Harrison J, et al: Cognitive behavioural therapy for older adults with depression: a review. J Ment Health 24(3):168–171, 2015 25358075
Jeyanantham K, Kotecha D, Thanki D, et al: Effects of cognitive behavioural therapy for depression in heart failure patients: a systematic review and meta-analysis. Heart Fail Rev 22(6):731–741, 2017 28733911
Jorge RE, Moser DJ, Acion L, Robinson RG: Treatment of vascular depression using repetitive transcranial magnetic stimulation. Arch Gen Psychiatry 65(3):268–276, 2008 18316673
Jorm AF: History of depression as a risk factor for dementia: an updated review. Aust N Z J Psychiatry 35(6):776–781, 2001 11990888
Kasckow J, Klaus J, Morse J, et al: Using problem solving therapy to treat veterans with subsyndromal depression: a pilot study. Int J Geriatr Psychiatry 29(12):1255–1261, 2014 24789736
Katz S: Assessing self-maintenance: activities of daily living, mobility, and instrumental activities of daily living. J Am Geriatr Soc 31(12):721–727, 1983 6418786
Kellner CH, Greenberg RM, Murrough JW, et al: ECT in treatment-resistant depression. Am J Psychiatry 169(12):1238–1244, 2012 23212054
Kendler KS, Gatz M, Gardner CO, Pedersen NL: Personality and major depression: a Swedish longitudinal, population-based twin study. Arch Gen Psychiatry 63(10):1113–1120, 2006 17015813
Kiosses DN, Alexopoulos GS: Problem-solving therapy in the elderly. Curr Treat Options Psychiatry 1(1):15–26, 2014 24729951
Klap R, Unroe KT, Unützer J: Caring for mental illness in the United States: a focus on older adults. Am J Geriatr Psychiatry 11(5):517–524, 2003 14506085
Kneebone II, Dunmore E: Psychological management of post-stroke depression. Br J Clin Psychol 39(1):53–65, 2000 10789028
Kocsis JH, Shaw ED, Stokes PE, et al: Neuropsychologic effects of lithium discontinuation. J Clin Psychopharmacol 13(4):268–275, 1993 8376614
Koenig HG, Meador KG, Cohen HJ, et al: Depression in elderly hospitalized patients with medical illness. Arch Intern Med 148(9):1929–1936, 1988 3415405
Koenig HG, Meador KG, Shelp F, et al: Major depressive disorder in hospitalized medically ill patients: an examination of young and elderly male veterans. J Am Geriatr Soc 39(9):881–890, 1991 1885863
Kok RM, Reynolds CF 3rd: Management of depression in older adults: a review. JAMA 317(20):2114–2122, 2017 28535241
Kok RM, Nolen WA, Heeren TJ: Efficacy of treatment in older depressed patients: a systematic review and meta-analysis of double-blind randomized controlled trials with antidepressants. J Affect Disord 141(2–3):103–115, 2012 22480823
Kornstein SG, Clayton AH, Soares CN, et al: Analysis by age and sex of efficacy data from placebo-controlled trials of desvenlafaxine in outpatients with major depressive disorder. J Clin Psychopharmacol 30(3):294–299, 2010 20473066
Kraaij V, de Wilde EJ: Negative life events and depressive symptoms in the elderly: a life span perspective. Aging Ment Health 5(1):84–91, 2001 11513018
Kraaij V, Kremers I, Arensman E: The relationship between stressful and traumatic life events and depression in the elderly. Crisis 18(2):86–88, 1997 9286132
Kraaij V, Pruymboom E, Garnefski N: Cognitive coping and depressive symptoms in the elderly: a longitudinal study. Aging Ment Health 6(3):275–281, 2002 12217096
Krabbendam L, Honig A, Wiersma J, et al: Cognitive dysfunctions and white matter lesions in patients with bipolar disorder in remission. Acta Psychiatr Scand 101(4):274–280, 2000 10782546

Krishnan KR, Hays JC, Blazer DG: MRI-defined vascular depression. Am J Psychiatry 154(4):497–501, 1997 9090336

Kroenke K, Spitzer RL, Williams JB: The PHQ-9: validity of a brief depression severity measure. J Gen Intern Med 16(9):606–613, 2001 11556941

Kunik ME, Veazey C, Cully JA, et al: COPD education and cognitive behavioral therapy group treatment for clinically significant symptoms of depression and anxiety in COPD patients: a randomized controlled trial. Psychol Med 38(3):385–396, 2008 17922939

Kutlubaev MA, Hackett ML: Part II: predictors of depression after stroke and impact of depression on stroke outcome: an updated systematic review of observational studies. Int J Stroke 9(8):1026–1036, 2014 25156411

Laidlaw K, Thompson LW, Dick-Siskin L: Cognitive Behaviour Therapy With Older People. New York, Wiley, 2003

Lenze EJ, Mulsant BH, Blumberger DM, et al: Efficacy, safety, and tolerability of augmentation pharmacotherapy with aripiprazole for treatment-resistant depression in late life: a randomised, double-blind, placebo-controlled trial. Lancet 386(10011):2404–2412, 2015 26423182

Lisanby SH, Husain MM, Rosenquist PB, et al: Daily left prefrontal repetitive transcranial magnetic stimulation in the acute treatment of major depression: clinical predictors of outcome in a multisite, randomized controlled clinical trial. Neuropsychopharmacology 34(2):522–534, 2009 18704101

Lustman PJ, Griffith LS, Freedland KE, et al: Cognitive behavior therapy for depression in type 2 diabetes mellitus. A randomized, controlled trial. Ann Intern Med 129(8):613–621, 1998 9786808

Lyness JM, Caine ED, King DA, et al: Depressive disorders and symptoms in older primary care patients: one-year outcomes. Am J Geriatr Psychiatry 10(3):275–282, 2002 11994214

Manning KJ, Chan G, Steffens DC: Neuroticism traits selectively impact long term illness course and cognitive decline in late-life depression. Am J Geriatr Psychiatry 25(3):220–229, 2017 27825555

Mathers SE, Chambers BR, Merory JR, et al: Subcortical arteriosclerotic encephalopathy: Binswanger's disease. Clin Exp Neurol 23:67–70, 1987 3665181

McClelland J, Mathys M: Evaluation of QTc prolongation and dosage effect with citalopram. Ment Health Clin 6(4):165–170, 2016 29955465

Meyer JP, Swetter SK, Kellner CH: Electroconvulsive therapy in geriatric psychiatry: a selective review. Psychiatr Clin North Am 41(1):79–93, 2018 29412850

Meyers BS, Kalayam B, Mei-Tal V: Late-onset delusional depression: a distinct clinical entity? J Clin Psychiatry 45(8):347–349, 1984 6746580

Meyers BS, Klimstra SA, Gabriele M, et al: Continuation treatment of delusional depression in older adults. Am J Geriatr Psychiatry 9(4):415–422, 2001 11739068

Miller MD, Cornes C, Frank E, et al: Interpersonal psychotherapy for late-life depression: past, present, and future. J Psychother Pract Res 10(4):231–238, 2001 11696649

Mittmann N, Herrmann N, Einarson TR, et al: The efficacy, safety and tolerability of antidepressants in late life depression: a meta-analysis. J Affect Disord 46(3):191–217, 1997 9547117

Mojtabai R, Olfson M: Major depression in community-dwelling middle-aged and older adults: prevalence and 2- and 4-year follow-up symptoms. Psychol Med 34(4):623–634, 2004 15099417

Montgomery SA, Henry J, McDonald G, et al: Selective serotonin reuptake inhibitors: meta-analysis of discontinuation rates. Int Clin Psychopharmacol 9(1):47–53, 1994 8195583

Morse JQ, Lynch TR: A preliminary investigation of self-reported personality disorders in late life: prevalence, predictors of depressive severity, and clinical correlates. Aging Ment Health 8(4):307–315, 2004 15370047

Mottram P, Wilson K, Strobl J: Antidepressants for depressed elderly. Cochrane Database Syst Rev (1):CD003491, 2006 16437456

Murphy E: Social origins of depression in old age. Br J Psychiatry 141:135–142, 1982 7116052

Nardone R, Tezzon F, Höller Y, et al: Transcranial magnetic stimulation (TMS)/repetitive TMS in mild cognitive impairment and Alzheimer's disease. Acta Neurol Scand 129(6):351–366, 2014 24506061

Nasreddine ZS, Phillips NA, Bédirian V, et al: The Montreal Cognitive Assessment, MoCA: a brief screening tool for mild cognitive impairment. J Am Geriatr Soc 53(4):695–699, 2005 15817019

Ownby RL, Crocco E, Acevedo A, et al: Depression and risk for Alzheimer disease: systematic review, meta-analysis, and metaregression analysis. Arch Gen Psychiatry 63(5):530–538, 2006 16651510

Park JH, Jeon BH, Lee JS, et al: CADASIL as a useful medical model and genetic form of vascular depression. Am J Geriatr Psychiatry 25(7):719–727, 2017 28434675

Pertl MM, Sooknarine-Rajpatty A, Brennan S, et al: Caregiver choice and caregiver outcomes: a longitudinal study of Irish spousal dementia caregivers. Front Psychol 10:1801, 2019 31456713

Piek E, Nolen WA, van der Meer K, et al: Determinants of (non-)recognition of depression by general practitioners: results of the Netherlands Study of Depression and Anxiety. J Affect Disord 138(3):397–404, 2012 22353380

Pollock BG: Geriatric psychiatry: psychopharmacology: general principles, in Kaplan and Sadock's Comprehensive Textbook of Psychiatry, 8th Edition. Edited by Sadock BJ, Sadock VA. Baltimore, MD, Williams & Wilkins, 2000, pp 3086–3090

Price TR, McAllister TW: Safety and efficacy of ECT in depressed patients with dementia: a review of clinical experience. Convuls Ther 5(1):61–74, 1989 11940996

Prigerson HG, Reynolds CF 3rd, Frank E, et al: Stressful life events, social rhythms, and depressive symptoms among the elderly: an examination of hypothesized causal linkages. Psychiatry Res 51(1):33–49, 1994 8197270

Prince MJ, Harwood RH, Thomas A, Mann AH: A prospective population-based cohort study of the effects of disablement and social milieu on the onset and maintenance of late-life depression. The Gospel Oak Project VII. Psychol Med 28(2):337–350, 1998 9572091

Rao V, Lyketsos CG: The benefits and risks of ECT for patients with primary dementia who also suffer from depression. Int J Geriatr Psychiatry 15(8):729–735, 2000 10960885

Raskin J, Xu JY, Kajdasz DK: Time to response for duloxetine 60 mg once daily versus placebo in elderly patients with major depressive disorder. Int Psychogeriatr 20(2):309–327, 2008 17588276

Raue PJ, Schulberg HC, Heo M, et al: Patients' depression treatment preferences and initiation, adherence, and outcome: a randomized primary care study. Psychiatr Serv 60(3):337–343, 2009 19252046

Raue PJ, Weinberger MI, Sirey JA, et al: Preferences for depression treatment among elderly home health care patients. Psychiatr Serv 62(5):532–537, 2011 21532080

Raue PJ, Ghesquiere AR, Bruce ML: Suicide risk in primary care: identification and management in older adults. Curr Psychiatry Rep 16(9):466, 2014 25030971

Reijnders JS, Ehrt U, Weber WE, et al: A systematic review of prevalence studies of depression in Parkinson's disease. Mov Disord 23(2):183–189, quiz 313, 2008 17987654

Reppermund S, Zhuang L, Wen W, et al: White matter integrity and late-life depression in community-dwelling individuals: diffusion tensor imaging study using tract-based spatial statistics. Br J Psychiatry 205(4):315–320, 2014 25147370

Reynolds CF 3rd, Frank E, Perel JM, et al: Nortriptyline and interpersonal psychotherapy as maintenance therapies for recurrent major depression: a randomized controlled trial in patients older than 59 years. JAMA 281(1):39–45, 1999a 9892449

Reynolds CF 3rd, Miller MD, Pasternak RE, et al: Treatment of bereavement-related major depressive episodes in later life: a controlled study of acute and continuation treatment with nortriptyline and interpersonal psychotherapy. Am J Psychiatry 156(2):202–208, 1999b 9989555

Robinson RG, Kubos KL, Starr LB, et al: Mood disorders in stroke patients. Importance of location of lesion. Brain 107(Pt 1):81–93, 1984 6697163

Robinson RG, Jorge RE, Moser DJ, et al: Escitalopram and problem-solving therapy for prevention of poststroke depression: a randomized controlled trial. JAMA 299(20):2391–2400, 2008 18505948
Rod NH, Bordelon Y, Thompson A, et al: Major life events and development of major depression in Parkinson's disease patients. Eur J Neurol 20(4):663–670, 2013 23114037
Roose SP, Nelson JC, Salzman C, et al: Open-label study of mirtazapine orally disintegrating tablets in depressed patients in the nursing home. Curr Med Res Opin 19(8):737–746, 2003 14687445
Royall DR, Schillerstrom JE, Piper PK, et al: Depression and mortality in elders referred for geriatric psychiatry consultation. J Am Med Dir Assoc 8(5):318–321, 2007 17570311
Rutherford B, Sneed J, Miyazaki M, et al: An open trial of aripiprazole augmentation for SSRI non-remitters with late-life depression. Int J Geriatr Psychiatry 22(10):986–991, 2007 17340654
Saraf AA, Petersen AW, Simmons SF, et al: Medications associated with geriatric syndromes and their prevalence in older hospitalized adults discharged to skilled nursing facilities. J Hosp Med 11(10):694–700, 2016 27255830
Schindler AE: Thyroid function and postmenopause. Gynecol Endocrinol 17(1):79–85, 2003 12724022
Schoevers RA, Beekman AT, Deeg DJ, et al: Risk factors for depression in later life: results of a prospective community based study (AMSTEL). J Affect Disord 59(2):127–137, 2000 10837881
Schulz R, Beach SR, Ives DG, et al: Association between depression and mortality in older adults: the Cardiovascular Health Study. Arch Intern Med 160(12):1761–1768, 2000 10871968
Scogin F, Jamison C, Gochneaur K: Comparative efficacy of cognitive and behavioral bibliotherapy for mildly and moderately depressed older adults. J Consult Clin Psychol 57(3):403–407, 1989 2738212
Scott J, Teasdale JD, Paykel ES, et al: Effects of cognitive therapy on psychological symptoms and social functioning in residual depression. Br J Psychiatry 177:440–446, 2000 11059998
Shear MK, Ghesquiere A, Glickman K: Bereavement and complicated grief. Curr Psychiatry Rep 15(11):406, 2013 24068457
Sheffrin M, Driscoll HC, Lenze EJ, et al: Pilot study of augmentation with aripiprazole for incomplete response in late-life depression: getting to remission. J Clin Psychiatry 70(2):208–213, 2009 19210951
Shulman KI, Tohen M, Satlin A, et al: Mania compared with unipolar depression in old age. Am J Psychiatry 149(3):341–345, 1992 1536272
Sobieraj DM, Martinez BK, Hernandez AV, et al: Adverse effects of pharmacologic treatments of major depression in older adults. J Am Geriatr Soc 67(8):1571–1581, 2019 31140587
Song F, Freemantle N, Sheldon TA, et al: Selective serotonin reuptake inhibitors: meta-analysis of efficacy and acceptability. BMJ 306(6879):683–687, 1993 8471919
Spira AP, Rebok GW, Stone KL, et al: Depressive symptoms in oldest-old women: risk of mild cognitive impairment and dementia. Am J Geriatr Psychiatry 20(12):1006–1015, 2012 22015706
Staab JP, Evans DL: Efficacy of venlafaxine in geriatric depression. Depress Anxiety 12 (suppl 1):63–68, 2000 11098416
Starkstein SE, Robinson RG, Price TR: Comparison of cortical and subcortical lesions in the production of poststroke mood disorders. Brain 110(Pt 4):1045–1059, 1987 3651794
Steffens DC: Vascular depression: is an old research construct finally ready for clinical prime time? Biol Psychiatry 85(6):441–442, 2019 30777170
Steffens DC, Skoog I, Norton MC, et al: Prevalence of depression and its treatment in an elderly population: the Cache County study. Arch Gen Psychiatry 57(6):601–607, 2000 10839339
Steuer JL, Mintz J, Hammen CL, et al: Cognitive-behavioral and psychodynamic group psychotherapy in treatment of geriatric depression. J Consult Clin Psychol 52(2):180–189, 1984 6715645

Sullivan MD, LaCroix AZ, Baum C, et al: Functional status in coronary artery disease: a one-year prospective study of the role of anxiety and depression. Am J Med 103(5):348–356, 1997 9375701

Tamashiro JH, Zung S, Zanetti MV, et al: Increased rates of white matter hyperintensities in late-onset bipolar disorder. Bipolar Disord 10(7):765–775, 2008 19032708

Tampi RR, Balderas M, Carter KV, et al: Citalopram, QTc prolongation, and torsades de pointes. Psychosomatics 56(1):36–43, 2015 25619672

Tariq SH, Tumosa N, Chibnall JT, et al: Comparison of the Saint Louis University mental status examination and the mini-mental state examination for detecting dementia and mild neurocognitive disorder—a pilot study. Am J Geriatr Psychiatry 14(11):900–910, 2006 17068312

Taylor MP, Reynolds CF 3rd, Frank E, et al: Which elderly depressed patients remain well on maintenance interpersonal psychotherapy alone? Report from the Pittsburgh study of maintenance therapies in late-life depression. Depress Anxiety 10(2):55–60, 1999 10569127

Taylor WD: Clinical practice. Depression in the elderly. N Engl J Med 371(13):1228–1236, 2014 25251617

Taylor WD, Doraiswamy PM: A systematic review of antidepressant placebo-controlled trials for geriatric depression: limitations of current data and directions for the future. Neuropsychopharmacology 29(12):2285–2299, 2004 15340391

Teresi J, Abrams R, Holmes D, et al: Prevalence of depression and depression recognition in nursing homes. Soc Psychiatry Psychiatr Epidemiol 36(12):613–620, 2001 11838834

Teri L, Gallagher-Thompson D: Cognitive-behavioral interventions for treatment of depression in Alzheimer's patients. Gerontologist 31(3):413–416, 1991 1879719

Thakur M, Hays J, Krishnan KR: Clinical, demographic and social characteristics of psychotic depression. Psychiatry Res 86(2):99–106, 1999 10397412

Tham A, Jonsson U, Andersson G, et al: Efficacy and tolerability of antidepressants in people aged 65 years or older with major depressive disorder—a systematic review and a meta-analysis. J Affect Disord 205:1–12, 2016 27389296

Thorlund K, Druyts E, Wu P, et al: Comparative efficacy and safety of selective serotonin reuptake inhibitors and serotonin-norepinephrine reuptake inhibitors in older adults: a network meta-analysis. J Am Geriatr Soc 63(5):1002–1009, 2015 25945410

van Schaik A, van Marwijk H, Adèr H, et al: Interpersonal psychotherapy for elderly patients in primary care. Am J Geriatr Psychiatry 14(9):777–786, 2006 16943174

Venna N, Mogocsi S, Jay M, et al: Reversible depression in Binswanger's disease. J Clin Psychiatry 49(1):23–26, 1988 3335486

Verwijk E, Comijs HC, Kok RM, et al: Short- and long-term neurocognitive functioning after electroconvulsive therapy in depressed elderly: a prospective naturalistic study. Int Psychogeriatr 26(2):315–324, 2014 24280446

Weihs KL, Settle EC Jr, Batey SR, et al: Bupropion sustained release versus paroxetine for the treatment of depression in the elderly. J Clin Psychiatry 61(3):196–202, 2000 10817105

Weissman MM, Markowitz JC, Klerman GL: Comprehensive Guide to Interpersonal Psychotherapy. New York, Basic Books, 2000

Williams BR, Sawyer Baker P, Allman RM, et al: Bereavement among African American and white older adults. J Aging Health 19(2):313–333, 2007 17413138

Yesavage JA, Brink TL, Rose TL, et al: Development and validation of a geriatric depression screening scale: a preliminary report. J Psychiatr Res 17(1):37–49, 1982–1983 7183759

PART VIII

Additional Perspectives on Mood Disorder

CHAPTER 39

Depression in Primary Care

Larry Culpepper, M.D., M.P.H.

Since the introduction of second-generation antidepressants in 1988, the role of primary care clinicians in mental health care has increased in importance. In 2002, the U.S. Preventive Services Task Force (USPSTF) first recommended screening for depression based on evidence that it could lead to improved outcomes. For primary care clinicians, major depressive disorder (MDD) served as a gateway condition that led to increased competency in recognition, treatment, and management of common psychiatric disorders. In many communities, primary care clinicians now provide the majority of depression care.

In this chapter I explore the roles of primary care at the population level of screening and surveillance, and at the clinical level of managing chronic illnesses in individual patients. I then describe practice-level activities required to carry out these roles. Many of these activities, including collaborative practice and use of measurement-based treatment, are also relevant in the care of patients with psychiatric conditions other than depression.

Primary Care Responsibilities at the Population Health Level

Primary care differs from other specialties in that it maintains a continuing relationship with patients without regard to health status. During times of health, the focus is on preventive care and encouraging health-promoting behaviors. During times of illness, and continuously for chronic illness, the focus extends to managing conditions, including collaboration and coordination with other health care professionals and integration of care for multiple conditions. An important quality of primary care is its sensitivity to the social and environmental context of the individual, including the family (in this chapter, "family" encompasses nontraditional relationships). Because of this continuing context-sensitive relationship, primary care clinicians are well positioned to engage in activities focused on entire populations. For depression, the population-level focus is on recognizing the illness and then maintaining affected individuals in care over the life span.

Screening

The USPSTF in 2016 updated its recommendations to include routine screening for depression in the general adult population, in pregnant and postpartum women, and in adolescents (Siu and U.S. Preventive Services Task Force 2016). The goal of screening is to identify individuals with unrecognized MDD in the total practice population as the first step in bringing them into effective care.

Of note, the USPSTF found no evidence to support a recommendation for repeated screening for MDD or for an optimal interval between screenings. Instead, the USPSTF suggested a pragmatic approach that includes screening patients who have not been previously screened and "using clinical judgment in consideration of risk factors, comorbid conditions, and life events to determine if additional screening of high-risk patients is warranted" (Siu and U.S. Preventive Services Task Force 2016, p. 382). However, promoted by quality metrics and reimbursement incentives, this practice population–focused goal is routinely displaced by the goal of annually screening the subset of patients who visit the practice. Yet, among members of a population who identify a primary care practice as their source of care, only one-half to two-thirds visit their primary care provider during any year, and about one-fifth to one-quarter have not visited for 3 years or longer (Bartholomeeusen et al. 2005; Cherkin et al. 1982; Ridley et al. 2020; Smith and Mazure 2021). Concentrating screening efforts on patients who are visiting (usually only during non-acute-care visits) results in those at highest risk of unrecognized depression being those least likely to be screened. For instance, despite the fact that patients in low-income and minority groups are three times more likely than nonminority patients with high incomes to be depressed (Ridley et al. 2020; Shao et al. 2016; Smith and Mazure 2021), many of these patients, because of financial, cultural, and stigma-related barriers, visit their primary care provider very infrequently, and then only for urgent needs. Depressive symptoms, including negative cognitive biases (Culpepper 2015), can themselves contribute to patients' reluctance to visit their primary care provider, even when they have other problems.

A reconceptualization of practice approaches that is in line with the USPSTF recommendations (Siu and U.S. Preventive Services Task Force 2016) is likely to engage more individuals in effective care for MDD. Such an approach continues to emphasize screening of all adults and adolescents when they initially become patients of a practice. However, after a confirmatory second negative screen in a patient who is not at increased risk, screening frequency can be reduced (e.g., to every 5–10 years), and practice resources can be redirected to case finding, which might increase the portion of a practice's population engaged in care for depression. Such case finding might occur during patient visits and at other contacts. A major change for most practices, risk-based case finding emphasizes outreach to patients with risk factors who have not visited within an arbitrary interval (e.g., a year). Such an approach shifts staff effort from

TABLE 39–1. Risk factors for and common presentations of depression in primary care

Risk factors for depression
Previous episodes of depression
Current or past anxiety disorders or substance use disorders
Persistent depressive disorder (dysthymia)
History of postpartum mood disorder
Recent bereavement or loss (e.g., death or divorce)
Family history of depression
Chronic medical illness
Traumatic event (e.g., car accident)
Major life change (e.g., job change, financial difficulties)
Stressful life event (e.g., job or geographic change)
Perimenopausal status
Low-income status
Spouse or partner with depressive illness
Common presentations of depression in primary care
Five or more medical visits per year
Multiple unexplained symptoms
Chronic medical illness
Fatigue
Pain syndromes
Sleep disturbance
Weight gain or loss
Memory and other cognitive complaints (e.g., difficulty concentrating or making decisions)
Dementia
Dampened affect
Complaints of stress or mood disturbance
Work or relationship dysfunction
Changes in interpersonal relationships

low-yield repeated screening of visiting patients to targeted outreach to patients more likely to have unrecognized depression. (Chapter 4 in this textbook, "Rating Scales and Structured Diagnostic Interviews for Mood Disorders," discusses instruments validated for screening and for periodic measurement of symptom severity.) The Patient Health Questionnaire (PHQ; Kroenke et al. 2001) is commonly used in primary care and is available in many languages (www.phqscreeners.com).

Case Finding

Table 39–1 outlines risk factors for depression and common presentations of depression. Familiarity with these characteristic presentations can help practice staff or clinicians to identify patients who may be depressed and prompt them to conduct an assessment for concurrent depression without regard to a patient's stated reason for visiting. Discrete data regarding many of the depression risk factors shown in Table 39–1 are available in electronic medical records. These can be used to generate prompts and alerts, facilitating targeted case-finding surveillance, including through outreach. Among the listed risk factors, a history of MDD, a serious traumatic event, and recent bereavement all convey major risk for depression. A single previous episode of MDD is associated with a 50% risk of recurrence within 5 years, two previous episodes convey a 70% risk, and three or more episodes convey a 90% risk (Consensus Development Panel 1985). Among individuals who have experienced or witnessed a serious traumatic event, 30%–40% will develop MDD—a risk similar to that of developing posttraumatic stress disorder (Flory and Yehuda 2015; Sartor et al. 2012). Recent bereavement carries a significant risk for depression, especially among elderly persons (Kendler et al. 2008). In 40%–60% of patients with MDD, a major life change preceded their first episode (Stroud et al. 2008, 2011).

Most depressed patients in primary care practices have multiple comorbidities, and most chronic medical illnesses are associated with a twofold or greater increased risk of concurrent depressive illness (Egede 2007). These chronic illnesses include cardiovascular, endocrine (diabetes and thyroid), respiratory, and neurological conditions as well as less-well-defined illness groups such as those associated with chronic pain, insomnia, or inflammatory conditions. Both at the time of initial diagnosis of these medical conditions and periodically during their care, assessment for depression may be beneficial. Case-finding efforts should also be deployed at times when treatment needs to be altered or intensified (e.g., increased disease severity, increased stress, or poor adherence to treatment).

For primary care practices located in low-income communities, in which most individuals are at increased risk of depression, there is little evidence to guide case finding. Routine assessment of all visiting patients may be reasonable to simplify office procedures. However, especially in these high-risk communities, concentrating effort on outreach to nonvisiting patients will likely have a high yield in identifying individuals with depression, other psychiatric conditions, and concurrent illness.

Primary Care Responsibilities at the Individual Patient Level

The roles of primary care clinicians caring for depressed patients, listed in Table 39–2, encompass a range of responsibilities, extending from initial recognition of depression to assistance with long-term functional recovery. The primary care clinician's prior knowledge of and ongoing connection with patients and families facilitate many of these roles.

The USPSTF has recommended that routine screening of all patients be implemented only in practices having systems and clinical staff in place to ensure that patients who screen positive for depression are accurately diagnosed and treated with evidence-based interventions or referred for care (U.S. Preventive Services Task Force 2009). The collaborative care model (van Eck van der Sluijs et al. 2018) provides an evidence-based strategy for organizing primary care practices to diagnose and treat depression. This model (Unützer et al. 2002) uses a multidisciplinary team consisting of the following:

TABLE 39–2. Responsibilities of primary care clinicians at the individual patient level

Assess type and severity of depression.
Assess relevant comorbidities.
Help patients and families understand and accept the diagnosis.
Educate the patient and family.
Promote active participation of the patient and family in planning and management of measurement-based care throughout the continuum of acute, continuation, and maintenance treatment.
Engage patients and families with psychiatric consultants, other mental health care providers, and community resources.
Integrate depression care with care of other chronic diseases and health-promoting care.
Encourage supportive lifestyle changes such as exercise and behavioral activation.
Identify and respond to any recurrences.
Optimize immediate and long-term functional recovery and other desired outcomes.

- Primary care clinicians who provide evidence-based depression care and use standardized instruments to screen for depression and monitor symptom severity, response to treatment plan, and remission.
- A care manager who tracks patients, reminds them of visits, and monitors treatment adherence and effectiveness, thus facilitating treatment changes and relapse prevention.
- A team member (often the care manager) who helps provide education and self-management support to patients.
- A psychiatrist who frequently and regularly communicates with the primary care team regarding patients under clinical supervision and provides direct patient visits as needed.

Randomized trials have demonstrated that the collaborative care model improves treatment adherence, quality of life, and depression outcomes (including reduced suicidality) (Archer et al. 2012; Katon and Seelig 2008). The model is also effective for treating depression during pregnancy and the postpartum period (Gjerdingen and Yawn 2007). The Improving Mood: Promoting Access to Collaborative Treatment (IMPACT) study randomly assigned 1,801 primary care patients to collaborative care or usual care, with follow-up for up to 4 years, and demonstrated cost savings of $3,363 per patient over the 4-year period (Unützer et al. 2008). Studies examining the workplace impact of collaborative care treatment of depression have shown that employers receive a significant return on their investment, with increased productivity and decreased absenteeism, as well as continued gains in year 2 (Lo Sasso et al. 2006; Rost et al. 2004).

Clinicians have reported the collaborative care model to be beneficial, as was demonstrated in the IMPACT study (Unützer et al. 2008). After implementation of the IMPACT model, 90% of the primary care physicians described the program as helpful; 93% were at least somewhat satisfied with the resources available for treatment using the model, compared with 61% for usual care (Levine et al. 2005). Clinicians identified the model's most helpful features as proactive patient follow-up and patient education; 94% rated the care managers as somewhat or very helpful, and 82% indicated that the IMPACT program improved their patients' clinical outcomes (Levine et al. 2005).

From Recognition of Depression to Treatment Initiation

Patients newly presenting to psychiatrists usually already suspect or know that they have a psychiatric disorder. In contrast, the most common depression presentations in primary care are for somatic symptoms. Consequently, many newly diagnosed patients in primary care are not immediately accepting of the diagnosis. Using a scale for screening or case finding and explaining to patients that such assessments are routine may be an initial step in reducing perceived stigma and educating patients. Although such instruments identify 80%–90% of individuals who are experiencing a major depressive episode, in most primary care practices, one-third to one-half of individuals who screen positive for depression are not experiencing a major depressive episode (Kroenke et al. 2001). On further assessment, many such patients will be found to have another condition (e.g., an adjustment, anxiety, or trauma-related disorder) or to be under situational stress that might benefit from care. Further assessment also is necessary to identify individuals with bipolar depression or substance use disorders and to evaluate the status of any chronic medical illnesses present, including pain and sleep disorders.

The therapeutic alliance can have a greater effect on outcomes than the treatment selected (psychotherapy vs. pharmacotherapy) and can have a large effect even when pharmacotherapy is used. Educating and reaching agreement with the patient (and family) on a biological model of a brain disease that includes the impact of stress and accounts for potential future episodes can be helpful. Parallels with chronic diseases may be helpful, because patients who mistakenly consider depression to be analogous to self-limited conditions such as headache or infection may stop taking their prescribed medication when their symptoms improve. Prognosis is usually a major concern for patients and families, and providing a realistic but positive overview of the anticipated course and impact of treatment can help engage them in care. Many patients have concerns based on misperceptions regarding psychiatric medications. Correcting these misperceptions often is essential to long-term adherence.

The depressed patient's low motivation, low energy, pessimism, and sense of social isolation often lead to nonadherence. Motivational interviewing may be beneficial. Eliciting and recording a patient's treatment priorities and goals also helps engage and motivate patients to adhere to recommendations. These interviewing techniques reassure patients that they have been heard and understood and that the clinician anticipates improvement. An essential component of motivational interviewing is evaluating current and premorbid functioning (work, family, social), coping effectiveness and coping strategies, and related problems. A natural extension of this process is reaching agreement with the patient on measurement tools to be used in monitoring symptoms and functional status, including frequency and modality (e.g., phone, internet, in-person visit). Recording and subsequently querying and counseling patients about their efforts to attain their goals provides additional individualization of care.

Patient education is an important responsibility of the primary care team and helps patients understand their options and resources. Given potential depression-related cognitive alterations, education, motivational support, and management planning activities often need to be continued over multiple visits for patients to fully comprehend and participate in their own care. Referring patients to web-based, print, and community resources may help in this process. The care team should ask whether a family member or person of the patient's choosing is available to be included in the education process. Important education components have been well described (Trangle et al. 2016). Key messages for patients and families include the following: 1) depression is a medical illness, not a character defect; 2) treatment is effective for most patients; 3) the aim of treatment is remission; and 4) relapse prevention is an essential component of care.

Selecting Treatment and Planning Management

One role of the primary care physician, possibly in consultation with a psychiatrist, is to select the intervention most suited to each patient for initial treatment, for treatment modifications, and for long-term maintenance treatment if needed. Other chapters in this textbook address somatic and psychotherapeutic treatments, depression subtypes, and additional factors important in treatment and management.

In the discussion with the patient about treatment choices, patient preferences need to be considered, and clinicians need to recognize the importance of cultural and family influences. Optimally, the patient and the clinician will reach agreement on the best treatment, although at times the clinician will need to explain why he or she is recommending a treatment that does not align with the patient's preferences. Studies have shown that reaching agreement on the selected treatment improves adherence and attainment of remission. In one study, 22.2% of patients who preferred medication but received psychotherapy achieved remission, versus 45.5% of those who received medication per their preference. Patients who preferred psychotherapy but were prescribed medication had a 7.7% remission rate, versus a rate of 50.0% for those who received psychotherapy per their preference (Kocsis et al. 2009).

Some patients obtain optimal benefit with a combination of pharmacotherapy and psychotherapy delivered either concurrently or at different times. Pharmacotherapy provides more rapid improvement, but psychotherapy may lengthen the time before relapse or recurrence (Biesheuvel-Leliefeld et al. 2015). Acute-phase-only cognitive-behavioral therapy without maintenance antidepressants may be equal in efficacy to maintaining patients on antidepressants for 6–18 months after remission (Cuijpers et al. 2013). Psychotherapy also may help patients alter dysfunctional patterns of relating to others, including at work.

The primary care physician may be aware of patient characteristics that impact the selection of treatment. In addition to knowledge of antidepressants that were effective in previous episodes and those that previously caused side effects, attention to the specific symptoms present, including those from comorbidities, may be of value in the choice of medication (e.g., selecting duloxetine for patients with pain; avoiding sedating antidepressants in patients with fatigue or somnolence; avoiding activating antidepressants such as bupropion in patients with insomnia or agitation). Comorbidities may be relevant (e.g., avoiding antidepressants that worsen cardiovascular or diabetes risks), and lifestyle may also be pertinent (e.g., selecting a long-half-life antidepressant for patients with irregular schedules or adherence challenges; using bupropion for smokers). The need to avoid drug interactions may make desvenlafaxine a good choice. The selegiline patch may be appropriate for patients who wish to avoid oral medications.

Integrating Depression Care With Care of Other Chronic Diseases

A first principle for treatment of patients who have multiple comorbidities and are taking multiple medications is to make one adjustment at a time and evaluate its effect before making additional changes. However, for patients with depression, this approach produces suboptimal results both for MDD and for medical comorbidities. Studies demonstrate that multi-comorbidity collaborative care management using concurrent measurement and treatment adjustment for depression, hypertension, diabetes, and lipid abnormalities leads to improvement in all outcomes (Katon et al. 2010; Lin et al. 2012). In this approach, a single treatment team and care manager provide integrated management of all conditions. For instance, one report (Katon et al. 2010) described the use of an integrated patient dashboard to monitor 214 patients with multiple chronic conditions, with the care manager working with each patient to control risk factors associated with each condition. This intervention resulted in enhanced disease recognition, increased rates of measurement-based treatment adjustments, and improved outcomes. In comparison with patients who received usual care ($n=108$), those who received integrated care ($n=106$) had greater 12-month improvement in glycated hemoglobin (HbA1c) levels (difference, 0.58%), low-density lipoprotein cholesterol levels (difference, 6.9 mg per deciliter), systolic blood pressure (difference, 5.1 mm Hg), and 20-item Hopkins Symptom Checklist depression scale (SCL-20; Williams et al. 2004) scores (difference, 0.40 point) ($P<0.001$), and they also reported better quality of life ($P<0.001$) and greater satisfaction with care for diabetes, coronary heart disease, and depression ($P<0.001$) (Katon et al. 2010; Lin et al. 2012). Multi-comorbidity collaborative care management using concurrent measurement and treatment adjustment significantly improved the process of care, including pharmacotherapy initiation and adjustment. Pharmacotherapy initiation and adjustment rates for patients receiving integrated care were sixfold higher for antidepressants (relative rate [RR]=6.20; $P<0.001$), threefold higher for insulin (RR=2.97; $P<0.001$), and nearly twofold higher for antihypertensives (RR=1.86; $P<0.001$) compared with rates for patients receiving usual care (Lin et al. 2012). In another study of primary care practices using an integrated care strategy ($N=180$), 60.9% of patients receiving the active intervention achieved HbA1c levels of less than 7% (vs. 35.7% of patients receiving usual care; $P<0.001$), and 58.7% experienced remission of depression (vs. 30.7% for usual care; $P<0.001$) (Bogner et al. 2012). Of note, these studies demonstrate the value of frequent proactive contact with patients and of frequent treatment adjustment.

Promoting Physical Activity and Behavioral Activation

Physical Activity

Physical activity at a dose consistent with public health recommendations might ease MDD symptoms, but its overall value in improving depressive symptoms or quality of life is uncertain (Dunn et al. 2005; Krogh et al. 2017; Schuch and de Almeida Fleck

2013), including for those whose depression is treatment resistant (Rethorst et al. 2017). When prescribing exercise, the clinician should consider the individual circumstances of each patient. Exercise may be blended with activation strategies that encourage patients to engage with others in exercise they find enjoyable. Aerobic exercise and resistance training (e.g., weight lifting) are equally effective in improving depression; however, mixed aerobic and resistance training may provide more benefit for depression than either alone (Cooney et al. 2013; Cusimano and VandenBerg 2020; Rethorst and Trivedi 2013). In regard to exercise benefit, total calories expended may be more important than frequency of exercise. The antidepressant effects of exercise do not persist after it is discontinued (Silveira et al. 2013).

Behavioral Activation

Depressed patients often avoid pleasurable or even routine activities as a result of negative outlooks that make social contact with others undesirable. Such avoidance of activities may increase depressive symptoms. The goal of behavioral activation is to interrupt this process and improve symptoms by increasing positive interactions with others. Behavioral activation is similar in efficacy to psychotherapy for depression and may be as effective as pharmacotherapy. Moreover, symptom improvements from behavioral activation persist after treatment is discontinued (Cuijpers et al. 2007). Given its benefits, its few risks, and the ease of combining behavioral activation with other treatments, behavioral activation should be used routinely in depression care. It is useful for clinicians to ask patients about activities they previously enjoyed, as well as about activities they are currently avoiding (e.g., time with friends, hobbies, housework, parenting, professional work). Activity scheduling is helpful for some patients. For example, participation in a senior day care program or participation in nursing home activities may help reduce depressive symptoms in older patients (Cuijpers et al. 2007).

The Institute for Clinical Systems Improvement (Trangle et al. 2016) has offered the following guidance for clinicians seeking to engage patients in behavioral activation:

- The clinician's role is to help patients resume or increase their exposure to the positive experiences they engaged in prior to becoming depressed.
- Goals should be focused on behaviors (e.g., resuming activities patients have avoided) rather than on ideation (e.g., motivation to change).
- Clinicians should help patients to prioritize their short- and long-term goals and to plan the steps needed to accomplish them.
- Clinicians should discourage patients from adopting ambitious new life or health goals (e.g., smoking cessation, weight loss), which may set patients up for failure and frustration.
- At follow-up appointments, clinicians should ask patients about progress on their goals and help them problem-solve any areas of difficulty encountered.

Long-Term Management of Depression

The probability of recurrence of MDD symptoms is about 25% after 1 year, 42% after 2 years, and 60% after 5 years, and each recurrence increases the risk of subsequent episodes by 16% (Solomon et al. 2000). Whereas initial episodes are usually associated with major stressors, later ones often occur without such precipitants. Consequently, when used, antidepressants should be continued for 2–3 years after the second episode, and indefinitely after an additional episode or in patients who had severe initial episodes. However, without proactive support, patients do not routinely adhere to such long-term treatment. Premature discontinuation of antidepressant treatment can be related to inadequate education about MDD, failure to set goals for and continue care management follow-up, psychosocial factors, and/or adverse side effects. Ongoing collaborative care can increase remission rates to as much as 76% by 2 years (Schoenbaum et al. 2001). Exercise and behavioral activation may also help prevent depression recurrence.

For patients in whom discontinuation is planned, the medication dosage can be gradually tapered over a period of weeks to months, with close monitoring for symptom recurrence in the months and then years after cessation. Medication discontinuation should not be undertaken during periods of increased stress or anticipated transitions. In women, planning monthly dosage decreases to correspond with menstrual cycles may facilitate interpretation of any related symptoms.

Anticipatory counseling, reinforcing education, and increased monitoring for depressive symptoms may be helpful during life transitions (e.g., leaving home, coping with an "empty nest," changing jobs, marriage or divorce, pregnancy, retirement). Anticipatory counseling should include identifying and managing family consequences of depression and mobilizing family support.

New Horizons in Primary Care of Patients With Depression

Beyond symptom remission, patients seek full recovery. They view recovery as including positive mental health—for example, optimism, energy, self-confidence, feeling like their normal (pre-depression) self, and feeling that they are in control of their emotions. Patients also highly value a return to their premorbid level of functioning at work, home, or school, including participating in, and enjoying, relationships with family and friends (Zimmerman et al. 2006).

As patients respond to treatment, clarifying their premorbid status and perceived shortfalls in attaining recovery may allow the clinician to be of further help. This includes identifying residual symptoms of both the depressive illness and the comorbid conditions (especially chronic pain or insomnia) that might be amenable to treatment. Use of functional assessment scales (see Chapter 4 in this textbook) may be helpful in evaluating and monitoring patients' functional status.

Cognitive impairments related to depression may have a major impact on recovery of function but be inadequately measured by depression symptom scales. Twenty percent to 40% of depressed individuals have significant impairments in at least one cognitive domain, most frequently in executive function, attention, working memory, or psychomotor processing (McIntyre et al. 2013). Patients with MDD frequently have negative cognitive biases, expressed as negative interpretations of sensory inputs and experiences, increased focus on negative information, decreased attention to positive information, and greater difficulty inhibiting negative thought processing (Culpepper 2015). Use of the subjective Perceived Deficits Questionnaire (PDQ-5, PDQ-20, or PDQ-D; Fehnel et al. 2016) or of rapid objective measures of cognitive function such as the Digit Symbol Substitution Test (DSST) is feasible in primary care settings and can help identify patients with cognitive impairment (McIntyre et al. 2013). These questionnaires and measures can provide useful information in the initial assessment of an episode and in follow-up assessments of patients with continued functional impairments. They also may be informative for patients considering taking leave from work or returning to work, since the cognitive demands of the workplace may differ from those in other realms of patients' lives. However, some workplaces may provide benefit by increasing activation and social contact.

Because MDD-associated cognitive dysfunction may respond to certain antidepressants, a treatment trial may be warranted. Certain psychotherapies also may lead to improvement and may be particularly helpful in altering the brain network processes underlying negative cognitive biases. In addition, behavioral activation and physical exercise may be helpful.

Practice-Level Activities for Management of Depression

A Catch-22 in primary care is that depressed patients usually present with multiple other problems that are viewed by primary care clinicians, patients, or their families as being of higher priority than the depression in allocating visit time. However, the comorbid depression often complicates care of these other conditions. Multiple meta-analyses have found that the presence of MDD worsens adherence (by threefold or more) to clinical recommendations for comorbid conditions, including recommendations regarding medication, diet, exercise, smoking cessation, and program participation (e.g., cardiac rehabilitation). Attention to organizing the practice can minimize the effort required with individual patients and is critical to sustainable and reliable management of MDD. Optimization of depression management is especially important for patients with multiple comorbidities—a group that includes the majority of depressed patients in primary care. Table 39–3 outlines the processes and resources required at the practice level to optimize primary practice management of patients with depression. Adopting an established practice guideline (Trangle et al. 2016) and then involving all members of the team in adapting the guideline and clarifying roles within the practice are important initial and ongoing activities.

Of particular importance in preparing practices to effectively manage patients with depression is developing the care manager roles and tools, both for population surveillance and relating to individual patients. Care managers often form important therapeutic relationships with patients and families, and the nuances of communication with patients and within the team may be critical to optimizing outcomes.

Of similar importance in preparing practices to effectively manage patients with depression are identifying collaborating psychiatrist(s) and other professionals (e.g., psychiatric social workers, psychologists) and reaching agreement on their roles and methods of interacting with the primary care team, whether embedded in the practice or located elsewhere. These professionals should be engaged throughout the process of discussing practice routines, staff roles and development, and communication strategies. One of the functions of the psychiatrist is as a coach to the physician and other team members. Experienced teams find that over time, the skills of the team in-

TABLE 39–3. Primary care practice preparation for care of patients with depression

Processes	Examples of resources
Identify collaborative care team composition	– Practice staff members – Area hospital and psychiatric providers
Develop orientation and training for current and new staff	– Training library and online resources
Select and adapt depression guideline • Methods of integrating comorbidity care into guideline • Specify team member roles	– Primary care–oriented depression guidelines (e.g., ICSI, CANMAT, NICE) – Guidelines for comorbid medical and psychiatric conditions – Standing orders
Select tools for • Screening and measurement • Case management • Telehealth	– PHQ, QIDS, PDQ, DSST, SDS; see Chapter 4) – Population screening and disease registries – Acute-, continuation-, and maintenance-phase treatment management tools – Recall tickler systems and tracking systems
Adapt electronic medical record • Forms • Presentation and risk identification • Record release consent and depression care summary forms	– Embedded PHQ, prescriptions, other tools – Clinical decision support systems – Automated search capabilities – Templates
Establish communication processes and identify participants • Daily flow, routine (e.g., screen response) • Urgent situations, suicidality, intoxication • Psychiatric consultation and referrals	– Before-session and during-session huddles, warm hand-offs – Weekly/monthly case management – External (e.g., hospital) notification, consent, and record exchange
Identify and engage community resources • Professional • Exercise, activity, and social support • Financial, housing, food, transportation	– Psychotherapists, social workers, visiting nurses, pharmacy, hospital – Procedural providers (e.g., ECT, rTMS, ketamine)
Outreach modalities	– Practice web portal, email, text, video contact, phone
Education and support • Practice-based groups • Community groups • Regional and national	– Online and practice-based reading material library – NAMI, ADAA, WebMD

Note. ADAA=Anxiety and Depression Association of America; CANMAT=Canadian Network for Mood and Anxiety Treatments; DSST=Digit Symbol Substitution Test; ECT=electroconvulsive therapy; ICSI=Institute for Clinical Systems Improvement; NAMI=National Alliance On Mental Illness; NICE=National Institute for Health and Care Excellence; PDQ=Perceived Deficits Questionnaire; PHQ=Patient Health Questionnaire; QIDS=Quick Inventory of Depressive Symptomatology; rTMS=repetitive transcranial magnetic stimulation; SDS=Zung Self-Rating Depression Scale.

crease, the complexity of care the team provides grows, and the scope and focus of case management meetings and in-person psychiatric consultations evolve.

A number of strategies can improve the sustainability of collaborative care. Such strategies include identifying a "physician champion"; selecting care managers with strong professional and interpersonal skills; educating the team about the collaborative care model and what it requires of them; adopting robust systems for communication, including regular face-to-face interaction; and attending to reimbursement for extra work and expenses (Overbeck et al. 2016).

Developing the procedures and resources of a primary care practice related to psychiatric care is an iterative process. Primary care practices may benefit from addressing care components or patient situations that create uncertainty or difficulty for team members. Standard quality-improvement approaches (e.g., a process map sketching out how a patient with suicidal ideation or behavior of varying severity should be managed) may be useful. Developing the necessary procedures and resources may be facilitated by adopting practice goals and metrics to prioritize and guide practice evolution.

Conclusion

Primary care clinicians, who provide a large portion of the care of individuals with depressive illness, must use a number of strategies that differ from ones used routinely in psychiatric practices. Since a majority of depressed primary care patients do not initially attribute their symptoms to psychiatric illness, screening and case finding strategies are critical to the recognition and then diagnosis of such patients. Once diagnosed, these patients (and their families) must be educated about depressive illness. Adherence and outcomes of treatment improve when the clinician and educated patient reach agreement on the goals and treatment selection. Patients often benefit from medication and psychotherapy, and these may be enhanced by use of behavioral activation and regular exercise. A majority of depressed primary care patients have comorbid medical conditions. When treatment and follow-up of depression activities are integrated with those of comorbid conditions, outcome of all generally improve in comparison to strategies that treat them separately. Primary care clinicians must use active management strategies or their depressed patients often do not improve. Organization of practices, including through adoption of collaborative care strategies involving a care manager, psychiatrist, and other professionals and preparing practice resources is important to the ability of primary care clinicians to routinely and effectively provide the necessary active management of depressed patients.

References

Archer J, Bower P, Gilbody S, et al: Collaborative care for depression and anxiety problems. Cochrane Database Syst Rev (10):CD006525, 2012 23076925

Bartholomeeusen S, Kim CY, Mertens R, et al: The denominator in general practice, a new approach from the Intego database. Fam Pract 22(4):442–447, 2005 15964863

Biesheuvel-Leliefeld KE, Kok GD, Bockting CL, et al: Effectiveness of psychological interventions in preventing recurrence of depressive disorder: meta-analysis and meta-regression. J Affect Disord 174:400–410, 2015 25553400

Bogner HR, Morales KH, de Vries HF, et al: Integrated management of type 2 diabetes mellitus and depression treatment to improve medication adherence: a randomized controlled trial. Ann Fam Med 10(1):15–22, 2012 22230826

Cherkin DC, Berg AO, Phillips WR: In search of a solution to the primary care denominator problem. J Fam Pract 14(2):301–309, 1982 7057151

Consensus Development Panel: NIMH/NIH Consensus Development Conference statement. Mood disorders: pharmacologic prevention of recurrences. Am J Psychiatry 142(4):469–476, 1985 3976921

Cooney GM, Dwan K, Greig CA, et al: Exercise for depression. Cochrane Database Syst Rev (9):CD004366, 2013 24026850

Cuijpers P, van Straten A, Warmerdam L: Behavioral activation treatments of depression: a meta-analysis. Clin Psychol Rev 27(3):318–326, 2007 17184887

Cuijpers P, Sijbrandij M, Koole SL, et al: The efficacy of psychotherapy and pharmacotherapy in treating depressive and anxiety disorders: a meta-analysis of direct comparisons. World Psychiatry 12(2):137–148, 2013 23737423

Culpepper L: Cognition in MDD: implications for primary care, in Cognitive Impairment in Major Depressive Disorder: Clinical Relevance, Biological Substrates, and Treatment Opportunities. Edited by McIntyre RS. New York, Cambridge University Press, 2015, pp 30–46

Cusimano J, VandenBerg A: Low-hanging fruit for getting back on your feet: a critical review of diet and exercise interventions for depression. Journal of Affective Disorders Reports 1:100019, 2020. Available at: https://doi.org/10.1016/j.jadr.2020.100019. Accessed September 26, 2021.

Dunn AL, Trivedi MH, Kampert JB, et al: Exercise treatment for depression: efficacy and dose response. Am J Prev Med 28(1):1–8, 2005 15626549

Egede LE: Major depression in individuals with chronic medical disorders: prevalence, correlates and association with health resource utilization, lost productivity and functional disability. Gen Hosp Psychiatry 29(5):409–416, 2007 17888807

Fehnel SE, Forsyth BH, DiBenedetti DB, et al: Patient-centered assessment of cognitive symptoms of depression. CNS Spectr 21(1):43–52, 2016 24067243

Flory JD, Yehuda R: Comorbidity between post-traumatic stress disorder and major depressive disorder: alternative explanations and treatment considerations. Dialogues Clin Neurosci 17(2):141–150, 2015 26246789

Gjerdingen DK, Yawn BP: Postpartum depression screening: importance, methods, barriers, and recommendations for practice. J Am Board Fam Med 20(3):280–288, 2007 17478661

Katon WJ, Seelig M: Population-based care of depression: team care approaches to improving outcomes. J Occup Environ Med 50(4):459–467, 2008 18404019

Katon WJ, Lin EH, Von Korff M, et al: Collaborative care for patients with depression and chronic illnesses. N Engl J Med 363(27):2611–2620, 2010 21190455

Kendler KS, Myers J, Zisook S: Does bereavement-related major depression differ from major depression associated with other stressful life events? Am J Psychiatry 165(11):1449–1455, 2008 18708488

Kocsis JH, Leon AC, Markowitz JC, et al: Patient preference as a moderator of outcome for chronic forms of major depressive disorder treated with nefazodone, cognitive behavioral analysis system of psychotherapy, or their combination. J Clin Psychiatry 70(3):354–361, 2009 19192474

Kroenke K, Spitzer RL, Williams JB: The PHQ-9: validity of a brief depression severity measure. J Gen Intern Med 16(9):606–613, 2001 11556941

Krogh J, Hjorthøj C, Speyer H, et al: Exercise for patients with major depression: a systematic review with meta-analysis and trial sequential analysis. BMJ Open 7(9):e014820, 2017 28928174

Levine S, Unützer J, Yip JY, et al: Physicians' satisfaction with a collaborative disease management program for late-life depression in primary care. Gen Hosp Psychiatry 27(6):383–391, 2005 16271652

Lin EH, Von Korff M, Ciechanowski P, et al: Treatment adjustment and medication adherence for complex patients with diabetes, heart disease, and depression: a randomized controlled trial. Ann Fam Med 10(1):6–14, 2012 22230825

Lo Sasso AT, Rost K, Beck A: Modeling the impact of enhanced depression treatment on workplace functioning and costs: a cost-benefit approach. Med Care 44(4):352–358, 2006 16565636

McIntyre RS, Cha DS, Soczynska JK, et al: Cognitive deficits and functional outcomes in major depressive disorder: determinants, substrates, and treatment interventions. Depress Anxiety 30(6):515–527, 2013 23468126

Overbeck G, Davidsen AS, Kousgaard MB: Enablers and barriers to implementing collaborative care for anxiety and depression: a systematic qualitative review. Implement Sci 11(1):165, 2016 28031028

Rethorst CD, Trivedi MH: Evidence-based recommendations for the prescription of exercise for major depressive disorder. J Psychiatr Pract 19(3):204–212, 2013 23653077

Rethorst CD, South CC, Rush AJ, et al: Prediction of treatment outcomes to exercise in patients with nonremitted major depressive disorder. Depress Anxiety 34(12):1116–1122, 2017 28672073

Ridley M, Rao G, Schilbach F, Patel V: Poverty, depression, and anxiety: causal evidence and mechanisms. Science 370(6522):eaay0214, 2020 33303583

Rost K, Smith JL, Dickinson M: The effect of improving primary care depression management on employee absenteeism and productivity. A randomized trial. Med Care 42(12):1202–1210, 2004 15550800

Sartor CE, Grant JD, Lynskey MT, et al: Common heritable contributions to low-risk trauma, high-risk trauma, posttraumatic stress disorder, and major depression. Arch Gen Psychiatry 69(3):293–299, 2012 22393221

Schoenbaum M, Unützer J, Sherbourne C, et al: Cost-effectiveness of practice-initiated quality improvement for depression: results of a randomized controlled trial. JAMA 286(11):1325–1330, 2001 11560537

Schuch FB, de Almeida Fleck MP: Is exercise an efficacious treatment for depression? A comment upon recent negative findings. Front Psychiatry 4:20, 2013 23565097

Shao Z, Richie WD, Bailey RK: Racial and ethnic disparity in major depressive disorder. J Racial Ethn Health Disparities 3(4):692–705, 2016 27294764

Silveira H, Moraes H, Oliveira N, et al: Physical exercise and clinically depressed patients: a systematic review and meta-analysis. Neuropsychobiology 67(2):61–68, 2013 23295766

Siu AL, U.S. Preventive Services Task Force: Screening for depression in adults: US Preventive Services Task Force recommendation statement. JAMA 315(4):380–377, 2016 26813211

Smith MV, Mazure CM: Mental health and wealth: depression, gender, poverty, and parenting. Annu Rev Clin Psychol 17:181–205, 2021 33962537

Solomon DA, Keller MB, Leon AC, et al: Multiple recurrences of major depressive disorder. Am J Psychiatry 157(2):229–233, 2000 10671391

Stroud CB, Davila J, Moyer A: The relationship between stress and depression in first onsets versus recurrences: a meta-analytic review. J Abnorm Psychol 117(1):206–213, 2008 18266498

Stroud CB, Davila J, Hammen C, Vrshek-Schallhorn S: Severe and nonsevere events in first onsets versus recurrences of depression: evidence for stress sensitization. J Abnorm Psychol 120(1):142–154, 2011 21171724

Trangle M, Gursky J, Haigh TR, et al: Adult depression in primary care. Institute for Clinical Systems Improvement, March 2016. Available at: www.icsi.org/wp-content/uploads/2019/01/Depr.pdf. Accessed December 20, 2020.

Unützer J, Katon W, Callahan CM, et al: Collaborative care management of late-life depression in the primary care setting: a randomized controlled trial. JAMA 288(22):2836–2845, 2002 12472325

Unützer J, Katon WJ, Fan MY, et al: Long-term cost effects of collaborative care for late-life depression. Am J Manag Care 14(2):95–100, 2008 18269305

U.S. Preventive Services Task Force: Screening for depression: recommendations and rationale. Ann Intern Med 136(10):760–764, 2002 12020145

U.S. Preventive Services Task Force: Screening for depression in adults: U.S. Preventive Services Task Force recommendation statement. Ann Intern Med 151(11):784–792, 2009 19949144

van Eck van der Sluijs JF, Castelijns H, Eijsbroek V, et al: Illness burden and physical outcomes associated with collaborative care in patients with comorbid depressive disorder in chronic medical conditions: a systematic review and meta-analysis. Gen Hosp Psychiatry 50:1–14, 2018 28957682

Williams JW Jr, Stellato CP, Cornell J, Barrett JE: The 13- and 20-item Hopkins Symptom Checklist Depression Scale: psychometric properties in primary care patients with minor depression or dysthymia. Int J Psychiatry Med 34(1):37–50, 2004 15242140

Zimmerman M, McGlinchey JB, Posternak MA, et al: How should remission from depression be defined? The depressed patient's perspective. Am J Psychiatry 163(1):148–150, 2006 16390903

CHAPTER 40

Depression in Medical Illness

James K. Rustad, M.D.
Vanessa Padilla, M.D.
Mitchell Rovner, M.D.
Dominique L. Musselman, M.D., M.S.C.R.

In a pioneering article published in the *American Journal of Psychiatry* in 1937, Benjamin Malzberg reported findings indicating that patients with severe depression had a higher rate of mortality, mostly attributable to cardiovascular disease, in comparison with the general population (Malzberg 1937). Studies conducted during the 1960s revealed an increased prevalence of depression in patients with endocrine disorders; psychobiological investigators in the 1970s and 1980s discovered dysregulation of the hypothalamic-pituitary-adrenal (HPA), hypothalamic-pituitary-thyroid (HPT), and other hypothalamic-pituitary–end organ axes in patients with major mood disorders (Gillespie and Nemeroff 2005), as well as elevated prevalence rates of depression in persons with serious medical disorders (Table 40–1).

Also during the 1970s and 1980s, inclusion of psychometric rating instruments within large-scale epidemiological studies such as the first National Health and Nutrition Examination Survey (NHANES I) in 1971 (Egede et al. 2005) and the NHANES I Epidemiologic Follow-up Study in 1982 (Anda et al. 1993) allowed for eventual quantification of the negative impact of depression symptoms on population health. During the 1980s and 1990s, clinical researchers began to understand the multidimensional deleterious effects of depression in people who had undergone a myocardial infarction (MI) or stroke, been diagnosed with cancer, or contracted a new infectious disease, human immunodeficiency virus (HIV).

During the 1990s, however, with the advent of high-resolution structural and functional neuroimaging, the longed-for "windows into the brain" became a reality. In the ensuing years, it was hoped that the promise of "big data" techniques such as ge-

TABLE 40–1. Prevalence of depression in medically ill individuals

Patient population	Prevalence
Coronary heart disease	15%–30% (Lichtman et al. 2014)
Type 2 diabetes	15%–19% (Roy and Lloyd 2012; Wang et al. 2019)
Poststroke	28%–35% (Hackett and Pickles 2014)
Cancer	8%–24% (Krebber et al. 2014)
Hepatitis C	18%–33% (Adinolfi et al. 2017)
HIV	20%–50% (Bing et al. 2001)

nome-wide association studies (GWAS), metabolomics, and proteomics would allow further discrimination of the true mechanistic pathways underlying neurobehavioral symptoms in medically ill individuals, rather than merely revealing associations between biological epiphenomena and mood disorders (Table 40–2). Today, the hope is that these techniques will reveal new therapeutic targets to help solve age-old patient self-care challenges, diagnostic conundrums, and treatment impasses.

Epidemiology and Diagnosis

There is no overall agreement on the definition of major depressive disorder (MDD) in epidemiological research. Some studies use cutoff scores on structured dimensional questionnaires—for example, the Montgomery-Åsberg Depression Rating Scale (MADRS; Montgomery and Åsberg 1979)—to define "clinically significant depression." Although lengthy and time-consuming to complete, structured clinical interviews remain the gold standard for diagnosis in psychiatric research, but they can only reasonably be administered in clinical research settings (Carney and Freedland 2017). By contrast, self-report symptom questionnaires such as the 9-item Patient Health Questionnaire (PHQ-9; Kroenke et al. 2001) are efficient, practical screening measures designed for use within busy clinical settings.

In clinical populations of persons with major medical disorders, MDD can be challenging to diagnose. A patient with medical illness may experience anorexia, insomnia, and other neurovegetative symptoms that are frequently attributed to depression, but these symptoms may in fact be a consequence of disease progression and/or treatment (Caruso et al. 2017a, 2017b). Decades of debate have failed to yield a consensus on the most precise and reliable method of diagnosing depression in medically ill people. Some have advocated use of an exclusive diagnostic approach (Guan et al. 2013) that ignores somatic symptoms and uses only cognitive and affective symptoms to make a diagnosis. Others have recommended an inclusive approach that counts all relevant symptoms toward the diagnosis of depression without attempting to determine whether symptoms should be attributed to depression or to medical illness, so as to avoid "false negatives." Notably, the inclusive approach has not been shown to "overestimate" the diagnosis of depression in medically ill people (Simon and Von Korff 2006; Walker and Sharpe 2014).

TABLE 40–2. Biological mechanisms by which depression can influence disease

Cardiovascular disease	Cancer	Diabetes	Stroke	HIV
• Cortisol exacerbates atherosclerosis by making changes in lipids and increasing vessel fragility • SNS and PNS dysregulation (e.g., increased heart rate, decreased HRV) • Increased platelet reactivity • Endothelial dysfunction	• Inflammatory stimulation of CRH release • Shunting of tryptophan metabolism toward kynurenine formation • Oxidative damage	• Stress-induced release of counterregulatory hormones, resulting in hyperglycemia • Insulin resistance	• Alterations in monoamine neurotransmitter pathways • Increased release of pro-inflammatory cytokines • HPA axis dysfunction • Stroke-induced immune response leading to changes in neuroplasticity	• HPA axis dysregulation that can negatively affect the immune response • Stress-induced declines in lymphocyte subsets

Note. SNS=sympathetic nervous system, PNS=parasympathetic nervous system, CRH=corticotropin-releasing hormone; HPA=hypothalamic-pituitary-adrenal; HRV=heart rate variability.

Guo et al. (2006) developed a novel biostatistical strategy for identifying items from the observer-rated Hamilton Rating Scale for Depression (HAM-D) that would optimize the diagnosis of depression among patients with cancer. The diagnostic tool they found to be most optimal contained six HAM-D items (late-onset insomnia, agitation, psychic anxiety, diurnal mood variation, depressed mood, and reduced libido) and showed a relatively high sensitivity and specificity (Guo et al. 2006). Another approach to identifying treatable symptoms involves characterization of specific clusters of neurobehavioral symptoms that most accurately reflect disease course and allow isolation of neurobiological pathways of adverse treatment effects, thereby stimulating targeted interventions to reduce patient burden and improve quality of life (Capuron et al. 2002).

Cardiovascular Disease and Depression

Epidemiology

In 1988, Carney showed that in comparison with nondepressed persons who had undergone a cardiac catheterization for coronary artery disease, depressed patients who had undergone a cardiac catheterization had an increased risk of angioplasty, coronary bypass surgery, MI, and death within the next 12 months (Carney et al. 1988). In a 1990s study examining whether a diagnosis of MDD in patients hospitalized after an MI would have an effect on cardiac mortality during the first 6 months after discharge, Frasure-Smith and colleagues at the Montreal Heart Institute found that in comparison with nondepressed post-MI patients, post-MI patients with MDD (diagnosed ~7 days after the MI with the modified version of the National Institute of Mental Health Diagnostic Interview Schedule [Robins et al. 1981]) had a three- to fourfold increased cardiac mortality rate over the 18-month follow-up (Frasure-Smith et al. 1993). The lethal effect of depression was most evident in depressed patients with 10 or more premature ventricular contractions (PVCs) per hour (Frasure-Smith et al. 1995). Multiple research teams have subsequently replicated Frasure-Smith's early findings. Meijer et al. (2013) conducted a meta-analysis of 16 studies of post-acute MI patients (N=10,175) and confirmed that after adjustment for cardiac-related variables (i.e., history of MI, left ventricular ejection fraction [LVEF], Killip class), depression remained independently associated with a 13% increased risk of cardiovascular events and a 22% increased risk of all-cause mortality. Mean follow-up time was 1,151 days (3.2 years), with a range of 350 days to 2,428 days (Meijer et al. 2013).

Large-scale community-based epidemiological studies, as well as other studies conducted in the United States and abroad, have also confirmed that depression acts as an independent risk factor for incident coronary heart disease (CHD). A meta-analysis by Gan et al. (2014) that included 893,850 participants in 30 prospective cohort studies (with 40 independent reports) found that depressed patients with no evidence of CHD at baseline exhibited a significantly increased risk of 30% for development of CHD and MI over follow-up periods ranging from 2 to 37 years. The association remained after adjustment (when possible) for the usual risk factors for CHD, including smoking, high BMI, diabetes, hypertension, physical inactivity, high cholesterol, and low socioeconomic status (Gan et al. 2014).

More recent clinical investigations have explored other relevant questions, including the following:

- Is the prevalence of depression greater in certain types of heart disease (or therapeutic intervention)?
- How impactful is the presence of depression compared with other prognostic cardiac risk factors in relation to an acute cardiac event?
- Is the prevalence and/or severity of depression associated with the severity of cardiac disease?
- Is the timing of the onset of depression (i.e., before or after an acute cardiac event) independently predictive of morbidity and mortality?

Individuals who require catheterization due to unstable angina represent a model wherein depression and underlying cardiac disease interact most acutely, and these patients have prevalence rates of diagnosed MDD as high as 42% (Hance et al. 1996). Lespérance et al. (2000) confirmed depression in 41% of patients with unstable angina, which was on average greater than rates of depression observed in congestive heart failure (22% [Rutledge et al. 2006]), post-acute MI (20% [Thombs et al. 2006]), post–coronary artery bypass surgery (20% [Connerney et al. 2001]), and stable coronary artery disease (7% [Frasure-Smith and Lespérance 2008]). In a meta-analysis of 20 studies ($N \geq 11{,}000$) involving patients with a wider range of unstable angina or angiographically validated coronary artery disease, Barth et al. (2004) found that the risk of dying during the 2 years following a cardiac event was two times higher for patients with depressive symptoms or MDD compared with nondepressed patients. A meta-analysis of 22 studies ($N=6{,}367$ MI patients) demonstrated that depression also carries increased risk for mortality among post-MI patients (van Melle et al. 2004). Depressed post-MI patients were found to have a 2.4-fold increased risk (unadjusted) for all-cause mortality relative to nondepressed post-MI patients (van Melle et al. 2004).

Another meta-analysis found that depression at the time of a cardiac event was independently predictive of increased cardiac morbidity and mortality risk, regardless of whether depression onset occurred before or after the onset of acute cardiac illness (Leung et al. 2012). However, for patients with no depression at the time of a cardiac event, having a history of one or more episodes of depression before an index acute cardiac event was not predictive of adverse outcomes (Leung et al. 2012)

Although severity of cardiac disease/dysfunction is not routinely measured in many studies (Freeland and Carney 2013), results from the Dutch clinical MIND-IT (Myocardial Infarction and Depression–Intervention Trial) study showed that in patients who had experienced an index MI ($N=1{,}989$), the prevalence and severity of depression were significantly related to the severity of cardiac dysfunction and the risk of developing congestive heart failure (van Melle et al. 2005).

Treatment of Depression in Patients With Cardiovascular Disease

Three randomized, placebo-controlled trials (Glassman et al. 2002; Lespérance et al. 2007; van Melle et al. 2007) have been conducted to evaluate the effectiveness and tolerability of antidepressant treatment for individuals with MDD with an acute coronary syndrome (ACS; i.e., MI or unstable angina). In the Sertraline Antidepressant Heart Attack Randomized Trial (SADHART), Glassman et al. (2002) evaluated the safety and efficacy of 6 months of treatment with the selective serotonin reuptake inhibitor (SSRI) sertraline (n=186) versus placebo (n=183) for MDD in individuals hospitalized for an ACS. The investigators documented an incidence of severe cardiovascular adverse events of 14.5% with sertraline and 22.4% with placebo. In the total randomized sample, scores on the Clinical Global Impression—Improvement (CGI-I) subscale (P=0.049) favored sertraline, but scores on the HAM-D (P=0.14) did not. The CGI-I responder rates were significantly higher with sertraline than with placebo for patients in the total sample (67% vs. 53%; P=0.01), for patients with at least one prior episode of depression (72% vs. 51%; P=0.003), and for patients with at least one prior episode of depression and greater current severity of depressive symptoms (HAM-D score ≥18) (78% vs. 45%; P=0.001). In the latter two groups, both CGI-I and HAM-D scores were significantly better for patients assigned to sertraline compared with those assigned to placebo (Glassman et al. 2002). SADHART (Glassman et al. 2002) found no evidence of harm with sertraline treatment in cardiac populations, and the incidence of severe cardiac adverse events was numerically lower (although not statistically significant) with sertraline versus placebo. The Canadian Cardiac Randomized Evaluation of Antidepressant and Psychotherapy Efficacy (CREATE) trial showed that the SSRI citalopram, with or without cognitive-behavioral therapy (CBT), was superior to placebo in reducing 12-week HAM-D scores in patients with coronary artery disease and MDD, with a small to medium effect size of 0.33 (Lespérance et al. 2007). The Dutch MIND-IT study examined whether the presynaptic α_2-adrenergic receptor antagonist mirtazapine improved long-term depression and cardiac prognosis after an acute MI (van Melle et al. 2007). First-choice treatment consisted of placebo-controlled pharmacotherapy with mirtazapine; in the event of refusal or insufficient response after 8 weeks, open-label treatment with citalopram was offered as an alternative. No differences were observed between the intervention and control groups in mean Beck Depression Inventory (Beck and Steer 1987) scores, and the cardiac event rate was also similar between the intervention group and the control group (van Melle et al. 2007).

Interestingly, two large randomized controlled trials (RCTs) by O'Connor et al. (2010) (N=469) and by Angermann et al. (2016) (N=372) of depressed patients with New York Heart Association class II–IV heart failure and reduced left ventricular fraction (≤45% and <45%, respectively) found that neither sertraline (initial dosage of 50 mg/day, up to 200 mg/day) nor escitalopram (dosage of 10–20 mg/day) was better than placebo in improving depression.

Psychotherapy, not just antidepressant treatment, has also been used as a therapeutic intervention in depressed post-MI patients. The large-scale randomized Enhancing Recovery in Coronary Heart Disease Patients (ENRICHD) trial (N=2,482) utilized individual or group CBT to treat post-MI patients with depression and/or low social support. In comparison with patients who received usual medical care, patients who received CBT showed statistically significant improvement in depressive symptoms (mean [SD] change in HAM-D score, −10.1 [7.8] in the CBT group vs. −8.4 [7.7] in the usual care group (P<0.001]) (Berkman et al. 2003). Of note is that CBT did not improve survival in the intervention group, a result similar to that found in other randomized clinical trials that showed limited or no improvement in important cardiac-related outcomes (e.g., rehospitalizations, mortality) in response to psychological interventions (Baumeister et al. 2011).

Comorbid depression has been shown to impair self-care in patients with CHD, which is another "pathway" whereby depression is associated with increased risk of medical complications and mortality (Katon et al. 2010). Collaborative care models for management of mental health conditions in patients with cardiovascular illness were reviewed by Huffman et al. (2018). Such models utilize a nonphysician care manager to identify depression (and/or other psychiatric conditions), obtain recommendations from a team psychiatrist, and relay the treatment plan to the prescribing primary medical provider and the patient (Huffman et al. 2018). Although collaborative care models can be effective in improving mood, anxiety, social functioning, and mental health–related quality of life in patients with cardiovascular disease, to date these models have shown only a limited positive effect on medical outcomes (e.g., cardiac-related readmissions) (Huffman et al. 2018).

Finally, Rutledge et al. (2013) performed a meta-analysis (N=9,896) to evaluate mental health–focused care (psychotherapy and antidepressant medication) and cardiac rehabilitation therapies for reducing secondary events and improving depression severity in individuals with CHD. They found that the mental health therapies showed moderate efficacy in reducing CHD events and had a medium effect size in improving depression, although these treatments did not reduce total mortality. In contrast, cardiac rehabilitation (typically consisting of supervised graded exercise) showed efficacy similar to that of mental health therapies in improving depression and reducing CHD events—and, importantly, also reduced total mortality. Rutledge et al. (2013) concluded that their findings supported a continued role for psychotherapy and pharmacotherapy in tandem with a greater role for cardiac rehabilitation interventions (e.g., exercise-based) in mental health treatment of individuals with CHD and comorbid depression.

Diabetes and Depression

Epidemiology

The first meta-analysis to demonstrate an increased prevalence of depression among patients with diabetes was published by Anderson et al. in 2001. In their analysis, Anderson et al. (2001) estimated the odds and prevalence of depression in diabetes from 39 studies (N=20,218) and found that diabetes doubled the odds of having depression (OR=2.0, 95% CI: 1.8–2.2). In the studies examined, the reported prevalence of depression varied by patient gender (28% in woman with diabetes vs. 18% in men with diabetes), study design (30% in uncontrolled vs. 21% in controlled studies), patient source (32% in clinical samples vs. 20% in community samples), and depression assessment method used (31% in self-report vs. 11% with diagnostic interview). Surprisingly, despite differences in clinical onset of illness (i.e., younger onset in persons with type 1 diabetes) and in management of disease (i.e., typically more complex treatment regimens in persons with type 1 diabetes), the prevalence rates of depression in persons with type 1 diabetes (21.3%) versus type 2 diabetes (27%) were statistically similar (Anderson et al. 2001). Also in 2001, a meta-analysis of 27 studies (N=5,374 adult patients with type 1 or type 2 diabetes) by de Groot et al. (2001) found that depression was significantly associated with a variety of diabetes complications (e.g., retinopathy, nephropathy, neuropathy, macrovascular complications, sexual dysfunction). In a systematic review and meta-analysis of 10 large-scale controlled, community-based cross-sectional studies (N=51,331), Ali et al. (2006) confirmed that rates of depression in adults with type 2 diabetes (18%) were significantly higher than rates in control subjects (10%). Moreover, Wang et al. (2019), in a meta-analysis of 26 studies (8 cohort, 8 cross-sectional epidemiological, 10 case-control) (N=96,842), reported a point prevalence for MDD of 14.5% in individuals with type 2 diabetes. Patients with type 2 diabetes were more likely to have MDD than were individuals in the general population. Along with study site, diagnostic criteria, and age, study type significantly moderated the prevalence of MDD. For example, in the 10 case-control studies examined, the point prevalence of MDD was 9.2% (95% CI: 3.2–23.7; I^2=99.2%) in the type 2 diabetes group compared with 4.3% (95% CI: 1.2–14.1; I^2=99.9%) in the general population. Conversely, a meta-analysis by Vancampfort et al. (2015) showed that patients with MDD (10 studies; N=154,366) had a significantly increased risk of type 2 diabetes relative to general population control subjects (10 studies; N=2,098,063). This increased risk for type 2 diabetes among individuals with MDD remained even after adjustment for the usual risk factors for type 2 diabetes.

Similar to findings in studies examining depression and heart disease, other meta-analyses of large-scale, community-based studies have found that depression is an independent risk factor for the development of incident type 2 diabetes (Mezuk et al. 2008; Rotella and Mannucci 2013; Yu et al. 2015), even after adjustment for demographic characteristics (e.g., age, sex, race, socioeconomic indicators, marital status/household composition) or for prominent effect modifiers (i.e., family history of diabetes; health behaviors such as excess caloric intake, smoking, physical inactivity, adiposity). In a meta-analysis of 33 articles examining individuals with depression (N=2,411,641), Yu et al. (2015) documented that depressed people have a 41% increased risk for developing diabetes mellitus and a 32% increased risk for developing type 2 diabetes.

Depression in Patients With Diabetes as a Risk Factor for Diabetes-Related Morbidity and Mortality

As is the case in heart disease, nonadherence to self-care is one way that depression leads to negative health outcomes in patients with diabetes and other medical disorders (Gonzalez et al. 2008a, 2008b). Compared with nondepressed patients with diabetes, depressed diabetic patients tend to be less adherent to diabetes self-care guidelines and to experience greater glycemic dyscontrol (even at subclinical levels of depression) (Gonzalez et al. 2007), exhibit more functional disability (Egede 2004), have longer hospital stays (Davydow et al. 2011), and have a higher prevalence of end-organ diabetic disease (e.g., retinopathy, nephropathy, neuropathy, sexual dysfunction, macrovascular complications) (Coleman et al. 2013), including cognitive decline and dementia (Exalto et al. 2013; Katon et al. 2015; Sullivan et al. 2013), with the accumulated burden of these negative outcomes conferring a lower life expectancy (Egede et al. 2005).

Pathophysiology of Depression in Diabetes

Potential pathways through which depression may mediate or moderate type 2 diabetes include activation of the HPA axis (i.e., increased cortisol release) and the sympathetic nervous system (i.e., increased catecholamine release) as well as poor health behaviors (i.e., decreased physical activity and increased caloric intake) (Golden 2007; Roose et al. 2006).

Treatment of Depression in Patients With Diabetes

Three types of therapeutic modalities have been utilized to ameliorate depression in patients with diabetes: psychotherapy, antidepressant pharmacotherapy, and collaborative care models. Van der Feltz-Cornelis et al. (2010) conducted a meta-analysis of 14 RCTs (N=1,724) evaluating the efficacy of interventions designed to treat depression in patients with diabetes. The effect size was large (–0.581) for improvement in depressive symptoms in response to psychotherapeutic interventions in tandem with educational interventions focused on diabetes self-care and was moderate (–0.467) for symptom improvement in response to pharmacological interventions (five of the six pharmacotherapy studies used antidepressants only, while Lustman et al. [1997] used glucometer training plus nortriptyline versus placebo). All five of the psychotherapy interventions were associated with significant improvements in glycemic control; however, three of these studies also featured interventions aimed at improving self-management of diabetes, a confounding variable that makes it difficult to identify which treatment was most helpful, and the small overall number of participants limits generalizability. In an RCT conducted by Lustman et al. (1998), 51 patients with type 2 diabetes and depression were randomly assigned to 10 weeks of either individual CBT or a control condition involving no specific antidepressant treatment. Both groups of patients participated in a diabetes education program, and at the end of treatment, hemoglobin A1c (HbA1c) levels were not different between the groups. However, at 6-month follow-up, mean HbA1c levels were better in the CBT group than in the control group (9.5% vs. 10.9%, respectively; P=0.03). Pharmacotherapy (6 studies, N=281), like collaborative care models (3 studies; N=1,133), reduced depressive symptoms but, aside from the sertraline-versus-placebo study (Echeverry et al. 2009), had no effect on glycemic control (van der Feltz-Cornelis et al. 2010). In their 6-month double-blind RCT examining the effect of pharmacotherapy with sertraline on HbA1c levels in patients with diabetes (n=87 patients with type 2 and n=2 with type 1), Echeverry et al. (2009) found significant reductions in HbA1c levels from baseline to 6 months in both sertraline-treated and placebo-treated patients; however, reductions in the sertraline group were more than twice as great as those in the placebo group (–2.0%±2.1 vs. –0.9%±2.0; P=0.003).

Unfortunately, alleviating depressive symptoms does not reliably confer improvements in self-care and glycemic control (Katon et al. 2004) when depression treatment does not specifically target adherence to diabetes treatment (Padilla et al. 2017). Of relevance in this regard is that collaborative care models are designed to provide "co-treatment" of depression and chronic medical illnesses such as diabetes. A meta-analysis of seven short- to medium-term RCTs examining collaborative care for depression in adults with comorbid depression and chronic illness (i.e., diabetes, coronary heart disease, or both conditions), conducted predominantly in the United States (N=1,895 participants), showed that for depression, the difference in the standardized mean depression score was −0.32 (95% CI: −0.53 to −0.11; I^2=79%), and for HbA1c level, the weighted mean difference was −0.33% (95% CI: −0.66% to −0.00%; I^2=72.9%), compared with control conditions (Atlantis et al. 2014). Depression remission did not predict improved glycemic control across studies. Notably, consensus groups have proposed thresholds for what constitutes "clinically significant change" in depression (i.e., reduction of 3 or more points [or > 50% decrease from baseline] on the HAM-D; National Institute for Health and Clinical Excellence 2009) and in diabetes (i.e., 0.5% decrease from baseline in HbA1c levels; [Little et al. 2011]).

Stroke and Depression

Epidemiology

Stroke is the fifth-leading cause of death in the United States (Xu et al. 2018) and is a major cause of disability worldwide (Mozaffarian et al. 2016), with most of the burden occurring in low-income and middle-income countries (Feigin et al. 2017). As the definition of stroke has not been consistently established (Easton et al. 2009), the Stroke Council of the American Heart Association/American Stroke Association now defines a central nervous system infarction ("stroke") as a "brain, spinal cord, or retinal cell death attributable to ischemia, based on neuropathological, neuroimaging, and/or clinical evidence of permanent injury." Stroke occurs over a clinical spectrum including intracerebral hemorrhage and subarachnoid hemorrhage (Sacco et al. 2013). Statistical projections have shown that by 2030, an additional 3.4 million U.S. adults older than 18 years (3.9% of the adult population) will have had a stroke, a 20.5% increase in stroke prevalence compared with 2012. The highest increase (29%) is projected to occur among White Hispanic males (Ovbiagele et al. 2013).

Stroke is a major circulatory disease condition mediated by cardiovascular health status. Around 90% of stroke risk can be attributed to modifiable risk factors, such as high blood pressure, obesity, and hyperglycemia (O'Donnell et al. 2016). Up to 74% of the risk can be attributed to specific modifiable behavioral risk factors, such as smoking, alcohol use, sedentary lifestyle, and poor diet (Benjamin et al. 2019; GBD 2016 Disease and Injury Incidence and Prevalence Collaborators 2016). Globally, the risk of stroke has also been attributed to air pollution (Babatola et al. 2018; Stafoggia et al. 2014).

With proper identification and emergency treatment following a stroke, the chances of individual long-term survival increase. Poststroke depression affects approximately one-third of all stroke survivors (Hackett and Pickles 2014) and usually appears within the first 3 months after a stroke; among patients who experience poststroke depression, 15%–57% recover from the depression within 1 year following their stroke (Ayerbe et al. 2013). Individuals with poststroke depression exhibit poorer functional outcomes (Kutlubaev and Hackett 2014), worsened quality of life (Kim et al. 2018), and higher mortality rates in comparison with nondepressed stroke patients (Bartoli et al. 2018).

Thus, in 2017, the American Heart Association Stroke Council's Scientific Statements Oversight Committee and the American Heart Association's Manuscript Oversight Committee appointed an expert group to develop the first scientific statement from the American Heart Association about poststroke depression. The group created a specific summary of findings as an available tool for clinicians to further understand the causes, predisposing factors, epidemiology, screening, treatment, and prevention of poststroke depression, as well as management implications for clinical practice (Towfighi et al. 2017).

Pathophysiology of Poststroke Depression

The pathophysiology of poststroke depression has been described as multifactorial and complex because the depression is thought to involve a combination of neurobiological dysfunction and psychosocial factors. From a neurobiological perspective, poststroke depression could be mediated by monoamine pathway alterations, increased pro-inflammatory cytokines, HPA axis dysfunction, and stroke-induced immune/inflammatory response leading to changes in neuroplasticity (Villa et al. 2018). The vascular depression hypothesis posited that even silent cerebral lesions can disrupt the cortico-striato-pallido-thalamo-cortical pathways, resulting in depressive symptoms, which could explain the biological pathogenesis of poststroke depression (Alexopoulos et al. 1999; Feng et al. 2014). In an attempt to understand the complex neurobiological pathogenesis of poststroke depression, researchers have explored neuroanatomical factors such as lesion location and size (Feng et al. 2014; Nickel and Thomalla 2017). Systematic methodological limitations (Bhogal et al. 2004) have hampered efforts to find a clear association between poststroke depression and lesion location, and these limitations may explain why many studies have found no relationship between poststroke depression and lesion location (Aben et al. 2006; Caeiro et al. 2006; Nickel and Thomalla 2017; Snaphaam et al. 2009). However, an association has been suggested between poststroke depression and the size of the infarction (i.e., total volume of the brain affected, irrespective of location), although no definitive impact has been established (Nickel and Thomalla 2017; Nys et al. 2005; Vataja et al. 2004; Zhang et al. 2012).

A 2017 meta-analytic review of 36 studies found that a history of mental illness (i.e., depression and/or anxiety) was the highest-ranking risk factor for poststroke depression; other risk factors included a family history of mental illness, age greater than 70 years, female gender, greater stroke severity, and the presence of neuroticism (Shi et al. 2017). Also contributing to risk was the level of handicap (which reflects the degree of disability as well as the degree of brain damage) during the first 3 months after stroke.

Screening and Prevention of Poststroke Depression

A 2014 meta-analysis of 24 studies (N=2,907) found the Center for Epidemiological Studies Depression Scale (CES-D; Radloff 1977), the HAM-D, and the PHQ-9 to be the most optimal screening tools for poststroke depression (Meader et al. 2014). Further studies are needed to determine whether screening for poststroke depression in addition to early interventions and follow-up improves outcomes for those at higher risk of poststroke depression.

Given the increased burden, morbidity, and mortality associated with poststroke depression, preventive interventions are a key component of treatment. In 2008, a Cochrane review of 14 RCTs involving 1,515 subjects found that antidepressants did not prevent poststroke depression; however, a small but significant beneficial effect was identified for psychotherapy (Hackett et al. 2008). In contrast, a 2012 meta-analysis of eight RCTs including 776 initially nondepressed stroke patients described the efficacy of using antidepressants as a prophylactic pharmacological intervention against poststroke depression. In this investigation, pooled analyses showed that the likelihood of developing poststroke depression was reduced in stroke patients who received active antidepressant treatment if such treatment was initiated within the first few months after a stroke (Salter et al. 2013). In regard to antidepressant classes, this meta-analysis examined four trials (*N*=401), with each RCT finding a benefit for antidepressant over placebo, and with SSRI use associated with a significant reduction in the risk for poststroke depression (Salter et al. 2013). Furthermore, a 2016 meta-analysis (11 studies; 1,258 participants) that specifically examined the protective role of sertraline against poststroke depression found that the incidence was significantly lower in the sertraline group compared with the control group (Feng et al. 2018). The appropriate timing and duration of psychopharmacological treatment required to confer the most effective prevention against poststroke depression remains unclear.

Treatment of Poststroke Depression

In addition to examining the utility of screening and preventive interventions for poststroke depression, studies have explored antidepressants and alternatives to pharmacological management for the treatment of poststroke depression (Paolucci 2008; Villa et al. 2018), including psychosocial interventions (e.g., CBT) and neuromodulation (Towfighi et al. 2017).

Most of the available clinical evidence regarding treatment of poststroke depression is related to the use of antidepressants, although there are insufficient data to conduct a meta-analysis examining specific medications. CBT has been the most widely used psychosocial intervention, despite inconclusive data due to lack of high-quality RCTs. A 2018 meta-analysis including 23 CBT studies (*N*=1,972) found positive effects for CBT alone (vs. attention intervention and routine rehabilitation), CBT combined with antidepressants (vs. antidepressants alone), and CBT with or without antidepressants (vs. placebo with or without antidepressants), with significantly higher rates of response and remission of poststroke depression in all of these active conditions (Wang et al. 2018).

Antidepressants have also been studied for their potential role in motor recovery after ischemic stroke, mediated by their effects on serotonergic and dopaminergic pathways (Cramer 2015). Among classes of psychotropic medications, a 2010 narrative review suggested moderate evidence for SSRIs, tricyclic antidepressants, and stimulants, with no evidence for atypical antipsychotics or mood stabilizers in the treatment of poststroke depression (Capaldi and Wynn 2010). The FLAME study, an RCT including 118 patients, found that in patients with ischemic stroke and moderate to severe motor deficits, early prescription of fluoxetine with physiotherapy improved motor recovery after 3 months (Chollet et al. 2011).

Among stroke patients, the role and efficacy of stimulants has been mostly described in case reports, open-label trials, and a small RCT. Stimulants such as methylphenidate have been used for treatment of depression and fatigue in medically ill individuals, to augment response to SSRIs, and to improve poststroke motor recovery

(Grade et al. 1998; Lazarus et al. 1992; Martinsson and Eksborg 2004; Walker-Batson et al. 1995, 2016). In general, stimulants in poststroke depression should be used with caution over a short period of time, at the minimum needed dosage, with slow titration, and while monitoring for potential side effects (Capaldi and Wynn 2010).

Neuromodulation techniques such as electroconvulsive therapy (ECT), transcranial direct current stimulation (tDCS), and repetitive transcranial magnetic stimulation (rTMS) are commonly used to target severe depressive symptoms; however, the role of these techniques in poststroke depression is not well established despite recent emerging evidence (Bucur and Papagno 2018; Liu et al. 2019; Shen et al. 2017). Currently, there are no published RCTs documenting the utility or efficacy of ECT in poststroke depression. The first published systematic review and meta-analysis of the use of rTMS for treatment of poststroke depression (Shen et al. 2017) reviewed 22 RCTs (N= 1,764 patients). rTMS was found to improve depression response rates (50% or more reduction in the baseline HAM-D score at the end of treatment), stroke severity, and activities of daily living in poststroke depression, whereas no significant difference from the control conditions was found related to remission rates (predefined HAM-D-based remission criteria from each individual trial) (Shen et al. 2017). A 2019 meta-analysis of 17 RCTs (N=1,053) exploring the efficacy and safety of high-frequency rTMS for patients with poststroke depression (Liu et al. 2019) found significant positive effects on depression, with adequate response and remission rates in comparison with control groups. Because poststroke depression negatively affects functional outcomes and recovery while increasing morbidity and mortality, it is crucial to study and understand the mechanisms modulating poststroke depression to further identify appropriate and effective therapeutic intervention modalities after stroke survival.

Cancer and Depression

Epidemiology

Receiving a diagnosis of cancer is a significant psychosocial stressor that can precipitate emergence of a depressive disorder. Depression in patients with cancer often goes undetected in clinical practice, and diagnostic factors are an important cause of this underrecognition (Caruso et al. 2017a). The concept of depressive spectrum disorders has been proposed as a helpful model to address the different manifestations of depression in patients with cancer, including MDD, persistent depressive disorder (dysthymia), and subsyndromal depression (Caruso et al. 2017b). A large-scale prospective study (N=8,387) that examined the risk of developing significant depressive symptoms after a new diagnosis of one of seven different medical conditions (cancer, diabetes, hypertension, heart disease, arthritis, chronic lung disease, or stroke) found that within 2 years of the initial diagnosis, individuals with cancer had the highest risk of depressive symptoms, followed by individuals with chronic lung disease and those with heart disease (Polsky et al. 2005). Prevalence rates of depression generally increase in the context of neoplastic progression and high levels of pain; in addition, immunotherapy agents (including interferon-α) used in some cancers (e.g., melanoma) have been reported to cause depression in up to 50% of patients (Smith 2015]).

Pancreatic, oropharyngeal, and lung cancer are associated with the highest rates of depression, with prevalences averaging 33%–50%, 22%–57%, and 11%–44%, respectively (Massie 2004). Risk of suicide also differs with certain types of cancer. In a retrospective population-based study of data for 8,651,569 patients with cancer in the Surveillance, Epidemiology, and End Results program conducted over the years 1973 to 2014, Zaorsky et al. (2019) found that 13,311 of these patients died by suicide. The standardized mortality ratio (SMR) of suicide was 4.44 (95% CI: 4.33–4.55); that is, patients with cancer were four times more likely than people in the general population to kill themselves. Patients with cancers of the lung, head and neck, testes, or bladder and those with Hodgkin's lymphoma had the highest SMRs (>5–10), and those who died by suicide were largely older than 50 years (particularly white, unmarried males) and had a diagnosis of cancer of the prostate, lung, bladder, or colon/rectum.

In a meta-analysis of 25 studies of patients with cancer (N=2,097), depression was associated with a 25% higher mortality rate in patients experiencing depressive symptoms and a 39% higher mortality rate in patients with DSM-IV (American Psychiatric Association 1994) minor depression or MDD (Satin et al. 2009). Adjustment for usual prognostic factors did not reduce the deleterious effects of depression on cancer survival (Satin et al. 2009).

In contrast to the extant literature focused on depression as a risk factor for heart disease, diabetes, and stroke, evidence suggesting that depression may be a risk factor for the incidence of cancer is mixed. Although some large-scale studies suggest that depression is a risk factor for cancer (Gross et al. 2010; Penninx et al. 1998), other studies have found no such association (Dalton et al. 2002; Linkins and Comstock 1990; Oerlemans et al. 2007). These discrepant findings might be explained by differences in follow-up time, sample size, assessment methods, and chronicity of depression or by failure to control for confounding variables (Currier and Nemeroff 2014).

Treatment of Depression in Patients With Cancer

Antidepressant treatment for patients with cancer has involved psychotherapy (Okuyama et al. 2017), psychopharmacotherapy (Ostuzzi et al. 2018), and collaborative care models. Okuyama et al. (2017) performed a meta-analysis of 12 RCTs (N=1,067) that compared psychotherapy against control conditions (e.g., treatment as usual) for treatment of depression in patients with advanced, incurable cancer. Psychotherapy was associated with moderate decreases in depression scores, but the authors of the meta-analysis concluded that there was not enough high-quality evidence to support the effectiveness of psychotherapy for patients with cancer who had clinically diagnosed depression. Noted limitations on generalizability included the focus on non-terminally-ill patients with advanced cancer with depressive symptomatology (rather than a clinical diagnosis of MDD). Moreover, a review by Barrera and Spiegel (2014) noted that study findings were mixed regarding how psychotherapeutic interventions affect survival rate, with some studies demonstrating that psychotherapy slowed disease progression and others documenting no survival benefit for those treated with psychotherapy.

With regard to psychopharmacological treatments, a Cochrane review meta-analysis found very-low-quality evidence for an effect of antidepressants as a class on symptoms of depression in patients with cancer compared with placebo when measured as a continuous outcome (five RCTs, N=266) (Ostuzzi et al. 2018). On subgroup analysis by cancer site, the effect size was greater for antidepressants versus placebo in patients with breast cancer (two RCTs, N=90) relative to patients with other cancer types (three RCTs, N=176). Subgroup analysis by cancer stage indicated a greater effect size for antidepressant treatment (vs. placebo) for patients with late-stage cancer (one RCT, N=24) relative to patients with early-stage cancer (one RCT, N=69). Ostuzzi et al. (2018) concluded that the use of antidepressants in people with cancer should be considered on a patient-by-patient basis, and the choice of which agent to prescribe may be based on efficacy data for the general population of individuals with MDD, taking into consideration drug-drug interactions and the positive safety profile of SSRIs. In summary, current evidence suggests that psychotherapy and antidepressant medications are no more effective than placebo in depressed patients with cancer (Okuyama et al. 2017; Ostuzzi et al. 2018). Further studies are clearly needed to break down treatment response to psychotherapy and pharmacotherapy approaches by important covariables such as pain levels and tumor location and stage.

Li et al. (2017) recently performed a meta-analysis comparing the efficacy of collaborative care (four RCTs, N=1,989) and pharmacological (eight RCTs, N=722) and psychological (nine RCTs, N=786) treatments. Collaborative care interventions were significantly more effective than usual care in reducing depression scores (SMD=−0.49; P=0.003), and the reduction in scores was sustained at 12 months. By comparison, short-term (up to 12 weeks) but not longer-term effectiveness was demonstrated for both psychological and pharmacological interventions (Li et al. 2017). Remaining to be determined is whether collaborative care interventions can routinely and effectively reduce depression in patients with cancer over sustained periods of time and extend survival in these patients (Pinquart and Duberstein 2010).

HIV and Depression

Epidemiology

Depression has been considered the most common neuropsychiatric disorder in persons living with HIV (Rabkin 2008; Simoni et al. 2011), with this mood disorder often comorbid with substance use disorders. Depression not only is a risk factor for becoming HIV positive (Perry et al. 1990) but is also associated with an increased rate of HIV progression to AIDS (Leserman et al. 2002), resulting in reduced survival among HIV-positive depressed people accessing antiretroviral therapy (ART) (Lima et al. 2007). Depression, like substance misuse, plausibly acts as a "vector" for dissemination of HIV by increasing risky behaviors that promote HIV transmission (e.g., unprotected sex [van Empelen et al. 2003]), impairing ART adherence, and inhibiting the ability of individuals with HIV to navigate each stage of the HIV care cascade: diagnosis of HIV infection, linkage to care, retention in care, receipt of antiretroviral therapy, and achievement of HIV suppression.

Conversely, the prevalence of MDD among persons living with HIV infection appears to be twice that among HIV-negative individuals, as suggested by a meta-analysis of 10 studies (N=2,596 persons) (Ciesla and Roberts 2001). Approximately

20%–50% of HIV-infected individuals in the United States and abroad experience depressive symptoms (Bing et al. 2001). Wang et al. (2018) recently analyzed 74 observational studies involving 20,635 persons living with HIV in China, producing a prevalence of depression or depressive symptoms of 51% among HIV-positive individuals who were not intravenous drug users.

Furthermore, systemic illnesses comorbid with or secondary to HIV infection, such as hepatitis, *Pneumocystis carinii* pneumonia, CNS disease (intracerebral infection or malignancy), endocrinopathies (adrenal insufficiency, hypogonadism and hypothyroidism), and malnourishment (particularly with deficiencies in vitamins B_6 and B_{12}), can mimic depression. The ART efavirenz (frequently prescribed for patients with HIV [combined with emtricitabine and tenofovir disoproxil fumarate in one pill taken once daily]) can also cause mood disturbances. HIV-positive patients experience pain from a variety of sources that can create depressive symptoms. Over time, the pathophysiology of HIV can damage subcortical and cortical areas of the brain and produce HIV dementia, resulting in symptoms that are frequently mistaken for clinical depression.

Unfortunately, nearly all chronic health conditions increase suicide risk, and individuals with multiple (two or more) chronic health conditions have at least a twofold increased suicide risk in comparison with individuals with none or only one chronic health condition. Compared with people not diagnosed with HIV/AIDS, people living with HIV/AIDS have a twofold increased risk of suicide (Ahmedani et al. 2017).

Pathophysiology of Depression in HIV

In acute infection, CNS immune activation after HIV entry into brain is associated with depression (Hellmuth et al. 2017). As reviewed by Rivera-Rivera et al. (2016), the pathophysiology of depression during chronic HIV-1 infection is maintained by the release of proinflammatory cytokines, thereby activating the HPA axis and leading to cortisol and monoamine imbalance.

Depression also alters the immune response in HIV, especially in the presence of severe stress, via decline in lymphocyte subsets (e.g., $CD16^+$ and $CD56^+$ natural killer cells, $CD8^+$ cytotoxic/suppressor T cells) (Leserman et al. 1997). That immune perturbations resulting from increased cortisol and a heightened sympathetic response to stress and depression impact disease progression of HIV in humans is less clear (Leserman et al. 2002). Depression is a risk factor for both HIV viral load increase and $CD4^+$ cell count decline, even after controlling for adherence to ART (Ironson et al. 2015). Thus, in addition to facilitating behavioral transmission, depression accelerates HIV disease progression (Nanni et al. 2015). Moreover, depression is associated with increased risk for all-cause mortality in persons with HIV, as reported in a recent cohort study of U.S. military veterans (N=129,140), in which elevated depressive symptoms ascertained via the PHQ-9 were found to be associated with a significantly increased mortality risk among veterans with HIV infection (24% increased risk) but not among those without HIV infection (nonsignificant 4% increased risk) (So-Armah et al. 2019).

Of note is that an incremental relationship between symptoms of depression and risk for treatment nonadherence, observable at both lower and higher levels of depression severity, does not support the idea that depression becomes a risk factor for nonadherence only when it reaches the threshold for a clinical diagnosis (Gonzalez et al. 2011). Instead, a greater amount of time spent with depression was associated in a dose-response fashion with a higher risk of missing appointments for HIV primary care, a higher risk of having a detectable viral load, and higher mortality rates (Pence et al. 2018).

Treatment of Depression in Patients With HIV

In a meta-analysis of 29 controlled studies (published through 2012) of 12,243 individuals living with HIV/AIDS, Sin and DiMatteo (2014) examined the effect of depression treatment on ART adherence. In this analysis, depression treatment was broadly defined as any intervention aimed at alleviating depressive symptoms or psychological distress (e.g., psychotherapy, antidepressant medication, CBT for stress management). Although the average effect size for depression treatment was modest ($r=0.15$, $P<0.001$) in comparison with the effect sizes for the control conditions (e.g., standard care, wait-list control, psychoeducational program), individuals with HIV exhibited an 83% increased odds of adherence to ART if they were treated for depression and a 35% greater risk of nonadherence if they were not treated for depression (Sin and DiMatteo 2014).

In a subsequent systematic review, Eshun-Wilson et al. (2018) examined 10 RCTs (conducted between January 1, 1980, and April 18, 2017) of antidepressant therapy compared with placebo only (2 studies) or compared with placebo and another antidepressant drug class (8 studies). Overall, 709 depressed adults living with HIV were included in the review, and outcomes were assessed with HAM-D scores or CGI-I scores. Pooled data from the 6 studies ($N=357$) that compared mean change in HAM-D scores showed moderate improvement in depression, with a greater reduction in HAM-D scores among participants receiving antidepressants than among those receiving placebo (Eshun-Wilson et al. 2018).

Another recent meta-analysis (involving 5,095 participants recruited from 1997 to 2013 into 43 RCTs) examined the utility of psychosocial interventions in improving ART adherence in persons living with HIV (Spaan et al. 2020). Intervention characteristics included treatment type (CBT, peer/social support, or counseling), provider (psychologist/psychiatrist, counselor, nurse, peer, health care professional, or other), setting (individual, group, or both), and use of cognitive and/or behavioral techniques, motivational interviewing, or relaxation. The overall effect size indicated a small to moderate positive effect (Hedges' $g=0.37$) of psychosocial interventions on medication adherence in people living with HIV (Spaan et al. 2020). Study and intervention characteristics were investigated as moderators; many different forms of psychosocial treatment in many different settings were effective, possibly due to common effective factors such as the therapeutic alliance. Interestingly, objective measures (e.g., pill count, monitoring device) that did not rely on patient recall might have been more sensitive to changes in adherence than subjective measures that relied on self-report (Spaan et al. 2020).

Treatment of depression is of paramount importance for people living with HIV. Treatment-naive HIV-positive persons who have recently started ART and who are nonadherent and experiencing significant depressive symptoms (i.e., a CES-D score >16) show the highest mortality in comparison with depressed persons who are able to be adherent to their ART (Lima et al. 2007). Therefore, the challenge is arguably to offer effective (and tolerable) depression treatment to HIV-positive persons, with concomitant tracking and support of ART compliance in order to reduce HIV-related morbidity and mortality (Wagner et al. 2014).

Conclusion

Large-scale epidemiological studies continue to document that depression is an independent risk factor for the development of heart disease, stroke, and diabetes, and that it contributes to the transmission of HIV and the accelerated progression of HIV to AIDS. Although depressed individuals can struggle with adherence to medical treatments, thereby incurring increased risk for morbidity, reduced survival, and diminished quality of life, the underlying pathophysiology of depression, especially inflammation and pain, may also reduce the effectiveness of "antidepression" pharmacotherapies and psychotherapies aimed at relieving the suffering of patients with congestive heart failure or cancer. Conversely, secondary interventions designed to prevent the onset of depression after an index event—for example, the use of antidepressants or psychotherapy for persons at risk of poststroke depression—appear most promising at this juncture. Unfortunately, alleviation of depression is not always associated with improvement in glycemic control or hypertension; therefore, integrated or collaborative care models in real-world clinical settings may offer an advantage over short-term, placebo-controlled psychopharmacology or psychotherapy trials for individuals with multiple medical conditions. Moreover, ongoing and future studies targeting depression "early in the game" offer additional hope for patients and researchers alike, as pathophysiological alterations related to depression can contribute to prediabetes, hyperlipidemia, and hypertension prior to the onset of diabetes, myocardial infarction, and cerebrovascular events. When preemptive antidepressant treatment is able to reduce the incidence of these "end-stage" conditions, depression's "mind-body" connection as a clinical risk factor will be ultimately confirmed.

References

Aben I, Lodder J, Honig A, et al: Focal or generalized vascular brain damage and vulnerability to depression after stroke: a 1-year prospective follow-up study. Int Psychogeriatr 18(1):19–35, 2006 16403249

Adinolfi LE, Nevola R, Rinaldi L, et al: Chronic hepatitis C virus infection and depression. Clin Liver Dis 21(3):517–534, 2017 28689590

Ahmedani BK, Peterson EL, Hu Y, et al: Major physical health conditions and risk of suicide. Am J Prev Med 53(3):308–315, 2017 28619532

Alexopoulos GS, Bruce ML, Silbersweig D, et al: Vascular depression: a new view of late-onset depression. Dialogues Clin Neurosci 1(2):68–80, 1999 22033775

Ali S, Stone MA, Peters JL, et al: The prevalence of co-morbid depression in adults with type 2 diabetes: a systematic review and meta-analysis. Diabet Med 23(11):1165–1173, 2006 17054590

American Psychiatric Association: Diagnostic and Statistical Manual of Mental Disorders, 4th Edition. Washington, DC, American Psychiatric Association, 1994

Anda R, Williamson D, Jones D, et al: Depressed affect, hopelessness, and the risk of ischemic heart disease in a cohort of U.S. adults. Epidemiology 4(4):285–294, 1993 8347738

Anderson RJ, Freedland KE, Clouse RE, et al: The prevalence of comorbid depression in adults with diabetes: a meta-analysis. Diabetes Care 24(6):1069–1078, 2001 11375373

Angermann CE, Gelbrich G, Störk S, et al: Effect of escitalopram on all-cause mortality and hospitalization in patients with heart failure and depression: the MOOD-HF randomized clinical trial. JAMA 315(24):2683–2693, 2016 27367876

Atlantis E, Fahey P, Foster J: Collaborative care for comorbid depression and diabetes: a systematic review and meta-analysis. BMJ Open 4(4):1–10, 2014. Available at: https://bmjopen.bmj.com/content/bmjopen/4/4/e004706.full.pdf. Accessed October 26, 2021.

Ayerbe L, Ayis S, Wolfe CD, et al: Natural history, predictors and outcomes of depression after stroke: systematic review and meta-analysis. Br J Psychiatry 202(1):14–21, 2013 23284148

Babatola SS: Global burden of diseases attributable to air pollution. J Public Health Afr 9(3):813, 2018 30687484

Barrera I, Spiegel D: Review of psychotherapeutic interventions on depression in cancer patients and their impact on disease progression. Int Rev Psychiatry 26(1):31–43, 2014 24716499

Barth J, Schumacher M, Herrmann-Lingen C: Depression as a risk factor for mortality in patients with coronary heart disease: a meta-analysis. Psychosom Med 66(6):802–813, 2004 15564343

Bartoli F, Di Brita C, Crocamo C, et al: Early post-stroke depression and mortality: meta-analysis and meta-regression. Front Psychiatry 9:530, 2018 30443225

Baumeister H, Hutter N, Bengel J: Psychological and pharmacological interventions for depression in patients with coronary artery disease. Cochrane Database Syst Rev 9(9):CD008012, 2011 21901717

Beck AT, Steer RA: Beck Depression Inventory: Manual. New York, Harcourt Brace Jovanovich, 1987

Benjamin EJ, Muntner P, Alonso A, et al: Heart disease and stroke statistics—2019 update: a report from the American Heart Association. Circulation 139(10):e56–e528, 2019 30700139

Berkman LF, Blumenthal J, Burg M, et al: Effects of treating depression and low perceived social support on clinical events after myocardial infarction: the Enhancing Recovery in Coronary Heart Disease Patients (ENRICHD) randomized trial. JAMA 289(23):3106–3116, 2003 12813116

Bhogal SK, Teasell R, Foley N, et al: Lesion location and poststroke depression: systematic review of the methodological limitations in the literature. Stroke 35(3):794–802, 2004 14963278

Bing EG, Burnam MA, Longshore D, et al: Psychiatric disorders and drug use among human immunodeficiency virus-infected adults in the United States. Arch Gen Psychiatry 58(8):721–728, 2001 11483137

Bucur M, Papagno C: A systematic review of noninvasive brain stimulation for post-stroke depression. J Affect Disord 238:69–78, 2018 29860185

Caeiro L, Ferro JM, Santos CO, et al: Depression in acute stroke. J Psychiatry Neurosci 31(6):377–383, 2006 17136215

Capaldi VF 2nd, Wynn GH: Emerging strategies in the treatment of poststroke depression and psychiatric distress in patients. Psychol Res Behav Manag 3:109–118, 2010 22110334

Capuron L, Gumnick JF, Musselman DL, et al: Neurobehavioral effects of interferon-alpha in cancer patients: phenomenology and paroxetine responsiveness of symptom dimensions. Neuropsychopharmacology 26(5):643–652, 2002 11927189

Carney RM, Freedland KE: Depression and coronary heart disease. Nat Rev Cardiol 14(3):145–155, 2017 27853162

Carney RM, Rich MW, Freedland KE, et al: Major depressive disorder predicts cardiac events in patients with coronary artery disease. Psychosom Med 50(6):627–633, 1988 2976950

Caruso R, GiuliaNanni M, Riba MB, et al: Depressive spectrum disorders in cancer: diagnostic issues and intervention. A critical review. Curr Psychiatry Rep 19(6):33, 2017a 28488207

Caruso R, Nanni MG, Riba M, et al: Depressive spectrum disorders in cancer: prevalence, risk factors and screening for depression: a critical review. Acta Oncol 56(2):146–155, 2017b 28140731

Chollet F, Tardy J, Albucher JF, et al: Fluoxetine for motor recovery after acute ischaemic stroke (FLAME): a randomised placebo-controlled trial. Lancet Neurol 10(2):123–130, 2011 21216670

Ciesla JA, Roberts JE: Meta-analysis of the relationship between HIV infection and risk for depressive disorders. Am J Psychiatry 158(5):725–730, 2001 11329393

Coleman SM, Katon W, Lin E, et al: Depression and death in diabetes; 10-year follow-up of all-cause and cause-specific mortality in a diabetic cohort. Psychosomatics 54(5):428–436, 2013 23756124

Connerney I, Shapiro PA, McLaughlin JS, et al: Relation between depression after coronary artery bypass surgery and 12-month outcome: a prospective study. Lancet 358(9295):1766–1771, 2001 11734233

Cramer SC: Drugs to enhance motor recovery after stroke. Stroke 46(10):2998–3005, 2015 26265126

Currier MB, Nemeroff CB: Depression as a risk factor for cancer: from pathophysiological advances to treatment implications. Annu Rev Med 65:203–221, 2014 24215332

Dalton SO, Mellemkjaer L, Olsen JH, et al: Depression and cancer risk: a register-based study of patients hospitalized with affective disorders, Denmark, 1969–1993. Am J Epidemiol 155(12):1088–1095, 2002 12048222

Davydow DS, Russo JE, Ludman E, et al: The association of comorbid depression with intensive care unit admission in patients with diabetes: a prospective cohort study. Psychosomatics 52(2):117–126, 2011 21397103

de Groot M, Anderson R, Freedland KE, et al: Association of depression and diabetes complications: a meta-analysis. Psychosom Med 63(4):619–630, 2001 11485116

Easton JD, Saver JL, Albers GW, et al: Definition and evaluation of transient ischemic attack: a scientific statement for healthcare professionals from the American Heart Association/American Stroke Association Stroke Council; Council on Cardiovascular Surgery and Anesthesia; Council on Cardiovascular Radiology and Intervention; Council on Cardiovascular Nursing; and the Interdisciplinary Council on Peripheral Vascular Disease. Stroke 40(6):2276–2293, 2009 19423857

Echeverry D, Duran P, Bonds C, et al: Effect of pharmacological treatment of depression on A1C and quality of life in low-income Hispanics and African Americans with diabetes: a randomized, double-blind, placebo-controlled trial. Diabetes Care 32(12):2156–2160, 2009 19729522

Egede LE: Diabetes, major depression, and functional disability among U.S. adults. Diabetes Care 27(2):421–428, 2004 14747223

Egede LE, Nietert PJ, Zheng D: Depression and all-cause and coronary heart disease mortality among adults with and without diabetes. Diabetes Care 28(6):1339–1345, 2005 15920049

Eshun-Wilson I, Siegfried N, Akena DH, et al: Antidepressants for depression in adults with HIV infection. Cochrane Database Syst Rev (1):CD008525, 2018 25355886

Exalto LG, Biessels GJ, Karter AJ, et al: Risk score for prediction of 10 year dementia risk in individuals with type 2 diabetes: a cohort study. Lancet Diabetes Endocrinol 1(3):183–190, 2013 24622366

Feigin VL, Norrving B, Mensah GA: Global burden of stroke. Circ Res 120(3):439–448, 2017 28154096

Feng C, Fang M, Liu XY: The neurobiological pathogenesis of poststroke depression. Scientific World Journal 2014:531349, 2014 27744682

Feng R, Wang P, Gao C, et al: Effect of sertraline in the treatment and prevention of poststroke depression: a meta-analysis. Medicine (Baltimore) 97(49):e13453, 2018 30544429

Frasure-Smith N, Lespérance F: Depression and anxiety as predictors of 2-year cardiac events in patients with stable coronary artery disease. Arch Gen Psychiatry 65(1):62–71, 2008 18180430

Frasure-Smith N, Lespérance F, Talajic M: Depression following myocardial infarction. Impact on 6-month survival. JAMA 270(15):1819–1825, 1993 8411525

Frasure-Smith N, Lespérance F, Talajic M: Depression and 18-month prognosis after myocardial infarction. Circulation 91(4):999–1005, 1995 7531624

Freedland KE, Carney RM: Depression as a risk factor for adverse outcomes in coronary heart disease. BMC Med 11:131, 2013 23675637

Gan Y, Gong Y, Tong X, et al: Depression and the risk of coronary heart disease: a meta-analysis of prospective cohort studies. BMC Psychiatry 14:371, 2014 25540022

Gillespie CF, Nemeroff CB: Hypercortisolemia and depression. Psychosom Med 67 (suppl 1):S26–S28, 2005 15953796

Glassman AH, O'Connor CM, Califf RM, et al: Sertraline treatment of major depression in patients with acute MI or unstable angina. JAMA 288(6):701–709, 2002 12169073

GBD 2016 Disease and Injury Incidence and Prevalence Collaborators: Global, regional, and national incidence, prevalence, and years lived with disability for 328 diseases and injuries for 195 countries, 1990–2016: a systematic analysis for the Global Burden of Disease Study 2016. Lancet 390(10100):1211–1259, 2017 28919117

Golden SH: A review of the evidence for a neuroendocrine link between stress, depression and diabetes mellitus. Curr Diabetes Rev 3(4):252–259, 2007 18220683

Gonzalez JS, Safren SA, Cagliero E, et al: Depression, self-care, and medication adherence in type 2 diabetes: relationships across the full range of symptom severity. Diabetes Care 30(9):2222–2227, 2007 17536067

Gonzalez JS, Safren SA, Delahanty LM, et al: Symptoms of depression prospectively predict poorer self-care in patients with type 2 diabetes. Diabet Med 25(9):1102–1107, 2008a 19183315

Gonzalez JS, Peyrot M, McCarl LA, et al: Depression and diabetes treatment nonadherence: a meta-analysis. Diabetes Care 31(12):2398–2403, 2008b 19033420

Gonzalez JS, Batchelder AW, Psaros C, et al: Depression and HIV/AIDS treatment nonadherence: a review and meta-analysis. J Acquir Immune Defic Syndr 58(2):181–187, 2011 21857529

Grade C, Redford B, Chrostowski J, et al: Methylphenidate in early poststroke recovery: a double-blind, placebo-controlled study. Arch Phys Med Rehabil 79(9):1047–1050, 1998 9749682

Gross AL, Gallo JJ, Eaton WW: Depression and cancer risk: 24 years of follow-up of the Baltimore Epidemiologic Catchment Area sample. Cancer Causes Control 21(2):191–199, 2010 19885645

Guan NC, Sulaiman AH, Zainal NZ, et al: Diagnostic criteria for major depressive disorder in cancer patients: a review. Int J Psychiatry Med 45(1):73–82, 2013 23805605

Guo Y, Musselman DL, Manatunga AK, et al: The diagnosis of major depression in patients with cancer: a comparative approach. Psychosomatics 47(5):376–384, 2006 16959925

Hackett ML, Pickles K: Part I: frequency of depression after stroke: an updated systematic review and meta-analysis of observational studies. Int J Stroke 9(8):1017–1025, 2014 25117911

Hackett ML, Anderson CS, House A, Halteh C: Interventions for preventing depression after stroke. Cochrane Database Syst Rev (3):CD003689, 2008 18646094

Hance M, Carney RM, Freedland KE, Skala J: Depression in patients with coronary heart disease. A 12-month follow-up. Gen Hosp Psychiatry 18(1):61–65, 1996 8666215

Hellmuth J, Colby D, Valcour V, et al; RV254/SEARCH 010 Study Group: Depression and anxiety are common in acute HIV infection and associate with plasma immune activation. AIDS Behav 21(11):3238–3246, 2017 28484888

Huffman JC, Adams CN, Celano CM: Collaborative care and related interventions in patients with heart disease: an update and new directions. Psychosomatics 59(1):1–18, 2018 29078987

Ironson G, O'Cleirigh C, Kumar M, et al: Psychosocial and neurohormonal predictors of HIV disease progression (CD4 cells and viral load): a 4 year prospective study. AIDS Behav 19(8):1388–1397, 2015 25234251

Katon WJ, Von Korff M, Lin EHB, et al: The Pathways Study: a randomized trial of collaborative care in patients with diabetes and depression. Arch Gen Psychiatry 61(10):1042–1049, 2004 15466678

Katon W, Lin EH, Von Korff M, et al: Integrating depression and chronic disease care among patients with diabetes and/or coronary heart disease: the design of the TEAMcare study. Contemp Clin Trials 31(4):312–322, 2010 20350619

Katon W, Pedersen HS, Ribe AR, et al: Effect of depression and diabetes mellitus on the risk for dementia: a national population-based cohort study. JAMA Psychiatry 72(6):612–619, 2015 25875310

Kim ES, Kim JW, Kang HJ, et al: Longitudinal impact of depression on quality of life in stroke patients. Psychiatry Investig 15(2):141–146, 2018 29475223

Krebber AMH, Buffart LM, Kleijn G, et al: Prevalence of depression in cancer patients: a meta-analysis of diagnostic interviews and self-report instruments. Psychooncology 23(2):121–130, 2014 24105788

Kroenke K, Spitzer RL, Williams JB: The PHQ-9: validity of a brief depression severity measure. J Gen Intern Med 16(9):606–613, 2001 11556941

Kutlubaev MA, Hackett ML: Part II: predictors of depression after stroke and impact of depression on stroke outcome: an updated systematic review of observational studies. Int J Stroke 9(8):1026–1036, 2014 25156411

Lazarus LW, Winemiller DR, Lingam VR, et al: Efficacy and side effects of methylphenidate for poststroke depression. J Clin Psychiatry 53(12):447–449, 1992 1487474

Leserman J, Petitto JM, Perkins DO, et al: Severe stress, depressive symptoms, and changes in lymphocyte subsets in human immunodeficiency virus-infected men. A 2-year follow-up study. Arch Gen Psychiatry 54(3):279–285, 1997 9075469

Leserman J, Petitto JM, Gu H, et al: Progression to AIDS, a clinical AIDS condition and mortality: psychosocial and physiological predictors. Psychol Med 32(6):1059–1073, 2002 12214787

Lespérance F, Frasure-Smith N, Juneau M, et al: Depression and 1-year prognosis in unstable angina. Arch Intern Med 160(9):1354–1360, 2000 10809041

Lespérance F, Frasure-Smith N, Koszycki D, et al: Effects of citalopram and interpersonal psychotherapy on depression in patients with coronary artery disease: the Canadian Cardiac Randomized Evaluation of Antidepressant and Psychotherapy Efficacy (CREATE) trial. JAMA 297(4):367–379, 2007 17244833

Leung YW, Flora DB, Gravely S, et al: The impact of premorbid and postmorbid depression onset on mortality and cardiac morbidity among patients with coronary heart disease: meta-analysis. Psychosom Med 74(8):786–801, 2012 23001393

Li M, Kennedy EB, Byrne N, et al: Systematic review and meta-analysis of collaborative care interventions for depression in patients with cancer. Psychooncology 26(5):573–587, 2017 27643388

Lichtman JH, Froelicher ES, Blumenthal JA, et al: Depression as a risk factor for poor prognosis among patients with acute coronary syndrome: systematic review and recommendations: a scientific statement from the American Heart Association. Circulation 129(12):1350–1369, 2014 24566200

Lima VD, Geller J, Bangsberg DR, et al: The effect of adherence on the association between depressive symptoms and mortality among HIV-infected individuals first initiating HAART. AIDS 21(9):1175–1183, 2007 17502728

Linkins RW, Comstock GW: Depressed mood and development of cancer. Am J Epidemiol 132(5):962–972, 1990 2239911

Little RR, Rohlfing CL, Sacks DB; National Glycohemoglobin Standardization Program (NGSP) Steering Committee: Status of hemoglobin A1c measurement and goals for improvement: from chaos to order for improving diabetes care. Clin Chem 57(2):205–214, 2011 21148304

Liu C, Wang M, Liang X, et al: Efficacy and safety of high-frequency repetitive transcranial magnetic stimulation for poststroke depression: a systematic review and meta-analysis. Arch Phys Med Rehabil 100(10):1964–1975, 2019 31002813

Lustman PJ, Griffith LS, Clouse RE, et al: Effects of nortriptyline on depression and glycemic control in diabetes: results of a double-blind, placebo-controlled trial. Psychosom Med 59(3):241–250, 1997 9178335

Lustman PJ, Griffith LS, Freedland KE, et al: Cognitive behavior therapy for depression in type 2 diabetes mellitus. A randomized, controlled trial. Ann Intern Med 129(8):613–621, 1998 9786808

Malzberg B: Mortality among patients with involution melancholia. Am J Psychiatry 93:1231–1238, 1937

Martinsson L, Eksborg S: Drugs for stroke recovery: the example of amphetamines. Drugs Aging 21(2):67–79, 2004 14960125
Massie MJ: Prevalence of depression in patients with cancer. J Natl Cancer Inst Monogr (32):57–71, 2004 15263042
Meader N, Moe-Byrne T, Llewellyn A, et al: Screening for poststroke major depression: a meta-analysis of diagnostic validity studies. J Neurol Neurosurg Psychiatry 85(2):198–206, 2014 23385849
Meijer A, Conradi HJ, Bos EH, et al: Adjusted prognostic association of depression following myocardial infarction with mortality and cardiovascular events: individual patient data meta-analysis. Br J Psychiatry 203(2):90–102, 2013 23908341
Mezuk B, Eaton WW, Albrecht S, et al: Depression and type 2 diabetes over the lifespan: a meta-analysis. Diabetes Care 31(12):2383–2390, 2008 19033418
Montgomery SA, Åsberg M: A new depression scale designed to be sensitive to change. Br J Psychiatry 134:382–389, 1979 444788
Mozaffarian D, Benjamin EJ, Go AS, et al: Heart disease and stroke statistics—2016 update: a report from the American Heart Association. Circulation 133(4):e38–e360, 2016 26673558
Nanni MG, Caruso R, Mitchell AJ, et al: Depression in HIV infected patients: a review. Curr Psychiatry Rep 17(1):530, 2015 25413636
National Institute for Health and Clinical Excellence: Depression in adults: recognition and management. Clinical guideline CG90. Published 28 October 2009. Available at: https://www.nice.org.uk/guidance/cg90. Accessed September 1, 2021.
Nickel A, Thomalla G: Post-stroke depression: impact of lesion location and methodological limitations—a topical review. Front Neurol 8:498, 2017 28983281
Nys GM, van Zandvoort MJ, van der Worp HB, et al: Early depressive symptoms after stroke: neuropsychological correlates and lesion characteristics. J Neurol Sci 228(1):27–33, 2005 15607207
O'Connor CM, Jiang W, Kuchibhatla M, et al: Safety and efficacy of sertraline for depression in patients with heart failure: results of the SADHART-CHF (Sertraline Against Depression and Heart Disease in Chronic Heart Failure) trial. J Am Coll Cardiol 56(9):692–699, 2010 20723799
O'Donnell MJ, Chin SL, Rangarajan S, et al: Global and regional effects of potentially modifiable risk factors associated with acute stroke in 32 countries (INTERSTROKE): a case-control study. Lancet 388(10046):761–775, 2016 27431356
Oerlemans ME, van den Akker M, Schuurman AG, et al: A meta-analysis on depression and subsequent cancer risk. Clin Pract Epidemiol Ment Health 3:29, 2007 18053168
Okuyama T, Akechi T, Mackenzie L, Furukawa TA: Psychotherapy for depression among advanced, incurable cancer patients: a systematic review and meta-analysis. Cancer Treat Rev 56:16–27, 2017 28453966
Ostuzzi B, Matcham F, Dauchy S, et al: Antidepressants for the treatment of depression in people with cancer. Cochrane Database Syst Rev (4):CD011006, 2018 29683474
Ovbiagele B, Goldstein LB, Higashida RT, et al: Forecasting the future of stroke in the United States: a policy statement from the American Heart Association and American Stroke Association. Stroke 44(8):2361–2375, 2013 23697546
Padilla VL, Rustad JK, Harvey PD, et al: Neurocognitive impairment in patients with comorbid diabetes mellitus and depression. Personalized Medicine in Psychiatry 1:2–10, 2017. Available at: https://www.personalizedmedpsych.com/article/S2468-1717(16)30017-5/fulltext. Accessed October 26, 2021.
Paolucci S: Epidemiology and treatment of post-stroke depression. Neuropsychiatr Dis Treat 4(1):145–154, 2008 18728805
Pence BW, Mills JC, Bengtson AM, et al: Association of increased chronicity of depression with HIV appointment attendance, treatment failure, and mortality among HIV-infected adults in the United States. JAMA Psychiatry 75(4):379–385, 2018 29466531
Penninx BW, Guralnik JM, Pahor M, et al: Chronically depressed mood and cancer risk in older persons. J Natl Cancer Inst 90(24):1888–1893, 1998 9862626
Perry S, Jacobsberg LB, Fishman B, et al: Psychiatric diagnosis before serological testing for the human immunodeficiency virus. Am J Psychiatry 147(1):89–93, 1990 2293794

Pinquart M, Duberstein PR: Depression and cancer mortality: a meta-analysis. Psychol Med 40(11):1797–1810, 2010 20085667

Polsky D, Doshi JA, Marcus S, et al: Long-term risk for depressive symptoms after a medical diagnosis. Arch Intern Med 165(11):1260–1266, 2005 15956005

Rabkin JG: HIV and depression: 2008 review and update. Curr HIV/AIDS Rep 5(4):163–171, 2008 18838056

Radloff LS: The CES-D scale: a self-report depression scale for research in the general population. Appl Psychol Meas 1(3):385–401, 1977

Rivera-Rivera Y, Vázquez-Santiago FJ, Albino E, et al: Impact of depression and inflammation on the progression of HIV disease. J Clin Cell Immunol 7(3):423, 2016 27478681

Robins LN, Helzer JE, Croughan J, et al: National Institute of Mental Health Diagnostic Interview Schedule. Its history, characteristics, and validity. Arch Gen Psychiatry 38(4):381–389, 1981 6260053

Roose SP, Glassman A, Mathew SJ, et al: Managing patients with vascular disease and depression. J Clin Psychiatry 67:1633–1644, 2006

Rotella F, Mannucci E: Depression as a risk factor for diabetes: a meta-analysis of longitudinal studies. J Clin Psychiatry 74(1):31–37, 2013 23419223

Roy T, Lloyd CE: Epidemiology of depression and diabetes: a systematic review. J Affect Disord 142 (suppl):S8–S21, 2012 23062861

Rutledge T, Reis VA, Linke SE, et al: Depression in heart failure a meta-analytic review of prevalence, intervention effects, and associations with clinical outcomes. J Am Coll Cardiol 48(8):1527–1537, 2006 17045884

Rutledge T, Redwine LS, Linke SE, et al: A meta-analysis of mental health treatments and cardiac rehabilitation for improving clinical outcomes and depression among patients with coronary heart disease. Psychosom Med 75(4):335–349, 2013 23630306

Sacco RL, Kasner SE, Broderick JP, et al: An updated definition of stroke for the 21st century: a statement for healthcare professionals from the American Heart Association/American Stroke Association. Stroke 44(7):2064–2089, 2013 23652265

Salter KL, Foley NC, Zhu L, et al: Prevention of poststroke depression: does prophylactic pharmacotherapy work? J Stroke Cerebrovasc Dis 22(8):1243–1251, 2013 22554569

Satin JR, Linden W, Phillips MJ: Depression as a predictor of disease progression and mortality in cancer patients: a meta-analysis. Cancer 115(22):5349–5361, 2009 19753617

Shen X, Liu M, Cheng Y, et al: Repetitive transcranial magnetic stimulation for the treatment of post-stroke depression: a systematic review and meta-analysis of randomized controlled clinical trials. J Affect Disord 211:65–74, 2017 28092847

Shi Y, Yang D, Zeng Y, et al: Risk factors for post-stroke depression: a meta-analysis. Front Aging Neurosci 9:218, 2017 28744213

Simon GE, Von Korff M: Medical co-morbidity and validity of DSM-IV depression criteria. Psychol Med 36(1):27–36, 2006 16202189

Simoni JM, Safren SA, Manhart LE, et al: Challenges in addressing depression in HIV research: assessment, cultural context, and methods. AIDS Behav 15(2):376–388, 2011 21046221

Sin NL, DiMatteo MR: Depression treatment enhances adherence to antiretroviral therapy: a meta-analysis. Ann Behav Med 47(3):259–269, 2014 24234601

Smith HR: Depression in cancer patients: pathogenesis, implications and treatment (Review). Oncol Lett 9(4):1509–1514, 2015 25788991

Snaphaan L, Van Der Werf S, Kanselaar K, De Leeuw FE: Post-stroke depressive symptoms are associated with post-stroke characteristics. Cerebrovasc Dis 28:551–557, 2009 19844094

So-Armah K, Gupta SK, Kundu S, et al: Depression and all-cause mortality risk in HIV-infected and HIV-uninfected US veterans: a cohort study. HIV Med 20(5):317–329, 2019 30924577

Spaan P, van Luenen S, Garnefski N, et: Psychosocial interventions enhance HIV medication adherence: a systematic review and meta-analysis. J Health Psychol 25(10-11):1326–1340, 2020 29417851

Stafoggia M, Cesaroni G, Peters A, et al: Long-term exposure to ambient air pollution and incidence of cerebrovascular events: results from 11 European cohorts within the ESCAPE project. Environ Health Perspect 122(9):919–925, 2014 24835336

Sullivan MD, Katon WJ, Lovato LC, et al: Association of depression with accelerated cognitive decline among patients with type 2 diabetes in the ACCORD-MIND trial. JAMA Psychiatry 70(10):1041–1047, 2013 23945905
Thombs BD, Bass EB, Ford DE, et al: Prevalence of depression in survivors of acute myocardial infarction. J Gen Intern Med 21(1):30–38, 2006 16423120
Towfighi A, Ovbiagele B, El Husseini N, et al: Poststroke depression: a scientific statement for healthcare professionals from the American Heart Association/American Stroke Association. Stroke 48(2):e30–e43, 2017 27932603
Vancampfort D, Mitchell AJ, De Hert M, et al: Type 2 diabetes patients with major depressive disorder: a meta-analysis of prevalence estimates and predictors. Depress Anxiety 32(10):763–773, 2015 26114259
van der Feltz-Cornelis CM, Nuyen J, Stoop C, et al: Effect of interventions for major depressive disorder and significant depressive symptoms in patients with diabetes mellitus: a systematic review and meta-analysis. Gen Hosp Psychiatry 32(4):380–395, 2010 20633742
van Empelen P, Kok G, van Kesteren NM, et al: Effective methods to change sex-risk among drug users: a review of psychosocial interventions. Soc Sci Med 57(9):1593–1608, 2003 12948569
van Melle JP, de Jonge P, Spijkerman TA, et al: Prognostic association of depression following myocardial infarction with mortality and cardiovascular events: a meta-analysis. Psychosom Med 66(6):814–822, 2004 15564344
van Melle JP, de Jonge P, Ormel J, et al: Relationship between left ventricular dysfunction and depression following myocardial infarction: data from the MIND-IT. Eur Heart J 26(24):2650–2656, 2005 16143708
van Melle JP, de Jonge P, Honig A, et al: Effects of antidepressant treatment following myocardial infarction. Br J Psychiatry 190:460–466, 2007 17541103
Vataja R, Leppävuori A, Pohjasvaara T, et al: Poststroke depression and lesion location revisited. J Neuropsychiatry Clin Neurosci 16(2):156–162, 2004 15260366
Villa RF, Ferrari F, Moretti A: Post-stroke depression: mechanisms and pharmacological treatment. Pharmacol Ther 184:131–144, 2018 29128343
Wagner GJ, Ngo V, Glick P, et al: INtegration of DEPression Treatment into HIV care in Uganda (INDEPTH-Uganda): study protocol for a randomized controlled trial. Trials 15:248, 2014 24962086
Walker J, Sharpe M: Integrated management of major depression for people with cancer. Int Rev Psychiatry 26(6):657–668, 2014 25553783
Walker-Batson D, Smith P, Curtis S, et al: Amphetamine paired with physical therapy accelerates motor recovery after stroke. Further evidence. Stroke 26(12):2254–2259, 1995 7491646
Walker-Batson D, Mehta J, Smith P, et al: Amphetamine and other pharmacological agents in human and animal studies of recovery from stroke. Prog Neuropsychopharmacol Biol Psychiatry 64:225–230, 2016 25896190
Wang SB, Wang YY, Zhang QE, et al: Cognitive behavioral therapy for post-stroke depression: a meta-analysis. J Affect Disord 235:589–596, 2018 29704854
Wang F, Wang S, Zong QQ, et al: Prevalence of comorbid major depressive disorder in type 2 diabetes: a meta-analysis of comparative and epidemiological studies. Diabet Med 36(8):961–969, 2019 31127631
Xu JQ, Murphy SL, Kochanek KD, et al: Deaths: final data for 2016. Natl Vital Stat Rep 67(5):1–76, 2018 30248015
Yu M, Zhang X, Lu F, et al: Depression and risk for diabetes: a meta-analysis. Can J Diabetes 39(4):266–272, 2015 25773933
Zaorsky NG, Zhang Y, Tuanquin L, et al: Suicide among cancer patients. Nat Commun 10(1):207, 2019 30643135
Zhang T, Jing X, Zhao X, et al: A prospective cohort study of lesion location and its relation to post-stroke depression among Chinese patients. J Affect Disord 136(1–2):e83–e87, 2012 21763001

CHAPTER 41

Mood Disorders and Substance Use

Edward Nunes, M.D.
Eric Rubin, M.D., Ph.D.
Kenneth Carpenter, Ph.D.
Deborah Hasin, Ph.D.

The use of addictive substances has been ubiquitous in human cultures since the dawn of civilization and remains almost universal across a wide variety of contemporary cultures, especially when one considers caffeine and nicotine in addition to alcohol and harder drugs. Substance use disorders (SUDs) are among the most common mental disorders in the general population (Grant et al. 2004). Furthermore, the presence of a mood disorder at least doubles the odds of having an SUD in general population surveys in which this issue has been examined (Grant 1995; Grant and Harford 1995; Grant et al. 2004, 2005, 2015, 2016; Hasin et al. 2005, 2018; Kessler et al. 1994; Regier et al. 1990). This strong and consistent association raises the question of what the relationships may be between these two sets of disorders.

SUDs are in some respects the best-understood mental disorders in terms of pathophysiology and neuropharmacology. What addictive substances have in common, and what sets them apart from all other drugs and compounds, is that they target brain reward circuitry centered on mesolimbic and mesocortical dopamine projections (Gard-

This work was supported in part by grants P50 DA09236, R01 DA12271, R01 DA08950, and K02 DA00288 from the National Institute on Drug Abuse and grant K05 AA00161 from the National Institute on Alcohol Abuse and Alcoholism.

The authors are grateful to Carrie Davies, Richard Malkin, Elizabeth Costello, and Valerie Richmond for assistance in preparation of the manuscript and to Eve Vagg and Rachel Yarmolinsky for assistance with illustration.

ner 1997). The understanding of drugs as positive reinforcers, and of their effects on and relation to the brain reward circuitry, has led to a rich array of animal models (Johanson and Schuster 1981; Robbins and Everitt 2002) that, arguably, come closer to modeling the actual human disorder than do animal models of other common psychiatric disorders. The addictive substances all affect mood and have euphorigenic effects during intoxication and often dysphorigenic effects during withdrawal, suggesting relationships at the level of brain circuitry between mood regulation and substance use. Thus, we argue that any clinical framework for understanding mood disorders is incomplete without consideration of substance use and SUDs. Not only are SUDs prevalent among individuals with mood disorders, presenting a significant clinical problem, but insights into the pathophysiology of addiction are also likely to improve our approach to mood disorders, and vice versa. The benefit of a convergent, transdiagnostic approach is well illustrated by our growing clinical and neurobiological understanding of the states of anhedonia (Rømer Thomsen et al. 2015) and reward responsiveness (Sharma et al. 2017), which figure importantly in both substance abuse and mood regulation.

In this chapter, we review the pathophysiology and phenomenology of SUDs and the epidemiological evidence regarding their co-occurrence with mood disorders. We then discuss various lines of research evidence (e.g., longitudinal and family genetic studies, behavioral and neurobiological studies, and treatment studies) relevant to an understanding of the potential relationships between mood disorders and SUDs. We conclude the chapter with sections on approaches to clinical evaluation and treatment in patients with co-occurring mood and substance-related disorders.

Overview of Pathophysiology of Substance Use Disorders

The brain reward system was conceptualized in the 1950s, when it was found that electrical stimulation of specific sites in the medial forebrain was highly positively reinforcing. Animals would work intensely to self-administer direct stimulation of these regions. Subsequently, the circuitry has been described in detail, as reviewed by Gardner (1997). Figure 41–1 shows Gardner's summary of brain reward circuitry, modified to highlight points of overlap with regions involved in mood regulation. The core of the system consists of mesolimbic and mesocortical projections that originate from dopaminergic cells in the ventral tegmental area of the brain stem. These fibers course rostrally to an array of targets, including the nucleus accumbens (a portion of the ventral striatum), the amygdala, and the frontal cortex. These targets of the brain stem dopaminergic projection sit within frontal and limbic circuitry that mediates executive cognitive functioning, as well as emotional and motivational functioning (Heimer 2003). The involvement of these same frontal and limbic circuits in the regulation of mood (Drevets 2000; see also Chapter 11, "Brain Imaging," in this volume) provides an ample neurobiological substrate for interactions between the effects of abused substances and long-term mood regulation.

Microiontophoretic studies have documented that addictive substances have a wide variety of pharmacological actions and effects. For example, alcohol is a tranquil-

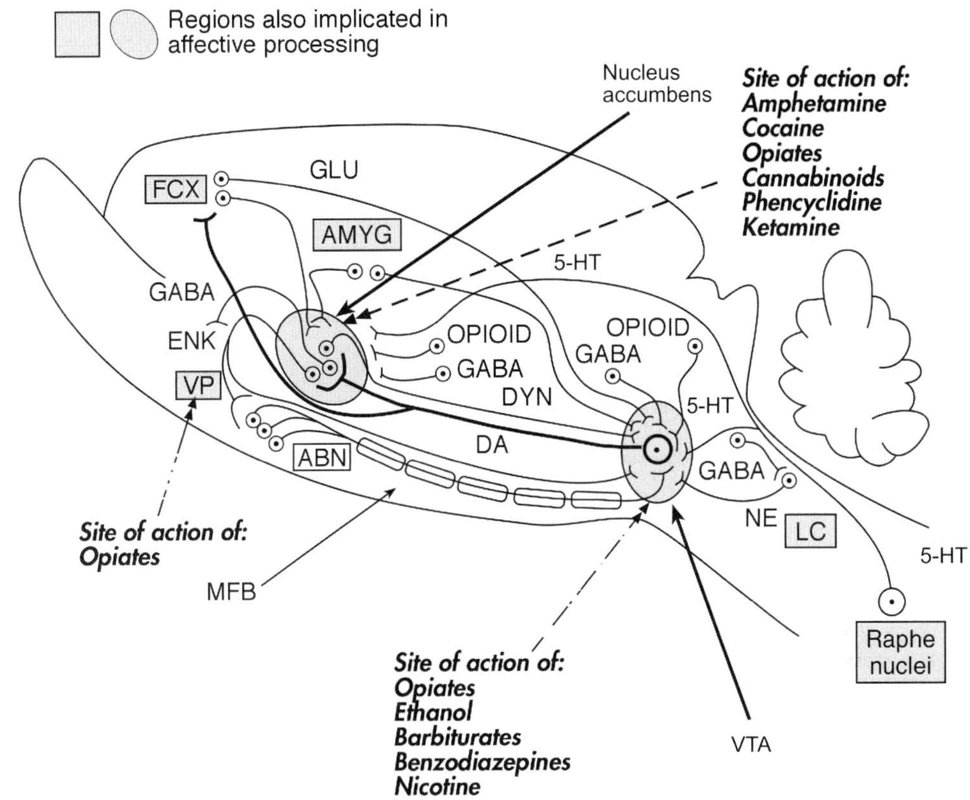

FIGURE 41–1. **Presumed neural substrate for interactions between substance abuse and mood regulation.**

Illustration shows anatomical pathways and regional neurotransmitter mechanisms involved in brain reward and in effects of addictive drugs. The core of the system comprises two components: myelinated fibers of the median forebrain bundle (MFB), which provide input to dopaminergic (DA) cells in the ventral tegmental area (VTA), and axons of the VTA cells (indicated with *bold line*) that ascend to provide dopaminergic input to the nucleus accumbens (mesolimbic fibers), frontal cortex (FCX) (mesocortical fibers), and other targets not detailed. Sites at which various addictive substances are thought to act on the reward system are indicated. Data on drug effects are derived primarily from invasive studies in laboratory animals and hence are presented on a drawing of the rat brain, although the essential features have been verified in primate studies (Volkow et al. 2013). *Shaded regions (ovals and boxes)* indicate structures whose homologues in the human brain are likely involved in the regulation of emotion and affect. Data regarding brain mechanisms for human mood regulation derive primarily from functional imaging studies in humans during induced mood states or in clinical mood disorders (see Drevets 2000 and Chapter 11, "Brain Imaging," in this volume).

ABN=anterior bed nuclei of median forebrain bundle; AMYG=amygdala; DYN=dynorphin; ENK=enkephalin; GABA=γ-aminobutyric acid; GLU=glutamate; 5-HT=5-hydroxytryptamine (serotonin); LC=locus coeruleus; NE=norepinephrine; OPIOID=endogenous opioid peptide systems; VP=ventral pallidum.

Source. Adapted from Gardner 1997.

izer used in diverse social settings as a social lubricant. Stimulants, such as cocaine, nicotine, and caffeine, have been used throughout history to promote productivity. Yet despite this diversity of effects, these substances all have actions on the mesolimbic and mesocortical dopamine systems. They enhance the release of dopamine from the mesolimbic and mesocortical projections in their target areas. Stimulants such as cocaine and amphetamines act directly on dopaminergic synapses. Other drugs, such as nicotine, opiates, and cannabis, act through systems that impinge on and modulate the physiology of the dopamine release. Each of these substances has diverse pharmacological effects related to its unique pharmacology.

Several animal models have advanced our understanding of the pathophysiology of addictive disorders (Johanson and Schuster 1981; Robbins and Everitt 2002). Important findings from such models include the following: 1) drugs that are addictive for humans are likely to be self-administered by laboratory animals, functioning in a behaviorally lawful way as positive reinforcers; 2) different genetic strains of animals vary in their propensity to self-administer different drugs; and 3) animals will work hard to obtain doses of drugs and, in some instances, will endure substantial adversity (e.g., starvation) to self-administer drugs.

A useful model for understanding the mechanism of addiction has been the model of brain stimulation reward (Gardner 1997). In this model, a microelectrode is situated within the brain reward system of an animal, and the animal is allowed to work (e.g., press a lever) for electrical stimulation at that site. The stimulation strength is then gradually reduced until a threshold is reached at which the animal will no longer work for stimulation. This is called the threshold for brain stimulation reward. Acute doses of addictive drugs lower the brain stimulation threshold—that is, they appear to sensitize the brain reward system to the effects of electrical stimulation. However, chronic administration of addictive drugs has the opposite effect—namely, of raising the threshold for brain stimulation reward. This finding appears to model the state of tolerance that occurs in response to most addictive drugs (i.e., larger doses are needed over time to achieve the same effects). Tolerance is likely transduced via neuronal intracellular adaptations at the levels of second messengers and gene expression (Nestler 1993). Tolerance is also consistent with a state of anhedonia, in which the brain reward system becomes less responsive to natural reinforcers, such as food and social interaction. The substance becomes the most salient positive reinforcer. This intersection between the substrates for drug tolerance and anhedonia within the brain reward system indicates a fundamental relationship with mood disorders, via the core symptom of anhedonia (Rømer Thomsen et al. 2015).

Withdrawal states that occur when the addictive substance is withheld are negative affective states that substantially overlap with mood disorder symptoms, a relationship that is emphasized in contemporary formulations of the neurobiology of addiction. Opioid withdrawal, for example, in addition to symptoms of autonomic overdrive (e.g., tachycardia, tremor, intestinal cramping), typically involves fatigue, anorexia, insomnia, dysphoria, anxiety, and irritability, symptoms that also typify depression and anxiety disorders. This sets up a negative reinforcement mechanism in which more drug is taken to alleviate withdrawal (Koob 2015), leading to what has been described as a vicious circle between opioid addiction and mood dysregulation mediated via the endogenous opioid system (Emery and Akil 2020). Cannabis withdrawal, a withdrawal syndrome not previously recognized, was identified in the mid-2000s (Budney et al. 2004) and added to DSM-5 in 2013 (American Psychiatric Association 2013; Hasin et al. 2013).

Advances in delineating the underlying neurocircuitry and neurochemistry of addiction suggest that dysregulation occurs in three interconnected systems:

1. The incentive salience system and dopamine circuitry in the ventral striatum and basal ganglia mediating hedonic response, which becomes desensitized in addiction;
2. Negative affective states mediated through the stress system and extended amygdala that involve corticotropin-releasing hormone (CRH) and dynorphin, among other transmitters, which become activated during addiction; and
3. Deficits in executive functioning circuits based in the prefrontal cortex and insula, which exert control over the reward and stress systems (Koob and Volkow 2016; Uhl et al. 2019).

The overlap with systems implicated in mood disorders is evident.

Phenomenology of Substance-Related Disorders

The major substance-related disorders include intoxication, withdrawal, and substance use disorders. General psychiatrists should be familiar with the various intoxication and withdrawal syndromes produced by addictive substances. These syndromes, well summarized in DSM-5, include several symptoms that overlap phenotypically with mood disorders, including manic-level euphoria, depression, anxiety, appetite disturbances, sleep disturbances, excess energy, and lack of energy. Familiarity with such effects is important for making the differential diagnosis between a mood disorder and intoxication or withdrawal (Nunes and Weiss 2014). To some extent, the intoxication syndromes can be viewed as mimicking hypomania, whereas the withdrawal states mimic depressive or anxiety symptoms. This overlap in symptoms again suggests fundamental common ground between the pathophysiology of SUDs and mood disorders and invites inquiry into how substance intoxication and withdrawal states might serve as models of mood disorders.

SUD represents a chronic, maladaptive patterns of the use of substances. The DSM-5 criteria are summarized in Table 41–1. As can be seen in the table, the criteria fall into four broad categories: 1) loss of control, 2) psychosocial impairment, 3) continued use despite risk or medical or psychological consequences, and 4) physiological symptoms (tolerance and withdrawal). SUDs are highly comorbid—that is, a history of one SUD substantially increases the risk of having others (Grant 1995; Grant and Harford 1995; Grant et al. 2004, 2015, 2016; Hasin et al. 2018; Kessler et al. 1994, Regier et al. 1990).

SUD has a typical natural history, with onset most commonly in the early to mid-teenage years. It may remit as young individuals make the transition into adulthood, with its occupational and familial responsibilities. However, among some, SUD has a chronic, relapsing course. These individuals may enter and leave treatment repeatedly, despite the availability (contrary to popular belief) of many effective treatments (see later sections of this chapter). Despite the prevalence of this course, however, it is worth noting that SUD onset can occur at any age, even among the elderly population.

Several well-established risk factors promote the development of SUD, including availability of substances, without which use and use disorder cannot occur. Other risk factors include family history of SUD, which reflects a moderate degree of genetic

TABLE 41–1. Summary of DSM-5 criteria for substance use disorder

A maladaptive pattern of substance use leading to clinically significant impairment or distress, as manifested by two or more of the following, occurring at any time in the same 12-month period (two or three criteria is considered "mild," four or five criteria is considered "moderate," and six or more criteria is considered "severe"):

Loss of control over substance use*

- Substance is often taken in larger amounts or over a longer period than was intended
- There is a persistent desire or unsuccessful efforts to cut down or control substance use
- A great deal of time is spent in activities necessary to obtain the substance
- Craving to use substances is present

Impairment of social functioning*

- Failure to fulfill major role obligations at work, school, or home as a result of recurrent substance use
- Persistent or recurrent social or interpersonal problems that are exacerbated by substance use or continued use of substance despite these problems
- Important social, occupational, or recreational activities are given up or reduced because of substance use

Continued use despite risk or medical-psychological consequences*

- Substance use in physically hazardous situations
- Substance use is continued despite knowledge of having a persistent or recurrent physical or psychological problem that is likely to have been caused or exacerbated by the substance

Physiological effects*

- Tolerance: increased amounts of substance needed to achieve desired effects, and/or diminished effects with continue use of the same amount
- Withdrawal: symptoms of substance withdrawal syndrome; substance taken to avoid withdrawal

*Subcategories of criteria (loss of control, impairment, continued use despite consequence, and physiological effects) added for emphasis.

Source. Adapted from American Psychiatric Association 2013.

influence; childhood externalizing disorders, such as conduct disorder; and childhood temperamental features, including aggressiveness, impulsivity, and inattention. Adverse events in childhood, such as parental loss (Kendler et al. 2002) or being physically or sexually abused (Kendler et al. 2000), have been implicated as risk factors as well. Stress is a risk factor that has been shown both to increase self-administration of substances in animal models and to increase risk of SUDs in human populations. The role of stress and trauma in the etiology of both SUDs and mood disorders represents another point of common ground between the two sets of disorders.

The diagnostic category of SUD has undergone change across different versions of the DSM criteria. Prior to DSM-5, SUDs were divided into two categories—substance abuse and substance dependence. DSM-IV-TR (American Psychiatric Association 2000) conceptualized substance abuse as a distinct category representing a repeated pattern of use that results in dangerous or life-threatening consequences (most often, driving after drinking too much) (Hasin and Paykin 1999) or severe psychosocial impairment. However, problems with the prior DSM approach led to the elimination of the abuse and dependence diagnoses, combining them into a unified disorder in

DSM-5. A common assumption about alcohol abuse was that it was a prodromal condition to dependence; however, longitudinal studies of substance abuse indicated that it often resolved without recurrence or development into dependence (Grant et al. 2001; Hasin et al. 1997; Schuckit et al. 2000). Dependence, on the other hand, is more likely to have a chronic, relapsing course, and many individuals with dependence did not meet criteria for abuse, especially women and minorities (Hasin and Grant 2004). In contrast to the notion of it representing a milder prodrome, substance abuse could be quite serious, with potentially life-threatening consequences such as motor vehicle accidents and violent deaths. Finally, studies done during the development of DSM-5, using item response theory, showed that the criteria for DSM-IV (American Psychiatric Association 1994) abuse and dependence fell along a single dimension and were best conceptualized as part of a single disorder (Hasin et al. 2013). Hence the criteria for DSM-IV abuse and dependence were in effect combined into DSM-5 SUD. Craving was added to the DSM-5 criteria due to evidence and consensus around its importance as a feature of the use disorder syndrome, and the legal problems criterion, previously part of the substance abuse criteria, was removed (Hasin et al. 2013).

Comorbidity of Mood Disorders and Substance Use Disorders

Clinical Samples and Issues in Diagnostic Assessment

With the introduction of contemporary psychiatric diagnostic criteria, prevalence studies of mood disorders among patients in treatment for SUD began to appear in the literature (for a review, see Hasin et al. 2004). These studies included alcohol-, opiate-, and cocaine-dependent samples. Lifetime rates of major depressive disorder (MDD) in several early studies were in the 30%–50% range, whereas current rates ranged from 10% to 30%. Because the rates were high, concerns were raised that this result actually represented diagnostic confusion with symptoms of intoxication or withdrawal rather than true mood disorders (Schuckit 1986).

To avoid such misdiagnosis, some early investigators focused on *primary depression,* defined as depression whose lifetime onset predated the onset of the SUD. Studies that used this definition found lower lifetime rates of primary depression, in the range of 10%–20% (Nunes et al. 2004). However, the natural history of MDD indicates a later lifetime onset than the onset of SUD. Hence, basing the diagnosis entirely on initial lifetime onset may cause true depressions among people with SUDs to be overlooked. DSM-IV created a category of substance-induced mood disorder to provide an updated way to address this diagnostic challenge without relying on the order of lifetime onset, and DSM-5 has retained this approach. In DSM-5, substance-induced mood disorders are those occurring among people using substances in whom the mood disorder cannot be established as independent of the substance use (i.e., mood disorder has always occurred in the setting of substance use) but whose symptoms clearly exceed the expected intoxication and withdrawal symptoms of the drugs being used. The DSM-5 substance-induced category provides recognition of the potential clinical importance of mood disorders among individuals who use alcohol or drugs or meet criteria for a use disorder.

Another criticism of these data is that the elevated rates of depression may be a manifestation of Berkson's bias or the clinician's illusion (Cohen and Cohen 1984), whereby patients with multiple disorders are more likely to seek treatment, so the elevated rate of comorbidity is an artifact of treatment-seeking rather than a reflection of a true relation between the two disorders. However, the consistent finding that considerable comorbidity is found between substance-related and other psychiatric disorders in general population surveys suggests that Berkson's bias is not the reason for the elevated rates of depression seen in clinical settings.

The importance of identifying depressive disorders among people with SUDs is highlighted by the relatively consistent finding that a mood disorder, particularly MDD, predicts poor prognosis and treatment outcome among substance-dependent patients. In a review by Hasin et al. (2004), prospective studies of the effect of depression on the course of SUD were divided into two groups: 1) studies that used mood symptom scales and 2) studies that diagnosed mood disorders with standardized diagnostic criteria and structured interviews. Mood disorders identified by diagnostic criteria (e.g., Greenfield et al. 1998; Hasin et al. 2002) consistently predicted poor outcomes for the SUDs, whereas the prognostic effect of low mood assessed by symptom scales was much less consistent. Similarly, a lifetime diagnosis of MDD among nicotine-dependent patients reduces the likelihood of sustained smoking cessation (Glassman 1993). This evidence indicates that the occurrence of depression in substance-dependent patients is a significant clinical problem and supports the importance of careful clinical diagnosis.

Data on the occurrence of bipolar illness with SUD emerge mainly from studies of patients hospitalized or admitted to psychiatric treatment with a primary diagnosis of bipolar illness. Prevalence rates of bipolar illness in substance-dependent patients have been relatively low and variable (for a review, see Hasin et al. 2004), reflecting both the relatively low prevalence of bipolar disorder in the general population and confusion about how to distinguish symptoms of bipolar illness from euphoria, impulsivity, and poor judgment related to substance intoxication. However, studies among samples of patients with bipolar disorder (Salloum and Brown 2017) suggest that SUDs, particularly alcohol and cocaine use disorder, are highly prevalent among patients with bipolar disorder and are associated with worse outcomes.

General Population Surveys

The Epidemiologic Catchment Area (ECA) study (Regier et al. 1990), the National Comorbidity Survey (NCS) (Kessler et al. 1994), the National Longitudinal Alcohol Epidemiologic Survey (NLAES) (Grant 1995; Grant and Harford 1995), the National Epidemiological Survey of Alcohol and Related Conditions (NESARC) (Grant et al. 2005; Hasin et al. 2005), and the NESARC-III (Grant et al. 2015, 2016) were five studies undertaken with the aim of determining the prevalence of psychiatric disorders in large samples representative of the general population. A major advantage of these studies in terms of evaluating comorbidity is that they avoided concerns about Berkson's bias because the samples were not treatment-seeking. The potential for diagnostic confusion remains; however, in each study, the structured interviewing methods used included features that attempted to help interviewers distinguish true mood disorders from substance-related toxicity or withdrawal effects.

Alcohol or drug use disorders (lifetime prevalence in the 15%–25% range) and mood disorders are both prevalent in the general population. Table 41–2 displays the odds ratios (ORs) that represent the degree of association between SUDs and mood disorders. (Recall that an OR of 1.0 represents no association; an OR >1.0 indicates association, generally considered of a meaningful magnitude when the OR is ≥2.0.) As can be seen from the table, ORs reflecting a degree of association between mood disorders and SUDs are relatively consistent across studies. The data suggest that the presence of an SUD at least doubles the odds of MDD, and the associations of SUDs and bipolar disorders are even larger. The associations are also generally larger for current disorders than for lifetime disorders. The associations are similar for men and women. In summary, the data from these community surveys confirm that the high rate of co-occurrence between mood disorders and SUDs is not simply an artifact of treatment-seeking but instead reflects some fundamental relations between these syndromes.

Relationships Between Mood and Substance Use Disorders

Types of Relationships

As has been previously elucidated (Meyer 1986), several types of relationships between two comorbid syndromes are theoretically possible. These are summarized in Table 41–3, along with the types of evidence that would support each relationship. Mood disorders may function as a causal risk factor for SUDs. One mechanism for this could be self-medication (Khantzian 1985), whereby a patient with a mood disorder takes addictive substances to elevate or control his or her mood. For example, regular drug or alcohol use might be initiated or maintained to relieve the low mood, low energy, or insomnia associated with depression. Alcohol might be used to control excessive energy during mania. However, evidence for such mechanisms has been inconsistent (Aharonovich et al. 2001). Also, the pathophysiology of mood disorders might predispose a patient to SUDs at a neurochemical level. Conversely, SUDs could function as a causal risk factor for mood disorders. Substance use might trigger the onset of mood disorders or promote dysregulation in neural systems that regulate mood. In some instances, substance use or an SUD may be a consequence of the impulsivity and poor judgment of bipolar illness, which resolves once mania resolves (Schuckit 1986). Toxic effects of substances may be mistaken for the symptoms of a depressive disorder, resulting in diagnostic confusion (Schuckit 1986). However, a study of a national sample of former drinkers, most of them abstinent for many years, refuted this as a full explanation (Hasin and Grant 2002). In this study, a history of past, remitted DSM-IV alcohol dependence increased the risk of current MDD fourfold when use of other drugs and nicotine was controlled. In this study, even the most protracted withdrawal would have had time to resolve, suggesting that some other factor was causing the association between alcohol dependence and MDD.

Mood disorders and SUDs might share common underlying risk factors. Several analyses of twin studies have suggested common genetic liabilities (Fu et al. 2002;

TABLE 41–2. Increased risk (OR) for substance use disorders among individuals with mood disorders (or vice versa) in community surveys

	ECA[a]		NCS[a]		NESARC[b]		NESARC-III[c]	
	Alcohol	Drug	Alcohol	Drug	Alcohol	Drug	Alcohol	Drug
Lifetime								
Major depressive disorder	1.9	3.5	1.9	2.4	1.7	2.0	1.3	1.3
Dysthymia	2.0	3.2	2.1	2.3	–	–		
Bipolar disorder (mania)	4.6	7.4	4.9	4.9	–	–	3.0	5.5
Current[d]								
Major depressive disorder	2.7	3.4	2.6	3.0	3.7	9.0	1.2	1.5
Dysthymia	1.7	2.0	1.8	4.3	2.8	11.3		
Bipolar disorder (mania)	3.8	3.2	5.6	5.7	5.7	13.9	5.0	5.3

Note. ECA=Epidemiologic Catchment Area study; NCS=National Comorbidity Survey; NESARC=National Epidemiological Survey of Alcohol and Related Conditions.
[a]Data for ECA and NCS are from Kessler 1995. ECA ORs calculated on the subsample of participants younger than age 55 years for comparability with the NCS sample.
[b]Data for NESARC are from Grant et al. 2005 and Hasin et al. 2005.
[c]Data for NESARC-III are from Grant et al. 2015 and Grant et al. 2016.
[d]Current disorders are past 6 months for ECA and NCS.

TABLE 41–3. Potential relations between mood disorders and substance use disorders (SUDs)

Relation	Supporting evidence
Mood disorder is a causal risk factor for SUD (e.g., self-medication).	Mood disorder precedes onset of SUD (mood disorder is chronologically primary). Mood disorder is associated with greater severity, worse outcome of SUD. Treatment of mood disorder improves substance use.
SUD is a causal risk factor for mood disorder.	SUD precedes onset of mood disorder (mood disorder is chronologically secondary). Substance use is associated with greater severity, worse prognosis for mood disorder (e.g., in bipolar illness). Treatment of substance use disorder improves mood disorder.
Substance toxicity or withdrawal mimics symptoms of mood disorder (i.e., diagnostic confusion).	Mood symptoms resolve with abstinence.
Mood disorders and SUDs share common risk factors.	Twin studies show common genetic factors predisposing to both sets of disorders. Stress is a risk factor for both.
Mood disorders and SUDs occur together but are independent disorders.	Both are common and will co-occur by chance.
Mood disorders and SUDs become linked over time.	Co-occurrence is associated with greater severity and worse outcome, suggesting interaction. Moods as conditioned cues trigger craving and drug-seeking behavior.

Kendler et al. 1993a, 1993b) that predispose individuals to both sets of disorders. Life events and social stress are environmental risk factors that have been associated with both mood disorders and addictive disorders (Dohrenwend et al. 1992), as are adverse childhood experiences (Elliott et al. 2014; Fenton et al. 2013; Keyes et al. 2012, 2014; Meyers et al. 2018).

Finally, in some individuals, mood disorders and SUDs may be independent but co-occur by chance. However, this cannot explain the substantial rates of co-occurrence (see Table 41–2). Even if the initial occurrence of the two disorders is independent, they may become associated within an individual over time (Meyer et al. 1986). One mechanism for this could be classical conditioning, whereby external environmental stimuli or internal sensations become conditioned cues that trigger drug use behavior. Unpleasant moods, particularly anger and sadness, have been shown to function as conditioned cues that trigger craving for opiates in opiate-dependent patients (Childress et al. 1994). This association could gradually amplify a link between depression and substance use.

In the following sections, we review various types of evidence that bear on the relation between mood disorders and SUDs, including longitudinal studies, family and genetic studies, behavioral and neurobiological evidence, and treatment studies of co-occurring mood and substance use disorders.

Longitudinal Studies

Longitudinal studies that follow up cohorts of individuals from childhood into adolescence and adulthood seeking to uncover risk factors for SUDs (Brook et al. 1990; Kellam et al. 1983; Martin et al. 1994; Moss et al. 1994) consistently identify childhood externalizing disorders, such as conduct disorder, as strong risk factors, but they also identify an anxious-depressive temperament in early childhood as a risk factor. Striking evidence subsequently emerged that early-onset nicotine (Breslau et al. 1993) and marijuana use (Brook et al. 2002; Fergusson et al. 2002; Patton et al. 2002) increased the subsequent risk for anxiety and depressive disorders. Taken together, these studies suggested a potentially complex bidirectional relation between mood disorders and SUDs during development.

In adults, some studies have suggested that cannabis use increases subsequent risk for depression (Bovasso 2001; Kuo et al. 2001). Various longitudinal studies have found that a current mood disorder increases the risk for poor course and outcome of SUDs (for review, see Hasin et al. 2004). For example, a history of MDD reduces the odds of successfully quitting smoking (Glassman 1993) and increases the risk of relapse to alcohol or drug use disorder (Greenfield et al. 1998; Hasin et al. 1996a, 2002). Similarly, psychiatric disorders, including depression, have been found to be associated with a worse prognosis in samples of opiate- (Rounsaville et al. 1986b), alcohol- (Rounsaville et al. 1987), and cocaine-dependent patients (Carroll et al. 1993), and SUD worsens prognosis in bipolar disorder (Sonne and Brady 1999).

Conversely, among opiate-dependent patients, depression has been found to be transient over long-term follow-up, suggesting that some depressions in this population represent either responses to substance toxicity and withdrawal or responses to psychosocial stress, to which this population is particularly vulnerable (De Leon et al. 1973; Rounsaville et al. 1986a). Similarly, among alcohol-dependent (Brown et al.

1995; Liappas et al. 2002) and cocaine-dependent patients (Satel et al. 1991; Weddington et al. 1990), it has been shown that most mood symptoms resolve after detoxification and a brief period of abstinence, again suggesting that these symptoms represent toxic or withdrawal effects. These latter findings relate mainly to depressive symptoms rather than to depressive disorders, which have more clear adverse prognostic effects (Hasin et al. 2004).

In summary, the longitudinal studies, taken together, suggest a complex bidirectional relation between the two sets of disorders—mood disorders may function as a risk factor for SUDs, and, conversely, SUDs function as a risk factor for mood disorders.

Family and Genetic Studies

Early family studies (Winokur and Coryell 1992) suggested that depressive disorders could be divided into two types: pure depressive disorder and depression spectrum disorder, the latter of which includes a mixture of depression, alcoholism, and other comorbid disorders that appear to aggregate in some families. Family studies have found increased rates of depression among families with alcohol (Schuckit 1986) or drug dependence (Rounsaville et al. 1991), but the pattern suggests various interpretations, including that the disorders aggregate in families but are causally independent. Such a pattern could result from assortative mating, the increased likelihood of individuals with one condition to marry and have children with individuals who have the other disorder.

Adoption studies (Goodwin 1979; Sigvardsson et al. 1996) provided the initial basis for the genetic study of alcoholism by clarifying that among those adopted away at a very early age, alcoholism in the biological but not the adoptive parents predicted alcoholism in the adoptee. However, attempts in adoption studies to identify a subtype of alcohol use disorder partially defined by accompanying depressive or anxious traits (Cloninger 1987) were not supported in subsequent research (Babor et al. 1992). Some twin studies (Kendler et al. 1993a, 1993b) have suggested patterns consistent with common genetic risk factors that underlie both SUDs and MDD. Other studies suggested that genetic factors for internalizing disorders (including depression) and externalizing disorders (including SUDs) are largely distinct (Kendler et al. 2003). One study suggested that the common genetic risk may be mediated by antisocial personality traits (Fu et al. 2002), consistent with a typology of alcohol dependence proposed by Babor et al. (1992). These issues may be resolved more clearly when specific genetic polymorphisms are studied.

Identifying specific genes involved in the risk for complex disorders such as SUDs and MDD has been a challenge, but the progress in understanding the genetic etiology of alcohol use disorder is advancing rapidly. Because GABA transmission mediates several effects of alcohol, GABA receptor genes have been investigated in several studies. Whole-genome surveys (Long et al. 1998; Reich et al. 1998) implicated the *GABRB1* gene on chromosome 4, as did a study that used brain oscillations measured by electroencephalogram (EEG-β), a trait associated with alcoholism (Porjesz et al. 2002). A study of single-nucleotide polymorphisms in the four genes of chromosome 4 that encode subunits of the $GABA_A$ receptor found evidence that variation in the *GABRA2* gene influenced both alcohol dependence and EEG-β (Edenberg et al. 2004). Studies designed to generate a similar line of research for MDD (Holmans et al. 2004;

Levinson et al. 2003) are now under way. A linkage study of an "either/or" phenotype (alcohol dependence or MDD) in alcoholic probands and their relatives suggested linkage in an area of chromosome 1 that also has been implicated in linkage studies of affective disorders (Nurnberger et al. 2001).

Perspectives From Behavioral Science

Behavioral models of substance use and depression emphasize the role of environmental contingencies (e.g., reinforcement and punishment) in both disorders. Drug use disorder is associated with significant psychosocial deficits (e.g., unemployment, lower education) that restrict access to alternative, nondrug positive reinforcement and increase the rate of negative life events, both of which increase the probability of SUDs and depressive disorders (Dohrenwend et al. 1992; Kessler 1997). Human and animal laboratory studies indicated that the presence of alternative, nondrug reinforcers reduced the probability of drug use across a wide range of substances (Carroll 1996; Hart et al. 2000), and clinical interventions that increased the accessibility of alternative, nondrug reinforcement reduced both drug use (Iguchi et al. 1997) and depressive symptoms (Jacobson et al. 1996; Lewinsohn and Graf 1973).

Although the amount of positive reinforcement and punishment in the environment can be an important link between depression and drug use disorder, the two disorders also may be linked by changes in the hedonic value of previous reinforcers. As noted earlier, addictive substances function as positive reinforcers, and models of both classical and operant conditioning afford powerful explanatory schemes for these disorders. During development of tolerance to an addictive drug, the hedonic value of that drug, as well as the hedonic value of all natural reinforcers, is gradually reduced, as reflected in the model of altered brain stimulation reward thresholds (Gardner 1997). The addictive substance engages the brain reward system so powerfully that the system is rendered less responsive to natural reinforcers, producing an anhedonic state that also could be viewed as a model of depression. The demonstrated shifts in the subjective value of reinforcers in the context of SUDs have also been captured in the programmatic line of research assessing the extent to which individuals discount future rewards (e.g., delayed discounting). The rate of temporally discounting rewards has been shown to be different across substance-using and nonsubstance-using groups (e.g., Businelle et al. 2010). These findings suggest that SUDs are associated with a propensity to choose more immediate rewards of lesser value over rewards of greater value that will not be obtainable until a later time. This dynamic can be exacerbated as the number of competing nondrug rewards decreases and rewards become more delayed, thus leaving substance use as the more immediately accessible and reinforced behavior. Furthermore, it has been suggested that a quantification of temporal discounting may serve as an important marker for tracking shifts in self-control over time (Bickel et al. 2014) and an important process in understanding the neural substrates of decision making and its link to psychopathology (Lempert et al. 2019).

Behavioral formulations of depression also have featured the loss of reinforcer effectiveness as a central factor (Costello 1972). Experimental studies show that individuals with depressive disorders have a blunted response to pleasurable stimuli compared with people without depression (Berenbaum and Oltmanns 1992; Sloan et al. 2001), and depressive disorders have been associated with a greater discounting of future rewards (e.g., Pulcu et al. 2014). Moody et al. (2016) demonstrated that individuals with a comorbid depressive disorder and SUD evidenced greater discounting of future rewards than substance users with no comorbidity, suggesting a compounded trend to choose more immediate rewards instead of larger rewards that are more temporally distant in the context of comorbidity.

Corresponding animal models, such as the forced swim test, are useful in predicting the efficacy of antidepressant medications. The inability to escape aversive conditions is a model of psychological stress, and similar stress that has been modeled in animals has been found to increase the propensity of animals to self-administer various drugs (Goeders 2003). Thus, similarities between behavioral models of mood disorders and behavioral models of addiction emerge with respect to environmental contingencies (e.g., positive reinforcement), response to stress, and status of the brain reward system. Pathophysiological models of depression have tended to focus on neurochemical deficits, such as serotonin system deficits (Malone and Mann 1993) or CRH excess (Nemeroff 1992). The notion of depression as a disorder of the brain reward system has received less attention but is an implication of the comorbidity of mood disorders and SUDs that may represent a promising direction for future research (see Naranjo et al. 2001).

Neurobiological Commonalities

Markou et al. (1998) and Volkow et al. (2013), among others, have reviewed derangements in a wide variety of neurochemical and neurohumoral systems across patient populations with depression and substance dependence. These reviews demonstrated substantial concordance—that is, derangements that tended to point in the same direction—in both sets of disorders. Such findings strengthen the argument for a pathophysiological common ground.

Brain imaging offers another framework to elucidate neuroanatomical and neurochemical relations between SUDs and other psychiatric disorders (Koob and Volkow 2016; Volkow 2001). Broadly speaking, human brain imaging studies of regional neural activity (PET, structural and functional MRI) indicate overlap in the brain pathways involved in the symptomatic expression of SUD and depression (see Figure 41–1). Delineation of shared circuitry, even without yet specifying shared neurochemical abnormalities, establishes brain network commonality between SUDs and mood disorders. Such functional and structural imaging studies have identified deficits in the frontal lobes in association with various forms of SUD (Goldstein and Volkow 2002). Frontal deficits also have been implicated in depressive disorders (Drevets 2000; see Chapter 11, "Brain Imaging," in this volume). Overall, the human functional imaging data implicate frontal-striatal-limbic circuitry in the executive, motivational, and emotional functioning of both humans and laboratory animals (Heimer 2003; Volkow et al. 2013). Common deficits in these brain systems observed in mood disorders and SUDs suggest pathophysiological common ground for further exploration and treatment possibilities.

Less consensus emerges from the literature on brain imaging studies of specific transmitter systems implicated in human SUDs and mood disorders. Striatal D_2 dopamine receptor availability has been documented in association with SUDs

may be useful (Levin et al. 2004), the most important tool is a careful clinical history that seeks evidence of substance use, or use disorder, according to DSM-5 criteria. Practice with the Structured Clinical Interview for DSM-5 Disorders (SCID-5; First et al. 2015), the Psychiatric Research Interview for Substance and Mental Disorders (PRISM; Hasin et al. 1996b, 2002), or similar structured instruments can be useful training on how to ask about these symptoms. It is important to inquire about substance use and SUD symptoms in an accepting and nonjudgmental fashion because SUDs are stigmatized, and patients may be defensive and motivated to conceal or minimize the extent of substance use. Gentle inquiry with an accepting stance is recommended to overcome this. Biological testing using urine toxicology or breath-alcohol levels may be used if concealment is suspected.

As part of the evaluation process, it is important to anticipate potential intoxication and withdrawal symptoms that may confuse the diagnostic picture. Also, if the patient is abstinent, withdrawal symptoms may emerge and need to be treated. Withdrawal symptoms are often benign and can be treated in an office setting. However, alcohol and sedative-hypnotic withdrawal can be quite serious or even life-threatening, and opiate withdrawal is extremely unpleasant and almost invariably leads to relapse unless treated aggressively.

Evaluation of Mood Disorders in Patients With Substance Use Disorders

The essential problem is that of distinguishing true mood disorders from mood symptoms that represent substance toxicity or withdrawal, and distinguishing DSM-5 primary or independent mood disorders from what DSM-5 calls substance-induced mood disorders (Nunes and Weiss 2014). No sure method exists for solving this problem, as reflected in the results of the meta-analysis discussed earlier in the "Treatment Studies of Co-Occurring Mood and Substance Use Disorders" section (Nunes and Levin 2004); subsequent trials (Kranzler et al. 2006) showed that despite efforts at careful clinical diagnosis, high placebo response rates consistent with the selection of transient mood disturbances were a problem in some of the trials. Various approaches have been developed to address this problem (Nunes et al. 2004), many of which are integrated in the DSM-IV and DSM-5 constructs of independent and substance-induced depression.

In brief, a DSM-5 primary or independent syndrome is one that has been shown to occur independently of substance use over time; that is, during abstinence from substances. A substance-induced mood syndrome is one that has never occurred independent of substance use but in which the symptoms are in excess of what would be expected given the toxic and withdrawal effects of the substances alone. SUDs often have an early onset and a chronic course, making it difficult to find a period of abstinence in the history during which to inquire about mood disorders. The substance-induced category recognizes that depression in this setting still may be clinically significant. Both primary and substance-induced depression are to be distinguished from usual and expected toxic or withdrawal effects of substances.

The DSM-5 criteria for primary depression are straightforward and can be determined by taking a careful parallel history of mood and substance problems over the lifetime, but DSM-5 is less clear on specific criteria for substance-induced mood disorder, leaving this to the clinician's judgment. The PRISM is a structured clinical interview that provides a reliable method for diagnosing primary and substance-induced depression among substance-dependent patients. Predictive validity has been established in that both PRISM-identified primary and substance-induced depressions have been shown to have adverse prognostic effects among substance-dependent patients (Hasin et al. 2002). Clinicians might be encouraged to practice interviewing with the PRISM as a way of developing interviewing skills with dual-diagnosis patients. Other historical features to look for include severity or chronicity of depressive symptoms, suicidality, and other comorbid disorders, such as anxiety or personality syndromes (Nunes et al. 2004). Such features would suggest that the mood syndrome is in excess of what would be expected from routine toxic or withdrawal symptoms from substances. The surest method of diagnosing a mood disorder is to have the patient become abstinent for a period of time before making a final evaluation. Thus, all such patients should be encouraged to achieve abstinence. Hospitalization to achieve abstinence is less of an option in the current health care system. However, treatment for the SUD, with the goal of abstinence, should be initiated on an outpatient basis in any case, including both counseling and medications if indicated (methadone, buprenorphine, or injection naltrexone for opioid use disorder; naltrexone or disulfiram for alcohol use disorder). Despite initiating such treatment, clinicians are still often left with a patient who is actively using substances and has a mood syndrome that needs diagnostic assessment and treatment planning.

Another important step in the evaluation of a patient with mood symptoms and an SUD is to look for other co-occurring mental disorders. PTSD, ADHD, and anxiety disorders each commonly co-occur with both depression and SUD, and these disorders have specific treatment implications that would be important in treatment planning (Nunes and Weiss 2014).

Treatment of Substance Use Disorder in Patients With Mood Disorders

Complete coverage of the treatment of SUDs is well beyond the scope of this chapter. Excellent textbooks exist (e.g., Ries et al. 2014). Nonetheless, substance use or SUD is likely to worsen mood symptoms, which may resolve if abstinence is achieved, and substance use increases suicide risk (Aharonovich et al. 2002; Levy and Deykin 1989; Murphy et al. 1992). Therefore, treatment of SUDs should be a high priority from the outset in patients with a mood disorder who present with substance use or SUD. We believe that all clinicians should be familiar with the basic tools for treating SUDs.

Psychosocial and Behavioral Methods

Several psychosocial and behavioral methods are likely to be particularly useful to general clinicians and those working with patients with mood disorders. Even simple advice from a physician to quit substance use can be an effective intervention (Fleming et al. 1997). For patients with ambivalence or resistance to giving up drugs or alcohol (which is to be expected), motivational interviewing is a useful tool that shows substantial evidence of efficacy (Miller and Rollnick 2002). Motivational interviewing shifts the clinician away from an authoritarian stance and toward an empathic and collaborative approach, in which they seek to elicit the patient's own point of view, concerns about substances, and reasons for quitting. Recent studies have investigated an integrated treatment approach in which motivational interviewing strategies are employed to help increase change talk in terms of substance use, as well as client language directly linked to the availability of non-substance-related competing reinforcement and the temporal availability of these reinforcers (Ladd et al. 2021). This combined strategy provides a platform to bring the conceptual lenses of behavioral economic theory to bear on clinical conversations and leverage the power of competing reinforcement as an important agent of change.

Self-help groups, such as Alcoholics Anonymous, have a strong tradition, and most communities have active groups of this type. Evidence suggests that referral to 12-step groups is effective (Project MATCH Research Group 1997), and it is useful for clinicians to be familiar with their principles and procedures to encourage patients to participate (Emrick and Tonigan 2004). In the Combining Medications and Behavioral Interventions for Alcoholism (COMBINE) study, a multisite randomized trial examining outpatient treatment of alcohol use disorder with naltrexone or acamprosate versus placebo and medical management or cognitive therapy in a factorial design, the best alcohol use outcome was among patients receiving medical management plus naltrexone (Anton et al. 2006). Medical management (Pettinati et al. 2005) provides a straightforward structure for brief visits between a physician or other medical clinician and patient, emphasizing adherence to medication, adherence to other aspects of the treatment plan, and participation in 12-step meetings (e.g., Alcoholics Anonymous).

Other useful techniques include cognitive-behavioral relapse prevention, which is based on social learning theory and seeks to help patients see the connections between events within themselves and their environment that trigger substance use (Carroll et al. 2004), and the use of positive reinforcement with voucher incentives (Carroll and Weiss 2017; Higgins et al. 1993; Silverman et al. 1996).

Cognitive-behavioral therapy (CBT) and contingency management are now available on web-based or smartphone app–based platforms, such as Computer-Based Training for Cognitive Behavioral Therapy (CBT4CBT; Carroll et al. 2008) and Therapeutic Education System (Campbell et al. 2014), now marketed as reSET (Pear Therapeutics). This may make it more feasible for physicians and other clinicians in a range of practice settings to make these behavioral treatments available to their patients without needing to directly deliver the treatments.

Pharmacotherapy

For nicotine, alcohol, and opiate use disorders, a general psychiatrist should be familiar with and relatively comfortable in using several effective medication treatments. As a general rule, such medications are more effective when used in concert with some form of psychosocial intervention.

Nicotine use disorder is common among psychiatric patients and can be effectively treated with nicotine-replacement products, including nicotine-containing chewing gum and nicotine patches (Hughes et al. 1996), which are available over the counter. Patients should be encouraged to set a quit date on which they will apply the nicotine patch and chew nicotine gum at times when they experience craving for a cigarette. If patients fail to quit or relapse to smoking, it is best to praise their effort and suggest that they try again. This positive, encouraging approach is important in the treatment of any SUD. Furthermore, in the case of nicotine use disorder, the statistics suggest that any single quit attempt has a low likelihood of success, but patients who try to quit repeatedly are likely to succeed eventually. Noradrenergic antidepressant medications, including bupropion (Hurt et al. 1997) and nortriptyline (Hall et al. 1998), are also effective for smoking cessation; they should be started several weeks before the determined quit date and can be used in concert with nicotine replacement. Interestingly, these medications may work by reducing the dysphoric symptoms that often follow smoking cessation (Hall et al. 1998). The typical recommendation would be to discontinue the antidepressant several months after successful quitting, although evidence now shows that continuation of the medication has a role in preventing relapse (Hays et al. 2001). It is important to be aware that MDD may emerge after a successful quit attempt (Glassman 1993). Varenicline, a nicotine receptor partial agonist, is also effective for smoking cessation (Ebbert et al. 2010).

Detoxification from alcohol is usually benign and can be treated supportively or with a tapering schedule of a long-acting benzodiazepine, such as chlordiazepoxide. For prevention of alcohol relapse, disulfiram is a clinical tool that is rarely used, even though it can be extremely effective if its daily ingestion is monitored by a significant other (Schuckit and Tapert 2004). Disulfiram impairs the metabolism of acetaldehyde, a toxic by-product of alcohol metabolism, such that any drinking produces an unpleasant reaction. The opiate antagonist naltrexone is also modestly effective for alcohol use disorder (Kranzler and Van Kirk 2001), particularly in combination with relapse prevention therapy. Again, involvement of a significant other to monitor the medication is likely to be helpful. Interestingly, naltrexone may act by blunting the reinforcing effects of alcohol or may interfere with the role of moods, both positive and negative, in triggering drinking behavior (Kranzler et al. 2004). Naltrexone and disulfiram have been found to be safe and effective for patients with co-occurring mood and alcohol use disorders (Petrakis et al. 2005)

For opiate use disorder, methadone maintenance is a powerful treatment (Schottenfeld 2004), although it is for the most part little known and poorly understood by general clinicians. Methadone is an orally bioavailable, long-acting opiate agonist that terminates opiate withdrawal and, when given at sufficiently high doses over a prolonged period, induces tolerance and blockade of the effects of other opiates. By law, methadone maintenance can be administered only by specially licensed clinics. Buprenorphine, a long-acting partial opiate agonist, is an alternative to methadone maintenance and can be prescribed by any physician who has taken a brief training course and received certification. It is hoped that this will increase the involvement of general physicians in the treatment of opiate use disorder and attract more opiate-dependent patients into treatment (Li et al. 2014). Extended-release injected formulations of buprenorphine are now available (Haight et al. 2019; Lofwall et al. 2018; Walsh et al. 2017), providing an additional tool for patients for whom adherence to daily medication is a challenge. The opiate antagonist naltrexone is an effective maintenance treatment for opiate use disorder as long as patients take it; drawbacks include the fact that it requires detoxification from opiates before it can be safely started (otherwise it precipitates withdrawal). Compliance with the oral formulation taken daily has been poor (O'Brien and Kampman 2004), which is a limiting factor even in the presence of intensive behavioral therapy to promote adherence (Nunes et al. 2006; Rothenberg et al. 2002). However, development of an extended-release monthly injection of naltrexone (Vivitrol) circumvents the need for adherence to daily dosing and has produced effectiveness close to that of buprenorphine in clinical trials (Lee et al. 2018; Tanum et al. 2017)

Treatment of Mood Disorders in Patients With Substance Use Disorders

Depression

The evidence on treatment of depression among patients with SUDs, reviewed earlier in this chapter in the section "Treatment Studies of Co-Occurring Mood and Substance Use Disorders," suggests that depressive syndromes, carefully diagnosed by clinical history according to standard diagnostic criteria, respond to antidepressant medications (Nunes and Levin 2004; Torrens et al. 2005). The placebo response rates reported were often high, reflecting either diagnostic confusion and poor selection of patients or favorable effects of concurrent psychotherapy. Some of the largest antidepressant effects were seen in studies that required a period of abstinence from substances prior to diagnosis of depression. In view of this evidence, the most prudent clinical approach is to start by encouraging abstinence and offering psychosocial methods or pharmacotherapy to help initiate abstinence. After a period of treatment for the SUD and an effort to achieve abstinence, if the depression persists, it should be treated with either antidepressant medication or specific psychotherapy (Nunes and Weiss 2014). It is important not to delay treatment of depression beyond a reasonable period, even if abstinence is not achieved, because such depression may have adverse prognostic effects (Hasin et al. 2002) and risk of suicide (Aharonovich et al. 2002; Levy and Deykin 1989; Murphy et al. 1992). Finally, the evidence from clinical trials suggests that treatment of depression, even in the setting of active substance use, can be effective (Nunes and Levin 2004).

Although tricyclic antidepressants show more evidence of efficacy among the published clinical trials (Nunes and Levin 2004; Torrens et al. 2005), selective serotonin reuptake inhibitors (SSRIs) have shown efficacy in several trials (Cornelius et al. 1997; Roy 1998). SSRIs can be recommended as the first treatment of choice in dually diagnosed patients because of the good tolerability and low toxicity of these agents. If an SSRI fails, then antidepressant agents with alternative mechanisms should be considered. Agents with antianxiety or soporific effects (e.g., tricyclic antidepressants, mirtazapine, or trazodone) may be considered, particularly for patients with substantial anxiety or insomnia as a component of their depression. As always, the potential risks of combining therapeutic medications with addictive substances need to be weighed.

More research is needed on the use of psychotherapeutic techniques that have been designed specifically for the treatment of depression or for combined depression plus SUDs, but existing studies suggest the promise of this approach (Brown et al. 1997; Lydecker et al. 2010). For example, the inverse relationship between depression severity and engaging in pleasant activities has been previously highlighted (Lewinsohn 1975) and has served as a basis for depression-focused treatments that aim to increase pleasant life events (Lewinsohn et al. 1984) or activities that promote a rewarding life (e.g., behavioral activation [Martell et al. 2001]). More recent findings suggest that use of behavioral activation can also be an effective strategy for the treatment of SUDs (Daughters et al. 2018), suggesting that treatment frameworks that focus on increasing an individual's contact with meaningful reinforcement may provide an important platform for addressing these comorbid conditions.

Bipolar Disorder

As noted earlier, controlled trials of treatments for bipolar illness among substance-dependent patients are limited (Brady and Malcolm 2004). Small, controlled trials suggest that both lithium (Geller et al. 1998) and the anticonvulsant carbamazepine (Brady et al. 2002) are effective among such patients. The anticonvulsants valproate and lamotrigine have also shown promise in controlled trials (for review, see Salloum and Brown 2017). The second-generation antipsychotic quetiapine has been tested in three controlled trials as an add-on to other mood stabilizers, demonstrating improvement in mood compared with placebo but not in substance use (for a review, see Salloum and Brown 2017). Thus, medications used to treat bipolar disorder appear to be helpful overall in the setting of co-occurring substance use, suggesting the importance of optimizing treatment for the mood disorder, although the SUD may persist and require independent treatment. Medication treatments for alcohol use disorder, naltrexone and disulfiram, have shown promise for improving alcohol outcome among patients with a mixture of mood disorders, including some with bipolar disorder (Salloum and Brown 2017). Psychotherapy approaches targeting the combination of bipolar disorder and SUDs have also shown positive results in reducing substance use among individuals with bipolar disorder (Salloum et al. 2008; Weiss et al. 2000).

Future Directions

The comorbidity of mood disorders and SUDs has been a long-standing source of controversy for the field. Clinicians at one time were polarized into camps, either viewing SUD as the predominant force among comorbid patients, with mood symptoms representing mainly toxic effects, or viewing the mood disturbance as predominant and substance use as a response to it, as in self-medication. Research from recent decades, reviewed here, suggests a multiplicity of possible relationships between these disorders (see Table 41–3), the high prevalence of comorbidity clinically, and potential common ground at the neurobiological level. A challenge for the future will be to design more research that seeks to translate findings and insights back and forth across basic and clinical disciplines and across disorders, and it is hoped that this chapter has stimulated interest in the potential of this approach.

At the clinical level, clinicians, services, and treatment systems remain, in many instances, polarized into those that provide care for mood and other psychiatric disorders and those that provide care for SUDs, and the availability of treatment for mood disorders in settings that treat SUDs remains uneven (Petrakis et al. 2003). The challenge here is to place evaluation and treatment of substance use, as well as of mood disorders, among the core skills of psychiatrists and allied mental health professionals and to design more integrated systems of care.

References

Aharonovich E, Nguyen HT, Nunes EV: Anger and depressive states among treatment-seeking drug abusers: testing the psychopharmacological specificity hypothesis. Am J Addict 10(4):327–334, 2001 11783747

Aharonovich E, Liu X, Nunes E, et al: Suicide attempts in substance abusers: effects of major depression in relation to substance use disorders. Am J Psychiatry 159(9):1600–1602, 2002 12202286

American Psychiatric Association: Diagnostic and Statistical Manual of Mental Disorders, 4th Edition. Washington, DC, American Psychiatric Association, 1994

American Psychiatric Association: Diagnostic and Statistical Manual of Mental Disorders, 4th Edition, Text Revision. Washington, DC, American Psychiatric Association, 2000

American Psychiatric Association: Diagnostic and Statistical Manual of Mental Disorders, 5th Edition. Arlington, VA, American Psychiatric Association, 2013

Anton RF, O'Malley SS, Ciraulo DA, et al: Combined pharmacotherapies and behavioral interventions for alcohol dependence: the COMBINE study: a randomized controlled trial. JAMA 295(17):2003–2017, 2006 16670409

Babor TF, Hofmann M, DelBoca FK, et al: Types of alcoholics, I. Evidence for an empirically derived typology based on indicators of vulnerability and severity. Arch Gen Psychiatry 49(8):599–608, 1992 1637250

Bardo MT: Neuropharmacological mechanisms of drug reward: beyond dopamine in the nucleus accumbens. Crit Rev Neurobiol 12(1–2):37–67, 1998 9444481

Berenbaum H, Oltmanns TF: Emotional experience and expression in schizophrenia and depression. J Abnorm Psychol 101(1):37–44, 1992 1537971

Bickel WK, Landes RD, Kurth-Nelson Z, et al: A quantitative signature of self-control repair: rate-dependent effects of successful addiction treatment. Clin Psychol Sci 2:685–695, 2014

Bovasso GB: Cannabis abuse as a risk factor for depressive symptoms. Am J Psychiatry 158(12):2033–2037, 2001 11729021

Brady KT, Malcolm RJ: Substance use disorders and co-occurring Axis I psychiatric disorders, in The American Psychiatric Publishing Textbook of Substance Abuse Treatment, 3rd Edition. Edited by Galanter M, Kleber HD. Arlington, VA, American Psychiatric Publishing, 2004, pp 529–537

Brady KT, Halligan P, Malcolm RJ: Dual diagnosis, in The American Psychiatric Press Textbook of Substance Abuse Treatment, 2nd Edition. Edited by Galanter M, Kleber HD. Washington, DC, American Psychiatric Press, 1999, pp 475–483

Brady KT, Sonne SC, Malcolm RJ, et al: Carbamazepine in the treatment of cocaine dependence: subtyping by affective disorder. Exp Clin Psychopharmacol 10(3):276–285, 2002 12233988

Breslau N, Kilbey MM, Andreski P: Nicotine dependence and major depression. New evidence from a prospective investigation. Arch Gen Psychiatry 50(1):31–35, 1993 8422219

Brook DW, Brook JS, Zhang C, et al: Drug use and the risk of major depressive disorder, alcohol dependence, and substance use disorders. Arch Gen Psychiatry 59(11):1039–1044, 2002 12418937

Brook JS, Brook DW, Gordon AS, et al: The psychosocial etiology of adolescent drug use: a family interactional approach. Genet Soc Gen Psychol Monogr 116(2):111–267, 1990 2376323

Brown RA, Evans DM, Miller IW, et al: Cognitive-behavioral treatment for depression in alcoholism. J Consult Clin Psychol 65(5):715–726, 1997 9337490

Brown SA, Inaba RK, Gillin JC, et al: Alcoholism and affective disorder: clinical course of depressive symptoms. Am J Psychiatry 152(1):45–52, 1995 7802119

Budney AJ, Hughes JR, Moore BA, et al: Review of the validity and significance of cannabis withdrawal syndrome. Am J Psychiatry 161(11):1967–1977, 2004 15514394

Businelle MS, McVay MA, Kendzor D, et al: A comparison of delay discounting among smokers, substance abusers, and non-dependent controls. Drug Alcohol Depend 112(3):247–250, 2010 20696538

Campbell AN, Nunes EV, Matthews AG, et al: Internet-delivered treatment for substance abuse: a multisite randomized controlled trial. Am J Psychiatry 171(6):683–690, 2014 24700332
Carroll KM, Weiss RD: The role of behavioral interventions in buprenorphine maintenance treatment: a review. Am J Psychiatry 174(8):738–747, 2017 27978771
Carroll KM, Power ME, Bryant K, et al: One-year follow-up status of treatment-seeking cocaine abusers. Psychopathology and dependence severity as predictors of outcome. J Nerv Ment Dis 181(2):71–79, 1993 8426174
Carroll KM, Ball SA, Martino S: Cognitive, behavioral, and motivational therapies, in The American Psychiatric Publishing Textbook of Substance Abuse Treatment, 3rd Edition. Edited by Galanter M, Kleber HD. Arlington, VA, American Psychiatric Publishing, 2004, pp 365–376
Carroll KM, Ball SA, Martino S, et al: Computer-assisted delivery of cognitive-behavioral therapy for addiction: a randomized trial of CBT4CBT. Am J Psychiatry 165(7):881–888, 2008 18450927
Carroll ME: Reducing drug abuse by enriching the environment with alternative reinforcers, in Advances in Behavioral Economics, Vol 3: Substance Use and Abuse. Edited by Green L, Kagel JH. Norwood, NJ, Ablex Publishing, 1996, pp 37–68
Childress AR, Ehrman R, McLellan AT, et al: Can induced moods trigger drug-related responses in opiate abuse patients? J Subst Abuse Treat 11(1):17–23, 1994 8201629
Cloninger CR: Neurogenetic adaptive mechanisms in alcoholism. Science 236(4800):410–416, 1987 2882604
Cohen P, Cohen J: The clinician's illusion. Arch Gen Psychiatry 41(12):1178–1182, 1984 6334503
Cornelius JR, Salloum IM, Ehler JG, et al: Fluoxetine in depressed alcoholics. A double-blind, placebo-controlled trial. Arch Gen Psychiatry 54(8):700–705, 1997 9283504
Costello CG: Depression: loss of reinforcers or loss of reinforcer effectiveness? Behav Ther 3:240–247, 1972 27816073
Cousins MS, Roberts DC, de Wit H: GABA(B) receptor agonists for the treatment of drug addiction: a review of recent findings. Drug Alcohol Depend 65(3):209–220, 2002 11841892
Daughters SB, Magidson JF, Anand D, et al: The effect of a behavioral activation treatment for substance use on post-treatment abstinence: a randomized controlled trial. Addiction 113(3):535–544, 2018 28963853
De Leon G, Skodol A, Rosenthal MS: Phoenix House. Changes in psychopathological signs of resident drug addicts. Arch Gen Psychiatry 28(1):131–135, 1973 4405119
Dohrenwend BP, Levav I, Shrout PE, et al: Socioeconomic status and psychiatric disorders: the causation-selection issue. Science 255(5047):946–952, 1992 1546291
Drevets WC: Neuroimaging studies of mood disorders. Biol Psychiatry 48(8):813–829, 2000 11063977
Ebbert JO, Wyatt KD, Hays JT, et al: Varenicline for smoking cessation: efficacy, safety, and treatment recommendations. Patient Prefer Adherence 4:355–362, 2010 21049087
Edenberg HJ, Dick DM, Xuei X, et al: Variations in GABRA2, encoding the alpha 2 subunit of the GABA(A) receptor, are associated with alcohol dependence and with brain oscillations. Am J Hum Genet 74(4):705–714, 2004 15024690
Elliott JC, Stohl M, Wall MM, et al: The risk for persistent adult alcohol and nicotine dependence: the role of childhood maltreatment. Addiction 109(5):842–850, 2014 24401044
Emery MA, Akil H: Endogenous opioids at the intersection of opioid addiction, pain, and depression: the search for a precision medicine approach. Annu Rev Neurosci 43(1):355–374, 2020 32109184
Emrick CD, Tonigan JS: Alcoholics Anonymous and other 12-step groups, in The American Psychiatric Publishing Textbook of Substance Abuse Treatment, 3rd Edition. Edited by Galanter M, Kleber HD. Arlington, VA, American Psychiatric Publishing, 2004, pp 433–443
Fenton MC, Geier T, Keyes K, et al: Combined role of childhood maltreatment, family history, and gender in the risk for alcohol dependence. Psychol Med 43(5):1045–1057, 2013 22883538

Fergusson DM, Horwood LJ, Swain-Campbell N: Cannabis use and psychosocial adjustment in adolescence and young adulthood. Addiction 97(9):1123–1135, 2002 12199828
First MB, Williams JBW, Karg RS, Spitzer RL: Structured Clinical Interview for DSM-5 Disorders (SCID-5-CV): Clinician Version. Arlington, VA, American Psychiatric Association, 2015
Fleming MF, Barry KL, Manwell LB, et al: Brief physician advice for problem alcohol drinkers. A randomized controlled trial in community-based primary care practices. JAMA 277(13):1039–1045, 1997 9091691
Fu Q, Heath AC, Bucholz KK, et al: Shared genetic risk of major depression, alcohol dependence, and marijuana dependence: contribution of antisocial personality disorder in men. Arch Gen Psychiatry 59(12):1125–1132, 2002 12470129
Gardner EL: Brain reward mechanisms, in Substance Abuse: A Comprehensive Textbook. Edited by Lowinson JH, Ruiz P, Millman RB, et al. Baltimore, MD, Williams & Wilkins, 1997, pp 51–85
Geller B, Cooper TB, Sun K, et al: Double-blind and placebo-controlled study of lithium for adolescent bipolar disorders with secondary substance dependency. J Am Acad Child Adolesc Psychiatry 37(2):171–178, 1998 9473913
Gerasimov MR, Ashby CR Jr, Gardner EL, et al: Gamma-vinyl GABA inhibits methamphetamine, heroin, or ethanol-induced increases in nucleus accumbens dopamine. Synapse 34(1):11–19, 1999 10459167
Glassman AH: Cigarette smoking: implications for psychiatric illness. Am J Psychiatry 150(4):546–553, 1993 8465868
Goeders NE: The impact of stress on addiction. Eur Neuropsychopharmacol 13(6):435–441, 2003 14636959
Goldstein RZ, Volkow ND: Drug addiction and its underlying neurobiological basis: neuroimaging evidence for the involvement of the frontal cortex. Am J Psychiatry 159(10):1642–1652, 2002 12359667
Goodwin DW: Alcoholism and heredity. A review and hypothesis. Arch Gen Psychiatry 36(1):57–61, 1979 367310
Grace AA: Dysregulation of the dopamine system in the pathophysiology of schizophrenia and depression. Nat Rev Neurosci 17(8):524–532, 2016 27256556
Grant BF: Comorbidity between DSM-IV drug use disorders and major depression: results of a national survey of adults. J Subst Abuse 7(4):481–497, 1995 8838629
Grant BF, Harford TC: Comorbidity between DSM-IV alcohol use disorders and major depression: results of a national survey. Drug Alcohol Depend 39(3):197–206, 1995 8556968
Grant BF, Stinson FS, Harford TC: Age at onset of alcohol use and DSM-IV alcohol abuse and dependence: a 12-year follow-up. J Subst Abuse 13(4):493–504, 2001 11775078
Grant BF, Stinson FS, Dawson DA, et al: Prevalence and co-occurrence of substance use disorders and independent mood and anxiety disorders: results from the National Epidemiologic Survey on Alcohol and Related Conditions. Arch Gen Psychiatry 61(8):807–816, 2004 15289279
Grant BF, Stinson FS, Hasin DS, et al: Prevalence, correlates, and comorbidity of bipolar I disorder and Axis I and II disorders: results from the National Epidemiologic Survey on Alcohol and Related Conditions. J Clin Psychiatry 66(10):1205–1215, 2005 16259532
Grant BF, Goldstein RB, Saha TD, et al: Epidemiology of DSM-5 alcohol use disorder: results from the National Epidemiologic Survey on Alcohol and Related Conditions III. JAMA Psychiatry 72(8):757–766, 2015 26039070
Grant BF, Saha TD, Ruan WJ, et al: Epidemiology of DSM-5 drug use disorder: results from the National Epidemiologic Survey on Alcohol and Related Conditions–III. JAMA Psychiatry 73(1):39–47, 2016 26580136
Greenfield SF, Weiss RD, Muenz LR, et al: The effect of depression on return to drinking: a prospective study. Arch Gen Psychiatry 55(3):259–265, 1998 9510220
Haight BR, Learned SM, Laffont CM, et al: Efficacy and safety of a monthly buprenorphine depot injection for opioid use disorder: a multicentre, randomised, double-blind, placebo-controlled, phase 3 trial. Lancet 393(10173):778–790, 2019 30792007

Hall SM, Reus VI, Muñoz RF, et al: Nortriptyline and cognitive-behavioral therapy in the treatment of cigarette smoking. Arch Gen Psychiatry 55(8):683–690, 1998 9707377

Hart CL, Haney M, Foltin RW, et al: Alternative reinforcers differentially modify cocaine self-administration by humans. Behav Pharmacol 11(1):87–91, 2000 10821213

Hasin DS, Grant BF: Major depression in 6050 former drinkers: association with past alcohol dependence. Arch Gen Psychiatry 59(9):794–800, 2002 12215078

Hasin DS, Grant BF: The co-occurrence of DSM-IV alcohol abuse in DSM-IV alcohol dependence: results of the National Epidemiologic Survey on Alcohol and Related Conditions on heterogeneity that differ by population subgroup. Arch Gen Psychiatry 61(9):891–896, 2004 15351767

Hasin D, Paykin A: DSM-IV alcohol abuse: investigation in a sample of at-risk drinkers in the community. J Stud Alcohol 60(2):181–187, 1999 10091956

Hasin DS, Tsai WY, Endicott J, et al: Five-year course of major depression: effects of comorbid alcoholism. J Affect Disord 41(1):63–70, 1996a 8938207

Hasin DS, Trautman KD, Miele GM, et al: Psychiatric Research Interview for Substance and Mental Disorders (PRISM): reliability for substance abusers. Am J Psychiatry 153(9):1195–1201, 1996b 8780425

Hasin DS, Van Rossem R, McCloud S, Endicott J: Differentiating DSM-IV alcohol dependence and abuse by course: community heavy drinkers. J Subst Abuse 9:127–135, 1997 9494944

Hasin D, Liu X, Nunes E, et al: Effects of major depression on remission and relapse of substance dependence. Arch Gen Psychiatry 59(4):375–380, 2002 11926938

Hasin D, Nunes E, Meydan J: Comorbidity of alcohol, drug and psychiatric disorders: epidemiology, in Dual Diagnosis and Treatment: Substance Abuse and Comorbid Disorders, 2nd Edition. Edited by Kranzler HR, Tinsley JA. New York, Marcel Dekker, 2004, pp 1–34

Hasin DS, Goodwin RD, Stinson FS, et al: Epidemiology of major depressive disorder: results from the National Epidemiologic Survey on Alcoholism and Related Conditions. Arch Gen Psychiatry 62(10):1097–1106, 2005 16203955

Hasin DS, O'Brien CP, Auriacombe M, et al: DSM-5 criteria for substance use disorders: recommendations and rationale. Am J Psychiatry 170(8):834–851, 2013 23903334

Hasin DS, Sarvet AL, Meyers JL, et al: Epidemiology of adult DSM-5 major depressive disorder and its specifiers in the United States. JAMA Psychiatry 75(4):336–346, 2018 29450462

Hays JT, Hurt RD, Rigotti NA, et al: Sustained-release bupropion for pharmacologic relapse prevention after smoking cessation. a randomized, controlled trial. Ann Intern Med 135(6):423–433, 2001 11560455

Heimer L: A new anatomical framework for neuropsychiatric disorders and drug abuse. Am J Psychiatry 160(10):1726–1739, 2003 14514480

Hetherington HP, Pan JW, Telang F, et al: Reduced brain GABA levels in cocaine abusers (abstract no. 523). Paper presented at the Proceedings of the International Society of Magnetic Resonance Medicine, Denver, CO, April 3–7, 2000

Higgins ST, Budney AJ, Bickel WK, et al: Achieving cocaine abstinence with a behavioral approach. Am J Psychiatry 150(5):763–769, 1993 8480823

Holmans P, Zubenko GS, Crowe RR, et al: Genomewide significant linkage to recurrent, early onset major depressive disorder on chromosome 15q. Am J Hum Genet 74(6):1154–1167, 2004 15108123

Hughes JR, Fiester S, Goldstein M, et al: Practice guideline for the treatment of patients with nicotine dependence. Am J Psychiatry 153(10 suppl):1–31, 1996 8831466

Hurt RD, Sachs DP, Glover ED, et al: A comparison of sustained-release bupropion and placebo for smoking cessation. N Engl J Med 337(17):1195–1202, 1997 9337378

Iguchi MY, Belding MA, Morral AR, et al: Reinforcing operants other than abstinence in drug abuse treatment: an effective alternative for reducing drug use. J Consult Clin Psychol 65(3):421–428, 1997 9170765

Iovieno N, Tedeschini E, Bentley KH, et al: Antidepressants for major depressive disorder and dysthymic disorder in patients with comorbid alcohol use disorders: a meta-analysis of placebo-controlled randomized trials. J Clin Psychiatry 72(8):1144–1151, 2011 21536001

Jacobson NS, Dobson KS, Truax PA, et al: A component analysis of cognitive-behavioral treatment for depression. J Consult Clin Psychol 64(2):295–304, 1996 8871414
Johanson CE, Schuster CR: Animal models of drug self-administration, in Advances in Substance Abuse, Vol 2. Edited by Mello NK. Greenwich, CT, JAI Press, 1981, pp 219–297
Kellam SG, Brown CH, Rubin BR, et al: Paths leading to teenage psychiatric symptoms and substance use: developmental epidemiological studies in Woodlawn, in Childhood Psychopathology and Development. Edited by Guze SB, Earls FJ, Barrett JE. New York, Raven, 1983, pp 17–51
Kendler KS, Heath AC, Neale MC, et al: Alcoholism and major depression in women. A twin study of the causes of comorbidity. Arch Gen Psychiatry 50(9):690–698, 1993a 8357294
Kendler KS, Neale MC, MacLean CJ, et al: Smoking and major depression. A causal analysis. Arch Gen Psychiatry 50(1):36–43, 1993b 8422220
Kendler KS, Bulik CM, Silberg J, et al: Childhood sexual abuse and adult psychiatric and substance use disorders in women: an epidemiological and cotwin control analysis. Arch Gen Psychiatry 57(10):953–959, 2000 11015813
Kendler KS, Sheth K, Gardner CO, et al: Childhood parental loss and risk for first-onset of major depression and alcohol dependence: the time-decay of risk and sex differences. Psychol Med 32(7):1187–1194, 2002 12420888
Kendler KS, Prescott CA, Myers J, et al: The structure of genetic and environmental risk factors for common psychiatric and substance use disorders in men and women. Arch Gen Psychiatry 60(9):929–937, 2003 12963675
Kessler RC: Epidemiology of psychiatric comorbidity, in Textbook in Psychiatric Epidemiology. Edited by Tsuang MT, Tohen M, Zahner GEP. New York, Wiley, 1995, pp 179–197
Kessler RC: The effects of stressful life events on depression. Annu Rev Psychol 48:191–214, 1997 9046559
Kessler RC, McGonagle KA, Zhao S, et al: Lifetime and 12-month prevalence of DSM-III-R psychiatric disorders in the United States. Results from the National Comorbidity Survey. Arch Gen Psychiatry 51(1):8–19, 1994 8279933
Keyes KM, Eaton NR, Krueger RF, et al: Childhood maltreatment and the structure of common psychiatric disorders. Br J Psychiatry 200(2):107–115, 2012 22157798
Keyes KM, Shmulewitz D, Greenstein E, et al: Exposure to the Lebanon War of 2006 and effects on alcohol use disorders: the moderating role of childhood maltreatment. Drug Alcohol Depend 134:296–303, 2014 24262650
Khantzian EJ: The self-medication hypothesis of addictive disorders: focus on heroin and cocaine dependence. Am J Psychiatry 142(11):1259–1264, 1985 3904487
Koob GF: The dark side of emotion: the addiction perspective. Eur J Pharmacol 753:73–87, 2015 25583178
Koob GF, Volkow ND: Neurobiology of addiction: a neurocircuitry analysis. Lancet Psychiatry 3(8):760–773, 2016 27475769
Kranzler HR, Van Kirk J: Efficacy of naltrexone and acamprosate for alcoholism treatment: a meta-analysis. Alcohol Clin Exp Res 25(9):1335–1341, 2001 11584154
Kranzler HR, Armeli S, Feinn R, et al: Targeted naltrexone treatment moderates the relations between mood and drinking behavior among problem drinkers. J Consult Clin Psychol 72(2):317–327, 2004 15065964
Kranzler HR, Mueller T, Cornelius J, et al: Sertraline treatment of co-occurring alcohol dependence and major depression. J Clin Psychopharmacol 26(1):13–20, 2006 16415699
Kuo WH, Gallo JJ, Tien AY: Incidence of suicide ideation and attempts in adults: the 13-year follow-up of a community sample in Baltimore, Maryland. Psychol Med 31(7):1181–1191, 2001 11681544
Ladd BO, Murphy JG, Borsari B: Integration of motivational interviewing and behavioral economic theories to enhance brief alcohol interventions: rationale and preliminary examination of client language. Exp Clin Psychopharmacol 29(1):90–98, 2021 32191069
Lee JD, Nunes EV Jr, Novo P, et al: Comparative effectiveness of extended-release naltrexone versus buprenorphine-naloxone for opioid relapse prevention (X:BOT): a multicentre, open-label, randomised controlled trial. Lancet 391(10118):309–318, 2018 29150198

Lempert KM, Steinglass JE, Pinto A, et al: Can delay discounting deliver on the promise of RDoC? Psychol Med 49(2):190–199, 2019 30070191
Levin FR, Gunderson EW, Levounis P: Medical education, in The American Psychiatric Publishing Textbook of Substance Abuse Treatment, 3rd Edition. Edited by Galanter M, Kleber HD. Arlington, VA, American Psychiatric Publishing, 2004, pp 597–609
Levinson DF, Zubenko GS, Crowe RR, et al: Genetics of recurrent early onset depression (GenRED): design and preliminary clinical characteristics of a repository sample for genetic linkage studies. Am J Med Genet B Neuropsychiatr Genet 119B(1):118–130, 2003 12707949
Levy JC, Deykin EY: Suicidality, depression, and substance abuse in adolescence. Am J Psychiatry 146(11):1462–1467, 1989 2817119
Lewinsohn PM: Engagement in pleasant activities and depression level. J Abnorm Psychol 84(6):729–731, 1975 1194539
Lewinsohn PM, Graf M: Pleasant activities and depression. J Consult Clin Psychol 41(2):261–268, 1973 4147832
Lewinsohn PM, Antonuccio DO, Brekenridge JS, et al: The Coping with Depression Course. Eugene, OR, Castalia Publishing, 1984
Li X, Shorter D, Kosten TR: Buprenorphine in the treatment of opioid addiction: opportunities, challenges and strategies. Expert Opin Pharmacother 15(15):2263–2275, 2014 25171726
Liappas J, Paparrigopoulos T, Tzavellas E, et al: Impact of alcohol detoxification on anxiety and depressive symptoms. Drug Alcohol Depend 68(2):215–220, 2002 12234651
Lofwall MR, Walsh SL, Nunes EV, et al: Weekly and monthly subcutaneous buprenorphine depot formulations vs daily sublingual buprenorphine with naloxone for treatment of opioid use disorder: a randomized clinical trial. JAMA Intern Med 178(6):764–773, 2018 29799968
Long JC, Knowler WC, Hanson RL, et al: Evidence for genetic linkage to alcohol dependence on chromosomes 4 and 11 from an autosome-wide scan in an American Indian population. Am J Med Genet 81(3):216–221, 1998 9603607
Lydecker KP, Tate SR, Cummins KM, et al: Clinical outcomes of an integrated treatment for depression and substance use disorders. Psychol Addict Behav 24(3):453–465, 2010 20853931
Malone K, Mann JJ: Serotonin and depression, in Biology of Depressive Disorders, Part A: A Systems Perspective. Edited by Mann JJ, Kupfer DJ. New York, Plenum, 1993, pp 29–49
Markou A, Kosten TR, Koob GF: Neurobiological similarities in depression and drug dependence: a self-medication hypothesis. Neuropsychopharmacology 18(3):135–174, 1998 9471114
Martell CR, Addis ME, Jacobson NS: Depression in Context: Strategies for Guided Action. New York, WW Norton, 2001
Martin CS, Earleywine M, Blackson TC, et al: Aggressivity, inattention, hyperactivity, and impulsivity in boys at high and low risk for substance abuse. J Abnorm Child Psychol 22(2):177–203, 1994 8064028
Meyer RE: How to understand the relationship between psychopathology and addictive disorders: another example of the chicken and the egg, in Psychopathology and Addictive Disorders. Edited by Meyer RE. New York, Guilford, 1986, pp 3–16
Meyers JL, Sartor CE, Werner KB, et al: Childhood interpersonal violence and adult alcohol, cannabis, and tobacco use disorders: variation by race/ethnicity? Psychol Med 48(9):1540–1550, 2018 29310741
Miller WR, Rollnick S: Motivational Interviewing: Preparing People for Change, 2nd Edition. New York, Guilford, 2002
Moody L, Franck C, Bickel WK: Comorbid depression, antisocial personality, and substance dependence: relationship with delay discounting. Drug Alcohol Depend 160:190–196, 2016 26846198
Moss HB, Majumder PP, Vanyukov M: Familial resemblance for psychoactive substance use disorders: behavioral profile of high risk boys. Addict Behav 19(2):199–208, 1994 8036966
Murphy GE, Wetzel RD, Robins E, et al: Multiple risk factors predict suicide in alcoholism. Arch Gen Psychiatry 49(6):459–463, 1992 1599370
Naranjo CA, Tremblay LK, Busto UE: The role of the brain reward system in depression. Prog Neuropsychopharmacol Biol Psychiatry 25(4):781–823, 2001 11383978

Nemeroff CB: New vistas in neuropeptide research in neuropsychiatry: focus on corticotropin-releasing factor. Neuropsychopharmacology 6(2):69–75, 1992 1610487
Nestler EJ: Cellular responses to chronic treatment with drugs of abuse. Crit Rev Neurobiol 7(1):23–39, 1993 8385579
Nunes EV, Levin FR: Treatment of depression in patients with alcohol or other drug dependence: a meta-analysis. JAMA 291(15):1887–1896, 2004 15100209
Nunes EV, Weiss RD: Co-occurring addictive and mood disorders, in The ASAM Principles of Addiction Medicine, 5th Edition. Edited by Ries RK, Fiellin DA, Miller SC, Saitz R. Philadelphia, PA, Lippincott Williams & Wilkins, 2014, pp 1300–1332
Nunes E, Hasin D, Blanco C: Overview of diagnostic methods: diagnostic criteria, structured and semi-structured interviews, and biological markers, in Dual Diagnosis and Psychiatric Treatment: Substance Abuse and Disorders, 2nd Edition. Edited by Kranzler HR, Tinsley JA. New York, Marcel Dekker, 2004, pp 53–86
Nunes EV, Rothenberg JL, Sullivan MA, et al: Behavioral therapy to augment oral naltrexone for opioid dependence: a ceiling on effectiveness? Am J Drug Alcohol Abuse 32(4):503–517, 2006 17127538
Nurnberger JI Jr, Foroud T, Flury L, et al: Evidence for a locus on chromosome 1 that influences vulnerability to alcoholism and affective disorder. Am J Psychiatry 158(5):718–724, 2001 11329392
O'Brien CP, Kampman KM: Opioids: antagonists and partial agonists, in The American Psychiatric Publishing Textbook of Substance Abuse Treatment, 3rd Edition. Edited by Galanter M, Kleber HD. Arlington, VA, American Psychiatric Publishing, 2004, pp 305–319
Patton GC, Coffey C, Carlin JB, et al: Cannabis use and mental health in young people: cohort study. BMJ 325(7374):1195–1198, 2002 12446533
Petrakis IL, Leslie D, Rosenheck R: The use of antidepressants in alcohol-dependent veterans. J Clin Psychiatry 64(8):865–870, 2003 12926999
Petrakis IL, Poling J, Levinson C, et al: Naltrexone and disulfiram in patients with alcohol dependence and comorbid psychiatric disorders. Biol Psychiatry 57(10):1128–1137, 2005 15866552
Pettinati HM, Weiss RD, Dundon W, et al: A structured approach to medical management: a psychosocial intervention to support pharmacotherapy in the treatment of alcohol dependence. J Stud Alcohol Suppl (15):170–178, 2005 16223068
Porjesz B, Almasy L, Edenberg HJ, et al: Linkage disequilibrium between the beta frequency of the human EEG and a GABAA receptor gene locus. Proc Natl Acad Sci USA 99(6):3729–3733, 2002 11891318
Prisciandaro JJ, Schacht JP, Prescot AP, et al: Brain glutamate, GABA, and glutamine levels and associations with recent drinking in treatment-naïve individuals with alcohol use disorder versus light drinkers. Alcohol Clin Exp Res 43(2):221–226, 2019 30537347
Project MATCH Research Group: Matching Alcoholism Treatments to Client Heterogeneity: Project MATCH posttreatment drinking outcomes. J Stud Alcohol 58(1):7–29, 1997 8979210
Pulcu E, Trotter PD, Thomas EJ, et al: Temporal discounting in major depressive disorder. Psychol Med 44(9):1825–1834, 2014 24176142
Regier DA, Farmer ME, Rae DS, et al: Comorbidity of mental disorders with alcohol and other drug abuse. Results from the Epidemiologic Catchment Area (ECA) Study. JAMA 264(19):2511–2518, 1990 2232018
Reich T, Edenberg HJ, Goate A, et al: Genome-wide search for genes affecting the risk for alcohol dependence. Am J Med Genet 81(3):207–215, 1998 9603606
Ries RK, Fiellin DA, Miller SC, et al: The ASAM Principles of Addiction Medicine, 5th Edition. Philadelphia, PA, Lippincott Williams & Wilkins, 2014
Robbins TW, Everitt BJ: Limbic-striatal memory systems and drug addiction. Neurobiol Learn Mem 78(3):625–636, 2002 12559840
Rømer Thomsen K, Whybrow PC, Kringelbach ML: Reconceptualizing anhedonia: novel perspectives on balancing the pleasure networks in the human brain. Front Behav Neurosci 9:49, 2015 25814941

Rothenberg JL, Sullivan MA, Church SH, et al: Behavioral naltrexone therapy: an integrated treatment for opiate dependence. J Subst Abuse Treat 23(4):351–360, 2002 12495797

Rounsaville BJ, Kosten TR, Kleber HD: Long-term changes in current psychiatric diagnoses of treated opiate addicts. Compr Psychiatry 27(5):480–498, 1986a 3757496

Rounsaville BJ, Kosten TR, Weissman MM, et al: Prognostic significance of psychopathology in treated opiate addicts. A 2.5-year follow-up study. Arch Gen Psychiatry 43(8):739–745, 1986b 3729668

Rounsaville BJ, Dolinsky ZS, Babor TF, et al: Psychopathology as a predictor of treatment outcome in alcoholics. Arch Gen Psychiatry 44(6):505–513, 1987 3579499

Rounsaville BJ, Kosten TR, Weisman MM, et al: Psychiatric disorders in relatives of probands with opiate addiction. Arch Gen Psychiatry 48(1):33–42, 1991 3579499

Roy A: Placebo-controlled study of sertraline in depressed recently abstinent alcoholics. Biol Psychiatry 44(7):633–637, 1998 9787889

Salloum IM, Brown ES: Management of comorbid bipolar disorder and substance use disorders. Am J Drug Alcohol Abuse 43(4):366–376, 2017 28301219

Salloum IM, Douaihy AB, Kelly TM, et al: Integrating pharmacotherapy and a novel individual counseling for alcoholism with bipolar disorder. Alcohol Clin Exp Res 32:260A, 2008

Sanacora G, Mason GF, Krystal JH: Impairment of GABAergic transmission in depression: new insights from neuroimaging studies. Crit Rev Neurobiol 14(1):23–45, 2000 11253954

Satel SL, Price LH, Palumbo JM, et al: Clinical phenomenology and neurobiology of cocaine abstinence: a prospective inpatient study. Am J Psychiatry 148(12):1712–1716, 1991 1957935

Schottenfeld RS: Opioids: maintenance treatment, in The American Psychiatric Publishing Textbook of Substance Abuse Treatment, 3rd Edition. Edited by Galanter M, Kleber HD. Arlington, VA, American Psychiatric Publishing, 2004, pp 291–304

Schuckit MA: Genetic and clinical implications of alcoholism and affective disorder. Am J Psychiatry 143(2):140–147, 1986 3511739

Schuckit MA, Tapert S: Alcohol, in The American Psychiatric Publishing Textbook of Substance Abuse Treatment, 3rd Edition. Edited by Galanter M, Kleber HD. Arlington, VA, American Psychiatric Publishing, 2004, pp 151–166

Schuckit MA, Smith TL, Landi NA: The 5-year clinical course of high-functioning men with DSM-IV alcohol abuse or dependence. Am J Psychiatry 157(12):2028–2035, 2000 11097971

Schür RR, Draisma LW, Wijnen JP, et al: Brain GABA levels across psychiatric disorders: a systematic literature review and meta-analysis of (1)H-MRS studies. Hum Brain Mapp 37(9):3337–3352, 2016 27145016

Sharma A, Wolf DH, Ciric R, et al: Common dimensional reward deficits across mood and psychotic disorders: a connectome-wide association study. Am J Psychiatry 174(7):657–666, 2017 28135847

Sigvardsson S, Bohman M, Cloninger CR: Replication of the Stockholm Adoption Study of alcoholism. Confirmatory cross-fostering analysis. Arch Gen Psychiatry 53(8):681–687, 1996 8694681

Silverman K, Higgins ST, Brooner RK, et al: Sustained cocaine abstinence in methadone maintenance patients through voucher-based reinforcement therapy. Arch Gen Psychiatry 53(5):409–415, 1996 8624184

Sloan DM, Strauss ME, Wisner KL: Diminished response to pleasant stimuli by depressed women. J Abnorm Psychol 110(3):488–493, 2001 11502092

Sonne SC, Brady KT: Substance abuse and bipolar comorbidity. Psychiatr Clin North Am 22(3):609–627, 1999 10550858

Tanum L, Solli KK, Latif ZE, et al: Effectiveness of injectable extended-release naltrexone vs daily buprenorphine-naloxone for opioid dependence: a randomized clinical noninferiority trial. JAMA Psychiatry 74(12):1197–1205, 2017 29049469

Torrens M, Fonseca F, Mateu G, et al: Efficacy of antidepressants in substance use disorders with and without comorbid depression. A systematic review and meta-analysis. Drug Alcohol Depend 78(1):1–22, 2005 15769553

Tundo A, de Filippis R, De Crescenzo F: Pramipexole in the treatment of unipolar and bipolar depression. A systematic review and meta-analysis. Acta Psychiatr Scand 140(2):116–125, 2019 31111467

Uhl GR, Koob GF, Cable J: The neurobiology of addiction. Ann NY Acad Sci 1451(1):5–28, 2019 30644552

Volkow ND: Drug abuse and mental illness: progress in understanding comorbidity. Am J Psychiatry 158(8):1181–1183, 2001 11481146

Volkow ND, Wang GJ, Tomasi D, et al: Unbalanced neuronal circuits in addiction. Curr Opin Neurobiol 23(4):639–648, 2013 23434063

Walsh SL, Comer SD, Lofwall MR, et al: Effect of buprenorphine weekly depot (CAM2038) and hydromorphone blockade in individuals with opioid use disorder: a randomized clinical trial. JAMA Psychiatry 74(9):894–902, 2017 28655025

Weddington WW, Brown BS, Haertzen CA, et al: Changes in mood, craving, and sleep during short-term abstinence reported by male cocaine addicts. A controlled, residential study. Arch Gen Psychiatry 47(9):861–868, 1990 2393345

Weiss RD, Griffin ML, Greenfield SF, et al: Group therapy for patients with bipolar disorder and substance dependence: results of a pilot study. J Clin Psychiatry 61(5):361–367, 2000 10847311

Winokur G, Coryell W: Familial subtypes of unipolar depression: a prospective study of familial pure depressive disease compared to depression spectrum disease. Biol Psychiatry 32(11):1012–1018, 1992 1467381

Zubieta JK, Ketter TA, Bueller JA, et al: Regulation of human affective responses by anterior cingulate and limbic mu-opioid neurotransmission. Arch Gen Psychiatry 60(11):1145–1153, 2003 14609890

CHAPTER 42

Depression in Women

Alison Myoraku, M.S.
Lexi Nutkiewicz, B.A.
Teresa Lanza di Scalea, M.D., Ph.D.
Natalie Rasgon, M.D., Ph.D.
D. Jeffrey Newport, M.D., M.S.

This chapter focuses on the various subcategories of depression in women across the life span. While it is well established that major depressive episodes are more common in women than in men, there are also a number of types of depression that are specific to females. Briefly, this chapter covers the neurobiology of depression in women, as well as new findings about sex differences in response to depression treatments. Other sections are devoted to different types of depression in women, including peripartum depression, premenstrual dysphoric disorder, and perimenopausal depression, which focus on the pathophysiology and current treatment options for each respective type.

Sex Differences in Depression

Prevalence of Depression

Depression is one of the most common mental disorders in the United States, affecting 19.4 million adults (National Institute of Mental Health 2019). Major depressive disorder (MDD) is diagnosed based on the following criteria: a period of at least 2 weeks when a person experiences depressed mood or loss of interest in daily activities, as well as other specified symptoms such as loss of appetite, fatigue, feelings of worthlessness, and slowing of physical movement. Although depression can occur at any age, common risk factors include a family history of depression, major life changes, and certain physical illnesses (e.g., diabetes, cancer). A major depressive episode can cause severe impairment, preventing the individual from carrying out everyday tasks and major life activities. Depression also takes different forms. Persistent depressive disorder (dysthymia) is characterized by a depressed mood that lasts for at least 2 years. MDD with seasonal pattern (also called seasonal affective disorder) is characterized by symptoms of social withdrawal, increased sleep, and weight gain that most commonly emerge during the winter months, when there is less natural sunlight.

Although MDD has an estimated prevalence of 7.8% in the U.S. adult population, major depressive episodes are more common in adult females (prevalence of 9.6%) than in adult males (prevalence of 6.0%) (National Institute of Mental Health 2019). This difference in prevalence between females and males can be attributed not only to environmental and society-driven risk factors but also to biological factors. Certain types of depression are specific to women. Premenstrual dysphoric disorder (PMDD) is typically experienced during the weeks before menstruation. Peripartum depression strikes pregnant and postpartum mothers and hinders them from fulfilling daily care responsibilities for themselves and their babies (Rapkin et al. 2002). In addition to these specific disorders, hormonal fluctuations and changes associated with the menstrual cycle and the menopause transition can exacerbate existing mood disorders in women. For example, in a study of adults with bipolar disorder, women more frequently reported depression and large fluctuations in mood (specifically across the menstrual cycle) than did men (Rasgon et al. 2005). Similarly, during the transition to menopause and beyond, women ages 45–55 years with bipolar disorder were found to experience more depressive symptoms and episodes than did men of similar age with bipolar disorder (Marsh et al. 2008, 2009). These sex-specific depressive disorders and periods of increased vulnerability to depression can be explained by changes in ovarian hormones and may contribute to the increased prevalence of depression in females (Albert 2015).

Neurobiology of Depression

Studying the neurobiology of depression enables researchers to discover the etiology behind this common mental disorder. Generally, the biological mechanisms of depression, including increased stress response, reduced neuroplasticity, and inflammation, are reciprocally connected with each other and with neurochemical pathways, such as monoamines, glutamate, and brain-derived neurotrophic factor (BDNF) (Dean and Keshavan 2017).

Neurophysiology

The monoamine hypothesis of depression posited that alterations or impairments in monoamine neurotransmission are a cause of depression because of the role monoamine neurotransmission plays in regulating complex behaviors and emotions (Delgado 2000). Serotonin, one of the monoamine neurotransmitters, is multifaceted in its effects, as it helps modulate learning, memory, reward, and cognition. Serotonin deficiency is also linked to depression, but serotonin depletion is insufficient to induce depression on its own (Shors and Leuner 2003). Glutamate, an excitatory neurotransmitter, promotes the flow of signals between nerve cells. Dysfunction of glutamate synapses in the central nervous system can lead to depression (Sanacora et al. 2012). BDNF is responsible for supporting the survival of existing neurons and encouraging growth and differentiation of new neurons and synapses. A reduction in BDNF expression or activity in the hippocampus can cause impairment of neuronal plasticity, which is one of the biological causes of MDD (Lee and Kim 2010). However, there are sex differences in neurobiological risk factors for depression. In a systematic review of biological sex differences in MDD, researchers found that women with MDD showed greater reductions in BDNF- and GABA-related genes than did men with MDD (Labaka et al. 2018).

Neuroendocrinology

Researchers have also discovered that depressed women have higher leptin and interleukin 6 (IL-6) levels than do depressed men. Although researchers have found higher levels of leptin in depressed females compared with healthy control females, studies examining the association between leptin and depression have yielded discrepant findings (Ge et al. 2018). A potential reason for these differing results was the presence in study samples of patients with elevated BMIs, which made it difficult to establish a positive link between leptin and depression. IL-6 is an endogenous chemical that plays an active role in inflammation. Higher IL-6 levels have a significant association with the subsequent development of depressive symptoms and are typically seen in patients with elevated BMIs (Miller et al. 2002; Valkanova et al. 2013).

Sex Hormones

Researchers have additionally looked at the effects of sex hormones on depression. Estrogen, the primary female sex hormone, is responsible for the development and regulation of the female reproductive system and other sex characteristics. In women, depression most commonly occurs during menses, during the post-pregnancy period, and during and after menopause (Shors and Leuner 2003). During the luteal phase of the menstrual cycle, estrogen and progesterone levels decrease, in some women triggering symptoms such as depression and irritability that disappear at or soon after the onset of menses.

Treatment Response

In addition to sex differences in risk of experiencing a major depressive episode, response to antidepressant treatment also varies for men and women. A clear consensus on sex differences in treatment response remains elusive because of several significant confounds in clinical studies. Even in some meta-analyses, the studies did not use the same criteria for deciding what constituted a significant response to treatment. Studies in female patients recruited a range of ages, which is problematic because women have varying levels of female sex hormones at different stages of the reproductive life cycle. The extensive list of potential factors that can contribute to sex differences in antidepressant efficacy include both patient factors (e.g., medication adherence, adiposity, neuromonoamine functioning, interactions between estrogen and serotonin in the brain) and medication factors (e.g., differences in side-effect profiles). Because of these multiple variables, treatment must be individualized on the basis of the patient's medical record.

Nevertheless, there is some consistency between studies. Multiple studies have shown that women respond better to selective serotonin reuptake inhibitors (SSRIs) than do men. For example, in a large-scale study investigating sex differences in response to the SSRI citalopram, women responded better than men to the antidepressant treatment (Young et al. 2009). In one study, premenopausal women specifically appeared to have a better response than males to SSRIs, suggesting that female hormones might improve the efficacy of serotonergic antidepressants (Sramek et al. 2016). As discussed previously, low serotonin levels can lead to depression symptoms such as changes in appetite, sleep, and arousal, as well as increased anxiety and aggression. SSRIs increase serotonin activity in the brain by blocking the reuptake of serotonin into neurons, which makes more serotonin available to improve transmission of neuron messages (Neill and Kulkarni 2011). Additionally, serotonin is thought to mediate the positive feedback exerted by estrogen when there is a preovulatory surge in luteinizing hormone. In the presence of estrogen, serotonin stimulates the release of luteinizing hormone and triggers ovulation (Amin et al. 2005).

In several studies, males responded better to imipramine and other tricyclic antidepressants (TCA) than did females (Raskin 1974). Other studies found that women were slower to respond to TCAs and were less likely to achieve a response (Montoya et al. 2016; Raskin 1974). Most TCAs, particularly imipramine and desipramine, are predominantly noradrenergic reuptake inhibitors. Noradrenergic reuptake inhibitors act by inhibiting the reuptake of norepinephrine and/or epinephrine (Montoya et al. 2016). This action increases both cortical arousal and energy levels. The clinical benefits of TCAs are most likely due to the neuroadaptive changes produced by these medications.

It is difficult to concisely list all of the differences in treatment response between the sexes. However, some conclusions can be drawn from the numerous studies that have examined treatment response. Findings from several studies suggest that females respond better to serotonergic antidepressants, such as SSRIs, than do males. Postmenopausal females do not respond to serotonergic antidepressants as well as younger females do, a finding that has been linked to elevated levels of follicle-stimulating hormone (FSH) after menopause (Pae et al. 2009). In order to effectively research these sex differences, studies must use consistent methodology and consider additional factors such as age. More studies that maintain consistency will help us to better understand what is contributing to different responses to treatment.

Peripartum Depression

History, Prevalence, and Diagnostic Criteria

The syndrome of postpartum depression has been recognized for more than 2,000 years, with the earliest extant documentation provided by Hippocrates circa 400 B.C. (Hamilton 1962) and Trotula in the twelfth century A.D. (Trotula of Salerno 1940). Interest in postpartum mental illness was rekindled in the nineteenth century with the publication of Esquirol's case reports and a seminal treatise by Marcé, who postulated that postpartum depression was a consequence of biological perturbations in the female reproductive system following childbirth (Hamilton 1962).

With the introduction and evolution of the American Psychiatric Association's *Diagnostic and Statistical Manual of Mental Disorders* (DSM) during the twentieth century, a variety of diagnostic specifiers were introduced for mood disorders in an effort "to increase diagnostic specificity and create more homogeneous subgroups, assist in treatment selection, and improve the prediction of prognosis" (American Psychiatric Association 1994, p. 318). The incorporation of "with postpartum onset" as a diagnostic specifier for DSM-IV mood disorders bore witness to the long-standing recognition and continuing clinical relevance of postpartum depression while also defining it as a subtype of DSM-IV mood disorder (MDD) or mood episode (i.e., major depressive or manic) rather than a distinct syndrome (in contrast to PMDD). Postpartum depression affects 10%–22% of adult mothers and up to 26% of teen mothers (Stowe and Nemeroff 1995; Troutman and Cutrona 1990), leading to a dramatic rise in psychiatric hospitalization during the postpartum period (Duffy 1983; Kendler et al. 1993).

Nevertheless, despite the fact that it has been recognized since antiquity, is known to have a high prevalence, and has been the focus of extensive research dating to the mid-nineteenth century, the syndrome of postpartum depression, including its relationship to other types of MDD, remains enigmatic. For example, even the appropriate time window following childbirth that constitutes a postpartum onset lacks consensus. In DSM-IV, the mood disorder specifier "with postpartum onset" could be applied if the onset of mood symptoms occurred within the first 4 weeks after childbirth (American Psychiatric Association 1994), and in DSM-5, the specifier "with peripartum onset" could be applied to mood symptoms that occurred during pregnancy as well as within the 4 weeks following delivery. By contrast, in ICD-10 and ICD-11, the category "mental or behavioral disorders associated with pregnancy, childbirth, and the puerperium, not elsewhere classified" could be applied to mood symptoms with onset up to 6 weeks after delivery (World Health Organization 1992). Other studies have indicated that susceptibility to postpartum depression extends to 6 months postpartum (Stowe et al. 2005; Wisner et al. 2004). In addition, although the symptomatology of postpartum depression largely parallels that of other MDD subtypes, certain clinical features are unique to postpartum depression. In particular, intrusive ego-dystonic thoughts (often manifesting as obsessions regarding violence directed toward the newborn child) are common, with one study indicating that more than 48% of women with postpartum depression also struggled with obsessions and/or compulsions (Miller et al. 2015). In addition, a longitudinal study of women experiencing MDD both during the postpartum period and later found that women were less likely to experience anhedonia and more likely to experience guilt and worry in periods of depression during the peripartum period than in periods of depression after the peripartum period (Fox et al. 2018).

Despite folklore characterizing pregnancy as a time of emotional well-being, rates of depression among pregnant women are as high as rates among nonpregnant women (Buesching et al. 1986; Cutrona 1983; Kumar and Robson 1984; Manly et al. 1982; O'Hara et al. 1982; Watson et al. 1984). Indeed, two large studies, collectively comprising 122,400 women, reported a 14%–20% incidence of depression during pregnancy (Marcus et al. 2003; Oberlander et al. 2006). In addition, one study found that among women presenting for evaluation of postpartum depression (N=209), 11% actually experienced symptom onset during gestation (Stowe et al. 2005).

Pathophysiology

A burgeoning line of research on depression and anxiety disorders has recently focused on alterations in the activity of numerous neurosteroids, including allopregnanolone, pregnenolone, and dehydroepiandrosterone (DHEA), which interact with various receptors involved in emotion regulation, including GABA type A ($GABA_A$), serotonin, and sigma-1 receptors (Perkins and Newport 2018).

Neurophysiology

Although there is evidence of neurosteroid dysfunction in numerous depressive and anxiety disorders, neurosteroid systems may prove particularly important in elucidating the pathophysiology of depression in women, given that fluctuations in reproductive hormones are accompanied by adaptive changes in neurosteroid levels and structural modifications in the receptors with which they interact. Specifically, alterations in $GABA_A$ receptor subunits, which modulate the receptor's sensitivity to neurosteroids, may occur as a compensatory mechanism during periods of marked change in reproductive hormones (Hauser et al. 1996). Some researchers have posited that defects in the homeostatic adjustment of $GABA_A$ subunits to fluctuating levels of reproductive hormones may contribute to the pathophysiology of depression in women (Brot et al. 1997; Hauser et al. 1996).

Indeed, $GABA_A$ plasticity during pregnancy is modulated by neurosteroids (Concas et al. 1999). In pregnant mice, reduced expression of $GABA_A$ is associated with an increase in allopregnanolone levels, which revert to baseline within 48 hours of delivery (Ferando and Mody 2013). Sudden withdrawal from estradiol following parturition in a rat model of postpartum depression produced increases in DHEA sulfate, which in turn is thought to contribute to reductions in $GABA_A$ activity and behavioral disturbance (Maayan et al. 2005). In humans, low allopregnanolone levels have been associated with depression in late pregnancy (Hellgren et al. 2014, 2017) as well as postpartum "blues" (Nappi et al. 2001). Such data led to clinical trials examining the efficacy of brexanolone, an aqueous solution of allopregnanolone suitable for intravenous administration.

Neuroendocrinology

Peripartum depression is also associated with neuroimmune and neuroendocrine alterations that have been described in nonpuerperal depression. Although these findings do not discriminate peripartum depression from other forms of MDD, they may elucidate the mechanisms whereby depression during pregnancy is associated with an array of adverse outcomes. Inflammation during human pregnancy is complex and subject to misunderstanding. Evidence of inflammation is normally present during the earliest (implantation) and latest (parturition) phases of pregnancy, playing a critical role in the initial viability of gestation and the timing of delivery. However, heightened inflammation typically is not present during the lengthy middle phase (growth and development) of gestation. Several groups have reported aberrant immune activation—notably, increased concentrations of tumor necrosis factor-α (TNF-α) and IL-6 as well as decreased concentrations of anti-inflammatory IL-10—during the middle phase of pregnancy in the context of prenatal depression or heightened psychosocial stress (Chang et al. 2018; Christian 2012; Christian et al. 2009; Coussons-Read et al. 2005, 2007; Lahti-Pulkkinen et al. 2020; Osborne et al. 2018).

Steroid Hormones

Prenatal elevations in corticotropin-releasing hormone (CRH), beyond the increases normally observed during gestation, have been observed in association with prenatal depression (Rich-Edwards et al. 2008) and have been implicated as a predictor of postpartum depression (Meltzer-Brody et al. 2011). Moreover, prenatal depression is associated with altered expression of glucocorticoid chaperone proteins, resulting in decreased glucocorticoid receptor sensitivity (Katz et al. 2012).

Pregnancy Outcomes

The role of aberrant neuroimmune and neuroendocrine activation in the pathogenesis of adverse pregnancy outcomes has been the focus of intense scrutiny for more than two decades. Both clinical and preclinical evidence points to increased concentrations of proinflammatory cytokines, including IL-1β, IL-6, and TNF-α; increased levels of C-reactive protein (CRP); and decreased concentrations of the anti-inflammatory cytokine IL-10, in the pathophysiology of preterm birth, preeclampsia, and gestational diabetes (Cappelletti et al. 2016; Harmon et al. 2016; Wei et al. 2010; Xu et al. 2014). Furthermore, elevated serum CRH concentrations have been associated with preterm birth (Mohamed et al. 2018; Ruiz et al. 2016; Smith et al. 2009). Similarly, preeclampsia has been associated with heightened placental production of CRH (Ng et al. 2003; Perkins et al. 1995; Petsas et al. 2012) and altered methylation of genes regulating glucocorticoid signaling in the placenta (Hogg et al. 2013). These biological perturbations may constitute the mechanism whereby prenatal depression is linked to adverse pregnancy outcomes.

Safety Data for Antidepressant Use During Pregnancy and Lactation

Long deemed authoritative resources for reproductive safety, pregnancy safety classification schemes such as those produced by the FDA have numerous shortcomings. First, the frequency and severity of safety alerts may vary widely for medications with the same safety rating. Moreover, the volume and reliability of the safety data for agents within the same classification may also vary widely. For example, because pregnant and breastfeeding women do not participate in premarketing clinical trials, initial safety ratings for newly introduced medications are established with scant supporting data. Consequently, newer medications, even those with favorable ratings, may carry as-yet-unidentified risks. Nor does a safety rating identify the window of risk for a particular adverse outcome. Furthermore, medication safety ratings have not been subjected to regularly scheduled reevaluations; instead, reassessment of a medication's reproductive safety often is undertaken haphazardly, triggered by events such as the manufacturer's application for approval of a new indication or formulation. Finally, neurodevelopmental outcomes, important when considering safety profiles for centrally acting medications, are seldom factored into the classification assignment.

Clinical decisions demand a more comprehensive awareness of the risk profiles provided by a safety category. It is critical to understand the specific risks—such as birth defects, obstetrical complications, neonatal or nursing complications, and neurodevelopmental sequelae—encountered within specific windows of exposure. In light of the shortcomings of safety rating schemes, a standard pregnancy and lactation reference by Briggs et al. (2017) has adopted a considerably broader and more descriptive classification system, and the FDA has enacted plans to eliminate pregnancy ratings altogether, replacing them with a narrative summary of the risk profile for each medication (U.S. Food and Drug Administration 2014). Unfortunately, numerous obstacles have delayed widespread implementation of the new FDA reproductive safety information scheme. A synopsis of the reproductive safety data for commonly used antidepressants is presented in the following subsections.

Selective Serotonin Reuptake Inhibitors

A meta-analysis of birth defect risks associated with SSRIs (Grigoriadis et al. 2013) found no evidence of increased risk for congenital malformations (OR=0.93; 95% CI: 0.85–1.02), major malformations (OR=1.07; 95% CI: 0.99–1.17), or ventricular septal defects (OR=1.54; 95% CI: 0.71–3.33), although there were increases in the risk for any cardiovascular defect (OR=1.36; 95% CI: 1.08–1.71) and any septal defect (OR=1.40; 95% CI: 1.10–1.77). Among individuals agents, paroxetine was associated with an increased risk of any cardiovascular malformation (OR=1.43, 95% CI: 1.08–1.88), which should not be surprising, given that this risk had previously been reported by the manufacturer (Williams and Wooltorton 2005). Nevertheless, caution should be used in interpreting these results, because another meta-analysis (Bar-Oz et al. 2007) observed that antidepressant-exposed infants underwent twice as many echocardiograms as nonexposed infants, raising the specter of a surveillance bias.

Findings from studies examining SSRI risk for hypertensive disorders of pregnancy, including preeclampsia, are decidedly mixed, with three studies reporting an association between SSRIs and hypertensive disorders (De Vera and Bérard 2012; Toh et al. 2009; Zakiyah et al. 2018) but four finding no association (Palmsten et al. 2012, 2013; Malm et al. 2015; Newport et al. 2016). Closer inspection of two of the positive studies (De Vera and Bérard 2012; Zakiyah et al. 2018) suggested that the association was largely attributable to paroxetine, which has been shown to block norepinephrine reuptake (Gilmor et al. 2002), casting doubt on any link between SSRIs and hypertension during pregnancy.

Studies examining the impact of SSRI exposure on fetal growth have been largely reassuring. Four studies (El Marroun et al. 2014; Hannerfors et al. 2015; Viktorin et al. 2016; Wisner et al. 2009) observed no difference in rates of low birthweight among SSRI-exposed newborns. Slight increases in the risk for small-for-gestational-age infants have been reported (Oberlander et al. 2006; Sujan et al. 2017), but this finding was not sustained in a paired-sibling analysis (Sujan et al. 2017).

Studies of miscarriage risk have also been reassuring, with three of four studies reporting no association of miscarriages with SSRI exposure (Andersen et al. 2014; Ban et al. 2012; Diav-Citrin et al. 2008; Johansen et al. 2015); however, the relationship between SSRI exposure and preterm birth risk is unclear. Whereas four studies found an association between SSRIs and risk of preterm birth (El Marroun et al. 2014; Hannerfors et al. 2015; Oberlander et al. 2006; Sujan et al. 2017), five studies did not (Şahingöz et al. 2014; Venkatesh et al. 2016; Viktorin et al. 2016; Wisner et al. 2009; Yonkers et al. 2012). Interpretation of these mixed results is further complicated by the numerous reports linking maternal depression itself with preterm birth (Liu et al. 2016; Orr et al. 2002; Şahingöz et al. 2014; Steer et al. 1992; Uguz et al. 2013; Venkatesh et al. 2016).

A transient syndrome of neonatal distress, often called poor neonatal adaptation, has been widely reported and variably characterized as including irritability, restlessness, respiratory distress, abnormal crying, poor feeding, hypoglycemia, jaundice, tremors, jitteriness, and convulsions. Poor characterization of this syndrome has made it difficult to derive an accurate estimate of its frequency in SSRI-exposed neonates, with one study reporting a prevalence of 20%–77% (Kieviet et al. 2013) and another an odds ratio of 3.0 (95% CI: 2.0–4.4) (Moses-Kolko et al. 2005). There is agreement that the syndrome is transient and nonemergent, resolving with supportive measures.

The relationship between SSRI exposure and a more severe neonatal syndrome, persistent pulmonary hypertension of the newborn (PPHN), continues to be debated. The first study to examine the effect of SSRIs on PPHN (Chambers et al. 2006) estimated a 1% prevalence of PPHN among SSRI-exposed neonates, leading the FDA to issue a warning (U.S. Food and Drug Administration 2006). Inconsistent results in subsequent studies led the FDA to retract the PPHN warning 5 years later (U.S. Food and Drug Administration 2011). A recent meta-analysis of nine studies estimated an odds ratio of 1.52 (95% CI: 1.04–2.00) for PPHN following SSRI exposure (Ng et al. 2019). A large case-control study using the Swedish national registry suggested that the magnitude of risk is small, with approximately 1 in 680 SSRI-exposed neonates developing PPHN (versus 1 in 2,000 nonexposed neonates) (Källén and Olausson 2008).

Finally, numerous studies have attempted to examine the neurodevelopmental effects of fetal SSRI exposure. With one exception (Brown et al. 2016), studies of intellectual development in young children have consistently failed to show any adverse impact from prenatal SSRI exposure (Austin et al. 2013; Casper et al. 2003; El Marroun et al. 2017; Eriksen et al. 2015; Nulman et al. 1997, 2002, 2012; Oberlander et al. 2004), and some have instead shown an association between intellectual deficits and maternal depression (El Marroun et al. 2017; Nulman et al. 2002). Findings from investigations of child motor development have been mixed, with some studies demonstrating no effect from SSRI exposure (Brown et al. 2016; Nulman et al. 1997, 2002; Oberlander et al. 2004) and others revealing lower motor development scores for SSRI-exposed children (Casper et al. 2003, 2011; Handal et al. 2016; Hanley et al. 2013). The limited magnitude of the motor score differences in the positive studies suggests that any functional impact would be minimal.

A series of studies examining the risk for autism spectrum disorder (ASD) among children exposed to SSRIs or other antidepressants during pregnancy have yielded inconsistent findings (Boukhris et al. 2016; Morales et al. 2018; Rai et al. 2017). A recent meta-analysis, however, indicated that evidence potentially linking antidepressant exposure to ASD in some of the studies was a consequence of an ascertainment bias arising from ethnicity-based differences in health care access; family-based analyses eliminated this bias and demonstrated that SSRI exposure was not associated with risk for ASD (OR=0.76, 95% CI: 0.50–1.16) (Vega et al. 2020).

Published reports on lactation exposure to SSRIs exceed reports for any other medication class, with only a few isolated adverse effects reported. Long-term neurobehavioral studies of infants exposed to SSRIs during lactation warrant continued examination. For SSRIs, pharmacokinetic profiles of breast milk excretion indicate that quantitative infant exposure during lactation is considerably lower than fetal exposure during pregnancy (Stowe et al. 1997, 2000, 2003; Suri et al. 2002).

Serotonin-Norepinephrine Reuptake Inhibitors

In many respects, the prenatal risk profiles for serotonin-norepinephrine reuptake inhibitors (SNRIs) largely parallel those for SSRIs; however, the volume of safety data for SNRIs is considerably lower than that for SSRIs, often precluding definitive conclusions. The best-studied agents among the SNRIs are venlafaxine and its active metabolite, desvenlafaxine, followed by duloxetine. Scant safety data are available for levomilnacipran and milnacipran.

Three controlled studies demonstrated no evidence of increased birth defects with SNRI exposure (Einarson et al. 2001, 2012; Huybrechts et al. 2014). However, one study did report increased rates of atrial septal defects and anencephaly with venlafaxine exposure (Polen et al. 2013), although sample sizes were small in this study.

A pattern that warrants concern is emerging in regard to SNRIs and risk of hypertensive disorders of pregnancy. To date, three studies have reported significantly higher rates of gestational hypertension in association with SNRI treatment during pregnancy (Newport et al. 2016; Lupattelli et al. 2017; Zakiyah et al. 2018). Although one study reported a sixfold higher rate of hypertension during pregnancy with venlafaxine at dosages of 225 mg/day or greater (Newport et al. 2016), a more recent study did not observe an association between duloxetine exposure and hypertension during pregnancy (Huybrechts et al. 2020).

Two recent studies failed to demonstrate any association between venlafaxine (Richardson et al. 2019) or duloxetine (Huybrechts et al. 2020) and spontaneous abortion, preterm birth, or low birth weight.

As with SSRIs, poor neonatal adaptation has been reported following intrauterine SNRI exposure (Convertino et al. 2016). Of note, two studies have not demonstrated an association between SNRI exposure and PPHN (Bérard et al. 2017; Huybrechts et al. 2015).

Neurodevelopmental data from children exposed to SNRIs prenatally are sparse. In one study, venlafaxine-exposed children exhibited no evidence of cognitive deficiencies (Nulman et al. 2012). Neither of the two studies that conducted independent analyses of prenatal SNRI exposure found an association with ASD in exposed children (Boukhris et al. 2016; Brown et al. 2017). For SNRIs, the limited data available on pharmacokinetic profiles of breast milk excretion indicate that quantitative infant exposure during lactation is considerably lower than fetal exposure during pregnancy, and there have been only a few reports of adverse effects.

Other Antidepressants

The first class of antidepressants subjected to systematic evaluation of reproductive safety—that is, the TCAs—has safety profiles in pregnancy and lactation that are similar to those for SSRIs and SNRIs. Given that TCAs are now seldom used in pregnancy or otherwise, their safety data are not reviewed here. Because monoamine oxidase inhibitors (MAOIs) and recently introduced antidepressants such as vilazodone and vortioxetine have so seldom been used in pregnancy and breastfeeding, there are virtually no reproductive safety data for these agents.

There are limited pregnancy and lactation safety data for bupropion and mirtazapine. Studies examining the risk of birth defects among children with first-trimester exposure to bupropion (Boshier et al. 2003; Chun-Fai-Chan et al. 2005; GlaxoSmithKline 2008) or to mirtazapine (Djulus et al. 2006; Smit et al. 2016; Winterfeld et al. 2015) have estimated birth defect prevalences of 2.8% and 2.2%, respectively, rates that are well within population norms. Reports of other adverse reproductive outcomes in association with bupropion or mirtazapine are too sparse to draw even preliminary conclusions. It bears noting, however, that women who develop preeclampsia during gestation should be advised to discontinue bupropion therapy due to seizure risk.

Principles of Treatment

Sound decision making weighs the risks, to mother and child, posed by both peripartum depression and antidepressant exposure. The fundamentals of peripartum depression treatment depend on a proper balancing of the competing dangers of peripartum depression and antidepressant exposure. These fundamentals are perhaps best conveyed as responses to a series of questions frequently encountered in the clinical setting.

Question 1: Is It Safe to Take an Antidepressant During Pregnancy?

Among patients and clinicians alike, many individuals reduce peripartum depression decision making to this single question; however, choices predicated solely on this criterion are wholly inadequate. First, this question ignores the risk posed by peripartum depression itself. In addition, it fails to recognize that no antidepressant can be declared categorically safe because none has been, or will ever be, so exhaustively studied that all possible risks are eliminated from consideration. This question, therefore, might be better reframed as "What plan provides an expectant mother *and* her baby with the best chance for a safe pregnancy?" Reframing the question in this manner, however, invites additional questions.

Question 2: What Are the Risks Associated With Peripartum Depression?

This question is not unique to peripartum depression but should be asked when a pregnant or nursing mother experiences any illness. If an illness poses little risk to mother and infant (e.g., allergic rhinitis), then medicine used to treat that illness should also pose little risk. Conversely, using a medication with considerable risk may be acceptable when the illness it treats poses grave danger to a mother or her child (e.g., epilepsy, HIV).

The volume of data regarding the risks of peripartum depression has steadily accrued over several decades. Depression during pregnancy has been associated with poor adherence to recommended obstetrical care and greater exposure to both prescription and nonprescription medications and habit-forming substances (Newport et al. 2012; Zuckerman et al. 1989). Prenatal depression has also been associated with numerous adverse obstetrical and neonatal outcomes, including poor maternal weight gain and greater risk for preeclampsia, preterm delivery, low birth weight, and smaller neonatal head circumference (Jarde et al. 2016; Marcus et al. 2009). Finally, prenatal depression has been associated with adverse neurodevelopmental effects on child cognition, language, and motor activity (Kingston et al. 2012). Similarly, maternal depression during the postpartum period has been linked to an array of detrimental effects in children, including poor attachment (Lovejoy et al. 2000) and deficits in cognitive, language, and emotional development (Goodman et al. 2011; Grace et al. 2003; Liu et al. 2017).

Question 3: How Likely Is the Depression to Return During Pregnancy if the Antidepressant Is Stopped?

Newly pregnant women with histories of depression often face the difficult decision of whether to continue taking an antidepressant. Contrary to popular lore that visualizes pregnancy as a time of emotional well-being, the most extensive study to date (N=201) found that 68% of pregnant women who stopped antidepressant treatment experienced a relapse, compared with 26% of women who continued antidepressant therapy (Cohen et al. 2006). Of course, this finding indicates that nearly one-third (32%) of the women who discontinued antidepressant treatment remained euthymic during pregnancy. Although there are as yet no data to reliably identify the subset of pregnant women likely to remain well after stopping antidepressant treatment, our experience suggests that clinicians should consider the patient's prior psychiatric history. For example, women with a history of fewer or less frequent depressive episodes or of periods of sustained euthymia in the absence of antidepressant therapy may have a better chance of remaining euthymic if they discontinue antidepressant treatment after learning they are pregnant.

Question 4: How Safe and Effective Are Nonmedication Treatments for Depression?

Because psychotherapy has demonstrated benefit for peripartum depression (Curry et al. 2019) and carries minimal risk during gestation, it should be a standard treatment recommendation, either in combination with or in lieu of antidepressant medication. The best-studied psychotherapies for peripartum depression are interpersonal therapy (IPT) (Sockol 2018) and cognitive-behavioral therapy (CBT) (Sockol 2015). Complementary low-risk treatments such as exercise (Coll et al. 2019; Perales et al. 2015), prenatal yoga (Davis et al. 2015), and meditation (Pan et al. 2019) may also be considered, although data supporting these treatments' efficacy for depression are scant. However, naturopathic supplements (e.g., St. John's wort, *Rhodiola rosea*, saffron, lavender, Maharishi Amrit Kalash, Mentat) are not recommended for peripartum depression, given the absence of data on their safety during pregnancy or lactation.

Question 5: What Is the Preferred Antidepressant for Peripartum Depression?

It depends. A patient-centered approach to treatment selection, considering both the patient's treatment history and current preferences, is advised. Moreover, the ideal antidepressant balances safety and efficacy. All too often, clinicians, understandably focused on antidepressant safety, lose sight of the need for an efficacious treatment. Choosing an ineffective antidepressant, even one with a favorable safety profile, cannot be justified. Obtaining a comprehensive treatment history and documenting the efficacy, tolerability, dosage level, and treatment duration for previous antidepressants are helpful in narrowing the list of medication choices. Particularly important is the effectiveness of an antidepressant during or immediately following a previous pregnancy.

After identifying antidepressants with a reasonable likelihood of efficacy and tolerability, safety considerations enter the decision-making process. It is important to review the reproductive safety profiles of medications deemed likely to provide therapeutic benefit. The ideal antidepressant lies at the intersection of this efficacy and safety survey.

Time-Dependent Decision Making

Just as the treatment choices for peripartum depression differ for each patient, the clinical concerns and therefore the suitability of particular treatment options may also vary depending on the gestational timing of the decision. We recommend a time-dependent approach to peripartum depression treatment decisions, as outlined in the following subsections.

Preconception Planning

Because nearly one-half of U.S. pregnancies are unplanned (Finer and Zolna 2016), there may be no opportunity for a formal preconception planning discussion. Thus, it is wise to always be mindful of the possibility of an unanticipated pregnancy when choosing antidepressant therapy for a woman of childbearing age. When there is an opportunity for a preconception planning visit, the discussion should begin with maternal health behavior counseling, which should include advising women before they conceive to start a prenatal vitamin and to avoid alcohol, tobacco, caffeine, and herbal remedies. They should be encouraged to consume ample amounts of water and to engage in moderate daily exercise unless otherwise directed by their obstetrician. In addition, laboratory screening to rule out subclinical hypothyroidism (American College of Obstetricians and Gynecologists 2007) and vitamin D insufficiency (American College of Obstetricians and Gynecologists 2011) should be performed, given that these conditions, which increase the risk for adverse pregnancy outcomes, are more prevalent among women with depressive symptoms (Siegmann et al. 2018; Williams et al. 2016).

For patients of childbearing age who are taking antidepressants, the first decision is whether to conceive at all, remembering that the only risk-free option is choosing not to conceive. If the patient elects to proceed with planning a pregnancy, her next decision is whether to continue or discontinue her antidepressant treatment before conceiving. In making this decision, the woman must consider the competing dangers of untreated depression versus antidepressant exposure, as well as the likelihood of her depression recurring if antidepressant treatment is stopped. Finally, if she decides to continue antidepressant treatment, she may want to consider whether she should switch to an alternative antidepressant with a better safety profile. Switching antidepressants may be the preferred choice when the current antidepressant 1) conveys risks that can be avoided by switching (e.g., paroxetine carries heart defect risks; bupropion carries seizure risk for women with a history of preeclampsia) or 2) is a recently marketed antidepressant with very limited reproductive safety data (e.g., vortioxetine) relative to older agents.

Early-Pregnancy Decisions

When a patient first seeks clinical advice during early pregnancy, having missed the opportunity for preconception counseling, a sense of urgency arises, because offspring exposure is actively unfolding while choices are being deliberated. Early-pregnancy consultations typically come about in one of two ways.

Sometimes a woman learns she is pregnant while she is being treated with an antidepressant and seeks advice from her physician as to whether she should continue the antidepressant. As with preconception decisions regarding medication, the continue/discontinue decision in early pregnancy rests upon an appraisal of the woman's likelihood of relapse if the antidepressant is discontinued as well as the relative dangers posed by antidepressant exposure versus prenatal depression. However, unlike choices contemplated prior to conception, switching antidepressants in early pregnancy is seldom advisable, because this choice incurs additional risks while seldom affording any improvement in safety. Specifically, switching antidepressants after the patient is already pregnant exposes the baby to yet another medication and may inadvertently increase the likelihood of depressive relapse in the mother (because the new medication may be less effective). However, an early-pregnancy consultation is usually too late to protect the baby from birth defect concerns. For example, the window of concern for heart defects begins during the fifth week of pregnancy. Consequently, whereas a woman treated with paroxetine would likely be counseled during a preconception visit to switch to an alternative antidepressant, it is typically too late to protect a child from paroxetine-associated heart defect risks during a pregnancy consultation. In addition, some clinicians are tempted to reduce the antidepressant dosage after learning that a patient is pregnant; however, such an action is seldom wise, because it runs the risk of subjecting the mother and child to subtherapeutic dosing. Subtherapeutic dosing is the worst possible medication scenario in pregnancy and should be avoided at all costs, as it continues to expose the baby to the medication while undermining the medication's effectiveness, thereby leaving the baby more vulnerable to the risks of the underlying illness.

Some early-pregnancy consultations are scheduled after a patient has already discontinued antidepressant therapy. In these cases, it is important to remember that the baby was already exposed to an antidepressant during the first weeks of pregnancy. Thus, if antidepressant treatment is resumed, restarting the previous antidepressant is preferred for the reasons stated above. Typically, a pregnant woman seeking advice after having stopped antidepressant treatment has already experienced a recurrence of depression—in fact, it is likely the return of her depression that drives her to seek the clinical evaluation. The risks posed by depression to both mother and child therefore warrant resumption of the antidepressant treatment. In a less common scenario, the expectant mother who has discontinued her antidepressant is still euthymic at the time of the early-pregnancy consultation. In this situation, the potential timing for future resumption of antidepressant treatment (e.g., for postpartum prophylaxis) should be discussed with the patient.

Late-Pregnancy Decisions

Treatment issues encountered in the later weeks of pregnancy include safeguarding neonatal outcomes and monitoring symptoms to determine whether antidepressant dosage adjustments are necessary.

Numerous pharmacokinetic changes occurring during pregnancy—including increases in hepatic metabolism, renal clearance, and blood volume—combine to lower medication concentrations. Declining medication levels may, in turn, necessitate dosage increases to maintain efficacy (DeVane et al. 2006; Hodge and Tracy 2007; Sit et al. 2008), particularly during the late second or early third trimester. When a dosage adjustment is needed, a single stepwise dose increment is often sufficient to sustain patient well-being.

The possibility of pregnancy and neonatal complications also influences late-pregnancy decisions. For example, bupropion treatment should be discontinued in women who develop preeclampsia due to the attendant seizure risk. In addition, the potential adverse neonatal effects of serotonergic antidepressants must be considered in late-pregnancy treatment decisions. In the past, euthymic pregnant women at risk for peripartum depression were often counseled to start antidepressant prophylaxis several weeks before delivery; however, growing concerns regarding adverse neonatal effects of serotonergic antidepressants have led many clinicians to prefer postponing initiation of antidepressant prophylaxis until after delivery. This approach is supported by a sertraline clinical trial indicating that beginning antidepressant therapy after delivery provided effective prophylaxis against postpartum depression (Wisner et al. 2004); however, this approach was ineffective in a similar study with nortriptyline (Wisner et al. 2001).

Finally, concerns about risk to the neonate have led some to recommend discontinuing antidepressant therapy several weeks prior to delivery; however, such recommendations are seldom tenable due to the considerable risks to mother and child of depression coupled with the likelihood of depressive relapse if those who were unable to stop antidepressant treatment earlier in pregnancy were to attempt to do so proximate to delivery.

Peripartum and Postpartum Decisions

Two clinical concerns arise during the postpartum period: 1) worsening or recurrence of depression and 2) antidepressant safety during lactation. These issues are interrelated in that treatment changes necessitated by worsening depression may in turn affect breastfeeding safety considerations.

For many women with histories of depression, maximizing antidepressant safety during breastfeeding is the paramount consideration during the postpartum period. When an antidepressant has been used and found effective during pregnancy, it should be continued into the postpartum period when the risk for depression remains high. In such cases, there is little reason to discourage breastfeeding. Breastfeeding only continues to expose the nursing infant to the same medication at a fraction of prenatal exposure levels at a time when the child is presumably less susceptible to untoward developmental effects. There are occasions, however, in which a new mother develops postpartum depression following a euthymic antidepressant-free pregnancy. When this occurs, the need to introduce an antidepressant brings the advisability of lactation into question. Given the overall favorable safety profile for antidepressant use during lactation, some women will choose to continue breastfeeding, while others may opt to discontinue breastfeeding in order to avoid infant medication exposure. Both are reasonable choices; however, postponing treatment and thus remaining depressed in order to continue breastfeeding is not recommended in light of the long-term effects of maternal depression on child development.

Depression during the postpartum period has afforded opportunities to explore novel treatments whose use would be imprudent during pregnancy. For example, experimental evidence suggests that precipitously falling estrogen levels following delivery may contribute to the vulnerability to postpartum depression in some women (Bloch et al. 2000). A randomized clinical trial of transdermal estradiol for postpartum depression reported significantly greater reductions in depressive symptoms among women randomly assigned to estradiol versus placebo; however, the effect size was modest, with only a 4-point difference in Edinburgh Postnatal Depression Scale scores between the two groups (Gregoire et al. 1996). A second controlled trial of transdermal estradiol was initiated nearly 20 years later but was abandoned when it was discovered that the estradiol patches were not producing the expected changes in circulating estrogen levels (Wisner et al. 2015). Thus, to date, data do not support routine use of estrogen supplementation when treating postpartum depression. Moreover, estrogen therapy precludes breastfeeding.

In 2019, brexanolone, a formulation of allopregnanolone that renders it soluble in aqueous solutions and thus suitable for intravenous administration, became the first medication to be approved by the FDA specifically for treating postpartum depression. In an initial Phase II trial for postpartum depression, brexanolone, which acts as a positive allosteric modulator of the $GABA_A$ receptor, produced a statistically significant and robust 12.2-point greater reduction in Hamilton Rating Scale for Depression (HAM-D) scores than placebo, with no serious adverse events in the brexanolone-treated group (Kanes et al. 2017). In two subsequent Phase III trials, brexanolone also produced statistically significant (albeit less robust) 2.5- to 5.5-point greater reductions in HAM-D scores than placebo, with two brexanolone-treated participants experiencing serious adverse events (i.e., suicide attempt in one patient; syncope and altered level of consciousness in the other) (Meltzer-Brody et al. 2018). While brexanolone has opened the door to a truly novel biological approach to treating postpartum depression, at present, clinical use of brexanolone is limited by its exorbitant cost, the black box warning regarding risk of excessive sedation and loss of consciousness, and the requirement for a 60-hour hospitalization to complete the intravenous infusion, with requisite suspension of breastfeeding. A functionally similar agent suitable for oral administration, zuranolone, produced a statistically significant 7-point greater reduction in HAM-D scores than placebo in a Phase II trial for adults with MDD (Gunduz-Bruce et al. 2019). As of December 2021, zuranolone is in Phase III trials for postpartum depression and MDD as well as Phase II trials for a number of other indications. If zuranolone is approved, the regimen for treatment of depression will consist of 30 mg/day taken for a 2-week period.

Premenstrual Dysphoric Disorder

PMDD is defined in DSM-5 (American Psychiatric Association 2013) by a combination of clinically significant psychological, neurovegetative, and physical symptoms that begin in the final week before the onset of menses, start to improve within a few days after the onset of menses, and become minimal or absent in the week postmenses, as confirmed by prospective daily ratings during at least two symptomatic cycles. To receive the diagnosis, a woman must have experienced a total of five symptoms during most menstrual cycles in the preceding year, which must come from two different categories: 1) Criterion B symptoms (marked affective lability, irritability or anger, depressed mood, or anxiety; and 2) Criterion C symptoms (diminished interest, difficulty concentrating, low energy, changes in sleep or appetite, sense of being overwhelmed or out of control, or premenstrual physical symptoms). Affective lability and irritability are the most common psychological symptoms (Hartlage et al. 2012). Other organizations have proposed nuanced definitions of premenstrual conditions (American College of Obstetricians and Gynecologists 2014; Kadian and O'Brien 2012), and the World Health Organization recently added PMDD to ICD-11 (World Health Organization 2020), in line with the DSM-5 criteria.

Epidemiology

The prevalence of PMDD has been estimated at between 1.2% and 6.4% of premenopausal women (Epperson et al. 2012). By contrast, a much larger percentage of women experience menstrual cycle–related symptom exacerbations (85%) or premenstrual syndrome (PMS) (20%–25%), a condition less severe than PMDD and defined by less rigid criteria (Clayton 2008).

Diagnosis

Prospective rating of symptoms (i.e., ratings taken over at least two menstrual cycles) is required for diagnosis, unlike any other disorders in DSM. The most commonly used tool is the Likert-rated Daily Record of Severity of Problems (DRSP; Endicott et al. 2006). Although prospective symptom tracking remains the gold standard, it is time-consuming and challenging, and a retrospective symptom rating tool—the Premenstrual Symptoms Screening Tool (PSST)—has been developed and validated (Steiner et al. 2003). More recently, the Carolina Premenstrual Assessment Scoring System (C-PASS) was developed to improve prospective diagnosis reliability (Eisenlohr-Moul et al. 2017).

Clinical Features

PMDD produces functional impairment comparable to that produced by other depressive disorders (Halbreich et al. 2003). The natural history of PMDD has not been extensively investigated. An older 10-year prospective study reported worsening premenstrual symptoms with age (Merikangas et al. 1993); however, a larger but shorter 2-year prospective study reported stable symptom severity in PMDD (Wittchen et al. 2002). In comparison with healthy control subjects, women with PMDD are more likely to have experienced prior trauma with or without PTSD (Bertone-Johnson et al. 2014; Perkonigg et al. 2004; Pilver et al. 2011), with one study showing the strongest association with sexual abuse during childhood (Perkonigg et al. 2004). Although the mechanism underlying this association is not fully understood, one theory suggested that early abuse causes specific changes in autonomic and neuroendocrine functioning that confer vulnerability to developing PMDD. For example, studies of women with histories of abuse have reported greater peripheral vascular resistance and blood pressure (Girdler et al. 2007) and elevated triiodothyronine (T_3) concentrations (Bunevicius et al. 2012) in women with PMDD relative to those without PMDD.

Retrospective assessments have shown that PMS/PMDD increases the odds of depressive symptoms in the peripartum period (Pataky and Ehlert 2020) and during the menopause transition (Freeman et al. 2004; Harlow et al. 1999). Studies that follow women with prospectively confirmed PMDD across the life span are needed to better elucidate the relationship of PMDD with other disorders of the female reproductive life cycle.

Pathogenesis

Otherwise physiological gonadal hormonal concentrations have been associated with symptom exacerbation in women with PMDD (Schmidt et al. 1998), but the nature of this vulnerability is not fully known. A relevant current theory has focused on the role of allopregnanolone, a metabolite of progesterone and a strong positive modulator of the $GABA_A$ receptor, which is implicated (alongside other neurosteroids) in the pathophysiology of disorders across the female reproductive life cycle (Perkins and Newport 2018). This theory posits that women with PMDD have an altered sensitivity of the GABA system to allopregnanolone (Timby et al. 2016), and a study testing whether inhibition of allopregnanolone, through use of the $GABA_A$ receptor–modulating steroid antagonist Sepranolone, could improve PMDD symptoms reported reductions in negative mood from this treatment versus placebo (Bixo et al. 2017). Maladaptive response (i.e., reduced sensitivity) of the $GABA_A$ receptor also at the benzodiazepine site has been shown in PMS (Sundström et al. 1997). Notably, this maladaptive effect does not appear to occur in postpartum depression, as suggested by the significant reductions in depressive symptoms after infusion of brexanolone, a proprietary formulation of allopregnanolone. Other proposed etiological mechanisms in PMDD include serotonin system alterations (Steege et al. 1992), a polymorphism in the estrogen receptor 1 (*ESR1*) gene (Huo et al. 2007), and abnormal responses in emotion processing and regulation, as demonstrated in fMRI studies involving emotion-regulating tasks (Petersen et al. 2018).

Treatment of PMDD

The two main pharmacological strategies for PMDD aim to suppress ovulation or to modulate the serotonin system. FDA-approved medications for PMDD include the SSRIs fluoxetine, sertraline, and paroxetine (continuous and luteal-phase dosing) and oral contraceptives containing drospirenone 3 mg and ethinyl estradiol 20 mcg, taken for 24 days of a 28-day cycle. SSRIs are considered the first-line treatment choice (Ismaili et al. 2016; Royal College of Obstetricians and Gynaecologists 2016) and produce response rates between 60% and 70%. Symptom-onset SSRI dosing (i.e., starting pills at symptom onset and continuing into the first few days of menses) has been tested (Yonkers et al. 2015) and appears to be beneficial. This strategy may be preferred for women with menses irregularity, which would hinder luteal dosing. Low dosages of clomipramine (both continuous and intermittent dosing) (Sundblad et al. 1993) or venlafaxine (continuous dosing) (Cohen et al. 2004) have been found to be effective. SSRIs have demonstrated greater efficacy than have antidepressants with limited serotonergic activity (such as maprotiline [Eriksson et al. 1999], desipramine [Freeman et al. 1999], and bupropion [Pearlstein et al. 1995]). Some evidence exists for the beneficial effect of buspirone (Landén et al. 2001) and for short-term use of alprazolam (Freeman et al. 1995). Among medications used for mood stabilization, quetiapine sustained release (SR) with luteal dosing was shown to be more effective than placebo as an adjunct to SSRI/SNRI therapy in a small sample of patients with inadequate response to SSRIs/SNRIs (Jackson et al. 2015), but lithium monotherapy has not been found to be efficacious (Steiner et al. 1993).

Medical and surgical methods for suppressing ovulation have been shown to be effective. Gonadotropin-releasing hormone agonists have been recommended for PMS/PMDD symptoms that are severe or life-threatening and have not responded to SSRIs (Ismaili et al. 2016); given the risk of PMDD recurrence (Wyatt et al. 2004), the lowest possible dose of hormonal add-back should be used (Ismaili et al. 2016). Administration via the levonorgestrel-releasing intrauterine system (LNG-IUS) has been suggested as a possible way to minimize symptom recurrence, given its minimal systemic absorption (Leminen et al. 2012); however, evidence is limited. Anovulation can also be achieved with estrogen at inhibitory dosages (Studd 2012) or with danazol; however, the latter is rarely favored due to its androgenic effects (Ismaili et al. 2016). Hysterectomy with bilateral oophorectomy is the final step when medical management has failed (Ismaili et al. 2016). Despite the limited evidence available, hormonal contraceptives are commonly used, with shorter hormone-free intervals preferred over longer intervals to limit hormonal fluctuation (Freeman et al. 2012). An oral contraceptive containing ethinyl estradiol 20 mcg and drospirenone 3 mg administered as 24 days of active pills followed by 4 days of inert pills was shown to be more effective than placebo (Lopez et al. 2012), whereas the use of a shorter active phase (i.e., 21 days) was not (Freeman 2002). Drospirenone's anti-aldosterone activity may underlie its beneficial effect. Use of an oral contraceptive containing drospirenone is recommended for mild to moderate PMS/PMDD (Ismaili et al. 2016). Head-to-head comparisons are needed with other oral contraceptives or with serotonergic agents. In line with the limitations of the serotonergic literature, data are lacking on long-term efficacy of, recommended treatment duration for, and predictors of response to serotonergic agents. Among the best-studied complementary medicine strategies are complex carbohydrates (Freeman et al. 2002), calcium supplementation (Yonkers et al. 2013), and *Vitex agnus-castus* (Verkaik et al. 2017). CBT has shown benefit, and its use is recommended (Ismaili et al. 2016; Ussher and Perz 2017).

Perimenopausal Depression

The hormonal changes that occur at specific points throughout a woman's life span, especially during the menopause transition, represent windows of vulnerability to mental illness. During *perimenopause* (defined as the time from the first clinical manifestation of menopause until there has been an absence of menses for 12 months, and characterized by a marked drop in estrogen), many women experience a constellation of symptoms including mood swings, increased irritability and anger, and vasomotor symptoms. Researchers have investigated perimenopausal depression in an effort to correlate these symptoms with specific neural and/or hormonal signatures expressed in perimenopausal women. Given that perimenopausal depressive symptoms differ from symptoms of PMDD and peripartum depression, it is also important to consider how different treatment options affect patients with perimenopausal depression.

Clinical Presentation and Etiology

During the menopausal transition, women experience numerous symptoms, including vasomotor symptoms (e.g., hot flashes, flushing, night sweats) that can interrupt sleeping patterns, anger and irritability, paranoia, and increased energy (Kulkarni et al. 2018; Maki et al. 2018; Zappert and Rasgon 2007). In addition to these physiological symptoms, perimenopausal women undergo a number of endocrine changes, including fluctuations in levels of endogenous estrogen and of FSH, alterations of the hypothalamic-pituitary-gonadal (HPG) and hypothalamic-pituitary-adrenal (HPA) axes, and changes in levels of anti-Mullerian hormone and inhibin B (Kulkarni et al. 2018).

Steroids

In 2015, Gordon and colleagues published a meta-analysis in which they proposed a model of perimenopausal depression that involves the interaction of reproductive steroids and neurosteroids as mediated by GABA and HPA axis function (Gordon et al. 2015). These researchers also conducted a thorough investigation of potential risk factors for perimenopausal depression and found that a history of MDD was the strongest predictor, alongside stress, financial strain, and lack of social support.

Estrogen

In a more recent study, Gordon et al. (2019) examined the relationship of perimenopausal estradiol (E2) levels to depressive symptoms and stress in 15 perimenopausal women. E2 levels were measured indirectly by collecting urine samples and analyzing them for the E2 metabolite estrone-3-glucuronide (E1G). Study participants also completed the Trier Social Stress Test (TSST) (Kirschbaum et al. 1993), the Center for Epidemiologic Studies—Depression Scale (CES-D) (Radloff 1977), and the Positive and Negative Affect Schedule—Expanded Form (PANAS-X) (Watson and Clark 1999). The researchers found that greater fluctuations of E1G were associated with higher weekly scores for PANAS-X negative affect and for CES-D anhedonia (Gordon et al. 2019).

Neurophysiology

In a study by a team of scientists from Mongolia (Guo et al. 2018) that examined the relationship between depression and levels of serum inflammatory factors and BDNF in depressed and nondepressed perimenopausal women, the investigators found that peripheral BDNF was significantly lower in the depressed group than in the nondepressed group. Conversely, they found that CRP, IL-6, and TNF-α were all significantly higher in the depressed group (Guo et al. 2018).

Neuroimaging

Finally, some researchers are focusing on characterizing perimenopausal depression from a neuroimaging standpoint. Wang et al. (2019) used MEGA-PRESS, a type of magnetic resonance spectroscopy (MRS), in a longitudinal study to measure the levels of GABA in the anterior cingulate cortex of women going through the menopause transition who were either healthy or presented with symptoms of anxiety or depression. The women were followed for 18–24 months and upon reaching menopause, were divided into a control group, an anxiety group, and a depression group. The results from this study indicate that postmenopausal women with depression had significantly lower levels of GABA than when they were premenopausal. These women also exhibited significantly lower levels of GABA in comparison with the healthy controls and the women with anxiety. GABA, the main inhibitory neurotransmitter in the central nervous system, is proposed to mediate stress by limiting the extent and duration of the HPA axis response (Wang et al. 2019).

Currently, there are not many studies that have investigated perimenopausal depression specifically from a functional neuroimaging perspective. While the limbic and striatal regions, as well as the default mode, salience, and sensorimotor networks, have been identified as key players in MDD, the literature lacks comparable information regarding perimenopausal depression (Stickel et al. 2019). One study that followed women across the menopause transition did identify abnormal activation of the right temporal-parietal-occipital (TPO) junction and a correlation between degree of TPO activation and Beck Depression Inventory (BDI; Beck et al. 1961) scores, but the majority of neuroimaging studies within the field have focused primarily on MDD, PMDD, or peripartum depression (Berent-Spillson et al. 2017). Imaging studies conducted solely in women with perimenopausal depression could contribute to a better understanding of the disorder and how it differs from MDD.

Assessment

Although MDD and perimenopausal depression share many symptoms, important differences between the two disorders suggest the need for a validated scale specifically designed to rate the severity of symptoms of perimenopausal depression. Kulkarni et al. (2018) utilized literature reviews, clinical observation, and focus groups to identify 12 different symptom areas: energy, paranoia, irritability, self-esteem, isolation, anxiety, somatic symptoms, sleep, weight, sexual interest, memory, and concentration. Factor analysis then identified five subgroups of symptoms: self, somatic, cognition, sexual, and sleep. This new questionnaire, known as the Meno-D, can either be used as a self-report tool or be administered by a clinical professional (Kulkarni et al. 2018). Access to a diagnostic tool tailored to perimenopausal depression will aid in earlier diagnosis, which in turn is hoped to contribute to more effective treatment.

Treatment

Several studies have focused on the efficacy of different therapies in perimenopausal depression, although up-to-date literature appears to be lacking. From the standpoint of pharmacotherapy, one study found that desvenlafaxine was equally effective for perimenopausal and postmenopausal women with depression (Kornstein et al. 2010). Some studies found that SNRIs were more effective than SSRIs in treating perimenopausal depression, while other studies found no difference between the two (Kornstein et al. 2014; Soares et al. 2010).

While studies examining the efficacy of combination estrogen and progesterone therapy for perimenopausal depression have not yet been conducted, a significant body of literature suggests that hormone therapy is largely ineffective for postmenopausal women with depression (Morrison et al. 2004; Rudolph et al. 2004). However, some studies have shown that hormone therapy could potentially play a protective role against development of depressive symptoms for women in the perimenopausal and early postmenopausal phases (Burt et al. 1998; Gordon et al. 2018; Schmidt et al. 2000). Gordon and Girdler (2014) found that transdermal estrogen was more effective in alleviating depressive symptoms among perimenopausal women than among postmenopausal women (Gordon and Girdler 2014). Another study revealed the effectiveness of estrogen replacement therapy in women with perimenopause-related depression, with or without the accompaniment of antidepressants (Rasgon et al. 2002).

Additionally, some researchers have investigated other methods of therapy to treat perimenopausal depression as an alternative to pharmacotherapy or hormone therapy. One study found that while CBT was effective for treating depression related to the menopause transition, the treatment effect was not significantly different between perimenopausal and postmenopausal women (Brandon et al. 2013). Additional treatment include techniques such as transcranial magnetic stimulation (TMS), as employed by Dubin et al. (2016) in their study investigating the effects of TMS on GABA levels in the brain. These researchers found that stimulation of the medial prefrontal cortex resulted in higher levels of GABA, which is correlated with improvement in depressive symptoms (Dubin et al. 2016).

In summary, current literature supports the conclusion that perimenopausal depression is distinct from other forms of depression that arise during reproductive windows in a woman's lifetime. Researchers believe that women undergoing perimenopause are particularly vulnerable to the development of depression due to a combination of psychological, social, and biological changes that occur in that phase of life. From a neurochemical perspective, there are a number of potential markers, including GABA and BDNF, that have been correlated to perimenopausal depressive symptoms. Imaging studies within this population are severely lacking and could lead to new insights about specific regions and networks that may be causing symptoms of the disorder. In an effort to treat perimenopausal depression, researchers have conducted several trials of pharmacotherapy, hormone therapy, and behavioral therapy, with varying results. Further research will allow researchers to improve upon the current understanding of the disorder and will ultimately allow for more effective prevention and treatment.

Conclusion

Depression in women is diverse and is especially likely to occur during periods of increased vulnerability across the life span. These different types of depression (peripartum depression, premenstrual dysphoric disorder, perimenopausal depression) are distinct and require treatment tailored to each woman's symptoms and the severity of the depression at that specific stage in life. Pregnant women in particular face difficult decisions regarding treatment of their depression. While depression in women, and especially perimenopausal depression, can be heterogeneous and varied, researchers and clinicians in the field are actively working to better define these different types of depression in order to provide the highest-quality care to their patients.

References

Albert PR: Why is depression more prevalent in women? J Psychiatry Neurosci 40(4):219–221, 2015 26107348
American College of Obstetricians and Gynecologists: Subclinical hypothyroidism in pregnancy. ACOG Committee Opinion No. 381. Obstet Gynecol 110:959–960, 2007 17906045
American College of Obstetricians and Gynecologists: Vitamin D: screening and supplementation during pregnancy. ACOG Committee Opinion No. 495. Obstet Gynecol 118:197–198, 2011 21691184
American College of Obstetricians and Gynecologists: Guidelines for Women's Health Care: A Resource Manual, 4th Edition. Washington, DC, American College of Obstetricians and Gynecologists, 2014, pp 607–613
American Psychiatric Association: Diagnostic and Statistical Manual of Mental Disorders, 4th Edition. Washington, DC, American Psychiatric Association, 1994
American Psychiatric Association: Diagnostic and Statistical Manual of Mental Disorders, 5th Edition. Arlington, VA, American Psychiatric Association, 2013
Amin Z, Canli T, Epperson CN: Effect of estrogen-serotonin interactions on mood and cognition. Behav Cogn Neurosci Rev 4(1):43–58, 2005 15886402
Andersen JT, Andersen NL, Horwitz H, et al: Exposure to selective serotonin reuptake inhibitors in early pregnancy and the risk of miscarriage. Obstet Gynecol 124(4):655–661, 2014 25198261
Austin MP, Karatas JC, Mishra P, et al: Infant neurodevelopment following in utero exposure to antidepressant medication. Acta Paediatr 102(11):1054–1059, 2013 23927695
Ban L, Tata LJ, West J, et al: Live and non-live pregnancy outcomes among women with depression and anxiety: a population-based study. PLoS One 7(8):e43462, 2012 22937052
Bar-Oz B, Einarson T, Einarson A, et al: Paroxetine and congenital malformations: meta-analysis and consideration of potential confounding factors. Clin Ther 29(5):918–926, 2007 17697910
Beck AT, Ward CH, Mendelson M, et al: An inventory for measuring depression. Arch Gen Psychiatry 4:561–571, 1961 13688369
Bérard A, Sheehy O, Zhao JP, et al: SSRI and SNRI use during pregnancy and the risk of persistent pulmonary hypertension of the newborn. Br J Clin Pharmacol 83(5):1126–1133, 2017 27874994
Berent-Spillson A, Marsh C, Persad C, et al: Metabolic and hormone influences on emotion processing during menopause. Psychoneuroendocrinology 76:218–225, 2017 27622993
Bertone-Johnson ER, Whitcomb BW, Missmer SA, et al: Early life emotional, physical, and sexual abuse and the development of premenstrual syndrome: a longitudinal study. J Womens Health (Larchmt) 23(9):729–739, 2014 25098348
Bixo M, Ekberg K, Poromaa IS, et al: Treatment of premenstrual dysphoric disorder with the GABAA receptor modulating steroid antagonist Sepranolone (UC1010)—a randomized controlled trial. Psychoneuroendocrinology 80:46–55, 2017 28319848
Bloch M, Schmidt PJ, Danaceau M, et al: Effects of gonadal steroids in women with a history of postpartum depression. Am J Psychiatry 157(6):924–930, 2000 10831472
Boshier A, Wilton LV, Shakir SA: Evaluation of the safety of bupropion (Zyban) for smoking cessation from experience gained in general practice use in England in 2000. Eur J Clin Pharmacol 59(10):767–773, 2003 14615857
Boukhris T, Sheehy O, Mottron L, Bérard A: Antidepressant use during pregnancy and the risk of autism spectrum disorder in children. JAMA Pediatr 170(2):117–124, 2016 26660917
Brandon AR, Minhajuddin A, Thase ME, Jarrett RB: Impact of reproductive status and age on response of depressed women to cognitive therapy. J Womens Health (Larchmt) 22(1):58–66, 2013 23305218

Briggs GG, Freeman RK, Towers CV, et al: Drugs in Pregnancy and Lactation: A Reference Guide to Fetal and Neonatal Risk, 11th Edition. Philadelphia, PA, Wolters Kluwer, 2017

Brot MD, Akwa Y, Purdy RH, et al: The anxiolytic-like effects of the neurosteroid allopregnanolone: interactions with GABA(A) receptors. Eur J Pharmacol 325(1):1–7, 1997 9151931

Brown AS, Gyllenberg D, Malm H, et al: Association of selective serotonin reuptake inhibitor exposure during pregnancy with speech, scholastic, and motor disorders in offspring. JAMA Psychiatry 73(11):1163–1170, 2016 27732704

Brown HK, Ray JG, Wilton AS, et al: Association between serotonergic antidepressant use during pregnancy and autism spectrum disorder in children. JAMA 317(15):1544–1552, 2017 28418480

Buesching DP, Glasser ML, Frate DA: Progression of depression in the prenatal and postpartum periods. Women Health 11(2):61–78, 1986 3751082

Bunevicius A, Leserman J, Girdler SS: Hypothalamic-pituitary-thyroid axis function in women with a menstrually related mood disorder: association with histories of sexual abuse. Psychosom Med 74(8):810–816, 2012 23001392

Burt VK, Altshuler LL, Rasgon N: Depressive symptoms in the perimenopause: prevalence, assessment, and guidelines for treatment. Harv Rev Psychiatry 6(3):121–132, 1998 10372280

Cappelletti M, Della Bella S, Ferrazzi E, et al: Inflammation and preterm birth. J Leukoc Biol 99(1):67–78, 2016 26538528

Casper RC, Fleisher BE, Lee-Ancajas JC, et al: Follow-up of children of depressed mothers exposed or not exposed to antidepressant drugs during pregnancy. J Pediatr 142(4):402–408, 2003 12712058

Casper RC, Gilles AA, Fleisher BE, et al: Length of prenatal exposure to selective serotonin reuptake inhibitor (SSRI) antidepressants: effects on neonatal adaptation and psychomotor development. Psychopharmacology (Berl) 217(2):211–219, 2011 21499702

Chambers CD, Hernandez-Diaz S, Van Marter LJ, et al: Selective serotonin-reuptake inhibitors and risk of persistent pulmonary hypertension of the newborn. N Engl J Med 354(6):579–587, 2006 16467545

Chang JP, Lin CY, Lin PY, et al: Polyunsaturated fatty acids and inflammatory markers in major depressive episodes during pregnancy. Prog Neuropsychopharmacol Biol Psychiatry 80(Pt C):273–278, 2018 28536068

Christian LM, Franco A, Glaser R, Iams JD: Depressive symptoms are associated with elevated serum proinflammatory cytokines among pregnant women. Brain Behav Immun 23(6):750–754, 2009 19258033

Christian LM: Psychoneuroimmunology in pregnancy: immune pathways linking stress with maternal health, adverse birth outcomes, and fetal development. Neurosci Biobehav Rev 36(1):350–361, 2012 21787802

Chun-Fai-Chan B, Koren G, Fayez I, et al: Pregnancy outcome of women exposed to bupropion during pregnancy: a prospective comparative study. Am J Obstet Gynecol 192(3):932–936, 2005 15746694

Clayton AH: Symptoms related to the menstrual cycle: diagnosis, prevalence, and treatment. J Psychiatr Pract 14(1):13–21, 2008 18212599

Cohen LS, Soares CN, Lyster A, et al: Efficacy and tolerability of premenstrual use of venlafaxine (flexible dose) in the treatment of premenstrual dysphoric disorder. J Clin Psychopharmacol 24(5):540–543, 2004 15349012

Cohen LS, Altshuler LL, Harlow BL, et al: Relapse of major depression during pregnancy in women who maintain or discontinue antidepressant treatment. JAMA 295(5):499–507, 2006 16449615

Coll CVN, Domingues MR, Stein A, et al: Efficacy of regular exercise during pregnancy on the prevention of postpartum depression: the PAMELA randomized clinical trial. JAMA Netw Open 2(1):e186861, 2019 30646198

Concas A, Follesa P, Barbaccia ML, et al: Physiological modulation of GABA(A) receptor plasticity by progesterone metabolites. Eur J Pharmacol 375(1–3):225–235, 1999 10443579

Convertino I, Sansone AC, Marino A, et al: Neonatal adaptation issues after maternal exposure to prescription drugs: withdrawal syndromes and residual pharmacological effects. Drug Saf 39(10):903–924, 2016 27289228
Coussons-Read ME, Okun ML, Schmitt MP, Giese S: Prenatal stress alters cytokine levels in a manner that may endanger human pregnancy. Psychosom Med 67(4):625–631, 2005 16046378
Coussons-Read ME, Okun ML, Nettles CD: Psychosocial stress increases inflammatory markers and alters cytokine production across pregnancy. Brain Behav Immun 21(3):343–350, 2007 17029703
Curry SJ, Krist AH, Owens DK, et al; U.S. Preventive Services Task Force: Interventions to prevent perinatal depression: U.S. Preventive Services Task Force Recommendation Statement. JAMA 321(6):580–587, 2019 30747971
Cutrona CE: Causal attributions and perinatal depression. J Abnorm Psychol 92(2):161–172, 1983 6863731
Davis K, Goodman SH, Leiferman J, et al: A randomized controlled trial of yoga for pregnant women with symptoms of depression and anxiety. Complement Ther Clin Pract 21(3):166–172, 2015 26256135
Dean J, Keshavan M: The neurobiology of depression: an integrated view. Asian J Psychiatr 27:101–111, 2017 28558878
Delgado PL: Depression: the case for a monoamine deficiency. J Clin Psychiatry 61 (suppl 6):7–11, 2000 10775018
DeVane CL, Stowe ZN, Donovan JL, et al: Therapeutic drug monitoring of psychoactive drugs during pregnancy in the genomic era: challenges and opportunities. J Psychopharmacol 20(4 suppl):54–59, 2006 16785271
De Vera MA, Bérard A: Antidepressant use during pregnancy and the risk of pregnancy-induced hypertension. Br J Clin Pharmacol 74(2):362–369, 2012 22435711
Diav-Citrin O, Shechtman S, Weinbaum D, et al: Paroxetine and fluoxetine in pregnancy: a prospective, multicentre, controlled, observational study. Br J Clin Pharmacol 66(5):695–705, 2008 18754846
Djulus J, Koren G, Einarson TR, et al: Exposure to mirtazapine during pregnancy: a prospective, comparative study of birth outcomes. J Clin Psychiatry 67(8):1280–1284, 2006 16965209
Dubin MJ, Mao X, Banerjee S, et al: Elevated prefrontal cortex GABA in patients with major depressive disorder after TMS treatment measured with proton magnetic resonance spectroscopy. J Psychiatry Neurosci 41(3):E37–E45, 2016 26900793
Duffy CL: Postpartum depression: identifying women at risk. Genesis 11:21, 1983
Einarson A, Fatoye B, Sarkar M, et al: Pregnancy outcome following gestational exposure to venlafaxine: a multicenter prospective controlled study. Am J Psychiatry 158(10):1728–1730, 2001 11579012
Einarson A, Smart K, Vial T, et al: Rates of major malformations in infants following exposure to duloxetine during pregnancy: a preliminary report. J Clin Psychiatry 73(11):1471, 2012 23218163
Eisenlohr-Moul TA, Girdler SS, Schmalenberger KM, et al: Toward the reliable diagnosis of DSM-5 premenstrual dysphoric disorder: the Carolina Premenstrual Assessment Scoring System (C-PASS). Am J Psychiatry 174(1):51–59, 2017 27523500
El Marroun H, White TJ, van der Knaap NJ, et al: Prenatal exposure to selective serotonin reuptake inhibitors and social responsiveness symptoms of autism: population-based study of young children. Br J Psychiatry 205(2):95–102, 2014 25252317
El Marroun H, White TJ, Fernandez G, et al: Prenatal exposure to selective serotonin reuptake inhibitors and non-verbal cognitive functioning in childhood. J Psychopharmacol 31(3):346–355, 2017 27624153
Endicott J, Nee J, Harrison W: Daily record of severity of problems (DRSP): reliability and validity. Arch Women Ment Health 9(1):41–49, 2006 16172836
Epperson CN, Steiner M, Hartlage SA, et al: Premenstrual dysphoric disorder: evidence for a new category for DSM-5. Am J Psychiatry 169(5):465–475, 2012 22764360

Eriksen HL, Kesmodel US, Pedersen LH, Mortensen EL: No association between prenatal exposure to psychotropics and intelligence at age five. Acta Obstet Gynecol Scand 94(5):501–507, 2015 25711407

Eriksson E, Hedberg MA, Andersch B, et al: The serotonin reuptake inhibitor paroxetine is superior to the noradrenaline reuptake inhibitor maprotiline in the treatment of premenstrual syndrome. Arch Gen Psychiatry 56(10):932–939, 1999 10530636

Ferando I, Mody I: Altered gamma oscillations during pregnancy through loss of delta subunit-containing GABA(A) receptors on parvalbumin interneurons. Front Neural Circuits 7:144, 2013 24062647

Finer LB, Zolna MR: Declines in unintended pregnancy in the United States, 2008–2011. N Engl J Med 374(9):843–852, 2016 26962904

Fox M, Sandman CA, Davis EP, Glynn LM: A longitudinal study of women's depression symptom profiles during and after the postpartum phase. Depress Anxiety 35(4):292–304, 2018 29394510

Freeman EW: Evaluation of a unique oral contraceptive (Yasmin) in the management of premenstrual dysphoric disorder. Eur J Contracept Reprod Health Care 7 (suppl 3):27–34, discussion 42–43, 2002 12659404

Freeman EW, Rickels K, Sondheimer SJ, Polansky M: A double-blind trial of oral progesterone, alprazolam, and placebo in treatment of severe premenstrual syndrome. JAMA 274(1):51–57, 1995 7791258

Freeman EW, Rickels K, Sondheimer SJ, Polansky M: Differential response to antidepressants in women with premenstrual syndrome/premenstrual dysphoric disorder: a randomized controlled trial. Arch Gen Psychiatry 56(10):932–939, 1999 10530636

Freeman EW, Stout AL, Endicott J, Spiers P: Treatment of premenstrual syndrome with a carbohydrate-rich beverage. Int J Gynaecol Obstet 77(3):253–254, 2002 12065140

Freeman EW, Sammel MD, Liu L, et al: Hormones and menopausal status as predictors of depression in women in transition to menopause. Arch Gen Psychiatry 61(1):62–70, 2004 14706945

Freeman EW, Halbreich U, Grubb GS, et al: An overview of four studies of a continuous oral contraceptive (levonorgestrel 90 mcg/ethinyl estradiol 20 mcg) on premenstrual dysphoric disorder and premenstrual syndrome. Contraception 85(5):437–445, 2012 22152588

Ge T, Fan J, Yang W, et al: Leptin in depression: a potential therapeutic target. Cell Death Dis 9(11):1096, 2018 30367065

Ghaemi SN: Feeling and time: the phenomenology of mood disorders, depressive realism, and existential psychotherapy. Schizophr Bull 33(1):122–130, 2007 17122410

Gilmor ML, Owens MJ, Nemeroff CB: Inhibition of norepinephrine uptake in patients with major depression treated with paroxetine. Am J Psychiatry 159(10):1702–1710, 2002 12359676

Girdler SS, Leserman J, Bunevicius R, et al: Persistent alterations in biological profiles in women with abuse histories: influence of premenstrual dysphoric disorder. Health Psychol 26(2):201–213, 2007 17385972

GlaxoSmithKline: The Bupropion Pregnancy Registry: Final Report, 1 September 1997 through 31 March 2008. Wilmington, NC, Kendle International Inc., August 2008. Available at: https://pregnancyregistry.gsk.com/documents/bup_report_final_2008.pdf. Accessed December 13, 2021.

Goodman SH, Rouse MH, Connell AM, et al: Maternal depression and child psychopathology: a meta-analytic review. Clin Child Fam Psychol Rev 14(1):1–27, 2011 21052833

Gordon JL, Girdler SS: Hormone replacement therapy in the treatment of perimenopausal depression. Curr Psychiatry Rep 16(12):517, 2014 25308388

Gordon JL, Girdler SS, Meltzer-Brody SE, et al: Ovarian hormone fluctuation, neurosteroids, and HPA axis dysregulation in perimenopausal depression: a novel heuristic model. Am J Psychiatry 172(3):227–236, 2015 25585035

Gordon JL, Rubinow DR, Eisenlohr-Moul TA, et al: Efficacy of transdermal estradiol and micronized progesterone in the prevention of depressive symptoms in the menopause transition: a randomized clinical trial. JAMA Psychiatry 75(2):149–157, 2018 29322164

Gordon JL, Peltier A, Grummisch JA, Sykes Tottenham L: Estradiol fluctuation, sensitivity to stress, and depressive symptoms in the menopause transition: a pilot study. Front Psychol 10:1319, 2019 31244722

Grace SL, Evindar A, Stewart DE: The effect of postpartum depression on child cognitive development and behavior: a review and critical analysis of the literature. Arch Women Ment Health 6(4):263–274, 2003 14628179

Gregoire AJ, Kumar R, Everitt B, et al: Transdermal oestrogen for treatment of severe postnatal depression. Lancet 347(9006):930–933, 1996 8598756

Grigoriadis S, VonderPorten EH, Mamisashvili L, et al: Antidepressant exposure during pregnancy and congenital malformations: is there an association? A systematic review and meta-analysis of the best evidence. J Clin Psychiatry 74(4):e293–e308, 2013 23656855

Gunduz-Bruce H, Silber C, Kaul I, et al: Trial of SAGE-217 in patients with major depressive disorder. N Engl J Med 381(10):903–911, 2019 31483961

Guo L, Ren L, Zhang C: Relationship between depression and inflammatory factors and brain-derived neurotrophic factor in patients with perimenopause syndrome. Exp Ther Med 15(5):4436–4440, 2018 29849779

Halbreich U, Borenstein J, Pearlstein T, Kahn LS: The prevalence, impairment, impact, and burden of premenstrual dysphoric disorder (PMS/PMDD). Psychoneuroendocrinology 28 (suppl 3):1–23, 2003 12892987

Hamilton JA: Postpartum Psychiatric Problems. St. Louis, MO, Mosby Harwin, 1962

Handal M, Skurtveit S, Furu K, et al: Motor development in children prenatally exposed to selective serotonin reuptake inhibitors: a large population-based pregnancy cohort study. BJOG 123(12):1908–1917, 2016 26374234

Hanley GE, Brain U, Oberlander TF: Infant developmental outcomes following prenatal exposure to antidepressants, and maternal depressed mood and positive affect. Early Hum Dev 89(8):519–524, 2013 23384962

Hannerfors AK, Hellgren C, Schijven D, et al: Treatment with serotonin reuptake inhibitors during pregnancy is associated with elevated corticotropin-releasing hormone levels. Psychoneuroendocrinology 58:104–113, 2015 25978816

Harlow BL, Cohen LS, Otto MW, et al: Prevalence and predictors of depressive symptoms in older premenopausal women: the Harvard Study of Moods and Cycles. Arch Gen Psychiatry 56(5):418–424, 1999 10232296

Harmon AC, Cornelius DC, Amaral LM, et al: The role of inflammation in the pathology of preeclampsia. Clin Sci (Lond) 130(6):409–419, 2016 26846579

Hartlage SA, Freels S, Gotman N, Yonkers K: Criteria for premenstrual dysphoric disorder: secondary analyses of relevant data sets. Arch Gen Psychiatry 69(3):300–305, 2012 22393222

Hauser CA, Wetzel CH, Rupprecht R, Holsboer F: Allopregnanolone acts as an inhibitory modulator on alpha1- and alpha6-containing GABA-A receptors. Biochem Biophys Res Commun 219(2):531–536, 1996 8605022

Hellgren C, Åkerud H, Skalkidou A, et al: Low serum allopregnanolone is associated with symptoms of depression in late pregnancy. Neuropsychobiology 69(3):147–153, 2014 24776841

Hellgren C, Comasco E, Skalkidou A, Sundström-Poromaa I: Allopregnanolone levels and depressive symptoms during pregnancy in relation to single nucleotide polymorphisms in the allopregnanolone synthesis pathway. Horm Behav 94:106–113, 2017 28666923

Hodge LS, Tracy TS: Alterations in drug disposition during pregnancy: implications for drug therapy. Expert Opin Drug Metab Toxicol 3(4):557–571, 2007 17696806

Hogg K, Blair JD, McFadden DE, et al: Early onset pre-eclampsia is associated with altered DNA methylation of cortisol-signalling and steroidogenic genes in the placenta. PLoS One 8(5):e62969, 2013 23667551

Huo L, Straub RE, Roca C, et al: Risk for premenstrual dysphoric disorder is associated with genetic variation in ESR1, the estrogen receptor alpha gene. Biol Psychiatry 62(8):925–933, 2007 17599809

Huybrechts KF, Palmsten K, Avorn J, et al: Antidepressant use in pregnancy and the risk of cardiac defects. N Engl J Med 370(25):2397–2407, 2014 24941178

Huybrechts KF, Bateman BT, Palmsten K, et al: Antidepressant use late in pregnancy and risk of persistent pulmonary hypertension of the newborn. JAMA 313(21):2142–2151, 2015 26034955

Huybrechts KF, Bateman BT, Pawar A, et al: Maternal and fetal outcomes following exposure to duloxetine in pregnancy: cohort study. BMJ 368:m237, 2020 32075794

Ismaili E, Walsh S, O'Brien PMS, et al; Consensus Group of the International Society for Premenstrual Disorders: Fourth consensus of the International Society for Premenstrual Disorders (ISPMD): auditable standards for diagnosis and management of premenstrual disorder. Arch Women Ment Health 19(6):953–958, 2016 27378473

Jackson C, Pearson B, Girdler S, et al: Double-blind, placebo-controlled pilot study of adjunctive quetiapine SR in the treatment of PMS/PMDD. Hum Psychopharmacol 30(6):425–434, 2015 26193781

Jarde A, Morais M, Kingston D, et al: Neonatal outcomes in women with untreated antenatal depression compared with women without depression: a systematic review and meta-analysis. JAMA Psychiatry 73(8):826–837, 2016 27276520

Johansen RL, Mortensen LH, Andersen AM, et al: Maternal use of selective serotonin reuptake inhibitors and risk of miscarriage—assessing potential biases. Paediatr Perinat Epidemiol 29(1):72–81, 2015 25382157

Kadian S, O'Brien S: Classification of premenstrual disorders as proposed by the International Society for Premenstrual Disorders. Menopause Int 18(2):43–47, 2012 22611220

Källén B, Olausson PO: Maternal use of selective serotonin reuptake inhibitors and persistent pulmonary hypertension of the newborn. Pharmacoepidemiol Drug Saf 17(8):801–806, 2008 18314924

Kanes S, Colquhoun H, Gunduz-Bruce H, et al: Brexanolone (SAGE-547 injection) in postpartum depression: a randomised controlled trial. Lancet 390(10093):480–489, 2017 28619476

Katz ER, Stowe ZN, Newport DJ, et al: Regulation of mRNA expression encoding chaperone and co-chaperone proteins of the glucocorticoid receptor in peripheral blood: association with depressive symptoms during pregnancy. Psychol Med 42(5):943–956, 2012 21995950

Kendler KS, Kessler RC, Neale MC, et al: The prediction of major depression in women: toward an integrated etiologic model. Am J Psychiatry 150(8):1139–1148, 1993 8328557

Kieviet N, Dolman KM, Honig A: The use of psychotropic medication during pregnancy: how about the newborn? Neuropsychiatr Dis Treat 9:1257–1266, 2013 24039427

Kingston D, Tough S, Whitfield H: Prenatal and postpartum maternal psychological distress and infant development. Child Psychiatry Hum Dev 43(5):683–714, 2012 22407278

Kirschbaum C, Pirke KM, Hellhammer DH: The "Trier Social Stress Test"—a tool for investigating psychobiological stress responses in a laboratory setting. Neuropsychobiology 28(1–2):76–81, 1993 8255414

Kornstein SG, Jiang Q, Reddy S, et al: Short-term efficacy and safety of desvenlafaxine in a randomized, placebo-controlled study of perimenopausal and postmenopausal women with major depressive disorder. J Clin Psychiatry 71(8):1088–1096, 2010 20797382

Kornstein SG, Pedersen RD, Holland PJ, et al: Influence of sex and menopausal status on response, remission, and recurrence in patients with recurrent major depressive disorder treated with venlafaxine extended release or fluoxetine: analysis of data from the PREVENT study. J Clin Psychiatry 75(1):62–68, 2014 24345717

Kulkarni J, Gavrilidis E, Hudaib AR, et al: Development and validation of a new rating scale for perimenopausal depression—the Meno-D. Transl Psychiatry 8(1):123, 2018 29955034

Kumar R, Robson KM: A prospective study of emotional disorders in childbearing women. Br J Psychiatry 144:35–47, 1984 6692075

Labaka A, Goñi-Balentziaga O, Lebeña A, Pérez-Tejada J: Biological sex differences in depression: a systematic review. Biol Res Nurs 20(4):383–392, 2018 29759000

Lahti-Pulkkinen M, Girchenko P, Robinson R, et al: Maternal depression and inflammation during pregnancy. Psychol Med 50(11):1839–1851, 2020 31439060

Landén M, Eriksson O, Sundblad C, et al: Compounds with affinity for serotonergic receptors in the treatment of premenstrual dysphoria: a comparison of buspirone, nefazodone and placebo. Psychopharmacology (Berl) 155(3):292–298, 2001

Lee B-H, Kim Y-K: The roles of BDNF in the pathophysiology of major depression and in antidepressant treatment. Psychiatry Investig 7(4):231–235, 2010 21253405

Leminen H, Heliövaara-Peippo S, Halmesmäki K, et al: The effect of hysterectomy or levonorgestrel-releasing intrauterine system on premenstrual symptoms in women treated for menorrhagia: secondary analysis of a randomized controlled trial. Acta Obstet Gynecol Scand 91(3):318–325, 2012 22168810

Liu C, Cnattingius S, Bergström M, et al: Prenatal parental depression and preterm birth: a national cohort study. BJOG 123(12):1973–1982, 2016 26786413

Liu Y, Kaaya S, Chai J, et al: Maternal depressive symptoms and early childhood cognitive development: a meta-analysis. Psychol Med 47(4):680–689, 2017 27834159

Lopez LM, Kaptein AA, Helmerhorst FM: Oral contraceptives containing drospirenone for premenstrual syndrome. Cochrane Database Syst Rev (2):CD006586, 2012 22336820

Lovejoy MC, Graczyk PA, O'Hare E, Neuman G: Maternal depression and parenting behavior: a meta-analytic review. Clin Psychol Rev 20(5):561–592, 2000 10860167

Lupattelli A, Wood M, Lapane K, et al: Risk of preeclampsia after gestational exposure to selective serotonin reuptake inhibitors and other antidepressants: a study from The Norwegian Mother and Child Cohort Study. Pharmacoepidemiol Drug Saf 26(10):1266–1276, 2017 28815791

Maayan R, Strous RD, Abou-Kaoud M, Weizman A: The effect of 17 beta estradiol withdrawal on the level of brain and peripheral neurosteroids in ovarectomized rats. Neurosci Lett 384(1–2):156–161, 2005 15927368

Maki PM, Kornstein SG, Joffe H, et al; Board of Trustees for The North American Menopause Society (NAMS) and the Women and Mood Disorders Task Force of the National Network of Depression Centers: Guidelines for the evaluation and treatment of perimenopausal depression: summary and recommendations. Menopause 25(10):1069–1085, 2018 30179986

Malm H, Sourander A, Gissler M, et al: Pregnancy complications following prenatal exposure to SSRIs or maternal psychiatric disorders: results from population-based national register data. Am J Psychiatry 172(12):1224–1232, 2015 26238606

Manly PC, McMahon RJ, Bradley CF, Davidson PO: Depressive attributional style and depression following childbirth. J Abnorm Psychol 91(4):245–254, 1982 7130519

Marcus SM: Depression during pregnancy: rates, risks and consequences—Motherisk Update 2008. Can J Clin Pharmacol 16(1):e15–e22, 2009 19164843

Marcus SM, Flynn HA, Blow FC, Barry KL: Depressive symptoms among pregnant women screened in obstetrics settings. J Womens Health (Larchmt) 12(4):373–380, 2003 12804344

Marsh WK, Templeton A, Ketter TA, Rasgon NL: Increased frequency of depressive episodes during the menopausal transition in women with bipolar disorder: preliminary report. J Psychiatr Res 42(3):247–251, 2008 17266987

Marsh WK, Ketter TA, Rasgon NL: Increased depressive symptoms in menopausal age women with bipolar disorder: age and gender comparison. J Psychiatr Res 43(8):798–802, 2009 19155021

Meltzer-Brody S, Stuebe A, Dole N, et al: Elevated corticotropin releasing hormone (CRH) during pregnancy and risk of postpartum depression (PPD). J Clin Endocrinol Metab 96(1):E40–E47, 2011 20943787

Meltzer-Brody S, Colquhoun H, Riesenberg R, et al: Brexanolone injection in post-partum depression: two multicentre, double-blind, randomised, placebo-controlled, phase 3 trials. Lancet 392(10152):1058–1070, 2018 30177236

Merikangas KR, Foeldenyi M, Angst J: The Zurich Study, XIX: patterns of menstrual disturbances in the community: results of the Zurich Cohort Study. Eur Arch Psychiatry Clin Neurosci 243(1):23–32, 1993 8399407

Miller ES, Hoxha D, Wisner KL, Gossett DR: Obsessions and compulsions in postpartum women without obsessive compulsive disorder. J Womens Health (Larchmt) 24(10):825–830, 2015 26121364

Miller GE, Stetler CA, Carney RM, et al: Clinical depression and inflammatory risk markers for coronary heart disease. Am J Cardiol 90(12):1279–1283, 2002 12480034

Mohamed SA, El Andaloussi A, Al-Hendy A, et al: Vitamin D and corticotropin-releasing hormone in term and preterm birth: potential contributions to preterm labor and birth outcome. J Matern Fetal Neonatal Med 31(21):2911–2917, 2018 28780891

Montoya A, Bruins R, Katzman MA, Blier P: The noradrenergic paradox: implications in the management of depression and anxiety. Neuropsychiatr Dis Treat 12:541–557, 2016 27042068

Morales DR, Slattery J, Evans S, Kurz X: Antidepressant use during pregnancy and risk of autism spectrum disorder and attention deficit hyperactivity disorder: systematic review of observational studies and methodological considerations. BMC Med 16(1):6, 2018 29332605

Morrison MF, Kallan MJ, Ten Have T, et al: Lack of efficacy of estradiol for depression in postmenopausal women: a randomized, controlled trial. Biol Psychiatry 55(4):406–412, 2004 14960294

Moses-Kolko EL, Bogen D, Perel J, et al: Neonatal signs after late in utero exposure to serotonin reuptake inhibitors: literature review and implications for clinical applications. JAMA 293(19):2372–2383, 2005 15900008

Nappi RE, Petraglia F, Luisi S, et al: Serum allopregnanolone in women with postpartum "blues." Obstet Gynecol 97(1):77–80, 2001 11152912

National Institute of Mental Health: Major depression. Data from the 2019 National Survey on Drug Use and Health (NSDUH). Available at: https://www.nimh.nih.gov/health/statistics/major-depression#part_155721. Accessed December 19, 2021.

Neill JC, Kulkarni J (eds): Biological Basis of Sex Differences in Psychopharmacology (Current Topics in Behavioral Neurosciences, Vol 8; Geyer M, Ellenbroek B, Marsden C, series eds). New York, Springer, 2011

Newport DJ, Ji S, Long Q, et al: Maternal depression and anxiety differentially impact fetal exposures during pregnancy. J Clin Psychiatry 73(2):247–251, 2012 22152400

Newport DJ, Hostetter AL, Juul SH, et al: Prenatal psychostimulant and antidepressant exposure and risk of hypertensive disorders of pregnancy. J Clin Psychiatry 77(11):1538–1545, 2016 28076672

Ng EK, Leung TN, Tsui NB, et al: The concentration of circulating corticotropin-releasing hormone mRNA in maternal plasma is increased in preeclampsia. Clin Chem 49(5):727–731, 2003 12709362

Ng QX, Venkatanarayanan N, Ho CYX, et al: Selective serotonin reuptake inhibitors and persistent pulmonary hypertension of the newborn: an update mate-analysis. J Womens Health (Larchmt) 28(3):331–338, 2019 30407100

Nulman I, Rovet J, Stewart DE, et al: Neurodevelopment of children exposed in utero to antidepressant drugs. N Engl J Med 336(4):258–262, 1997 8995088

Nulman I, Rovet J, Stewart DE, et al: Child development following exposure to tricyclic antidepressants or fluoxetine throughout fetal life: a prospective, controlled study. Am J Psychiatry 159(11):1889–1895, 2002 12411224

Nulman I, Koren G, Rovet J, et al: Neurodevelopment of children following prenatal exposure to venlafaxine, selective serotonin reuptake inhibitors, or untreated maternal depression. Am J Psychiatry 169(11):1165–1174, 2012 23128923

Oberlander TF, Misri S, Fitzgerald CE, et al: Pharmacologic factors associated with transient neonatal symptoms following prenatal psychotropic medication exposure. J Clin Psychiatry 65(2):230–237, 2004 15003078

Oberlander TF, Warburton W, Misri S, et al: Neonatal outcomes after prenatal exposure to selective serotonin reuptake inhibitor antidepressants and maternal depression using population-based linked health data. Arch Gen Psychiatry 63(8):898–906, 2006 16894066

O'Hara MW, Rehm LP, Campbell SB: Predicting depressive symptomatology: cognitive-behavioral models and postpartum depression. J Abnorm Psychol 91(6):457–461, 1982 7153419

Orr ST, James SA, Blackmore Prince C: Maternal prenatal depressive symptoms and spontaneous preterm births among African-American women in Baltimore, Maryland. Am J Epidemiol 156(9):797–802, 2002 12396996

Osborne S, Biaggi A, Chua TE, et al: Antenatal depression programs cortisol stress reactivity in offspring through increased maternal inflammation and cortisol in pregnancy: the Psychiatry Research and Motherhood—Depression (PRAM-D) Study. Psychoneuroendocrinology 98:211–221, 2018 30033161

Pae CU, Mandelli L, Kim TS, et al: Effectiveness of antidepressant treatments in pre-menopausal versus post-menopausal women: a pilot study on differential effects of sex hormones on antidepressant effects. Biomed Pharmacother 63(3):228–235, 2009 18502089

Palmsten K, Setoguchi S, Margulis AV, et al: Elevated risk of preeclampsia in pregnant women with depression: depression or antidepressants? Am J Epidemiol 175(10):988–997, 2012 22442287

Palmsten K, Huybrechts KF, Michels KB, et al: Antidepressant use and risk for preeclampsia. Epidemiology 24(5):682–691, 2013 23873072

Pan WL, Chang CW, Chen SM, Gau ML: Assessing the effectiveness of mindfulness-based programs on mental health during pregnancy and early motherhood—a randomized control trial. BMC Pregnancy Childbirth 19(1):346, 2019 31601170

Pataky EA, Ehlert U: Longitudinal assessment of symptoms of postpartum mood disorder in women with and without a history of depression. Arch Women Ment Health 23(3):391–399, 2020 31350668

Pearlstein TB, Stone AB, Lund SA, et al: Comparison of fluoxetine, bupropion, and placebo in the treatment of premenstrual dysphoric disorder. Neuropsychopharmacology 12(2):167–176, 1995 7779245

Perales M, Refoyo I, Coteron J, et al: Exercise during pregnancy attenuates prenatal depression: a randomized controlled trial. Eval Health Prof 38(1):59–72, 2015 24872442

Perkins AV, Linton EA, Eben F, et al: Corticotrophin-releasing hormone and corticotrophin-releasing hormone binding protein in normal and pre-eclamptic human pregnancies. Br J Obstet Gynaecol 102(2):118–122, 1995 7756202

Perkins EC, Newport DJ: Neurosteroids in the pathophysiology and treatment of mood and anxiety disorders. Curr Treat Options Psychiatry 5(4):377–400, 2018

Perkonigg A, Yonkers KA, Pfister H, et al: Risk factors for premenstrual dysphoric disorder in a community sample of young women: the role of traumatic events and posttraumatic stress disorder. J Clin Psychiatry 65(10):1314–1322, 2004 15491233

Petersen N, Ghahremani DG, Rapkin AJ, et al: Brain activation during emotion regulation in women with premenstrual dysphoric disorder. Psychol Med 48(11):1795–1802, 2018 29145910

Petsas G, Jeschke U, Richter DU, et al: Aberrant expression of corticotropin-releasing hormone in pre-eclampsia induces expression of FasL in maternal macrophages and extravillous trophoblast apoptosis. Mol Hum Reprod 18(11):535–545, 2012 22763913

Pilver CE, Levy BR, Libby DJ, Desai RA: Posttraumatic stress disorder and trauma characteristics are correlates of premenstrual dysphoric disorder. Arch Women Ment Health 14(5):383–393, 2011 21786081

Polen KN, Rasmussen SA, Riehle-Colarusso T, Reefhuis J; National Birth Defects Prevention Study: Association between reported venlafaxine use in early pregnancy and birth defects, national birth defects prevention study, 1997–2007. Birth Defects Res A Clin Mol Teratol 97(1):28–35, 2013 23281074

Radloff LS: The CES-D scale: a self-report depression scale for research in the general population. Appl Psychol Meas 1(3):385–401, 1977

Rai D, Lee BK, Dalman C, et al: Antidepressants during pregnancy and autism in offspring: population based cohort study. BMJ 358:j2811, 2017 28724519

Rapkin AJ, Mikacich JA, Moatakef-Imani B, Rasgon N: The clinical nature and formal diagnosis of premenstrual, postpartum, and perimenopausal affective disorders. Curr Psychiatry Rep 4(6):419–428, 2002 12441021

Rasgon NL, Altshuler LL, Fairbanks LA, et al: Estrogen replacement therapy in the treatment of major depressive disorder in perimenopausal women. J Clin Psychiatry 63 (suppl 7):45–48, 2002 11995778

Rasgon N, Bauer M, Grof P, et al: Sex-specific self-reported mood changes by patients with bipolar disorder. J Psychiatr Res 39(1):77–83, 2005 15504425

Raskin A: Age-sex differences in response to antidepressant drugs. J Nerv Ment Dis 159(2):120–130, 1974 4850465

Ratcliffe M: The phenomenology of depression and the nature of empathy. Med Health Care Philos 17(2):269–280, 2014 23775337

Rich-Edwards JW, Mohllajee AP, Kleinman K, et al: Elevated midpregnancy corticotropin-releasing hormone is associated with prenatal, but not postpartum, maternal depression. J Clin Endocrinol Metab 93(5):1946–1951, 2008 18303075

Richardson JL, Martin F, Dunstan H, et al: Pregnancy outcomes following maternal venlafaxine use: a prospective observational comparative cohort study. Reprod Toxicol 84:108–113, 2019 30639403

Royal College of Obstetricians and Gynaecologists: Premenstrual Syndrome, Management (Green-top Guideline No. 48). Published: 01/12/2016. Available at: https://www.rcog.org.uk/en/guidelines-research-services/guidelines/gtg48/. Accessed December 19, 2021.

Rudolph I, Palombo-Kinne E, Kirsch B, et al: Influence of a continuous combined HRT (2 mg estradiol valerate and 2 mg dienogest) on postmenopausal depression. Climacteric 7(3):301–311, 2004 15669555

Ruiz RJ, Gennaro S, O'Connor C, et al: CRH as a predictor of preterm birth in minority women. Biol Res Nurs 18(3):316–321, 2016 26512053

Şahingöz M, Yuksel G, Karsidag C, et al: Birth weight and preterm birth in babies of pregnant women with major depression in relation to treatment with antidepressants. J Clin Psychopharmacol 34(2):226–229, 2014 24525643

Sanacora G, Treccani G, Popoli M: Towards a glutamate hypothesis of depression: an emerging frontier of neuropsychopharmacology for mood disorders. Neuropharmacology 62(1):63–77, 2012 21827775

Schmidt PJ, Nieman LK, Danaceau MA, et al: Differential behavioral effects of gonadal steroids in women with and in those without premenstrual syndrome. N Engl J Med 338(4):209–216, 1998 9435325

Schmidt PJ, Nieman L, Danaceau MA, et al: Estrogen replacement in perimenopause-related depression: a preliminary report. Am J Obstet Gynecol 183(2):414–420, 2000 10942479

Schreiber R: Wandering in the dark: women's experiences with depression. Health Care Women Int 22(1–2):85–98, 2001 11813799

Shors TJ, Leuner B: Estrogen-mediated effects on depression and memory formation in females. J Affect Disord 74(1):85–96, 2003 12646301

Siegmann EM, Müller HHO, Luecke C, et al: Association of depression and anxiety disorders with autoimmune thyroiditis: a systematic review and meta-analysis. JAMA Psychiatry 75(6):577–584, 2018 29800939

Sit DK, Perel JM, Helsel JC, Wisner KL: Changes in antidepressant metabolism and dosing across pregnancy and early postpartum. J Clin Psychiatry 69(4):652–658, 2008 18426260

Smit M, Dolman KM, Honig A: Mirtazapine in pregnancy and lactation—a systematic review. Eur Neuropsychopharmacol 26(1):126–135, 2016 26631373

Smith R, Smith JI, Shen X, et al: Patterns of plasma corticotropin-releasing hormone, progesterone, estradiol, and estriol change and the onset of human labor. J Clin Endocrinol Metab 94(6):2066–2074, 2009 19258402

Soares CN, Thase ME, Clayton A, et al: Desvenlafaxine and escitalopram for the treatment of postmenopausal women with major depressive disorder. Menopause 17(4):700–711, 2010 20539246

Sockol LE: A systematic review of the efficacy of cognitive behavioral therapy for treating and preventing perinatal depression. J Affect Disord 177:7–21, 2015 25743368

Sockol LE: A systematic review and meta-analysis of interpersonal psychotherapy for perinatal women. J Affect Disord 232:316–328, 2018 29501991

Sramek JJ, Murphy MF, Cutler NR: Sex differences in the psychopharmacological treatment of depression. Dialogues Clin Neurosci 18(4):447–457, 2016 28179816
Steege JF, Stout AL, Knight DL, Nemeroff CB: Reduced platelet tritium-labeled imipramine binding sites in women with premenstrual syndrome. Am J Obstet Gynecol 167(1):168–172, 1992 1442921
Steer RA, Scholl TO, Hediger ML, Fischer RL: Self-reported depression and negative pregnancy outcomes. J Clin Epidemiol 45(10):1093–1099, 1992 1474405
Steiner M, Haskett RF, Osmun JN, et al: Treatment of premenstrual tension with lithium carbonate. A pilot study. Arch Gen Psychiatry 50(6):467–473, 1993 8498881
Steiner M, Macdougall M, Brown E: The Premenstrual Symptoms Screening Tool (PSST) for clinicians. Arch Women Ment Health 6(3):203–209, 2003 12920618
Stickel S, Wagels L, Wudarczyk O, et al: Neural correlates of depression in women across the reproductive lifespan—an fMRI review. J Affect Disord 246:556–570, 2019 30605874
Stowe ZN, Nemeroff CB: Women at risk for postpartum-onset major depression. Am J Obstet Gynecol 173(2):639–645, 1995 7645646
Stowe ZN, Owens MJ, Landry JC, et al: Sertraline and desmethylsertraline in human breast milk and nursing infants. Am J Psychiatry 154(9):1255–1260, 1997 9286185
Stowe ZN, Cohen LS, Hostetter A, et al: Paroxetine in human breast milk and nursing infants. Am J Psychiatry 157(2):185–189, 2000 10671385
Stowe ZN, Hostetter AL, Owens MJ, et al: The pharmacokinetics of sertraline excretion into human breast milk: determinants of infant serum concentrations. J Clin Psychiatry 64(1):73–80, 2003 12590627
Stowe ZN, Hostetter AL, Newport DJ: The onset of postpartum depression: implications for screening in obstetrical and primary care. Am J Obstet Gynecol 192(2):522–526, 2005 15695997
Studd J: Treatment of premenstrual disorders by suppression of ovulation by transdermal estrogens. Menopause Int 18(2):65–67, 2012 22611224
Sujan AC, Rickert ME, Öberg AS, et al: Associations of maternal antidepressant use during the first trimester of pregnancy with preterm birth, small for gestational age, autism spectrum disorder, and attention-deficit/hyperactivity disorder in offspring. JAMA 317(15):1553–1562, 2017 28418479
Sundblad C, Hedberg MA, Eriksson E: Clomipramine administered during the luteal phase reduces the symptoms of premenstrual syndrome: a placebo-controlled trial. Neuropsychopharmacology 9(2):133–145, 1993 8216696
Sundström I, Nyberg S, Bäckström T: Patients with premenstrual syndrome have reduced sensitivity to midazolam compared to control subjects. Neuropsychopharmacology 17(6):370–381, 1997 9397425
Suri R, Stowe ZN, Hendrick V, et al: Estimates of nursing infant daily dose of fluoxetine through breast milk. Biol Psychiatry 52(5):446–451, 2002 12242061
Timby E, Bäckström T, Nyberg S, et al: Women with premenstrual dysphoric disorder have altered sensitivity to allopregnanolone over the menstrual cycle compared to controls—a pilot study. Psychopharmacology (Berl) 233(11):2109–2117, 2016 26960697
Toh S, Mitchell AA, Louik C, et al: Selective serotonin reuptake inhibitor use and risk of gestational hypertension. Am J Psychiatry 166(3):320–328, 2009 19122006
Troisi A, Moles A: Gender differences in depression: an ethological study of nonverbal behavior during interviews. J Psychiatr Res 33(3):243–250, 1999 10367990
Trotula of Salerno: The Disease of Women: A Translation of Passionibus Mulierum Curandorum. Translated by Mason-Hohl E. Los Angeles, CA, Ward Ritchie Press, 1940
Troutman BR, Cutrona CE: Nonpsychotic postpartum depression among adolescent mothers. J Abnorm Psychol 99(1):69–78, 1990 2307769
Uguz F, Şahingöz M, Sonmez EO, et al: The effects of maternal major depression, generalized anxiety disorder, and panic disorder on birth weight and gestational age: a comparative study. J Psychosom Res 75(1):87–89, 2013 23751245

U.S. Food and Drug Administration: Public Health Advisory: Treatment challenges of depression in pregnancy and the possibility of persistent pulmonary hypertension in newborns. 2006. Available at: https://wayback.archive-it.org/7993/20170112032454/http://www.fda.gov/Drugs/DrugSafety/PostmarketDrugSafetyInformationforPatientsandProviders/ucm124348.htm. Accessed October 26, 2021.

U.S. Food and Drug Administration: FDA Drug Safety Communication: Selective serotonin reuptake inhibitor (SSRI) antidepressant use during pregnancy and reports of a rare heart and lung condition in newborn babies. 2011. Available at: https://www.fda.gov/Drugs/DrugSafety/ucm283375.htm. Accessed December 22, 2020.

U.S. Food and Drug Administration: Content and format of labeling for human prescription drug and biological products; requirements for pregnancy and lactation labeling: final rule. Fed Regist 79(233):72064–72103, 2014 PMID: 25509060

Ussher JM, Perz J: Evaluation of the relative efficacy of a couple cognitive-behaviour therapy (CBT) for premenstrual disorders (PMDs), in comparison to one-to-one CBT and a wait list control: a randomized controlled trial. PLoS One 12(4):e0175068, 2017 28419170

Valkanova V, Ebmeier KP, Allan CL: CRP, IL-6 and depression: a systematic review and meta-analysis of longitudinal studies. J Affect Disord 150(3):736–744, 2013 23870425

Vega ML, Newport GC, Bozhdaraj D, et al: Implementation of advanced methods for reproductive pharmacovigilance in autism: a meta-analysis of the effects of prenatal antidepressant exposure. Am J Psychiatry 177(6):506–517, 2020 32375539

Venkatesh KK, Riley L, Castro VM, et al: Association of antenatal depression symptoms and antidepressant treatment with preterm birth. Obstet Gynecol 127(5):926–933, 2016 27054941

Verkaik S, Kamperman AM, van Westrhenen R, Schulte PFJ: The treatment of premenstrual syndrome with preparations of Vitex agnus castus: a systematic review and meta-analysis. Am J Obstet Gynecol 217(2):150–166, 2017 28237870

Viktorin A, Lichtenstein P, Lundholm C, et al: Selective serotonin re-uptake inhibitor use during pregnancy: association with offspring birth size and gestational age. Int J Epidemiol 45(1):170–177, 2016 26748846

Wang D, Wang X, Luo MT, et al: Gamma-aminobutyric acid levels in the anterior cingulate cortex of perimenopausal women with depression: a magnetic resonance spectroscopy study. Front Neurosci 13:785, 2019 31481863

Watson D, Clark LA: The PANAS-X: Manual for the Positive and Negative Affect Schedule—Expanded Form. Ames, IA, The University of Iowa, 1999

Watson JP, Elliott SA, Rugg AJ, Brough DI: Psychiatric disorder in pregnancy and the first postnatal year. Br J Psychiatry 144:453–462, 1984 6733369

Wei SQ, Fraser W, Luo ZC: Inflammatory cytokines and spontaneous preterm birth in asymptomatic women: a systematic review. Obstet Gynecol 116(2 Pt 1):393–401, 2010 20664401

Williams JA, Romero VC, Clinton CM, et al: Vitamin D levels and perinatal depressive symptoms in women at risk: a secondary analysis of the mothers, omega-3, and mental health study. BMC Pregnancy Childbirth 16(1):203, 2016 27485050

Williams M, Wooltorton E: Paroxetine (Paxil) and congenital malformations. CMAJ 173(11):1320–1321, 2005 16272192

Winterfeld U, Klinger G, Panchaud A, et al: Pregnancy outcome following maternal exposure to mirtazapine: a multicenter, prospective study. J Clin Psychopharmacol 35(3):250–259, 2015 25830592

Wisner KL, Perel JM, Peindl KS, et al: Prevention of recurrent postpartum depression: a randomized clinical trial. J Clin Psychiatry 62(2):82–86, 2001 11247106

Wisner KL, Perel JM, Peindl KS, et al: Prevention of postpartum depression: a pilot randomized clinical trial. Am J Psychiatry 161(7):1290–1292, 2004 15229064

Wisner KL, Sit DK, Hanusa BH, et al: Major depression and antidepressant treatment: impact on pregnancy and neonatal outcomes. Am J Psychiatry 166(5):557–566, 2009 19289451

Wisner KL, Sit DK, Moses-Kolko EL, et al: Transdermal estradiol treatment for postpartum depression: a pilot, randomized trial. J Clin Psychopharmacol 35(4):389–395, 2015 26061609

Wittchen HU, Becker E, Lieb R, Krause P: Prevalence, incidence and stability of premenstrual dysphoric disorder in the community. Psychol Med 32(1):119–132, 2002 11883723

World Health Organization: The International Statistical Classification of Diseases and Related Health Problems, 10th Revision. Geneva, World Health Organization, 1992

World Health Organization: International Statistical Classification of Diseases and Related Health Problems, 11th Revision (ICD-11). Geneva, World Health Organization, 2020. Available at: https://icd.who.int/. Accessed May 7, 2021.

Wyatt KM, Dimmock PW, Ismail KM, et al: The effectiveness of GnRHa with and without "add-back" therapy in treating premenstrual syndrome: a meta analysis. BJOG 111(6):585–593, 2004 15198787

Xu J, Zhao YH, Chen YP, et al: Maternal circulating concentrations of tumor necrosis factor-alpha, leptin, and adiponectin in gestational diabetes mellitus: a systematic review and meta-analysis. ScientificWorldJournal 2014:926932, 2014 25202741

Yonkers KA, Norwitz ER, Smith MV, et al: Depression and serotonin reuptake inhibitor treatment as risk factors for preterm birth. Epidemiology 23(5):677–685, 2012 22627901

Yonkers KA, Pearlstein TB, Gotman N: A pilot study to compare fluoxetine, calcium, and placebo in the treatment of premenstrual syndrome. J Clin Psychopharmacol 33(5):614–620, 2013 23963058

Yonkers KA, Kornstein SG, Gueorguieva R, et al: Symptom-onset dosing of sertraline for the treatment of premenstrual dysphoric disorder: a multi-site, double-blind, randomized, placebo-controlled trial. JAMA Psychiatry 72(10):1037–1044, 2015 26351969

Young EA, Kornstein SG, Marcus SM, et al: Sex differences in response to citalopram: a STAR*D report. J Psychiatr Res 43(5):503–511, 2009 18752809

Zakiyah N, Ter Heijne LF, Bos JH, et al: Antidepressant use during pregnancy and the risk of developing gestational hypertension: a retrospective cohort study. BMC Pregnancy Childbirth 18(1):187, 2018 29843629

Zappert LN, Rasgon NL: Biological and psychosocial correlates of perimenopausal depression: implications for treatment. Depress Mind Body 3(2):50–56, 2007. Available at: https://www.cecentral.com/assets/393/MEN07334_1.pdf. Available at: December 19, 2021.

Zuckerman B, Amaro H, Bauchner H, Cabral H: Depressive symptoms during pregnancy: relationship to poor health behaviors. Am J Obstet Gynecol 160(5 pt 1):1107–1111, 1989 2729387

CHAPTER 43

Depression Across Cultures

An Ecosocial Approach

Laurence J. Kirmayer, M.D.
G. Eric Jarvis, M.D.
Ana Gómez-Carrillo, M.D.

Depression is now recognized as a global health problem, with estimates that it accounts for up to 10% of years lost to disability in low- and middle-income countries (Desjarlais et al. 1995; Murray and Lopez 1997; World Health Organization 2017). Global disability due to depression has increased over the past two decades, especially for women (GBD 2017 DALYs and HALE Collaborators 2018). Given this widespread prevalence and social impact, there is a pressing need to examine cross-cultural differences in the causes, course, and treatment of depression (Scott and Dickey 2003; Steel et al. 2014). At the same time, responding to the health disparities associated with cultural diversity is increasingly recognized as an important issue in high-income countries, creating new challenges for mental health care (Napier et al. 2014; U.S. Surgeon General 2002).

Cultural psychiatry is concerned with the impact of variations in ways of life on psychiatric disorders and their treatment (Kleinman 1988). Among the questions it seeks to address are the following: How does culture shape the experience and expression of human suffering? What are the most effective methods of interpreting and responding to suffering in a given social or clinical context? Are the forms of distress identified in current psychiatric nosology similar around the globe? More specifically, can mood disorders be recognized across diverse cultures, and do they have similar symptoms, courses, treatment responses, and outcomes? These questions raise complex epistemological and methodological problems for psychiatric research and practice (Kirmayer and Ban 2013). The answers are crucial to the advancement of research, the design of health care systems, and the delivery of clinical care in societies facing increasing cultural diversity (Kirmayer and Jarvis 2019).

Much of what we know about the role of culture in psychopathology comes from qualitative ethnographic research in clinical settings and in the community (Kirmayer 1989; Kleinman 1986, 1988). Conventional psychiatric research is ill-suited to explore the cultural meaning of distress because it tends to reduce the complexity of illness narratives down to checklists of symptoms and signs of disorder. However, a growing body of epidemiological research informed by ethnography goes beyond parochial assumptions to identify clinically important cultural variation. In this chapter, we review some of what is known about cultural variations in the prevalence, clinical presentation, mechanisms, and treatment of depressive disorders and address some of the broader conceptual issues that are central to meaningful research and effective clinical intervention.

Defining Culture

Culture encompasses all the forms of knowledge and practices that make up a way of life, with its social roles, norms, values, and institutions. This includes the ways in which social groups are marked off from one another in terms of ethnicity, racialized identity, religion, or emerging social categories. The definition of a group is always vis-à-vis some other, and hence the meanings of ethnicity, race, and other culturally constructed aspects of identity change depending on the larger social context.

Older notions of cultures as homogeneous, self-contained, homeostatic systems have given way to a view of culture as an abstraction based on fluid, ever-changing constructions that emerge from interactions between individuals, communities, and social institutions, which in turn are embedded in global systems (Kirmayer 2006). Individuals use resources available in their local social worlds to construct durable and culturally valued identities and competent selves. At the same time, individuals and groups are constrained by the ways in which culture frames and defines their options and experience. In the contemporary world, migration and electronic communication allow individuals to position themselves within multiple cultural worlds, resulting in cultural hybridization or creolization.

Emerging work in cognitive science views culture in terms of embodied and enacted ways of engaging particular social niches that present individuals with social and cultural affordances, which are available and accessible possibilities for action (Kirmayer and Ramstead 2017). A growing body of work explores how the brain and the social environment interact across development (Kirmayer et al. 2020). Despite increasing recognition of the importance of culture in shaping mental disorders, most psychiatric research and practice continues to employ outmoded concepts of culture. Cross-national studies tend to use geographic location as a proxy for culture, ignoring local cultural diversity. In the United States, most studies refer to ethnoracial blocs (African American, Asian American, Native American, Latino, white), which are heterogeneous categories constructed by the census. Epidemiological research tends to use these population-level categories, while specialized clinical texts offer chapters on specific ethnocultural groups with case examples or generalizations that may inadvertently lead to stereotypes. In this chapter, we aim to move beyond these static, essentializing notions of culture to consider more dynamic views that can inform research and clinical practice.

The Problem of Cross-Cultural Equivalence

Studying any psychiatric disorder across cultures presupposes that we can accurately identify or measure the same construct across different social and cultural contexts. This is not simply a technical problem of establishing psychometric equivalence, for which there are established methods (Kirmayer and Ban 2013), but is also a conceptual problem that involves translating vocabularies, experiences, and expressions of distress and establishing that they have similar clinical and pathological significance across cultures. Thus, it may be possible to identify people who fit conventional psychiatric criteria for depression in diverse settings, but this may not be the best or only way to understand and describe their problem, and unknown numbers of people may exist who have related forms of distress but whose symptoms do not fit the conventional categories and criteria of mood disorders (Kendler et al. 2018). Kleinman (1977) termed this potentially misleading application of categories across different cultural contexts "the category fallacy."

One way to avoid the category fallacy is to step back from the received categories of psychiatric nosology and conduct ethnographic research on local ways of expressing distress. This type of research can uncover idioms of distress that include local cultural models and metaphors for distress that emerge from the interaction of biology and culture-specific understandings of affliction (Lewis-Fernández and Kirmayer 2019). Such work may identify symptoms and behaviors that are culturally salient and can be investigated alongside the established symptoms of depression. Standard diagnostic instruments can be employed to provide an anchor point for comparison, but they need to be supplemented with an expanded symptom pool based on ethnographic research. This strategy generates clinical and epidemiological data that may confirm the validity of existing categories and criteria or suggest alternative ways of categorizing distress that have greater utility in predicting treatment response and outcome.

Several efforts have been made to develop culturally sensitive measures of depression and related forms of demoralization or emotional distress (see Table 43–1). Most of these are self-report scales that tap nonspecific dimensions of depression, anxiety, and common somatic symptoms of distress. For example, Abas et al. (1998) developed the Caribbean Culture–Specific Screening questionnaire for emotional distress, incorporating common expressions for dysphoria and depression among older African-Caribbean adults (e.g., "Have you felt pressured, like pressure is rising in your head? Have you had lots of pain or gas in the belly or the pit of your stomach? Have you been feeling empty or spiritless inside?"). A validation study comparing the screening measure with standard and culturally adapted diagnostic interviews found that the culture-specific measure did not perform any better than the standard Geriatric Depression Scale (GDS) in identifying clinical depression (Sheikh and Yesavage 1986); the authors noted that the sensitivity and overall performance of the GDS could be improved by lowering its cutoff. Thus, it appeared that African-Caribbean

TABLE 43–1. Examples of culture-specific measures of depression and related forms of distress

Scale	Target population (languages)	Characteristics
Vietnamese Depression Scale (Kinzie et al. 1982)	Vietnamese (in U.S.)	15-item scale derived from a clinical sample
Four Measures of Mental Health (Beiser and Fleming 1986)	Vietnamese (in Canada)	15-item depression scale
Indochinese Hopkins Symptom Checklist (HSCL)–25 (Mollica et al. 1987)	Cambodian, Laotian, Vietnamese	25 items from the HSCL-58
Phan Vietnamese Psychiatric Scale (Phan et al. 2004)	Vietnamese (in Australia)	26-item depression subscale (also anxiety and somatization scales), good psychometrics
Amritsar Depression Inventory (Singh et al. 1974)	Punjabi-speaking patients in India	30-item depression scale
Bradford Somatic Inventory (Mumford et al. 1981)	Pakistani, Urdu	44-item scale of common somatic symptoms developed simultaneously in Pakistan and the United Kingdom
Enugu Somatization Scale (Ebigbo 1982, 1986)	Nigeria	65-item somatic symptom inventory
Shona Symptom Questionnaire (Patel et al. 1997)	Shona-speaking primary care users in Zimbabwe	14-item common mental disorder scale
Self-Reporting Questionnaire (SRQ-20) (Fischer et al. 2019)	Rufumbira-speaking women from rural Uganda ages 18–35 years	20-item "Yes or No" screening questionnaire for common mental disorders in community settings modified for use in Sub-Saharan Africa
Caribbean Culture-Specific Screen (Abas et al. 1998)	Older (>60 years) African-Caribbean primary care users in South London	13-item depression scale
International Depression Symptom Scale–General version (IDSS-G) (Haroz et al. 2017a)	Nonpsychotic clinic patients older than 18 years of age from Yangon, Myanmar	29-item self-report instrument derived from symptoms common to multiple geographical regions and cultural settings
Indonesian Depression Checklist (IDC) (Widiana et al. 2018)	Indonesians (Yogyakarta, Java)	19 items in five clusters: physical symptoms, affect, cognition, social engagement, religiosity

patients might be significantly depressed even when they report only a small number of symptoms of depression.

Notwithstanding these attempts at developing culture-specific measures of distress, most epidemiological research on depression has used only standard instruments constructed for and validated in Euro-American and European populations. Moreover, studies published to date do not consider the internal cultural variation of countries and hence cannot determine the significance of cultural variables for the prevalence, course, or outcome of mood disorders. Some researchers have drawn attention to the fact that most studies lack rigor and are of poor quality and therefore may produce misleading findings (Kohrt et al. 2014). Future research will depend on culturally validated measures and, most importantly, on unpacking the meaning of cultural variation within and across countries in terms of social, psychological, and biological processes that interact in the cause and course of depression.

The Cultural Epidemiology of Depression

International research over the past several decades has found that depression can be identified in all countries, regions, and cultures that have been studied (Kessler and Bromet 2013; Sartorius et al. 1980; Weissman et al. 1996). Even with standard epidemiological methods, depression can be found around the world (World Health Organization 1983) and has an especially high prevalence in some low-income countries (Desjarlais et al. 1995; Fischer et al. 2019; Orley and Wing 1979; Vorcaro et al. 2001). Despite this apparent universality, wide variations in prevalence, symptomatology, and clinical presentation are evident (Kleinman and Good 1985), and social factors, such as income inequality, have been linked to a higher prevalence of major depressive episodes (Cifuentes et al. 2008).

The World Health Organization (WHO) Collaborative Study on the Assessment of Depressive Disorders compared patients seeking help for depressive symptoms at clinics in cities from four countries (Canada, Switzerland, Iran, and Japan) using a standardized interview instrument (Sartorius et al. 1980). The most common symptoms across sites were sadness, joylessness, anxiety, tension, and lack of energy (Jablensky et al. 1981). Other common symptoms included loss of interest, loss of ability to concentrate, and ideas of oneself as insufficient, inadequate, and worthless. Feelings of guilt and self-reproach varied in frequency across sites: 68% in Basle, 58% in Montreal, 48% in Tokyo, 41% in Nagasaki, and 32% in Tehran. Suicidal ideation also varied substantially, ranging from 70% in Montreal and Nagasaki to 41% in Tokyo. Somatic symptoms (e.g., vegetative symptoms of anorexia, weight loss, loss of libido, and constipation) were most common in Tehran (57%) and least frequent in Montreal (27%).

The WHO Cross-National Study of Mental Disorders in Primary Care studied clinical samples at 15 centers in 14 countries. In a two-stage design, 25,916 primary care patients were screened with the 12-item General Health Questionnaire, and the diagnosis of depression was made with the Composite International Diagnostic Interview (CIDI; Ustün and Sartorius 1995). As summarized in Table 43–2, the prevalence of major depressive disorder varied 11-fold across centers. There was a similar pattern of symptom covariation and threshold behavior across sites (Simon et al. 2002). However, at the higher-prevalence centers, depression was associated with lower levels of

TABLE 43–2. **World Health Organization Cross-National Study of Mental Disorders in Primary Care: Prevalence of Major Depressive Disorder**

Country (center)	Point prevalence rate (%)	Female	Male	Gender ratio, F:M
Brazil (Rio de Janeiro)	15.8	19.6	5.8	3.4
Chile (Santiago)	29.5	36.8	11.2	3.3
China (Shanghai)	4.0	4.4	3.3	1.3
France (Paris)	13.7	18.7	9.3	2.0
Germany (Berlin)	6.1	7.7	3.7	2.1
Germany (Mainz)	11.2	12.3	9.8	1.3
Greece (Athens)	6.4	6.4	6.5	1.0
India (Bangalore)	9.1	13.3	4.8	2.8
Italy (Verona)	4.7	5.5	3.2	1.7
Japan (Nagasaki)	2.6	2.8	2.3	1.2
Netherlands (Groningen)	15.9	17.9	13.0	1.4
Nigeria (Ibadan)	4.2	3.8	5.3	0.7
Turkey (Ankara)	11.6	12.5	9.8	1.3
USA (Seattle)	6.3	6.5	6.0	1.1
UK (Manchester)	16.9	18.3	13.9	1.3

Source. Data adapted from Ustün and Sartorius 1995.

disability, suggesting that people with milder cases were seeking help. This may account for some of the variation in prevalence across clinical sites. This study illustrates how identical measures and diagnostic criteria may, in fact, identify different levels of depression severity in different countries or cultures.

In Table 43–3, cross-national comparisons of the community prevalence of affective disorders have been made possible by data from surveys using the Diagnostic Interview Schedule (DIS) (Robins et al. 1985) in the United States, Canada, Puerto Rico, West Germany, Taiwan, Korea, and New Zealand (Weissman et al. 1996). The annual prevalence of depression varied widely, from less than 1% in Taiwan to almost 6% in Christchurch, New Zealand. Lifetime prevalence varied from 1.5% in Taiwan to 11.6% in Christchurch, 12.4% in Florence, 16.4% in Paris, and 19% in Beirut. The exceptionally low rates in Taiwan remain unexplained but may reflect both underreporting of distress and positive effects of social support and family function. Lifetime rates of bipolar disorder showed much less variability (from 0.3% to 1.5%) but were also consistently lower in Asian countries.

Cross-national comparison with the DIS found that the most common symptoms of depression (reported by ≥60% of individuals with major depressive disorder) were insomnia, loss of energy, thoughts of death, suicidal ideation, and concentration problems (Weissman et al. 1996). Feelings of worthlessness were less common in Puerto Rico, Beirut, and Taiwan. Poor appetite was common only in Beirut, Taiwan, and Korea.

Data from comparative studies using the CIDI (Wittchen et al. 1991) confirmed the wide variation found in earlier studies. The International Consortium for Psychiatric

TABLE 43–3. Cross-national comparative community studies of depression

Sites	Lifetime prevalence rates, %	Annual prevalence rates, %	Gender ratio, F:M
Cross-national comparison with Diagnostic Interview Schedule (Weissman et al. 1996)			
Canada (Edmonton)	9.6	5.2	1.9
France (Paris)	16.4	4.5	2.1
Italy (Florence)	12.4	—	2.0
Korea	2.9	2.3	1.6
Lebanon (Beirut)	19.0	—	1.6
New Zealand (Christchurch)	11.6	5.8	2.1
Puerto Rico	4.3	3.0	1.8
Taiwan	1.5	0.8	1.6
United States	5.2	3.0	2.6
West Germany	9.2	5.0	3.1
International Consortium in Psychiatric Epidemiology Study with Composite International Diagnostic Interview (Andrade et al. 2003)			
Brazil	12.6	5.8	2.1
Canada	8.3	4.3	2.0
Chile	9.0	5.6	2.1
Czech Republic	7.8	2.0	1.2
Germany	11.5	5.2	2.3
Japan	3.0	1.2	2.5
Mexico	8.1	4.5	1.9
Netherlands	15.7	5.9	1.9
Turkey	6.3	3.5	2.3
United States	16.9	10.0	2.0
World Mental Health Survey with Composite International Diagnostic Interview—selected countries (Bromet et al. 2011; Kessler and Bromet 2013)			
France	21.0	5.9	1.7
Israel	10.2	6.1	1.6
Japan	6.6	2.2	2.3
United States	19.2	8.3	1.7
Brazil	18.4	10.4	2.6
India	9.0	4.5	1.9
China	6.5	3.8	1.2
South Africa	9.8	4.9	2.2

Epidemiology compared data from community surveys in 10 different countries (Andrade et al. 2003). As shown in Table 43–3, lifetime rates of depression indicated great variability, with Asian countries showing the lowest rates, as in the earlier consortium study (from 3.0% in Japan to 16.9% in the United States). In all countries, women had higher rates than men, and the sex ratio varied only slightly. Comparison of the prevalence ratios of 12-month to lifetime and 30-day to 12-month also suggests differences in the course of depression across countries. Data from the WHO World Mental Health (WMH) Survey essentially confirmed many of these findings 10 years later (Bromet et al. 2011). Of note, the data for Nigeria were excluded from the WMH Survey due to an extremely low prevalence of depression, raising the question of the applicability of the CIDI in some settings.

Although these are some of the best data available for cross-national comparisons, many methodological problems remain (Ferrari et al. 2013). The probe flow sheet of the CIDI, designed to establish the clinical significance of depressive symptoms, relies on a series of criteria for severity that includes medical help-seeking, use of medication, and interference with daily activities. Variations in context may render these probes insensitive and result in biased estimates of prevalence (Hicks 2002; Van Ommeren et al. 2000). Of course, diagnostic interviews only canvas symptoms already identified as criteria of depression. Although Simon et al. (2002) claimed that their item response analysis of the CIDI shows that large cross-national variations in depression cannot be attributed to a category fallacy, in fact, the lack of locally developed measures means that existing studies cannot resolve basic questions, including the following: 1) Is there undetected morbidity in the community or in the clinic that is not captured by the current measures of depression but is related to it in some way (e.g., by similar mechanisms, symptomatic networks or overlap, or other features)? 2) Can people with mild to moderate depression identified by the CIDI be better understood and treated in terms of different local or indigenous categories?

Broad comparisons across countries also do not address the important issue of variations across ethnocultural groups within each region. For example, in the United States, major depressive disorder and suicide have been found to be significantly less common among African Americans than among other groups; however, these differences may in part reflect the impact of stereotypes and different modes of expressing distress that influence diagnostic practices (Barnes et al. 2013; Jarvis 2012; Kessler et al. 2003; Schwartz et al. 2019; Zhang and Snowden 1999). Rates also may vary across specific subpopulations; for example, mood disorders may be more prevalent among Caribbean immigrants to the United States (Williams et al. 2007). In the United States, rates of depression among Euro-Americans may be increasing more quickly than rates in some minorities (Weinberger et al. 2018). Depression is less prevalent among Mexican immigrants with indigenous Indian heritage but increases with acculturation to approximate that of the general population (Alderete et al. 2000; Vega et al. 1998). The reasons for these variations are poorly understood but do not appear to be purely methodological artifacts and may be related to cultural differences in values and identity, as well as family and social support. Studies in the United Kingdom have found that South Asian (i.e., Indian and Pakistani) immigrants had lower rates of depression than the general U.K. population (Bhui 1999). However, ethnographic studies find significant levels of distress, suggesting underrecognition of distress in research measures or some form of sampling bias. Surveys in Pakistan using culturally adapted instruments have found high levels of depression (Mumford et al. 1997). Of course, the prevalence of any disorder in immigrant populations need not reflect that of their country of origin, since migration itself involves many selection biases. However, a study in the United Kingdom that used a culturally adapted measure found higher levels of depression among Punjabi immigrants, particularly women, compared with their white U.K. counterparts (Bhui et al. 2004). This underscores the need for culturally adapted measures that are sensitive to expressions of distress that may otherwise be unreported or unrecognized.

Cultural Constructions of Affect and Depression

Although there are cross-cultural universals of affective meaning (Osgood et al. 1975), these rudimentary feelings may reflect the evolutionarily adaptive capacity to rapidly evaluate events as potentially helpful or harmful (Barrett et al. 2007). The everyday experience of emotion involves a process of interpretation and categorization that is guided by embodied knowledge and social context (Barrett 2006). Hence, over the course of development, the so-called basic emotions are built into more complex feelings or sentiments that refer to social situations with specific antecedents and consequences (Lebois et al. 2020). Emotion terms thus reference bodily states, behaviors, feelings, and social situations (Shweder and Haidt 2000). Through the course of development, even the simplest bodily experiences are imbued with specific cultural meanings (Kirmayer 1992). Emotions then can be understood as metaphoric elaborations of bodily feelings and social events, framed in terms of cognitive schemas, scripts, or scenarios, and as discursive or rhetorical practices that contribute to the cultural construction of the person and the social world (Atzil and Barrett 2017; Barrett 2017; White 2000).

The etymology of emotion terms in each language reflects a cultural history that centers on prototypical social situations (White 2000). Like other concepts, emotions are based on metaphors with both universal and culture-specific connotations (Hoemann et al. 2019; Kövecses 2003; Lakoff 1987). The emotional lexicon therefore encodes the socially and morally significant values of a cultural community (Levy 1978; Lutz 1988; Rosaldo 1980; Shweder and Haidt 2000).

Like emotions, the concept and experience of depression—whether as a feeling, an idiom of distress, a syndrome, or diagnostic construct—is deeply rooted in cultural narratives, models, and metaphors (Kirmayer et al. 2017). Jackson (1996) traced the history of the emergence of the modern concept of depression. The English term *acedia*, derived from the Latin *accidia*, meaning "heedlessness or torpor," was used to describe a condition common in medieval monks, characterized by "exhaustion, listlessness, sadness or dejection, restlessness, aversion to the cell and the ascetic life, and yearning for family and former life" (Jackson 1996, p. 66). The term *melancholia* (from the Latin for black bile) was invoked in humoral theories of temperament and affliction, but by the 1600s came to have positive connotations as an affliction of those with superior intelligence, sensitivity, and refinement (Radden 2000). The term *depression*, which only supplanted *melancholia* in the twentieth century, derives from the verb "to depress" (Latin *de primere,* "to press down"). In the fourteenth century, "to depress" had the meaning "to subjugate," and by the fifteenth century it also meant "to bring down in vigor or spirits" (Onions 1966).

Although *depression* is now readily used in English as a metaphor for everyday fluctuations in mood, as an everyday idiom of distress, and as the diagnostic label for a clinical disorder, the term has not had the same fate in other societies. A review of common cultural concepts of distress found only partial overlap with depression (Kohrt et al. 2014). Another review of qualitative research on cultural variations in de-

but also will uncover cultural resources that can complement and, at times, supplant conventional psychiatric treatment (Kirmayer et al. 2003).

The clinician's ability to understand local idioms of distress is crucial both for accurate diagnosis and to develop the communication necessary for a therapeutic alliance. At the same time, cultural idioms of distress provide a way for patients to safely initiate a therapeutic conversation. To understand this conversation, the clinician must think not only in terms of disorders but also in terms of life predicaments. Feelings of depression and despair may come from universally recognized losses or conflicts and from the failure to achieve or maintain deeply held cultural values.

Future work on culture in depression must advance on multiple fronts. Quantitative research on depression, especially randomized clinical trials, continues to exclude ethnic minority and low-income groups from participation in studies and when evaluating treatment effects (Polo et al. 2020). These oversights require immediate attention by the research community. In addition, careful qualitative and ethnographic research on illness experience and the social context of depression is needed to design culturally valid larger-scale longitudinal studies of course and outcome (Alarcón et al. 2002). Such studies must consider alternative configurations of distress that reflect indigenous categories to determine if these are better predictors of social course and treatment outcome. At the same time, study of indigenous forms of coping with loss, failure, and demoralization may identify new strategies for therapeutic intervention that can be supported locally and adapted for use in other cultural contexts. Ultimately, researchers need to revisit the construct of depression itself as it is enshrined in psychiatric nosology in order to facilitate the study of local cultural variations of dysphoria and distress. Although this is a challenging undertaking, it may yield better understanding of the meaning of patients' symptoms in context and allow clinicians to address potential Western cultural biases and the risk of medicalizing social suffering (Kirmayer et al. 2017).

Clinicians must engage in ongoing dialogue with patients that acknowledges and works with cultural difference rather than assuming that ethnic matching finesses the issues. There is much to be learned from the models of service developed in different countries (Kirmayer and Minas 2000). In situations with high levels of diversity, a model of cultural consultation that employs multilingual, multicultural clinicians and culture brokers may be a useful supplement to routine care and improve clinicians' cultural competence (Kirmayer et al. 2003).

Psychiatry has had a complex and complicit relationship with the pharmaceutical industry that has undermined professional autonomy (Cristea et al. 2017). New standards in research, publishing, and the regulation of the profession aim to ensure that the evidence on which clinical practice is based is not biased by commercial interests and that clinicians are able to choose from a wide array of interventions based on their demonstrated efficacy and cost-effectiveness (Cosgrove and Vaswani 2019).

Social marketing and media campaigns, as well as the poignant testimonials of writers, artists, and figures of popular culture, can do much to reduce the stigma attached to depression. At the same time, it is important to look at the causes and contexts of depression more critically. Distress may serve as a barometer of wider social problems attached to certain features of modernity, particularly consumerism, that need to be named and confronted, even as clinicians strive to help the afflicted person before them. The profound challenges associated with climate change are likely to be major drivers of mental health problems including depression in the years to come (Evans 2019; Majeed and Lee 2017; Obradovich et al. 2018).

References

Abas MA, Broadhead JC: Depression and anxiety among women in an urban setting in Zimbabwe. Psychol Med 27(1):59–71, 1997 9122309

Abas MA, Phillips C, Carter J, et al: Culturally sensitive validation of screening questionnaires for depression in older African-Caribbean people living in south London. Br J Psychiatry 173:249–254, 1998 9926102

Adeponle A, Groleau D, Kola L, et al: Perinatal depression in Nigeria: perspectives of women, family caregivers and health care providers. Int J Ment Health Syst 11(1):27, 2017 28428813

Ahmad F, Maule C, Wang J, Fung WLA: Symptoms and experience of depression among Chinese communities in the West: a scoping review. Harv Rev Psychiatry 26(6):340–351, 2018 30407233

Alarcón RD, Bell CC, Kirmayer LJ, et al: Beyond the funhouse mirrors: research agenda on culture and psychiatric diagnosis, in A Research Agenda for DSM-V. Edited by Kupfer DJ, First MB, Regier DA. Washington, American Psychiatric Press, 2002, pp 219–289

Alderete E, Vega WA, Kolody B, et al: Effects of time in the United States and Indian ethnicity on DSM-III-R psychiatric disorders among Mexican Americans in California. J Nerv Ment Dis 188(2):90–100, 2000 10695837

Alegría M, Chatterji P, Wells K, et al: Disparity in depression treatment among racial and ethnic minority populations in the United States. Psychiatr Serv 59(11):1264–1272, 2008 18971402

Allan BA, Campos ID, Wimberley TE: Interpersonal psychotherapy: a review and multicultural critique. Couns Psychol Q 29(3):253–273, 2016

American Psychiatric Association: Diagnostic and Statistical Manual of Mental Disorders, 5th Edition. Arlington, American Psychiatric Association, 2013

Andrade L, Caraveo-Anduaga JJ, Berglund P, et al: The epidemiology of major depressive episodes: results from the International Consortium of Psychiatric Epidemiology (ICPE) surveys. Int J Methods Psychiatr Res 12(1):3–21, 2003 12830306

Anonymous: Spirit of the age: malignant sadness is the world's great hidden burden. The Economist, December 19, 1998, pp 115–123

Antoniades J, Mazza D, Brijnath B: Efficacy of depression treatments for immigrant patients: results from a systematic review. BMC Psychiatry 14(1):176, 2014 24930429

Araya R, Lewis GH, Rojas G, et al: "Patient knows best"—detection of common mental disorders in Santiago, Chile: cross sectional study. BMJ 322(7278):79–81, 2001 11154620

Araya R, Rojas G, Fritsch R, et al: Treating depression in primary care in low-income women in Santiago, Chile: a randomised controlled trial. Lancet 361(9362):995–1000, 2003 12660056

Asendorpf JB, Ostendorf F: Is self-enhancement healthy? Conceptual, psychometric, and empirical analysis. J Pers Soc Psychol 74(4):955–966, 1998 9569653

Atzil S, Barrett LF: Social regulation of allostasis: commentary on "Mentalizing Homeostasis: The Social Origins of Interoceptive Inference" by Fotopoulou and Tsakiris. Neuropsychoanalysis 19(1):29–33, 2017

Barnes DM, Keyes KM, Bates LM: Racial differences in depression in the United States: how do subgroup analyses inform a paradox? Soc Psychiatry Psychiatr Epidemiol 48(12):1941–1949, 2013 23732705

Barrett LF: Solving the emotion paradox: categorization and the experience of emotion. Pers Soc Psychol Rev 10(1):20–46, 2006 16430327

Barrett LF: The theory of constructed emotion: an active inference account of interoception and categorization. Soc Cogn Affect Neurosci 12(1):1–23, 2017 27798257

Barrett LF, Mesquita B, Ochsner KN, et al: The experience of emotion. Annu Rev Psychol 58:373–403, 2007 17002554

Bass J, Neugebauer R, Clougherty KF, et al: Group interpersonal psychotherapy for depression in rural Uganda: 6-month outcomes: randomised controlled trial. Br J Psychiatry 188(6):567–573, 2006 16738348

Bauman Z: Globalization: The Human Consequences. New York, Columbia University Press, 1998

Beiser M: A study of depression among traditional Africans, urban North Americans, and Southeast Asian refugees, in Culture and Depression. Edited by Kleinman A, Good B. Berkeley, CA, University of California Press, 1985, pp 272–298

Beiser M: Strangers at the Gate: The "Boat People's" First Ten Years in Canada. Toronto, ON, University of Toronto Press, 1999

Beiser M, Fleming JAE: Measuring psychiatric disorder among Southeast Asian refugees. Psychol Med 16(3):627–639, 1986 3763777

Bhugra D, Mastrogianni A: Globalisation and mental disorders. Overview with relation to depression. Br J Psychiatry 184:10–20, 2004 14702222

Bhui K: Common mental disorders among people with origins in or immigrant from India and Pakistan. Int Rev Psychiatry 11:136–144, 1999

Bhui K, Bhugra D, Goldberg D, et al: Assessing the prevalence of depression in Punjabi and English primary care attenders: the role of culture, physical illness and somatic symptoms. Transcult Psychiatry 41(3):307–322, 2004 15551723

Bolton P, Haroz EE: Experience versus diagnosis as the appropriate basis for assessment of depression: a reply to the commentary from Kirmayer et al. (2017). Soc Sci Med 232:432–433, 2019 29329943

Bolton P, Bass J, Neugebauer R, et al: Group interpersonal psychotherapy for depression in rural Uganda: a randomized controlled trial. JAMA 289(23):3117–3124, 2003 12813117

Borsboom D: A network theory of mental disorders. World Psychiatry 16(1):5–13, 2017 28127906

Borsboom D, Cramer AO: Network analysis: an integrative approach to the structure of psychopathology. Annu Rev Clin Psychol 9:91–121, 2013 23537483

Bracken P, Thomas P, Timimi S, et al: Psychiatry beyond the current paradigm. Br J Psychiatry 201(6):430–434, 2012 23209088

Bröer C, Besseling B: Sadness or depression: making sense of low mood and the medicalization of everyday life. Soc Sci Med 183:28–36, 2017 28458072

Bromet E, Andrade LH, Hwang I, et al: Cross-national epidemiology of DSM-IV major depressive episode. BMC Med 9:90, 2011 21791035

Chen Y, Bennett D, Clarke R, et al: Patterns and correlates of major depression in Chinese adults: a cross-sectional study of 0.5 million men and women. Psychol Med 47(5):958–970, 2017 27919307

Chentsova-Dutton YE, Ryder AG: Cultural models of normalcy and deviancy. Asian J Soc Psychol 23(2):187–204, 2020

Chowdhary N, Jotheeswaran AT, Nadkarni A, et al: The methods and outcomes of cultural adaptations of psychological treatments for depressive disorders: a systematic review. Psychol Med 44(6):1131–1146, 2014 23866176

Cifuentes M, Sembajwe G, Tak S, et al: The association of major depressive episodes with income inequality and the human development index. Soc Sci Med 67(4):529–539, 2008 18524442

Cooper S: Global mental health and its critics: moving beyond the impasse. Crit Public Health 26(4):355–358, 2016

Cosgrove L, Vaswani A: The influence of pharmaceutical companies and restoring integrity to psychiatric research and practice, in Critical Psychiatry: Controversies and Clinical Implications. Edited by Steingard S. New York, Springer, 2019, pp 71–96

Cristea IA, Gentili C, Pietrini P, et al: Sponsorship bias in the comparative efficacy of psychotherapy and pharmacotherapy for adult depression: meta-analysis. Br J Psychiatry 210(1):16–23, 2017 27810891

Cross S, Bhugra D: Management and culture—psychopharmacology. Psychiatry 8(9):365–367, 2009

Cross-National Collaborative Group: The changing rate of major depression. Cross-national comparisons. JAMA 268(21):3098–3105, 1992 1433741
Desjarlais RR: Presence, in The Performance of Healing. Edited by Laderman C, Roseman M. New York, Routledge, 1996, pp 143–164
Desjarlais R, Eisenberg L, Good B, et al: World Mental Health: Problems and Priorities in Low-Income Countries. New York, Oxford University Press, 1995
De Vaus J, Hornsey MJ, Kuppens P, et al: Exploring the East-West divide in prevalence of affective disorder: a case for cultural differences in coping with negative emotion. Pers Soc Psychol Rev 22(3):285–304, 2018 29034806
Dressler WW, Balieiro MC, dos Santos JE: Agency, cultural consonance and depressive symptoms: a Brazilian example. Ethos 47(2):148–167, 2019
Ebigbo PO: Development of a culture specific (Nigeria) screening scale of somatic complaints indicating psychiatric disturbance. Cult Med Psychiatry 6(1):29–43, 1982 7105787
Ebigbo PO: A cross sectional study of somatic complaints of Nigerian females using the Enugu Somatization Scale. Cult Med Psychiatry 10(2):167–186, 1986 3487415
Ehrenberg A: La Fatigue d'Etre Soi. Dépression et société [The Fatigue of Being Oneself: Depression and Society]. Paris, Éditions Odile Jacob, 1998
Ehrenberg A: The Weariness of the Self: Diagnosing the History of Depression in the Contemporary Age. Kingston, ON, McGill-Queen's Press, 2016
Eisenbruch M: "Wind illness" or somatic depression? A case study in psychiatric anthropology. Br J Psychiatry 143:323–326, 1983 6626850
Escobar JI, Gomez J, Tuason VB: Depressive phenomenology in North and South American patients. Am J Psychiatry 140(1):47–51, 1983 6847984
Evans GW: Projected behavioral impacts of global climate change. Annu Rev Psychol 70:449–474, 2019 29975596
Ferrari AJ, Somerville AJ, Baxter AJ, et al: Global variation in the prevalence and incidence of major depressive disorder: a systematic review of the epidemiological literature. Psychol Med 43(3):471–481, 2013 22831756
Fischer M, Ramaswamy R, Fischer-Flores L, et al: Measuring and understanding depression in women in Kisoro, Uganda. Cult Med Psychiatry 43(1):160–180, 2019 30105653
Ford BQ, Dmitrieva JO, Heller D, et al: Culture shapes whether the pursuit of happiness predicts higher or lower well-being. J Exp Psychol Gen 144(6):1053–1062, 2015 26347945
Fuchs C, Lee JK, Roemer L, Orsillo SM: Using mindfulness- and acceptance-based treatments with clients from nondominant cultural and/or marginalized backgrounds: clinical considerations, meta-analysis findings, and introduction to the special series. Cognit Behav Pract 20(1):1–12, 2013
García-Campayo J, Lobo A, Pérez-Echeverría MJ, et al: Three forms of somatization presenting in primary care settings in Spain. J Nerv Ment Dis 186(9):554–560, 1998 9741561
GBD 2017 DALYs and HALE Collaborators: Global, regional, and national disability-adjusted life-years (DALYs) for 359 diseases and injuries and healthy life expectancy (HALE) for 195 countries and territories, 1990–2017: a systematic analysis for the Global Burden of Disease Study 2017. Lancet 392(10159):1859–1922, 2018 30415748
Good BJ, Good MJD, Moradi R: The interpretation of Iranian depressive illness and dysphoric affect, in Culture and Depression. Edited by Kleinman A, Good B. Berkeley, CA, University of California Press, 1985, pp 369–428
Groleau D, Kirmayer LJ: Sociosomatic theory in Vietnamese immigrants' narratives of distress. Anthropol Med 11(2):117–133, 2004 26868197
Grote NK, Swartz HA, Geibel SL, et al: A randomized controlled trial of culturally relevant, brief interpersonal psychotherapy for perinatal depression. Psychiatr Serv 60(3):313–321, 2009 19252043
Guinness EA: Brief reactive psychosis and the major functional psychoses: descriptive case studies in Africa. Br J Psychiatry 160 (suppl 16):24–41, 1992 1389028
Gupta R, Singh P, Verma S, Garg D: Standardized Assessment of Depressive Disorders: a replicated study from northern India. Acta Psychiatr Scand 84(4):310–312, 1991 1746278

Gureje O, Nortje G, Makanjuola V, et al: The role of global traditional and complementary systems of medicine in the treatment of mental health disorders. Lancet Psychiatry 2(2):168–177, 2015 26359753

Hacking I: The Social Construction of What? Cambridge, MA, Harvard University Press, 1999

Hall GCN, Ibaraki AY, Huang ER, et al: A meta-analysis of cultural adaptations of psychological interventions. Behav Ther 47(6):993–1014, 2016 27993346

Hari J: Lost Connections: Uncovering the Real Causes of Depression—and the Unexpected Solutions. New York, Bloomsbury, 2019

Haroz EE, Bass J, Lee C, et al: Development and cross-cultural testing of the International Depression Symptom Scale (IDSS): a measurement instrument designed to represent global presentations of depression. Glob Ment Health (Camb) 4:e17, 2017a 29230313

Haroz EE, Ritchey M, Bass JK, et al: How is depression experienced around the world? A systematic review of qualitative literature. Soc Sci Med 183:151–162, 2017b 28069271

Harper Shehadeh M, Heim E, Chowdhary N, et al: Cultural adaptation of minimally guided interventions for common mental disorders: a systematic review and meta-analysis. JMIR Ment Health 3(3):e44, 2016 27670598

Heim E, Wegmann I, Maercker A: Cultural values and the prevalence of mental disorders in 25 countries: a secondary data analysis. Soc Sci Med 189:96–104, 2017 28793240

Heine SJ, Lehman DR, Markus HR, et al: Is there a universal need for positive self-regard? Psychol Rev 106(4):766–794, 1999 10560328

Heine SJ, Lehman DR, Ide E, et al: Divergent consequences of success and failure in Japan and North America: an investigation of self-improving motivations and malleable selves. J Pers Soc Psychol 81(4):599–615, 2001 11642348

Heinrich LM, Gullone E: The clinical significance of loneliness: a literature review. Clin Psychol Rev 26(6):695–718, 2006 16952717

Hicks MH-R: Validity of the CIDI probe flow chart for depression in Chinese American women. Transcult Psychiatry 39(4):434–451, 2002

Hoemann K, Xu F, Barrett LF: Emotion words, emotion concepts, and emotional development in children: a constructionist hypothesis. Dev Psychol 55(9):1830–1849, 2019 31464489

Hofmann SG, Sawyer AT, Witt AA, et al: The effect of mindfulness-based therapy on anxiety and depression: a meta-analytic review. J Consult Clin Psychol 78(2):169–183, 2010 20350028

Hsu FLK: Psychosocial homeostasis and jen: conceptual tools for advancing psychological anthropology. Am Anthropol 173:23–44, 1971

Ifabumuyi OI: The dynamics of central heat in depression. Psychopathologie Africaine 17:127–133, 1981

Jablensky A, Sartorius N, Gulbinat W, et al: Characteristics of depressive patients contacting psychiatric services in four cultures. A report from the WHO Collaborative Study on the Assessment of Depressive Disorders. Acta Psychiatr Scand 63(4):367–383, 1981 7315484

Jackson S: Melancholia and Depression: From Hippocratic to Modern Times. New Haven, CT, Yale University Press, 1996

Jacob KS, Kuruvilla A: Psychotherapy across cultures: the form-content dichotomy. Clin Psychol Psychother 19(1):91–95, 2012 22232048

Jarvis GE: Changing psychiatric perception of African-Americans with affective disorders. J Nerv Ment Dis 200(12):1031–1040, 2012 23197118

Jenkins JH, Cofresi N: The sociosomatic course of depression and trauma: a cultural analysis of suffering and resilience in the life of a Puerto Rican woman [see comment]. Psychosom Med 60(4):439–447, 1998 9710289

Joiner T, Coyne JC (eds): The Interactional Nature of Depression. Washington, DC, American Psychological Association, 1999

Kalibatseva Z, Leong FT: A critical review of culturally sensitive treatments for depression: recommendations for intervention and research. Psychol Serv 11(4):433–450, 2014 25383996

Kasser T: The High Price of Materialism. Cambridge, MA, MIT Press, 2002

Katz MM: Evaluating drug and other therapies across cultures, in Cross-Cultural Counseling and Psychotherapy. Edited by Marsella A, Pedersen P. New York, Pergamon, 1981

Kendler KS, Aggen SH, Flint J, et al: The centrality of DSM and non-DSM depressive symptoms in Han Chinese women with major depression. J Affect Disord 227:739–744, 2018 29179144
Kessler RC, Bromet EJ: The epidemiology of depression across cultures. Annu Rev Public Health 34:119–138, 2013 23514317
Kessler RC, Berglund P, Demler O, et al: The epidemiology of major depressive disorder: results from the National Comorbidity Survey Replication (NCS-R). JAMA 289(23):3095–3105, 2003 12813115
Khoury B, Lecomte T, Fortin G, et al: Mindfulness-based therapy: a comprehensive meta-analysis. Clin Psychol Rev 33(6):763–771, 2013 23796855
Khoury B, Knäuper B, Schlosser M, et al: Effectiveness of traditional meditation retreats: a systematic review and meta-analysis. J Psychosom Res 92:16–25, 2017 27998508
Kinzie JD, Manson SM, Vinh DT, et al: Development and validation of a Vietnamese-language depression rating scale. Am J Psychiatry 139(10):1276–1281, 1982 7124979
Kinzie JD, Leung P, Boehnlein JK, et al: Antidepressant blood levels in Southeast Asians. Clinical and cultural implications. J Nerv Ment Dis 175(8):480–485, 1987 3625187
Kirmayer LJ: Cultural variations in the response to psychiatric disorders and emotional distress. Soc Sci Med 29(3):327–339, 1989 2669146
Kirmayer LJ: The body's insistence on meaning: metaphor as presentation and representation in illness experience. Med Anthropol Q 6(4):323–346, 1992
Kirmayer LJ: Psychopharmacology in a globalizing world: the use of antidepressants in Japan. Transcult Psychiatry 39(3):295–312, 2002
Kirmayer LJ: The cultural diversity of healing: meaning, metaphor and mechanism. Br Med Bull 69:33–48, 2004 15226195
Kirmayer LJ: Beyond the "new cross-cultural psychiatry": cultural biology, discursive psychology and the ironies of globalization. Transcult Psychiatry 43(1):126–144, 2006 16671396
Kirmayer LJ: Mindfulness in cultural context. Transcult Psychiatry 52(4):447–469, 2015 26264787
Kirmayer LJ, Ban L: Cultural psychiatry: research strategies and future directions. Adv Psychosom Med 33:97–114, 2013
Kirmayer LJ, Jarvis GE: Culturally responsive services as a path to equity in mental healthcare. Healthc Pap 18(2):11–23, 2019 31596698
Kirmayer LJ, Minas H: The future of cultural psychiatry: an international perspective. Can J Psychiatry 45(5):438–446, 2000 10900523
Kirmayer LJ, Ramstead MJD: Embodiment and enactment in cultural psychiatry, in Embodiment, Enaction, and Culture: Investigating the Constitution of the Shared World. Edited by Durt C, Fuches T, Tewes C. Cambridge, MA, MIT Press, 2017, pp 397–422
Kirmayer LJ, Robbins JM: Patients who somatize in primary care: a longitudinal study of cognitive and social characteristics. Psychol Med 26(5):937–951, 1996 8878327
Kirmayer LJ, Young A: Culture and somatization: clinical, epidemiological, and ethnographic perspectives. Psychosom Med 60(4):420–430, 1998 9710287
Kirmayer LJ, Robbins JM, Dworkind M, et al: Somatization and the recognition of depression and anxiety in primary care. Am J Psychiatry 150(5):734–741, 1993 8480818
Kirmayer LJ, Young A, Robbins JM: Symptom attribution in cultural perspective. Can J Psychiatry 39(10):584–595, 1994 7828110
Kirmayer LJ, Dao THT, Smith A: Somatization and psychologization: understanding cultural idioms of distress, in Clinical Methods in Transcultural Psychiatry. Edited by Okpaku S. Washington, American Psychiatric Press, 1998, pp 233–265
Kirmayer LJ, Groleau D, Guzder J, et al: Cultural consultation: a model of mental health service for multicultural societies. Can J Psychiatry 48(3):145–153, 2003 12728738
Kirmayer LJ, Gomez-Carrillo A, Veissière S: Culture and depression in global mental health: an ecosocial approach to the phenomenology of psychiatric disorders. Soc Sci Med 183:163–168, 2017 28478959
Kirmayer LJ, Worthman CM, Kitayama S, et al (eds): Culture, Mind, and Brain: Emerging Concepts, Models, Applications. New York, Cambridge University Press, 2020
Kitanaka J: Depression in Japan: Psychiatric Cures for a Society in Distress. Princeton, NJ, Princeton University Press, 2011

Kitayama S, Markus HR: The pursuit of happiness and the realization of sympathy: cultural patterns of self, social relations, and well-being, in Culture and Subjective Well-Being. Edited by Diener E, Suh EM. Cambridge, MA, MIT Press, 2000, pp 113–161

Kitayama S, Markus HR, Matsumoto H, et al: Individual and collective processes in the construction of the self: self-enhancement in the United States and self-criticism in Japan. J Pers Soc Psychol 72(6):1245–1267, 1997 9177018

Kleinman AM: Depression, somatization and the "new cross-cultural psychiatry." Soc Sci Med 11(1):3–10, 1977 887955

Kleinman A: Social Origins of Distress and Disease: Depression, Neurasthenia, and Pain in Modern China. New Haven, CT, Yale University Press, 1986

Kleinman A: Rethinking Psychiatry. New York, Free Press, 1988

Kleinman A, Becker AE: "Sociosomatics": the contributions of anthropology to psychosomatic medicine. Psychosom Med 60(4):389–393, 1998 9710283

Kleinman AM, Good B (eds): Culture and Depression. Berkeley, CA, University of California Press, 1985

Kleinman A, Kleinman J: Somatization: the interconnections among culture, depressive experiences, and the meanings of pain. A study in Chinese society, in Culture and Depression. Edited by Kleinman A, Good B. Berkeley, CA, University of California Press, 1985, pp 132–167

Klerman GL, Lavori PW, Rice J, et al: Birth-cohort trends in rates of major depressive disorder among relatives of patients with affective disorder. Arch Gen Psychiatry 42(7):689–693, 1985 4015310

Kohrt BA, Rasmussen A, Kaiser BN, et al: Cultural concepts of distress and psychiatric disorders: literature review and research recommendations for global mental health epidemiology. Int J Epidemiol 43(2):365–406, 2014 24366490

Kövecses Z: Metaphor and Emotion: Language, Culture, and Body in Human Feeling. New York, Cambridge University Press, 2003

Kroenke K, Jackson JL, Chamberlin J: Depressive and anxiety disorders in patients presenting with physical complaints: clinical predictors and outcome. Am J Med 103(5):339–347, 1997 9375700

Kroll J, Linde P, Habenicht M, et al: Medication compliance, antidepressant blood levels, and side effects in Southeast Asian patients. J Clin Psychopharmacol 10(4):279–283, 1990 2286700

Lakoff G: Women, Fire, and Dangerous Things. Chicago, IL, University of Chicago Press, 1987

Law RW, Sbarra DA: The effects of church attendance and marital status on the longitudinal trajectories of depressed mood among older adults. J Aging Health 21(6):803–823, 2009 19535821

Lebois LA, Wilson-Mendenhall CD, Simmons WK, et al: Learning situated emotions. Neuropsychologia 145:106637, 2020 29330097

Lee S: Estranged bodies, simulated harmony, and misplaced cultures: neurasthenia in contemporary Chinese society. Psychosom Med 60(4):448–457, 1998 9710290

Levy RI: Tahitians: Mind and Experience in the Society Islands. Chicago, IL, University of Chicago Press, 1978

Lewinsohn PM, Mischel W, Chaplin W, et al: Social competence and depression: the role of illusory self-perceptions. J Abnorm Psychol 89(2):203–212, 1980 7365132

Lewis-Fernández R, Kirmayer LJ: Cultural concepts of distress and psychiatric disorders: understanding symptom experience and expression in context. Transcult Psychiatry 56(4):786–803, 2019 31347476

Lin KM: Biological differences in depression and anxiety across races and ethnic groups. J Clin Psychiatry 62 (suppl 13):13–19, discussion 20–21, 2001 11434414

Lin K-M, Lau JKC, Yamamoto J, et al: Hwa-byung. A community study of Korean Americans. J Nerv Ment Dis 180(6):386–391, 1992 1593273

Littlewood R: An indigenous conceptualization of reactive depression in Trinidad. Psychol Med 15(2):275–281, 1985 4023132

Liu CY, Wang SJ, Teng EL, et al: Depressive disorders among older residents in a Chinese rural community. Psychol Med 27(4):943–949, 1997 9234471

Lock M: Encounters With Aging: Mythologies of Menopause in Japan and North America. Berkeley, CA, University of California Press, 1993

Lock M, Wakewich-Dunk P: Nerves and nostalgia: expression of loss among Greek immigrants in Montreal. Can Fam Physician 36:253–258, 1990 21234036

Low S: Embodied metaphors: nerves as lived experience, in Embodiment and Experience: The Existential Ground of Culture and Self. Edited by Csordas T. New York, Cambridge University Press, 1994, pp 139–162

Lund C, Breen A, Flisher AJ, et al: Poverty and common mental disorders in low and middle income countries: a systematic review. Soc Sci Med 71(3):517–528, 2010 20621748

Lutz CA: Unnatural Emotions. Chicago, IL, University of Chicago Press, 1988

Ma SH, Teasdale JD: Mindfulness-based cognitive therapy for depression: replication and exploration of differential relapse prevention effects. J Consult Clin Psychol 72(1):31–40, 2004 14756612

Majeed H, Lee J: The impact of climate change on youth depression and mental health. Lancet Planet Health 1(3):e94–e95, 2017 29851616

Marazziti D, Mucci F, Avella MT, et al: The increasing challenge of the possible impact of ethnicity on psychopharmacology. CNS Spectr 26(3):222–231, 2020 32115000

Markus HR, Kitayama S: Culture and the self: implications for cognition, emotion, and motivation. Psychol Rev 98(2):224–253, 1991

Marsella AJ: Thoughts on cross-cultural studies on the epidemiology of depression. Cult Med Psychiatry 2(4):343–357, 1978 729393

Mausner-Dorsch H, Eaton WW: Psychosocial work environment and depression: epidemiologic assessment of the demand-control model. Am J Public Health 90(11):1765–1770, 2000 11076247

McMullen LM, Conway JB: Conventional metaphors for depression, in The Verbal Communication of Emotions: Interdisciplinary Perspectives. Edited by Fussell S. Mahwah, NJ, Lawrence Erlbaum, 2002, pp 167–181

Metzl JM, Angel J: Assessing the impact of SSRI antidepressants on popular notions of women's depressive illness. Soc Sci Med 58(3):577–584, 2004 14652053

Metzl JM, Hansen H: Structural competency: theorizing a new medical engagement with stigma and inequality. Soc Sci Med 103:126–133, 2014 24507917

Miller L, Wickramaratne P, Gameroff MJ, et al: Religiosity and major depression in adults at high risk: a ten-year prospective study. Am J Psychiatry 169(1):89–94, 2012 21865527

Miranda J, Chung JY, Green BL, et al: Treating depression in predominantly low-income young minority women: a randomized controlled trial. JAMA 290(1):57–65, 2003a 12837712

Miranda J, Azocar F, Organista KC, et al: Treatment of depression among impoverished primary care patients from ethnic minority groups. Psychiatr Serv 54(2):219–225, 2003b 12556604

Mollica RF, Wyshak G, de Marneffe D, et al: Indochinese versions of the Hopkins Symptom Checklist-25: a screening instrument for the psychiatric care of refugees. Am J Psychiatry 144(4):497–500, 1987 3565621

Moncrieff J: Psychiatric drug promotion and the politics of neo-liberalism. Br J Psychiatry 188(4):301–302, 2006 16582053

Mumford DB: The "Dhat syndrome": a culturally determined symptom of depression? Acta Psychiatr Scand 94(3):163–167, 1996 8891081

Mumford DB, Bavington JT, Bhatnagar KS, et al: The Bradford Somatic Inventory. A multiethnic inventory of somatic symptoms reported by anxious and depressed patients in Britain and the Indo-Pakistan subcontinent. Br J Psychiatry 158:379–386, 1991 2036538

Mumford DB, Saeed K, Ahmad I, et al: Stress and psychiatric disorder in rural Punjab. A community survey. Br J Psychiatry 170:473–478, 1997 9307700

Murphy HBM: Comparative Psychiatry: The International and Intercultural Distribution of Mental Illness. New York, Springer-Verlag, 1982

Murray CJ, Lopez AD: Global mortality, disability, and the contribution of risk factors: Global Burden of Disease Study. Lancet 349(9063):1436–1442, 1997 9164317

Nair RL, Roche KM, White RMB: Acculturation gap distress among Latino youth: prospective links to family processes and youth depressive symptoms, alcohol use, and academic performance. J Youth Adolesc 47(1):105–120, 2018 29030790
Napier AD, Ancarno C, Butler B, et al: Culture and health. Lancet 384(9954):1607–1639, 2014 25443490
Ng CH, Bousman CA: Cross-cultural psychopharmacotherapy, in Textbook of Cultural Psychiatry. Edited by Bhugra D, Bhui K. New York, Cambridge University Press, 2018, pp 432–440
Ngoma MC, Prince M, Mann A: Common mental disorders among those attending primary health clinics and traditional healers in urban Tanzania. Br J Psychiatry 183:349–355, 2003 14519614
Nickerson C, Schwarz N, Diener E, et al: Zeroing in on the dark side of the American Dream: a closer look at the negative consequences of the goal for financial success. Psychol Sci 14(6):531–536, 2003 14629682
Nortje G, Oladeji B, Gureje O, et al: Effectiveness of traditional healers in treating mental disorders: a systematic review. Lancet Psychiatry 3(2):154–170, 2016 26851329
Obeyesekere G: Depression, Buddhism, and the work of culture in Sri Lanka, in Culture and Depression. Edited by Kleinman AM, Good B. Berkeley, CA, University of California Press, 1985, pp 134–152
Obradovich N, Migliorini R, Paulus MP, Rahwan I: Empirical evidence of mental health risks posed by climate change. Proc Natl Acad Sci U S A 115(43):10953–10958, 2018 30297424
Ohaeri JU, Odejide OA: Somatization symptoms among patients using primary health care facilities in a rural community in Nigeria. Am J Psychiatry 151(5):728–731, 1994 8166315
O'Nell TD: Disciplined Hearts: History, Identity, and Depression in an American Indian Community. Berkeley, CA, University of California Press, 1996
Onions CT (ed): The Oxford Dictionary of English Etymology. New York, Oxford University Press, 1966
Orley J, Wing JK: Psychiatric disorders in two African villages. Arch Gen Psychiatry 36(5):513–520, 1979 373664
Osgood CE, May WH, Miron MS: Cross-Cultural Universals of Affective Meaning. Urbana, IL, University of Illinois Press, 1975
Pang KYC: Hwabyung: the construction of a Korean popular illness among Korean elderly immigrant women in the United States. Cult Med Psychiatry 14(4):495–512, 1990 2276269
Parker G, Cheah YC, Roy K: Do the Chinese somatize depression? A cross-cultural study. Soc Psychiatry Psychiatr Epidemiol 36(6):287–293, 2001 11583458
Patel V: Mental health: in the spotlight but a long way to go. Int Health 11(5):324–326, 2019 31529114
Patel V, Simunyu E, Gwanzura F, et al: The Shona Symptom Questionnaire: the development of an indigenous measure of common mental disorders in Harare. Acta Psychiatr Scand 95(6):469–475, 1997 9242841
Patel V, Chowdhary N, Rahman A, et al: Improving access to psychological treatments: lessons from developing countries. Behav Res Ther 49(9):523–528, 2011 21788012
Perry A, Gardener C, Oliver JE, et al: Exploring the cultural flexibility of the ACT model as an effective therapeutic group intervention for Turkish speaking communities in East London. The Cognitive Behaviour Therapist 12:e2, 2019
Phan T, Silove D: An overview of indigenous descriptions of mental phenomena and the range of traditional healing practices amongst the Vietnamese. Transcult Psychiatry 36(1):79–94, 1999
Phan T, Steel Z, Silove D: An ethnographically derived measure of anxiety, depression and somatization: the Phan Vietnamese Psychiatric Scale. Transcult Psychiatry 41(2):200–232, 2004 15446721
Phung TH: The family in Vietnam and its social life, in An Introduction to Indo-Chinese History, Culture, Language and Life. Edited by Withmore JK. Ann Arbor, MI, Center for South and Southeast Asian Studies, University of Michigan, 1979, pp 77–84

Piccinelli M, Simon G: Gender and cross-cultural differences in somatic symptoms associated with emotional distress. An international study in primary care. Psychol Med 27(2):433–444, 1997 9089835

Polo AJ, Makol BA, Castro AS, et al: Diversity in randomized clinical trials of depression: a 36-year review. Clin Psychol Rev 67:22–35, 2020 30292439

Radden J (ed): The Nature of Melancholy: From Aristotle to Kristeva. New York, Oxford University Press, 2000

Raguram R, Weiss MG, Channabasavanna SM, et al: Stigma, depression, and somatization in South India. Am J Psychiatry 153(8):1043–1049, 1996 8678173

Rathod S, Kingdon D: Cognitive behaviour therapy across cultures. Psychiatry 8(9):370–371, 2009

Ravitz P, Wondimagegn D, Pain C, et al: Psychotherapy knowledge translation and interpersonal psychotherapy: using best-education practices to transform mental health care in Canada and Ethiopia. Am J Psychother 68(4):463–488, 2014 26453347

Robins LN, Helzer JE, Orvaschel H: The Diagnostic Interview Schedule, in Epidemiologic Field Methods in Psychiatry. Edited by Eaton WW, Kessler LG. Orlando, FL, Academic Press, 1985, pp 143–170

Rodriguez E, Frongillo EA, Chandra P: Do social programmes contribute to mental well-being? The long-term impact of unemployment on depression in the United States. Int J Epidemiol 30(1):163–170, 2001 11171879

Rosaldo MZ: Knowledge and Passion: Ilongot Notions of Self and Social Life. Cambridge, UK, Cambridge University Press, 1980

Rothbaum F, Pott M, Azuma H, et al: The development of close relationships in Japan and the United States: paths of symbiotic harmony and generative tension. Child Dev 71(5):1121–1142, 2000 11108082

Ruscio AM: Normal versus pathological mood: Implications for diagnosis. Annu Rev Clin Psychol 15:179–205, 2019 31067413

Ryder AG, Chentsova-Dutton YE: Depression in cultural context: "Chinese somatization," revisited. Psychiatr Clin North Am 35(1):15–36, 2012 22370488

Sartorius N, Jablensky A, Gulbinat W, et al: Application of WHO scales for the assessment of depressive states in different cultures. Acta Psychiatr Scand 62:204–211, 1980

Sayar K, Kirmayer LJ, Taillefer SS: Predictors of somatic symptoms in depressive disorder. Gen Hosp Psychiatry 25(2):108–114, 2003 12676424

Schwartz B: Self-determination. The tyranny of freedom. Am Psychol 55(1):79–88, 2000 11392868

Schwartz EK, Docherty NM, Najolia GM, et al: Exploring the racial diagnostic bias of schizophrenia using behavioral and clinical-based measures. J Abnorm Psychol 128(3):263–271, 2019 30762376

Scott J, Dickey B: Global burden of depression: the intersection of culture and medicine. Br J Psychiatry 183:92–94, 2003 12893658

Sheikh JA, Yesavage GA: Geriatric Depression Scale (GDS): recent findings and development of a shorter version, in Clinical Gerontology: A Guide to Assessment and Intervention. Edited by Brink TL. New York, Haworth Press, 1986, pp 182–214

Shweder RA: Menstrual pollution, soul loss, and the comparative study of emotions, in Culture and Depression. Edited by Kleinman A, Good B. Berkeley, University of California Press, 1985, pp 182–214

Shweder RA, Haidt J: The cultural psychology of the emotions: ancient and new, in Handbook of Emotions. Edited by Lewis M, Haviland-Jones JM. New York, Guilford, 2000, pp 397–414

Shweder RA, Much NC, Mahapatra M, et al: The "big three" of morality (autonomy, community, divinity) and the "big three" explanations of suffering, in Morality and Health. Edited by Brandt A, Rozin P. New York, Routledge, 1997, pp 119–126

Simon GE, VonKorff M, Piccinelli M, et al: An international study of the relation between somatic symptoms and depression. N Engl J Med 341(18):1329–1335, 1999 10536124

Simon GE, Goldberg DP, Von Korff M, et al: Understanding cross-national differences in depression prevalence. Psychol Med 32(4):585–594, 2002 12102373

Singh G, Verma HC, Kaur H: A new depressive inventory. Indian J Psychiatry 16:183–188, 1974
Singla DR, Kohrt BA, Murray LK, et al: Psychological treatments for the world: lessons from low- and middle-income countries. Annu Rev Clin Psychol 13:149–181, 2017 28482687
Skultans V: From damaged nerves to masked depression: inevitability and hope in Latvian psychiatric narratives. Soc Sci Med 56(12):2421–2431, 2003 12742605
Slote WH: The intrapsychic locus of power and personal determination in a Confucian society: the case of Vietnam, in The Psycho-Cultural Dynamics of the Confucian Family: Past and Present. Edited by Slote WH. Seoul, Korea, International Cultural Society of Korea, 1986
Smith R, Alkozei A, Killgore WDS, et al: Nested positive feedback loops in the maintenance of major depression: an integration and extension of previous models. Brain Behav Immun 67:374–397, 2018 28943294
Steel Z, Marnane C, Iranpour C, et al: The global prevalence of common mental disorders: a systematic review and meta-analysis 1980–2013. Int J Epidemiol 43(2):476–493, 2014 24648481
Svob C, Wickramaratne PJ, Reich L, et al: Association of parent and offspring religiosity with offspring suicide ideation and attempts. JAMA Psychiatry 75(10):1062–1070, 2018 30090928
Sweet E: "Like you failed at life": debt, health and neoliberal subjectivity. Soc Sci Med 212:86–93, 2018 30025383
Teasdale JD, Segal ZV, Williams JM, et al: Prevention of relapse/recurrence in major depression by mindfulness-based cognitive therapy. J Consult Clin Psychol 68(4):615–623, 2000 10965637
Tennant C: Work-related stress and depressive disorders. J Psychosom Res 51(5):697–704, 2001 11728512
Tompar-Tiu A, Sustento-Seneriches J: Depression and Other Mental Health Issues: The Filipino American Experience. San Francisco, CA, Jossey-Bass, 1995
U.S. Surgeon General: Mental Health: Culture, Race, and Ethnicity. Rockville, MD, U.S. Department of Health and Human Services, 2002
Ustün TB, Sartorius N (eds): Mental Illness in General Health Care: An International Study. Hoboken, NJ, John Wiley & Sons, 1995
Van Ommeren M, Sharma B, Makaju R, et al: Limited cultural validity of the Composite International Diagnostic Interview's probe flow chart. Transcult Psychiatry 37(1):119–129, 2000
Vega WA, Kolody B, Aguilar-Gaxiola S, et al: Lifetime prevalence of DSM-III-R psychiatric disorders among urban and rural Mexican Americans in California. Arch Gen Psychiatry 55(9):771–778, 1998 9736002
Verdeli H, Clougherty K, Bolton P, et al: Adapting group interpersonal psychotherapy for a developing country: experience in rural Uganda. World Psychiatry 2(2):114–120, 2003 16946913
Vorcaro CM, Lima-Costa MF, Barreto SM, et al: Unexpected high prevalence of 1-month depression in a small Brazilian community: the Bambui Study. Acta Psychiatr Scand 104(4):257–263, 2001
Wakefield JC, Horwitz AV, Lorenzo-Luaces L: Uncomplicated depression as normal sadness: rethinking the boundary between normal and disordered depression, in The Oxford Handbook of Mood Disorders. Edited by DeRubeis RJ, Strunk DR. New York, Oxford University Press, 2017, pp 83–94
Weinberger AH, Gbedemah M, Martinez AM, et al: Trends in depression prevalence in the USA from 2005 to 2015: widening disparities in vulnerable groups. Psychol Med 48(8):1308–1315, 2018 29021005
Weissman MM, Bland RC, Canino GJ, et al: Cross-national epidemiology of major depression and bipolar disorder. JAMA 276(4):293–299, 1996 8656541
White GM: Representing emotional meaning: category, metaphor, schema, discourse, in Handbook of Emotions. Edited by Lewis M, Haviland-Jones JM. New York, Guilford, 2000, pp 30–44

Widiana HS, Simpson K, Manderson L: Cultural expressions of depression and the development of the Indonesian Depression Checklist. Transcult Psychiatry 55(3):339–360, 2018 29633909

Wierzbicka A: Imprisoned in English: The Hazards of English as a Default Language. Oxford University Press, 2013

Williams DR, González HM, Neighbors H, et al: Prevalence and distribution of major depressive disorder in African Americans, Caribbean blacks, and non-Hispanic whites: results from the National Survey of American Life. Arch Gen Psychiatry 64(3):305–315, 2007 17339519

Wittchen H-U, Robins LN, Cottler LB, et al: Cross-cultural feasibility, reliability and sources of variance of the Composite International Diagnostic Interview (CIDI). Br J Psychiatry 159:645–653, 658, 1991 1756340

Wittenborn AK, Rahmandad H, Rick J, et al: Depression as a systemic syndrome: mapping the feedback loops of major depressive disorder. Psychol Med 46(3):551–562, 2016 26621339

World Health Organization: Depressive Disorders in Different Cultures: Report on the WHO Collaborative Study on Standardized Assessment of Depressive Disorders. Geneva, World Health Organization, 1983

World Health Organization: Depression and Other Common Mental Disorders: Global Health Estimates (WHO/MSD/MER/2017.2). Geneva, World Health Organization, 2017. Available at: https://apps.who.int/iris/bitstream/handle/10665/254610/WHO-MSD-MER-2017.2-eng.pdf. Accessed September 17, 2021.

Yamaguchi A, Kim MS, Akutsu S: The effects of self-construals, self-criticism, and self-compassion on depressive symptoms. Pers Individ Dif 68:65–70, 2014

Yen S, Robins CJ, Lin N: A cross-cultural comparison of depressive symptom manifestation: China and the United States. J Consult Clin Psychol 68(6):993–999, 2000 11142551

Zandi T, Havenaar JM, Smits M, et al: First contact incidence of psychotic disorders among native Dutch and Moroccan immigrants in the Netherlands: influence of diagnostic bias. Schizophr Res 119(1–3):27–33, 2010 20332065

Zhang AY, Snowden LR: Ethnic characteristics of mental disorders in five U.S. communities. Cultur Divers Ethnic Minor Psychol 5(2):134–146, 1999 15605683

Zhou X, Peng Y, Zhu X, et al: From culture to symptom: testing a structural model of "Chinese somatization." Transcult Psychiatry 53(1):3–23, 2016 26076689

Zhu W, Wang CD, Chong CC: Adult attachment, perceived social support, cultural orientation, and depressive symptoms: a moderated mediation model. J Couns Psychol 63(6):645–655, 2016 27584034

CHAPTER 44

Mood Disorders and Sleep

Zhixing Yao, M.D.
Trevor Mooney, M.D.
William V. McCall, M.D., M.S.

Sleep and watchfulness, both of them, when immoderate, constitute disease.... In whatever disease sleep is laborious, it is a deadly symptom....

—Hippocrates (1939)

Recognition of the importance of sleep for health is as old as Hippocrates, but the modern science of sleep began with a sleep nosology naming four main categories of sleep disorders: the insomnias, the hypersomnias, the parasomnias, and the circadian rhythm disorders (Thorpy and Diagnostic Classification Steering Committee 1990). In this chapter we examine the association between sleep and mood disorders, focusing on insomnia, hypersomnias, parasomnias, and circadian rhythm disorders in both major depressive disorder (MDD) and bipolar disorder.

Definitions of the sleep disorders vary slightly, depending on the nosology used, but the key terms are defined as follows:

- *Insomnia*: dissatisfaction with the quantity or quality of sleep, despite adequate opportunity to sleep, associated with adverse daytime consequences such as fatigue, poor concentration, irritability, and/or inability to fulfill normal domestic, social, or vocational obligations.
- *Hypersomnia*: inability to maintain a normal level of alertness during times that alertness would be expected, leading to adverse consequences such as lapses of attention and unexpected sleep episodes, associated with inability to fulfill normal domestic, social, or vocational obligations, or endangerment related to sleep lapses.

- *Parasomnia*: Abnormal behavior or abnormal physiology that occurs exclusively—or reliably worsens—during sleep, causing distress, impairment, or disease. Examples include sleepwalking, nocturnal reflux, and sleep-related exacerbation of asthma. In this chapter the only parasomnia we will discuss is nightmares.
- *Circadian rhythm disorder*: Problems in the timing of sleep and wakefulness (as opposed to the amount of sleep and wakefulness), leading to fatigue, poor concentration, lapses of attention, irritability, and/or inability to fulfill normal domestic, social, or vocational obligations.

Establishing the presence of insomnia, hypersomnia, parasomnia, or circadian rhythm disorder is accomplished by clinical interview and does not require sleep laboratory or other physiological testing, although specific sleep disorders such as obstructive sleep apnea do require testing. The population prevalence of chronic insomnia in developed countries is 6%–10% (Roth 2007), with the respective rates of hypersomnia, parasomnia, and circadian rhythm disorders at 4%–10%, 5%, and less than 1% (Li et al. 2010; Mignot 2008; Takaesu et al. 2016). The fact that the prevalence of these sleep disorders among individuals with mood disorders is much higher raises questions about the role of sleep problems in the onset and maintenance of mood disorders, and associated complications. We examine these questions in the following sections, which are divided topically by major mood disorders.

Major Depressive Disorder

Insomnia in Major Depressive Disorder

Insomnia Preceding MDD

Epidemiological data have shown that the persistence of insomnia for a year or more is associated with a higher rate of first-episode MDD than the rate seen in adults whose insomnia resolves within a year, with an estimated relative risk (RR) ratio of 2–30 (Dryman and Eaton 1991; Ford and Kamerow 1989). The exact nature of the relationship between insomnia and incident MDD is not known. Whereas some have speculated that insomnia simply represents the leading edge of a major depressive episode (MDE) that is already under way, others have suggested that insomnia is a risk factor for MDD that is subject to modification, a theory that potentially opens an avenue for interrupting incident MDEs.

Insomnia During Major Depressive Episodes

Insomnia and hypersomnia are among the nine DSM-5 symptoms of MDD, but neither is mandatory for a diagnosis of MDD (American Psychiatric Association 2013). Insomnia or hypersomnia must be present nearly every day to be counted toward the diagnostic criteria of MDD. Reported rates of insomnia in MDD depend on the setting. Insomnia is seen in up to 70% of individuals with MDD in the community (Ohayon et al. 2000; Weissman et al. 1996) and in 80% of individuals will MDD in inpatient psychiatric care (McCall et al. 2000). MDD-associated insomnia in older patients manifests higher rates of early-morning awakening compared with insomnia in younger patients with MDD (Gillin et al. 1981). Patients with MDD have very poor quality of life, worse than that seen with the most common conditions seen in primary care (Wells et al. 1989). The presence of insomnia adds an additional burden over and above that carried by the other symptoms of MDD (McCall et al. 1999, 2000, 2010a; O'Brien et al. 2011; Roth et al. 2006). Of greater importance, a higher intensity of insomnia symptoms is associated with increased rates and severity of suicidal ideation, suicidal behavior, and suicide death, even after adjustment for the other symptoms of MDD (McCall et al. 2010a). There are multiple possible mechanisms linking insomnia to suicide risk, including diminished decision-making capacity related to insomnia (McCall and Black 2013).

Hypersomnia in Major Depressive Disorder

The proportion of patients with MDD who report hypersomnia (23%–27%) is lower than the proportion who report insomnia (Yates et al. 2004). In comparison with healthy control subjects, patients with MDD who complain of hypersomnolence do indeed sleep longer at night and take more naps during the day, but they have normal latencies to the onset of rapid eye movement (REM) sleep (Plante et al. 2017). Notably, MDD with hypersomnia shows no evidence of the irresistible, uncontrollable daytime sleepiness that characterizes sleep disorders such as narcolepsy or severe sleep apnea. The frequency of hypersomnia complaints is greater among patients with MDD who are young adults and women, and also among patients with bipolar depression (Dauvilliers et al. 2013). Compared with nondepressed individuals with narcolepsy, depressed persons with hypersomnia generally have normal findings on measures of daytime sleepiness as determined by the Multiple Sleep Latency Test (MSLT) (Nofzinger et al. 1991). The prolonged time in bed and the lengthy time spent asleep may be in part due to a desire to not be awake to avoid experiencing depressive affect. Like insomnia, hypersomnia independently predicts suicidal ideation (McCall et al. 2015). Hypersomnia in MDD with atypical features is likely to persist even after other symptoms have remitted, confers a 2.5–2.9 times increased risk for a subsequent MDE, and may be biologically mediated by decreased sensitivity to corticotropin-releasing hormone (Kaplan and Harvey 2009).

Nightmare Parasomnia in Major Depressive Disorder

Nightmares are characterized by unpleasant mentation during sleep that involves a narrative, high visual content, and wakening from the mental content. Individuals with mood disorders have high rates of nightmares (OR > 15 relative to healthy control subjects) (Li et al. 2010). Nightmares are also associated with a high risk of suicidal ideation, suicidal behavior, and suicide death (McCall et al. 2013). In addition to classic nightmares, patients with MDD may also report "bad dreams" that do not meet the definition of a nightmare. The bad dreams in MDD are low in visual content, more contemplative than narrative, and characterized by depressive themes (Cartwright 1996).

Polysomnography in Major Depressive Disorder

Polysomnographic Abnormalities in MDD

Individuals without MDD who have chronic insomnia show abnormalities on polysomnography that include delayed onset of sleep, increased wake time after sleep onset, reduced total sleep time, and increased percentage of light sleep (stage N1). Sleep disturbances among individuals with MDD are characterized by additional abnormalities, including reduced slow-wave sleep (stage N3), shortened time between sleep onset and REM sleep onset (i.e., decreased REM sleep latency), redistribution of REM sleep toward the earlier portion of the sleeping period, and increased numbers of eye movements per minute of REM sleep (i.e., increased REM sleep density) (Kupfer and Foster 1972). REM latency (RL) is defined as the time elapsed from sleep onset to the first REM sleep period. In a study in which all participants completed 2 consecutive nights of sleep recording and the shortest RL was used for comparison, an RL value less than 70 minutes had a sensitivity of 82% and a specificity of 69% in separating patients with MDD from nondepressed control subjects (Akiskal et al. 1982). By contrast, an RL value less than 52 minutes had a sensitivity and specificity of 34% and 92%, respectively, in distinguishing MDD patients from control subjects

Neural control of REM sleep is very complex, with separate brain stem nuclei controlling REM sleep–related desynchronized electroencephalogram (EEG) activity, rapid eye movements, and skeletal muscle atonia. Cholinergic systems coordinate these different elements at the onset of REM sleep; thus, a decreased RL value suggests potentiated cholinergic activity. Additionally, cholinergic orchestration of REM sleep onset is inhibited by noradrenergic systems (Héricé et al. 2019). Thus, the finding of a short RL in MDD is consistent with the premise of a CNS imbalance between cholinergic and noradrenergic systems that favors cholinergic systems.

RL abnormalities in MDD partially resolve with remission of the MDE (i.e., from 20 minutes to 60 minutes) but do not necessarily move into the normal range (i.e., 90 minutes in adults) (Rush et al. 1986). REM sleep abnormalities in patients with MDD may persist even after remission of the MDE, in the absence of medications, suggesting that REM sleep abnormalities may be at least partially a trait characteristic of MDD (Rush et al. 1986). This phenomenon has been described as a "partial state, partial trait" (Kupfer and Ehlers 1989), suggesting that a short RL is a biomarker of risk for MDD that becomes progressively more abnormal as the patient moves from euthymia into an MDE. As the patient moves back into euthymia, the continuing biological vulnerability for relapse can be demonstrated in the sleep laboratory by giving an intravenous dose of arecoline (an acetylcholine partial agonist). Patients with MDD and healthy control subjects both demonstrate dose-dependent REM induction with arecoline (versus placebo infusions); however, arecoline-induced RL was significantly shorter in nearly euthymic, medication-free patients with MDD in comparison with control participants without MDD (Gillin et al. 1991). We interpret this finding as showing that the "REM-on" system remains "twitchy" (i.e., the mechanisms that govern REM sleep remain hypersensitive to perturbation) during near-remission, perhaps reflecting the ongoing risk for relapse.

Given the familial risk for MDD, it is not surprising that first-degree relatives of patients with MDD with reduced RLs are more likely to have a low RL, as compared with the first-degree relatives of patients with MDD without reduced RLs (Giles et al. 1998).

Polysomnography as a Tool for Distinguishing MDD From Dementia

Advanced dementia can often be challenging to distinguish from pseudodementia (due to MDD) on mental status exam alone. Polysomnography can provide useful data to discriminate the underlying pathophysiology, given that dementia is associated with lowered acetylcholine levels leading to prolonged RL values and decreased REM sleep density, whereas MDD has the exact opposite profile: reduced RL values and increased REM sleep density (Kohl et al. 2000; Reynolds et al. 1985, 1988).

Actigraphic Circadian Rhythm Abnormalities in Major Depressive Disorder

Actigraphy uses an accelerometer for the longitudinal recording of motor activity, commonly recorded from the nondominant wrist. The captured activity data can be linked to clock time, allowing for analysis of activity data in relationship to the 24-hour circadian cycle. Often, the data are analyzed by proprietary software that calculates estimates of time to sleep onset, time awake in the middle of the night, and total sleep time. Although many individuals with insomnia, including those with MDD, have actigraphically determined reductions in estimated sleep (McCall and McCall 2012a), actigraphy is subject to errors, in that some individuals with insomnia lie very still in bed while awake, leading to the erroneous conclusion that they are asleep when in fact they are not (McCall and McCall 2012b). This pitfall can be avoided by looking at the raw actigraphy data and interpreting it as activity data, rather than inferring that it indicates wake versus sleep. The activity data can be examined principally as an indicator of circadian phase (i.e., the timing of activity) rather than an indicator of amount of sleep (Lundeen et al. 2018). Actigraphic rest-activity rhythms are closely correlated with patients' self-reports of whether they judge themselves to be "larks" or "owls" (Lundeen et al. 2018). Persons who have significant delay in the timing of their major rest period (i.e., "owls" with an "eveningness" chronotype, as assessed by the Morningness-Eveningness Questionnaire [Horne and Ostberg 1976]), are more likely to experience depression and more likely to be suicidal than persons with a "morningness" chronotype (Rumble et al. 2018). Similarly, reduced peak-to-trough variations in activity across the day are also seen in patients with MDD. Remarkably, patients with MDD who have later rest-activity rhythms may have a superior response to antidepressants (McCall 2015). Depressed patients with MDD show decreased sleep efficiency, increased wake time after sleep onset, and less daily activity than do healthy control subjects (Tazawa et al. 2019). In patients with MDD, treatment results in decreased sleep-onset latency and increased sleep efficiency (Tazawa et al. 2019). MDD patients who have achieved symptom remission show no actigraphic differences from healthy control subjects (Tazawa et al. 2019). Interpretation of the timing of rest-activity data must take into account the individual patient's age, because the timing of the rest period tends to advance to earlier times across the life cycle (McCall et al. 2012).

Effects of Antidepressant Treatments on Sleep

Pharmacotherapy for MDD

Tricyclic antidepressants. The tricyclic antidepressant (TCA) amitriptyline heralded the modern era of MDD pharmacotherapy. TCAs have an immediate, first-night effect on lengthening (normalizing) reduced RLs in patients with MDD (Kupfer et al. 1978, 1982). Slow-wave (N3) sleep is enhanced by TCAs (Kupfer et al. 1978;

Reynolds et al. 1997a). The effects of TCAs on sleep continuity are more variable than their effects on RL values but tend more in the direction of improvements in sleep continuity. The effects of TCAs on RL values are consistent with the enhancement of bioaminergic neurotransmitters and the blockade of cholinergic receptors by TCAs. Depression-targeted psychotherapies do not have the early effects on MDD-associated insomnia that are seen with TCAs (DiMascio et al. 1979). Patients with MDD with baseline abnormalities in REM sleep, such as reduced RL and increased REM sleep density, were found to respond preferentially to antidepressants (TCAs or selective serotonin reuptake inhibitors) (Rush et al. 1989) and to respond poorly to a course of psychotherapy (Thase et al. 1996, 1997). Long-term treatment with TCAs is associated with persistent lengthening of RL values (Kupfer et al. 1982). Abrupt cessation of a TCA is quickly followed by a rebound of all REM sleep phenomena, which normalize over 1–2 weeks (Dunleavy et al. 1972); this finding suggests that TCAs do not eliminate the need for REM sleep but instead merely postpone the expression of REM sleep until such time that the TCA is removed.

Monoamine oxidase inhibitors, selective serotonin reuptake inhibitors, and serotonin-norepinephrine reuptake inhibitors. Monoamine oxidase inhibitors (MAOIs), selective serotonin reuptake inhibitors (SSRIs), and serotonin-norepinephrine reuptake inhibitors (SNRIs) have effects on REM sleep that vary in degree but are otherwise similar to the effects of TCAs on REM sleep (Landolt et al. 2001; van Bemmel et al. 1993; Winokur et al. 2003). The effects of SSRIs on sleep continuity in patients with MDD are mixed, with some patients experiencing deterioration, including an increased wake time, a higher percentage of EEG light sleep, and a loss of EEG deep sleep (Jindal et al. 2003; Levitan et al. 2000; Luthringer et al. 1996; Winokur et al. 2003). Although most patients with MDD report less insomnia while taking an SSRI or SNRI, the rate of treatment-emergent insomnia is higher among patients taking these medications (Brecht et al. 2008). Indeed, patients with MDD who take SSRIs or SNRIs may report some improvement in insomnia symptoms, while at the same time, their polysomnography findings show objective deterioration in sleep continuity (Gillin et al. 1997). A prospective study of a successful trial of an SSRI (fluoxetine) leading to depression remission found that insomnia was the most common residual symptom (Nierenberg et al. 1999), and residual insomnia has been linked to relapse of MDD in some (Reynolds et al. 1997b) but not all studies (Iovieno et al. 2011). There are only three antidepressant medications that have no REM sleep–suppressing effects: bupropion, nefazodone, and trimipramine (Gillin et al. 1997; Hohagen et al. 1994; Ott et al. 2004).

Mirtazapine. Mirtazapine is similar in efficacy to TCAs and produces improvements in sleep efficiency, total sleep time, and sleep quality in individuals with MDD (Dolder et al. 2012). Mirtazapine has been shown to increase slow-wave (N3) sleep, increase RL, and reduce wake time after sleep onset (Shen et al. 2006). Furthermore, it appears not only to improve subjective sleep quality but also to reverse the polysomnographic effects of MDD-associated insomnia (Schittecatte et al. 2002; Shen et al. 2006). Individuals with insomnia, MDD, and suicidal ideation who receive treatment with mirtazapine have shown improvements in sleep and reductions in suicidal ideation (Gandotra et al. 2018).

Neurostimulation for Treatment-Resistant Depression

Electroconvulsive therapy (ECT) and repetitive transcranial magnetic stimulation (rTMS) are effective treatments for treatment-resistant depression, and successful ECT and successful rTMS are both associated with improvement in insomnia symptoms. However, there does not appear to be a direct anti-insomnia effect of either ECT or rTMS, apart from the overall syndromal antidepressant effect of these treatments (McCall et al. 2018; Rosenquist et al. 2013). ECT is associated with increases in EEG total sleep time and in EEG deep sleep (Göder et al. 2016). In common with TCAs, MAOIs, SSRIs, and SNRIs, ECT has a REM sleep–suppressing effect (Coffey et al. 1988), but with an important difference: after a course of ECT, there is no REM sleep rebound, which may indicate that ECT produces a more complete and durable effect on REM sleep than is produced by pharmacotherapies.

Forced Sleep Deprivation for Treatment-Resistant Depression

Individuals living with treatment-resistant depression can sometimes get stuck in the feeling that "nothing works"—an understandable response when multiple treatments have been futile. Forced sleep deprivation (FSD) is a powerful and rapid-acting therapy that can be beneficial in certain cases. Response rates can be as high as 50%, and effectiveness is similar for total (36 hours awake) and partial (3–4 hours of sleep followed by forced wakefulness for 20–21 hours) deprivation strategies, as long as the deprivation occurs in the later part of the night (Boland et al. 2017). Although FSD is not a permanent solution (because the antidepressant effect of sleep deprivation is transient [Ioannou et al. 2021]), a positive response to this therapy can engender hope in patients (that "at least something can work"), help build rapport, and provide evidence that nonpharmacological interventions can have a profound effect on symptoms (which may be useful to improve patient buy-in for therapies such as cognitive-behavioral therapy).

Targeted Treatment for Insomnia in Major Depressive Disorder

Residual insomnia symptoms after treatment with SSRIs or SNRIs often leads to a need for supplemental, targeted treatment of insomnia. Targeted treatment of insomnia can be accomplished with cognitive-behavioral therapy for insomnia (CBT-I) or with pharmacotherapy. CBT-I is the preferred approach for treating chronic insomnia, according to the American College of Physicians (Qaseem et al. 2016). Although CBT-I has been most extensively tested in insomnia not associated with MDD, there is evidence to support its application in MDD-associated insomnia, with the understanding that the onset of effect may not be as rapid as that afforded by hypnotic medications (Manber et al. 2008, 2016).

Among patients with MDD taking an SSRI, the addition of a bedtime medication to manage insomnia symptoms is common; in one study, up to 60% of patients using sertraline or fluoxetine were also using a bedtime soporific (Cook and Conner 1995). Although low-dosage trazodone was the preferred pharmacological treatment of

MDD-associated insomnia for many years (Nierenberg and Keck 1989; Nierenberg et al. 1994), zolpidem has recently overtaken the use of trazodone (Bertisch et al. 2014). Head-to-head comparisons of trazodone and zolpidem show a short-term advantage for zolpidem in insomnia (Walsh et al. 1998). Among patients with MDD, short-term, 6- to 8-week trials of hypnotics have led to improvements in insomnia, quality of life, and suicidal ideation (McCall et al. 2010b). In one study, patients with concurrent MDD, insomnia, and suicidal ideation who received zolpidem in addition to their SRRI treatment showed greater reductions in suicidality than did patients who received placebo with their SSRI treatment (McCall et al. 2019a). This effect was larger in patients with more severe insomnia (McCall et al. 2019a). Remarkably, after 6–8 weeks of concurrent treatment with an SSRI, the hypnotic can be abruptly discontinued without incurring a protracted rebound insomnia (Krystal et al. 2007).

Primary Sleep Disorders in Patients With Major Depressive Disorder

Apart from insomnia, the most common primary sleep disorders are obstructive sleep apnea (OSA), restless legs syndrome (RLS), and periodic limb movement disorder (PLMD). Whereas OSA has a prevalence of 4% in the general adult population (Partinen and Telakivi 1992), its prevalence in clinical populations of patients with MDD is much higher, 36.3% (*N*=522) (Stubbs et al. 2016). In population cohort studies, the prevalence of OSA in MDD is 19.8% (*N*=359,378) (Stubbs et al. 2016). In a study of suicidal MDD outpatients with insomnia, the rates of previously unsuspected OSA—approximately 14%–17%—were higher than rates in the general population (McCall et al. 2019b). The presence of OSA will inhibit the antidepressant effects of SNRIs (Waterman et al. 2016), and treatment of the OSA will reduce depression symptoms (Balcan et al. 2019). RLS has a population prevalence of 5%–10% in adults, and individuals with RLS have higher rates of MDD compared with those without RLS (Koo et al. 2016). Treatment with SSRIs may induce or aggravate RLS (OR=15.9), an effect that may perhaps explain some of the insomnia symptoms seen with SSRI treatment (Perez-Lloret et al. 2012). The prevalence of PLMD in depressed patients is unknown; however, antidepressant therapy in patients with PLMD will need to be tailored, as SSRIs are associated with increased periodic limb movements in sleep (Picchietti and Winkelman 2005). Bupropion is a reasonable alternative with associated benefit for PLMD (Nofzinger et al. 2000). The current evidence base for primary sleep disorders in patients with MDD does not support a recommendation for routine sleep testing of all patients with MDD; however, emergence of treatment-resistant depression or worsening of sleep symptoms in a patient should prompt the clinician to consider sleep testing.

The pathophysiology of OSA is mediated by several mechanical and neuromuscular factors, including anatomy, obesity, muscle tone, inflammation, and ventilation control via proprioceptive and chemoreceptor feedback (Dempsey et al. 2010). Classically, OSA consists of sleep-induced hypotonia of the upper airway, leading to hypoxia and repeated transient arousals from sleep. Consequent mood dysregulation appears to be attributable to these repeated awakenings, given that disruptions in sleep continuity have been shown to negatively impact mood (Finan et al. 2015). In addition, hypoxia may itself be depressogenic, given that hypoxia during sleep is a risk factor for developing depression and is predictive of greater depression severity (Szabó and Ihász 2019), lower quality of life (Akashiba et al. 2002), and impaired decision making under conditions involving ambiguous risk (Iowa Gambling Task) (Delazer et al. 2016).

Bipolar Disorder

> *The attacks of manic-depressive insanity are invariably accompanied by all kinds of bodily changes. By far the most striking are the disorders of sleep and general nourishment. In mania sleep is in the more severe states of excitement always considerably encroached upon; sometimes there is even almost complete sleeplessness, at most interrupted for a few hours, which may last for weeks, even months.... In the states of depression in spite of great need for sleep, it is for the most part sensibly encroached upon; the patients lie for hours, sleepless in bed,...although even in bed they find no refreshment.*
>
> —Emil Kraepelin (1921)

Sleep disturbance can be a core feature in manic episodes as well as MDEs in both bipolar I and bipolar II disorder (Gold and Sylvia 2016). Sleep disturbances, which can manifest in all phases of illness (including euthymic phases), negatively affect the illness course, the symptom burden, the patient's quality of life and functioning, and treatment outcomes of bipolar disorder (Gold and Sylvia 2016). For this reason, it is imperative to understand and treat sleep disturbances to reduce the morbidity and mortality of bipolar disorder.

A classic symptom of hypomania and mania is a reduced need for sleep (American Psychiatric Association 2013). However, sleep disturbances are also prevalent in the depressive, interepisode, and prodromal phases of bipolar disorder. As previously described, sleep disturbances include insomnias, hypersomnias, circadian rhythm dysfunctions, and parasomnias (Cormier 1990). With the exception of parasomnias (for which conclusive data in bipolar disorder are lacking), we will briefly examine how these sleep disturbances commonly manifest in each phase of bipolar disorder.

Insomnia in Bipolar Disorder

A decreased need for sleep is acknowledged as a core, pervasive feature of symptomatic mania. However, insomnia (defined as a subjective dissatisfaction with the quantity or quality of sleep) is also common in mania. Whereas the majority of individuals with bipolar disorder report a reduced need for sleep (which is not insomnia) during manic or hypomanic episodes, some report difficulties in falling asleep or staying asleep (i.e., insomnia) during these episodes (Gold and Sylvia 2016). Insomnia is also commonly reported in euthymic patients with bipolar disorder at rates ranging from 14% to 50% (Soehner et al. 2013).

Hypersomnia in Bipolar Disorder

During bipolar MDEs, sleep disturbances often take the form of hypersomnia, with reported rates varying from 38% to 78% among patients with bipolar disorder (Kaplan et al. 2015). For this reason, some clinicians suggest that hypersomnia may help differentiate bipolar depression from MDD, a distinction with clearly important implications for treatment (Bowden 2005). Hypersomnia is also commonly reported by euthymic patients with bipolar disorder; in one study, 25% of patients with bipolar disorder (N=56) reported experiencing hypersomnia during an interepisode period (Kaplan et al. 2011). A meta-analysis examining hypersomnia in individuals with bipolar disorder (N=1,824) estimated an overall prevalence of 29.9% (95% CI: 25.8–34.1%; P<0.05) (Grigolon et al. 2019). Hypersomnia was not significantly related to mood polarity, bipolar disorder type, medication use, or age, but its presence did indicate risk of relapse to MDEs or manic/hypomanic episodes (Grigolon et al. 2019).

Circadian Rhythm Dysfunction in Bipolar Disorder

The body's circadian rhythms are controlled by the suprachiasmatic nucleus of the hypothalamus, a so-called master clock that responds to photic and nonphotic cues. The genes that underlie the circadian clock mechanism have been well described, and some potential pathophysiological mechanisms have been proposed; however, studies examining circadian rhythm dysfunction in patients with bipolar disorder remain limited (Ketchesin et al. 2020).

A key biomarker of bipolar disorder is a dysfunctional sleep-wake cycle (Gold and Kinrys 2019; Gold and Sylvia 2016). In fact, evidence suggests that bipolar disorder may primarily originate from a disorder of circadian rhythms (Soreca 2014). According to this unifying "circadian rhythm disruption model," patients with bipolar disorder have "weakly entrained" circadian rhythms that are vulnerable to disruption by life stressors (social *zeitgebers*), leading to mood episodes (Soreca 2014). Laboratory evidence supports this model; euthymic patients with bipolar disorder secrete less melatonin than do healthy control subjects (Nurnberger et al. 2000), and depressed and hypomanic patients with bipolar disorder secrete more cortisol than do healthy control subjects (Cervantes et al. 2001). Moreover, a number of circadian genes (e.g., *CLOCK, TIMELESS, DBP, ARNTL2*) have been associated with circadian phenotypes identified in patients with bipolar disorder (Shi et al. 2008).

The prevalence of circadian rhythm sleep-wake disorders (CRSWDs) in euthymic patients with bipolar disorder was shown in one study to be 32.4% (N=104 outpatients of Tokyo Medical University with either bipolar I or II disorder meeting DSM-5 criteria), compared with a prevalence of 0.13% in the general Japanese population and 0.17% in the general Norwegian population (Takaesu et al. 2016). The presence of CRSWD is significantly associated with younger age at onset of bipolar disorder and a family history of suicide (Takaesu et al. 2016). Circadian rhythm disruption has been widely demonstrated in bipolar disorder and includes sleep-wake rhythm abnormalities, "eveningness" chronotype, melatonin dysregulation, *CLOCK* gene differences, and social time cue irregularities (Takaesu 2018). Sleep-wake rhythm irregularities—especially CRSWD, delayed sleep phase type—are prominent in bipolar disorder, even in the euthymic state (Takaesu 2018). Biological rhythm disturbance has a "dose-dependent" correlation with depression severity in patients with bipolar disorder and is an independent predictor of functional impairment (Pinho et al. 2016). Patients with bipolar disorder are more likely than healthy control subjects to have an "eveningness" chronotype (Melo et al. 2017); however, the relationship between chronotype and risk of mood symptoms is unclear (Takaesu 2018). In the manic phase, melatonin peak time is advanced and melatonin secretion is increased, whereas in the depressive and euthymic phases, melatonin peak time is delayed and secretion is decreased (Takaesu 2018).

Relationship Between Sleep and Mood in Bipolar Disorder

In all phases of bipolar disorder, sleep is disturbed relative to sleep in healthy control subjects. Sleep disturbance can take many forms, including insomnia, hypersomnia, sleep-wake cycle dysfunction, and parasomnias, as well as the ability to maintain energy despite decreased sleep. For the clinician, acknowledging the ubiquity of sleep disturbances in patients with bipolar disorder is extremely important, because sleep disruption can cause functional impairment even in the absence of mood problems and can negatively affect the course of illness (Gold and Sylvia 2016; Harvey et al. 2015; Plante and Winkelman 2008). We next examine how sleep disturbance can signal, or even trigger, mood episodes in bipolar disorder.

Prior to the initial mood episode, bipolar patients commonly undergo a "prodromal" period, lasting on average around 2 years, in which they experience subclinical symptoms such as insomnia, decreased need for sleep, and other sleep disturbances (Van Meter et al. 2016). The same subclinical symptoms, lasting for a much shorter period (reported range of 0.5–1.3 months in studies), also precede a mood episode recurrence (Van Meter et al. 2016).

Bipolar disorder is characterized partly by its burden of subsyndromal symptomatology between episodes (Sachs 2003). Thus, it is not surprising that sleep problems persist even after resolution of syndromal mood episodes. Up to 70% of euthymic patients with bipolar disorder experience clinically significant sleep disturbance (Harvey et al. 2005). Additionally, in comparison with healthy individuals, euthymic patients with bipolar disorder exhibit greater sleep variability, longer sleep durations, longer sleep-onset latencies, more nighttime awakenings, and poorer sleep efficiency (Millar et al. 2004; Soehner et al. 2013). There is some evidence that patients with bipolar disorder experience increased REM sleep density during interepisode periods (Eidelman et al. 2010).

But sleep problems are more than just a residual symptom of remitted bipolar disorder. Research evidence in three areas strongly suggests that sleep disturbance is also a precipitant of future mood episodes in bipolar disorder (Gruber et al. 2009):

1. *Reports of common precipitants of mood changes*—Anecdotal reports abound of patients switching into mania in the context of social rhythm disruption—for example, during drug use, transmeridian travel, postpartum states, and bereavement (Plante and Winkelman 2008). Circadian rhythm disruptions such as jet lag or shift work can also trigger mood episodes or worsen symptoms (Ketchesin et al. 2020). Jet lag is particularly problematic because of the imbalance between the internal preset circadian timing tuned to the departure time zone and the desired timing

needed to acclimate to the external cues of the destination time zone (Roach and Sargent 2019). Eastward transmeridian travel has been associated with an increased risk of manic/hypomanic episodes, while westward travel may carry an increased risk of MDEs (Inder et al. 2016).

2. *Longitudinal studies of sleep and mood*—Research that longitudinally examined sleep parameters and mood in patients with bipolar disorder has demonstrated that increased sleep is inversely correlated with subsequent manic symptoms (Bauer et al. 2006; Leibenluft et al. 1996; Wehr et al. 1982).
3. *Experimental sleep deprivation studies*—Studies using experimentally induced sleep deprivation in both patients with unipolar depression and patients with bipolar depression have established a causal relationship between sleep and mood in bipolar disorder (Plante and Winkelman 2008). Experimentally induced sleep deprivation in bipolar depression produces manic and hypomanic switch rates comparable to those produced by antidepressant drug treatments (Colombo et al. 1999).

Taken together, these lines of evidence indicate that disturbed sleep is a valuable therapeutic target for preventing syndromal mood episodes over the course of bipolar disorder. Indeed, sleep reduction has been identified by some as the "final common pathway" in the development of mania (Wehr et al. 1987).

Objectifying Sleep in Bipolar Disorder: Actigraphy and Polysomnography

Actigraphic Circadian Rhythm Abnormalities in Bipolar Disorder

Patients with bipolar disorder show several actigraphic differences from healthy control patients. A meta-analysis of actigraphic studies that measured activity changes and sleep patterns in bipolar patients and healthy control subjects found that patients with bipolar disorder were less active during the day, slept longer but less efficiently, had longer sleep-onset latencies, and spent more time awake after sleep onset than did control subjects (De Crescenzo et al. 2017). This meta-analysis included data from studies of euthymic and depressed patients; however, subgroup analyses of depressed patients showed no substantial differences. In contrast to patients with MDD whose symptoms are in remission, who show no sleep pattern differences from healthy control subjects, patients with bipolar disorder whose symptoms are in remission continue to show longer sleep-onset latencies, longer sleep durations with lower efficiency, and longer wake times after sleep onset (Geoffroy et al. 2015). Patients with bipolar disorder whose symptoms are in remission also display decreased daily activity between episodes (Ng et al. 2015). Patients with bipolar disorder experiencing an MDE likewise have reduced daily activity, longer total sleep times, and longer wake times after sleep onset (Tazawa et al. 2019). As with treatment of patients with MDD, treatment of depression in patients with bipolar disorder results in decreased sleep-onset latency and increased sleep efficiency (Tazawa et al. 2019). Patients experiencing a manic episode have longer sleep-onset latencies and longer wake times after sleep onset than do healthy control subjects (Tazawa et al. 2019).

Polysomnographic Abnormalities in Bipolar Disorder

Polysomnography during mood episodes. Sleep in bipolar depression shares many polysomnographic similarities with sleep in MDD: disturbed sleep continuity, decreased slow-wave (N3) sleep, reduced RL, and increased REM sleep density (Gold and Sylvia 2016; Plante and Winkelman 2008; Riemann et al. 2002). Sleep is more curtailed in mania, but it still overlaps with the polysomnographic features of unipolar depression (Hudson et al. 1992; Riemann et al. 2002). Strong polysomnographic similarities between unipolar and bipolar depression may represent common biological underpinnings of both disorders (Asaad et al. 2016). Nonetheless, in their review of the literature, Gold and Sylvia (2016) highlighted some of the more subtle differences in sleep architecture between patients with bipolar and unipolar depression: in bipolar depression compared with unipolar depression, studies have demonstrated heightened fragmentation of REM sleep (especially in patients with bipolar I disorder), longer sleep-onset latencies, a trend toward an increased number of EEG spindles, a greater percentage of awakenings, and greater REM sleep density (Gold and Sylvia 2016).

Polysomnography between mood episodes. The research literature suggests that REM sleep disturbances may be a marker of affective vulnerability (Eidelman et al. 2010). Sitaram et al. (1982) found increased REM sleep density and reduced RL values in euthymic individuals with bipolar disorder compared with healthy control subjects. Furthermore, studies of healthy relatives of patients with mood disorders have shown increased REM sleep density in these subjects compared with control subjects (Modell et al. 2003). More recently, Eidelman et al. (2010) studied sleep architecture in interepisode periods, finding greater REM sleep density in the bipolar disorder group relative to nonpsychiatric control subjects. While this study did not show any correlation between sleep architecture and concurrent mood symptoms, it demonstrated strong correlations between sleep architecture in euthymic patients with bipolar disorder and future mood symptoms at 3-month follow-up—specifically, a longer duration of the first REM sleep period and decreased N2 sleep were positively associated with future manic symptoms, while increased REM sleep density was positively associated with future depressive symptoms (Eidelman et al. 2010).

Effects of Medications for Bipolar Disorder on Sleep

Mood Stabilizers

The efficacy of lithium in bipolar disorder may be due to its effect of stabilizing circadian rhythms (Geoffroy et al. 2014). Lithium has been associated with lengthened circadian rhythms (Johnsson et al. 1983) and phase delay (Kripke et al. 1979). Lithium also modulates the retinal-hypothalamic-pineal pathway and has been shown to reduce melatonin sensitivity to light (i.e., nocturnal light suppresses melatonin secretion, and lithium reversed this effect in healthy control subjects [Hallam et al. 2005a]). Lithium improves sleep efficiency in patients with bipolar I disorder during the euthymic phase (Geoffroy et al. 2016). Valproic acid, similar to lithium, decreases sensitivity of melatonin to light (Hallam et al. 2005b) but does not affect sleep architecture in healthy adults (Jain and Glauser 2014). Valproic acid may induce central sleep apnea (Guichard et al. 2019; Revol et al. 2020). Carbamazepine in healthy adults resulted in reduced sleep latency and arousals and increased sleep efficiency and N3 sleep (Jain and Glauser 2014).

Antipsychotics

In patients with mania, clozapine is primarily a non–REM sleep enhancer, increasing N2 sleep and slow-wave (N3) sleep (Armitage et al. 2004). Of note, clozapine is effective for circadian phase advancement, promoting more sleep at the beginning of the night (Armitage et al. 2004). In a head-to-head comparison trial between haloperidol and olanzapine, both were equally effective in treating mania; however, olanzapine was superior for promoting sleep, increasing sleep efficiency, reducing total wake time, and decreasing time awake after sleep onset (Moreno et al. 2007). Patients with bipolar depression who are treated with quetiapine report improvements in both quality of sleep and quality of life (Endicott et al. 2007), and they show increased sleep efficiency (Kim et al. 2014). Ziprasidone increases RL values, lengthens durations of slow-wave (N3) sleep, and improves sleep continuity in bipolar depression (Baskaran et al. 2013).

Hypothalamic-Pituitary-Adrenal Axis Dysregulation in Bipolar Disorder

There is a bidirectional influence between the hypothalamic-pituitary-adrenal (HPA) axis and sleep, with HPA axis activation generally being associated with arousal and (conversely) sleep leading to HPA axis suppression (Nicolaides et al. 2000). Overall meta-analytic findings suggest that bipolar disorder is associated with hypercortisolism, with higher basal and post-dexamethasone cortisol levels (Belvederi Murri et al. 2016). However, there is significant heterogeneity among studies. The discrepancies in outcomes may be explained by nonhomogeneous pathophysiology among bipolar disorder subtypes. For example, patients selected specifically for "anergic bipolar depression" did not show typical bipolar disorder polysomnography findings (i.e., these patients had normal RL values and sleep continuity) and had low levels of baseline cortisol and low rates of nonsuppression with dexamethasone (Thase et al. 1989). Some patients with bipolar disorder have relative hypocortisolism while others have relative hypercortisolism, as indicted by dexamethasone suppression testing; both states are associated with worse depression and lower quality of life (Maripuu et al. 2014). In particular, suicide risk is correlated with cortisol nonsuppression (Jokinen et al. 2008, 2009). HPA axis dysfunction may also evolve over time, as individuals with bipolar disorder may switch from hypercortisolism to hypocortisolism as the disease progresses (Maripuu et al. 2017). Lithium may confer some protective effect on the HPA axis, as lithium appears to prevent the development of hypocortisolism (Maripuu et al. 2017).

Primary Sleep Disorders in Patients With Bipolar Disorder

Apart from insomnia (which has been addressed separately), the most common primary sleep disorders are OSA, RLS, and PLMD. Aside from anecdotal findings linking atypical antipsychotics to RLS, conclusive data on the relationship between bipolar disorder and RLS or PLMD are limited. By contrast, there is a stronger body of evidence suggesting that OSA is more prevalent in individuals with bipolar disorder than in healthy control subjects. In general, patients with severe mental illness—which includes MDD, bipolar disorder, and schizophrenia spectrum disorders—are less physically healthy than the general population (Stubbs et al. 2016). Individuals with bipolar disorder are particularly vulnerable to OSA risk factors, particularly obesity (Stubbs et al. 2016). It is important to keep in mind that obesity in bipolar disorder may be iatrogenic, as many psychotropics prescribed for bipolar disorder induce weight gain (Devlin et al. 2000). While the prevalence of OSA in bipolar disorder is lower than that in MDD, OSA rates in bipolar disorder (24.5%; 95% CI: 10.6–47.1, n=681) (Stubbs et al. 2016) appear to be higher than rates in the general population (4% [Partinen and Telakivi 1992]). It has been reported that OSA can contribute to treatment-resistant mania (Strakowski et al. 1991); however, it is unclear whether this effect is due to the sleep disturbance itself or to other mechanisms. These findings suggest the importance of identifying and treating OSA in patients with bipolar disorder (Stubbs et al. 2016).

Treatment of Circadian Rhythm Disruption in Bipolar Disorder

Interpersonal and social rhythm therapy (IPSRT) (Frank et al. 2007) has a component that aims to stabilize circadian rhythm by teaching patients to structure meals, sleep/wake times, and patterns of daily activity. IPSRT has been shown to be effective in stabilizing social rhythms, aids resolution of depression and mania, and reduces the risk of recurrent mood episodes in patients with bipolar disorder (Gold and Kinrys 2019). Other therapies that incorporate social rhythm training are also available, such as Facilitated Integrated Mood Management (Miklowitz et al. 2012); however, IPSRT is better supported by current evidence. Evidence suggests that lithium can delay sleep-wake phase rhythm and promote regularity in daily activities by interacting with the circadian genes that regulate melatonin (Gold and Kinrys 2019). Other interventions such as light exposure, exercise, and melatonin can either advance or delay the sleep cycle, depending on timing of the intervention relative to time of minimum core body temperature (CBTmin). Direct measurement of CBTmin is often precluded by cost/invasiveness concerns; however, CBTmin can be estimated to be reached around 3 hours prior to waking in a person who typically sleeps 8 hours (Roach and Sargent 2019). Light exposure administered approximately 12 hours after CBTmin, melatonin ingestion a few hours prior to CBTmin, and exercise timed for about 9 hours after CBTmin will produce phase advancement; the converse timing relative to CBTmin produces phase delay (Roach and Sargent 2019). Administration time is especially important in the context of transmeridian travel, as timing is relative to the preset CBTmin in the departure time zone, not the destination time zone. Westward travel requires phase delay and eastward travel requires phase advancement to synchronize with local time. Natural sunlight may not always result in the desired phase shift. For example, when traveling eastward, a person may be exposed to morning sunlight in advance of the CBTmin, leading to unwanted phase delay. Melatonin and exercise must similarly be timed to the CBTmin, rather than to the destination "bedtime," to achieve the desired effect.

Targeted Treatment of Insomnia in Bipolar Disorder

Similar to standard CBT-I, there is a targeted cognitive-behavioral therapy for insomnia in bipolar disorder (CBTI-BP). This therapy incorporates some behavioral circadian rhythm strategies as well as cognitive elements to support sleep. CBTI-BP has been shown to increase insomnia remission and lower the risk of mood episodes in comparison with standard psychoeducation (Gold and Kinrys 2019).

Light Therapy in Seasonal-Pattern Mood Episodes

In DSM-5, seasonal affective disorder (SAD) is denoted with a specifier ("with seasonal pattern") that can be applied to both depressive disorders and bipolar and related disorders (American Psychiatric Association 2013). The most common presentation of SAD is as a recurrent depression that appears during the fall and winter, with remission or manic switching in the spring and summer (Menculini et al. 2018). Individuals with SAD have circadian rhythms that are offset from environmental photoperiods, as evidenced by delayed temperature rhythms in comparison with healthy individuals when controlled for routine, light exposure, and exogenous circadian cues (Kaplan and Harvey 2009). HPA axis dysregulation may also play a role in SAD, given that thyroid-stimulating hormone is significantly decreased in patients who respond to morning light therapy (Kaplan and Harvey 2009).

Study findings suggest that darkness functions as a mood stabilizer, as light influences intrinsically photosensitive retinal ganglion cells to suppress melatonin. These cells are most sensitive to blue light, and blue light–blocking lenses have been shown to reduce mania (Gold and Kinrys 2019). In bipolar disorder depressive episodes, light therapy is an effective antidepressant, but it does carry a risk of polarity switching at a rate similar to that associated with antidepressant medications (Tseng et al. 2016). Bright-light therapy has also been shown to improve hypersomnia and depressive symptoms in individuals with SAD, with morning timing being superior to evening treatment (Kaplan and Harvey 2009).

Forced Sleep Deprivation as a Treatment for Bipolar Depression

FSD is effective for treating bipolar depression (e.g., efficacy of 37.7% [N=177] in a meta-analysis of 7 studies); however, this treatment carries the risk of inducing a polarity switch into mania/hypomania (Boland et al. 2017). Reported rates of switching vary widely, from approximately 5% (Colombo et al. 1999) to around 30% (Boland et al. 2017). The efficacy of FSD is enhanced by light therapy (Tseng et al. 2016). The combination of FSD, light therapy, and lithium has been shown to rapidly decrease suicidality in otherwise drug-resistant bipolar depression and may potentiate subsequent response to lithium monotherapy (Benedetti et al. 2014).

Conclusion

Sleep is not unlike the "canary in the coal mine"—when a patient is sleeping poorly, or reports a sudden change in sleep, it often heralds the onset of psychiatric illness.

There is a bidirectional relationship between sleep disturbances and mood disorders. Left unaddressed, sleep disturbances can exacerbate underlying mood disorders. For instance, in MDD, the presence of insomnia significantly elevates the risk of suicide; in bipolar disorder, sleep deprivation is known to induce manic episodes. The inverse is also true—unaddressed mood disorders can perpetuate disordered sleep. Moreover, the spectrum of sleep problems associated with mood disorders is far broader than just reduced total sleep—for instance, circadian rhythm dysfunction has been implicated in the pathogenesis of bipolar disorder, and many individuals with bipolar disorder experience hypersomnia between manic episodes. In fact, it is not uncommon for sleep disturbances to persist in the individuals even after MDD or bipolar disorder is in remission. Thus, in this chapter we have discussed a number of targeted therapies for sleep disturbances in mood disorders, including both pharmacological measures (e.g., hypnotics) and nonpharmacological measures (e.g., light therapy, CBT-I), which may have value even in euthymic patients. It is important to remember that treatment-resistant mood disorders may indicate the presence of a primary sleep disorder such as OSA, and patients in whom a primary sleep disorder is suspected should receive appropriate screening.

References

Akashiba T, Kawahara S, Akahoshi T, et al: Relationship between quality of life and mood or depression in patients with severe obstructive sleep apnea syndrome. Chest 122(3):861–865, 2002 12226024

Akiskal HS, Lemmi H, Yerevanian B, et al: The utility of the REM latency test in psychiatric diagnosis: a study of 81 depressed outpatients. Psychiatry Res 7(1):101–110, 1982 6957895

American Psychiatric Association: Diagnostic and Statistical Manual of Mental Disorders, 5th Edition. Arlington, VA, American Psychiatric Association, 2013

Armitage R, Cole D, Suppes T, et al: Effects of clozapine on sleep in bipolar and schizoaffective disorders. Prog Neuropsychopharmacol Biol Psychiatry 28(7):1065–1070, 2004 15610918

Asaad T, Sabry W, Rabie M, et al: Polysomnographic characteristics of bipolar hypomanic patients: comparison with unipolar depressed patients. J Affect Disord 191:274–279, 2016 26688496

Balcan B, Thunström E, Strollo PJ Jr, et al: Continuous positive airway pressure treatment and depression in adults with coronary artery disease and nonsleepy obstructive sleep apnea. A secondary analysis of the RICCADSA trial. Ann Am Thorac Soc 16(1):62–70, 2019 30130421

Baskaran A, Summers D, Willing SL, et al: Sleep architecture in ziprasidone-treated bipolar depression: a pilot study. Ther Adv Psychopharmacol 3(3):139–149, 2013 24167686

Bauer M, Grof P, Rasgon N, et al: Temporal relation between sleep and mood in patients with bipolar disorder. Bipolar Disord 8(2):160–167, 2006 16542186

Belvederi Murri M, Prestia D, Mondelli V, et al: The HPA axis in bipolar disorder: systematic review and meta-analysis. Psychoneuroendocrinology 63:327–342, 2016 26547798

Benedetti F, Riccaboni R, Locatelli C, et al: Rapid treatment response of suicidal symptoms to lithium, sleep deprivation, and light therapy (chronotherapeutics) in drug-resistant bipolar depression. J Clin Psychiatry 75(2):133–140, 2014 24345382

Bertisch SM, Herzig SJ, Winkelman JW, et al: National use of prescription medications for insomnia: NHANES 1999–2010. Sleep (Basel) 37(2):343–349, 2014 24497662

Boland EM, Rao H, Dinges DF, et al: Meta-analysis of the antidepressant effects of acute sleep deprivation. J Clin Psychiatry 78(8):e1020–e1034, 2017 28937707

Bowden CL: A different depression: clinical distinctions between bipolar and unipolar depression. J Affect Disord 84(2–3):117–125, 2005 15708408

Brecht S, Kajdasz D, Ball S, Thase ME: Clinical impact of duloxetine treatment on sleep in patients with major depressive disorder. Int Clin Psychopharmacol 23(6):317–324, 2008 18854719

Cartwright R: Dreams and adaptation to divorce, in Trauma and Dreams. Edited by Barrett D. Cambridge, MA, Harvard University Press, 1996, pp 179–185

Cervantes P, Gelber S, Kin FN, et al: Circadian secretion of cortisol in bipolar disorder. J Psychiatry Neurosci 26(5):411–416, 2001 11762208

Coffey CE, McCall WV, Hoelscher TJ, et al: Effects of ECT on polysomnographic sleep: a prospective investigation. Convuls Ther 4(4):269–279, 1988 11940976

Colombo C, Benedetti F, Barbini B, et al: Rate of switch from depression into mania after therapeutic sleep deprivation in bipolar depression. Psychiatry Res 86(3):267–270, 1999 10482346

Cook M, Conner J: Retrospective review of hypnotic use in combination with fluoxetine and sertraline. Clinical Drug Investigation 9:212–216, 1995

Cormier RE: Sleep disturbances, in Clinical Methods: The History, Physical, and Laboratory Examinations, 3rd Edition. Edited by Walker HK, Hall WD, Hurst JW. Boston, MA, Butterworths, 1990

Dauvilliers Y, Lopez R, Ohayon M, et al: Hypersomnia and depressive symptoms: methodological and clinical aspects. BMC Med 11:78, 2013 23514569

De Crescenzo F, Economou A, Sharpley AL, et al: Actigraphic features of bipolar disorder: a systematic review and meta-analysis. Sleep Med Rev 33:58–69, 2017 28185811

Delazer M, Zamarian L, Frauscher B, et al: Oxygen desaturation during night sleep affects decision-making in patients with obstructive sleep apnea. J Sleep Res 25(4):395–403, 2016 26899164

Dempsey JA, Veasey SC, Morgan BJ, et al: Pathophysiology of sleep apnea. Physiol Rev 90(1):47–112, 2010 20086074

Devlin MJ, Yanovski SZ, Wilson GT: Obesity: what mental health professionals need to know. Am J Psychiatry 157(6):854–866, 2000 10831462

DiMascio A, Weissman MM, Prusoff BA, et al: Differential symptom reduction by drugs and psychotherapy in acute depression. Arch Gen Psychiatry 36(13):1450–1456, 1979 518245

Dolder CR, Nelson MH, Iler CA: The effects of mirtazapine on sleep in patients with major depressive disorder. Ann Clin Psychiatry 24(3):215–224, 2012 22860241

Dryman A, Eaton WW: Affective symptoms associated with the onset of major depression in the community: findings from the US National Institute of Mental Health Epidemiologic Catchment Area Program. Acta Psychiatr Scand 84(1):1–5, 1991 1927557

Dunleavy DL, Brezinova V, Oswald I, et al: Changes during weeks in effects of tricyclic drugs on the human sleeping brain. Br J Psychiatry 120(559):663–672, 1972 4339630

Eidelman P, Talbot LS, Gruber J, et al: Sleep architecture as correlate and predictor of symptoms and impairment in inter-episode bipolar disorder: taking on the challenge of medication effects. J Sleep Res 19(4):516–524, 2010 20408930

Endicott J, Rajagopalan K, Minkwitz M, et al: A randomized, double-blind, placebo-controlled study of quetiapine in the treatment of bipolar I and II depression: improvements in quality of life. Int Clin Psychopharmacol 22(1):29–37, 2007 17159457

Finan PH, Quartana PJ, Smith MT: The effects of sleep continuity disruption on positive mood and sleep architecture in healthy adults. Sleep (Basel) 38(11):1735–1742, 2015 26085289

Ford DE, Kamerow DB: Epidemiologic study of sleep disturbances and psychiatric disorders. An opportunity for prevention? JAMA 262(11):1479–1484, 1989 2769898

Frank E, Swartz HA, Boland E: Interpersonal and social rhythm therapy: an intervention addressing rhythm dysregulation in bipolar disorder. Dialogues Clin Neurosci 9(3):325–332, 2007 17969869

Gandotra K, Rajagopalan K, Minkwitz M, et al: Effective treatment of insomnia with mirtazapine attenuates concomitant suicidal ideation. J Clin Sleep Med 14(5):901–902, 2018 29734995

Geoffroy PA, Etain B, Sportiche S, Bellivier F: Circadian biomarkers in patients with bipolar disorder: promising putative predictors of lithium response. Int J Bipolar Disord 2(1):28, 2014 26092399

Geoffroy PA, Scott J, Boudebesse C, et al: Sleep in patients with remitted bipolar disorders: a meta-analysis of actigraphy studies. Acta Psychiatr Scand 131(2):89–99, 2015 25430914
Geoffroy PA, Samalin L, Llorca PM, et al: Influence of lithium on sleep and chronotypes in remitted patients with bipolar disorder. J Affect Disord 204:32–39, 2016 27318597
Giles DE, Kupfer DJ, Rush AJ, et al: Controlled comparison of electrophysiological sleep in families of probands with unipolar depression. Am J Psychiatry 155(2):192–199, 1998 9464197
Gillin JC, Duncan WC, Murphy DL, et al: Age-related changes in sleep in depressed and normal subjects. Psychiatry Res 4(1):73–78, 1981 6939001
Gillin JC, Sutton L, Ruiz C, et al: The cholinergic rapid eye movement induction test with arecoline in depression. Arch Gen Psychiatry 48(3):264–270, 1991 1996921
Gillin JC, Rapaport M, Erman MK, et al: A comparison of nefazodone and fluoxetine on mood and on objective, subjective, and clinician-rated measures of sleep in depressed patients: a double-blind, 8-week clinical trial. J Clin Psychiatry 58(5):185–192, 1997 9184611
Göder R, Hinrichsen I, Seeck-Hirschner M, et al: Sleep at baseline and after electroconvulsive therapy in patients with major depression. Psychiatry Res 246:683–687, 2016 27825788
Gold AK, Kinrys G: Treating circadian rhythm disruption in bipolar disorder. Curr Psychiatry Rep 21(3):14, 2019 30826893
Gold AK, Sylvia LG: The role of sleep in bipolar disorder. Nat Sci Sleep 8:207–214, 2016 27418862
Grigolon RB, Trevizol AP, Cerqueira RO, et al: Hypersomnia and bipolar disorder: a systematic review and meta-analysis of proportion. J Affect Disord 246:659–666, 2019 30611064
Gruber J, Harvey AG, Wang PW, et al: Sleep functioning in relation to mood, function, and quality of life at entry to the Systematic Treatment Enhancement Program for Bipolar Disorder (STEP-BD). J Affect Disord 114(1–3):41–49, 2009 18707765
Guichard K, Micoulaud-Franchi JA, McGonigal A, et al: Association of valproic acid with central sleep apnea syndrome: two case reports. J Clin Psychopharmacol 39(6):681–684, 2019 31725092
Hallam KT, Olver JS, Horgan JE, et al: Low doses of lithium carbonate reduce melatonin light sensitivity in healthy volunteers. Int J Neuropsychopharmacol 8(2):255–259, 2005a 15850501
Hallam KT, Olver JS, Norman TR: Effect of sodium valproate on nocturnal melatonin sensitivity to light in healthy volunteers. Neuropsychopharmacology 30(7):1400–1404, 2005b 15841104
Harvey AG, Schmidt DA, Scarnà A, et al: Sleep-related functioning in euthymic patients with bipolar disorder, patients with insomnia, and subjects without sleep problems. Am J Psychiatry 162(1):50–57, 2005 15625201
Harvey AG, Kaplan KA, Soehner AM: Interventions for sleep disturbance in bipolar disorder. Sleep Med Clin 10(1):101–105, 2015 25750600
Héricé C, Patel AA, Sakata S: Circuit mechanisms and computational models of REM sleep. Neurosci Res 140:77–92, 2019 30118737
Hippocrates: The Genuine Works of Hippocrates. Translated by Adams F. Baltimore, MD, Williams & Wilkins, 1939
Hohagen F, Montero RF, Weiss E, et al: Treatment of primary insomnia with trimipramine: an alternative to benzodiazepine hypnotics? Eur Arch Psychiatry Clin Neurosci 244(2):65–72, 1994 7948056
Horne JA, Ostberg O: A self-assessment questionnaire to determine morningness-eveningness in human circadian rhythms. Int J Chronobiol 4(2):97–110, 1976 1027738
Hudson JI, Lipinski JF, Keck PE Jr, et al: Polysomnographic characteristics of young manic patients. Comparison with unipolar depressed patients and normal control subjects. Arch Gen Psychiatry 49(5):378–383, 1992 1586273
Inder ML, Crowe MT, Porter R: Effect of transmeridian travel and jet lag on mood disorders: evidence and implications. Aust N Z J Psychiatry 50(3):220–227, 2016 26268923
Ioannou M, Wartenberg C, Greenbrook JTV, et al: Sleep deprivation as treatment for depression: systematic review and meta-analysis. Acta Psychiatr Scand 143(1):22–35, 2021 33145770

Iovieno N, van Nieuwenhuizen A, Clain A, et al: Residual symptoms after remission of major depressive disorder with fluoxetine and risk of relapse. Depress Anxiety 28(2):137–144, 2011 21284066

Jain SV, Glauser TA: Effects of epilepsy treatments on sleep architecture and daytime sleepiness: an evidence-based review of objective sleep metrics. Epilepsia 55(1):26–37, 2014 24299283

Jindal RD, Friedman ES, Berman SR, et al: Effects of sertraline on sleep architecture in patients with depression. J Clin Psychopharmacol 23(6):540–548, 2003 14624183

Johnsson A, Engelmann W, Pflug B, Klemke W: Period lengthening of human circadian rhythms by lithium carbonate, a prophylactic for depressive disorders. Int J Chronobiol 8(3):129–147, 1983 6862696

Jokinen J, Nordström A-L, Nordström P: ROC analysis of dexamethasone suppression test threshold in suicide prediction after attempted suicide. J Affect Disord 106(1–2):145–152, 2008 17662471

Jokinen J, Nordström A-L, Nordström P: CSF 5-HIAA and DST non-suppression—orthogonal biologic risk factors for suicide in male mood disorder inpatients. Psychiatry Res 165(1–2):96–102, 2009 19062105

Kaplan KA, Harvey AG: Hypersomnia across mood disorders: a review and synthesis. Sleep Med Rev 13(4):275–285, 2009 19269201

Kaplan KA, Gruber J, Eidelman P, et al: Hypersomnia in inter-episode bipolar disorder: does it have prognostic significance? J Affect Disord 132(3):438–444, 2011 21489637

Kaplan KA, McGlinchey EL, Soehner A, et al: Hypersomnia subtypes, sleep and relapse in bipolar disorder. Psychol Med 45(8):1751–1763, 2015 25515854

Ketchesin KD, Becker-Krail D, McClung CA: Mood-related central and peripheral clocks. Eur J Neurosci 51(1):326–345, 2020 30402924

Kim SJ, Lee YJ, Lee YJ, et al: Effect of quetiapine XR on depressive symptoms and sleep quality compared with lithium in patients with bipolar depression. J Affect Disord 157:33–40, 2014 24581825

Kohl FS, Pringuey D, Cherikh F, et al: Sleep polygraphy: diagnostic value in depressive pseudo-dementia. Attempt to improve visual scoring by digital periodic analysis [in French]. Encephale 26(6):3–10, 2000 11217536

Koo BB, Blackwell T, Lee HB, et al: Restless legs syndrome and depression: effect mediation by disturbed sleep and periodic limb movements. Am J Geriatr Psychiatry 24(11):1105–1116, 2016 27526989

Kraepelin E: Manic-Depressive Insanity and Paranoia. Translated by Barclay RM. Edinburgh, UK, Livingstone, 1921

Kripke DF, Judd LL, Hubbard B, et al: The effect of lithium carbonate on the circadian rhythm of sleep in normal human subjects. Biol Psychiatry 14(3):545–548, 1979 476235

Krystal A, Fava M, Rubens R, et al: Evaluation of eszopiclone discontinuation after cotherapy with fluoxetine for insomnia with coexisting depression. J Clin Sleep Med 3(1):48–55, 2007 17557453

Kupfer DJ, Ehlers CL: Two roads to rapid eye movement latency. Arch Gen Psychiatry 46(10):945–948, 1989 2679484

Kupfer DJ, Foster FG: Interval between onset of sleep and rapid-eye-movement sleep as an indicator of depression. Lancet 2(7779):684–686, 1972 4115821

Kupfer DJ, Spiker DG, Coble P, et al: Amitriptyline and EEG sleep in depressed patients, I: drug effect. Sleep 1(2):149–159, 1978 227029

Kupfer DJ, Spiker DG, Rossi A, et al: Nortriptyline and EEG sleep in depressed patients. Biol Psychiatry 17(5):535–546, 1982 7093390

Landolt HP, Raimo EB, Schnierow BJ, et al: Sleep and sleep electroencephalogram in depressed patients treated with phenelzine. Arch Gen Psychiatry 58(3):268–276, 2001 11231834

Leibenluft E, Albert PS, Rosenthal NE, Wehr TA: Relationship between sleep and mood in patients with rapid-cycling bipolar disorder. Psychiatry Res 63(2–3):161–168, 1996 8878312

Levitan RD, Shen JH, Jindal R, et al: Preliminary randomized double-blind placebo-controlled trial of tryptophan combined with fluoxetine to treat major depressive disorder: antidepressant and hypnotic effects. J Psychiatry Neurosci 25(4):337–346, 2000 11022398
Li SX, Zhang B, Li AM, et al: Prevalence and correlates of frequent nightmares: a community-based 2-phase study. Sleep 33(6):774–780, 2010 20550018
Lundeen J, McCall WV, Krystal A, Looney S: Validating functional data analysis measures from 24-h actigraphy data. Biological Rhythm Research 49(5):797–810, 2018
Luthringer R, Toussaint M, Schaltenbrand N, et al: A double-blind, placebo-controlled evaluation of the effects of orally administered venlafaxine on sleep in inpatients with major depression. Psychopharmacol Bull 32(4):637–646, 1996 8993085
Manber R, Edinger JD, Gress JL, et al: Cognitive behavioral therapy for insomnia enhances depression outcome in patients with comorbid major depressive disorder and insomnia. Sleep 31(4):489–495, 2008 18457236
Manber R, Buysse DJ, Edinger J, et al: Efficacy of cognitive-behavioral therapy for insomnia combined with antidepressant pharmacotherapy in patients with comorbid depression and insomnia: a randomized controlled trial. J Clin Psychiatry 77(10):e1316–e1323, 2016 27788313
Maripuu M, Wikgren M, Karling P, et al: Relative hypo- and hypercortisolism are both associated with depression and lower quality of life in bipolar disorder: a cross-sectional study. PLoS One 9(6):e98682, 2014 24932586
Maripuu M, Wikgren M, Karling P, et al: Hyper- and hypocortisolism in bipolar disorder—a beneficial influence of lithium on the HPA-axis? J Affect Disord 213:161–167, 2017 28237543
McCall C, McCall WV: Comparison of actigraphy with polysomnography and sleep logs in depressed insomniacs. J Sleep Res 21(1):122–127, 2012a 21447050
McCall C, McCall WV: Objective vs. subjective measurements of sleep in depressed insomniacs: first night effect or reverse first night effect? J Clin Sleep Med 8(1):59–65, 2012b 22334811
McCall WV: A rest-activity biomarker to predict response to SSRIs in major depressive disorder. J Psychiatr Res 64:19–22, 2015 25782717
McCall WV, Black CG: The link between suicide and insomnia: theoretical mechanisms. Curr Psychiatry Rep 15(9):389, 2013 23949486
McCall WV, Cohen W, Reboussin B, et al: Effects of mood and age on quality of life in depressed inpatients. J Affect Disord 55(2–3):107–114, 1999 10628879
McCall WV, Reboussin BA, Cohen W: Subjective measurement of insomnia and quality of life in depressed inpatients. J Sleep Res 9(1):43–48, 2000 10733688
McCall WV, Blocker JN, D'Agostino R Jr, et al: Insomnia severity is an indicator of suicidal ideation during a depression clinical trial. Sleep Med 11(9):822–827, 2010a 20478741
McCall WV, Blocker JN, D'Agostino R Jr, et al: Treatment of insomnia in depressed insomniacs: effects on health-related quality of life, objective and self-reported sleep, and depression. J Clin Sleep Med 6(4):322–329, 2010b 20726279
McCall WV, Gonzalez C, Deych E, et al: Age-related effects on circadian phase in the sleep of depressed insomniacs. Sleep (Basel) 35:A242, 2012
McCall WV, Batson N, Webster M, et al: Nightmares and dysfunctional beliefs about sleep mediate the effect of insomnia symptoms on suicidal ideation. J Clin Sleep Med 9(2):135–140, 2013 23372466
McCall WV, Ahn E, Benca R, et al: A preliminary report from the "REST IT" study: insomnia severity and hypersomnia severity each independently predict the intensity of suicidal ideation. Sleep (Basel) 38 (suppl):A339, 2015
McCall WV, Lisanby SH, Rosenquist PB, et al: Effects of a course of right unilateral ultrabrief pulse electroconvulsive therapy combined with venlafaxine on insomnia symptoms in elderly depressed patients. J Clin Psychiatry 79(2):16m11089, 2018 28742292

McCall WV, Benca RM, Rosenquist PB, et al: Reducing suicidal ideation through insomnia treatment (REST-IT): a randomized clinical trial. Am J Psychiatry 176(11):957–965, 2019a 31537089

McCall WV, Benca RM, Rumble ME, et al: Prevalence of obstructive sleep apnea in suicidal patients with major depressive disorder. J Psychiatr Res 116:147–150, 2019b 31238203

Melo MCA, Abreu RLC, Linhares Neto VB, et al: Chronotype and circadian rhythm in bipolar disorder: a systematic review. Sleep Med Rev 34:46–58, 2017 27524206

Menculini G, Verdolini N, Murru A, et al: Depressive mood and circadian rhythms disturbances as outcomes of seasonal affective disorder treatment: a systematic review. J Affect Disord 241:608–626, 2018 30172213

Mignot E: Excessive daytime sleepiness: population and etiology versus nosology. Sleep Med Rev 12(2):87–94, 2008 18342260

Miklowitz DJ, Price J, Holmes EA, et al: Facilitated Integrated Mood Management for adults with bipolar disorder. Bipolar Disord 14(2):185–197, 2012 22420594

Millar A, Espie CA, Scott J: The sleep of remitted bipolar outpatients: a controlled naturalistic study using actigraphy. J Affect Disord 80(2–3):145–153, 2004 15207927

Modell S, Huber J, Holsboer F, Lauer CJ: The Munich Vulnerability Study on Affective Disorders: risk factors for unipolarity versus bipolarity. J Affect Disord 74(2):173–184, 2003 12706519

Moreno RA, Hanna MM, Tavares SM, et al: A double-blind comparison of the effect of the antipsychotics haloperidol and olanzapine on sleep in mania. Braz J Med Biol Res 40(3):357–366, 2007 17334533

Ng TH, Chung KF, Ho FY, et al: Sleep-wake disturbance in interepisode bipolar disorder and high-risk individuals: a systematic review and meta-analysis. Sleep Med Rev 20:46–58, 2015 25060968

Nicolaides NC, Vgontzas AN, Kritikou I, Chrousos G: HPA axis and sleep, in Endotext [Internet]. Edited by Feingold KR, Anawalt B, Boyce A. South Dartmouth, MA, MDText.com, Inc., 2000. Last update: November 24, 2020. Available at: https://www.ncbi.nlm.nih.gov/books/NBK279071/. Accessed December 19, 2021.

Nierenberg AA, Keck PE Jr: Management of monoamine oxidase inhibitor-associated insomnia with trazodone. J Clin Psychopharmacol 9(1):42–45, 1989 2708555

Nierenberg AA, Adler LA, Peselow E, et al: Trazodone for antidepressant-associated insomnia. Am J Psychiatry 151(7):1069–1072, 1994 8010365

Nierenberg AA, Keefe BR, Leslie VC, et al: Residual symptoms in depressed patients who respond acutely to fluoxetine. J Clin Psychiatry 60(4):221–225, 1999 10221281

Nofzinger EA, Thase ME, Reynolds CF 3rd, et al: Hypersomnia in bipolar depression: a comparison with narcolepsy using the multiple sleep latency test. Am J Psychiatry 148(9):1177–1181, 1991 1882995

Nofzinger EA, Fasiczka A, Berman S, Thase ME: Bupropion SR reduces periodic limb movements associated with arousals from sleep in depressed patients with periodic limb movement disorder. J Clin Psychiatry 61(11):858–862, 2000 11105739

Nurnberger JI Jr, Adkins S, Lahiri DK, et al: Melatonin suppression by light in euthymic bipolar and unipolar patients. Arch Gen Psychiatry 57(6):572–579, 2000 10839335

O'Brien EM, Chelminski I, Young D, et al: Severe insomnia is associated with more severe presentation and greater functional deficits in depression. J Psychiatr Res 45(8):1101–1105, 2011 21306733

Ohayon MM, Shapiro CM, Kennedy SH: Differentiating DSM-IV anxiety and depressive disorders in the general population: comorbidity and treatment consequences. Can J Psychiatry 45(2):166–172, 2000 10742876

Ott GE, Rao U, Lin KM, et al: Effect of treatment with bupropion on EEG sleep: relationship to antidepressant response. Int J Neuropsychopharmacol 7(3):275–281, 2004 15122973

Partinen M, Telakivi T: Epidemiology of obstructive sleep apnea syndrome. Sleep 15 (6 suppl):S1–S4, 1992 1470800

Perez-Lloret S, Rey MV, Bondon-Guitton E, et al: Drugs associated with restless legs syndrome: a case/noncase study in the French Pharmacovigilance Database. J Clin Psychopharmacol 32(6):824–827, 2012 23131889

Picchietti D, Winkelman JW: Restless legs syndrome, periodic limb movements in sleep, and depression. Sleep 28(7):891–898, 2005 16124671

Pinho M, Sehmbi M, Cudney LE, et al: The association between biological rhythms, depression, and functioning in bipolar disorder: a large multi-center study. Acta Psychiatr Scand 133(2):102–108, 2016 26010130

Plante DT, Winkelman JW: Sleep disturbance in bipolar disorder: therapeutic implications. Am J Psychiatry 165(7):830–843, 2008 18483132

Plante DT, Cook JD, Goldstein MR: Objective measures of sleep duration and continuity in major depressive disorder with comorbid hypersomnolence: a primary investigation with contiguous systematic review and meta-analysis. J Sleep Res 26(3):255–265, 2017 28145043

Qaseem A, Kansagara D, Forciea MA, et al: Management of chronic insomnia disorder in adults: a clinical practice guideline from the American College of Physicians. Ann Intern Med 165(2):125–133, 2016 27136449

Revol B, Jullian-Desayes I, Guichard K, et al: Valproic acid and sleep apnoea: a disproportionality signal from the WHO pharmacovigilance database. Respirology 25(3):336–338, 2020 32000295

Reynolds CF 3rd, Kupfer DJ, Taska LS, et al: EEG sleep in elderly depressed, demented, and healthy subjects. Biol Psychiatry 20(4):431–442, 1985 3978175

Reynolds CF 3rd, Kupfer DJ, Houck PR, et al: Reliable discrimination of elderly depressed and demented patients by electroencephalographic sleep data. Arch Gen Psychiatry 45(3):258–264, 1988 3341880

Reynolds CF 3rd, Buysse DJ, Brunner DP, et al: Maintenance nortriptyline effects on electroencephalographic sleep in elderly patients with recurrent major depression: double-blind, placebo- and plasma-level-controlled evaluation. Biol Psychiatry 42(7):560–567, 1997a 9376452

Reynolds CF 3rd, Frank E, Houck PR, et al: Which elderly patients with remitted depression remain well with continued interpersonal psychotherapy after discontinuation of antidepressant medication? Am J Psychiatry 154(7):958–962, 1997b 9210746

Riemann D, Voderholzer U, Berger M: Sleep and sleep-wake manipulations in bipolar depression. Neuropsychobiology 45 (suppl 1):7–12, 2002 11893871

Roach GD, Sargent C: Interventions to minimize jet lag after westward and eastward flight. Front Physiol 10:927, 2019 31417411

Rosenquist PB, Krystal A, Heart KL, et al: Left dorsolateral prefrontal transcranial magnetic stimulation (TMS): sleep factor changes during treatment in patients with pharmacoresistant major depressive disorder. Psychiatry Res 205(1–2):67–73, 2013 23021320

Roth T: Insomnia: definition, prevalence, etiology, and consequences. J Clin Sleep Med 3 (5 suppl):S7–S10, 2007 17824495

Roth T, Jaeger S, Jin R, et al: Sleep problems, comorbid mental disorders, and role functioning in the national comorbidity survey replication. Biol Psychiatry 60(12):1364–1371, 2006 16952333

Rumble ME, Dickson D, McCall WV, et al: The relationship of person-specific eveningness chronotype, greater seasonality, and less rhythmicity to suicidal behavior: a literature review. J Affect Disord 227:721–730, 2018 29179142

Rush AJ, Erman MK, Giles DE, et al: Polysomnographic findings in recently drug-free and clinically remitted depressed patients. Arch Gen Psychiatry 43(9):878–884, 1986 3753165

Rush AJ, Giles DE, Jarrett RB, et al: Reduced REM latency predicts response to tricyclic medication in depressed outpatients. Biol Psychiatry 26(1):61–72, 1989 2655719

Sachs GS: Unmet clinical needs in bipolar disorder. J Clin Psychopharmacol 23 (3 suppl 1):S2–S8, 2003 12832943

Schittecatte M, Dumont F, Machowski R, et al: Effects of mirtazapine on sleep polygraphic variables in major depression. Neuropsychobiology 46(4):197–201, 2002 12566938

Shen J, Chung SA, Kayumov L, et al: Polysomnographic and symptomatological analyses of major depressive disorder patients treated with mirtazapine. Can J Psychiatry 51(1):27–34, 2006 16491981

Shi J, Wittke-Thompson JK, Badner JA, et al: Clock genes may influence bipolar disorder susceptibility and dysfunctional circadian rhythm. Am J Med Genet B Neuropsychiatr Genet 147B(7):1047–1055, 2008 18228528

Sitaram N, Nurnberger JI Jr, Gershon ES, et al: Cholinergic regulation of mood and REM sleep: potential model and marker of vulnerability to affective disorder. Am J Psychiatry 139(5):571–576, 1982 7072840

Soehner AM, Kaplan KA, Harvey AG: Insomnia comorbid to severe psychiatric illness. Sleep Med Clin 8(3):361–371, 2013 25302060

Soreca I: Circadian rhythms and sleep in bipolar disorder: implications for pathophysiology and treatment. Curr Opin Psychiatry 27(6):467–471, 2014 25211500

Strakowski SM, Hudson JI, Keck PE Jr, et al: Four cases of obstructive sleep apnea associated with treatment-resistant mania. J Clin Psychiatry 52(4):156–158, 1991 2016247

Stubbs B, Vancampfort D, Veronese N, et al: The prevalence and predictors of obstructive sleep apnea in major depressive disorder, bipolar disorder and schizophrenia: a systematic review and meta-analysis. J Affect Disord 197:259–267, 2016 26999550

Szabó K, Ihász F: The effect of reduced oxygen saturation during sleep on depression [in Hu]. Orv Hetil 160(20):780–783, 2019 31081357

Takaesu Y: Circadian rhythm in bipolar disorder: a review of the literature. Psychiatry Clin Neurosci 72(9):673–682, 2018 29869403

Takaesu Y, Inoue Y, Murakoshi A, et al: Prevalence of circadian rhythm sleep-wake disorders and associated factors in euthymic patients with bipolar disorder. PLoS One 11(7):e0159578, 2016 27442503

Tazawa Y, Wada M, Mitsukura Y, et al: Actigraphy for evaluation of mood disorders: a systematic review and meta-analysis. J Affect Disord 253:257–269, 2019 31060012

Thase ME, Himmelhoch JM, Mallinger AG, et al: Sleep EEG and DST findings in anergic bipolar depression. Am J Psychiatry 146(3):329–333, 1989 2919689

Thase ME, Simons AD, Reynolds CF 3rd: Abnormal electroencephalographic sleep profiles in major depression: association with response to cognitive behavior therapy. Arch Gen Psychiatry 53(2):99–108, 1996 8629894

Thase ME, Buysse DJ, Frank E, et al: Which depressed patients will respond to interpersonal psychotherapy? The role of abnormal EEG sleep profiles. Am J Psychiatry 154(4):502–509, 1997 9090337

Thorpy MJ; Diagnostic Classification Steering Committee: International Classification of Sleep Disorders: Diagnostic and Coding Manual. Rochester, MI, American Sleep Disorders Association, 1990

Tseng PT, Chen YW, Tu KY, et al: Light therapy in the treatment of patients with bipolar depression: a meta-analytic study. Eur Neuropsychopharmacol 26(6):1037–1047, 2016 26993616

van Bemmel AL, van den Hoofdakker RH, Beersma DG, et al: Changes in sleep polygraphic variables and clinical state in depressed patients during treatment with citalopram. Psychopharmacology (Berl) 113(2):225–230, 1993 7855186

Van Meter AR, Burke C, Youngstrom EA, et al: The bipolar prodrome: meta-analysis of symptom prevalence prior to initial or recurrent mood episodes. J Am Acad Child Adolesc Psychiatry 55(7):543–555, 2016 27343882

Walsh JK, Erman M, Erwin CW, et al: Subjective hypnotic efficacy of trazodone and zolpidem in DSM-III-R primary insomnia. Human Psychopharmacology: Clinical & Experimental 13(3):191–198, 1998

Waterman L, Stahl ST, Buysse DJ, et al: Self-reported obstructive sleep apnea is associated with nonresponse to antidepressant pharmacotherapy in late-life depression. Depress Anxiety 33(12):1107–1113, 2016 27636232

Wehr TA, Goodwin FK, Wirz-Justice A, et al: 48-hour sleep-wake cycles in manic-depressive illness: naturalistic observations and sleep deprivation experiments. Arch Gen Psychiatry 39(5):559–565, 1982 6124223

Wehr TA, Sack DA, Rosenthal NE: Sleep reduction as a final common pathway in the genesis of mania. Am J Psychiatry 144(2):201–204, 1987 3812788

Weissman MM, Bland RC, Canino GJ, et al: Cross-national epidemiology of major depression and bipolar disorder. JAMA 276(4):293–299, 1996 8656541

Wells KB, Stewart A, Hays RD, et al: The functioning and well-being of depressed patients. Results from the Medical Outcomes Study. JAMA 262(7):914–919, 1989 2754791

Winokur A, DeMartinis NA 3rd, McNally DP, et al: Comparative effects of mirtazapine and fluoxetine on sleep physiology measures in patients with major depression and insomnia. J Clin Psychiatry 64(10):1224–1229, 2003 14658972

Yates WR, Mitchell J, Rush AJ, et al: Clinical features of depressed outpatients with and without co-occurring general medical conditions in STAR*D. Gen Hosp Psychiatry 26(6):421–429, 2004 15567207

CHAPTER 45

Childhood Maltreatment and Mood Disorders

Elizabeth T.C. Lippard, Ph.D.
Charles B. Nemeroff, M.D., Ph.D.

Although the diatheses for major mood disorders are highly heritable, there has been minimal progress in identifying genetic markers for mood disorders. This scant progress is undoubtedly, in part, related to the polygenetic basis of mood disorders, as well as to the heterogeneity of the behavioral phenotypes of patients with bipolar disorder and unipolar depression. In addition, it is also now well established that environmental factors contribute to risk, onset, and disease course in mood disorders. More specifically, early-life stress, especially childhood maltreatment, is associated with long-lasting neural, somatic, and clinical consequences, including earlier illness onset, more frequent mood episode recurrence, and greater symptom severity in mood disorders. In this chapter we focus on the evidence that childhood maltreatment—defined as exposure to abuse and neglect (emotional, physical, and sexual) in children younger than 18 years—is a major contributor to higher disease risk, more severe illness course, and poorer treatment response in mood disorders. We additionally discuss the underlying neurobiology and gene-by-environment interactions that may contribute to the development of mood disorders following childhood maltreatment.

Effect of Childhood Maltreatment on Mood Disorder Prevalence, Onset, and Disease Course

According to the Centers for Disease Control and Prevention, one in seven children experienced childhood maltreatment in the last year (Fortson et al. 2016). Because maltreatment, especially emotional abuse and neglect, is often not reported, this rate is likely an underestimate of the true prevalence of maltreatment. In view of the fact that childhood maltreatment is well established as a risk factor for mood disorders, the high prevalence of maltreatment highlights a critical environmental factor that can be targeted for prevention/intervention strategies to substantially decrease both the presence of and disease burden in mood disorders. Higher rates of childhood maltreatment are reported by patients with unipolar depression and bipolar disorder in comparison with the general population. Childhood maltreatment was reported by 46% of patients with depression in one study (Nelson et al. 2017), and in another study in patients with bipolar disorder, the prevalence of childhood maltreatment was estimated at 57% (Post et al. 2013). Studies investigating the consequences of childhood maltreatment have found that maltreatment is associated with increased risk for and earlier onset of unipolar depression and bipolar disorder (Daruy-Filho et al. 2011; Nelson et al. 2017). Childhood maltreatment is also associated with a more virulent disease course, including more frequent mood episode recurrence and higher symptom severity (Agnew-Blais and Danese 2016; Nanni et al. 2012).

Although the majority of studies published to date on the role of childhood maltreatment in mood disorders have been cross-sectional, longitudinal investigations are now emerging with evidence showing the effects of childhood maltreatment on mood disorder risk, onset, and disease course (Scott et al. 2010). For example, childhood maltreatment in 676 children who were followed into adulthood was found to increase risk for unipolar depression (Widom et al. 2007), as well as an earlier age at onset. Another longitudinal study that followed patients with unipolar depression over a 3-year period found that a history of childhood maltreatment increased the risk of suicidal ideation and recurrent depressive episodes by 20%–30% (Gilman et al. 2013). Additionally, an association between childhood maltreatment and the development of mania was observed in a longitudinal study of 33,375 individuals from the National Epidemiologic Survey on Alcohol and Related Conditions. Specifically, childhood maltreatment increased the risk of first-onset and recurrent mania (Gilman et al. 2015). These longitudinal studies are critical to defining the long-lasting impact of childhood maltreatment because they avoid the recall bias and other study confounds that plague cross-sectional studies.

Childhood maltreatment is also associated with poor treatment response—defined as an inability to achieve symptom remission, or the need for a longer treatment duration before experiencing remission—to psychotherapy or pharmacotherapy. The majority of studies investigating treatment response following childhood maltreatment have assessed treatment response in unipolar depression. A history of childhood abuse and/or neglect is associated with poor treatment response to psychotherapy, pharmacotherapy, and combined therapy in unipolar depression (Nemeroff 2016). Although fewer studies have investigated treatment response in bipolar disorder in relation to a history of childhood maltreatment, one study reported a poor response to anticonvulsant medication, but not to lithium, in individuals with bipolar disorder, and specifically those with higher emotional and physical abuse scores on the Childhood Trauma Questionnaire (Cakir et al. 2016). Another study in patients with bipolar disorder reported that a history of childhood maltreatment was associated with less symptom improvement in response to treatment with benzodiazepines (Post et al. 2016), which are commonly prescribed in bipolar disorder to treat certain manic symptoms (e.g. restlessness, agitation, insomnia).

In addition to being associated with earlier mood episode onset, more frequent recurrence, higher symptom severity, and poorer treatment response, a history of childhood maltreatment is also associated with increased risk for comorbid anxiety disorders, posttraumatic stress disorder, and alcohol/substance use disorders; for atypical and psychotic depressive features; and for suicide attempts and completed suicide (Lippard and Nemeroff 2020). In light of the high risk of suicide attempts and completed suicide in mood disorders—as well as the fact that suicide is the second leading cause of death in youth, with increased rates over the last two decades (1999–2019) (Hedegaard et al. 2021)—the relation between childhood maltreatment and increased risk for suicide warrants greater emphasis. In 2001, the landmark Adverse Childhood Experiences (ACE) Study investigated the relationship between adverse childhood experiences (including childhood maltreatment) and suicide attempts in 17,337 adults (Dube et al. 2001). Childhood maltreatment was found to be associated with a two- to fivefold increase in risk of attempted suicide (Dube et al. 2001). Prospective longitudinal studies examining the relation between childhood maltreatment and suicide risk are emerging. A study that followed a cohort of 682 children and adolescents over a 3-year period found that a history of emotional maltreatment predicted suicidal ideation during follow-up (Miller et al. 2017). This relation remained significant after controlling for previous suicidal ideation and depression symptom severity. A more comprehensive understanding of the underlying mechanisms that contribute to the relationship between childhood maltreatment and risk for suicide attempts and completed suicide—as well as mechanisms that contribute to comorbid psychopathology and poor treatment response—is critically needed because these mechanisms, if identified, may serve as novel targets for interventions.

Potential Mediators of the Relationship Between Childhood Maltreatment and Risk for Mood Disorders and a More Pernicious Disease Course

Studies investigating biological mechanisms that may contribute to the increased risk for mood disorders and the more severe disease course conferred by childhood maltreatment have identified several potential mechanisms, including alterations in the hypothalamic-pituitary-adrenal (HPA) axis, structural and functional brain changes (observed on imaging scans), alterations in corticotropin-releasing hormone (CRH) brain circuits, and gene-by-environment interactions (both epigenetic changes and inflammation).

Alterations in Hypothalamic-Pituitary-Adrenal Axis

The HPA axis regulates endocrine, behavioral, immune, and autonomic responses to stress. Childhood maltreatment clearly alters HPA axis activity (Nemeroff 2016) and how individuals subsequently respond to stress. Stress sensitization models propose that childhood maltreatment alters the sensitivity of the HPA axis. This persistent increased sensitivity to stress later in life is believed to contribute to risk for earlier onset of mood disorders and episode recurrence. Individuals exposed to childhood maltreatment were found to have an increased risk of developing depression or mania following recent life stress in comparison with individuals not exposed to childhood maltreatment (Bandoli et al. 2017; Dienes et al. 2006). Additionally, there is evidence that even minor life stressors can induce a mood episode in individuals with a history of childhood maltreatment (Dienes et al. 2006; La Rocque et al. 2014). A study by Abercrombie et al. (2018) reported findings suggesting that interventions that increase cortisol signaling may be beneficial in treating depression in individuals with a history of emotional abuse. This study further supported the view that the HPA axis and brain circuits that mediate the stress response may be modifiable targets for future interventions.

Structural and Functional Changes in Brain Circuits

Brain circuits that mediate stress responses, in addition to other functions, including reward processing and higher-order cognitive functions, show long-lasting structural and functional changes as a consequence of childhood maltreatment (for reviews, see Lippard and Nemeroff 2020; Nemeroff 2016). Briefly, gray matter volume changes and altered functioning of prefrontal cortices (including the orbitofrontal and the anterior cingulate cortices) and of prefrontal limbic and striatal projection sites (including the hippocampus, insula, and striatum) have been found in individuals with a documented history of childhood maltreatment. Changes in white matter tracts that connect the prefrontal cortex with limbic and striatal regions and changes in functional connectivity between these regions have also been supported. Findings from multiple studies converge to suggest that childhood maltreatment is associated with lower gray matter volume and reduced cortical thickness in the aforementioned regions as well as lower structural integrity of their white matter tracts. Studies investigating altered function in these regions have emerged. Altered functioning in prefrontal-limbic systems in persons with a history of childhood maltreatment is associated with prodromal traits/symptoms—including impulsivity (Hallowell et al. 2019), poor inhibitory control (Zhai et al. 2019), and anxiety (Fonzo et al. 2016)—that may mediate the risk for mood disorder onset. Investigations employing functional connectivity methods are few but are emerging and suggest that altered connectivity within the dorsal attention networks and between the medial prefrontal cortex and striatum may contribute to mood disorder risk and disease course severity in individuals with a history of childhood maltreatment (Hanson et al. 2018; Yu et al. 2019). Decreased ventromedial prefrontal functional connectivity with the amygdala and hippocampus has been found to be associated with a history of childhood maltreatment in individuals with bipolar disorder (Souza-Queiroz et al. 2016).

It is important to note that because most studies to date that have investigated neural consequences of childhood maltreatment have been cross-sectional, results must be interpreted with caution, as these studies do not directly link childhood maltreatment–associated changes in the brain to future development of mood disorder (including initial onset and associated symptoms). However, longitudinal studies are emerging that are beginning to show evidence of such links. For example, a recent study of 110 patients with unipolar depression found that among depressed patients who had experienced childhood maltreatment, those who showed reductions in insula surface area were more likely to experience relapse of their depression during the follow-up period (Opel et al. 2019). Another study that followed 157 adolescents over a 2-year period reported that threat-related amygdala reactivity (as assessed via fMRI) increased with age and emerged before the onset of depressive symptoms not only in youths who were at high risk for depression based on family history, but also in youths with low familial risk who had experienced severe life stress (Swartz et al. 2015). Longitudinal studies are critical to improving our understanding of the biological mechanisms that contribute to the development of mood disorders and that influence symptom severity and mood episode recurrence, because such studies will help to disentangle mechanisms of risk from mechanisms of resiliency.

A few studies have suggested that some consequences of childhood maltreatment may be specific to, or more robust in, certain individuals, perhaps those with a genetic predisposition to mood disorders (Souza-Queiroz et al. 2016; Stevelink et al. 2018). However, currently this hypothesis has not been thoroughly tested because several potential confounds—such as treatment history and other clinical factors (e.g., a history of prior mood episodes)—cannot be ruled out. Likewise, findings that are more robust in or specific to individuals with mood disorders could be related to the higher rates and severity of maltreatment reported in patients with mood disorders. In order to test this hypothesis, we will need studies with sufficient power to investigate interactions with clinical history in individuals with mood disorders and a history of childhood maltreatment, as well as studies that incorporate a comparison group of healthy individuals who themselves also have greater rates of childhood maltreatment. Despite these confounds, there is a body of literature suggesting genetic vulnerability as a major contributor to detrimental outcomes after childhood maltreatment, as summarized in the following section.

Genetic and Epigenetic Contributions

Variations in certain genes very likely play a role in outcomes of childhood maltreatment, including risk for mood disorders. *Candidate gene studies* (a type of association study that focuses on associations between genetic variation in a predefined gene of interest and a disorder or outcome) have yielded findings that support the theory that some risk alleles interact with early-life stress to contribute to mood disorder risk and outcomes. Candidate gene studies have demonstrated that certain genetic variants (i.e., single nucleotide polymorphisms [SNPs]) are associated with greater risk for, or a more pernicious disease course in, mood disorders, but only if the individual is exposed to childhood maltreatment. In 2003, a hallmark study published by Caspi et al. (2003) reported that in comparison with adults who carried two long-arm alleles (i.e., homozygous L/L) in the *5HTTLPR* polymorphism in the promoter region of the serotonin transporter gene (*SLC6A4*), adults who carried the short allele (i.e., either S/S or S/L) exhibited more depressive symptoms, more diagnosable depression, and more suicidality if they had been exposed to childhood maltreatment. This study exemplified the now well-established concept of gene-by-environment interactions and disease vulnerability. Polymorphisms in other stress-related genes are also suggested to interact with childhood maltreatment and contribute to mood disorders. For example, one study found that differences in severity of depression symptoms among patients with a history of childhood maltreatment were associated with variants in the CRH receptor 1 (*CRHR1*) genotype (Heim et al. 2009). As illustrated in Figure 45–1, male patients

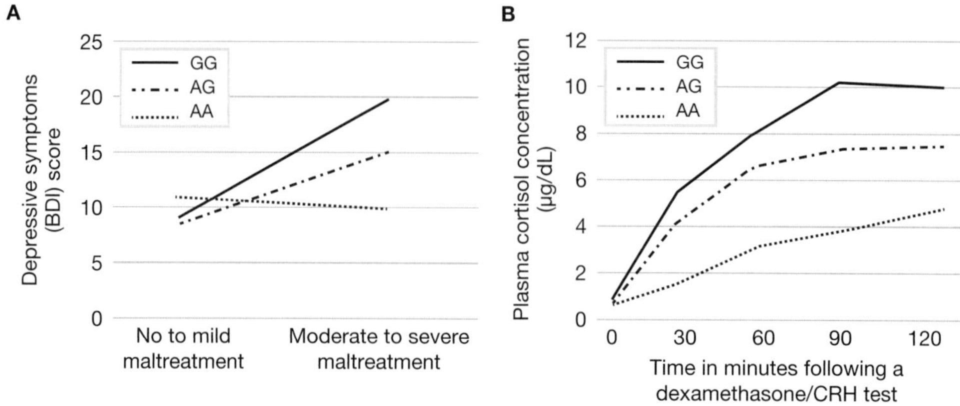

FIGURE 45–1. Findings from Heim et al. (2009) showing how genotype and exposure to childhood trauma interact to influence depressive symptoms and stress response.

(A) Higher scores on the Beck Depression Inventory (BDI), reflecting a greater number or severity of depression symptoms, were reported in individuals with a history of childhood maltreatment if they carried the G allele of a single nucleotide polymorphism (SNP) in the corticotropin-releasing hormone (CRH) receptor 1 gene (*CRHR1*). **(B)** The G allele was also associated with greater cortisol response following a dexamethasone/CRH test. *Solid black line* represents individuals with two copies of the G allele (genotype GG), *thick dashed line* represents individuals with one copy of the G allele (genotype AG), and *thin dashed line* represents individuals with two copies of the A allele (genotype AA).

Source. Adapted from Figures 1 and 3 in Heim C, Bradley B, Mletzko TC, et al.: "Effect of Childhood Trauma on Adult Depression and Neuroendocrine Function: Sex-Specific Moderation by CRH Receptor 1 Gene." *Frontiers in Behavioral Neuroscience* 3:41, 2009. Copyright © 2009 Heim, Bradley, Mletzko, Deveau, Musselman, Nemeroff, Ressler, and Binder. Used with permission.

with the G allele of a SNP in the *CRHR1* gene had more severe depression symptoms, but only if those patients had a history of childhood maltreatment, with the G allele also being associated with greater cortisol response following a dexamethasone/CRH test (an established method for assessing HPA axis function). Although null findings have been reported, many gene variants have been found to interact with environmental stressors, specifically with childhood maltreatment, to increase risk for mood disorders and contribute to a more pernicious disease course (Table 45–1).

Although gene-by-environment interactions are reported, these studies have suffered from a lack of replicability. A recent meta-analysis found no evidence of an interaction between the serotonin transporter gene promoter polymorphism (*5HTTLPR*) and stress that increases risk for depression (Culverhouse et al. 2018). Conflicting findings and a lack of reproducibility are likely related, in part, to methodological and conceptual issues (Dick et al. 2015). Additionally, studies suggest that complex mental disorders result from polygenetic causes. One study reported that the effects of childhood maltreatment on depression symptoms were moderated by gene-by-gene interactions between the *5HTTLPR* and *CHRH1* genotypes (Ressler et al. 2010). Future work is needed that extends beyond polymorphisms of single candidate genes to encompass investigation of polygenetic risk. Studies investigating the epigenetic consequences of early-life stress are also beginning to emerge (Kundakovic and Champagne 2015). *Epigenetics* refers to the modification of gene expression through DNA methylation and acetylation. Epigenetic modifications of the FK506 binding protein 5 gene (*FKBP5*) (Klengel et al. 2013), the glucocorticoid receptor gene ([*NR3C1*]) (McGowan et al.

TABLE 45–1. Gene variants for which there is evidence of gene-by-environment interactions affecting mood disorder outcomes in the context of childhood maltreatment

Genetic variants showing an interaction with childhood maltreatment	Function of gene	Associated outcomes
FK506 binding protein 5 (*FKBP5*) gene polymorphisms	Regulator of glucocorticoid effects and the CRH brain systems	Increased risk for unipolar depression, PTSD symptoms, and suicide attempts
5HTTLPR polymorphism in promoter region of the serotonin transporter gene (*SLC6A4*)	Regulator of the serotonergic system and contributor to stress regulation	Increased risk for mood disorders and decreased age at onset of mood disorders
Corticotropin-releasing hormone (CRH) receptor 1 gene (*CRHR1*) polymorphisms	Regulator of the stress hormone and CRH brain systems	Increased risk for syndromal depression and suicide attempts in adults
Brain-derived neurotrophic factor gene (*BDNF*) *Val66Met* polymorphism	Regulator of brain development, neural plasticity	Increased risk for depression and anxiety, with risk for depression mediated through reductions in hippocampal gray matter volume
Toll-like receptor 2 gene (*TLR2*) polymorphisms	Regulator of immune-mediated pathways	Decreased age at onset of bipolar disorder
Oxytocin receptor gene (*OXTR*) polymorphisms	Regulator of social behavior	Increased risk for depression and anxiety
Interleukin 6 gene (*IL-6*) and C-reactive protein gene (*CRP*) polymorphisms	Regulators of inflammation pathway	Increased risk for depression
Methylenetetrahydrofolate reductase gene (*MTHFR*) *C677T* polymorphism	Regulator of oxidative stress	Increased risk for depression

2009), and the serotonin 3A receptor gene (*5-HT3AR*) (Perroud et al. 2016) have been reported in individuals with a history of childhood maltreatment, and these changes are associated with altered stress hormone systems, increased suicide risk, and greater symptom severity.

Variations in the genes noted above are also associated with neural changes in prefrontal systems—changes that are similar to alterations reported in mood disorders. For example, variations in the *FKBP5* gene are associated with alterations in amygdala volume, amygdala reactivity to threat, and amygdala functional connectivity with the orbitofrontal cortex and hippocampus (Holz et al. 2015). Variations in the *5HTTLPR* polymorphism, including differences in methylation, are associated with volumetric differences in the hippocampus and orbitofrontal cortex as well as differences in amygdala and orbitofrontal cortex activity and amygdala functional connectivity during emotional processing (Little et al. 2014; Muehlhan et al. 2015; Nikolova et al. 2014). A few studies have suggested that structural and functional brain imaging alterations among individuals with a history of childhood maltreatment are moderated by genotype. For example, the *FKBP5* gene moderates the effects of childhood maltreatment on amygdala reactivity to stress (White et al. 2012), and the serotonin transporter gene (*SLC6A4*) moderates the effects of childhood maltreatment on hippocampal volume (Little et al. 2014). The brain-derived neurotrophic factor (BDNF) *Val66Met* polymorphism and a glutamate transporter polymorphism (*SLC1A2-181A>C*), respectively, have been reported to interact with childhood maltreatment to predict gray matter reductions in hippocampal volume and greater risk for depression (Gatt et al. 2009) and reduced hippocampal gray matter volume in patients with bipolar disorder (Poletti et al. 2014). Collectively, these studies suggest that gene-by-environment interactions may contribute to limbic system differences and, through these mechanisms, play a role in the development of both unipolar depression and bipolar disorder. More research is needed in this area to identify gene-brain-environment interactions, including polygenic risk and epigenetic changes, that may mediate the relationship between childhood maltreatment and risk for mood disorders, as these interactions may assist in identifying novel neurobiological targets for treatment to decrease risk or improve disease course in mood disorders.

Inflammation

Increased concentrations of inflammatory markers have been found in individuals with a history of childhood maltreatment and also in a subgroup of individuals with mood disorders. Meta-analyses have suggested that the observed increase in inflammation in depressed patients is in fact not due to depression per se, but rather is a consequence of childhood maltreatment (McDonnell et al. 2019). Individuals with a history of child abuse or neglect have been found to exhibit increased levels of C-reactive protein (CRP), tumor necrosis factor-alpha (TNF-α), and interleukin-6 (IL-6) (Nemeroff 2016; Pace et al. 2006). Longitudinal studies in this area are needed to further investigate the contribution of inflammation to mood disorder vulnerability and disease course following childhood maltreatment, because some, but not all, studies suggest a role for anti-inflammatory drugs in the treatment of depression (Miller and Raison 2015).

Other Factors to Consider: Severity, Type, Timing, and Duration of Maltreatment

Although childhood maltreatment that occurs during any developmental period—in isolation or combined with other forms of early-life stress—increases disease vulnerability and alters disease course, there is some evidence that early-life stress has an additive effect on disease vulnerability and that the timing and type of maltreatment experienced play an important role. For example, as seen in the hallmark ACE Study, a history of multiple early-life stressful events—specifically, having experienced four or more subtypes of early-life adverse events, including abuse but also parental loss, domestic violence, household substance abuse, and similar stressors—confers increased risk for psychiatric disorders such as depression, anxiety, alcohol/substance use disorders, and suicidality (Anda et al. 2006). Other researchers have found a dose-response relationship between the number of different types of childhood maltreatment experienced and the severity of illness in bipolar disorder (Sala et al. 2014).

Although studies suggest that the effects of early-life stress are cumulative, with burden growing as the number of different types of childhood maltreatment experienced increases, there is also evidence that different types of maltreatment may have different effects. Sexual abuse increases the risk for depression independently of other types of maltreatment (Maniglio 2010), and both physical and sexual abuse are reported to independently increase the risk for bipolar disorder and to contribute to a more severe disease course (Romero et al. 2009). In comparison with the large literature on physical and sexual abuse, fewer studies have investigated the consequences of neglect or emotional maltreatment. However, data suggesting differential clinical and neurobiological consequences for different types of neglect and emotional maltreatment are emerging (Shaffer et al. 2009; Teicher et al. 2018). One meta-analysis found that emotional abuse showed the strongest association with depression (Mandelli et al. 2015), and another study found that emotional abuse and neglect predicted depressive symptoms independently of physical and sexual abuse (Spertus et al. 2003). Individuals with bipolar disorder report high rates of emotional maltreatment (Saleptsi et al. 2004), and such maltreatment is associated with rapid cycling, comorbidities, and suicide (Dualibe and Osório 2017). Although these emerging studies suggest that specific subtypes of maltreatment can independently increase the risk for, and alter disease course in, mood disorders, it is important to note that maltreatment types do not occur in isolation, in that individuals who experience physical or sexual maltreatment most likely experience emotional maltreatment as well.

The consequences of childhood maltreatment are likewise suggested to be dependent on age at onset and duration of maltreatment experienced. In general, studies indicate that maltreatment that occurs during earlier stages of development and continues for a longer duration produces the worst outcomes (Dunn et al. 2018). For example, a study that retrospectively examined timing of childhood maltreatment and current depression and suicidal ideation in 15,701 young adults reported that depression during young adulthood was most strongly related to maltreatment if the maltreatment occurred during the preschool period (i.e., between 3 and 5 years of age) as compared with later developmental periods (Dunn et al. 2013). However, maltreatment that occurs later in development also increases the risk for mood disorders. Emotional abuse and neglect occurring during later childhood (between 8 and 9 years of age) and adolescence increased the risk for depression (Khan et al. 2015) and depressive symptoms (Schalinski et al. 2016). It is also worth emphasizing that emotional maltreatment extends beyond parental maltreatment to include victimization by peers (i.e., bullying). In a study of a longitudinal dataset, a history of bullying by peers increased the risk for depression, anxiety, and self-harm (Lereya et al. 2015). A relation between childhood bullying victimization and risk for suicide-related behaviors has also been reported (Campbell-Sills et al. 2017). The effects of bullying, including cyberbullying, are relatively understudied.

Conclusion

It is now well established that childhood maltreatment—physical, emotional, and sexual, including neglect—that occurs at any age increases the risk for, and alters disease course in, mood disorders. Consequences include increased frequency and severity of symptoms, increased comorbid psychopathology, increased risk for suicide-related behaviors, and increased risk of poor treatment response. Studies of biological mechanisms that may link childhood maltreatment with the development of mood disorders are emerging and suggest that alterations in the HPA axis and associated stress-related brain systems, genetics and epigenetics, and inflammation may be modifiable targets to improve outcomes among individuals exposed to childhood maltreatment. In addition, studies suggest that duration, type, and timing of maltreatment matters. Future longitudinal research using larger sample sizes and aimed at investigating modifiable targets is needed, because treatments that affect these modifiable targets may reduce disease burden by lowering the risk for developing mood disorders and improving outcomes among individuals who develop these disorders.

References

Abercrombie HC, Frost CP, Walsh EC, et al: Neural signaling of cortisol, childhood emotional abuse, and depression-related memory bias. Biol Psychiatry Cogn Neurosci Neuroimaging 3(3):274–284, 2018 29486869

Agnew-Blais J, Danese A: Childhood maltreatment and unfavourable clinical outcomes in bipolar disorder: a systematic review and meta-analysis. Lancet Psychiatry 3(4):342–349, 2016 26873185

Anda RF, Felitti VJ, Bremner JD, et al: The enduring effects of abuse and related adverse experiences in childhood. A convergence of evidence from neurobiology and epidemiology. Eur Arch Psychiatry Clin Neurosci 256(3):174–186, 2006 16311898

Bandoli G, Campbell-Sills L, Kessler RC, et al: Childhood adversity, adult stress, and the risk of major depression or generalized anxiety disorder in US soldiers: a test of the stress sensitization hypothesis. Psychol Med 47(13):2379–2392, 2017 28443533

Cakir S, Tasdelen Durak R, Ozyildirim I, et al: Childhood trauma and treatment outcome in bipolar disorder. J Trauma Dissociation 17(4):397–409, 2016 26683845

Campbell-Sills L, Kessler RC, Ursano RJ, et al: Associations of childhood bullying victimization with lifetime suicidal behaviors among new U.S. Army soldiers. Depress Anxiety 34(8):701–710, 2017 28370897

Caspi A, Sugden K, Moffitt TE, et al: Influence of life stress on depression: moderation by a polymorphism in the 5-HTT gene. Science 301(5631):386–389, 2003 12869766

Culverhouse RC, Saccone NL, Horton AC, et al: Collaborative meta-analysis finds no evidence of a strong interaction between stress and 5-HTTLPR genotype contributing to the development of depression. Mol Psychiatry 23(1):133–142, 2018 28373689

Daruy-Filho L, Brietzke E, Lafer B, et al: Childhood maltreatment and clinical outcomes of bipolar disorder. Acta Psychiatr Scand 124(6):427–434, 2011 21848703

Dick DM, Agrawal A, Keller MC, et al: Candidate gene-environment interaction research: reflections and recommendations. Perspect Psychol Sci 10(1):37–59, 2015 25620996

Dienes KA, Hammen C, Henry RM, et al: The stress sensitization hypothesis: understanding the course of bipolar disorder. J Affect Disord 95(1–3):43–49, 2006 16837055

Dualibe AL, Osório FL: Bipolar disorder and early emotional trauma: a critical literature review on indicators of prevalence rates and clinical outcomes. Harv Rev Psychiatry 25(5):198–208, 2017 28759479

Dube SR, Anda RF, Felitti VJ, et al: Childhood abuse, household dysfunction, and the risk of attempted suicide throughout the life span: findings from the Adverse Childhood Experiences Study. JAMA 286(24):3089–3096, 2001 11754674

Dunn EC, McLaughlin KA, Slopen N, et al: Developmental timing of child maltreatment and symptoms of depression and suicidal ideation in young adulthood: results from the National Longitudinal Study of Adolescent Health. Depress Anxiety 30(10):955–964, 2013 23592532

Dunn EC, Nishimi K, Gomez SH, et al: Developmental timing of trauma exposure and emotion dysregulation in adulthood: are there sensitive periods when trauma is most harmful? J Affect Disord 227:869–877, 2018 29254068

Fonzo GA, Ramsawh HJ, Flagan TM, et al: Early life stress and the anxious brain: evidence for a neural mechanism linking childhood emotional maltreatment to anxiety in adulthood. Psychol Med 46(5):1037–1054, 2016 26670947

Fortson B, Klevens J, Merrick M, et al: Preventing Child Abuse and Neglect: A Technical Package for Policy, Norm, and Programmatic Activities. Atlanta, GA, National Center for Injury Prevention and Control, Centers for Disease Control and Prevention, 2016. Available at: https://www.cdc.gov/violenceprevention/pdf/can-prevention-technical-package.pdf. Accessed October 26, 2021.

Gatt JM, Nemeroff CB, Dobson-Stone C, et al: Interactions between BDNF Val66Met polymorphism and early life stress predict brain and arousal pathways to syndromal depression and anxiety. Mol Psychiatry 14(7):681–695, 2009 19153574

Gilman SE, Trinh NH, Smoller JW, et al: Psychosocial stressors and the prognosis of major depression: a test of Axis IV. Psychol Med 43(2):303–316, 2013 22640506

Gilman SE, Ni MY, Dunn EC, et al: Contributions of the social environment to first-onset and recurrent mania. Mol Psychiatry 20(3):329–336, 2015 24751965

Hallowell ES, Oshri A, Liebel SW, et al: The mediating role of neural activity on the relationship between childhood maltreatment and impulsivity. Child Maltreat 24(4):389–399, 2019 30917694

Hanson JL, Knodt AR, Brigidi BD, Hariri AR: Heightened connectivity between the ventral striatum and medial prefrontal cortex as a biomarker for stress-related psychopathology: understanding interactive effects of early and more recent stress. Psychol Med 48(11):1835–1843, 2018 29248021

Hedegaard H, Curtin SC, Warner M: Suicide mortality in the United States, 1999–2019. NCHS Data Brief (398):1–8, 2021 33663651

Heim C, Bradley B, Mletzko TC, et al: Effect of childhood trauma on adult depression and neuroendocrine function: sex-specific moderation by CRH receptor 1 gene. Front Behav Neurosci 3:41, 2009 20161813

Holz NE, Buchmann AF, Boecker R, et al: Role of FKBP5 in emotion processing: results on amygdala activity, connectivity and volume. Brain Struct Funct 220(3):1355–1368, 2015 24756342

Khan A, McCormack HC, Bolger EA, et al: Childhood maltreatment, depression, and suicidal ideation: critical importance of parental and peer emotional abuse during developmental sensitive periods in males and females. Front Psychiatry 6:42, 2015 25870565

Klengel T, Mehta D, Anacker C, et al: Allele-specific FKBP5 DNA demethylation mediates gene-childhood trauma interactions. Nat Neurosci 16(1):33–41, 2013 23201972

Kundakovic M, Champagne FA: Early life experience, epigenetics, and the developing brain. Neuropsychopharmacology 40(1):141–153, 2015 24917200

La Rocque CL, Harkness KL, Bagby RM: The differential relation of childhood maltreatment to stress sensitization in adolescent and young adult depression. J Adolesc 37(6):871–882, 2014 24960433

Lereya ST, Copeland WE, Costello EJ, et al: Adult mental health consequences of peer bullying and maltreatment in childhood: two cohorts in two countries. Lancet Psychiatry 2(6):524–531, 2015 26360448

Lippard ETC, Nemeroff CB: The devastating clinical consequences of child abuse and neglect: increased disease vulnerability and poor treatment response in mood disorders. Am J Psychiatry 177(1):20–36, 2020 31537091

Little K, Olsson CA, Whittle S, et al: Association between serotonin transporter genotype, brain structure and adolescent-onset major depressive disorder: a longitudinal prospective study. Transl Psychiatry 4:e445, 2014 25226554

Mandelli L, Petrelli C, Serretti A: The role of specific early trauma in adult depression: a meta-analysis of published literature. Childhood trauma and adult depression. Eur Psychiatry 30(6):665–680, 2015 26078093

Maniglio R: Child sexual abuse in the etiology of depression: a systematic review of reviews. Depress Anxiety 27(7):631–642, 2010 20336807

McDonnell CG, Boan AD, Bradley CC, et al: Child maltreatment in autism spectrum disorder and intellectual disability: results from a population-based sample. J Child Psychol Psychiatry 60(5):576–584, 2019 30368827

McGowan PO, Sasaki A, D'Alessio AC, et al: Epigenetic regulation of the glucocorticoid receptor in human brain associates with childhood abuse. Nat Neurosci 12(3):342–348, 2009 19234457

Miller AB, Jenness JL, Oppenheimer CW, et al: Childhood emotional maltreatment as a robust predictor of suicidal ideation: a 3-year multi-wave, prospective investigation. J Abnorm Child Psychol 45(1):105–116, 2017 27032784

Miller AH, Raison CL: Are anti-inflammatory therapies viable treatments for psychiatric disorders? Where the rubber meets the road. JAMA Psychiatry 72(6):527–528, 2015 25853989

Muehlhan M, Kirschbaum C, Wittchen HU, et al: Epigenetic variation in the serotonin transporter gene predicts resting state functional connectivity strength within the salience network. Hum Brain Mapp 36(11):4361–4371, 2015 26303978

Nanni V, Uher R, Danese A: Childhood maltreatment predicts unfavorable course of illness and treatment outcome in depression: a meta-analysis. Am J Psychiatry 169(2):141–151, 2012 22420036

Nelson J, Klumparendt A, Doebler P, et al: Childhood maltreatment and characteristics of adult depression: meta-analysis. Br J Psychiatry 210(2):96–104, 2017 27908895

Nemeroff CB: Paradise lost: the neurobiological and clinical consequences of child abuse and neglect. Neuron 89(5):892–909, 2016 26938439

Nikolova YS, Koenen KC, Galea S, et al: Beyond genotype: serotonin transporter epigenetic modification predicts human brain function. Nat Neurosci 17(9):1153–1155, 2014 25086606

Opel N, Redlich R, Dohm K, et al: Mediation of the influence of childhood maltreatment on depression relapse by cortical structure: a 2-year longitudinal observational study. Lancet Psychiatry 6(4):318–326, 2019 30904126

Pace TW, Mletzko TC, Alagbe O, et al: Increased stress-induced inflammatory responses in male patients with major depression and increased early life stress. Am J Psychiatry 163(9):1630–1633, 2006 16946190

Perroud N, Zewdie S, Stenz L, et al: Methylation of serotonin receptor 3A in ADHD, borderline personality, and bipolar disorders: link with severity of the disorders and childhood maltreatment. Depress Anxiety 33(1):45–55, 2016 26350166

Poletti S, Locatelli C, Radaelli D, et al: Effect of early stress on hippocampal gray matter is influenced by a functional polymorphism in EAAT2 in bipolar disorder. Prog Neuropsychopharmacol Biol Psychiatry 51:146–152, 2014 24518437

Post RM, Altshuler L, Leverich G, et al: More stressors prior to and during the course of bipolar illness in patients from the United States compared with the Netherlands and Germany. Psychiatry Res 210(3):880–886, 2013 24021999

Post RM, Leverich GS, Kupka R, et al: Clinical correlates of sustained response to individual drugs used in naturalistic treatment of patients with bipolar disorder. Compr Psychiatry 66:146–156, 2016 26995248

Ressler KJ, Bradley B, Mercer KB, et al: Polymorphisms in CRHR1 and the serotonin transporter loci: gene x gene x environment interactions on depressive symptoms. Am J Med Genet B Neuropsychiatr Genet 153B(3):812–824, 2010 20029939

Romero S, Birmaher B, Axelson D, et al: Prevalence and correlates of physical and sexual abuse in children and adolescents with bipolar disorder. J Affect Disord 112(1–3):144–150, 2009 18538857

Sala R, Goldstein BI, Wang S, Blanco C: Childhood maltreatment and the course of bipolar disorders among adults: epidemiologic evidence of dose-response effects. J Affect Disord 165:74–80, 2014 24882181

Saleptsi E, Bichescu D, Rockstroh B, et al: Negative and positive childhood experiences across developmental periods in psychiatric patients with different diagnoses—an explorative study. BMC Psychiatry 4:40, 2004 15566566

Schalinski I, Teicher MH, Nischk D, et al: Type and timing of adverse childhood experiences differentially affect severity of PTSD, dissociative and depressive symptoms in adult inpatients. BMC Psychiatry 16:295, 2016 27543114

Scott KM, Smith DR, Ellis PM: Prospectively ascertained child maltreatment and its association with DSM-IV mental disorders in young adults. Arch Gen Psychiatry 67(7):712–719, 2010 20603452

Shaffer A, Yates TM, Egeland BR: The relation of emotional maltreatment to early adolescent competence: developmental processes in a prospective study. Child Abuse Negl 33(1):36–44, 2009 19167069

Souza-Queiroz J, Boisgontier J, Etain B, et al: Childhood trauma and the limbic network: a multimodal MRI study in patients with bipolar disorder and controls. J Affect Disord 200:159–164, 2016 27136413

Spertus IL, Yehuda R, Wong CM, et al: Childhood emotional abuse and neglect as predictors of psychological and physical symptoms in women presenting to a primary care practice. Child Abuse Negl 27(11):1247–1258, 2003 14637300

Stevelink R, Abramovic L, Verkooijen S, et al: Childhood abuse and white matter integrity in bipolar disorder patients and healthy controls. Eur Neuropsychopharmacol 28(7):807–817, 2018 29866576

Swartz JR, Williamson DE, Hariri AR: Developmental change in amygdala reactivity during adolescence: effects of family history of depression and stressful life events. Am J Psychiatry 172(3):276–283, 2015 25526599

Teicher MH, Anderson CM, Ohashi K, et al: Differential effects of childhood neglect and abuse during sensitive exposure periods on male and female hippocampus. Neuroimage 169:443–452, 2018 29288867

White MG, Bogdan R, Fisher PM, et al: FKBP5 and emotional neglect interact to predict individual differences in amygdala reactivity. Genes Brain Behav 11(7):869–878, 2012 22979952

Widom CS, DuMont K, Czaja SJ: A prospective investigation of major depressive disorder and comorbidity in abused and neglected children grown up. Arch Gen Psychiatry 64(1):49–56, 2007 17199054

Yu M, Linn KA, Shinohara RT, et al: Childhood trauma history is linked to abnormal brain connectivity in major depression. Proc Natl Acad Sci USA 116(17):8582–8590, 2019 30962366

Zhai ZW, Yip SW, Lacadie CM, et al: Childhood trauma moderates inhibitory control and anterior cingulate cortex activation during stress. Neuroimage 185:111–118, 2019 30342975